W0268029

HANDBUCH DER HAUT- UND GESCHLECHTSKRANKHEITEN

J. JADASSOHN

ERGÄNZUNGSWERK

BEARBEITET VON

G. ACHTEN · J. ALKIEWICZ · R. ANDRADE · R. D. AZULAY · H.-J. BANDMANN · L. M. BECHELLI M. BETETTO · H. H. BIBERSTEIN · R. M. BOHNSTEDT · G. BONSE · S. BORELLI · W. BORN · O. BRAUN-FALCO · J. BRODY · S. R. BRUNAUER · W. BURCKHARDT · J. CABRÉ · F.T. CALLOMON† C. CARRIÉ · H. CHIARI · G. B. COTTINI · G. J. CRAMER · R. DOEPFMER · CHR. EBERHARTINGER H. EBNER · G. EHRMANN · R. A. ELLIS · A. ENGELHARDT · F. FEGELER · E. FISCHER · H. FLEISCHHACKER · H. FRITZNIGGLI · H. GÄRTNER · O. GANS · M. GARZA TOBA · P. E. GEHRELS · H. GÖTZ · L. GOLDMAN · H. GOLDSCHMIDT · A. GREITHER · H. GRIMMER · P. GROSS · TH. GRÜNEBERG · J. HÄMEL · D. HARDER · W. HAUSER · E. HEERD · E. HEINKE · H.-J. HEITE · S. HELLERSTRÖM · A. HENSCHLER-GREIFELT · J. J. HERZBERG · J. HEWITT · G. VON DER HEYDT G. E. HEYDT · H. HILMER · H. HOBITZ · H. HOFF · G. HOPF · O. HORNSTEIN · L. ILLIG · W. JADASSOHN · M. JÄNNER · E. G. JUNG · R. KADEN · K. H. KÄRCHER · FR. KAIL · K. W. KALKOFF W. D. KEIDEL · PH. KELLER · J. KIMMIG · G. KLINGMÜLLER · N. KLÜKEN · W. KLUNKER A. G. KOCHS† · FR. KOGOJ · G. W. KORTING · E. KRÜGER-THIEMER · H. KUSKE · F. LATAPI · H. LAUSECKER† · P. LAVALLE · A. LEINBROCK · K. LENNERT · G. LEONHARDI · W. F. LEVER R. G. LIEBALDT · W. LINDEMAYR · K. LINSER · H. LÖHE† · L. J. A. LOEWENTHAL · A. LUGER E. MACHER · F. D. MALKINSON · C. MARCH · J. T. McCARTHY · R. T. McCLUSKEY · K. MEINICKE · W. MEISTERERNST · N. MELCZER · A. M. MEMMESHEIMER · J. MEYER-ROHN · A. MIESCHER · G. MIESCHER† · P. A. MIESCHER · A. MUSGER · TH. NASEMANN · FR. NEUWALD G. NIEBAUER · H. NIERMANN · W. NIKOLOWSKI · F. NÖDL · H. OLLENDORFF-CURTH · B. OSTERTAG · F. PASCHER · R. PFISTER · K. PHILIPP · A. PILLAT · H. PINKUS · W. POHLIT H. PORTUGAL · M. I. QUIROGA · W. RAAB · R. V. RAJAM · B. RAJEWSKY · J. RAMOS E SILVA H. REICH · R. RICHTER · G. RIEHL · H. RIETH · H. RÖCKL · N. F. ROTHFIELD · ST. ROTHMAN† T. ŠALAMON · S. A. P. SAMPAIO · R. SANTLER · E. SCHEICHER-GOTTRON · C. SCHIRREN C. G. SCHIRREN · H. SCHLIACK · W. SCHMIDT · R. SCHMITZ · W. SCHNEIDER · U. W. SCHNYDER · H. E. SCHREINER · H. SCHUERMANN† · K.-H. SCHULZ · R. SCHUPPLI · J. SCHWARZ M. SCHWARZ-SPECK · E. J. VAN SCOTT · H.-P.-R. SEELIGER · R. D. G. PH. SIMONS · J. SÖLTZ'-SZÖTS · C. E. SONCK · E. SOHER · H. W. SPIER · R. SPITZER · D. STARCK · Z. STARY · G. K. STEIGLEDER · H. STORCK · J. S. STRAUSS · G. STÜTTGEN · M. B. SULZBERGER · A. SZAKALL† A. TANAY · J. TAPPEINER · J. THEUNE · W. THIES · G. VELTMAN · J. VONKENNEL† · F. WACHSMANN · G. WAGNER · W. H. WAGNER · E. WALCH · G. WEBER · R. WEHRMANN · K. WEINGARTEN · G. G. WENDT · A. WIEDMANN · H. WILDE · A. WINKLER · D. WISE · A. WISKEMANN P. WODNIANSKY · KH. WOEBER · H. WÜST · K. WULF · L. ZALA · J. ZEITLHOFER · J. ZELGER P. ZIERZ · M. ZINGSHEIM · L. ZIPRKOWSKI

HERAUSGEGEBEN GEMEINSAM MIT

R. DOEPFMER · O. GANS · H. GÖTZ · H. A. GOTTRON · J. KIMMIG · A. LEINBROCK · G. MIESCHER† · TH. NASEMANN · H. RÖCKL · C. G. SCHIRREN · U. W. SCHNYDER · H. SCHUERMANN† · H. W. SPIER · G. K. STEIGLEDER · H. STORCK A. WIEDMANN

VON

A. MARCHIONINI†

ZWEITER BAND · TEIL II

SPRINGER-VERLAG

BERLIN · HEIDELBERG · NEW YORK

1965

ENTZÜNDLICHE DERMATOSEN II

BEARBEITET VON

S. R. BRUNAUER · P. GROSS · O. HORNSTEIN · E. G. JUNG
H. KUSKE · W. F. LEVER · C. MARCH · J. T. McCARTHY
R. T. McCLUSKEY · A. MIESCHER · P. A. MIESCHER · F. PASCHER
N. F. ROTHFIELD · R. SCHUPPLI · H. STORCK · M. B. SULZBERGER
L. ZALA

HERAUSGEGEBEN VON

G. MIESCHER† UND H. STORCK

MIT 239 TEILS FARBIGEN ABBILDUNGEN

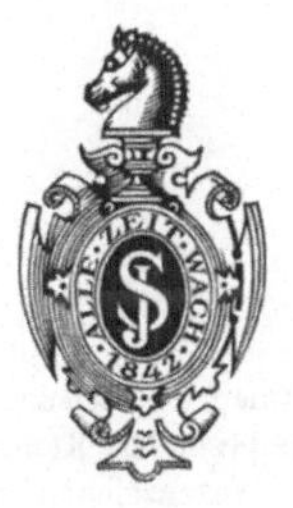

SPRINGER-VERLAG
BERLIN · HEIDELBERG · NEW YORK
1965

ISBN-13: 978-3-642-86597-8 e-ISBN-13: 978-3-642-86596-1
DOI: 10.1007/978-3-642-86596-1

softcover reprint of the hardcover 1st edition 1965

Library of Congress Catalog Card Number 28–17078

Titel-Nr. 5523

Vorwort

Im vorliegenden zweiten Halbband „Entzündliche Dermatosen" sind im Gegensatz zu vorher Krankheitsgruppen dargestellt, bei welchen gut erkennbare und experimentell erforschte allergische Mechanismen in den Hintergrund treten. Dafür sind aber zum Teil unbestimmte, vielleicht bakterielle, vielleicht autoimmunpathologische Reaktionen von Bedeutung. Es zeigt sich auch bei den vorliegenden Beiträgen, wie neben der althergebrachten exakten klinischen Beobachtung der Krankheitsveränderungen immer mehr biochemische, histopathologische und elektronenmikroskopische Forschungsmethoden und Resultate von Bedeutung werden, und wie dadurch ein großer Teil der krankhaften Hauterscheinungen mit Stoffwechsel und Funktionen innerer Organe zusammenhängt. Deshalb sind auch zunehmend Forscher und Kliniker anderer medizinischer Fachgebiete an Erkenntnis und therapeutischem Fortschritt von früher vorwiegend dermatologischen Krankheiten beteiligt. Dadurch entsteht eine gesunde Konkurrenz und eine Verpflichtung der Dermatologen, den Kontakt mit allgemeinmedizinischen Problemen zu pflegen, vor allem aber aufgeschlossen, großzügig und weitherzig die Probleme ihres Fachgebietes mit Kollegen anderer Richtungen zu diskutieren und zu bearbeiten („team-work"). Einige Mitarbeiter dieses Bandes haben erfolgreich versucht, sich im die neuen Erkenntnisse von Immunpathologie, innerer Medizin und Chirurgie und anderer Grenzgebiete ihres Themas selbst einzuarbeiten; andere ließen kompetente Fachkollegen zu Worte kommen, und ein sich hauptsächlich immunpathologisch und internistisch entwickelndes Wissensgebiet (visceraler Lupus erythematodes) wurde von einem Internisten bearbeitet.

Bei dem außergewöhnlichen Anwachsen der Literatur war es in einzelnen Gebieten nicht mehr möglich, den Handbuchcharakter zu wahren, und es mußte bei verschiedenen Spezialproblemen auf zusammenfassende Übersichtsarbeiten verwiesen werden. Es ist aber trotzdem zu hoffen, daß der Leser die Möglichkeit findet, sich über den heutigen Stand des Wissens oder der gültigen Ansichten über ihn interessierende Fragen der vorliegenden Hauptthemen genauestens zu orientieren. Bei dem raschen und voluminösen Fortschreiten der Forschung, sowie bei der in der Regel schweren täglichen Belastung der Mitarbeiter mit anderen Problemen war es leider auch diesmal nicht zu vermeiden, daß neben einzelnen termingerecht abgelieferten Beiträgen große Verspätungen auftraten. Es soll deshalb hier der besondere Dank an diejenigen Mitarbeiter gerichtet werden, welche die Mühe einer nochmaligen Überarbeitung ihrer rechtzeitig abgelieferten Beiträge auf den heutigen Stand bei Beendigung des gesamten Halbbandes nicht scheuten.

Wenige Beiträge, von heute in der USA wirkenden Mitarbeitern, sind aus technischen Gründen in englischer Sprache verfaßt; andere konnten trotz der vermehrten Schwierigkeiten deutsch geschrieben werden. Einzelne Überschneidungen durch Bearbeitung weniger Krankheitsbilder von verschiedenen Autoren unter verschiedenen Gesichtspunkten ließen sich nicht vermeiden, erleichtern aber vielleicht das Verständnis zusammenhängender Probleme aus einer Feder.

Erfreulicherweise spiegeln sich auch die großen therapeutischen Fortschritte mit Antibiotica, Antihistaminica und Corticosteroiden in der Behandlung eines großen Teils der hier dargestellten Krankheitsbilder.

Nur kurz zusammenfassend sei auf einige wesentliche Gesichtspunkte der einzelnen Beiträge hingewiesen:

Die eigentlich zu den Ekzemformen des vorangehenden Halbbandes gehörende Dermatitis seborrhoides (P. GROSS und J. T. McCARTHY, New York) wurde hauptsächlich hinsichtlich der mannigfaltigen biochemischen Probleme bearbeitet, mit Störung der Keratinisation, des Fettmantels, weniger des Säure- und Schweißmantels. Wahrscheinlich spielen Konstitution und polyätiologische Momente eine Rolle und führen zur cholesterinbildenden pathologischen Keratinisation, weniger zu Änderung des squalenhaltigen Talges. Mikrobielle Einflüsse geben keine genügende Erklärung; vielleicht aber sind Abnormitäten des Hypothalamus-Hypophysen-Nebennierenrindensystems, der Hormone, Vitamine und Nahrung pathogenetisch von Bedeutung. Mangels kausaler Therapie kann auch heute nur eine polyvalente, symptomatische Therapie Erfolg versprechen.

Die exsudative, discoide und lichenoide chronische Dermatose von SULZBERGER und GARBE wurde mit ihren vier Phasen, nämlich der exsudativen, der lichenoiden, der infiltrativen und schließlich der urticariellen von den Autoren selbst bearbeitet. An den bis anhin publizierten Fällen werden Klinik, Histologie und Verlauf geschildert mit Diskussion der nosologischen Stellung dieses noch etwas schwer abgrenzbaren Leidens sowie der Differentialdiagnose.

Die heute in vielem noch rätselhafte Gruppe entzündlicher, zum Teil granulomatöser Hautkrankheiten wie Erythema exsudativum multiforme, Erythema nodosum, Periarteriitis nodosa, Phlebitis saltans, Panniculitis, Cheilitis granulomatosa und Melkersson-Rosenthal-Syndrom, Granuloma annulare, Necrobiosis lipoidica diabeticorum, Granulomatosis disciformis, Necrobiosis maculosa (R. SCHUPPLI, Basel) ist pathogenetisch meist noch wenig geklärt, dies gilt besonders für die idiopathischen Formen, z.B. des Erythema exsudativum multiforme, weniger bei den symptomatischen, häufig allergischen Reaktionen. Die Ansichten über Identität verschiedener Formen geht noch auseinander, z.B. beim Erythema exsudativum betr. „Minor"- und „Major"-form, bei den verschiedenen Untergruppen der Periarteriitis nodosa, bei verschiedenen Panniculitiden, bei Cheilitis granulomatosa und Melkersson-Rosenthal-Syndrom, sowie bei den Granulomatosen der letzten Gruppen. Zum Teil legen charakteristische histologische Veränderungen eine Abgrenzung nahe, zum Teil sprechen Übergänge und der Wunsch nach Vereinheitlichung dagegen. Deutlichen Fortschritt brachte die Erkenntnis der histologisch pathognomonischen Radiärknötchen (MIESCHER) beim Erythema nodosum, die histologisch tuberkuloiden Strukturen bei Cheilitis granulomatosa, ohne daß aber hier ein engerer Zusammenhang mit Tuberkulose nachgewiesen werden konnte. Man muß die meisten Krankheitsbilder als polyätiologische, klinisch und histologisch mehr oder weniger scharf umrissene Hautmanifestationen auffassen.

Die Hautveränderungen rheumatischer Krankheiten (O. HORNSTEIN, Düsseldorf) wurden erstmals in diesem Handbuch von einem Dermatologen zusammenfassend bearbeitet und in die kompliziert gewordene Unterteilung der rheumatischen Krankheiten eingegliedert. Es kommen aber nur die Veränderungen bei eigentlichen rheumatischen Krankheiten (rheumatisches Fieber, primär-chronische Polyarthritis inklusive Morbus Felty, Still und Wissler-Fanconi) zur ausführlichen Darstellung, bei welchen die Hautveränderungen wie z.B. das Erythema annulare Lehndorff-Leiner zu den Kardinalsymptome gehören. Die sog. pararheumatischen Systemerkrankungen und die rheumatoiden Krankheiten werden differentialdiagnostisch berücksichtigt.

Die hämorrhagischen Diathesen (H. STORCK und E. G. JUNG, Zürich) sind ein außerordentlich vielschichtiges Problem geworden und wurden von den drei pathogenetisch wichtigen Gesichtspunkten der vasculären, thrombocytopenischen und koagulopathischen Genese aus einheitlich bearbeitet. Besonders berücksichtigt wurden die Physiopathologie der Blutstillung mit dem engen Ineinandergreifen von Gefäß-, Thrombocyten- und Gerinnungsfaktoren sowie die übergeordneten pathogenetischen Prinzipien, wie allergische Reaktionen, Shwartzman-Sanarelli-Phänomen und Genetik. Auch hier lassen Biochemie, Histologie und Elektronenmikroskopie in die Funktionen kleinster Dimensionen vordringen. Die Zahl der Krankheitsbilder in den einzelnen Krankheitsgruppen hat sich in letzter Zeit durch sorgfältige Differenzierung stark vermehrt, wobei vielleicht erst die Zukunft durch Aufdeckung von entscheidenden Gemeinsamkeiten das System vereinfachen lassen wird.

Die Fremdkörpergranulome (H. KUSKE, Bern) zeigen die verschiedensten Reaktionsmöglichkeiten der Haut zur Abkapselung oder Entfernung von Fremdkörpern, abgestuft in das erste Reaktionsstadium aus Blutbestandteilen, in das zweite histiocytäre Stadium und schließlich das dritte Narbenstadium mit einigen histologischen und lokalisatorischen Besonderheiten je nach eingedrungener Substanz.

Der Lupus erythematodes, nämlich die discoide (F. PASCHER, Brooklyn, N.Y.) und die viscerale Form (P. A. MIESCHER, R. T. MCCLUSKEY und R. E. ROTHFIELD, New York) bieten wohl heute interessanteste Probleme bezüglich Differenzierung, Krankheitsübergänge, autoimmunpathologischer Fragen sowie therapeutischer Probleme. Bei beiden Formen haben die Corticosteroide das therapeutische Feld erobert. Wie weit Antimalariamittel und andere Therapeutica bei der discoiden Form tatsächlich heilen oder nur die Krankheit unterdrücken, ist noch nicht gesichert. Ganz besonders interessant sind die vielseitigen immunologischen Abnormitäten bei der visceralen Form, von welchen nur einzelne antinucleäre Faktoren pathogenetisch für Leukopenie, Thrombopenie und Anämie von Bedeutung zu sein scheinen, nicht aber für andere systematische Schädigungen der gegen 18 beteiligten Gewebe und Organe. Offenbar sind Antikörper, Komplement und Fibrin für den Schaden von Bedeutung, vielleicht auch Antigen-Antikörperkomplexe, wobei aber das Antigen bis anhin nicht bekannt ist.

Ähnliche Probleme stellt die neuerdings durch Dermatologen besonders bearbeitete Dermatomyositis (F. PASCHER, Brooklyn, N.Y.) mit ihren Übergängen zum systematisierten Lupus erythematodes, zur generalisierten Sklerodermie, Periarteriitis nodosa sowie ihrer Differenzierung von anderen Myopathien. Das vermehrte Vorkommen von Malignomen bei älteren Patienten ist interessant, aber nicht geklärt. Auch hier haben sich die Corticosteroide therapeutisch als wirksam erwiesen.

Die aktinischen Dermatosen (H. KUSKE, Bern) sind zu einem der vielversprechendsten Gebiete der Dermatologie geworden, bei welchen sich mit den neu entwickelten Monochromatoren exakte Einblicke in Strahlenchemie und Gewebsreaktion gewinnen lassen. Es finden sich aber noch viele ungelöste Probleme bei den eigentlichen Lichtkrankheiten, bei den Photosensibilisierungen und bei den durch Licht fakultativ provozierten Dermatosen.

Die bullösen Dermatosen, nämlich die verschiedenen Formen des Pemphigus, des Pemphigoids, der Epidermolysis bullosa, der Akrodermatitis continua Hallopeau, der Impetigo herpetiformis, der Dermatitis herpetiformis, der subcornealen

Pustulosis und des Herpes gestationis (W. LEVER, Boston) haben in neuerer Zeit durch exakte histologische Abgrenzung der verschiedenen Krankheitsgruppen und durch die entscheidende Therapie mit Corticosteroiden wesentlich gewonnen. Die beiden Hauptformen Pemphigus vulgaris und Pemphigus foliaceus lassen sich exakt vom Pemphigoid und anderen nicht akantholytischen Blasenbildungen abtrennen. Ätiologisch ist man aber bei den meisten Gruppen nicht weiter gekommen. Genetisch interessante Probleme stellen die Fälle von Epidermolysis bullosa, bei welchen durch klinische und histologische Merkmale sowie durch Vererbungsmodus teils Zusammenlegung früherer Gruppen, teils Abtrennung neuerer Krankheitsbilder möglich wurde.

Bei den thermischen Schädigungen (H. KUSKE, Bern) vervollständigen die enormen Erfahrungen im zweiten Weltkrieg sowie bei den heute gehäuften Unfällen und Katastrophen die Kenntnis über Pathogenese, Schockbekämpfung und Lokaltherapie von Verbrennungen und Erfrierungen außerordentlich, wodurch ein neues Querschnittsfach zwischen Physiopathologie, Chirurgie, innerer Medizin und Dermatologie entstanden ist. Mit allen Vor- und Nachteilen haben sich für die Behandlung von Verbrennungen in einzelnen Ländern Zentren gebildet. Es ist wohl richtig, wenn auch der Dermatologe bei der umschriebenen oder generalisierten thermischen Schädigung seines Spezialorganes durch besonderes Wissen ein Mitspracherecht behält.

Zum Schluß sei besonders dankbar der umsichtigen Planung und Auswahl der Mitarbeiter durch meinen verehrten verstorbenen Lehrer, Vorgänger und Mitarbeiter GUIDO MIESCHER gedacht. Anerkennung gebührt wiederum dem *Springer-Verlag*, der wie stets durch minutiöse Drucklegung und sorgfältige Ausstattung die Herausgabe des Halbbandes in vorliegender Form ermöglichte.

Zürich, im Oktober 1964

H. STORCK

Inhaltsverzeichnis

Dermatitis Seborrhoides

By

Paul Gross and John T. McCarthy-New York

With 4 Figures in the Text (1 in Colour

1. Introduction

It is 33 years since WINKLER and UNNA wrote the chapter on "Seborrhoeic Eczema" in the JADASSOHN Handbuch. This treatise still remains a classic because of its authorship, the rich material presented and because of its investigative approach. Although much remains to be done to determine the etiology of this disease, progress has been made thanks to investigative work on the dermatosis, aptly called morbus Unna by some, and as a result of positive knowledge gained in other fields of dermatology and the basic sciences. A simple indicator of this progress is the change of the title of this supplemental chapter from Seborrhoeic Eczema to Dermatitis seborrhoides. The difference becomes less significant if we quote WINKLER and UNNA (page 446) saying that "UNNA chose the name Seborrhoeic Eczema because it also expresses the tendency of this disease to change to other forms of eczema". If we omit the word parasitic we can also use UNNA's definition of seborrhoeic eczema as "a chronic inflammation of the skin characterized by abnormal fat content of the superficial epidermal layers. Its chief symptoms are a habitual dryness, the sharp round or polycyclic outline of the lesions, the fairly constant picture of the disease and the fact that it can be easily influenced by certain therapeutic methods". The character of the inflammatory process and the special feature of fat formation in the epidermal cells assure the symptom complex a distinct nosologic position. If WINKLER and UNNA included some clinical manifestations which do not conform with their own definition and which we cannot accept today as forms of dermatitis seborrhoides, we may attribute this to the influence of DARIER's concept of eczematide and BROCQ's parakeratose psoriasiforme. After all, UNNA himself referred to the similarity of eczema seborrheicum and psoriasis, but made it quite clear that despite of clinical expressions ranging from an oozing eczema to the parakeratotic psoriasiform lesion, seborrheic eczema was a distinct clinical and histopathologic entity.

2. Definition

It is not only a question of nomenclature if GANS (1953) prefers the name of morbus Unna to seborrheic eczema because, as he declares, we are dealing here neither with seborrhea nor with eczema. The name chosen by BELISARIO (1952) of Dysseborrhoeic dermatitis may point in the right direction, but his definition of dysseborrhea as an abnormal flow of sebum puts the burden of dysfunction solely on the sebaceous glands, without stressing the complex nature of the skin surface fat and the abnormal lipid granules and droplets in the parakeratotic epidermis (CEDERKREUTZ 1912) and in the endothelium of the blood vessels of the papillae (KREIBICH 1927). The dyssebacia of SMITH, SMITH & CALLAWAY (1942) is significant inasmuch as it demonstrates a relationship of sebaceous glands and disturbances of general metabolism, in their cases produced by vitamin deficiency. Furthermore the distinction between seborrhea and dermatitis seborrhoides is born out by the fact that in acne which is partly due to dysfunction of sebaceous glands, one rarely finds a typical dermatitis seborrhoides (COHEN 1945). Pityriasis sicca is often found with acne. If there is a common denominator it is to be sought in the status seborrhoicus as conceived by ROST, INGRAM and others.

MARCHIONINI, MANZ and HUSS (1938) in their study of the skin surface findings of Dermatitis seborrhoides conclude that there is in Dermatitis seborrhoides a disturbance of cholesterol metabolism of the entire skin surface, but most in seborrheic sites and suggest that this is a pathochemical stigma of a special constitution of the skin (status seborrhoicus).

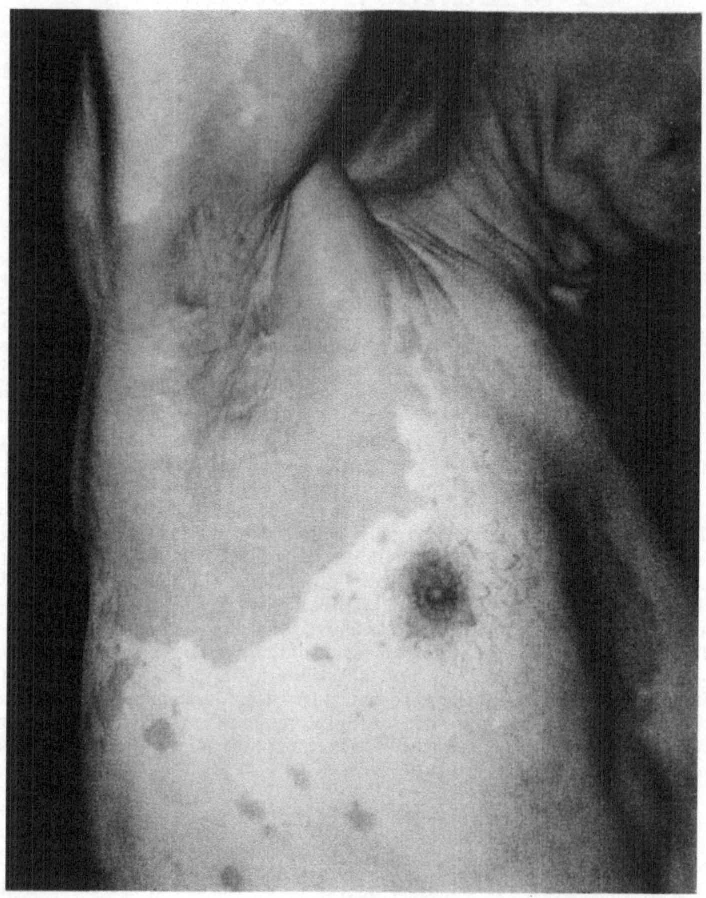

Fig. 1. Psoriasiform Dermatitis seborrhoides, type 1 spreading (NIKOLOWSKI). Centrifugal dissemination not bound to the sites of predilection. (Courtesy of Dr. LEWIS SKAPIRO, New York)

3. Clinical Picture

The primary efflorescence of uncomplicated Dermatitis seborrhoides is an erythematosquamous lesion. Even the follicular lesion, which NIKOLOWSKI (1953) considers to be probably the most important seborrheic reaction begins with a swelling of the follicle and a peripilar erythema and parakeratosis. It is possible that the superficial, configurated form of Dermatitis seborrhoides develops from multiple follicular lesions but at the time the patient consults the physician it has usually lost its follicular appearance. The true follicular type of seborrheic dermatitis is comparatively rare; it may be seen on the chest, midscapular region and occasionally in the nasolabial folds and chin.

The configurated type is the most typical form of Dermatitis seborrhoides. The yellowish color of the central portion and the slightly raised yellowish pink scaly border can best be seen in the midsternal and midscapular region, but also in the corona seborrheica of the forehead and mastoid region.

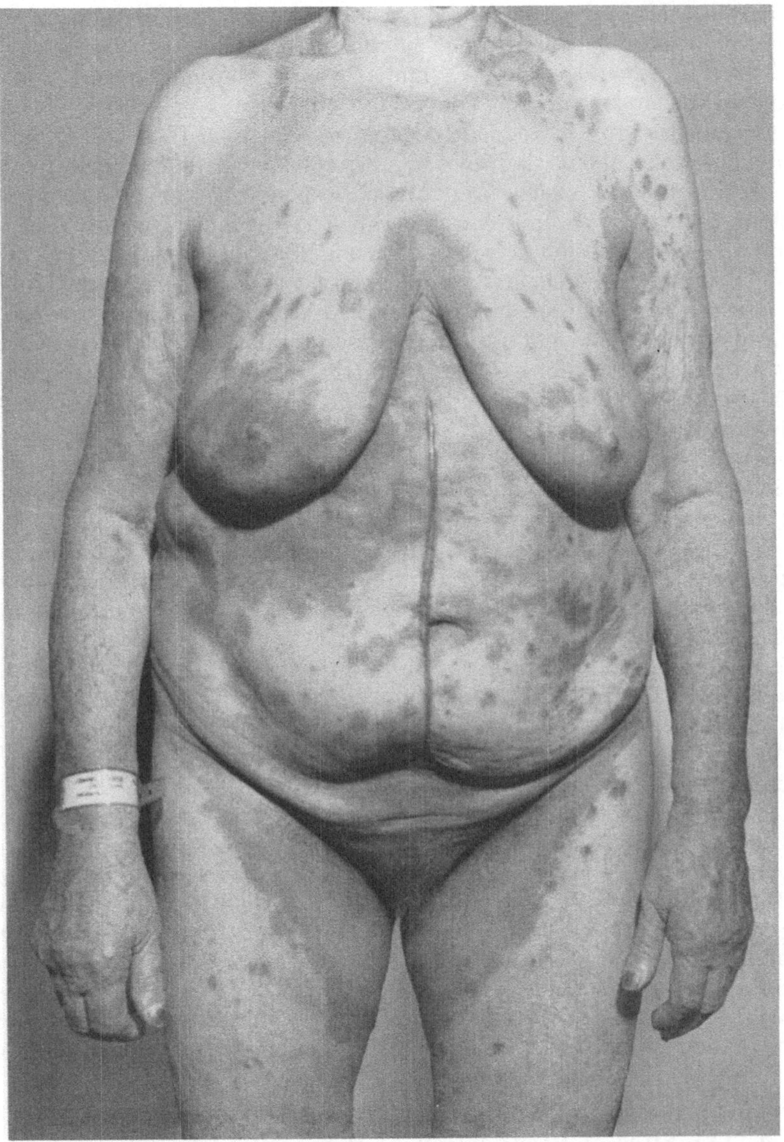

Fig. 2. Dermatitis seborrhoides, type 3 spreading (NIKOLOWSKI). With symmetrical distribution not bound to the sites of predilection (Eczematid of pityriasis rosea type). Female 62 years of age. Second hospital admission because of flare up and of Dermatitis seborrhoides oozing dermatitis in submammary folds and genito-crural region, followed by widespread dissemination (Microbid). (From the Department of Dermatology Columbia-Presbyterian Medical Center)

A classification and synonyms are given by DARIER (see DARIER, CIVATTE, TZANCK 1949).

1. Configurated steatoid eczematid, seborrheide mediothoracique (BROCQ), Pityriasis steatoides (SABOURAUD) Eczema acneique (BAZIN) Eczema flanellaire (older authors). Seborrhea corporis (DUHRING).

2. Psoriasiform eczematid. Pityriasiform seborrhoid, Parakeratose (Brocq), Pityriasis simplex (Sabouraud).

3. Eczematid of pityriasis rosea type (Pityriasis circinée Vidal).

Nicolowski (1953) describes three forms of spreading. a) asymetrical, centrifugal dissemination not bound to the sites of predilection. b) symmetrical type confined to sites of predilection. c) symmetrical distribution, appearing in crops, not bound to the sites of predilection. While there can be no doubt that type a and b dissemination are a frequent occurence in Dermatitis seborrhoides there are many questions about the factors precipitating the spreading. Regarding type c of Nikolowski which probably corresponds to the eczematid of the pityriasis rosea type, we would consider this a less common form of Dermatitis seborrhoides. One may see it as a dissemination of an intertriginous type or other forms of Dermatitis seborrhoides complicated by secondary microbial invasion or eczematization. It is necessary to question whether some of the cases referred to by Nikolowski would not fit better under the heading of autosensitization dermatitis (microbid reaction). Whether in the latter cases a seborrheic constitution determines the clinical picture of the "exanthem" can only be decided in the individual case.

In the seborrheic sites one finds more frequently the pityriasis sicca, the pityriasis steatoides and the configurated form of Dermatitis seborrhoides. The flexural sites more commonly present the psoriasiform type of lesions. As in true psoriasis, in these locations, scales are absent except when there is sufficient peripheral progression to involve areas not subject to maceration. In the midsternal region, in the scalp and the orifices of the ear canals the salmon color of Dermatitis seborrhoides may change to a deeper red and the scaling may be of a type which makes a differentiation from psoriasis quite difficult on first sight. Finally there is a phase which is spoken of as the exudative form of Dermatitis seborrhoides. One can see in such cases diffuse macerated, oozing, red lesions with crust formation on the border. The retroauricular region, the ear canal, the axillary vault, the submammary folds and genitocrural regions appear to be the sites of predilection for this form. Another type is a true eczematous dermatitis with oozing points and vesicular satellite lesions on a spreading border. It would be better to call this a complication of Dermatitis seborrhoides since we have ruled out the eczematous nature of the disease. To quote Miescher (1955) "In this discussion no mention was made of seborrheic eczema and neurodermatitis. Both are affections which are outside of the realm of true eczema, although they frequently become eczematized so that in some cases a clear distinction becomes difficult" (see also Gans 1953). This eczematization may occasionally be the result of a contact allergic reaction to topical therapeutics, but in the majority of cases it represents a secondary "microbial eczema".

4. The Sites of Predilection of Dermatitis Seborrhoides and Their Pathophysiological Significance

The recognition that Dermatitis seborrhoides is essentially an erythemato-squamous dermatosis is important for the understanding and diagnosis of this disease, but it is not a final diagnostic criterion. Only by stressing the sites of predilection (seborrheic and intertriginous) can we complete the definition of dermatitis seborrhoides. To quote Shelley (1959) "Seborrheic dermatitis is a chronic scaling inflammatory eruption in which the localization is the remarkable distinctive feature. It is the location of the lesions, rather than their clinical or microscopic appearance, which sets Dermatitis seborrhoides apart as true entity.

Certainly, we cannot culture or demonstrate any infectious or allergic causative agent. Despite the implications of the name, none of the epidermal appendages shows a unique change. It is not even a remarkable eczema either clinically or histologically. But always the localization stands as the singular feature."

It was part of UNNA's original concept of seborrheic eczema that not only the scalp was the site of this peculiar "dry" eczema but other areas of the trunk and extremities, as well.

The significance of the sites determining the distribution of dermatitis seborrhoides was brought into full focus by the extensive work of MARCHIONINI and his co-workers. The year 1938, thus marks a cornerstone in the clinical study of Dermatitis seborrhoides. MARCHIONINI, HAUSKNECHT, SCHMIDT and KIEFER (1938) demonstrated the higher values of p_H in the areas of the body, most of which coincide with the sites of predilection of Dermatitis seborrhoides. MARCHIONINI, MANZ and HUSS in the same year by determining quantitatively the free and esterified cholesterol in a chloroform dialysate, established the fact that the skin surface of the patient afflicted with Dermatitis seborrhoides in normal and affected areas showed a considerable elevation of total cholesterol and frequently changes in the ratio of free and esterified cholesterol. They considered the combination of this patho-chemical stigma with the relative decrease of acidity of the skin surface in several seborrheic sites of predilection as favorable conditions for the growth of bacteria and fungi. This they believed to be in support of the parasitic etiology and pathogenesis of seborrheic eczema. The factors which these authors thought to be responsible for the higher pH in certain sites were "1. the fact that the apocrine sweat which a priori is only slightly acid, neutral or slightly alkaline, becomes alkaline during evaporation. 2. the highly acid eccrine sweat becomes alkaline by ammoniacal formation if its evaporation is interfered with or prevented." They stressed the importance of the regional differences in the acid mantle of the skin for the variations in the defense against bacteria and the self disinfection of the skin.

The findings of increased pH in Dermatitis seborrhoides were confirmed by work using various refined methods (ANDERSON 1951, M. SCHMID 1952, BEARE, CHEESEMAN, GAILEY and NEILL 1958, MENEGHINI 1957, SCHIRREN and PAWLOWSKY 1956 and others).

The concept of the mechanism of normal pH is being dealt with by SZAKALL and SPIER, the function of the sebaceous glands by CARRIE and the microbiology of the healthy skin by RÖCKL in Volume I, part 4 of the Ergänzungs-Werk. Nevertheless, it is necessary for the understanding of the nature of seborrheic dermatitis and the implications of its localization to touch on some of these subjects. The change in the concept of the pH of the skin and its buffer capacity is revealed by the following statement of SPIER and PASCHER (1957) "The pH of the skin surface is the result of all dissociable components of the water solubles with relation to their dissociation constant. Stabilization and buffer capacity are mediated by the free amino acids, the sum total of which gives an approximately neutral reaction (contrary to a conventional hypothesis). As repeatedly stated, one must assume the existence of a more physical than chemical principle of autoregulation of the pH of the skin surface, or else one would have to be able to observe greater variations of the pH in view of the variable sweat secretion and the changing supply of a total of at least 27 substances which determine the pH or influence its stability."

Many of the complexities of this statement were understood by BURCKHARDT, SCHUPPLI, SCHMID, VERMEER, SZAKALL, EPPRECHT, SCHIRREN and PAWLOWSKY and others but more work is still needed to clarify the situation.

There is no contradiction to SPIER and PASCHER's concept of pH if HERMANN (1957) postulates two complex buffered systems, which are controlled by different, though not unrelated factors. One system is the superficial stratum corneum which maintains its pH by virtue of "autoregulatory" mechanisms and tends to stay near the isoelectric point of the keratinous structure. The second system is that upon the skin surface, where sweating is of utmost importance for the pH.

HERMANN, PROSE and SULZBERGER (1952) could show again in more recent experiments that "stimulation by acetylcholine or pilocarpine produces a considerably higher pH in the sweat, as well as on the skin surface than does thermal stimulation of ordinary intensity, though prolonged exposure to heat causes the pH to rise". It is evident that MARCHIONINI's stress on the role of sweat is still valid especially in some sites of predilection of Dermatitis seborrhoides. The fact that lactic acid and lactate and sometimes also CO_2 and the bicarbonate system, dissolved in the native sweat affect the pH of the skin (HERRMANN, SZAKALL and others) may be of significance in Dermatitis seborrhoides. This may explain the disappearance of pityrosporon ovale (optimum pH 5 for growth in SCOTT-MARTIN's culture media) when pityriasis sicca capitis changes to pityriasis "steatoides" with its subcorneal exudate. It certainly is an important reason why maceration of the lesions in the intertriginous areas increases the pH by liberating CO_2 from the deeper layers of the skin and in turn increases chances of secondary invasion of pathogenic bacteria.

The role which the free amino acids play in the regulation of the pH of the skin surface may give an explanation of the findings of BEARE, CHEESEMAN, et al. (1958) who found the skin of the children afflicted with seborrheic dermatitis more alkaline than in normal children *both in affected and normal skin.*

The problem of the skin surface involves other factors, namely, 1. the constituents of the lipid film, especially the free fatty acids, cholesterol and squalene, and 2. the interrelationship between the aqueous and lipid surface film. According to ROTHMAN (1954) "the main source of lipid material in this film are the sebaceous glands. The second source is the keratinizing epidermis; the invisible horny lamellae which are steadily cast off carry a great amount of lipid substances. Apocrine glands also excrete lipid droplets. Whether the eccrine glands contribute to the maintenance of the fatty film is rather doubtful. By definition, the term 'sebum' should be reserved to designate the product of sebaceous glands only".

This dual origin of the skin surface fat should be kept in mind when discussing the abnormal findings in Dermatitis seborrhoides. LOBITZ (1957) talking about the structure and function of the sebaceous glands in normal adults, psoriatics and patients with seborrheic dermatitis finds "that the most puzzling however is seborrheic dermatitis. Here the sebaceous glands are seemingly normal. There are normal sebum levels. In the composition of sebum the free fatty acids are normal, but the iodine number (which represents the total unsaturated fatty acids) in sebum is lowered. The squalene concentration is normal or slightly lowered. The cholesterol contents is raised. The cholesterol-squalene ratio is greatly altered. All this would indicate that there is a derangement of metabolism as a whole rather than a deficiency or excess in any one component, in particular a derangement in the cholesterol squalene ratio. This apparently is a constant abnormality."

Much of the puzzling situation can be explained by the fact that only a part, though a relatively great part, of this fat stems from sebaceous glands. The normal squalene concentration expresses the absence of pathological changes in the sebaceous glands, since this hydrocarbon is an intermediate in cholesterol biosynthesis which cannot be performed by the sebaceous gland (NICOLAIDES and

Rothman 1952, 1955; Boughton, Hodgson Jones, MacKenna et al. 1955, Boughton, Mackenna, Wheatley & Wormall 1959). On the other hand, most of the cholesterol is derived from the cornifying cells of epidermis. If we remember Marchionini's findings of disturbed ratio of free and esterified cholesterol we must agree with Rothman that these variations reflect variations in the keratinization process rather than changes in sebaceous gland function.

These considerations make it doubtful that in Dermatitis seborrhoides we are dealing primarily with a "dysseborrhoea" (Belisario 1953) but rather with a disturbance of metabolism in the epidermis, involving keratinization. This opinion was expressed by Sabouraud who attributed the fatty appearance of the scales in Dermatitis seborrhoides not to their fat content, but to an alteration of keratinization and speaks of dyskeratosis seborrhoiformis (quoted from Winkler and Unna 1927, page 486). A similarity to psoriasis is obvious, not withstanding the differences in the nosology, histopathology and histochemistry.

It will require histochemical and biochemical studies as extensive as those carried out in the last decade on psoriasis to reveal the metabolic disturbance in the affected and normal skin of the patient with "seborrheic dermatitis" which result in the abnormal behavior of the skin surface in its aqueous and lipid phase. That this plays an important role in the lowered antibacterial defense mechanism of the seborrheic cannot be doubted. On the other hand, undue stress on the antibacterial function of the skin surface can lead to a statement, which was made by Loewenthal (1954):

"Marchionini's work purported to map out areas of relative alkalinity or as he termed it gaps in the acid mantle of the skin. It is interesting to note that these areas are predominantly involved in acute bacterial eczema of the type described as producing an exuberant growth of staphylococci. Many dermatologists still prefer to attach the label 'seborrheic' to this clinical type."

The complexity of this mechanism is best demonstrated by Miescher's studies, summarized by him at the International Congress in Stockholm (1956). He explained the differences of the antibacterial action of sebum in vitro and in vivo by the inhibitory effect of the free amino acids. While the total amino-acids are inhibitory because of the inclusion of the alkaline amino-acids, the neutral amino-acids show only moderate inhibition and the acid amino-acids none or rather an enhancing effect. He concludes: "the antimicrobial effect of the skin surface evidently depends on conditions which are not constant and obviously the water content plays an important part."

5. Microbiology

Much has been written on the bacterial flora of the normal skin (Storck 1948, Evans 1950, Pillsbury 1954 and others). Most authors agree that there is a relatively harmless array of anaerobic and aerobic organisms present on the normal skin, plus a transient population of other organisms which may be saprophytes, facultative pathogens or highly virulent ones. Intact normal skin is highly resistant to bacterial invasion and some defect is ordinarily needed for bacterial propagation. The sebaceous glands of the normal skin and areas where these glands are numerous have a higher bacterial population than other areas of skin (Evans 1950). It is now well known that any exudative process encourages secondary bacterial contamination and subsequent bacterial infection. Dermatitis seborrhoides in its more acute and exudative forms provides an ideal climate for the establishment of bacterial infection. No discussion of Dermatitis seborrhoides can be complete without reference to the closely allied entity, microbial eczema.

The role of bacteria in the pathogenesis of eczema has been studied extensively. The investigative work by Robert (1935, 1937), Miescher (1949) and especially Storck (1948, 1950) has firmly established the importance of the microbial eczema. The complexities of the problem and the results of experimental studies are discussed in detail in part 1 of the second volume of this Ergänzungswerk by Miescher and Storck. Nevertheless, some reference has to be made to this field, since the parasitic etiology of dermatitis seborrhoides, created by Unna and upheld by and expanded by Sabouraud still has its adherents today. Gans

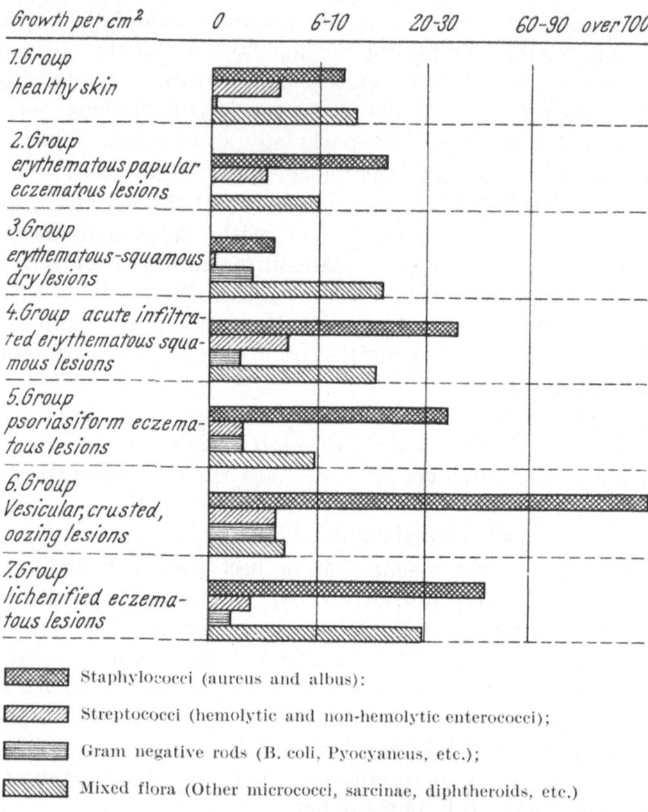

Fig. 3. Bacterial flora of erythemato-squamous lesions (group 3) shows no significant differences from that of the normal skin. (Compare with group 6 — vesicular, crusting and oozing eczema.) From H. Storck: Experimentelle Untersuchungen zur Frage der Bedeutung von Mikroben in der Ekzemgenese. Dermatologica (Basel) **96**, 177 (1948)

(1952) dismisses the role of the bacterial etiology of Dermatitis seborrhoides by saying that "in the acute oozing forms of morbus Unna we are not dealing with the pure form of morbus Unna but with a secondary infection. For the morbus Unna sui generis, i.e. for the dry type, the bacteriological findings and reactions (to patch tests) are of no significance. They only explain the inflammatory component, which may transform the quiescent morbus Unna, into the severe disease, known to all dermatologists". He finds himself in this respect on common ground with Barber (1948) who also had in recent papers attributed less and less importance to the much discussed triad of organisms, which thrive particularly well on the seborrheic skin.

No better proof for this concept can be found than in the work of Storck himself. Storck's ingenious studies of the quantitative rather than of the qualitative flora of various dermatoses graphically illustrates that no significant differences exist between the dry, typical forms of seborrheic dermatitis and normal skin, when measured by the quantity of staphylococcal and streptococcal colonies cultured in situ. Only the exudative form of Dermatitis seborrhoides shows a significant increase in the bacterial flora. Corresponding differences between the primary type of seborrheic dermatitis and the exudative lesions are demonstrated by the results of the patch tests with bacterial filtrates, as demonstrated by STORCK. He also raises the question, whether the exudative phase of Dermatitis seborrhoides is a true eczema in the sense of bacterial sensitization or a toxic effect. This question has been debated in the recent extensive study by MAIBACH & KLIGMAN (1962) on the biology of experimental human cutaneous moniliasis. These authors came to the conclusion that "the pathologic reaction in cutaneous moniliasis is mediated by endotoxin-like substances, released by the organisms on the surface. It was concluded that cutaneous moniliasis is a biological contact dermatitis of the *primary irritant type*". In the discussion of this paper SULZBERGER and WILSON do not agree that MAIBACH & KLIGMAN's thesis of a non-allergic reaction (of cutaneous moniliasis) has been fully proved. Without entering in this discussion we believe that on clinical grouns one could discern two types of exudative dermatitis seborrhoides, namely a toxic (primary irritant type) without microscopic vesiculation, and an eczematous type based on bacterial allergy. The latter would be characterized by vesicles, oozing points, loss of sharp outline, satellite lesions and occurrence of bacterial type autosensitization exanthems. This can only be proven by a purposeful clinical study of these two types of exudative dermatitis seborrhoides supported by the investigative methods as those used by ROBERT, MIESCHER and STORCK.

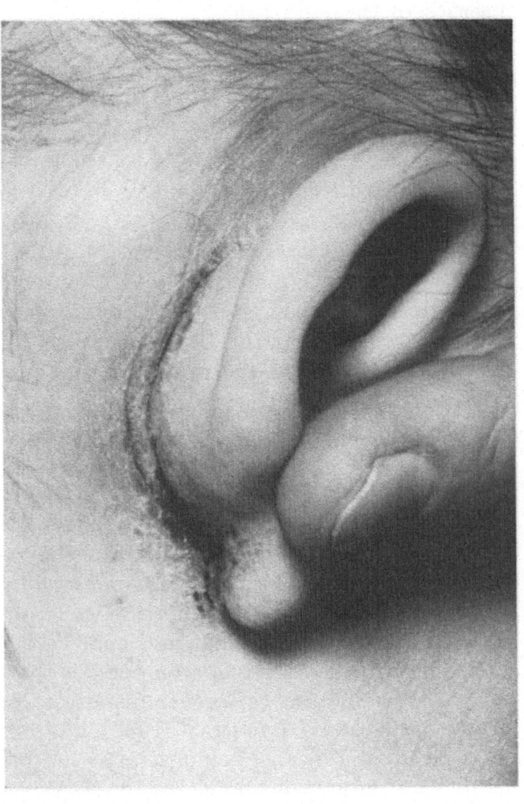

Fig. 4. Secondary Microbial Eczema, superimposed on dermatitis seborrhoides. Female $2^1/_2$ years of age. Persistent dermatitis seborrhoides and blepharitis since infancy. Bacteriology: Culture positive for Staphylococcus aureus haemolyticus. Responded to topical applications of Erythromycin ointment. (From the Department of Dermatology, Columbia-Presbyterian-Medical Center)

The observations of NIKOLOWSKI (1953) of "seborrhoid reactions following localized furuncles" also points up the fact that pathogenic staphylococci are the determining factors for an exanthematic dissemination of Dermatitis seborrhoides.

There is no direct proof that bacteria are the cause of Dermatitis seborrhoides but it appears that they play an important triple role in the evolution of its lesions:

1. They may produce secondary pyoderma.
2. They may act as primary irritants and aggravate the condition.
3. They may produce sensitization and subsequent absorption (autosensitization).

Bacteria alone probably do not cause primary irritation and sensitization in seborrheic dermatitis. But bacteria, plus local exudates, plus the degradation products of cells and exudates may well be irritants and occasionally may sensitize. We feel very strongly that our future understanding of many acute exudative diseases of the skin will rest upon the further study of the secondary effects of bacterial propagation on an injured skin.

Pityrosporon ovale a yeast like, lipophilic organism, discovered in 1874 has been the source of controversy and speculation to the present day.

MALASSEZ was the first to mention the presence of the organism and it is thus known by the historical name of the "spore of Malassez". It is difficult to precisely place credit for the first reliable culture of the organism because several authors have claimed to have obtained cultures but were subsequently unable to subculture the organism. TEMPLETON (1926) credits HUANG with the first true culture, while OTA and HUANG (1933) give credit to CASTELLANI. TEMPLETON cultured the organism on beefwort agar but was unable to subculture it. Authors, writing since 1939 credit BENHAM (1939) for her monumental work in defining the characteristics of the organism and giving detailed procedures for reliable culture. NIKOLOWSKI (1949) demonstrated a whitish-yellow fluorescence of the organism. MARTIN-SCOTT (1952) established that p. ovale survives best at a pH of 5 and LEONE (1952) convincingly demonstrated a direct correlation between p. ovale and the lipid content of the skin surface. The decrease in pityrosporon ovale as lesions become more acute and exudative may be due to a change in pH, a loss of lipids or competitive inhibition by other micro-organisms. A careful review of the literature reveals a distinct trend away from claims that pityrosporon ovale is the cause of Dermatitis seborrhoides. Not a single author claims that KOCH's postulates have been fulfilled and none give convincing proof that they have. We do not believe that pityrosporon ovale is the sole cause of Dermatitis seborrhoides but we are reluctant to forever dismiss the organism as a harmless saprophyte. STORCK (1948) and KLIGMAN (1962), the former utilizing staphylococci and the latter candida albicans, demonstrated the primary irritant action a microbe may have. Thus, organisms may damage skin, over and above their role as pathogenic invaders. It is premature to claim a primary irritant role for pityrosporon ovale in the pathogenesis of Dermatitis seborrhoides but further studies are warranted, using quantitative techniquies.

The greatest controversy involving pityrosporon ovale is centered around its possible etiologic role in dermatitis seborrhoides. UNNA, MALASSEZ, SABOURAUD, ENGMANN, HODARA, MARZINOWSKI, BOGRON, PEKELHARING, TEMPLETON, PANJA, MACLEOD, DOWLING, BENEDEK and others believe p. ovale to be important in the etiology of Dermatitis seborrhoides. JACQUET, RONDEAU, DARIER, TIECHE, OTA, MOORE, KILE, MACKEE, LEWIS, LEONE, MARTIN-SCOTT and many others believe p. ovale to be a harmless saprophyte. Several authors report a very high incidence of positive cultures from patients with seborrhea sicca (70—99%) and some have produced seborrheic lesions with local application of cultures of the organisms (MACLEOD and DOWLING 1928a, b). These two facts have been used as evidence to prove the etiological significance of pityrosporon ovale in dermatitis seborrhoides. Other authors note that the more acute and exudative the lesions of seborrheic dermatitis, the less likely one is to obtain pityrosporon ovale in significant numbers (McKEE and LEWIS, MARTIN-SCOTT). These same authors were unable to reproduce lesions employing pure cultures of the organism.

6. The Role of Metabolic Disturbances in the Etiology of Dermatitis Seborrhoides

Despite the stress which UNNA, WINKLER and others of their contemporaries laid on the parasitic etiology of seborrhoic eczema WINKLER states that "the alteration of keratinization (which prompted SABOURAUD to speak of dyskeratosis seborrhoiformis) manifests itself in the abnormal fat formation of the epidermal cells, and one cannot refute the idea that the excessive fat formation of the epidermis in seborrhoic eczema is connected with the action of micro-organisms as well as with a dysfunction of some endocrine glands. The pancreas, which plays a role in seborrhoea of infancy according to CRANSTON LOW and PEDRO RUEDA, may possibly have a bearing on the etiology of seborrhoic eczema" (quoted from WINKLER & UNNA, Hdb. 1927).

The search for the internal disturbances which may have an etiological role or at least predispose to the development of Dermatitis seborrhoides has continued up to the present time. There are many reasons why this search appears to have yielded disappointing results, despite the great advances in physiology, biochemistry and other basic sciences of the last 35 years. The fact that much of the work has by necessity been based on clinical observations and its inherent difficulties and shortcomings is one explanation. Another reason is the one sided approach which for instance, draws too sharp a line between infection and metabolic disturbance. The valuable lessons derived from the clinical and laboratory research on vitamin deficiencies have been overlooked. The intensive studies on the histochemistry of the psoriatic lesion and parakeratosis in general have not found a counterpart in the study of Dermatitis seborrhoides. The interrelationship of vitamins and cellular enzymes and hormones has only partially been appreciated. The broad concept of stress as outlined by SELYE has not been sufficiently correlated to the well established effects of emotional, physical, toxic and climatic factors on Dermatitis seborrhoides. Finally, it is at times difficult to evaluate the available findings and results because of the lack of distinction made between dandruff, seborrheic conditions (including acne, sycosis, etc.) and seborrheic dermatitis in a strict sense, despite the fact that Dermatitis seborrhoides is an "entité morbide" (GANS 1952). One may regard the epidermis as a vast holocrine gland secreting keratin on its surface, and, from invaginations in the dermis, hair, nails and sebum, (DESAUX 1932) but this anatomical and physiologic unitarianism does not prevent biochemical variations resulting from functional differentiation.

One cannot deny the fact or strong possibility that there is a common denominator for seborrhea, acne, dandruff, seborrheic dermatitis and calvities, which may be found in a constitutional background namely the status seborrhoicus. That "the whole problem of coarse hair, seborrhea, dandruff and of the seborrhoic eruptions rests basically on the fact that androgens stimulate the surface epithelium and the sebaceous glands and that oestrogens have a contrary action" (BARBER 1948) appears to be a somewhat doubtful simplification.

One can agree with BARBER, that the characteristic of DARIER's Kérose (DARIER 1928, 1936) are those of what is commonly termed "the seborrheic skin". DARIER described la kérose as a chronic morbid state of the skin, characterized clinically: 1. by a dirty yellow, bistrée, or greyish color. 2. by an accentuation of the pilosebaceous orifices. 3. by slight thickening of the integuement. The histopathology reveals: 1. a slight diffuse hypertrophy of the stratum corneum with a tendency to fine desquamation, and a modification of its fatty content: 2. hyperkeratosis of the pilo-sebaceous orifices (quoted from BARBER 1948). BARBER then continues to state that "It is now clear that the basic factor, upon which DARIER's

Kérose and its various manifestations depend is stimulation of the epidermis, hair follicles and sebaceous glands by androgens, derived either from the male gonad or from the adrenal cortex". Barber in discussing the effect of androgenic stimulation on the skin in eunuchs, eunuchoids and male castrates concludes that such results illustrate the stimulating action of androgens upon sebaceous activity and upon the formation of keratin in the follicles. In this connection one should remember that the fundamental studies of Hamilton (1941) in eunuchs clearly demonstrate that the result of androgen therapy only produces comedones, acne and changes in hair growth. Barber himself (1948, p. 129) makes it quite clear that "while admitting the roles of androgens and of individual predisposition, the development and severity of the inflammatory 'seborrhoeic' eruptions depend upon other factors". In his opinion these factors are diet, mode of life and perhaps emotional disturbances.

The concept of the seborrheic diathesis (seborrheic state) is well summarized by Ingram (1957) "there is perhaps no dermatological field that so completely involves the whole man and his adjustment to his whole environment. Every seborrheic subject presents an individual problem, whereas in this address I shall have to generalize, and he who generalizes generally lies. From a limited conception of infective skin disease propounded by the great Unna, we now realize that there is an underlying systemic motif to all these varied expressions. All systems are concerned in this symphony but especially the endocrine, nutritional and emotional. In the seborrheic certain fundamental instabilities and tendencies exist which are expressed through the skin but which are tied to humoral influences, particularly endocrine, emotional, nutritional or metabolic. Stress, acting through these and other channels, as through climatic and toxic influences, will particularly determine seborrheic disorders". Indeed, only a physician and scientist, who has thought and written for many years about the difficult problem of the seborrheic diathesis, will make such a fine distinction between the constitutional background, the humoral influences and the role of stress and the channels by which it exerts its effect.

7. Nutrition and Vitamins in Relation to Dermatitis Seborrhoides

"Seborrheic disorders are described in standard works on nutrition as evidence of deficiency and these particularly relate to deficiency of vitamin B complex, iron, and proteins—all essential constituents of epidermal enzyme systems."

This statement by Ingram, although subject to some modification, brings the role of vitamins and nutrition in proper focus. There is no question that dermatology has gained a better insight from the modern research on nutrition. The knowledge of the role of the vitamins as prosthetic groups of cellular enzymes, the biochemistry of the amino acids, lipids and lipoproteins have opened new fields for study and research. The skin manifestations of vitamin deficiencies in experimental animals have been instructive as far as the histopathology, cellular and general metabolism, liver damage and metal toxicity are concerned (Sullivan, Gross, Gans and others). The clinical implications of the experimental deficiencies in animals are limited. To quote Marrack (1948): "We can learn much about the effects of nutrients on other parts of the body from experiments on other animals, but human skin differs so profoundly from that of other animals in its structure and functions and in the way in which it is treated, that we can learn about it only from studies on human beings."

A case in point with special implications for seborrheic dermatitis is the history of Pyridoxine. It was the important discovery of Paul György (1935) that the acrodynia of the rat was due to a deficiency in a water soluble vitamin distinct from thiamin and riboflavin.

György designated this vitamin deficiency as a status seborrhoicus with dermatitis, oedema of the ears and paws, alopecia and erythroderma desquamativum like development in the advanced stages.

The synthesis of Pyridoxine by Harris & Folkers (1939) and the availability of a synthetic diet containing the optimal proportions of protein, carbohydrates, unsaturated fatty acids and vitamins (thiamin, riboflavin, panthotenic acid, etc.) also lead to the observation that these animals developed epileptic fits, muscle weakness and lesions in other organs. Experiments in human volunteers by Hawkins & Barsky (1948), kept on a Pyridoxine deficient diet for 54 days did not produce specific skin lesions. It required the use of the antagonist Desoxypyridoxine and a diet deficient in vitamin B complex to produce skin manifestations in human beings (Mueller & Vilter 1950). In further experiments Schreiner, Slinger, Hawkins and Vilter (1951) impressed by the similarity of the lesions produced by desoxypyridoxine to seborrheic dermatitis treated 11 patients with seborrheic dermatitis of "sicca type" with large doses of pyridoxine. They saw only slight improvement after as much as 600—1000 mg were administered parenterally. Despite this failure these authors did not eliminate the possibility that spontaneous seborrhea occurs because of local needs for pyridoxine. They found that the desoxypyridoxine induced lesions were relieved in 72 hours by applications of an ointment containing 10 mg. pyridoxine per gm. These negative findings raise considerable doubt about a relationship of Dermatitis seborrhoides and pyridoxine deficiency which Gyorgy had intimated (1941).

Pehl (1940) studies the effect of vitamin B 6 (Adermin) on the seborrheic dermatitis of infancy. It was only through the experience that infants fed a synthetic milk developed convulsions which were traced eventually to the lack of pyridoxine in the milk product that a true "spontaneous" vitamin B 6 deficiency in humans could be recognized (Snyderman, Holt et al. 1953, Molony and Parmelee 1954, Coursin 1954).

The use of unsaturated fatty acids in treatment of seborrheic dermatitis of infancy (Gay Prieto et al. 1953, Steinhardt 1956) may be based on the relationship of essential fatty acids and Pyridoxine (Birch 1938, Quackenbush, Platz and Steenbock 1939, and others). Gross (1940) showed that pyridoxine is effective in curing rat acrodynia only if the animals are also given essential fatty acids. The pyridoxine under these conditions has a sparing action on the unsaturated fatty acids. According to Lorincz (1954) it seems likely that vitamin B 6 functions in the biological synthesis of fats from protein.

György (1941) pointed out that the clinical manifestations of Biotin deficiency of the rat resemble the skin lesions of seborrheic dermatitis in infants and Leiner's disease. The histologic findings of Biotin deficiency in the rat as described by Sullivan & Nicholls (1942) can also be compared to those of Dermatitis seborrhoides. They consist of hyperkeratosis, some parakeratosis, acanthosis and edema. There is also an excessive amount of sudanophilic fat in the hyperkeratotic lamellae. The study of egg white injury of the rat (Boas 1924) by Parsons (1931) and further analysis of the curative effect of certain food stuffs on this rat dermatitis (Parsons & Lease 1934) leading to György's work on vitamin H (1935) and the final identification of vitamin H with Biotin by György, du Vigneaud and co-workers (1940) presents one of the most fascinating stories of nutritional research and biochemistry.

The deductions made from the clinical resemblance of vitamin H deficiency of the rat, produced by feeding raw egg white, to seborrheic dermatitis opened an era of indiscriminate use of a preparation containing the "Haut vitamin" in the treatment of seborrheic conditions including dandruff.

It was thanks to the careful investigations of Milbradt (1936) and Moncorps (1936) that the lack of value of this therapy was firmly established.

The clinical picture of Biotin deficiency in man differs considerably from seborrheic dermatitis as shown by Sydenstricker and co-workers (1942). They were able to produce in 4 human subjects fed a basic diet containing large amounts of dried raw egg white and supplemented by vitamins of the B complex, except biotin, a deficiency syndrome. The manifestations consisted of dryness of the skin with bran-like scales, anemia with lowered hemoglobin and decrease in red blood cells and other systemic symptoms. It took 7—10 weeks for the manifestations to appear and 3—5 weeks of daily injections of a biotin concentrate to correct the deficiency.

The mechanism of avidin, the active factor in egg white which inactivates biotin is based on the fact that this glycoprotein forms a complex with biotin, which cannot be absorbed from the intestinal tract.

The role which the intestinal flora plays in the biosynthesis (see also Majumdar 1958) of Biotin may explain the absence of a spontaneous biotin deficiency in man. On the other hand, the curative effect of biotin in erythrodermia desquamativa of Leiner reported by some authors after World War II (Thélin 1949, Švejcar and Homolka 1950, Kokil 1956, Steinhardt 1956, Vujašin and Petrovic 1952, Barker, Gross, McCarthy 1958) may find some explanation in the make up of the intestinal flora of the infant in the first few weeks of life, resulting in insufficient biosynthesis to satisfy the requirement (Kimmig 1957). The intrauterine hormonal influences, the quality of the skin of the first trimenon, and constitutional factors influence the clinical picture of the resulting syndrome, namely, dermatitis seborrhoides and Leiner's disease (Wolfram 1959).

A detailed discussion of dermatitis seborrhoides of infancy by Bandman will be found in Volume II, part 1 of the Ergänzungswerk.

Skin lesions resembling Dermatitis seborrhoides have also been observed in ariboflavinosis (Sebrell and Butler 1939), consisting of greasy desquamation in the naso-labial folds, on the alae nasi, in the vestibule of the nose, and in a few instances, on the ears and eyelids.

Hou (1941) also speaks of seborrheic dermatitis of the face in 4 of 10 pellagrins in refugee camps, responding to Riboflavin.

One may doubt whether one can classify these lesions of malnutrition as true Dermatitis seborrhoides especially if we consider the findings of Simons (1949) on prisoners of war in the Far East. He described some of the skin lesions of the scrotum, radix penis, pubis and seborrheic eczema of alae nasi, but found that "seborrheic eczema in the seborrheic regions (head, sternum, back) was not commoner perhaps even less so than in normal life". Sefton (1949) on the basis of experiences in a prisoner of war camp hospital in Singapore found seborrheic dermatitis to be a rare skin disorder.

The extensive erythemato-squamous eruptions which responded to intensive therapy with injections of crude liver extract, were not due to a primary nutritional deficiency (Gross 1941). Especially in the cases presenting a picture of dermatitis seborrhoides other factors of a constitutional type had to be postulated to explain a "conditioned malnutrition". Abnormal functions of the skin associated with gastric hypo or anacidity, anemia and a diet sufficient in calories but not properly balanced in food stuffs and vitamins were found to be present.

Even though the great advances in nutritional research and the study of the clinical manifestations and biochemical basis of vitamin deficiencies have not solved the etiology and therapy of dermatitis seborrhoides, they have given us a better insight into the pathogenesis of a group of dermatoses characterised by erythemato-squamous lesions. Merk (1925) recognized the similarity of the parakeratosis of Dermatitis seborrhoides and that of Pellagra and called this form of loose parakeratosis "Chaunokeratose".

The common denominator may be found in a metabolic disturbance of the skin, which in the case of pellagra and other avitaminoses is caused by nutritional deficiencies and in seborrheic dermatitis by a mechanism, so far unknown. The broader concepts of the KOEBNER phenomenon gained from the studies of BEAN, SPIES & VILTER (1944) in pellagra, the role of tissue deficiency (KRUSE 1943) predisposing to infection, the response of monilia intertrigo in diabetics, controlled by insulin, to injections of crude liver extracts (GROSS 1941) may give us a better understanding of some features of Dermatitis seborrhoides. SINCLAIR (1956) summarized the role of the vitamins in skin metabolism in these words: "It is reasonable to conclude that energy metabolism in the skin occurs as in most other tissues through glycolysis, the citric acid cycle and the cytochrome system. Therefore, the vitamins; nicotinic acid, riboflavin, thiamine and panthotenic acid are required. The extensive work upon the metabolism of protein and amino-acids in the skin cannot be reviewed here. Pyridoxine may be involved in this important turnover." The relationship of enzymes and vitamins to skin diseases was ably discussed by RUST (1958). He found constant values of Riboflavin in all groups of dermatoses but more pronounced fluctuations in total nicotinic acid, inasmuch as dermatitis seborrhoides and psoriasis showed higher levels than the allergic dermatoses. The arithmetical median values of the codehydrogenases in the blood were higher in psoriasis and Dermatitis seborrhoides than in controls, but not statistically significant. ROTHMAN and SCHAAF (1929) find that the skin is the first organ to display clinical disease particularly in deficiencies of B factors, required for carbohydrate metabolism.

ROTHMAN (1954) refers to the peculiarities of the carbohydrate metabolism of the skin as being the reason for the skin's being particularly vulnerable to inadequate nutrition.

8. Metabolism

The erythemato-squamous skin eruptions observed in human and animal deficiency diseases tend to demonstrate that metabolic disturbances rather than allergic sensitivity and infection are the basis of the pathological changes of the skin in Dermatitis seborrhoides. The studies of the abnormalities of the skin surface discussed in a previous chapter are the reflection not only of pathophysiological but also patho-chemical changes of the entire skin in Dermatitis seborrhoides. The question how far protein, sugar, fat, mineral and water metabolism of the skin are involved and what their relationship is to aberrations of general metabolism, has occupied dermatologists studying Dermatitis seborrhoides for many years. Some advances have been made, but much work is still to be done. The findings of MARCHIONINI, MANZ & HUSS (1938) demonstrated that the cholesterol content of the affected as well as the normal skin in Dermatitis seborrhoides is elevated.

LEONHARDI (GANS 1952) attempted to find out whether this condition on the skin surface was based on a general metabolic disturbance. In 12 cases of Dermatitis seborrhoides (morbus Unna) they determined the fasting values of the serum content in total lipids, total cholesterol, free cholesterol and lipid phosphorus. They found some increases in total lipids, cholesterol and lipid phosphorus, but the difference from the 13 control cases was not statistically significant. GANS concludes that with the present methods one cannot assume a general disturbance of fat metabolism in Dermatitis seborrhoides.

The studies of WALTER and OBTULOWICZ (1937, 1938, 1939) on the seborrheic diathesis and the distribution of lipids in the skin and serum of seborrhoics and rats would at least give a rational basis to the dietary measures advocated by BARBER (1948), SUTTON & SUTTON (1949) and others designed to correct the lipid disturbance in the skin of the seborrhoic. More clarity may come from studies of Dermatitis seborrhoides with the modern methods of determining the lipo proteins of the blood by ultracentrifuge and paper electrophoresis.

If and when these data will be available, they will offer some interesting comparisons with those already obtained in recent reports on psoriasis.

The findings regarding water and mineral metabolism in Dermatitis seborrhoides are equivocal. NATHAN and STERN (1928) found high water and chloride values in lesions of seborrheic dermatitis, lichen planus, pityriasis rosea and psoriasis in the acute and subacute phases. In chronic psoriasis NADEL (1932) found the water content of the lesions only moderately increased and the chloride content usually unchanged.

In lesions of chronic non exudative erythemato-squamous eruptions the changes in water and mineral content are very much less conspicuous than in acute inflammation (quoted from ROTHMAN 1954). URBACH (1945) studied extensively the influence of diet on metabolism of the skin and discussed in detail the antiretentional diet of FÖLDES (1933). BARBER (1939, 1948) supports the view of FÖLDES that water retention is a feature of the seborrheic diathesis. He concerns himself primarily with the influence of retention and mobilization of fluid on the growth of bacteria. According to him "wateriness" both of the skin and mucous membranes of the upper respiratory tract favors bacterial activity.

Various mechanisms have been claimed to be responsible for the anti-retention effect of the FÖLDES diet. FÖLDES attributes it to the diuretic action of proteins and especially nucleoproteins. STOKES, BEERMAN & INGRAM (1938) believe that the dehydrating action of high protein diet is attributable to its acid-ash properties.

Barber also points out that a high carbohydrate content of the diet increases the requirement for B complex vitamins. GROSS (1944) refers to the "carbohydrate menance" which reduces the intake of vitamin B complex containing foods. He finds it, therefore, understandable that beneficial effects can be obtained in acne and seborrheic dermatitis by a properly balanced diet and the administration of crude vitamin B complex cantaining substances, such as yeast, liver extract and wheat germ.

ROTHMAN (1954) states that the only clear cut clinical fact which can be related to the changed chemical composition of the skin in diabetes is the greatly increased susceptibility to staphylococci and monilial infections and the greater severity of these infections in diabetics. He refers to the experimental work of PILLSBURY & STERNBERG (1937), the interpretation of which is still controversial. Since PILLSBURY & KULCHAR (1935) had pointed out that some patients with severe diabetes may have an entirely normal resistance to infection and that thus the increased amount of glucose in the skin is apparently not the sole reason for the decreased resistance to infection. KULCHAR & ANDERSON (1936) supplied experimental support to the value of the antiretention diet (low in carbohydrate) in decreasing the susceptibility to infection. ROTHMAN finds that much more work is to be done in the domain of investigative dermatology, to reconcile these and other contradictions relating to the role of faulty sugar metabolism and infection. Based on his observations and those of SYDENSTRICKER, GEESLIN & WEAVER (1939) as well as RUDY and HOFFMAN (1942), GROSS (1944) believed that cutaneous eruptions observed in diabetics (monilia intertrigo, vulvitis) controlled by insulin are effectively treated by vitamins and injections of crude liver extract.

9. Hormonal Influences in Dermatitis Seborrhoides

GANS (1952) complains that the relationship of morbus Unna to and its dependence on the function of the endocrine glands respectively have barely been studied experimentally. He finds this even more surprising since there is general agreement that the true Morbus Unna only begins with puberty. One cannot but agree with GANS' statement, and one can add that the extensive experimental work concerned with the hormonal influences especially of estrogen, androgen and progesterone on the development and function of the sebaceous glands has clarified some misconceptions, but not added much to our knowledge of Dermatitis seborrhoides. The normal and pathologic physiology of the activity of sebaceous glands will be discussed by CARRIÉ in Vol. I, part 3, of the Handbuch supplement. Some puzzling problems of seborrhea and acne and possibly of seborrheic dermatitis may find clarification if and when the presence of a pituitary sebaceous gland tropic factor (LASHER, LORINCZ & ROTHMAN 1955, LORINCZ and LANCASTER 1957) in man has been established. The significant differences in the androgenic activity of the adrenal corticosteroids, which has become evident through the descending paper partition chromatography (MUNSON quoted by POCHI et al. 1962) of the 17 ketosteroids, will also provide new leads for experimental and clinical research.

BARBER (1948) believes that the influence of the sex hormones, of sexual evolution, of pregnancy and of the menopause, upon seborrhoea, acne, dandruff, seborrhoeic dermatitis and calvities, which was clear to SABOURAUD, can be explained by our present knowledge of the mechanism of their action. Two essential facts have been established 1. that androgens derived either from the male gonad or from the adrenal cortex stimulate the surface epithelium and the sebaceous glands, tending to produce hyperkeratosis and seborrhoea. 2. that estrogens have a contrary action in that they diminish keratinization and the activity of the sebaceous glands. That these facts explain the clinical and histologic findings of DARIER's kérose and its various manifestations is supported according to Barber, by presumptive evidence. This can be gained by studying skin of cases of frank virilism and of CUSHING's syndrome, and changes of the skin in women at or after the climacteric. The similarity of the effect of progesterone in the female to that of the testicular hormone in the male (HASKIN, LASHER, ROTHMAN 1953) has given impetus for further study and research in laboratory and clinic. Much interesting material can be found in the discussion of this problem by ROTHMAN (1954). He also gives credit to ARON BRUNETIERE (1952) for observing development of acne under the influence of progesterone therapy who, therefore, changed the usual androgen/estrogen ratio to androgen and progesterone/estrogen. These observations and the analysis of the acneiform eruptions resulting from corticosteroid therapy are important for the understanding of acne vulgaris. As far as the effect of the sex hormones on fungus growth and tinea capitis is concerned, deductions can hardly be valid if applied to the yeast family of fungi, including the pityrosporon ovale. It would be better to correlate the age incidence of pityriasis simplex with the possible hormonal influences on the growth of pityrosporon ovale. The findings of MARTIN-SCOTT (1952) of an abundance of p. ovale on the infantile scalp could be used as further support of the influence in this case of the maternal hormones on the skin surface fat and pityrosporon ovale. The reappearance of seborrheic dermatitis in women at menopause, who had the disease in early life, but were free from it after marriage and child bearing, or the experience that women develop a classic and severe seborrheic dermatitis for the first time after the menopause, may give a clue to the importance of the sex hormones in this disease (see BARBER 1948). Favorable results with estrogenic hormone therapy in the menopausal type of Dermatitis seborrhoides are an experience shared by many dermatologists. Finally there is evidence that Dermatitis seborrhoides may show a premenstrual flare up similar to the type frequently seen in acne vulgaris.

STOKES and STERNBERG (1939) attributed such premenstrual flares to water retention. The studies by SCHREUS and SCHULTEN (1953) may furnish an additional or different explanation of these premenstrual flares. Determination of the skin surface fat in 16 women during the entire menstrual cycle gave the following results: measured by the chrom-oxydation method the fat content was elevated in the second half of the cycle (premenstrual-menstrual) and declined regularly after the menstruation. The improvement of acne and seborrhoic diseases during pregnancy according to BRUN and RITZ (1958) is reflected in a decrease of sebaceous secretion. This is explained by the fact that the increased estrogen levels have an inhibitory effect on sebum secretion and cause retrogressive changes in the sebaceous glands, KOROLEV (1957) distinguishes 3 types of sebaceous secretion 1. thin flowing, 2. thick flowing, and 3. transitional type. The 17 ketosteroids (in blood and urine) are normal in type 1 but markedly increased in type 2.

10. Neurologic Diseases and Seborrhea

COHN (1920) described the first case of Dermatitis seborrhoides associated with postencephalitic Parkinsonism. Reports by STIEFLER (1921), KRESTIN (1927), WEIDMAN (1930) and RATTNER (1935) confirmed a definite association between encephalitic states and both increased sebum production and Dermatitis seborrhoides. Some controversy exists as to whether only postencephalitis PARKINSON's disease can cause the Dermatitis seborrhoides. KRESTIN (1927) noted cases of idiopathic or senile paralysis agitans producing the same findings. POCHI, STRAUSS & MESCON (1962) agreed with KRESTIN and added to the list of known associations between neurologic disorders and Dermatitis seborrhoides. SERRATI (1938) and many others since have reported cases of peripheral nerve injury resulting in increased sebaceous secretion. BETTLEY and MARTEN (1956) reported a case of unilateral seborrheic dermatitis following injury to the fifth cranial nerve and its sympathetic fibers. GRASSET (1959) reported a correlation between seborrheic dermatitis and epilepsy.

It thus appears that there is a definite association between widely disassociated neurologic disorders and increased sebaceous secretion, sometimes combined with Dermatitis seborrhoides. The cheek and forehead are most prominently involved and the disorder may often be unilateral.

Many early authors presumed that the association between Dermatitis seborrhoides and neurologic disorders lent weight to a direct innervation of the sebaceous gland or some indirect influence of the central nervous system on the gland. More recent authors tend to discount any direct innervation of the gland (MIESCHER, DOUPE, HODGSON-JONES, HURLEY, KLIGMAN, POCHI). POCHI et al. (1962) studied the possibility that androgens may produce the stimulus to increased sebaceous secretion in neurologic disorders but found no androgenic abnormalities. Sebotropic hormone has been demonstrated in hogs (LASHER, LORINCZ & ROTHMAN 1955) but not in the human, but being a product of the anterior pituitary may explain the sequelae of neurologic defects and increased sebum production. At present the mechanism is unknown.

POCHI and co-workers found in 5 cases of neurological disorders, thought to involve the basal ganglia, the mean sebum level of lipids to be slightly lower than the average of non-Parkinsonian neurological disorders and considerably lower than that of the patients with Parkinsonism. This suggests that damage to the basal ganglia, per se, is not specific for the development of glandular hyperplasia in Parkinsonism.

Rothman (in discussion of Pochi) finds the best explanation for the over production of sebum in diseases of the central nervous system to be that hypothalamic disease leads to an overproduction of the sebotropic factor of Lorincz. This concept would add strength to Marchionini's (1938) assumption that the disturbance in cholesterol metabolism of the skin is the result of changes in a regulatory center in the hypothalamus.

11. Dermatitis Seborrhoides and Stress

The role of the hypothalamus in psoriasis is described by Charpy (1950) as a hereditary or acquired specific fragility of the diencephalic centers. The well known precipitating factors of psoriatic attacks namely emotional disturbances, psychologic shock, adverse climatic conditions, injuries, etc. act through the hypothalamic, pituitary-adrenocortical pathway. Charpy defines psoriasis as a disease of adaptation in predisposed individuals and prefers to call psoriasis a corticosomatic rather than psychosomatic disease. Arnold (1953) speaking of stress dermatoses, a term used already by Selye (1947) considers their mechanism as one of depression of the pituitary-adrenal axis, which can be produced by foods, bacterial toxins, drugs, emotional tension or other stress agents.

It is interesting to note that Groover (1957) in studies on atherosclerosis found that increase in serum cholesterol and changes in lipoproteins can be brought about by emotional stress in predisposed individuals. Marchionini (1962) states that "the high U.V. content of the sun rays (in tropical and subtropical regions) and the intense summer heat produce conditions in the chemistry of the skin surface, which in preparing the soil favor the invasion of Staphylococci. The pH value declines (decreased protection of the acid mantle) the sugar content rises, the cellular structure loosens". Applied to dermatitis seborrhoides and particularly to the development of its microbial complications one can think of a chemical reaction of the skin surface precipitated by climatic stress. The role of sodium chloride loss and rapid decrease of ascorbic acid are other effects of tropical climate pointing to the role of the adrenal cortex.

Barber (1948) speaks of the influence of emotional disturbances on resistant seborrhoeic eruptions, which was studied in the second World War. He thinks that the influence of such disturbances as for example the anxiety state, is dependent upon fluid retention, the emotional stress acting on the hypothalamic pituitary mechanism.

Edgell (1953) acknowledging the hereditary tendency to the so-called seborrheic eruptions, enumerates the factors for activating a latent seborrheic eczema or dermatitis. He includes emotional stresses, nutritional deficiencies, superficial infections, chemicals and physical noxae. In a study of 100 cases he found that in 76 patients the onset of the skin trouble was preceded by some event which might have been upsetting to anybody. "The significance and possible etiological relevance of these events can be fully appreciated only if the uniformity of the emotional repercussions in the patients, their previous personalities, and their reactions to the disturbing events are taken into account."

This statement could well be taken as a compromise between a corticosomatic and a purely psychosomatic approach to the understanding of the skin diseases in which psychogenic factors are of particular importance.

Witkower and MacKenna (1947) believe that the seborrheic patient presents what is commonly called an obsessional character (difficulties in social contacts are the most prominent feature). This is due not to his skin affection, but because he feels and has always felt ostracized. This would make it appear that these authors are confirmed believers in personality profiles (DUNBAR). That this is not the case is shown by their admission, that only two thirds of their patients conformed to the personality type described. To answer this and the question, why individuals of this type under the impact of disturbing events (war) develop this particular skin disorder and not a nervous breakdown or any other psychosomatic affection, WITKOWER and MACKENNA say: "It must be assumed, that in the aetiology of seborrheic dermatitis multiple factors are at play and that a skin predisposition, possibly on a constitutional basis, or perhaps as a result of previous skin infections, prepares the soil for the eventual outbreak."

A critical evaluation of psychosomatic medicine in relation to dermatology is given by I. MACALPINE (1954). This author makes the point that psoriasis and acne vulgaris cannot be regarded as psychosomatic in the strict sense of that word. Investigations have been concerned with the acute stages and exacerbations; that these are influenced by emotional factors does not warrant the conditions being labelled psychosomatic.

OBERMAYER (1955) has never been impressed that patients with uncomplicated seborrheic dermatitis exhibit deviations of personality. When that cutaneous disorder becomes widespread and acute its sudden aggravation more likely represents the virus-pyogen sensitization sequence (STOKES) rather than constituting a somatic expression of an underlying neurosis. Regarding the effect of emotion on sebaceous secretion OBERMAYER finds the explanation for its increase resulting from fear or weeping by ROBIN and KEPECS (1953) plausible.

These authors suggested that the increase of the rate of sebaceous secretion observed in the general adaptation syndrome of SELYE offers an explanation of the results of their experiments as a reaction to stress.

This discussion would not be complete without a reference to STOKES (1930) who introduced the concept of the "tension frame of mind" as a psychosomatic factor in skin diseases. It is interesting to note that STOKES (1942) lists among the psychoneurogenous factors of acne vulgaris in first place "emotional effects on the thalamic control of sebaceous secretion".

The regional differences in the incidence of Dermatitis seborrhoides established by GANS & KIMMIG (1952) would indicate that the climate of the north German seaboard (Hamburg-Kiel) has an adverse effect on the seborrheic if compared to the conditions of the inland climate of Frankfurt a.M. and Breslau. Whether this indicates regional or climatic influences on the bacterial and fungus flora considered by GANS or whether climatic stress is responsible for the increase of acute and subacute attacks of Dermatitis seborrhoides cannot be decided.

The foregoing discussion leaves little doubt about the influence which stress, especially emotional and climatic, may exert on the course of seborrheic dermatitis. Much has to be learned yet about the mechanism of the adaptation syndrome as it relates to skin diseases, especially of non-allergic etiology. The danger of oversimplication and generalization can be seen when we examine the role of acute and chronic infection as a factor leading to exacerbations of seborrheic dermatitis. The acute or subacute-chronic dysseborrheic dermatitis, according to GANS (1952) is a secondary dermatitis, grafted on a hereditary or acquired constitutional anomaly. It is dependent in its development on bacterial, physical or chemical stimuli, in a broad sense, on climate, on milieu. The role of a septic focus has been discussed by STORCK, NIKOLOWSKI and others in connection with bacterial sensitization leading to exacerbations and dissemination of Dermatitis seborrhoides.

Of course, the exacerbation of an uncomplicated Dermatitis seborrhoides may be due to the action of bacterial toxins on the endocrine system or general metabolism, in other words a stress effect.

12. Association of Dermatitis Seborrhoides with Other Diseases

There is reference in text books and general articles on seborrheic dermatitis, that it may be associated with internal disease. PILLSBURY, SHELLEY and KLIGMAN (1956) find that this association is frequent enough to deserve comment. In addition to PARKINSON's disease, endocrine states with obesity, they mention that obese diabetics frequently have seborrheic dermatitis with intertriginous involvement. Both these conditions have been discussed in the preceding chapters.

Some of the cases of skin eruptions associated with macrocytic anemia reported by STRYKER and HALBEISEN (1945) could be interpreted as seborrheic dermatitis. PASTINSZKY and GESZTI (1955) describe 10 cases "resembling" dermatitis seborrhoides, which were associated with signs of macrocytic anemia, disturbed liver function and hypoprothrombinemia. Parallel with the improvement of the hemogram resulting from therapy with B 12 and Folic acid there was an essential improvement or disappearance of the skin manifestations. The importance of gastrointestinal disturbances in relation to Dermatitis seborrhoides has been stressed in a series of papers by VARGA V. KIBÉD (1939, 1942, 1948). Individualized approach consisting of nutritional therapy and correction of the various types of gastrointestinal difficulties is advocated by this author for the management of seborrheic eruptions.

That malabsorption is one of the mechanisms which explains the effect of gastrointestinal disturbances on the skin, is demonstrated by the occurence of seborrheic dermatitis in endemic sprue. The role which the liver plays in utilization and transport of vitamins and as a detoxifying agent may express itself by various skin manifestations, among which seborrheic dermatitis seems to be prominent.

The occurence of skin eruptions with features of Dermatitis seborrhoides following malaria prophylaxis with Quinacrine (NISBET 1947) and the seborrheic dermatitis like drug reactions following arsphenamine and gold therapy may also be explained by the hepatotoxic effect of these drugs. MILIAN (1936) interpreting seborrheic eczema like reactions under salvarsan therapy as "microbial activiation" also attributes this phenomenon to a decreased resistance of the macro-organism.

The relationship of allergic contact eczema and Dermatitis seborrhoides has been studied by HUG (1942). There was no significant difference between patients with Dermatitis seborrhoides and those afflicted with psoriasis when the sensitization index of various topical remedies (Resorcin, hydrargyrum ammoniatum, Balsam Peru, Mitigal) was observed. Both showed a relatively low tendency (Dermatitis seborrhoides 2.1%, Psoriasis 2.3%) to contact sensitization. This was further born out by experiments with the SULZBERGER technique of contact sensitization to 2—4 dinitrobenzol. The results showed that 66% of normals and 60% of patients with Dermatitis seborrhoides were sensitized. No flare up of the skin eruption was observed among the seborrheic cases.

On the other hand, statistics of 1028 cases revealed that persons affected with various degrees of seborrheic dermatitis represented 59% of patients developing allergic contact dermatitis against 23% of those with normal skin. Hug concludes that seborrhoics are more susceptible to contact allergic eczema under the complex and varied conditions of everyday life. GOLDSMITH and HELLIER (1954) state that patients with seborrheic dermatitis are very vulnerable to dusty, or hot work but the mere presence of greasy skin does not highten susceptibility to industrial dermatitis.

Undoubtedly, the seborrhoic constitution is a common denominator for acne and dermatitis seborrhoides. The distinction between those two diseases is illustrated by the fact that patients with acne rarely have a frank seborrheic dermatitis. As Cohn (1945) points out, acne and gross dandruff are frequently found together but not acne and dermatitis seborrhoides. Andrews, Post and Domonkos (1951) state that Dermatitis seborrhoides and acne are physiologically distinct. We can readily subscribe to this statement, since even pityriasis steatoides or mediothoracic seborrhoid are uncommon findings in acne patients.

The question of the simultaneous occurence of Dermatitis seborrhoides and psoriasis in one and the same patient is complicated by the similarity of the psoriasiform type of Dermatitis seborrhoides and the seborrheic form of psoriasis. The difficulty of this differential diagnosis has been stressed by many authors (J. Jadassohn, Kreibich 1929, Bernhard 1931, Tachau 1939, Freeman 1954, Sulzberger and co-authors 1961 and others). This is certainly true of the clinical manifestations, and at times even the most experienced histopathologist will confine himself to reporting a biopsy as psoriasiform dermatitis.

This is not a contradiction to the distinction between Dermatitis seborrhoides and psoriasis, which Gans (1952) draws on the basis of careful studies of the histopathology, histochemistry and oxidative metabolism of the skin. The occurrence of psoriasis in seborrheic sites is viewed by Shelley (1959) as a Koebner's phenomenon so that one does see psoriasis developing in seborrheic patches, whether they be on the scalp, face, chest or flexural areas. This statement of courses accept the possibility of coexistence of Dermatitis seborrhoides and psoriasis in one patient. This is supported by clinical observation including response to therapy and by the fact that psoriasis answers various stimuli with an isomorphous reaction only in the "eruptive stage".

That the metabolic disturbance characteristic of the seborrhoic diathesis, especially in the sites of predilection, may act as a stimulus for the isomorphous effect, resulting in manifestations of seborrheic dermatitis, is probable.

The observations of Zenner, Beutnagel and Friedrich (1951) include 17 cases of Dermatitis seborrhoides which were suspected to be aggravated by exposure to sun rays.

The case of "actinobiotropism" with acute seborrhoic manifestations following radiotherapy of epithelioma (Degos, Duverne and Picot 1961) may be viewed also in the same light. Finally, in the experiments by Kohlfahl (1954) with the nicotinic ester (Pyridin B carbonylic acid benzyl ester) tended to demonstrate an individual reaction type (Reaktionsbereitschaft) in 21.1% of "seborrhoid-microbial eczema".

13. Tinea amiantacea

Tinea amiantacea is a distinct entity, usually occuring in children, where the scalp reveals tightly matted whitish, grey, scales, not unlike asbestos. Alibert (1832) first described the disease and believed it was due to a fungus. Sabouraud (1920) discussed its differentiation from chronic impetiginous eruptions of the scalp. Becker and Muir (1929) gave a detailed clinical description of three cases and stated that, although the etiology was obscure seborrheic dermatitis and psoriasis were to be considered. Bernhardt raised the possibility that it was related to keratosis follicularis and Brown (1948) felt it was a form of neurodermatitis of the scalp. The hair is normal. Ammoniated mercury ointment or sulfur ointment is effective.

14. Blepharoconjunctivitis

Blepharitis and conjunctivitis often accompany Dermatitis seborrhoides when there is involvment of the supraorbital ridges. The diagnosis is made by observing the clinical presence of Dermatitis seborrhoides. GOTS, THYGERSON and WAISMAN (1947) found pityrosporon ovale in about $^{2}/_{3}$ of cases of seborrheic blepharitis and emphasized the possible appearance of keratitis, as well as blepharoconjunctivitis.

15. External Otitis

There is a vast and confusing literature on the subject of otitis externa. Several anatomic and physiologic considerations will aid in understanding the pathophysiology of this entity. The external auditory canal is a blind and tortuous cul de sac. Apocrine and sebaceous glands are present in quantity and the pH is somewhat more alkaline than on other areas of the skin (FABRICANT 1949). The factors noted contribute to bacterial propagation and may, in part, explain the predisposition to external otitis. Dermatitis seborrhoides is one of the multiple factors which may underly the clinical entity. Psoriasis, pyoderma, microbial eczema, neurodermatitis, contact dermatitis, and Dermatitis seborrhoides are commonly associated with otitis externa. RÖCKL (1956) emphasized the association with otitis media. The climate is ideal for mixed bacterial infection thus staphylococci, streptococci and pseudomonas aeruginosa are commonly found in this affliction. Much has been written regarding the mycotic origin of external otitis. NELSON and MCCARTHY (1959) obtained mycologic cultures from several hundred cases and were able to demonstrate a fungus in but one or two cases. The work of JONES and PERRY emphasizes the important secondary role bacteria play in otitis externa. Dermatitis seborrhoides must be placed among the contributing factors in the clinical entity of external otitis.

16. Histopathology

The histopathologic picture of Dermatitis seborrhoides is not diagnostic but is quite characteristic. The horny layer is not uniform (LAYMON, LEVER, GANS and STEIGLEDER) but does show parakeratosis and areas of hyperkeratosis. There is a moderate acanthosis and evidence of intracellular edema and spongiosis (LEVER 1961). MUNRO's microabscesses and migrating neutrophils, which are characteristic of psoriasis, are sometimes seen in Dermatitis seborrhoides and lend to the difficulty of differentiating the two diseases. The dermis shows evidence of a chronic non-specific inflammatory infiltrate. Dermatitis seborrhoides thus shows the histopathology of a dermatitis. The practical differentiation between psoriasis and Dermatitis seborrhoides is aided by the presence of spongiosis in Dermatitis seborrhoides especially on the border of the lesion and its usual absence in psoriasis (LAYMON 1950). Dermatitis seborrhoides is differentiated from neurodermatitis, in its many clinical forms, by the absence of pronounced acanthosis and hyperkeratosis.

The psoriasiform type of Dermatitis seborrhoides resembles psoriasis by the presence of lipophages which migrate from the blood vessels. STEIGLEDER who had studied the Nadi reaction and tetrazolium chloride reaction in psoriasis (1952) made comparative studies with this technique between psoriasis and typical seborrheic dermatitis. Typical Dermatitis seborrhoides showed staining which approximated that of the normal skin while the psoriasiform lesions showed essentially the same changes as psoriasis. There was a strong increase of the stain deposits in the acanthotic epithelium. Since the Nadi reaction gives information on the activity of oxidases and cytochrome oxidase and Tetrazolium chloride reaction shows up reducing substances including dehydrogenases and sulfhydril groups, these findings indicate a very lively metabolism in this type of acanthosis seen in psoriasis and psoriasiform Dermatitis seborrhoides. The studies of von Glasenapp and Gans (quoted from Gans 1952) on the QO_2 with Warburg apparatus showed a marked difference between psoriasis and Dermatitis seborrhoides. The average values for psoriasis were 3.0, for Dermatitis seborrhoides 1.45 and for normal skin 1.25—1.45. Thus there was no abnormal increase of cellular respiration in Dermatitis seborrhoides.

We see from these findings that much more remains to be done on the histochemistry of Dermatitis seborrhoides. The ingenious studies of Braun-Falco, Steigleder, Szakall, Flesh and Jackson-Esoda and others, which have thrown much light on the metabolic process involved in parakeratosis, should be extended to the investigation of Dermatitis seborrhoides in its classical manifestations.

17. Exfoliative Dermatitis and Dermatitis Seborrhoides

It is well known that seborrheic dermatitis may progress to a generalized exfoliative state. According to Pillsbury and co-authors (1956) it represents a real and ever present danger in severe seborrheic dermatitis. On the other hand, Darier, Civatte and Tzanck (1949) do not mention Dermatitis seborrhoides among the erythrodermic dermatoses. Needless to say, the best illustration of the progression of Dermatitis seborrhoides to a generalized disease is the erythrodermia desquamativa of Leiner. Surprisingly no special discussion of the development of exfoliative dermatitis in the adult afflicted with Dermatitis seborrhoides can be found in the literature. Case presentations like the one by Schönfeld before the 62nd meeting of the Southwest German Association of universal seborrheic eczema with partial alopecia (1936) are also rare. The significant findings of the subacute and chronic cases are the tendency to eczematization and the susceptibility to secondary pyogenic infections. In this respect they differ from psoriatic erythroderma, but a similarity exists in the type of healing. One can see after the involution of the erythroderma a reversion to the chronic form of Dermatitis seborrhoides with its typical sites of predilection, usually in the flexural and intertriginous regions.

The special aspects of the generalized exfoliative erythroderma of the adult are discussed by R. Richter in Volume III, part I of the Ergänzungs-Werk.

18. Heredity and Dermatitis Seborrhoides

Touraine (1955) discussing seborrhea and acne believes that while the external milieu has an undoubtful influence, the role of heredity is important. Stokes and King (1932) made a thorough study of the family background of seborrheic diseases. They find that the hereditary factors are probably complex and do not follow a simple mendelian distribution. Siemens (1929) studying the problem of heredity of acne in 47 pairs of monozygotic twins saw concordance in 22 pairs and of 32 pairs of dizygotic twins only in 8.

These data may apply to seborrheic conditions in general but specific findings on Dermatitis seborrhoides cannot be gathered from these studies. The fact that Stokes and King found a family background of atopy in 28% of cases of Dermatitis seborrhoides and only 13% in cases of acne only shows that fundamental differences exist in the "seborrheic diseases". A broader base in the study of heredity of Dermatitis seborrhoides including other diseases, for instance diabetes and constitutional types, and confined to the true morbus Unna is lacking. Therefore, we can only assume at present a hereditary factor for the "status seborrhoicus". According to ROST (1926) who deserves credit for his broad concept of the status seborrhoicus, we are dealing with a constitutional type presenting a dominant form of heredity.

19. Therapy of Dermatitis Seborrhoides

Significant changes have taken place in the treatment of dermatitis seborrhoides. This can be attributed to various factors. First of all there is the modern dermatologic approach of considering the patient as a whole, and not only the local changes in his skin. While there is no specific cure for the disease, general measures are of utmost importance. SHELLEY (1959) stresses the importance of general hygiene and the beneficial effect of simple psychotherapy. According to him, the three R's of anti-seborrheic routine are Rest, Reassurance, and Recreation. Correction of gastrointestinal disturbances is essential according to VARGA V. KIBÉD (1948). SCHOCH (1935) recommends dilute hydrochloric acid and pepsin preparations. Dietary measures include the antiretention diet of FÖLDES (1933) reduction of carbohydrates and fats (SUTTON and SUTTON 1940, SCOTT 1944 and others), and low caloric diets for obesity.

Advocates of parenteral therapy with liver extracts and oral administration of vitamin B complex were GROSS (1941), O'LEARY (1942), SAYER (1942), BALL (1947). Nicotinic acid was used by DESAUX, GOIFFON and PRÉTET (1939). MASHKILLEYSON and associates (1945) obtained good results with Riboflavin. Pyridoxine (Vitamin B 6) was used by PEHL (1940) and by SCARCELLA (1942) in Dermatitis seborrhoides of infancy, and by WRIGHT, SAMITZ and BRACON (1943) in adults. ERNST and SOLTZ-SZÖTS (1958) treated seborrheic alopecia with vitamin B 6. Since the publication of ANDREWS, POST and DOMONKOS (1950) who reported good results with parenteral vitamin B 12 this method was also found useful by NIEMAND-ANDERSSON (1952) who believed that vitamin B 12 has a regulatory effect on metabolic disturbances which form the basis of seborrheic diseases. BLUT (1954) obtained 3 cures and marked improvement in 13 cases of Dermatitis seborrhoides with bi-weekly injections of 30 micrograms of B 12. Increase to 1000 micrograms did not better the results. GONZALES DIAZ (1955) reports favorably on the effect of vitamin B 12 in Dermatitis seborrhoides of infants. Several authors have been impressed with the effect of Biotin in Dermatitis seborrhoides of infancy and in LEINER'S disease (MENDIHAHARZU and OYHENART (1944). THÉLIN (1949), VUJAŠIN and PETROVIC (1952), STEINHARDT (1956) and KOKIL (1956).

The effect of Biotin on seborrheic processes in general was studied by ALVAREZ (1939) by PRUSKI (1951) and TREGER, MOYS and MUZIKOVA (1953). GAY PRIETO, JAQUET and DEL PINAL (1953) used linoleic and linolenic acid in the treatment of seborrheic eczema in infants with satisfactory results. Therapy with choline found favor in studies by BÖHM and SPANYAR (1953 and 1958) and was used by BIAGINI (1951) in infants with seborrheic dermatitis. He observed a rise in the unsaturated fatty acids following this therapy. Finally, several authors were impressed with the action of vitamin A on seborrheic conditions (VARGA V. KIBÉD 1942, LUCA 1928 and HELLIER 1955).

The introduction of systemic corticosteroid therapy has lead to its use in seborrheic dermatitis. According to SHELLEY (1959) these drugs have played a significant role in reducing the morbidity of seborrheic dermatitis. The judicious use of either ACTH or the newer corticosteroids is indicated in the highly inflammatory extending seborrheic eruptions. Short courses with modest dosage are remarkably effective in averting serious extensive eruptions. SULZBERGER, WOLF and WITTEN (1961) believe that for the patient with severe widespread and incapacitating seborrheic dermatitis, a short course of systemic ACTH or corticosteroid therapy is often beneficial. We see that this form of therapy should be reserved for the severe cases and one may add, is especially useful in the control of the seborrheic type of dermatitis exfoliativa. The use of *short* courses of corticosteroid therapy is stressed by these and other authors. The need of simultaneous systemic antibiotic therapy to control a secondary microbial eczema and/or the microbid type of dissemination is evident. The high susceptibility of the generalized exfoliative dermatitis to pyogenic infection is an additional indication for antibiotic therapy.

The discovery of penicillin and especially of the broad spectrum antibiotics has also improved the internal therapy of Dermatitis seborrhoides even without the use of corticosteroid therapy. It is useful in the cases of intertriginous type, where there is evidence of massive bacterial invasion or microbial sensitization.

There have been advances in the local therapy of Dermatitis seborrhoides and again the proper selection of topical antibiotics alone or combined with corticosteroids incorporated in a suitable ointment base, has been an important addition to our therapeutic armamentarium.

The use of Salicylic acid $^1/_2$—1% and the cleansing solution consisting of salicylic acid 0.1%, Resorcin 1.0 Aqua distillata ad 100 (pH 4.2) originally introduced by ROST has found a sound rational in the pH findings of the seborrheic skin. MARCHIONINI (1934) recommends these formulas and the use of Aciderm, a cream of low pH for the treatment of Dermatitis seborrhoides. These simple remedies still deserve a place in the modern dermatologic therapy of the uncomplicated Dermatitis seborrhoides. The introduction of Vioform (Iodochlorhydroxyquin) has been a useful addition to dermatologic therapy (SULZBERGER and BAER 1948). It has a wide use in the various types of seborrheic dermatitis and it is especially the combination with hydrocortisone which will in many resistant cases produce a prompt response. Similar results can be obtained in Dermatitis seborrhoides with Sterosan and Sterosan hydrocortisone cream and ointment.

The usefulness of these two remedies is not based on their bacteriostatic and mycostatic properties alone. Their action on the psoriatic lesion compares favorably with other antisporiatics. We can assume that this effect is based as much on a specific action on the metabolic disturbance of the skin characteristics of seborrheic dermatitis. In analogy to mercury ammoniate and mercury oleate it may well be that this action is concerned with the parakeratotic process. The studies on British Antilewisite (BAL) have given us a better insight on the mechanism of certain topical remedies used in psoriasis and seborrheic dermatitis (VONKENNEL and SCHÖBERL 1949).

Finally the topical use of the corticosteroids in Dermatitis seborrhoides deserves to be mentioned. The comparative studies in various skin diseases may show up some differences between the hydrocortisone free alcohol and the various triamcinolones, but their outstanding merit is their anti-inflammatory effect. This action is reflected in their use in Dermatitis seborrhoides but it is undeniable that the combination of a topical corticosteroid with antibiotics or antiseborrheics (Vioform, Sterosan, mercury, tar, sulfur) yields better results. Of course, the antiflammatory effect of the corticosteroids also has an antibacterial action by improving the soil and their antipruritic action prevents scratching and secondary infection. These considerations are especially important in the treatment of otitis externa which ranges from simple seborrheic dermatitis to microbial eczema and chronic neurodermatitis.

Other new additions to the list of antiseborrheic remedies concerns mostly the therapy and control of pityriasis simplex and steatoides capitis. The following list will illustrate the wide variety of these remedies. Their pharmacological aspects can be found in Volume V, part 1 and 2 of the Ergänzungsband of the JADASSOHN's Handbuch.

Bituminous sulfonates (KLEINE-NATROP 1950).
Thiourea (MERCADAL & PINOL 1948).
Polythionic acid (FINNERUD & RIDDEL jr. 1951).
Selenium disulphide (Selsun) (SLINGER & HUBBARD 1951).
Colloidal Sulphur (Sulphanthrol dragees) (BRAUNER 1952).
Sodium sulfacetamide (DUEMLING 1954).
Phemerol (Vancide 89) (BALL 1955).
Cadmium sulfide suspension (Capsebon) (KIRBY 1957).
Sulfur iodatum (JUSTER and CHERAMY 1958).
Estrogen-amino acid compounds (LUBOWE 1958).
4-hydroxy 2-oxobenzoxathiol (Stepin) (UHLMAN 1958).
Tellurium dioxide suspension (R. GROSS & WRIGHT 1958).
Soropon (BIALKIN 1959).
Biphenamine hydrochloride (Alvinine) (LUBOWE 1960).

Many of these remedies have been used in the form of shampoos. The combination of salicylic acid and sulfur has also been popular both as ointment application to the scalp and as a shampoo (Fostex, Sebulex).

Literatur

ALVAREZ, G.: Influencia modificadora de la vitamine cutánea "H" en algunos procesos seborrheicos. Rev. Asoc. méd. **53**, 837 (1939). — ANDERSON, D. S.: Acid-base balance of the skin. Brit. J. Derm. **63**, 283 (1951). — ANDREWS, G. C., C. F. POST and A. N. DOMONKOS: Seborrheic dermatitis: Supplemental treatment with Vitamin B_{12}. N.Y. St. J. Med. **50**, 1921 (1950). — Advances in the treatment of seborrheic Dermatitis and acne vulgaris. Aust. J. Derm. **1**, 11 (1951). — ARNOLD jr., H. L.: Stress dermatoses. Arch. Derm. Syph. (Chic.) **67**, 566 (1953). — ARON-BRUNETIERE, R.: Essai d'interprétation physiopathologique de la seborrhée et de l'acné vulgaire. Conséquences thérapeutiques. Excerpta med. (Amst.), Sect. XIII **6**, No 1508 (1952).

BALL, F. I.: A new treatment for seborrheic dermatitis. A clinical investigation. Arch. Derm. **71**, 696 (1955). — BARBER, H. W.: The influence of the sex hormones on the skin and pilosebaceous system, with a discussion of the aetiology of "seborrhoeic" eruptions. In: R. M. B. MCKENNA ed., Modern trends in dermatology. New York: Hoeber 1948. — BEAN, W. B., T. D. SPIES and R. W. VILTER: Asymetrical cutaneous lesions in Pellagra. Arch. Derm. Syph. (Chic.) **49**, 335 (1944). — BEARE, J. M., E. A. CHEESEMAN, A. A. M. GAILEY and D. W. NEILL: The p_H of the skin surface of children with seborrhoeic dermatitis compared with unaffected children. Brit. J. Derm. **70**, 233 (1958). — BECKER, S. W., and K. B. MUIR: Tinea amiantacea. Arch. Derm. Syph. (Berl.) **20**, 45 (1929). — BELISARIO, J. C.: The pathogenesis of Eczema I. In: Proc. 10th Internat. Congr. Dermat. London 1952. London: Brit. Med. Assoc. 1953. — BENHAM, R. W.: The cultural characteristics of pityrosporon ovale, a lipophylic fungus. J. invest. Derm. **2**, 187 (1939). — BERGHEIM, O., and T. CORNBLEET: Acidity of the scalp, nature and possible relation to seborrhea. Arch. Derm. Syph. (Chic.) **56**, 448 (1947). — BERNHARDT, R.: Über das seborrhoische Ekzem und seine Beziehungen zu der Psoriasis. Acta derm.-venereol. (Stockh.) **12**, 301 (1931). — Porrigo amiantacea. Tinea amiantacea s. asbestina (ALIBERT) fausse teigne amiantaceé. Keratosis follicularis amiantacea (KIESS). Derm. Wschr. **105**, 884 (1937). — BETTLEY, R. R., and R. H. MARTEN: Unilateral seborrheic Dermatitis following a nerve lesion. Arch. Derm. **73**, 110 (1956). — BIAGINI, R.: Risultati del trattamento colinico nella dermatite seborroide e nell'eczema del lattante. Clin. pediat. (Bologna) **33**, 631 (1951). Cit. Excerpta med. (Amst.), Sect. XIII **7**, No 93 (1953). — BIALKIN, G.: Seborrhea capitis. Clinical effectiveness of a new therapeutic agent. Arch. Pediat. **76**, 328 (1959). — BLUT, F.: Erfahrungen mit Vitamin B_{12} (Cytobion) bei der Behandlung von Dermatosen, vornehmlich seborrhoischer Genese. Med. Klin. **49**, 1293 (1954). — BOAS, M. A.: An observation on the value of egg white as the sole source of nitrogen for young growing rats. Biochem. J. **18**, 422 (1924). — BOLLIGER, A., and R. GROSS: Water soluble compounds (non keratins) associated with the skin flakes of the human scalp. Aust. J. exp. Biol. med. Sci. **34**, 219 (1956). — BOUGHTON, B., I. S. HODGSON-JONES, R. M. B. MACKENNA, V. R. WHEATLEY and A. WORMALL: Some observations on the nature and possible function of the squalene and other hydrocarbons of human sebum. J. invest. Derm. **24**, 179 (1955). — BOUGHTON, B., R. M. B. MACKENNA, V. R. WHEATLEY and A. WORMALL: The fatty acid composition of the skin fats (sebum) in acne vulgaris and seborrheic dermatitis. J. invest. Derm. **33**, 57 (1959). — BRAUNER, F.: Erfahrungen mit kolloidalem Schwefel bei Dermatosen. Ther. Umsch. **9**, 33 (1952). Cit. Excerpta med. (Amst.), Sect. XIII **7**, No 1601 (1953). — BROWN, W. H.: Some observations on neurodermatitis of the scalp, with particular reference to tinea amiantacea. Brit. J. Derm. **60**, 81 (1948). — BRUN, R., and A. RITZ: Variation de la couche sébacée engendrées par la grossesse. (Durch Schwangerschaft bedingte Änderungen der Talgsekretion.) Dermatologica (Basel) **116**, 229 (1958). — BRUNNER, M. J.: Biologic basis of psychosomatic disease of the skin. Arch. Derm. Syph. (Chic.) **57**, 374 (1948). — BURCKHARDT, W.: Cutaneous resistance to alkalies, acids and commercial solvents. In: L. J. H. LOEWENTHAL, The eczemas. Edinburgh and London: E. S. Livingstone, Ltd. 1954. — BURTENSHAW, J. M. L.: The autogenous disinfection of the skin. In: R. M. B. MACKENNA, Modern trends in dermatology. New York: Hoeber 1948.

CARO, M. R.: Diagnostic pitfalls of dermal pathology. Arch. Derm. Syph. (Chic.) **67**, 18 (1953). — CEDERKREUTZ, A.: Über den Fettgehalt der Epidermiszellen bei der Parakeratose. Arch. Derm. Syph. (Vienna) **111**, 739 (1912). — CHARPY, J.: Essai-pathogénique du psoriasis. Un. méd. Can. **79**, 1436 (1950). Cit. Excerpta med. (Amst.), Sect. XIII **5**, No 1351 (1950). — CLARK, W. B.: Treatment of seborrheic blepharoconjunctivitis. Amer. J. Ophthal. **20**, 808 (1937). — COHEN, E. L.: Relationship of acne with dandruff and seborrheic dermatitis. Brit. J. Derm. **57**, 45 (1945). — COHN, T.: Encephalitis ohne Lethargie während der Grippeepidemie. Zbl. Neurochir. **39**, 260 (1920). — COURSIN, D. B.: Convulsive seizures in infants with Pyridoxinedeficient diet. J. Amer. med. Ass. **154**, 406 (1954).

DARIER, J.: Note sur la kérose. Nouvelle pratique dermatologic., vol. 7, p. 8. Paris: Masson & Cie. 1936. — DARIER, J., A. CIVATTE et A. TZANCK: Dermatologie. (Translation J. DARIER, Précis de dermatologie. Cinquième edit. par. A. CIVATTE.) Bern: Hans Huber 1949. — DEGOS, R., J. DUVERNE et C. PICOT: Actino biotropisme à manifestations séborrhéiques auguës après radiothèrapie pour épithélioma baso-cellulaire. Guerison par antibiotiques. Bull. Soc. franç. Derm. Syph. **68**, 225 (1961). — DESAUX, A.: Manuel pratique de dermatologie. Paris: Masson & Cie. 1932. — DESAUX, A., R. GOIFFON et H. PRÉTET: Note préliminaire sur l'emploi de la vitamine P.P. dans le traitement de la seborrhée et de acne. Bull. Soc. franç. Derm. Syph. **46**, 715 (1939). — DOUPE, J., and M. E. SHARP: Studies in denervation. G. Sebaceous secretion. J. Neurol. Psychiat., N.S. **6**, 133 (1943). — DOWLING, G. B.: Aetiology of seborrhoeic dermatitis. Brit. J. Derm. **51**, 1 (1939). — DUEMLING, W. W.: Sodium sulfacetamide in topical therapy. Arch. Derm. Syph. (Chic.) **69**, 75 (1954).

EAKIN, R. E., E. E. SNELL and R. J. WILLIAMS: The concentration and assay of avidin. The injury producing protein in raw egg white. J. biol. Chem. **140**, 535 (1941). — EDGELL: In: WITKOWER & RUSSELL, Emotional factors in skin diseases. New York: Hoeber 1953. — EFFERSØE, H.: The effect of topical application of pyridoxine ointment on the rate of sebaceous secretion in patients with seborrheic dermatitis. Acta derm.-venereol. (Stockh.) **34**, 272 (1954). Cit. Excerpta med. (Amst.), Sect. XIII **8**, No 2280 (1954). — EMMONS, C. W.: Isolation and pathogenecity of pityrosporon ovale. Publ. Hlth Rep. (Wash.) **55**, 1306 (1940). — ERNST, G., u. J. SÖLTZ-SZÖTS: Zur Behandlung des seborrhoischen Haarausfalles mit Vitamin B_6. Med. Kosmetik **7**, 201 (1958). — EVANS, C. A., W. M. SMITH, E. H. JOHNSTON and E. A. GIRBLETT: Bacterial flora of the normal human skin. J. invest. Derm. **15**, 305 (1950).

FABRICANT, N. D., and M. A. PERLSTEIN: The p_H of the cutaneous surface of the external auditory canal. Arch. Otolaryng. **49**, 201 (1949). — FINNERUD, C. W., and J. M. RIDDELL jr.: Polythionic acid in the therapy of acne vulgaris and seborrheic dermatitis. Arch. Derm. Syph. (Chic.) **63**, 373 (1951). — FLESCH, P., and E. C. JACKSON-ESODA: Defective epidermal protein metabolism in psoriasis. Arch. Derm. **76**, 393 (1957a). — Deficient water-binding in pathologic horny layers. J. invest. Derm. **28**, 5 (1957b). — FOELDES, E.: A new approach to dietetic therapy. Boston: Badger 1933. — FREEMAN, H. E.: Seborrhea-psoriasis syndrome. Sth. med. J. (Bgham, Ala.) **47**, 940 (1954).

GANS, O.: Zur Pathogenese des Eczems. II. Morbus Unna. Proc. 10th Internat. Congr. Dermat., London 1952, p. 30—54. London: Brit. Med. Assoc. 1953. — GAY PRIETO, J., G. JAQUETI y T. DEL PINAL: Los ácidos grasos insaturados en el tratamiento de los eczemas del lactante. Acta pediát. esp. **11**, 881 (1953). Cit. Excerpta med. (Amst.), Sect. XIII **9**, No 279 (1955). — GOLDSMITH, W. N., and F. F. HELLIER: Recent advances in dermatology, 2nd ed. New York: Blakiston Company 1954. — GONZALEZ DIAZ, I.: Effectos de la Vitamina B_{12} en el tratamiento de la dermatitis seborrheica del lactante. Act. dermo-sifiliogr. (Madr.) 47, 23 (1955). — GOTS, J. S., P. THYGERSON and M. WAISMAN: Observations on Pityrosporum ovale in seborrheic blepharitis and conjunctivitis. Amer. J. Ophthal. **30**, 1485 (1947). — GRANT PETERKIN, G. A.: Seborrheic dermatitis. In: L. J. A. LOEWENTHAL, ed., The eczemas, p. 127. Edinburgh and London: E. & S. Livingstone, Ltd. 1954. — GRASSET, N., et R. BRUN: Etude du film sebace de sujets sains et de patients attents d'epilepsie ou de maladie de Parkinson. Dermatologica (Basel) **119**, 232 (1959). — GROOVER, M. E.: Clinical evaluation of a public health program to prevent coronary artery disease. Trans. Coll. Phycns Philad. **24**, 105 (1957). — GROSS, P.: Role of unsaturated fatty acids in acrodynia (Vitamin B_6 deficiency) of the rat. J. invest. Derm. **3**, 505 (1940). — Nonpellagrous eruptions due to deficiency of Vitamin B-complex. Arch. Derm. Syph. (Chic.) **43**, 504 (1941). — The significance of nutritional deficiencies in the practice of dermatology. Clinics **3**, 789 (1944). — GROSS, R., and C. S. WRIGHT: Tellurium dioxide suspension in the treatment of seborrhea capitis. Arch. Derm. **78**, 92 (1958). — GYÖRGY, P.: Stoffwechsel und Immunobiologie der Haut. In: PFAUNDLER u. SCHLOSSMANN, Handbuch der Kinderheilkunde, vol. 10. Leipzig: F. C. W. Vogel 1935. — Dietary treatment of scaly desquamative dermatoses of seborrheic type; experimental foundation. Arch. Derm. Syph. (Chic.) **43**, 230 (1941). — GYÖRGY, P., D. B. MELVILLE, D. BUCK and V. DU VIGNEAUD: The possible identity of Vitamin H with Biotin and Coenzyme R. Science **91**, 243 (1940).

HALL-SMITH, S. P., and A. NORTON: Psychiatric survey of a random sample of skin outpatients. Brit. med. J. **1952 II**, 417. — HAMILTON, J. B.: Male hormone substance. A prime factor in acne. J. clin. Endocr. **1**, 570 (1941). — HASKIN, D., N. LASHER and S. ROTHMAN: Some effects of ACTH, cortisone, progesterone, and testosterone on sebaceous glands in the white rat. J. invest. Derm. **20**, 207 (1953). — HAWKINS, W. W., and J. BARSKY: Experiment on human Vitamin B_6 deprivation. Science **108**, 284 (1948). — HELLIER, F. F.: Seborrhoeic conditions. Med. Press **6053**, 433 (1955). — HERRMANN, F.: Some data concerning the aqueous and the lipid phase. Proc. 11th Internat. Congr. Dermat. Acta derm.-venereol. (Stockh.) **2**, 27 (1957). — HERRMANN, F., and PR. H. PROSE: Studies on the ether-soluble substances on the human skin. I. Quantity and "replacement sum". J. invest. Derm. **16**, 217 (1951). — HERRMANN, F., PH. H. PROSE and M. B. SULZBERGER: Studies on sweating. V. Studies of quantity and distribution of thermogenic sweat delivery to the skin. J. invest. Derm. **18**, 71 (1952). — HERZFELD, I.: Zur Behandlung der Seborrhoe des Gehörganges und des chronischen Ohrekzems mit Thorium-X-Degea. Mschr. Ohrenheilk. **70**, 1325 (1936). — HOU, H. C.: Riboflavin deficiency among Chinese. II. Cheilosis and seborrheic dermatitis. Chin. med. J. **59**, 314 (1941). Cit. Zbl. Haut- u. Geschl.-Kr. **68**, 393 (1942). — HUG, J.: Die Beziehungen des allergischen Kontaktekzems zum seborrhoischen Ekzem. Acta derm.-venereol. (Stockh.) **23**, 273 (1942). — HURLEY, H. J., W. B. SHELLEY and G. B. KOELLE: The distribution of cholinesterases in the skin with special reference to eccrine and apocrine sweat glands. J. invest. Derm. **21**, 139 (1953).

INGRAM, J. T.: The personality of the skin. Lancet **1933 I**, 889. — Seborrheic diathesis. Brit. med. J. **1939 II**, 5. — The seborrheic diathesis. Arch. Derm. **76**, 157 (1957).

JAEGER, H.: Erythrodermie exfoliative, secondaire à une dermatite séborrheique généralisée. Dermatologica (Basel) **94**, 189 (1947). — JEGHERS, H.: Skin changes of nutritional origin. New Engl. J. Med. **228**, 678, 714 (1943). — JESIONEK, A.: Eczema seborrhoicum. Derm. Z. **17**, 887 (1910). — JONES, E. H.: External Otitis. Med. Tms (Lond.) **89**, 496 (1961). — JONES, K. K., M. C. SPENSER and S. A. SANCHEZ: The estimation of rate of secretion of sebum in man. J. invest. Derm. **17**, 213 (1951). — JUSTER, E., et P. CHERAMY: Le soufre iodé dans le traitment de la seborrhée des alopècies detes séborrhéiques et del'acné (note preliminaire). Bull. Soc. franç. Derm. Syph. **65**, 517 (1958).

KENNEL, J. v., u. A. SCHÖBERL: Bal und die Behandlung der Syphilis und Psoriasis mit thiolopriven Substanzen. Med. Mschr. **3**, 561 (1949)- — KILE, R., and M. F. ENGMAN: Further studies of the relationship of Pityrosporon ovale to seborrheic eczema. Arch. Derm. **37**, 616 (1938). — KIMMIG, I.: Die Bedeutung der Vitamine für die Haut. Arch. klin. exp. Derm. **206**, 408 (1957). — KIRBY, W. I.: Cadmium sulfide suspension in seborrhea capitis. J. invest. Derm. **29**, 159 (1957). — KIRK, J. E.: The effect of biotin administration on the skin lipid secretion. Urol. cutan. Rev. **54**, 292 (1950). — KLEINE-NATROP, H. E.: Klinische Gesichtspunkte zu einer neuen Anwendungsform von Schieferölsulfonaten in der Oberflächentherapie. Dtsch. med. Wschr. **75**, 713 (1950). — KLIGMAN, A. M., and W. B. SHELLEY: An investigation of the biology of the human sebaceous gland. J. invest. Derm. **30**, 99 (1958). — KOHFAHL, M.: Physikalische und chemische Reize bei Ekzemkranken unter besonderer Berücksichtigung der individuellen Reaktionsbereitschaft. Arch. Derm. Syph. (Berl.) **197**, 557 (1954). — KOKIL, S.: Über die Anaemie bei Dermatitis seborrhoides und ihre Beeinflussung durch Biotin. Ann. paediat. (Basel) **186**, 79 (1956). Cit. Zbl. Haut- u. Geschl.-Kr. **96**, 332 (1956). — KOROLEV, Y. F.: Regarding clinical forms of seborrhea. Vestn. Derm. Vener. **31**, H. 3, 3 (1957). Cit. Zbl. Haut- u. Geschl.-Kr. **99**, 197

(1958). — Die Veränderungen der Zusammensetzung des Hautfetts bei Seborrhoe. Vestn. Derm. Vener. **32**, H. 4, 9 (1958). Cit. Zbl. Haut- u. Geschl.-Kr. **102**, 256 (1958/59). — KREIBICH, C.: Ekzeme und Dermatitiden. In: J. JADASSOHN, Handbuch der Haut- und Geschlechtskrankheiten, vol. VI/I, p. 136. Berlin: Springer 1927. — Seborrhoid. Dtsch. Derm. Ges. in der Tschech. Rep., Prag, **16** (1929). Cit. Zbl. Haut- u. Geschl.-Kr. **31**, 551 (1929). — KRESTIN, D.: The seborrhoeic facies as a manifestation of postencephalitic parkinsonism and allied disorders. Quart. J. Med. **21**, 177 (1927). — KRÜCKEN, H.: Studie über das sogenannte „mikrobielle" Ekzem. Zbl. Haut- u. Geschl.-Kr. **96**, 81 (1956). — KRUSE, H. D.: Medical evaluation of nutritional status. In: Handbook of nutrition. Chicago: Amer. Med. Assoc. 1943. — KULCHAR, G. V., and H. E. ALDERSON: Relation of water metabolism to experimental skin infections. Brit. J. Derm. **48**, 477 (1936). — KVORNING, S. A.: Excretion of skin lipids in patients with Parkinson syndrome. Acta derm.-venereol. (Stockh.) **32** (Suppl. 29), 201 (1952).

LASHER, N., A. L. LORINCZ and ST. ROTHMAN: Hormonal effects on sebaceous glands in the white rat. III. Evidence for the presence of a pituitary sebaceous gland tropic factor. J. invest. Derm. **24**, 499 (1955). — LAYMON, C. W.: Lesions of the scalp in certain scaly dermatoses. Arch. Derm. Syph. (Chic.) **62**, 181 (1950). — LEINER, C.: Hautkrankheiten im Säuglingsalter. In: J. JADASSOHNs Handbuch der Haut- und Geschlechtskrankheiten, Bd. XIV. Berlin: Springer 1930. — LEONE, R.: Presenza e significato del Pityrosporon ovalis, nella pitiriasi del cuoio capelluto, ne l'eczema seborroico figurato ed in dermatosi squamose varie. Nota I. Ricerche quantitative sulla presenza del Pityrosporon ovalis nella pityriasis del cuoio capelluto, nello eczema seborroico figurato ed in dermatosi squamose varie. Minerva derm. **27**, 93 (1952). Cit. Excerpta med. (Amst.), Sect. XIII **9**, No 1485 (1955). — LEONHARDI, G.: Seborrhoisches Ekzem. (Dysseborrhoische Dermatitis, Morbus Unna.) In: H. A. GOTTRON u. W. SCHÖNFELD, Dermatologie und Venerologie, Bd. III, Teil 1. Stuttgart: Georg Thieme 1959. — LEVER, W. F.: Histopathology of the skin. Philadelphia: J. B. Lippincott Company 1961. — LOBITZ jr., W. C.: The structure and function of the sebaceous glands. Arch. Derm. **76**, 162 (1957). — LOEWENTHAL, L. J. A. ed.: The Eczemas. Edinburgh and London: Livingstone 1954. — LORINCZ, A. L.: Nutritional influences. In: ROTHMAN, Physiology and biochemistry of the skin. Chicago: Chicago University Press 1954. — LORINCZ, A. L., and G. LANCASTER: Anterior pituitary preparation with tropic activity for sebaceous, preputials Harderian glands. Science **126**, 124 (1957). — LUBOWE, I. I.: Die Behandlung der Akne und der Seborrhoe des Kopfes unter Verwendung oestrogener Hormon-Aminosäureverbindungen. Med. Kosmetik **7**, 323 (1958). Cit. Zbl. Haut- u. Geschl.-Kr. **103**, 63 (1959). — Treatment of seborrhea capitis and associated diseases. Sth. med. J. (Bgham, Ala.) **54**, 350 (1961). — LUCA, M. DE: Cute e vitamin A: Ricerche clinico-sperimentali. Rif. med. **54**, 1189 (1938).

MACALPINE, I.: A critical evaluation of psychosomatic medicine in relation to dermatology. In: R. M. B. MACKENNA, Modern trends in dermatology. (Second ser.) New York: Hoeber 1954. — MACKEE, G. M., and G. M. LEWIS: Dandruff and seborrhea. I. Flora of normal and diseased scalps. J. invest. Derm. **1**, 131 (1938). — MACKEE, G. M., G. M. LEWIS, M. E. PINKERTON and M. E. HAPPER: Dandruff and seborrhea. II. J. invest. Derm. **2**, 31 (1939). — MACLEOD, J. M. H., and G. B. DOWLING: Cultures, preparations and cases illustrating the morphology, cultural characteristics and pathogenecity of the spore of Malassez. Proc. roy. Soc. Med. **21**, 9 (1928a). — An experimental study of pityrosporon of Mallassez: its morphology, cultivation and pathogenecity. Brit. J. Derm. **40**, 139 (1928b). — MAIBACH, H. I., and A. M. KLIGMAN: The biology of experimental human cutaneous moniliasis (Candida albicans). Arch. Derm. **85**, 233 (1962). — MAJUMDAR, T. D.: Vitaminmangelerscheinungen bei Hauterkrankungen und die Rolle der Biosynthese bei solchen Mangelzuständen. Arch. klin. exp. Derm. **206**, 476 (1958). — MARCHIONINI, A.: Untersuchungen über die Wasserstoffionenkonzentration der Haut. Arch. Derm. Syph. (Berl.) **158**, 290 (1929). — Säuresalbenbehandlung seborrhoischer Hauterkrankungen des Gesichtes. Dtsch. med. Wschr. **1**, 934 (1934). — Der Cholesterol-Stoffwechsel der Haut bei der Seborrhoe. Arch. Derm. Syph. (Berl.) **177**, 154 (1938). — Ist das seborrhoische Ekzem der Ausdruck einer Konstitutionsanomalie oder einer mikrobiellen Infektion der Haut. Ann. Hellen Derm. et Venerol. **1**, 177 (1939). Cit. Zbl. Haut- u. Geschl.-Kr. **64**, 611 (1940). — Untersuchungen zur geographischen Dermatologie in subtropischen und tropischen Regionen. Derm. tropic. **1**, 30 (1962). — MARCHIONINI, A., u. W. HAUSKNECHT: Säuremantel der Haut und Bakterienabwehr. I. Mitteilung. Die regionäre Verschiedenheit der Wasserstoffionenkonzentration der Hautoberfläche. Klin. Wschr. **17**, 663 (1938). — MARCHIONINI, A., E. MANZ u. F. HUSS: Der Cholesteringehalt der Hautoberschicht bei der Seborrhoe und bei Psoriasis. Arch. Derm. Syph. (Berl.) **176**, 613 (1938). — MARCHIONINI, A., R. SCHMIDT u. J. KIEFER: Säuremantel der Haut und Bakterienabwehr. II. Mitteilung über die regionäre Verschiedenheit der Bakterienabwehr und Desinfektionskraft der Hautoberfläche. Klin. Wschr. **17**, 736 (1938). — MARRACK, J. R.: Dermatology and nutrition. In: R. M. B. MACKENNA, ed., Modern trends in dermatology. New York: Hoeber 1948. — MARTIN-SCOTT, I.: The pityrosporon ovale. Brit. J. Derm. **64**, 257 (1952). — MASHKILLEYSON, L., E. BENYA-

MOVICH, E. KRICHEVSKAYA and L. SHATAMOVA: Role of vitamins in pathogenesis and treatment of skin diseases. Amer. Rev. Soviet. Med. **3**, 19 (1945). — MENDILAHARZU, J. R., y J. C. OYHENART: Estados seborreicos del lactante y su tratamiento por la vitamin H. Dia méd. **16**, 432 (1944). — MENEGHINI, C. I.: The buffer-capacity of the skin, measured by electrometric method, in normal and pathological conditions, with particular regard to occupational eczema. Proc. 11th Internat. Congr. Dermat. Stockh. 1957. Acta derm.-venereol. (Stockh.) **11**, 54. — MERCADAL, J., y J. PINOL: Nuestros resultados con el empleo de la tiourea en los estados seborreicos. Act. dermo-sifiliogr. (Madr.) **39**, 1003 (1948). Cit. Excerpta med. (Amst.), Sect. XIII **3**, No 1842 (1949). — MERK, L.: Die Pellagra. Z. Haut- u. Geschl.-Kr. **17**, 254 (1925). — MIESCHER, G.: Betrachtungen zur Ekzemfrage. Die Bedeutung der Mikrobenbesiedlung. Arch. Derm. Syph. (Berl.) **188**, 36 (1949). — Über das Wesen des Ekzems. In: Fortschritte der praktischen Dermatologie und Venerologie, p. 1. Berlin-Göttingen-Heidelberg: Springer 1955. — Antibacterial effects of Sebum and the inhibition of these effects by free amino-acids. Proc. 11th Internat. Congr. Dermat. Stockh. 1957. Acta derm.-venereol. (Stockh.) **2**, 9 (1957). — MIESCHER, G., u. A. SCHÖNBERG: Untersuchungen über die Funktion der Talgdrüsen. Bull. Schweiz. Akad. med. Wiss. **1**, 101 (1944). — MIESCHER, G., u. M. SPECK: Die Beeinflussung der bactericiden Wirkung des Hautfettes durch die Aminosäuren der Hautoberfläche. Naunyn-Schmiedeberg's Arch. exp. Path. Pharmak. **230**, 223 (1957). — MIESCHER, G., M. SPECK u. P. RINDERKNECHT: Untersuchungen zur Frage der Hemmung der antibakteriellen Wirkung des Hauttalges. Arch. klin. exp. Derm. **206**, 548 (1958). — MILBRADT, W.: Experimentelle Untersuchungen zur Frage der Bedeutung des H-Vitamins für die menschliche Pathologie. Derm. Wschr. **103**, 1402 (1936). — MILIAN, G.: Streptococcies. Nouvelle pratique dermatologic, vol. IV. Paris: Masson & Cie. 1936. — MILIAN, G., et M. LAUNAY: Parakératose a forme de Pityriasis rosea. Rev. franç. Derm. **5**, 17 (1929). Cit. Zbl. Haut- u. Geschl.-Kr. **30**, 731 (1929). — MOLONY, C. J., and A. H. PARMELEE: Convulsions in young infants as a result of Pyridoxine (Vitamin B_6) deficiency. J. Amer. med. Ass. **154**, 405 (1954). — MONACELLI, M., u. A. RIBUFFO: Der Hautzuckergehalt bei der Psoriasis. Hautarzt **3**, 498 (1952). — MONCORPS, C.: Zur Frage des Vitamin H. Derm. Wschr. **103**, 1230 (1936). — MOORE, M.: Cultivation and study of Pityrosporum ovale, so-called bottle bacillue of Unna. Arch. Derm. Syph. (Chic.) **31**, 661 (1935). — MOORE, M., A. L. KILE, M. F. ENGMAN jr. and M. F. ENGMAN: Pityrosporum ovale (bottle bacillus of Unna, Spore of Malassez) cultivation and possible role in seborrhoic dermatitis. Arch. Derm. Syph. (Chic.) **33**, 457 (1936). — MUELLER, J. F., and R. W. VILTER: Pyridoxine deficiency in human beings induced with desoxypyridoxine. J. clin. Invest. **29**, 193 (1950).

NADEL, A.: Chemische Studien an der menschlichen Haut. II. Untersuchungen an der normalen und pathologisehen Menschenhaut. Arch. Derm. Syph. (Berl.) **165**, 507 (1932). — NATHAN, E., u. F. STERN: Über den Mineralgehalt der Haut unter normalen und pathologischen Verhältnissen. III. Über den Kalium-Calcium- und Wassergehalt pathologisch veränderter Haut beim Menschen. Derm. Z. **54**, 232 (1928). — NEGRONI, P.: Microbiologia de la seborrea y sus complicaciones. Arch. argent. Derm. **6**, 159 (1956). Cit. Excerpta med. (Amst.), Sect. XIII **11**, No 2265 (1957). — NEGRONI, P., y C. B. DE NEGRONI: Estudios sobre la seborrea. III. Propiedades fisiologicas del Pityrosporon ovale. Rev. argent. Dermatosif. **42**, 103 (1958). Cit. Zbl. Haut- u. Geschl.-Kr. **107**, 333 (1960). — NELSON, C. T., and J. T. MCCARTHY: Pyodermas and their management. Med. Clin. N. Amer. **43**, 869 (1959). — NICOLAIDES, N., and ST. ROTHMAN: Studies on the chemical composition of human hair fat. I. The Squalene-cholesterol relationship. J. invest. Derm. **19**, 389 (1952). — The site of Sterol and Squalene synthesis in the human skin. J. invest. Derm. **24**, 125 (1955). — NIEMAND-ANDERSSEN, I.: Über eine neue Behandlungsmöglichkeit seborrhoischer Hautleiden. Derm. Wschr. **126**, 838 (1952). — NIKOLOWSKI, W.: Über die differentielle Morphogenese des sog. seborrhoischen Ekzems. Arch. Derm. Syph. (Berl.) **196**, 501 (1953). — NIKOLOWSKI, W., u. I. GASSER: Zur Früherfassung der Mikrosporie mittels des Woodlichtes, zugleich ein Beitrag hinsichtlich der Fluoreszenz des Pityrosporon Malassezii. Strahlentherapie **80**, 141 (1949). — NISBET, T. W.: Dermatitis due to Quinacrine hydrochloride (Atabrine). J. Amer. med. Ass. **134**, 446 (1947).

OBERMAYER, M. E.: Psychocutaneous medicine. Springfield, Ill.: Thomas 1955. — O'LEARY, P. A.: Vitamin therapy in dermatology and syphilology. Arch. Derm. Syph. (Chic.) **46**, 628 (1942). — OTA, M., et P. T. HUANG: Sur les champignons du genre Pityrosporum Sabouraud. Ann. Parasit. hum. comp. **11**, 49 (1933).

PACHTMAN, E. A., and E. E. VICHER: The bacteriologic flora in seborrheic dermatitis. J. invest. Derm. **22**, 389 (1954). — PASTINSZKY, I., u. GESZTI: Beiträge zur Pathogenese und Klinik der mit macrocytärer Anaemie verbundenen Fälle von Eczema seborrhoicum (Stryker-Halbeisensches Syndrom). Börgyögy. vener. Szle **9**, 46 (1955). Cit. Zbl. Haut- u. Geschl.-Kr. **92**, 351 (1955). — PEHL, W.: Über das Vitamin B_6 (Adermin) mit klinischen Versuchen bei der Säuglingsseborrhoe. Z. Kinderheilk. **61**, 613 (1940). — PERRY, E. T., and A. C. NICHOLS: Studies on the growth of bacteria in the human ear canal. J. invest. Derm. **27**, 165 (1956). —

PERUTZ, A., B. LUSTIG u. A. E. KLEIN: Zur zentralen Regulation des Fettstoffwechsels der Hautoberfläche. Arch. Derm. Syph. (Berl.) **170**, 511 (1934). — PIERINI, D., y E. S. BRAEGGER: Modificationes humorales en la seborrea, valores de lipidos y Vitamin A en sangre. Arch. argent. Derm. **6**, 153 (1956). Cit. Excerpta med. (Amst.), Sect. XIII **11**, No 1761 (1957). — PILLON: Poussee aigue généralisée consécutive à un traitement radiotherapique de deux placards d'eczema torpide. Bull. Soc. franç. Derm. Syph. **40**, 351 (1933). Cit. Z. Haut- u. Geschl.-Kr. **45**, 325 (1933). — PILLSBURY, D. M.: The pathogenesis of eczema. Proc. 10th Internat. Congr. of Dermat. London: Brit. Med. Ass. 1953. — PILLSBURY, D. M., and A. M. KLIGMAN: Some current problems in cutaneous bacteriology. In: R. M. B. MACKENNA, ed., Modern trends in dermatology. (Second ser.) New York: Hoeber 1954. — PILLSBURY, D. M., and G. V. KULCHAR: The relation of experimental skin infection to carbohydrate metabolism. The effect of hypertonic glucose and sodium chloride solutions injected intra peritoneally. Amer. J. med. Sci. **190**, 169 (1935). — PILLSBURY, D. M., W. B. SHELLEY and A. M. KLIGMAN: Dermatology. Philadelphia: W. B. Saunders Company 1956. — PILLSBURY, D. M., and T. H. STERNBERG: Relation of diet to cutaneous infection. Arch. Derm. Syph. (Chic.) **35**, 893 (1937). — POCHI, P. E., J. S. STRAUSS and H. MESCON: Sebum production and fractional 17-ketosteroid exeretion in Parkinsonism. J. invest. Derm. **38**, 45 (1962). — POPCHRISTOV, P., and I. BOGDANOV: Investigations on the microbial flora of the skin as a factor in its self protection against bacterial agents. Proc. 11th Internat. Congr. Dermat. Stockh. Acta derm.-venereol. (Stockh.) **3**, 172 (1957). — PRUSKI, P.: Efficacy of Vitamin H in seborrhoea. Przegl. lek. **7**, 121 (1951). Cit. Excerpta med. (Amst.), Sect. XIII **6**, No 2420 (1952). — PYMAN, C.: Otitis externa. Med. J. Aust. **46**, 534 (1959).

RABEAU, H., and M. FERRAND: Réactions secondes. 9th Internat. Dermat. Congr., Deliberations, 1935, I., p. 191. Leipzig: Johann Ambrosius Barth 1936. — RATTNER, H.: Changes in the skin in chronic encephalitis. Arch. Derm. **31**, 35 (1935). — REISS, H.: Zum Begriff des „seborrhoischen Ekzems“ und der parakeratotischen Diathese. Acta derm.-venereol. (Stockh.) **14**, 424 (1933). — REQUE, P. G., and J. E. TERRY: Seborrheic dermatitis of the scalp. Differential diagnosis. Sth. med. J. (Bgham, Ala.) **48**, 834 (1955). — RICKETTS, C. R., J. R. SQUIRE and E. TOPLEY: Human skin lipids with particular reference to the self-sterilizing power of the skin. Clin. Sci. **10**, 89 (1951). — RIDDLE, J. W., T. D. SPIES and N. P. HUDSON: A note on the interrelationship of deficiency diseases and resistance to infection. Proc. Soc. exp. Biol. (N.Y.) **45**, 361 (1940). — RIEHL jr., G.: Seborrhoe und Akne. Wien. klin. Wschr. **53**, 53 (1940). — ROBERT, P.: Beiträge zur Ekzemfrage. Untersuchungen über die Wirkung von Mikrobentoxinen auf die Haut. Arch. Derm. Syph. (Berl.) **173**, 267 (1935). — ROBIN, M., and J. G. KEPECS: The relationship between certain emotional states and the rate of secretion of sebum. J. invest. Derm. **20**, 373 (1953). — RÖCKL, H.: Untersuchungen zur Klinik und Pathogenese des mikrobiellen Ekzems. I. Mitteilung. Hautarzt **6**, 532 (1955). — Untersuchungen zur Klinik und Pathogenese des mikrobiellen Ekzems. II. Mitteilung. Hautarzt **7**, 14 (1956). — ROOK, A.: Seborrhoeic dermatitis. Practitioner **172**, 522 (1954). — ROST, G. A.: Hautkrankheiten. Berlin: Springer 1926. — ROTHMAN, ST.: Abnormalities in the chemical composition of the skin surface film in psoriasis. Arch. Derm. Syph. (Chic.) **62**, 814 (1950). — Physiology and biochemistry of the skin. Chicago: Chicago University Press 1954. — The lipid film of the skin surface. Proc. 11th Internat. Congr. Dermat. 1957. Acta derm.-venereol. (Stockh.) **2**, 38 (1957). — ROTHMAN, ST., u. F. SCHAAF: Die Chemie der Haut. In: JADASSOHNS Handbuch der Haut- und Geschlechtskrankheiten, Bd. I/2, S. 161. Berlin: Springer 1929. — RUDY, A., and R. HOFFMAN: Skin disturbances in diabetes mellitus: Their relation to vitamin deficiencies. New Engl. J. Med. **227**, 893 (1942). — RUST, S.: Beziehungen zwischen Fermenten und Vitaminen bei Hautkranken. Arch. Derm. (Berl.) **206**, 498 (1958).

SABOURAUD, R.: Diagnostic et traitement des affections du cuir cheveleu. Paris: Masson & Cie. 1932. — Seborrhée et états pré et post-séborrhéiques. Nouvelle pratique dermatologique, vol. 7, p. 27. Paris: Masson & Cie. 1936. — SATO, Y.: Studies on seborrhoea: especially the degree of the unsaturation of blood lipids. Jap. J. Derm. **66**, 501 (1956). Cit. Zbl. Haut- u. Geschl.-Kr. **98**, 13 (1957). — SAYER, A.: Newer concepts in the etiology and treatment of the seborrheic dermatoses. Urol. cutan. Rev. **46**, 719 (1942). — SCARCELLA, M.: La vitamine B_6 nel trattamento delle dermatiti seborrhoidi del lattante. Policlin. infant. **10**, 81 (1942). Cit. Zbl. Haut- u. Geschl.-Kr. **69**, 423 (1942/43). — SCHIRREN, C. G., u. H. PAWLOWSKY: Ist der p_H-Wert bei Eczematikern an der gesamten Hautoberfläche erhöht? Dermatologica (Basel) **112**, 225 (1956). — SCHMID, M.: Vergleichende Untersuchungen über die Säure-Basen-Verhältnisse auf der Haut. Dermatologica (Basel) **104**, 367 (1952). — SCHNAPKA, O.: Generalisierte superficielle Aspergilose unter dem Bilde einer „seborrhoischen Erythrodermie“. Z. Haut- u. Geschl.-Kr. **18**, 159 (1955). — SCHOCH, M. A.: Dilute hydrochloric acid and pepsin preparations. Schweiz. med. Wschr. **65**, 656 (1935). — SCHÖNFELD, A.: Universelles seborrhoisches Ekzem mit teilweisem Ausfall des Kopfhaares. Zbl. Haut- u. Geschl.-Kr. **57**, 246 (1937/38). — SCHREINER, A. W., W. SLINGER, V. R. HAWKINS and R. W. VILTER: Seborrheic dermatitis, a local metabolic defect involving pyridoxine. J. Lab. clin. Med. **38**, 948 (1951). — SCHREUS,

H. T., u. K. SCHULTEN: Hautfettbestimmungen in Abhängigkeit vom Zyklus. Arch. Derm. Syph. (Berl.) **196**, 422 (1953). — SCOTT, A.: The question of urinary hyperacidity in seborrhoeic dermatitis. Brit. J. Derm. **69**, 94 (1956). — SCOTT, J. A.: Seborrhoeic skin eruptions. Brit. J. Derm. **56**, 80 (1944). — SEBRELL jr., W. M., and R. E. BUTLER: Riboflavin deficiency in man (Ariboflavinosis). Publ. Hlth Rep. (Wash.) **54**, 2121 (1939). — SEFTON, L.: Some experiences in skin department of a prisoner of war camp hospital in Singapore. Brit. J. Derm. **59**, 159 (1947). — SELYE, H.: The alarm reaction and general adaptation syndrome. J. clin. Endocr. **6**, 117 (1947). — SERRATI, B.: Influenza del systema nervosa sulla secrezione sebacia. Osservazioni e ricerche cliniche. Riv. Pat. nerv.ment. **52**, 377 (1938). — SHELLEY, W. B.: Seborrheic dermatitis. In: T. H. STERNBERG, V. D. NEWCOMER, ed., Modern dermatologic therapy. New York: McGraw-Hill Book Co. 1959. — SIEMENS, H. W.: Die Vererbung in der Aetiologie der Hautkrankheiten. In: Handbuch der Haut- und Geschlechtskrankheiten, vol. III, p. 93. Berlin: Springer 1929. — SIMONS, R. D. G.: Nutritional disorders of the skin among prisoners of war in the Far East. Brit. J. Derm. **61**, 210 (1949). — SINCLAIR, H. M.: Vitamins and the skin. Brit. med. Bull. **12**, 24 (1956). — SLINGER, W. N., and D. M. HUBBARD: Treatment of seborrheic dermatitis with a shampoo containing selenium disulphide. Arch. Derm. Syph. (Chic.) **64**, 41 (1951). — SMITH, S. G., D. T. SMITH and J. L. CALLAWAY: Dysfunction of the sebaceous glands associated with pellagra. J. invest. Derm. **4**, 23 (1941). — SNYDERMAN, S. E., L. E. HOLT, R. CARRETERO and K. JACOBS: Pyridoxine deficiency in the human infant. J. clin. Nutr. **1**, 200 (1953). — SPIER, H. W., u. G. PASCHER: Analytische und physiologische Untersuchungen über die wasserlöslichen Inhaltsstoffe der peripheren Hornschicht (Hautoberfläche). Proc. 11th Internat. Congr. Dermat. Stockh. 1957. Acta derm.-venereol. (Stockh.) **2**, 14. — SPOOR, H. J., E. F. TRAUB and M. BELL: Pityrosporon ovale: types cultured from normal and seborrheic subjects. Arch. Derm. Syph. (Chic.) **69**, 323 (1954). — STEIFLER, G.: Die seborrhoeische Facies als ein Symptom der Encephalitis lethargica. J. Neurol. Psychiat. **73**, 455 (1921). — STEIGLEDER, G. K.: Histochemische Untersuchungen im psoriatischen Herd über Oxydation, Reduction und Lipoidstoffwechsel. Arch. Derm. Syph. (Berl.) **194**, 296 (1952). — Die Histochemie der Epidermis und ihrer Anhangsgebilde. Arch. klin. exp. Derm. **206**, 276 (1957a). — Kritische Analyse der parakeratotischen Hornschicht und der zugehörigen Epidermis mit besonderer Berücksichtigung der Perjodsäure-positiven. 11th Internat. Congr. of Dermat. Stockh. 1957b. Acta derm.-venereol. (Stockh.) **3**, 383. — STEINHARDT, M.: Dermatitis seborrhoides in children (with reference to the treatment of this condition with Biotin and Vitamin F). Diss. Bern 1956. Zit. Zbl. Haut- u. Geschl.-Kr. **96**, 272 (1956). — STOKES, J., H. BEERMAN and N. R. INGRAHAM jr.: Carbohydrate and water metabolism and the vitamins in skin inflammation (Dermatitis). Amer. J. med. Sci. **195**, 562 (1938). — STOKES, J., and A. D. KING: Acne vulgaris. Heredity in the etiologic background. Arch. Derm. Syph. (Chic.) **26**, 456 (1932). — STOKES, J., and T. H. STERNBERG: A factor analysis of the acne complex with therapeutic comment. Arch. Derm. Syph. (Chic.) **40**, 345 (1939). — STOKES, J. H.: Effect on the skin of emotional and nervous states. Masochism and other sex complexes in the background of neurogenous dermatitis. Amer. J. med. Sci. **179**, 69 (1930). — STOKES, J. H., and associates: A handbook of fundamental medical dermatology, 7th ed. Philadelphia: Department of Dermatology, Book Fund. 1942. — STORCK, H.: Experimentelle Untersuchungen zur Frage der Bedeutung von Mikroben in der Ekzemgenese. Dermatologica (Basel) **96**, 177 (1948). — Tierexperimentelle Untersuchungen zur Frage der ekzematösen Hautsensibilisierung. Dermatologica (Basel) **100**, 262 (1950). — The role of bacteria in eczema. In: L. S. A. LOEWENTHAL, ed., The eczemas. Edinburgh and London: E. S. Livingstone, Ltd. 1954. — STORCK, H., u. P. RINDERKNECHT: Über die Bedeutung der Hautbakterienflora beim Ekzem gemessen an der therapeutischen Wirkung von Aureomycin und Chloramphenicol. Dermatologica (Basel) **101**, 231 (1950). — STÜPEL, H., u. A. SZAKALL: Die Wirkung von Waschmitteln auf die Haut. Heidelberg: Dr. Alfred Hüthig 1957. — STRYKER, G. V., and W. A. HALBEISEN: Determination of macrocytic anemia as an aid in diagnosis of certain deficiency dermatoses. Arch. Derm. Syph. (Chic.) **51**, 116 (1945). — SULLIVAN, M., and J. NICHOLLS: Nutritional dermatoses in the rat. V. Signs and symptoms resulting from a diet containing unheated dried egg white as the source of protein. Arch. Derm. Syph. (Chic.) **45**, 295 (1942). — SULZBERGER, M. B., and R. L. BAER: Vioform in dermatologic therapy. Arch. Derm. Syph. (Chic.) **58**, 224 (1948). — SULZBERGER, M. B., J. WOLF, V. H. WITTEN and A. W. KAPF: Dermatology. Diagnosis and treatment, 2nd edit. Chicago: Year Book Publishers 1961. — SUTTON, R. L., and R. L. SUTTON jr.: Contribution to: Investigations concerning actual methods employed in the management of common dermatoses. J. invest. Derm. **3**, 152 (1940). — Handbook of diseases of the skin. St. Louis: C. V. Mosby Comp. 1949. — SYDENSTRICKER, V. P., L. E. GEESLIN and J. W. WEAVER: Avitaminosis occurring in diabetic patients under Insulin therapy. J. Amer. med. Ass. **113**, 2137 (1939). — SYDENSTRICKER, V. P., S. A. SINGAL, A. F. BRIGGS, N. M. DEVAUGHN and H. ISBELL: Observations on "Egg white injury" in man and its cure with Biotin concentrate. Science **95**, 176 (1942). Cit. J. Amer. med. Ass. **118**, 1199 (1942).

TACHAU, P.: Problems of so-called infantile eczema. III. Seborrhoic dermatitis (Psoriasoids, seborrheids) — general survey. Acta derm.-venereol. (Stockh.) **20**, 232 (1939). — TASLAKI, D.: Studies on the metabolism of lipids in skin diseases. Sequel 5-Seborrheic eczema. Jap. J. Derm. **66**, 246 (1956). Cit. Zbl. Haut- u. Geschl.-Kr. **97**, 154 (1957). — TEMPLETON, H. G.: A study of dandruff and of the pityrosporon of Malassez. Arch. Derm. Syph. (Chic.) **14**, 270 (1926). — THÉLIN, F.: Dermatite séborrhoide et biotine. Ann. paediat. (Basel) **172**, 193 (1949). — TOURAINE, A.: L'hérédité en medicine. Paris: Masson & Cie. 1955. — TRÉGER, J., A. MOYS and M. Z. MUZIKOVA: Intracutaneous biotin in seborrheic eczema. Bratisl. lek. Listy **31**, 562 (1951). Cit. Excerpta med. (Amst.), Sect. XIII **7**, No 94 (1953).

UHLMAN, W. J.: Beitrag zur Behandlung der Seborrhoe im Bereiche des Gesichtes. Medizinische **1958**, 1963. Cit. Zbl. Haut- u. Geschl.-Kr. **103**, 205 (1959). — URBACH, E.: Beitrag zu einer physiologischen und pathologischen Chemie der Haut. II. Mitt. Der Wasser-Kochsalz-Reststickstoff und Fettgehalt der Haut in der Norm und unter pathologischen Verhältnissen. Arch. Derm. Syph. (Berl.) **156**, 73 (1928). — Skin diabetes: hyperglycodermia without hyperglycemie. J. Amer. med. Ass. **129**, 438 (1945). — URBACH, E., and J. W. LENTZ: Carbohydrate metabolism and the skin. Arch. Derm. Syph. (Chic.) **52**, 301 (1945).

VARGA V. KIBÉD, A: Die Beteiligung des Vitamin A an den seborrhoischen Krankheitsbildern. Arch. Derm. Syph. (Berl.) **183**, 15 (1942). Cit. Zbl. Haut- u. Geschl.-Kr. **69**, 478 (1942/43). — Seborrhoea and nutrition. Orv. Lapja **4**, 518 (1948a). — La nutrition et la séborrhée. Ann. Derm. Syph. (Paris) 496 (1948b). — VERMEER, D. J., H. DE JONG and J. C. LENSTRA: The significance of amino-acids for the neutralization by the skin. Dermatologica (Basel) **103**, 1 (1951). — VONKENNEL, J., u. A. SCHÖBERL: BAL und die Behandlung der Syphilis und Psoriasis mit thiopriven Substanzen. Med. Mschr. **3**, 561 (1949). — VUJASIN, J., and D. PETROVIC: Biotin in some erythemato-squamous dermatoses of babies. Dermatologica (Basel) **105**, 180 (1952).

WALTER, F., and M. OBTULOWICZ: Seborrheic diathesis; distribution of lipoids in blood serum and skin of seborrheic patients and of rats. Przegl. Derm. Vener. **32**, 384 (1937). Cit. Zbl. Haut- u. Geschl.-Kr. **60**, 305 (1938). — Studien über den konstitutionellen seborrhoischen Zustand der Haut Przgl. Derm. Vener. **33**, 114 (1938). Cit. Zbl. Haut- und Geschl Kr. 62, 411 1939. — WEIDMAN, F. B.: Seborrheic dermatitis in a series of cases of post-epidemic encephalitis. Arch. Derm. **21**, 690 (1930). — WILLIAMS, H. L., H. MONTGOMERY and W. N. PORVELL: Dermatitis of ear. J. Amer. med. Ass. **113**, 641 (1939). — WITKOWER, E., and R. B. M. MACKENNA: Psychological aspects of seborrheic dermatitis. Brit. J. Derm. **59**, 281 (1947). — WITTKOWER, E., and B. RUSSELL: Emotional factors in skin disease. New York: Hoeber 1953. — WOLFRAM, G.: Zum Krankheitsbild der Dermatitis seborrhoides. Münch. med. Wschr. **101**, 1398 (1959). — WRIGHT, C. S., M. H. SAMITZ and H. BRACON: Vitamin B_6 (Pyridoxine) in dermatology. Arch. Derm. Syph. (Chic.) **47**, 651 (1943).

ZENNER, B., J. BEUTNAGEL u. M. L. FRIEDRICH: Zur Diagnose und Therapie lichtbedingter oder lichtverschlimmerter Hautkrankheiten. Dtsch. med. Wschr. **76**, 578 (1951).

Die exsudative discoide und lichenoide chronische Dermatose von Sulzberger und Garbe

Von

Marion B. Sulzberger-San Francisco, **Cyril March**

und

Stephan R. Brunauer-New York

Mit 8 Abbildungen (davon 2 farbige)

Historisches, Begriffsbestimmung

Die erste Beschreibung des als ,,Distinctive Exudative Discoid and Lichenoid Chronic Dermatosis" bezeichneten Krankheitsbildes erfolgte durch SULZBERGER und GARBE im Jahre 1937. Wohl waren schon vorher hierher zu rechnende Fälle ISADORE ROSEN durch ihre Eigenartigkeit aufgefallen, aber die eben erwähnte, detaillierte Beschreibung von neun Fällen war der *erste* Versuch, dieses Krankheitsbild aus der Gruppe der ekzemartigen Erkrankungen herauszuheben und von klinisch ähnlichen Affektionen abzugrenzen. Seither haben Krankenvorstellungen wie auch Publikationen die Zahl der in der Literatur niedergelegten Fälle auf 65 ansteigen lassen. Und kürzlich haben SULZBERGER-MARCH-GAY in einem Übersichtsartikel 41 Fälle von ,,exudative discoid and lichenoid chronic dermatosis" zusammenstellen können, die teils in ihrer Privatpraxis, teils im Department of Dermatology des Medical Center der New York University (im Bellevue Hospital und in der New York Skin and Cancer Unit) beobachtet, aber nicht veröffentlicht worden waren. Damit erhöht sich die Gesamtzahl der bisher berichteten einschlägigen Beobachtungen auf *106 Fälle.* Was hinsichtlich des Auftretens, der hauptsächlichen klinischen Charakteristika wie des Verlaufes der ,,exudative discoid and lichenoid chronic dermatosis" im Jahre 1937 hervorgehoben worden war, hat nicht nur durch wiederholte Nachuntersuchungen der ursprünglich beobachteten Fälle wie auch durch weitere einschlägige Beobachtungen anderer Autoren eine wesentliche Bestätigung und Unterstützung während der inzwischen vergangenen 25 Jahre erfahren. Die Wahrscheinlichkeit, daß dieses Krankheitsbild klinisch tatsächlich eine Dermatose sui generis ist, erscheint daher derzeit weitaus mehr begründet als damals; es hat auch den Anschein, daß diese Dermatose ,,populärer" geworden ist, denn wer einmal das voll entwickelte ,,klassische" Bild gesehen hat, kann späterhin ohne weiteres typische Fälle aus klinischen und grob morphologischen Gründen ebenso mühelos erkennen wie etwa typische Fälle von Psoriasis oder Lichen planus.

1. Klinisch charakteristische Merkmale der Distinctive Exsudative Discoid and Lichenoid Dermatosis

Obzwar ursprünglich angenommen worden war, daß die Dermatose nahezu ausschließlich bei Männern jüdischer Rassezugehörigkeit auftritt, hat es sich doch gezeigt, daß sie auch bei wenigen Frauen (12 in einer Gesamtzahl von 106 einschlägigen Fällen) und in einer ebenso geringen Anzahl von Patienten augenscheinlich nichtjüdischer Abstammung (12 von 106) beobachtet werden konnte (Tabelle 1). Die überwiegende Mehrzahl der Fälle betraf jedoch, wenigstens in New York City, Männer jüdischer Rasse, die, abgesehen von ihren Hauterscheinungen, einen gewöhnlich guten Gesundheitszustand aufwiesen. Das Alter der Patienten zu Beginn der Erkrankung lag zwischen 14 (Couperus) und 61 Jahren (Costello); der jüngste von Sulzberger-Garbe beobachtete Patient war 32 Jahre alt. Im Durchschnitt fiel der Krankheitsbeginn in den Anfang des 4. Lebensjahrzehnts, es ist aber immerhin möglich, daß in Wirklichkeit die ersten Anzeichen der Erkrankung in manchen Fällen schon früher auftraten, aber, wegen ihrer Geringfügigkeit oder Flüchtigkeit nicht beobachtet oder nicht erkannt, in den Krankengeschichten nicht verzeichnet wurden.

Die Identifizierung dieses Krankheitsbildes stützt sich in erster Linie auf bestimmte Charakteristika der Dermatose. Hier ist vor allem die *Chronizität* der Erkrankung hervorzuheben, zusammen mit dem oft überraschend schnellen Wandel im Bilde der klinischen Erscheinungen, die hierbei mehrere unterschiedliche Stadien durchlaufen oder auch während eines Rückfalles in ein früheres Stadium zurückkehren können.

Eine dominierende und immer vorhandene subjektive Klage ist der intensive und nahezu unerträgliche *Juckreiz*, der sich oft zu wahren Krisen steigert. Obwohl der Pruritus im exsudativen Stadium ganz besonders störend ist, bleibt er als Hauptsymptom während aller Krankheitsstadien bestehen, er kann sogar vorhanden sein, wenn der Patient praktisch keine sichtbaren Hauterscheinungen aufweist. Es ist nicht unwahrscheinlich, daß die so rasch auftretenden Veränderungen der Hauterscheinungen durch das heftige Kratzen und Reiben bedingt sind, wodurch die Kranken den Juckreiz zu stillen oder zu erleichtern versuchen. In Verbindung mit dem intensiven Pruritus wurden auch andere subjektive Symptome verzeichnet, so Frösteln (ohne begleitende Änderung der Körpertemperatur), Schmerzhaftigkeit und Brennen in den Brüsten und in der Umgebung der Brustwarzen (Sulzberger-Garbe).

Tabelle 1 zeigt eine Übersicht der klinischen Charakteristika dieser Dermatose, wie sie in den in der Literatur niedergelegten Beobachtungen beschrieben sind.

Tabelle 1

Zahl der in der Literatur beschriebenen Fälle von „exudative discoid and lichenoid chronic dermatosis“	106
Von diesen Fällen sind klinische oder anderweitige Einzelheiten nicht beschrieben in	17
	89
Zahl der erkrankten Frauen	12
Zahl der erkrankten Männer	77
Erkrankte nichtjüdischer Rasse	12
Klinische Charakteristika:	
Intensiver Juckreiz	88/89
Exsudative Phase	87/89
Lichenoide Phase	89/89
Infiltrative Phase	59/89
Urticarielle Ausbrüche (nicht erwähnt oder nicht beobachtet in 16 Fällen)	42/73
Penis-Läsionen (nicht erwähnt oder nicht beobachtet in 7 von 77 Männern)	65/70
Eosinophilie (nur in 61 Beobachtungen lag ein Hemogram vor)	51/61

Unter Benützung der in der Publikation von Sulzberger-March-Gay enthaltenen Tabelle 2.

2. Beginn und Frühstadien

In einer Anzahl von Fällen gehen den charakteristischen Eruptionen Hauterscheinungen voraus, die zuerst als primär-toxische Dermatitis oder allergische Kontaktdermatitis der Hände, Füße, Extremitäten, des Gesichts oder anderer Hautregionen anmuten. Die frühesten Phasen sind oft gekennzeichnet durch das

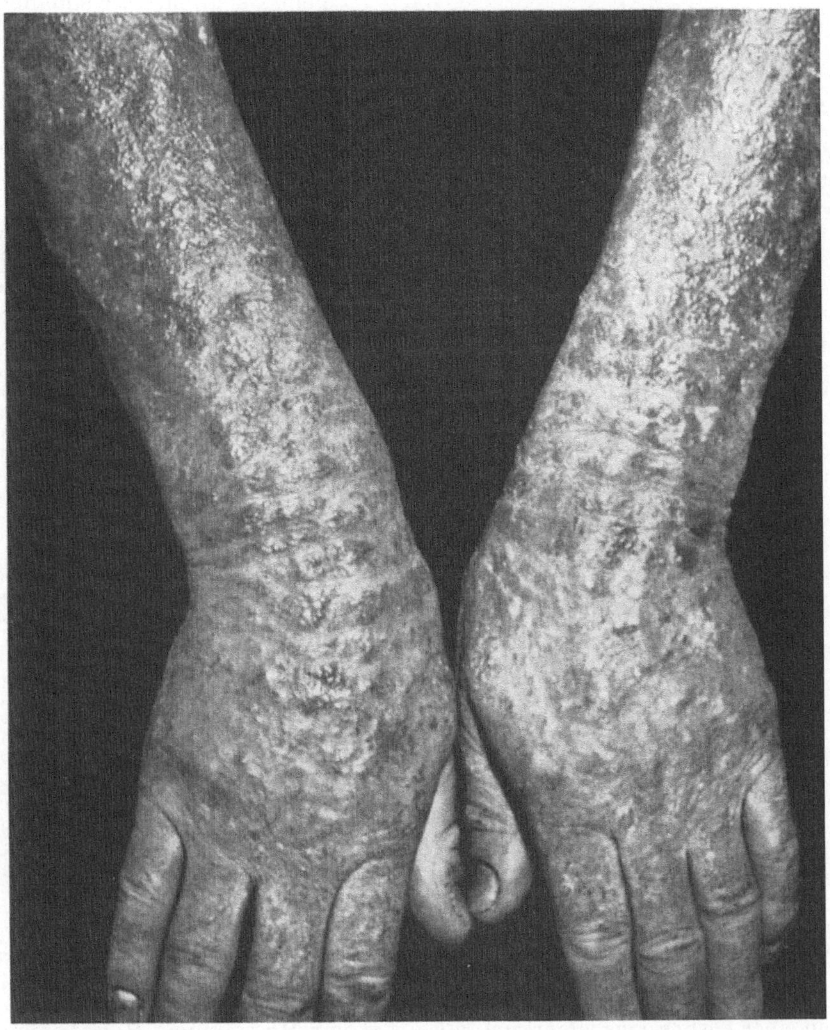

Abb. 1. Exsudative Phase. (Aus SULZBERGER-MARCH-GAY, Z. Haut- u. Geschl.-Kr. **27**, H. 8)

Auftreten ekzematöser, dyshidrosis-artiger Läsionen an den Händen und Füßen oder anderer Hautpartien, welchen sich zugleich oder etwas später disseminierte, scharf begrenzte, ovale und discoide, gelegentlich konfluierende Plaques hinzugesellen. Diese Plaques können in rascher Reihenfolge verschiedene Stadien durchlaufen und folgende Erscheinungsformen aufweisen: 1. elevierte, exsudative und verkrustende Typen, etwa dem nummulären Ekzem ähnelnd; 2. flache, trockene, schuppende Formen, etwa an Pityriasis rosea oder an seborrhoisches Ekzem erinnernd; 3. infiltrierte und lichenifizierte Plaques, etwa dem Lichen planus, der Neurodermatitis circumscripta (d.i. Lichen chronicus simplex), der Atopic-Dermatitis, den verschiedenen Prurigoformen u. a. gleichend. Diese Läsionen sind meistens am Stamm, den Oberarmen und Oberschenkeln lokalisiert, können aber auch an jedem anderen Teil der Hautoberfläche auftreten, so im Gesicht an der Nase, besonders „bridge of nose" (Koscard) und um die Lippen. Die Genitalien, insbesondere der Penis, sind fast regelmäßig befallen, meistens die glans penis, manchmal auch der Schaft (Niles). Befallensein des Scrotum erwähnen Mazzini-Calzetta, Schneider-Kesten, Sulzberger (in einer Diskussionsbemerkung zu einem von Rostenberg-Rostenberg jr. vorgestellten Falle). Häufig erscheinen auch die Füße befallen, wo sich namentlich zu Beginn der Erkrankung das klinische Bild von jenem anderer Körperstellen unterscheidet und an eine Dermatomykose denken läßt dadurch, daß an den Plantae Bläschen auftreten (Pascher), während klinisch wahrnehmbare Bläschenbildung an den übrigen Herden des Körpers fehlt. In einem von Sharlit beobachteten, hinsichtlich der Diagnose von Fred Wise bestätigten Falle begannen die klinischen Erscheinungen am Fußrücken.

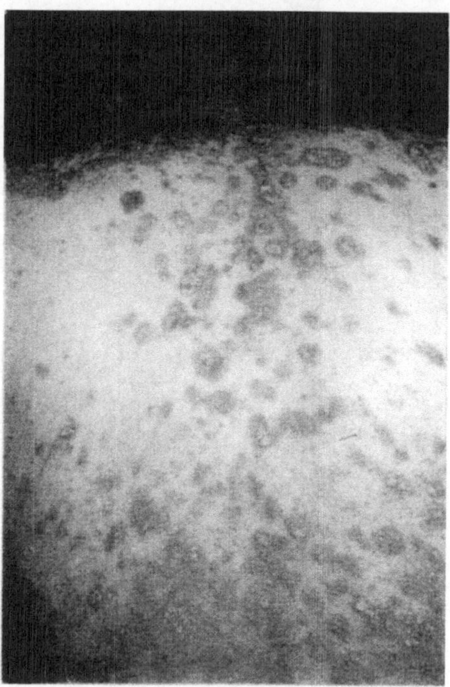

a b

Abb. 2a u. b. a Discoid-lichenoide Phase mit z. T. klein-papulösen, z. T. discoiden, lichenifizierten, mitunter pigmentierten Läsionen. (Aus Sulzberger-March-Gay, Z. Haut- u. Geschl.-Kr. **27**, H. 8). b An Pityriasis rosea erinnernde Anordnung der discoiden Efflorescenzen

Mitbefallensein der Schleimhäute ist bisher nicht beschrieben worden, weder bezüglich früher noch auch späterer Stadien der Dermatose. Eine Ausnahme bilden nur die „Haut-Schleimhaut-Übergänge", wie Lippenrot, Glans penis. Ob

Beobachtungen wie jene von Pigmentierungen (BETT) oder vom Auftreten weißlicher Herde an der Wangenschleimhaut (ROSTENBERG-ROSTENBERG jr.) zum Krankheitsbild der „exudative discoid and lichenoid dermatosis" gehören, muß dahingestellt bleiben.

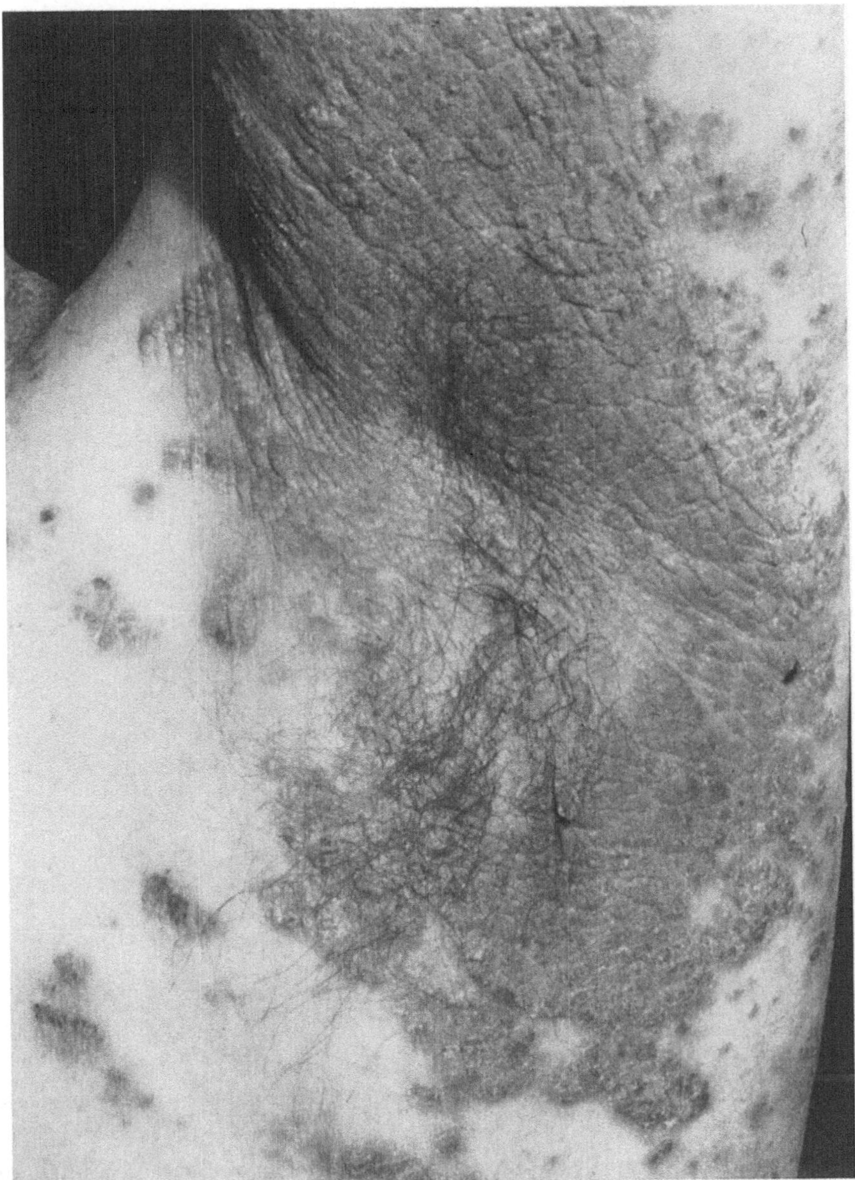

Abb. 3. Hypertrophisch-lichenifizierte, an Neurodermitis circumscripta erinnernde Plaque der Achselgegend. (Aus SULZBERGER-MARCH-GAY, Z. Haut- u. Geschl.-Kr. **27**, H. 8)

a) Exsudative und schuppende Hauterscheinungen

Das exsudative Stadium (Abb. 1) kann so rasch abklingen, daß es praktisch nur vorübergehend zu sein scheint, es kann aber auch einige Wochen andauern oder in unregelmäßigen Intervallen rezidivieren. Wie schon hervorgehoben, kann der Kranke nahezu plötzlich „trocken“ werden, oft aber nur, um in ein nässendes Stadium zurückzufallen. Akut exsudative Plaques können sich schließlich in flache, schuppende Herde umwandeln, die in ihrem Aussehen wie in ihrer Verteilung (entlang der Spaltlinien der Haut) an Pityriasis rosea erinnern und sich

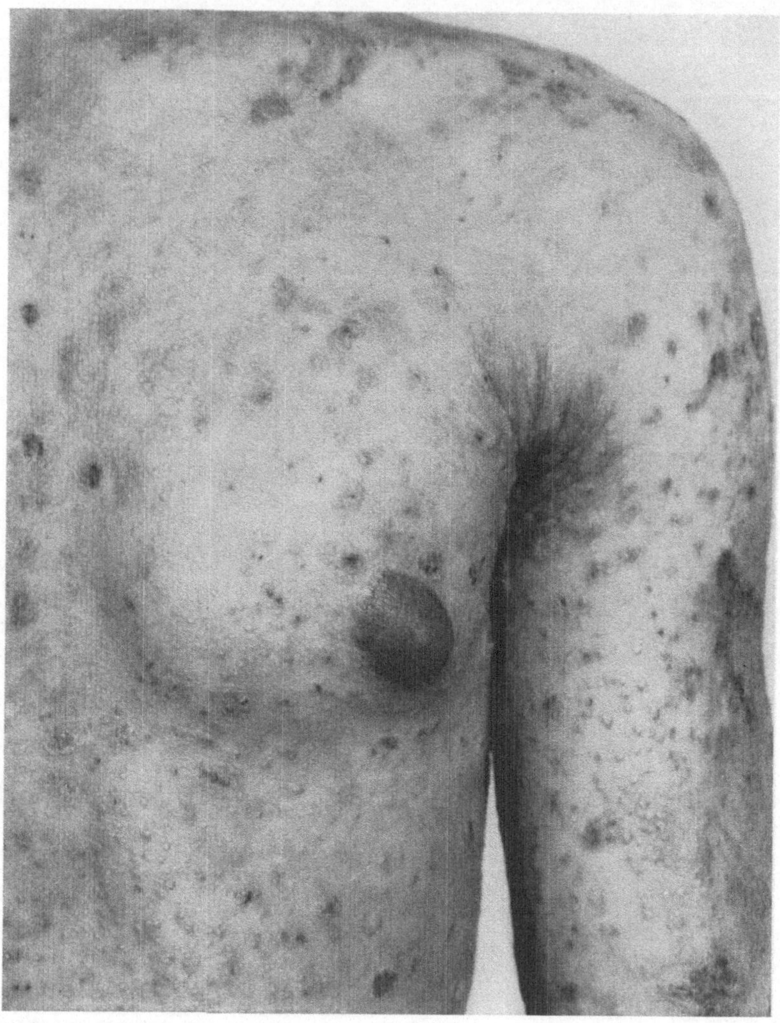

Abb. 4. Lichen planus-artige Veränderungen, besonders in der Mitte des linken Oberarmes, aber auch zusammen mit Erscheinungen der discoid-lichenoiden Phase am Rumpf. Schwellung und Infiltration der Brustwarze. (Aus SULZBERGER-MARCH-GAY, Z. Haut- u. Geschl.-Kr. **27**, H. 8)

entweder vollständig zurückbilden oder in das Stadium der Lichenifizierung übergehen (Abb. 2). Hyperpigmentierung der exsudativen Veränderungen kann während, meist aber nach erfolgter Heilung auftreten, ist mitunter durch ihre dunkelblau-braune Farbe besonders markant, ja entstellend und kann durch viele Monate, sogar durch Jahre bestehenbleiben (Abb. 3). KOCSARD berichtet eine deutliche Neigung zu Hyperpigmentierung, aber auch Depigmentierung in seinen drei in Shanghai beobachteten Fällen, die Pigmentverschiebungen traten aber in früher infiltrierten Gebieten auf.

b) Discoide und lichenoide Veränderungen

In der Regel ist der Beginn des nun folgenden, zweiten Stadiums der Dermatose dadurch gekennzeichnet, daß die exsudativen Veränderungen im Rückgang begriffen, Nässen und Krustenbildung fast vollständig geschwunden sind und papulöse sowie discoide licheninfizierte Herde (Abb. 4) das klinische Bild beherrschen. Diese Veränderungen entstehen entweder an der Stelle der vorangegangenen akuten Läsionen oder auf vorher normaler Haut und sind durch ihre, zumindest im Beginn follikuläre Entstehung wie auch durch ihre Chronizität gekennzeichnet. Disseminierte lichenoide Papeln können an verschiedenen Körperstellen auftreten, manche zerstreut, in regelmäßiger Anordnung, andere wiederum in Form kleinerer oder größerer Gruppen. Diese kleinen lichen-ähnlichen Efflorescenzen sind oft jenen des Lichen planus täuschend ähnlich (Abb. 6), obwohl sie meistens kleiner und weniger bläulich-rot sind, keinen wachsartigen Glanz aufweisen und keine Wickhamschen Striae erkennen lassen. Diffuse Lichenifizierung kann oft größere Areale einnehmen und an ausgedehnte Plaques von Lichen chronicus simplex (Neurodermitis circumscripta) erinnern (Abb. 3). Für die Diagnosenstellung in diesem Stadium der Erkrankung sind folgende Punkte von Bedeutung: 1. Trotz der deutlichen Lichenifizierung und Verdickung der Haut können die Läsionen innerhalb weniger Tage abklingen; 2. gerade in diesem Stadium treten Veränderungen am Penis auf (Abb. 5), die als „Puzzling persistent penile Plaques" beschrieben wurden (Sulzberger-Witten-Hunt) und welche hinsichtlich ihrer Abgrenzung von Lichen planus und Psoriasis oft Schwierigkeiten bereiten.

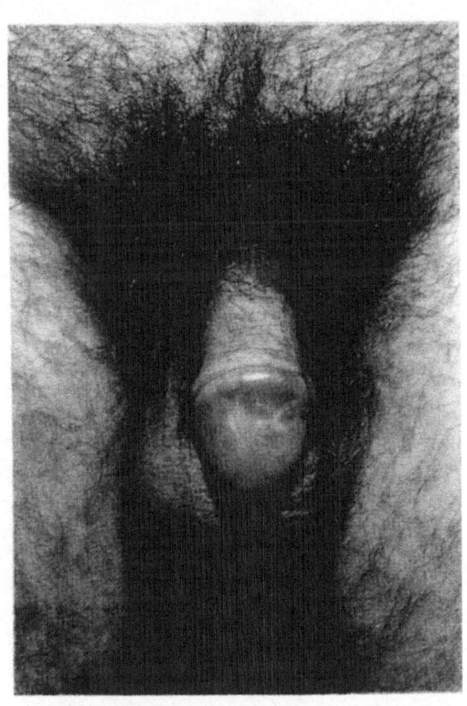

Abb. 5. Persistierende Plaques (discoide Efflorescenzen) am Penis

Wegen ihrer ausgesprochenen, mitunter sogar über Jahre sich erstreckenden Chronizität ist es gerade die lichenoide Phase der Erkrankung, die am häufigsten zur Beobachtung kommt. Hervorgehoben sei auch die hochgradige Cutis anserina (Gänsehaut), welche besonders in diesem Stadium in einem hohen Prozentsatz der Patienten auftritt, wenn sie relativ geringen Veränderungen der umgebenden Temperatur wie etwa Auskleiden in einem angenehm temperierten Raum ausgesetzt werden; auch Übererregbarkeit, Elevation, Schwellung, Brennen und Ekzematisation der Brustwarzen sei hier erwähnt (Abb. 4).

c) Infiltrative, an das prämykotische Stadium der Mycosis fungoides erinnernde Phase

Ein wiederum anderes klinisches Bild kann sich ergeben, wenn die Infiltration der Hautveränderungen so stark hervortritt, daß die elevierten ovalen oder discoiden Papeln und Plaques, die von einer Hyperplasie der regionalen Lymphknoten begleitet sein können, sehr an das prämykotische Stadium der Mycosis fungoides (oder auch an andere Krankheitsbilder der Gruppe der Lymphoblastome bzw. der Retikulosen) erinnern (Abb. 6). Histologische Untersuchungen derartiger Fälle berichteten fast immer von einer „chronischen Dermatitis" oder von Veränderungen, die „compatible", d.h., im Einklang mit der Sulzberger-Garbe-Dermatose sind, während die Biopsie der Lymphdrüsen lediglich chronisch entzündliche Veränderungen ergab.

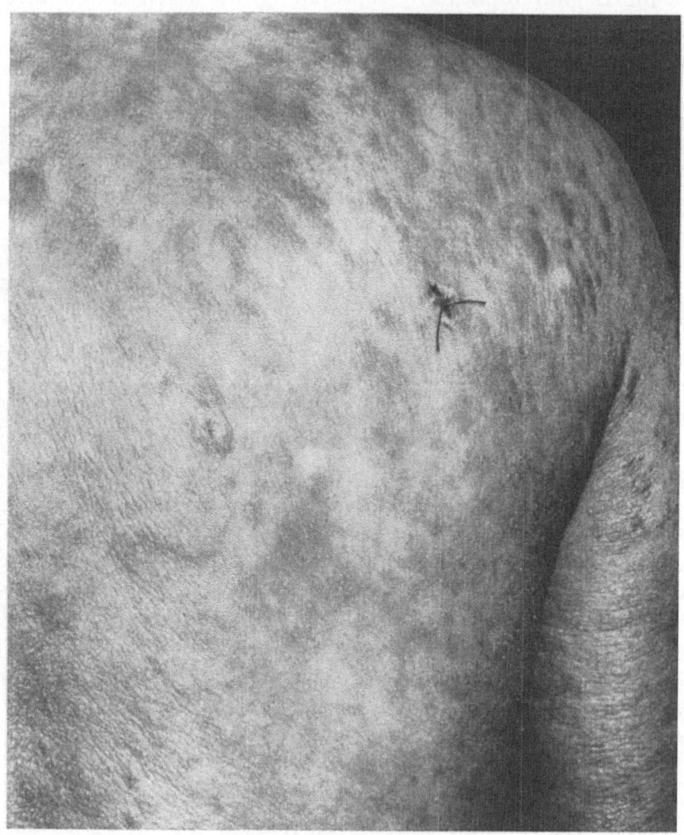

Abb. 6. Infiltrative Phase, die infolge der deutlich hervortretenden Infiltration an das prämykotische Stadium der Mycosis fungoides bzw. an andere Lymphoblastome oder Retikulosen erinnert. (Aus Sulzberger-March-Gay, Z. Haut- u. Geschl.-Kr. 27, H. 8)

In der Diskussion zu einem von Combes als „chronic discoid lichenoid Dermatitis associated with giant follicular Lymphadenopathy" vorgestellten Falle bestätigte Fred Wise die Richtigkeit der Diagnose der cutanen Manifestationen, wies aber darauf hin, daß dieser Befund nicht mit dem von Symmers als „Giant follicular adenopathy combined with polymorphous cell sarcoma of the lymphoid follicles" bezeichneten Bilde verwechselt werden dürfe. Von besonderer Wichtigkeit in solchen Fällen ist der nachdrückliche Hinweis auf die entscheidende Tatsache, daß nach längerer Beobachtungszeit bei *keinem* dieser Patienten eine *Veränderung des Blutbildes auftritt* und bei *allen schließlich eine mehr oder weniger vollkommene Heilung der Hautveränderungen mit völliger Rückbildung der regionalen Lymphdrüsenschwellungen erfolgt.*

d) Urticarielle Phasen

Schließlich treten in einer Anzahl (etwa der Hälfte) der beobachteten Fälle urticarielle Eruptionen auf. Diese können in jedem Stadium in Erscheinung treten, besonders während der lichenoiden Phase, sie sind jedoch charakteristischerweise während jener Perioden wahrnehmbar, in welchen alle oder fast alle anderen Hautveränderungen fehlen. Während im allgemeinen diese urticariellen Ausbrüche mitunter das Aussehen gewöhnlicher Nesseln aufweisen, erscheinen sie in diesen Perioden als eigenartige, tief sitzende, kleine, rundliche, etwas beständigere und eher an Prurigopapeln erinnernde Quaddeln, deren Auftreten oft eine Remission der übrigen Symptome dieser Dermatose ankündigt oder einleitet. BETT, CANNON, PASCHER erwähnen indes diese urticariellen Efflorescenzen zu Beginn eines Rückfalles.

3. Verlauf

Diejenige Läsion, welche die längste Bestandsdauer hat, ist meistens die exsudative Plaque am Penis, so daß viele Fälle eine solche solitäre, diagnostisch oft rätselhaft erscheinende Penisläsion selbst Jahre nach Verschwinden aller übrigen Manifestationen aufweisen. In der überweigenden Mehrzahl der Beobachtungen klingt die Dermatose vollständig oder fast vollkommen nach einem Verlauf von Monaten, öfters sogar nach Jahren (9—10 Jahren) allmählich ab. Oft bestehen noch für längere Zeit als Residuen der früheren Erkrankung die oben erwähnten urticaria-artigen Läsionen in Form von spärlichen, kleinen, rundlichen, tiefsitzenden Quaddeln, die durch ihre längere Bestandsdauer gewissermaßen an Prurigopapeln erinnern. Die verschiedenen, im Vorhergehenden getrennt aufgezählten Stadien können einander folgen, sind aber oft gleichzeitig vorhanden, wobei Übergänge von der exsudativen zur trockenen, schuppenden und dann zur lichenoiden Phase sowie weiterhin Rückfälle zum exsudativen Stadium in auffallend raschem Wechsel erfolgen können. In jedem Zeitpunkt des Krankheitsverlaufes können monate- oder jahrelang bestehende Remissionen eintreten, welchen ein plötzliches Wiederaufflammen eines einzigen oder aller genannten Stadien folgen kann. Während dieser Remissionen kann der Patient völlig erscheinungsfrei sein oder nur geringfügige Restzustände der Erkrankung wie etwa eine isolierte Penisplaque aufweisen. Eine Ursache der Rückfälle konnte niemals aufgedeckt werden, obwohl es in manchen Fällen den Anschein hatte, daß sie durch emotionelle Einflüsse (COSTELLO, KOCSARD) in anderen durch lokale Infektionsherde (NILES: Otitis media; SULZBERGER) ausgelöst worden waren. In der Aussprache zu einem von GOLDSTEIN-FERNANDEZ vorgestellten Falle meinte LIVINGOOD ein solches Wiederaufflammen nach einer Vaccinedarreichung sowie im Anschluß an eine Infektion der oberen Luftwege gesehen zu haben.

4. Laboratoriumsbefunde

Von den mannigfachen, bei Patienten mit „Exudative discoid and lichenoid chronic dermatosis“ durchgeführten Laboratoriumsuntersuchungen erscheint nur ein einziger Befund ziemlich konstant außerhalb der normalen Grenze zu liegen, nämlich eine deutliche Eosinophilie (6—60%). Wenn auch dieser Befund kaum als spezifisch angesehen werden kann, so vermag er immerhin bei der Diagnosenstellung von einigem Wert zu sein. Spektroskopisch erhöhte Werte für Kupfer werden von SULZBERGER und GARBE sowie von NILES erwähnt, von letzterem in der Diskussion zu einem von CANNON demonstrierten Fall. Die erstgenannten Autoren berichten auch, daß in den neun von ihnen beobachteten Fällen verschiedene Allergietests (scratch tests mit einer Anzahl von Nahrungsmitteln und staubbildenden Materialien, intracutane Tests sowie Läppchenproben mit routinemäßig gepüften Substanzen und mit Jodkali), Pilzuntersuchungen sowie intracutane Prüfung mit Trichophytin und Oidiomycin, wiederholte Untersuchungen von Urin und Faeces negative Resultate ergaben. Es zeigt sich also, daß Laboratoriumsuntersuchungen nur von geringem Wert hinsichtlich einer positiven Diagnosenstellung sind, aber doch insofern von Nutzen sein können, als der positive Ausfall von Pilzuntersuchungen, Patchtests, Jodkaliproben, Scratchtests eine Pilzerkrankung, bzw. Kontakt-Dermatitis, Duhrings disease oder eine atopic dermatitis annehmen, bzw. die Diagnose „Exudative discoid and lichenoid chronic dermatosis" ausschließen lassen.

5. Histopathologie

Die histologischen Veränderungen dieses Krankheitsbildes sind nicht „diagnostisch", nicht eindeutig genug, daß die mikroskopische Diagnose ohne weiteres gestellt werden kann. Immerhin gibt es in dem komplexen histologischen Bild eine Reihe von Merkmalen, welche bei der endgültigen Diagnosenstellung entscheidend sein können. Hier muß vor allem das Fehlen von Strukturen genannt werden, welche für die Diagnose der Dermatitis herpetiformis Duhring, Lichen planus, Psoriasis, Leukämie, Mycosis fungoides sprechen würden, d.h. jener Hauterkrankungen, welche bei der Abgrenzung der „Exudative discoid and lichenoid chronic Dermatosis" hauptsächlich in Betracht kommen.

Seit der ersten Beschreibung dieses Krankheitsbildes ist eine Reihe von Publikationen veröffentlicht worden, von welchen die Arbeiten von Sachs und Kirsch sowie von Sachs, Miller und Gray für den Dermatohistopathologen von besonderer Bedeutung sind. Die genannten Autoren betonen, daß entsprechend den in verschiedenen Stadien klinisch so verschiedenen Erscheinungsformen der Dermatose auch die histologischen Veränderungen der Epidermis verschieden sind, daß insbesondere die exsudative Phase der Erkrankung histologisch nur schwer von anderen Formen von exsudativem Ekzem wie nummular eczema und akuter Kontaktdermatitis unterschieden werden kann, während spätere Stadien mehr charakteristische Veränderungen in der Cutis aufweisen, sogar eine histologische Diagnose ermöglichen.

Das histologische Bild der *Epidermis* hängt den genannten Autoren zufolge ab von dem jeweiligen Stadium, in welchem die Untersuchung vorgenommen wurde, und läßt entweder interstitielles Ödem (Spongiosis), Bläschenbildung, Störungen in der Begrenzung der Basalschichte sowie fleckförmige Parakeratose erkennen oder aber ein Bild, das einer trockenen „neurodermatitischen Reaktion" (Sachs-Miller-Gray) ähnelt und irreguläre Akanthose sowie deutliche Körner- und Hornschichte erkennen läßt.

Mehr „diagnostische" Veränderungen sind, besonders in späteren Stadien in der *Cutis* vorhanden und weisen die folgenden, von Sachs-Kirsch als charakteristisch hervorgehobenen Merkmale auf: die Gefäße (Arteriolen) der oberen und mittleren Cutis sind erweitert, ihre Wandungen verdickt. Die Kerne der Intima erscheinen geschwollen. Die Capillaren, besonders jene des Papillarkörpers, sind erweitert. Die Arteriolen weisen einen perivasculären Mantel von kleinen Rundzellen und wandernden Bindegewebszellen, polymorphkernigen Leukocyten, Eosinophilen und zahlreichen Plasmazellen auf, gelegentlich auch die eine oder andere Epithelioidzelle, aber keine Riesenzellen. Die Plasmazellen, die sich zumeist in der nächsten Nähe der Gefäßwand befinden, können in den Frühstadien der Erkrankung fehlen, in welchen Fällen die histologische Diagnose nur eine tentative, eine Vermutungsdiagnose sein kann. Ödem ist allenthalben in der

Cutis vorhanden, interstitiell in ihren oberen Anteilen, aber innerhalb der Bindegewebsbündel in ihren tieferen Schichten. Die untere Cutis zeigt keine nennenswerten Veränderungen. In älteren Läsionen können Chromatophoren beobachtet werden. Kernverklumpungen, Mitosen, Kernzerfall („nuclear dust"), Mykosiszellen, PAUTRIERs Abscesse sowie ein Reticulum wurden nie gesehen. Abb. 7 und 8 illustrieren die geschilderten Veränderungen in einem discoid-lichenoiden Herd des vorliegenden Krankheitsbildes.

In ihren Ausführungen betonen SACHS-KIRSCH wie auch SACHS-MILLER-GRAY bei der Erörterung der *histologischen Differentialdiagnose*, wie schwierig es mit-

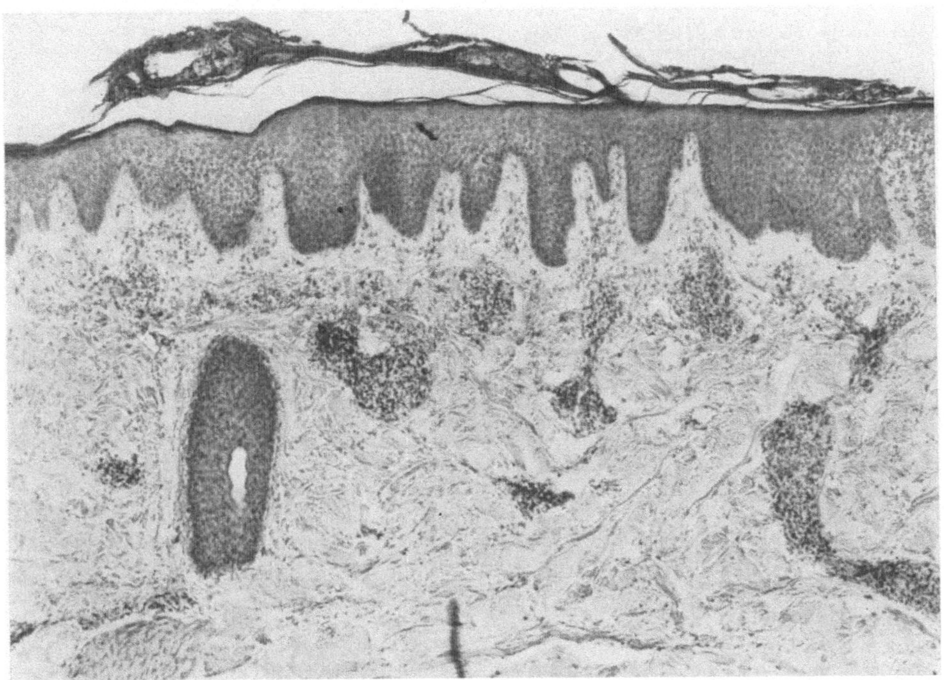

Abb. 7. Histologisches Bild eines discoid-lichenoiden Herdes (Übersichtsbild). Im *Epithel* unregelmäßige Acanthose, deutlich ausgeprägtes Stratum corneum und granulosum. In der *Cutis* umgeben buntzellige Infiltrate die meist erweiterten Gefäße. (Aus SULZBERGER-MARCH-GAY, Z. Haut- u. Geschl.-Kr. 27, H. 8)

unter sein kann, die „exudative discoid and lichenoid chronic dermatosis" von anderen Krankheitsbildern wie Jod- und Bromeruptionen gelegentlich auch von früh-sekundärer Syphilis abzugrenzen. In Jod- und Bromexanthemen bestehen die Infiltrate hauptsächlich aus polymorphkernigen Leukocyten und kleinen Rundzellen. Die Gefäßwandungen sind nicht verdickt. Späterhin erscheinen die Infiltrate dichter und aus verschiedenen Zelltypen zusammengesetzt, Colliquationsnekrosen und schließlich Granulationswucherungen beherrschen das Bild. In den Läsionen frühsekundärer Syphilis lassen tiefe wie oberflächliche Gefäße die gleichen Veränderungen erkennen, die Infiltrate sind nicht unbedingt herdförmig und bestehen hauptsächlich aus Plasmazellen. Die Gefäßlumina erscheinen verengt, mitunter nahezu obliteriert. Immerhin können die genannten Krankheitsprozesse klinisch sowie auf Grund anderer, nicht-histologischer Kriterien von der „exudative discoid and lichenoid chronic dermatosis" abgegrenzt werden. Gegen die Annahme einer lymphatischen Leukämie spricht das Fehlen eines einheitlich lymphocytären Infiltrates, gegen jene einer Mycosis fungoides das

Fehlen von PAUTRIERs Abscessen in der Epidermis, von Mitosen, Kernverklumpungen und Kernzerfall, Mykosiszellen sowie eines Reticulums.

Von besonderer Wichtigkeit ist die histopathologische Abgrenzung solitärer, persistierender Penisplaques gegenüber Manifestationen von Lichen planus, Psoriasis, Atopic Dermatitis und durch Arzneimittel bedingten Ausschlägen. Dies mag bei den beiden erstgenannten Dermatosen, deren histologisches Bild „diagnostisch" ist, unschwer gelingen. Gegenüber der Atopic Dermatitis, anderen ekzematösen Veränderungen, evtl. auch Arzneimittelausschlägen ist die Unterscheidung auf ausschließlich histologischen Gründen oft schwer, mitunter unmöglich. In solchen Fällen kann die eingehende klinische Untersuchung der Patienten, Fahnden nach etwa vorhandenen Veränderungen irgendwo an der Haut und an den Schleimhäuten wie auch sorgfältige, in Einzelheiten eingehende Nachforschungen hinsichtlich der Krankengeschichte zur Klärung der wahren Natur der vorliegenden „persistent penile plaque" beitragen (SULZBERGER-WITTEN-HUNT). Die therapeutisch wie prognostisch so wichtige Unterscheidung von der Erythroplasie Queyrat ist kürzlich von BLAU-HYMAN eingehend erörtert worden. Die echte präcanceröse bzw. canceröse Erythroplasie Queyrat mit ihren histologischen Veränderungen vom Charakter des Morbus Bowen oder bereits eines Plattenzellenkrebses ist histologisch unschwer zu erkennen, so daß eine Verwechslung wohl kaum vorkommen kann.

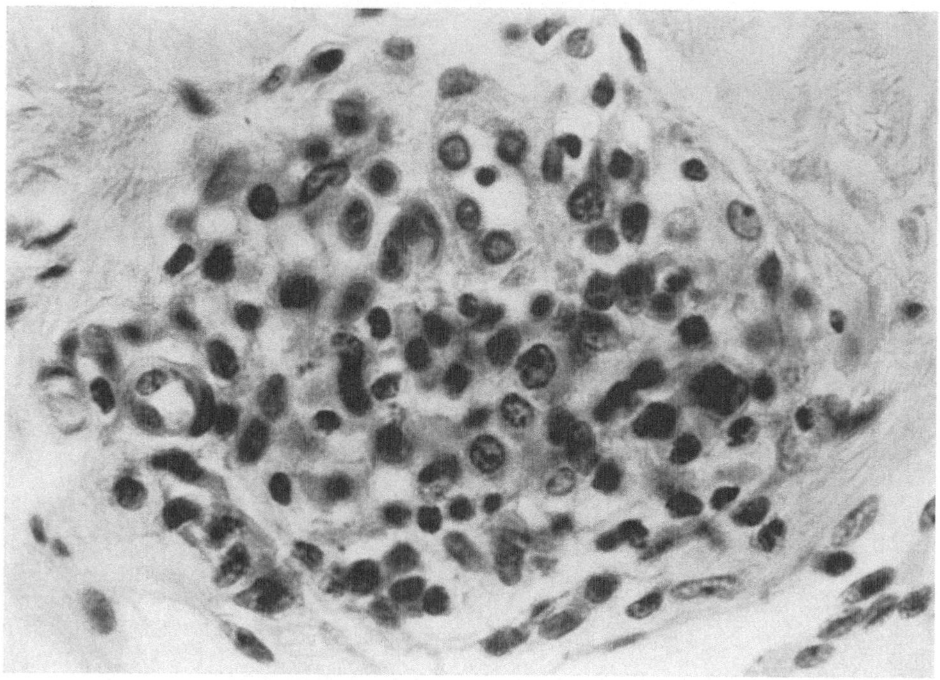

Abb. 8. Perivasculäres Infiltrat, bestehend aus kleinen Rundzellen, Bindegewebszellen, polymorphkernigen Leukocyten, Eosinophilen und zahlreichen Plasmazellen. (Aus SULZBERGER-MARCH-GAY, Z. Haut- u. Geschl.-Kr. 27, H. 8)

6. Differentialdiagnose

Wie bei einer Erkrankung mit so wechselnden klinischen Erscheinungsformen nicht anders erwartet werden kann, wechselt die Differentialdiagnose beträchtlich

Tabelle 2

zeigt zusammenfassend die verschiedenen Dermatosen, die *vor* der Diagnose „exudative discoid and lichenoid chronic dermatosis“ jeweils differentialdiagnostisch in Erwägung gezogen worden waren bei 83 einschlägigen Fällen, für welche von 106 in der Literatur niedergelegten Beobachtungen entsprechende Angaben vorliegen.

Mycosis fungoides, Lymphoblastom oder Leukämie	30/83
Contact Dermatitis	28/83
Dermatitis herpetiformis Duhring	13/83
Atopic Dermatitis	11/83
Psoriasis	11/83
Lichen planus	11/83
Seborrhoic Dermatitis	6/83
Parapsoriasis	4/83
Dermatophytosis and/or „Id“	4/83
Drug Eruption	3/83
Pityriasis rubra pilaris	3/83
Nummular Eczema	3/83
Erythrodermia	1/83

Unter Benützung der in der Publikation von SULZBERGER-MARCH-GAY enthaltenen Tabelle.

entsprechend dem jeweiligen Stadium, in welchem der Patient zur Beobachtung kommt. Tabelle 2 illustriert so zusammenfassend die verschiedenen Dermatosen, die jeweils in Erwägung gezogen wurden bei 83 einschlägigen Fällen, für welche von insgesamt 106 in der Literatur niedergelegten Beobachtungen entsprechende Angaben vorliegen.

Während der *exsudativen Phase* sind es hauptsächlich nummuläres Ekzem, Kontaktdermatitis, Dermatitis herpetiformis Duhring, Scabies, Dermatophytosis und Dermatophytide, welchen das Krankheitsbild der „exudative discoid and lichenoid chronic dermatosis“ weitgehendst ähneln kann, den letzteren namentlich, wenn Blasenbildungen an den Füßen vorhanden sind. Auch an eine Erythrodermie ist gedacht worden (NILES). Während des *lichenoiden und infiltrativen Stadiums* ähneln die papulösen Elemente wiederum jenen des Lichen planus, mitunter, wenn die Ausbreitung eine mehr diffuse ist, einer Atopic Dermatitis. Aber es sind vor allem das prämykotische Stadium der Mycosis fungoides oder Frühstadien der in die Gruppe der Lymphoblastome (Retikulosen) gehörenden Krankheitsbilder, welche zumeist als tentative Diagnosen genannt werden, wenn Patienten mit Erscheinungen der eben genannten Phase von „exudative discoid and lichenoid chronic dermatosis“ zur Diskussion oder aus diagnostischen Gründen vorgestellt werden.

Wichtiger als irgendwelche spezifischen positiven Erwägungen, die zur Diagnose der „exudative discoid and lichenoid chronic dermatosis“ führen, ist oft die Beobachtung des Krankheitsverlaufes über einen längeren Zeitraum zusammen mit dem Fehlen von Symptomen, die mit der Annahme des einen oder anderen der erwähnten Krankheitsbilder vereinbar sind. Bei der Abgrenzung vom *Eczema nummulare* sind die Ausdehnung der befallenen Hautgebiete, das lichenoide und das urticarielle Stadium, die Lokalisation der Veränderungen inklusive der persistierenden Plaques am Penis, der rasche Wechsel des klinischen Bildes und die Eosinophilie entscheidend. Die *Atopic Dermatitis* läßt sich meistens durch das Fehlen von Atopien in der Familienanamnese, den relativ späten Krankheitsbeginn und das Nichtvorhandensein sonstiger atopischer Merkmale ausschließen. Auch der Umstand, daß die Veränderungen der „exudative discoid and lichenoid chronic dermatosis“ meist in anderen Bereichen als an den Beugeflächen der Arme und Beine lokalisiert sind, mag von differentialdiagnostischer Bedeutung sein. Bei der Unterscheidung von *allergischer Kontaktdermatitis* muß in Betracht gezogen werden, daß die Veränderungen an nicht exponierten Hautflächen auftreten und auch nicht das Bild äußerer Einwirkung aufweisen, daß Läppchenproben mit den anamnestisch suspekten Substanzen meist negativ sind, Eosinophilie ziemlich konstant vorhanden ist, daß Versuche, einen allergisierenden Reizstoff ausfindig zu machen, erfolglos sind, schließlich, daß spontane Exacerbationen und Remissionen ohne wahrnehmbare Beziehung zu spezifischen äußeren Einwirkungen oder Vermeidung von solchen auftreten. *Dermatitis herpetiformis Duhring* kann, wenn man von den gelegentlich an den Fußsohlen beobachteten Bläschen absieht, durch das Fehlen persistierender vesiculöser Elemente, von Blasen oder Pusteln sowie von herpetiformen Hautblüten, das Vorliegen eines nicht der Dermatitis herpetiformis entsprechenden histologischen Bildes, das Ausbleiben von Narbenbildung, sowie durch den negativen Ausfall der Läppchenproben mit Jod- und Bromverbindungen ausgeschlossen werden. *Dermatophytosis mit id-Reaktion* kann nicht angenommen werden, wenn alle Pilzuntersuchungen negativ sind, Penisläsionen und intensiver Juckreiz vorhanden sind und jedwede antimykotische Therapie, einschließlich der oralen Verabreichung von Griseofulvin erfolglos ist. *Psoriasis* befällt im allgemeinen die Ellbogen, Knie, die behaarte Kopfhaut, öfters auch die Nägel, d.h. Lokalisationen, welche bei der „exudative discoid and lichenoid chronic dermatosis“ nicht öfters befallen erscheinen. Auch fehlt der intensive paroxysmale Juckreiz gewöhnlich bei Psoriasis. Der *Lichen planus* zeigt ein fast immer typisches Bild, das grundverschieden ist von jenem der „exudative discoid and lichenoid chronic dermatosis“. Der letzteren fehlen auch die für den Lichen planus charakteristische Dellenbildung der bläulich-roten, wachsartig glänzenden papulösen Effloreszenzen, die Wickhamschen Striae und das Befallensein der Schleimhäute. In Fällen, in welchen das klinische Bild an die Möglichkeit einer *Mycosis fungoides*, insbesondere ihres prämykotischen Stadiums oder an eine andere Erkrankung der Lymphoblastomgruppe denken läßt, werden der histologische Befund und das Blutbild die Entscheidung bringen, ebenso wie die Erfahrungstatsache, daß bei der „exudative discoid and lichenoid chronic dermatosis“ Röntgenbehandlungen nicht ungewöhnlich eher von einer Verschlimmerung als von einer Besserung gefolgt sind. Die ekzematöse, lichenoide und urticarielle Phase der „exudative, lichenoid and discoid chronic dermatosis“ haben mit dem prämykotischen Stadium keine Ähnlichkeit, was auch hinsichtlich der Penisläsionen zutrifft. Der *gutartige*, wenn auch chronische, durch Rückfälle unterbrochene Verlauf mit schließlich erfolgender *Heilung* sind letzten Endes der Beweis dafür, daß es sich nicht um eine Mycosis fungoides oder einen anderen Lymphoblastomtyp gehandelt hat.

Besonderer Erwähnung bedürfen noch jene Fälle, in welchen in irgendeinem Krankheitsstadium isolierte, persistente Penisplaques *ohne* sonstige Veränderungen am übrigen Körper beobachtet werden. Dieses Problem ist in einer Veröffentlichung unter dem Titel „Puzzling Persistent Penile Plaques“ erörtert worden (SULZBERGER-WITTEN-HUNT). Von primärer Wichtigkeit in solchen Fällen ist die Unterscheidung zwischen Veränderungen der „exudative discoid and lichenoid chronic dermatosis“ und jenen der echten Erythroplasie (QUEYRAT). In dem oben erwähnten Artikel wird auch die Unterscheidung der erstgenannten Dermatose von Penisläsionen bei Lichen planus und bei Psoriasis erörtert. Diese beiden letzteren stellen indes ein weitaus geringeres Problem dar als die echte Erythroplasie, bei welcher es darauf ankommt, endgültige Entscheidungen hinsichtlich der Prognose und der einzuschlagenden Therapie zu treffen. Es ist klar, daß es für den Patienten von besonderer Wichtigkeit ist, wenn bei Vorliegen einer solitären, persistierenden Plaque am Penis (besonders an der Glans) mit Merkmalen, die für eine Erythroplasie Queyrat verdächtig erscheinen, die Annahme oder Ablehnung der Diagnose Erythroplasie Queyrat nur mit größter Vorsicht und Sorgfalt erfolgt.

Ein Kriterium, das endlich bei der Diagnose der „exudative discoid and lichenoid chronic dermatosis“ in einer Anzahl von Fällen bedeutsam sein kann, ist das Ansprechen auf die Therapie. Wie später auch noch ausgeführt werden soll, spricht diese Dermatose auf orale Verabreichung von Corticosteroiden besonders gut an, therapeutische Erfolge werden ziemlich regelmäßig mit mittleren bis kleinen Dosen von Corticosteroiden erreicht und aufrecht erhalten. Bei der Mehrzahl der Erkrankungen dagegen, die hauptsächlich von der „exudative discoid and lichenoid chronic dermatosis“ differentialdiagnostisch abzugrenzen sind wie Dermatitis herpetiformis Duhring, nummuläres Ekzem, Lichen planus, Mycosis fungoides, sind die Erfolge mit mäßigen Corticosteroiddosen bestenfalls zweifelhaft, ein Umstand, der manchmal eine Diagnose „ex juvantibus“ erlaubt.

Tabelle 1 und 3 zeigen klinische Charakteristika und Befunde bei „exudative discoid and lichenoid chronic dermatosis“ (Tabelle 1), bzw. bei den „persistent penile plaques“ (Tabelle 4) dieser Erkrankung in Gegenüberstellung zu jenen der jeweils abzugrenzenden Krankheitsbilder.

7. Ätiologie

Die Ätiologie des uns hier beschäftigenden Krankheitsbildes ist unbekannt und von den verschiedentlich aufgestellten Hypothesen erscheint keine so wohlfundiert zu sein, daß sie anerkannt werden konnte. Zunächst glaubte man, daß die Erkrankung durch *Sensibilisierung* gegenüber Allergenen bedingt sei, die aus der Umgebung durch Kontakt oder auf anderem Wege wie etwa Inhalation in den Körper gelangen. So nahmen SULZBERGER eine Überempfindlichkeit gegen Staub („house dust“), ANDREWS gegen Orris root (einen aus der Wurzel von Iris florentina stammenden Zusatz zu Zahnpulver), CANNON gegenüber Pyrethrum (ein in den Vereinigten Staaten vielfach benütztes Insecticid) an, SHARLIT beschuldigte Seide und zur Färbung von Seidenmaterialien verwendete Farbstoffe als Krankheitsursache, MAX SCHEER glaubte in der Diskussion zu einem von COSTELLO vorgestellten Falle die Dermatose auf das in „moth balls“ enthaltene Naphthalin zurückführen zu sollen. Obwohl solche äußerlichen Kontakte in einzelnen Fällen vielleicht als „Trigger“- oder Verschlimmerungsfaktor wirken könnten, haben sie sich indes in Nachuntersuchungen oder späteren Beobachtungen als nicht stichhaltig erwiesen, vor allem nicht von fundamentaler kausaler Bedeutung für die Entstehung der Krankheit.

Einen weiten Raum in der Erörterung der Krankheitsursache der „exudative discoid and lichenoid chronic dermatosis“ nimmt die Annahme einer *psychosomatischen Ätiologie* ein. Dies ist nur allzu verständlich, weil in einer Reihe einschlägiger Beobachtungen immer wieder Abwegigkeiten der Psyche hervorgehoben werden. So sprechen beispielsweise BETT-WELLS von „anxiety and tension“, CANNON von „psychoneurotischen traits“, COSTELLO erwähnt „highstrung nervous disposition“ and „a profound psychic element bordering on anxiety neurosis“. KOCSARD betont das Vorhandensein von „neuropathic elements“, NILES das „neurotic temperament“ des von ihm beobachteten Patienten. In der Aussprache zu einem von SENEAR-PERLSTEIN beobachteten Falle weist ROTHMAN auf die Bedeutung des „strong psychic factors“ hin, und SMITH-GARRETT heben eine „underlying nervous instability“ hervor. Auch FRED WISE betont das Vorhandensein von „mental symptoms“, die mitunter mit Selbstmorddrohungen einhergehen. Von besonderer Bedeutung sind die Arbeiten von

Tabelle 3

	Exudative discoid and lichenoid chron. dermatosis	Mycosis fungoides	Dermatitis herpetiformis	Atopic dermatitis	Dermatophytosis und „Ids“	Allergic eczematous contact dermatitis
Alter	meist 30—60 Jahre	mittleres Alter	jedes Alter	jedes, Beginn im Kindesalter		
Rasse	meist jüdisch	jede	jede	jede		
Geschlecht	meist männlich	jedes	jedes	jedes		
Familiengeschichte	∅	∅	∅	Vorkommen von Atopien		
Frühere Ausbrüche	ja	nein	nein	Infantile eczema, Asthma, Heufieber		
Haut	vier charakteristische Phasen (exsudativ, discoid-lichenoid, infiltrativ, urticariell)	*prämykotisches Stadium:* verschiedene, herd- oder bandförmige Veränderungen, ekzemartig, psoriasiform, parapsoriasiform, oft bizarr. *Stadium der Tumorbildung*	Polymorphismus; Neigung zur Gruppenbildung der erythematösen, papulo-vesiculären oder urticariellen Efflorescenzen. Befallensein: meist Rumpf und Streckseiten	Symptome von Asthma, Heufieber, Rhinitis vasomotoria. Befallensein: meist Beugeseiten und Hals. Lichenifizierte und ekzematisierte Herde, diffuse Lichenifikation	zerstreute und/oder gruppierte papulöse und vesiculöse Efflorescenzen in verschiedenen Hautregionen. Schuppung an Händen und Füßen	Lokalisation an exponierten Stellen. Ekzematöse Veränderungen (klinisch und histologisch)
Lymphdrüsen	sekundär	Lymphadenopathie, Splenomegalie	eventuell (sekundär infolge Kratzen)	eventuell sekundär		
Schleimhäute	Befallensein bisher nicht beobachtet	können befallen sein	können befallen sein	frei	frei	
Nägel	glatt, glänzend, wie abgeschliffen (Kratzeffekt)	glatt, glänzend, wie abgeschliffen (Kratzeffekt)	∅		Nägel oft miterkrankt	
Penis	meist befallen			kann befallen sein		
Juckreiz	unerträglich	heftig	heftig	mäßig bis heftig	mäßig oder abwesend	mäßig

Andere subjektive Beschwerden	gering, z. B. Brennen (Brust, Mamilla)		Parästhesien	Verdauungs-, hormonale Störungen		
Blutbild	Eosinophilie (6—60%)	mitunter Monocytosis	Eosinophilie (im Hemogram und auch im Blaseninhalt)	Eosinophilie (5—10%)	normal	normal
Laboratorienbefunde	negativ	negativ	Patch-Tests mit Jodiden (und Bromiden) oft positiv	Patch-Tests negativ, Scratch-Tests und Intracutan-Sofortreaktion	positive Pilzbefunde in Haut, Nägeln, Haaren. Positive Intradermal-Tests mit Trichophytin	Patch-Tests positiv
Histologie	nicht diagnostisch, aber doch charakteristisch	charakteristisch: Pautrier-Abscesse in der Epidermis, Polymorphismus der Infiltrate, Mykosiszellen, Reticulum	charakteristisch: subepidermale Blasenbildung (besonders im Beginn), keine Acantholysis			
Erfolg der Therapie	oft günstig nach Lokal- und Allgemeinbehandlung mit Steroiden sowie nach Orts- und Umgebungswechsel. Sulfapyridin und Röntgentherapie unwirksam	Erfolge mit Arsen und Röntgen sowie mit Cytotoxicas	Sulfapyridin (oder ein anderes Sulfonamid), auch Arsen erfolgreich. In schweren Fällen Cortison	Besserung durch Orts- und Umgebungswechsel; Hospitalisierung, Steroide ,Antihistamins, Teer, etc.	äußerlich Antimycotica, evtl. Griseofulvin per os	Schutz gegen Kontakt, Hospitalisierung, Änderung der Umgebung oder sogar des Berufes, Antihistamins, Steroide
Verlauf	chronisch mit Rückfällen	progressiv	Rückfälle und Besserungen mit Neigung zu Pigmentierungen und Narbenbildung	chronisch	akut oder chronisch rezidivierend	akut oder rezidivierend oder chronisch
Ausgang	meist mit vollständigem Abklingen	Exitus letalis		günstig	günstig	günstig

Unter teilweiser Benützung der in der Publikation von SULZBERGER-GARBE enthaltenen verschiedenen Tabellen.

Tabelle 4. *Vergleichender Überblick über 4 Dermatosen, bei welchen die Differentialdiagnose der „Persistent penile Plaques" von besonderer Wichtigkeit ist*

	Exudative Discoid and Lichenoid Chronic Dermatosis	Erythroplasia	Lichen planus	Psoriasis
Alter	meist 30—60	Erwachsene	Erwachsene	jedes Alter
Rasse	vorwiegend jüdische Rasse	jede	jede	jede
Familiengeschichte (hinsichtlich der gleichen Erkrankung	∅	∅	∅	mitunter +
Einfluß einer vorangegangenen Verletzung (Trauma)	∅	∅	evtl. isomorph	evtl. isomorph
Frühere Ausbrüche	+	∅	+	+
Vorhandensein von Veränderungen irgendwo am Körper zur Zeit der Untersuchung der „Penile Plaques"				
1. Haut	oft	keine	gewöhnlich	gewöhnlich
2. Schleimhäute	nein	nein	oft	selten
3. Nägel	nein	nein	nein	oft „pitting of nails"
Charakteristika der Penisläsion:				
1. ekzematöse Phase	+	+	möglich	möglich
2. exsudative und discoide Phase	+	+	nicht wahrscheinlich	nicht wahrscheinlich
3. lichenoide Phase	+	∅	+	∅
4. Hinterlassung von Pigmentierung	oft	....	oft	selten
5. seröse Kruste	oft	oft	selten	selten
6. glimmerartige trockene Schuppung	∅	∅	∅	+
7. scharfe Begrenzung	ziemlich scharf	+	ziemlich scharf	+
8. Farbe	rot, feucht	samtartige Rötung	ziemlich bläulichrot	rot, manchmal charakteristisch schuppend
Blutbild	Eosinophilie	normal	normal	normal
Histopathologie	nicht diagnostisch	diagnostisch (Bowenoid)	diagnostisch	diagnostisch
Einfluß der Therapie	oft günstig beeinflußt durch lokal und/oder systematisch applizierte Corticosteroide	chirurgische Entfernung oder Zerstörung notwendig	wie bei den sonst vorhandenen Veränderungen	wie bei den sonst vorhandenen Veränderungen
Verlauf	oft durch Jahre bestehend; Rückfälle	persistierend	schließlich Ausgang in Heilung	schließlich Ausgang in Heilung
Ausgang	meist vollständige Rückbildung	wenn unbehandelt, immer bösartig (Ausgang in Stachelzellkrebs mit Metastasen)	meist vollständige Rückbildung	oft vollkommene Rückbildung

Unter Zugrundelegung der in der Publikation von Sulzberger-Witten-Hunt enthaltenen Tabelle.

Schneider-Kesten und von Shaffer-Beerman, in welchen die Annahme der psychosomatischen Ätiologie der „exudative discoid and lichenoid chronic dermatosis" diskutiert worden ist. Wenn wir auch die Möglichkeit nicht völlig ablehnen möchten, so ist doch unserer Meinung nach die Frage der etwaigen Rolle von psychischen Störungen hinsichtlich der Ätiologie dieses Krankheitsbildes noch ungeklärt. Es ist auch noch unentschieden, ob das Vorhandensein irgendwelcher psychologischer Abwegigkeiten, die bei manchen dieser Patienten bestehen, ein reiner Zufallsbefund ist oder aber die *Ursache*, das *Ergebnis oder nur ein Begleitsymptom* dieser Erkrankung darstellt.

Das Vorkommen der Mehrzahl der Beobachtungen bei Männern jüdischer Rasse ist auffallend und könnte vielleicht als Hinweis auf einen *rassisch* und *geschlechtsgebundenen* Krankheitstypus gedeutet werden. Es hat sich indes gezeigt, daß in einer bis jetzt immer noch kleinen Anzahl der Fälle auch Nichtjuden und Frauen Träger der Krankheitserscheinungen waren (vgl. Tabelle 3). Für *Heredität* und *familiäre Disposition* bestehen keine Anhaltspunkte, daß zwei Fälle der Erkrankung in irgendeiner Familie bei Blutsverwandten beobachtet worden wären, ist bisher nicht beschrieben worden. Costello berichtet über einen einschlägigen Fall, einen 62jährigen Mann mit den typischen Veränderungen des Krankheitsbildes, insbesondere mit „penile plaques", dessen 59jährige Ehefrau späterhin während eines Rückfalles ihres Gatten ebenfalls die charakteristischen Erscheinungen der „exudative discoid and lichenoid dermatosis" aufwies. Aufenthalt in Florida heilte beide Ehepartner. Nach H. W. Siemens spricht das Auftreten einer relativ seltenen Erkrankung unbekannter Ätiologie nacheinander bei beiden Ehegatten für äußere Einflüsse. Ob in der von Costello mitgeteilten Beobachtung die Ursache ein infectiöses Agens, ein Kontaktallergen oder psychologisch („folie à deux") bedingt war oder vielleicht nur ein lediglich zufälliges Vorkommen darstellt, muß unentschieden bleiben.

Die in Rede stehende Dermatose kann auch nicht als eine *atopische Affektion* angenommen werden, da bei den beobachteten Fällen weder die Familien- und Krankengeschichte noch auch die Untersuchung der Patienten mehr Hinweise oder atopische Merkmale ergaben als bei einer Kontrollgruppe der allgemeinen Bevölkerung. Endlich haben *hormonale Untersuchungen*, die in einschlägigen Beobachtungen durchgeführt worden waren (Kocsard), keinerlei Anhaltspunkte für das Bestehen einer abnormalen Schilddrüsen- oder Nebennierenrindenfunktion ergeben.

8. Geographisches Vorkommen

Beobachtungen von Fällen von „exudative discoid and lichenoid dermatosis" stammen fast ausschließlich aus Ländern der westlichen Hemisphäre, vor allem aus den United States, zum Teil auch aus Latein Amerika. Demgegenüber liegen, soweit die Durchsicht der Literatur erkennen läßt, nur ein Bericht von Bett-Wells über eine einschlägige Krankenvorstellung in der Royal Society of Medicine in London vor sowie eine von Gentele verfaßte Schilderung eines hierher gehörenden Falles in den Acta dermatovenereologica. Jessner betonte in der Diskussion zu einem von Goldstein-Fernandez gezeigten Fall von Sulzberger-Garbe disease, daß diese Erkrankung in Europa unbekannt war. Ob diese auffallende Erscheinung mit der vielfach, so von Marchionini, R. Spitzer u.a. betonten geographischen Verteilung der Hautkrankheiten erklärt werden kann, ist schwer zu sagen. Es mag aber auch sein, daß hierher gehörende Beobachtungen vielfach unter anderen Diagnosen aufscheinen, wie dies in der Einleitung zum Originalartikel schon seinerzeit hervorgehoben worden war. Auch heute noch wird mitunter die „exudative discoid and lichenoid chronic dermatosis" als entity sui generis angezweifelt, werden hier einzureihende Fälle mit anderen Diagnosen versehen. Diesen Standpunkt vertritt beispielsweise Témime gelegentlich der Erörterung der Abgrenzung des Lichen planus von dem Sulzberger-Garbe-Syndrom „dont l'individualisation n'a pas paru être nécessaire ou désirable en France".

9. Therapie

Ein Überblick über die zur Behandlung der „exudative discoid and lichenoid chronic dermatosis" in Anwendung gebrachten therapeutischen Maßnahmen läßt deutlich zwei Perioden erkennen. *Vor der Einführung des Cortison und seiner Derivative* hat es eigentlich keine regelmäßig einen Erfolg versprechende Behandlung dieser Krankheit gegeben. Vielmehr beschränkte man sich auf primär palliative Maßnahmen wie juckreizstillende Verbände, Schüttelmixturen und Salben sowie auf Verabreichung von Antihistaminen und Sedativa. Wegen des über lange Zeit sich erstreckenden und qualvollen Verlaufes der Erkrankung wie auch wegen der völligen Unkenntnis der Krankheitsursache wurden alle möglichen therapeutischen Methoden versucht wie diätetische Maßnahmen (einschließlich einer kalorienreichen Diät und Eliminationdiät), Injektionen von Calcium, Sodiumthiosulfat- und Strontiumbromidlösungen, Testosteronpräparaten, Bädern (Stärke-, Teer-, Schwefel- und Permanganatbädern), Entfernung der Tonsillen, Desensitisierungsversuche mit verschiedenen Allergenen und Vaccinen. Halbwegs befriedigende Resultate konnten jedoch mit allen üblichen Behandlungsarten kaum erreicht werden. Von älteren Methoden, mit welchen gelegentlich Besserungen und Remissionen erzielt werden konnten, stehen „change of milieu" (Umgebungs- oder Ortsveränderung) und Klimawechsel (besonders Aufenthalt in einem Klima mit niedriger relativer Feuchtigkeit) im Vordergrund, wie dies ja auch bei der Behandlung der atopic Dermatitis, Psoriasis sowie einer Anzahl anderer Haut- oder sonstiger Erkrankungen der Fall ist. Aber diese Besserungen werden keineswegs regelmäßig erzielt. Eine Übersicht über die *vor* dem Jahre 1951 beobachteten Patienten zeigt, daß sie mit oder ohne Behandlung an wiederholten akuten oder chronischen Schüben der Dermatose mit gelegentlichen Spontanremissionen zu leiden hatten, bis schließlich die Erkrankung „burned itself out", spontan allmählich an Intensität und Extensität verlor und nur geringfügige Residuen in Form einer Penisplaque oder von Schüben von tiefsitzenden, urticariellen Läsionen hinterließ. Abgesehen von der Wirksamkeit eines Umgebungswechsels erwähnen Pascher, Kocsard u.a. Erfolge mit der von Jessner empfohlenen intramusculären Anwendung von Natrium arsenicum. Aber auch die Arsentherapie erwies sich nicht oft erfolgreich, wie dies beispielsweise Andrews berichtet.

Seit der Einführung des Cortisons und der neueren cortisonartigen Steroide ist es nun möglich geworden, die meisten Fälle soweit unter Kontrolle zu bringen, daß die Patienten ihrer normalen Tätigkeit ungehindert nachgehen können. Die „exudative discoid and lichenoid chronicdermatosis" ist, wie Sulzberger betont, tatsächlich eine jener Dermatosen, die höchst dramatisch auf Cortison und cortisonartige Verbindungen ansprechen. Es kommen jedoch, wenn die Behandlung vor dem Abklingen der Krankheit, d.h. vor Eintreten der Spontanremission unterbrochen wird, die Symptome prompt wieder zum Vorschein. Die zur Zeit erfolgreichste Methode war unserer Erfahrung nach, mit einer angemessenen Dosis von Corticosteroiden, etwa eine tägliche orale Darreichung von 150—250 mg (3—5 Tabletten) Cortisonacetat (oder einer adequaten Dosis von anderen Corticosteroiden) zu beginnen und nach Unterdrückung der Krankheitserscheinungen die Dosis langsam zu verringern und zwar jede oder jede zweite Woche um 10% der vorhergehenden Dosis, bis sich wieder geringfügige Symptome bei einem bestimmten Dosierungsausmaß einstellen. Wird diese Dosis dann wieder um ein weniges gesteigert, so erreicht man die „Maintenance dosis“ oder „morbidistatische Dosis“. Die Patienten können dann durch viele Monate hindurch bei dieser Dosis mit periodischen Versuchen einer allmählichen Dosisreduktion gehalten werden, bis man schließlich zu ganz geringen Dosen gelangt (SULZBERGER, KANOF u.a.). Wir haben Patienten gesehen, die so präzis eingestellt waren, daß ein Wechsel von 10 mg *pro die* zu 7,5 mg *pro die* von Prednison einen Rückfall auslöste, während andere mit praktisch homöopathischen Dosen von 2 mg Triamcinolon oder Prednison *pro die* fast symptomfrei gehalten werden konnten, jedoch Rückfälle erlitten, wenn die Steroidtherapie vollständig ausgeschaltet wurde.

Der Gebrauch von Antihistaminpräparaten und Tranquilizers (Phenothiazinderivaten) hat sich gelegentlich als Zusatzbehandlung nützlich erwiesen. Für die Lokalbehandlung war, abgesehen von antipruriginösen Schüttelmixturen und Salben, die Anwendung von Hydrocortison und verwandten Steroiden in der Form von Trockenpinselungen, Cremes oder Salben, insbesondere bei weniger stark infiltrierten Läsionen und *namentlich* bei *Penisplaques* von gewissem Wert. Intradermale Infiltration von Suspensionen des unlöslichen Triamcinolon Acetonid (SQUIBB) (0,3 ml einer Aufschwemmung von 10 mg/ml) in isolierte persistent penile Plaques wurde kürzlich von ORENTREICH-MARCH als besonders erfolgreich beschrieben. Für diese Behandlungsmethode, bei welcher unter nur leichter Chloräthyl-Anaesthesie die genannte geringe Menge von Suspension mittels feiner Nadel injeziert wird, konnte auch Triamcinolon Diacetat (LEDERLE) benützt werden. Wahrscheinlich können auch andere, dem Hydrocortison verwandte Corticosteroide, lokal in analoger Weise verabfolgt, ähnliche Erfolge zeitigen. Okklusivverbände mit Cortico-Steroide, E. G. Triamcinolone, können für die Penis-Plaques therapeutisch recht wirksam sein (LEIDER, SULZBERGER).

Hinsichtlich der physikalischen Behandlung der „exudative discoid and lichenoid chronic dermatosis“ schwanken die Erfahrungen. Sicherlich gibt es Fälle, in welchen mit Ultraviolett-, Grenzstrahlen- oder mit Röntgenbehandlung Erfolge berichtet werden, wie beispielsweise ANDREWS das Schwinden der Hauterscheinungen nach Oberflächen-Röntgenbestrahlungen beobachten konnte. Unserer Erfahrung nach sprechen aber im allgemeinen die Läsionen der „exudative discoid and lichenoid chronic dermatosis“ auf Röntgenbehandlung nicht gut an, wir haben im Gegenteil in einer Anzahl von Fällen Exacerbationen der bestrahlten Gebiete beobachten können.

Literatur

ANDREWS, GEORGE C.: Chronic discoid and lichenoid dermatosis. Arch. Derm. Syph. (Chic.) **60**, 1004 (1949). — Diseases of the skin, 3. Aufl., S. 86. Philadelphia and London: W. B. Saunders Company 1946.

BERNSTEIN, EUGENE T.: Exudative discoid and lichenoid chronic dermatosis (Phase resembling leukotic dyscrasia). Arch. Derm. Syph. (Chic.) **41**, 1185 (1940). — BETT, D.C.G. (for G.C.WELLS): Exudative discoid and lichenoid chronic dermatosis of Sulzberger and Garbe. Brit. J. Derm. **70**, 184 (1958). — BLAU, S., and A.B. HYMAN: Erythroplasia of Queyrat. Acta derm. venereol. (Stockh.) **35**, 341 (1955).

CANNON, A. BENSON: Allergic dermatitis. Arch. Derm. Syph. (Chic.) **36**, 1269 (1937). — Allergic dermatosis simulating lymphoblastoma. Arch. Derm. Syph. (Chic.) **39**, 846 (1939). — Lichenoid exudative discoid dermatitis. Arch. Derm. Syph. (Chic.) **48**, 668 (1943). — COMBES, FRANK C.: Chronic discoid and lichenoid dermatitis associated with giant follicular lymphadenopathy. Arch. Derm. Syph. (Chic.) **45**, 1023 (1942). — COSTELLO, MAURICE J.: Exudative discoid and lichenoid chronic dermatosis. Arch. Derm. Syph. (Chic.) **51**, 145 (1945). — Chronic exudative lichenoid and discoid dermatosis treated successfully with intravenous injection of typhoid and paratyphoid vaccine, sunlight and salt water bathing. Arch. Derm. Syph. (Chic.) **59**, 359 (1949). — Chronic exudative, lichenoid and discoid dermatosis. Arch.

Derm. **76**, 376 (1957). — COUPERUS, M.: Exudative discoid lichenoid chronic dermatitis. Arch. Derm. Syph. (Chic.) **54**, 374 (1946).

GENTELE, H.: Exudative discoid and lichenoid chronic dermatosis of Sulzberger and Garbe. Acta derm.-venereolog. (Stockh.) **33**, 147 (1953). — GOLDSTEIN, L., and J. FERNANDEZ: Sulzberger-Garbe disease (?) (Exudative discoid and lichenoid dermatosis). Arch. Derm. Syph. (Chic.) **60**, 830 (1949).

KANOF, NORMAN B.: Exudative discoid and lichenoid chronic dermatosis (Sulzberger-Garbe) treated with Cortisone. Arch. Derm. Syph. (Chic.) **70**, 525 (1954). — KOCSARD, E.: Three cases of exudative chronic discoid and lichenoid dermatosis (Sulzberger and Garbe) in Shanghai. J. invest. Derm. **10**, 1 (1948).

MAZZINI, MIGUEL A., y D. CALZETTA: Dermatosis cronica exudativa discoide y liquenoide (SULZBERGER y GARBE, 1937). Rev. argent. Dermatosif. **39**, 340 (1955). Ref. Zbl. Haut- u. Geschl.-Kr. **103**, 57 (1958—1959).

NILES, HENRY D.: A case for diagnosis (Eczema? Chronic exudative lichenoid discoid dermatosis?). Arch. Derm. Syph. (Chic.) **42**, 954 (1940).

ORENTREICH, N., and C. MARCH: Intradermal triamcinolone acetonide and diacetate: Healing of persistent penile plaques due to distinctive exudative discoid and lichenoid chronic Dermatosis. J. Urol. (Baltimore) **85**, 827 (1961).

PASCHER, FRANCES: Exudative chronic discoid and lichenoid dermatitis (Sulzberger and Garbe). Treatment of five patients. Arch. Derm. Syph. (Chic.) **42**, 322 (1940). — PIERINI, L. E., A. ZURITA y J. ABULAFIA: Dermatosis exudativa discoide y liquenoide (Sulzberger-Garbe). Rev. argent. Dermatosif. **36**, 145 (1952).

ROSTENBERG, A., and A. ROSTENBERG jr.: A case for diagnosis. Arch. Derm. Syph. (Chic.) **35**, 509 (1937).

SACHS, W., and N. KIRSCH: Exudative discoid and lichenoid chronic dermatosis (Sulzberger-Garbe). Histopathologic study. J. invest. Derm. 8, 215 (1947). — SACHS, W., C. S. MILLER and M. B. GRAY: Neurodermatitic reaction. Arch. Derm. Syph. (Chic.) **54**, 397 (1946). — SCHNEIDER, E., and B. KESTEN: Polymorphic prurigo, psychosomatic study of three cases. J. invest. Derm. **10**, 205 (1948). — SENEAR, F. E., and O. MINNIO PERLSTEIN: Exudative discoid and lichenoid chronic dermatosis. Arch. Derm. Syph. (Chic.) **50**, 62 (1944). — SHAFFER, B., and H. BEERMAN: Lichen simplex chronicus and its variants. A discussion of certain pachydynamic mechanisms and chimical and histopathological considerations. Arch. Derm. Syph. (Chic.) **64**, 340 (1951). — SHARLIT, H.: Chronic exudative and lichenoid dermatitis. Arch. Derm. Syph. (Chic.) **45**, 776 (1942). — SMITH, LESLIE M., and H. D. GARRETT: Changes of climate and environment in treatment of dermatologic diseases: Effect on neurodermatitis and certain other chronic dermatoses. Arch. Derm. Syph. (Chic.) **68**, 28 (1953). — SULZBERGER, MARION B.: Exudative discoid and lichenoid chronic dermatosis. Arch. Derm. Syph. (Chic.) **40**, 288—291 (1939). — SULZBERGER, MARION B., and W. GARBE: Nine cases of a distinctive exudative discoid and lichenoid chronic dermatosis. Arch. Derm. Syph. (Chic.) **36**, 247 (1937). — SULZBERGER, MARION B., C. MARCH u. C. GAY: Besondere exsudative discoide und lichenoide chronische Dermatose. Z. Haut- u. Geschl.-Kr. **27**, 223 (1959). — SULZBERGER, MARION B., VICTOR H. WITTEN and JOHN A. HUNT: Puzzling persistent penile plaques. Arch. Derm. **73**, 101—109 (1956).

TÉMIME, P.: Aspect particulier d'un lichen plan cutanéo-muqueux de la lèvre inférieure prêtant à discussion avec un syndrome de Sulzberger et Garbe. Bull Soc. franç. Derm. **63**, 288—289 (1956).

WISE, F.: Exudative discoid and lichenoid chronic dermatosis. Arch. Derm. Syph. (Chic.) **40**, 287—288 (1939). — Exudative discoid and lichenoid chronic dermatosis. Arch. Derm. Syph. (Chic.) **55**, 273 (1947). — WRIGHT, C. S.: A case for diagnosis (Exudative discoid and lichenoid chronic dermatosis). Arch. Derm. Syph. (Chic.) **37**, 525 (1937).

Erythema exsudativum multiforme

Von

Rudolf Schuppli-Basel

Einleitung

Eine Übersicht über die sehr zahlreichen Arbeiten der letzten 3 Jahrzehnte, die sich mit dem Erythema exsudativum multiforme befassen, zeigt die Tendenz, dieses Krankheitsbild zu erweitern. Zwar bleibt das typische Erythema exsudativum multiforme, wie es HEBRA beschrieben hat, im großen und ganzen unverändert bestehen. Daneben aber gibt es zahlreiche Beobachtungen von Krankheitsbildern, die von der klassischen Beschreibung abweichen, aber wohl am ehesten in die Gruppe des Erythema exsudativum multiforme eingeordnet werden müssen. Auf diesem Gebiet des atypischen Erythema exsudativum multiforme ist die Verwirrung in den letzten Jahren eher größer als kleiner geworden. Drei Faktoren sind für die unbefriedigende Situation verantwortlich:

1. Das Fehlen genauerer Kenntnisse der Ätiologie und Pathogenese des Erythema exsudativum multiforme;

2. die Tatsache, daß sich auch Nicht-Dermatologen in vermehrtem Maße mit dem Krankheitsbild des Erythema exsudativum multiforme befassen, also Ärzte, die weniger Übung in der morphologischen Unterscheidung und Beschreibung von Hautveränderungen haben und oft auch mehr Wert auf den gesamten klinischen Verlauf einer Krankheit als auf Einzelheiten legen, und

3. der Umstand, daß verschiedene Syndrome von Haut- und Schleimhautveränderungen beschrieben worden sind, die gewisse Ähnlichkeiten mit dem klassischen Erythema exsudativum multiforme zeigen, deren Zugehörigkeit zu dieser Krankheitsgruppe aber unklar ist.

Es liegen eine ganze Reihe von gründlichen Arbeiten vor, die sich mit diesen Problemen befassen und die die Schwierigkeiten, die sich aus der Multiformität der klinischen Bilder ergeben, auf verschiedene Weise zu lösen suchen.

RUITER weist in mehreren Publikationen auf die Notwendigkeit hin, das eigentliche Erythema exsudativum multiforme von ähnlichen Krankheitsbildern zu unterscheiden. Er betont, daß der Begriff des Erythema exsudativum multiforme in den letzten Jahren viel zu weit gefaßt worden sei. Nicht nur die Internisten, sondern auch zahlreiche Dermatologen, speziell in Amerika, schienen sich kaum mehr bewußt zu sein, daß die Diagnose des Erythema exsudativum multiforme nur auf Grund klinisch-morphologischer Kennzeichen zu stellen sei und daß die Hautveränderungen ganz bestimmten Anforderungen genügen müßten. Er verlangt, daß man sich in dieser Hinsicht unbedingt an die seinerzeit von HEBRA aufgestellten Kriterien zu halten habe und daß diese Form des Erythema exsudativum multiforme scharf von den polymorphen Exanthemen toxischer oder bekannter Ätiologie abzutrennen sei. Auch TZANK und CORD äußern sich in ähnlichem Sinne, nämlich, daß die in das Bild des Erythema exsudativum multiforme gehörenden Eruptionen nur morphologisch klassiert werden können und daß alle

Versuche, diese nach ätiologischen Gesichtspunkten zu ordnen, bisher fehlgeschlagen haben. Man fasse daher sehr oft unter dem Begriff des Erythema exsudativum multiforme mindestens zwei vollkommen verschiedene Affektionen zusammen, nämlich eine infektiöse Krankheit und eine Reaktionsform der Haut auf ganz verschiedene Ursachen. Sie halten es für möglich, diese beiden Formen trotz weitgehender Identität ihres Bildes auf Grund einiger klinischer Kriterien, speziell des Juckreizes, zu unterscheiden. Sie trennen den Hebraschen Typus des Erythema exsudativum multiforme als Erythème polymorphe infectieux vom Erythème polymorphe réaction d'intolérance. Auch MANGANOTTI kommt zu den ähnlichen Schlußfolgerungen. Allerdings scheint es fraglich, ob damit sehr viel gewonnen ist, da die Bezeichnung infektiöses Erythème polymorphe eine Ätiologie impliziert, die noch völlig unbewiesen ist.

Demgegenüber besteht im angelsächsischen Sprachbereich allgemein eher die Tendenz einer einheitlichen Auffassung des ganzen Krankheitsbildes unter geringerer Beobachtung morphologischer Einzelheiten. So hält KEIL die ganze Krankheitsgruppe für eine einheitliche Affektion, die sich klinisch unter verschiedenen Formen manifestiert.

Auch einzelne europäische Autoren vertreten die Tendenz zur Vereinheitlichung. So sind KEINING und OLDACH der Auffassung, daß die Kennzeichnung der in Rede stehenden Hautveränderungen als multiforme Erytheme gegenüber Krankheitsbezeichnungen wie Erythema exsudativum multiforme vorzuziehen sei, weil unter diesem Oberbegriff eine bessere, weniger mißverständliche Gruppeneinteilung ätiologisch gleichgelagerter Krankheitsbilder möglich sei. Auch im französischen Schrifttum bürgert sich die Bezeichnung ,,polymorphe Erytheme" als Oberbegriff mehr und mehr ein.

Schwieriger als die klinische Differenzierung der erythematösen und exsudativen Hauterscheinungen ist die Frage zu entscheiden, ob verschiedene die Schleimhäute und die Haut befallende Krankheiten der Gruppe des Erythema exsudativum multiforme zugeordnet werden können. Es sei hier schon vorweggenommen, daß es sich um die vom Ophthalmologen FUCHS 1876 beschriebene Krankheit des Herpes iris conjunctivae, um die von FIESSINGER und RENDU 1917 beschriebene Ectodermose pluriorificielle, um das von den Pädiatern STEVENS und JOHNSON 1922 aufgestellte Syndrom und um die 1925 von BAADER beschriebene Dermatostomatitis handelt. Auch wird versucht, die Reitersche Krankheit (STEFANETTI) und den von HULUSI BEHÇET beschriebenen Trisymptomenkomplex in die gleiche Gruppe einzuordnen (MAURIELLO).

PROPPE hat diesen Fragen eine längere Studie gewidmet und äußert sich dahin, daß es auf Grund der großen Ähnlichkeit verschiedener akuter Syndrome untereinander wohl berechtigt sei, diese unter der Bezeichnung Syndroma mucocutaneo-oculare acutum (FUCHS) zusammenzufassen und daß es möglich sei, sie gegenüber den chronischen Syndromen abzugrenzen. Dieses akute Haut--Schleimhaut-Augensyndrom wiederum müsse vom Erythema exsudativum multiforme abgesondert werden, da es nicht angehe, ein derart unklar begrenztes Krankheitsbild wie das Erythema exsudativum multiforme mit einem so verschiedenen Krankheitsbild wie dem Fuchsschen Haut-Schleimhaut-Augen-Syndrom in Zusammenhang zu bringen, solange die Ätiologie dieser Syndrome noch unklar sei. HEBRA selbst hatte in seiner Beschreibung des Erythema exsudativa multiforme ja betont, daß weder Erscheinungen an den Schleimhäuten, noch an den serösen oder fibrösen Gebilden auftreten. Demgegenüber nimmt CERUTTI den entgegengesetzten Standpunkt ein, indem er es für ungerechtfertigt hält, diese Syndrome zu trennen, solange ihre Ätiologie nicht klar sei. Auch BOHNSTEDT schlägt vor, alle diese Syndrome unter dem Oberbegriff der multiformen Erytheme zusammenzufassen und den Typ Hebra auf reine Hautfälle zu beschränken. BRETT und SPRENGER sowie WOLFRAM et al. kommen zu ähnlichen Schlüssen. Eine vermittelnde Stellung nehmen englische Autoren ein. THOMAS glaubt, daß das Stevens-Johnson-Syndrom genügend sichere Zeichen aufweise, die es mit dem Erythema exsudativum multiforme in Verbindung bringen könnten und hält es lediglich für eine schwere Abart desselben. Er schlägt vor, die Krankheitsgruppe des Erythema exsudativum multiforme in zwei Formen einzuteilen, nämlich das Erythema exsudativum multiforme major (Stevens-Johnson-Syndrom) und minor (HEBRA). ASHBY und LAZAR halten zwar eine scharfe Trennung für unmöglich, rechnen aber doch auch alle Fälle in die Gruppe des Erythema exsudativum multiforme. Auch GINANDES möchte die Gruppe in die beiden Krankheitsbilder des Erythema exsudativum multiforme Typ Hebra und Typ Stevens-Johnson trennen.

In konsequenter Weise haben japanische Autoren das muco-cutaneo-oculäre Syndrom vom Erythema exsudativum multiforme abgetrennt. ITO unterscheidet darin zwei Formen, nämlich den akuten Typ Fuchs-Proppe und den chronischen Typ Gilbert-Behçet. NAKAMURA et al. unterteilen das Syndrom nach den klinischen Erscheinungen und nach dem Ansprechen auf Cortison und Antibiotica in fünf Typen. Die histologische Untersuchung zeigt immerhin, daß keine großen Unterschiede zwischen den einzelnen Typen bestehen (ITO) und daß die Art der Gefäßveränderungen, der Degeneration der kollagenen Fasern, der knötchenförmigen Zellinfiltrate (IWAI et al.) an eine gemeinsame allergische Ätiologie dieses Syndroms denken lassen.

Zusammenfassend kann festgestellt werden, daß es bisher nicht gelungen ist, eine einigermaßen befriedigende Einteilung der verschiedenen Formen des Erythema exsudativum multiforme vorzunehmen und daß dies wohl so lange nicht möglich sein wird, als die Ätiologie der verschiedenen Formen des Erythema exsudativum multiforme nicht besser bekannt ist. Man wird die Gruppe entweder als Einheit betrachten müssen und dann verschiedene Typen davon beschreiben, wie das z.B. COSTELLO (1948) tut, der sechs verschiedene Krankheitsgruppen bildet, nämlich 1. milder Typ (HEBRA), 2. pemphigoider Typ, 3. bullöser pluriorifizieller Typ (STEVENS-JOHNSON), 4. Erythema exsudativum multiforme bei Infektionskrankheiten, 5. Erythema exsudativum multiforme bei internen Affektionen, 6. Erythema exsudativum multiforme nach Medikamenten — oder aber sich an die ursprüngliche idiopathische, von HEBRA beschriebene Krankheitsform halten und alle Krankheitsbilder, die nicht mit dieser identifiziert werden können, als symptomatische Form bezeichnen. Beide Arten des Vorgehens sind unbefriedigend, da sie einer ganzen Reihe von Fällen nicht gerecht werden. Es wird aber bei der folgenden Diskussion über Klinik und Ätiologie der verschiedenen Formen des Erythema exsudativum multiforme immer wieder darauf hingewiesen werden müssen, daß die Grenzen zwischen den einzelnen Gruppen unscharf sind und daß deshalb einzelne Befunde nicht verallgemeinert werden können.

1. Klinisches Bild

a) Das idiopathische Erythema exsudativum multiforme

Nach TACHAU zeigt das idiopathische Erythema exsudativum multiforme, das von HEBRA beschrieben wurde, folgende hauptsächliche Kennzeichen: Nach unbestimmten Prodromen von 2—3 Tagen entsteht unvermittelt ein Exanthem, das immer zuerst Handrücken, dann auch andere Körperstellen befällt und aus einer Anzahl symmetrisch angeordneter, hellroter oder etwas livider Knötchen von oberflächlichem Sitz besteht. Innerhalb der nächsten 3—4 Tage dehnen sich diese Knötchen aus und bilden kreisrunde, in der Mitte eingesunkene Herde, die konfluieren können. Im Verlauf dieser Entwicklung kann sich der Entzündungsprozeß bis zur Blasenbildung steigern. Es können schubweise neue Efflorescenzen auftreten, wodurch ein mannigfaches Bild entsteht, das HEBRA zur Bezeichnung multiforme veranlaßte. Der schubweise Verlauf des Exanthems kann bis zu 4 Wochen betragen. Dann heilen die Efflorescenzen meist unter Pigmentierung ab. Schleimhauterscheinungen sind verschieden häufig, nach einer 272 Patienten umfassenden Statistik von BAIKOVA et al. in einem Drittel der Fälle, anzutreffen, wobei am häufigsten, d.h. in zwei Drittel der Fälle, die Lippenschleimhaut befallen ist. HEBRA allerdings hat Schleimhauterscheinungen nie erwähnt. Auch die Conjunctiva und die Genitalschleimhaut können Efflorescenzen zeigen. Hämorrhagische Bilder gehören nach TACHAU nicht zum Bilde des idiopathischen Erythema exsudativum multiforme. Ebenso fehlen Komplikationen durch schwere lebensgefährliche innere Erscheinungen. Häufig finden sich Rückfälle, deren Frequenz verschieden angegeben wird.

Aus den Ausführungsn TACHAUs geht nun bereits hervor, daß von diesem klassischen Typus zahlreiche Abweichungen beschrieben worden sind, so daß es schwer fällt, dem von HEBRA beschriebenen Bilde eine allgemeine Gültigkeit für die Diagnose des idiopathischen Erythema exsudativum multiforme zuzuerkennen. Auch im neueren Schrifttum finden sich entsprechende abweichende Beschreibungen, die z.T. die Lokalisation der Erscheinungen, z.T. ihre Morphologie, z.T. die Begleiterscheinungen betreffen. So beschreibt NADEL einen Fall von Erythema exsudativum multiforme, der sich durch atypische Lokalisation und exzessive Blasenbildung im Gesicht und am Genitale auszeichnete. Auch in einem Fall von FRÜHWALD fanden sich atypische, d.h. an den Handtellern und Fußsohlen lokalisierte bullöse Herde. KORTEN sah bei einem 13jährigen Knaben in jedem Frühjahr an den Handrücken rötlich-weiße, peripher wachsende Ringe auftreten, die in ihrer Konsistenz an Granuloma anulare erinnerten, aber unter innerlichen Salicylgaben jeweils rasch verschwanden. Auch OPPENHEIM beschreibt ähnliche Hauterscheinungen bei einer 30jährigen Frau. Histologisch ließ sich ein Granuloma anulare sicher ausschließen, da sich dichte, monomorphe Rundzellmäntel um die subpapillären und tiefen Gefäße und lockere Rundzellinfiltrate an einzelnen Stellen des Bindegewebes zeigten. KRUSPE demonstrierte einen Mann, bei dem stark gerötete, schmerzhafte Infiltrate mit kokardenförmigem Wachstum und zentraler Blasenbildung an den Handtellern auftraten, wobei das Zentrum der Blasen deutlich hämorrhagisch war. Einen besonders starken Befall des Gesichtes in Form großer Blasen bei gleichzeitigem Bestehen typischer Efflorescenzen an den Unterarmen erwähnte GRÜTZ. CARRIÉ sah in einem Fall derart starke Blasenbildung, daß zunächst ein Pemphigus diagnostiziert wurde und erst nach Auftreten typischer Efflorescenzen die richtige Diagnose gestellt werden konnte. Einen atypischen Heilungsverlauf zeigte ein von PRAKKEN erwähnter Fall. Der erste Schub hinterließ ein Leukoderm, während bei späteren Rezidiven keine Pigmentverschiebungen mehr auftraten.

Über schwerere interne Befunde bei typischem Erythema exsudativum multiforme berichtet SCHRANK. Er beobachtete den Fall eines Soldaten, der zugleich mit den Hauterscheinungen multiple Drüsenschwellungen zeigte, am 5. Krankheitstage eine Endokarditis und Nephritis durchmachte und komplikationslos heilte. ELIZADE und TURRO, ferner HÖLSCHER berichten, daß sich bei Säuglingen im Verlaufe eines Erythema multiforme oft atypische Pneumonien mit erhöhtem Kälteagglutinationstiter nachweisen lassen. LEMKE und BONSE fanden Hilusverschattungen, die am ehesten einer Viruspneumonie glichen und nach 10 Tagen vollständig zurückgebildet waren bei einem 51jährigen Kranken mit ausgeprägtem

Erythema exsudativum multiforme. CANTER und KATZ kommen auf Grund der Literatur zum Schluß, daß bei 30% aller Erythema exsudativum multiforme-Fälle Pneumonien vorkommen. LENGYEL et al. beschrieben Prodromalsymptome und allgemeine Symptome in Form von Fieber, Anämie, rheumatoiden und polyartikulären Schmerzen.

Die Tatsache, daß das Erythema exsudativum multiforme speziell an den dem Licht exponierten Stellen auftritt, führte zur Vermutung, daß Porphyrine eine gewisse Rolle spielen dürften. Tatsächlich wurden von HÜBNER erhöhte Porphyrinwerte im Urin gefunden. Demgegenüber konnte HÜLLSTRUNG keine erhöhte Porphyrinausscheidung konstatieren.

Einen großen Raum nimmt die Diskussion derjenigen Fälle von Erythema exsudativum multiforme ein, die mit Schleimhautveränderungen einhergehen. Wie schon erwähnt, hat HEBRA keine Schleimhautveränderungen in seinen Fällen gesehen, und deshalb sollten eigentlich — strenggenommen — alle die Schleimhäute befallenden Fälle separat behandelt werden. Nun aber sind Veränderungen der Mundschleimhaut ein derart häufiges Vorkommnis (ENKLING), daß die Gruppe des Erythema exsudativum multiforme Hebra wohl unzulässig eingeschränkt würde, wenn dieses negative Kriterium derart stark in Rechnung gezogen würde. Die Kasuistik über derartige Fälle ist so reichhaltig und ähnliche Beobachtungen in der Praxis sind so häufig, daß hier auf Zitierung einzelner Mitteilungen verzichtet werden kann. Wichtiger sind die Fälle, bei denen die Beteiligung der Haut und der Schleimhäute im Verlaufe verschiedener Rezidive beim gleichen Patient verschieden stark war. So beschreibt BECKER bei einer Frau sechs Attacken eines Erythema exsudativum multiforme, wobei zunächst bullöse Erscheinungen an den Lippen und Genitalien auftraten und erst später die typischen erythematösen Herde an Händen und Armen dazu kamen. BERGGREEN beschreibt einen Patienten, der in 6 Jahren 50 Rezidive eines Erythema exsudativum multiforme durchgemacht hatte. Meist zeigten sich typische Hautveränderungen, in einzelnen Fällen auch solche an Lippen und Wangenschleimhaut. Die Zunge war ungefähr in 2% der Rezidive mitbefallen. CROWLEY berichtete über einen Fall von Erythema exsudativum multiforme mit während 3 Jahren bestehender Stomatitis, die als chronische Plaut-Vincentsche Affektion gedeutet wurde und erst richtig erkannt werden konnte, als Hauterscheinungen an den Beinen auftraten. RETT und POTACS sahen bei einem 5jährigen Knaben in kurzer Zeit zwei Schübe eines Erythema exsudativum multiforme bzw. einer Ectodermose érosive pluriorificielle. Das erste Mal waren hauptsächlich Hauterscheinungen in Form eines typischen kokardenförmigen Exanthems vorhanden, das zweite Mal spielte sich der Schub in schwerer Form an den Schleimhäuten aller Körperöffnungen ab. Daß auch die Magenschleimhaut befallen sein kann, konstatierten CHEVALLIER et al. (1938) mittels Gastroskopie. Sie sahen starke Schleimabsonderung und Ödem der Schleimhaut. Auch in der Harnblase wurden kreisförmige Herde gefunden (BANDMANN et al.). OWREN beschreibt eine 23jährige Frau, die während vieler Jahre an einer ulcerösen rezidivierenden Stomatitis litt, später herpetiforme und vesiculöse Schleimhautgeschwüre an den Genitalien bekam und zuletzt an einer Conjunctivitis und Iritis zusammen mit einem typischen Erythema exsudativum multiforme erkrankte. Gleichzeitig bestanden Lungen- und Hilusveränderungen. FASAL sah einen besonders schweren Fall von Erythema exsudativum multiforme der Haut, wo sich nach dem Auftreten der Hauteffloreszenzen auch am harten und weichen Gaumen, am Pharynx und Larynx Erosionen zeigten, die von festhaftenden, weißlichen Membranen belegt waren. Es bestand eine schwere Conjunctivitis und Episkleritis. Er sah ferner eine Frau mit einem typischen Erythema exsudativum multiforme, die an den Ohrmuscheln Blasen zeigte und eine Stomatitis, Conjunctivitis und Vulvitis aufwies. Beide Fälle waren stark febril. Damit sollen die schweren Fälle des Erythema exsudativum multiforme besprochen werden, die speziell die Augen befallen und deshalb eine gesonderte Besprechung rechtfertigen.

b) Die muco-cutaneo-ocularen Syndrome

Während eine Beteiligung der Mundschleimhaut beim Erythema exsudativum multiforme in bis zu 60% der Fälle konstatiert wird (Trautmann) und deshalb wohl als regelmäßige Komplikation bezeichnet werden kann, nehmen diejenigen Fälle, bei denen Augensymptome im Vordergrund stehen, hauptsächlich wegen ihrer Schwere eine Sonderstellung ein. Es sind eine ganze Reihe solcher Krankheitsbilder beschrieben worden, die z.T. außerordentliche Ähnlichkeiten miteinander zeigen, so daß es wohl berechtigt erscheint, diese unter einer einheitlichen Bezeichnung zusammenzufassen. Es handelt sich hier um die vom Ophthalmologen Fuchs 1876 beschriebene Krankheit des Herpes iris conjunctivae, die wohl identisch sein dürfte mit der von Fiessinger und Rendu 1917 beschriebenen Ectodermose érosive pluriorificielle, mit dem von den Pädiatern Stevens und Johnson 1922 aufgestellten Syndrom, einer hochfebrilen Affektion, die mit erosiven Erscheinungen an Mund-, Genital- und Analschleimhaut einhergeht und Augensymptome verschiedener Schweregrade zeigt, und schließlich mit dem 1925 von Baader beschriebenen Krankheitsbild der Dermatostomatitis. Neuerdings wurde versucht, die Reitersche Krankheit (Stefanetti) und den von Hulusi Behçet beschriebenen Trisymptomenkomplex in die gleiche Gruppe einzuordnen (Mauriello).

Es sind nun speziell die Nicht-Dermatologen, die die Tendenz haben, alle Augen-Haut-Schleimhaut-Syndrome zusammenzufassen. Van der Meer et al. beschreiben Morbus Reiter, M. Rendu-Osler, M. Behçet, M. Stevens-Johnson als Varianten des Erythema exsudativum multiforme, da sie mehr verbindende als trennende Merkmale aufwiesen. Bleier hält den Morbus Behçet ebenfalls für eine Variante, nicht aber das Reitersche Syndrom. Behre, François, Magni möchten ebenfalls alle die Schleimhäute und die Haut befallenden Affektionen zusammenfassen. Aus vielen dieser Arbeiten geht — abgesehen von objektiv falschen Bezeichnungen, wie z.B. Morbus Rendu-Osler an Stelle der Ectodermose érosive pluriorificielle (Fiessinger u. Rendu) — die Tendenz hervor, die Morphologie der Hautveränderungen zu ignorieren. Daß diese Betrachtungsweise nur zur Verwirrung führen kann, ist jedem Dermatologen klar. Es sei nun von vornherein festgestellt, daß weder die Reitersche Krankheit noch der Trisymptomenkomplex von Hulusi Behçet in das Bild des Erythema exsudativum multiforme hineingehören. Wohl finden sich bei allen drei Krankheiten eine Urethritis zusammen mit Augen- und Hauterscheinungen. Die Hauterscheinungen sind aber in Morphologie und Verteilung derart different vom Erythema exsudativum multiforme, daß eine Erweiterung dieses Krankheitsbildes durch Einbeziehung dieser beiden Syndrome nicht angeht. So werden die Hauterscheinungen beim Behçetschen Trisymptomenkomplex als acneiform oder Erythema nodosum-ähnlich beschrieben. Auch die dabei meist auftretende Hypopyoniritis hat spezifischen Charakter. Weiter ist der chronische Verlauf beider Affektionen verschieden von demjenigen der sog. akuten muco-cutaneo-ocularen Syndrome Typ *Fuchs, Fiessinger-Rendu, Stevens-Johnson, Baader*.

Gemeinsam für diese Syndrome ist der akute Beginn, die schwere Störung des Allgemeinbefindens und die Kombination von Augen-, Schleimhaut- und Hautveränderungen. Die Augenveränderungen werden verschieden beschrieben. So sahen Sneddon, Ormea, Cheese, Tobiasch, Senra, Duggan, Friedmann et al.,

STORCK verschiedene Formen von Conjunctivitis, häufig als schwere, membranbildende Entzündung (NARÓK). PEREYRA beobachtete in drei Fällen nach Überstehen der Conjunctivitis beim Erythema exsudativum multiforme eine schrumpfende Vernarbung des Conjunctivalsackes und der Umschlagsfalten. COTTINI beschreibt das Auftreten von Knötchen auf der Conjunctiva, die sich histologisch durch Abschilferung des Epithels, durch proliferative Veränderungen im Bereich der Adventitia, der oberflächlichen und tiefen Gefäße und durch große Infiltrationsherde im Bindegewebe und in den peripheren Gefäßen auszeichneten. Auch WIRZ sah Papeln an den Conjunctiven. Schwere Hornhautveränderungen in Form von Ulcera beschrieben SPEKTOROV und SCHULZE. Auch kann es zu Erblindung infolge von Linsentrübungen (THIES), von Sekundärglaukom (MÜLLER et al.), von Keratitis (COSTELLO 1956) und chronischer Ophthalmie (THOMAS) kommen. Auch in der Originalarbeit von STEVENS und JOHNSON handelt es sich um einen solchen Fall.

Es dürfte vielleicht nicht abwegig sein, auch die von LORTAT-JACOB, GASTINEL und SOLENTE, ORMEA, OTTOLENGHI-LODIGIANI beschriebene schwere und fieberhafte Verlaufsform des Erythema exsudativum multiforme in diese Gruppe einzubeziehen, da sie weitgehend mit den anderen Formen übereinstimmt.

Die Hauterscheinungen bei diesen Syndromen zeigen verschiedene Ausdehnung und Schwere. Im allgemeinen treten sie als generalisiertes Exanthem auf, das sich aus verschieden großen erythematösen Herden zusammensetzt, die Bläschen verschiedener Größe, evtl. mit hämorrhagischer Komponente zeigen können. Typische Kokarden fehlen oft.

Einige wenige Mitteilungen lassen nun erkennen, daß bei dieser Form mit gewisser Regelmäßigkeit Befunde erhoben werden können, die es vielleicht gestatten, in Zukunft eine sicherere Basis für ihre Diagnose bzw. Differentialdiagnose zu haben. So haben LÖFFLER und MARTIN in ihren Fällen von muco-cutaneo-ocularem Syndrom regelmäßig eine flüchtige Monocytose von 18—26% gefunden, eine Feststellung, die schon STEIGER-KAZAL 1925 an zwei Fällen von allerdings nicht näher charakterisiertem Erythema exsudativum multiforme erhoben haben und die neuerdings von AGOSTAS et al. bestätigt wird. Es scheint auch eine Leukopenie vorzuliegen (TSUKADA et al.) im Gegensatz zur leichten Leukocytose (FASAL) und Lymphocytose der gewöhnlichen Form (LEIPNER). Auch die Berichte über das Vorhandensein von Kälteagglutinin im Blut beziehen sich wohl hauptsächlich auf Fälle von akutem muco-cutaneo-ocularem Syndrom (HUBER, SELVAAG).

Diese muco-cutaneo-ocularen Syndrome unterscheiden sich nun, abgesehen von der Schwere der Augenveränderungen, durch ihren Verlauf vom Erythema exsudativum multiforme, indem Rezidive selten sind, sowie durch relativ häufige innere Komplikationen. Diese betreffen meist die Lungen (SHORT, PAGÈS u. BOTREL, LOEWENTHAL et al.), doch können auch hämorrhagische Enteritis (EVANS, WEEKS et al., HUTSEBAUT), Colitis (BOE et al.), Nierenkomplikationen (SHORT, COMAISH et al.), Polyarthritis, Orchitis (WEEKS et al.), Pankreatitis necrotica (VAN DER MEIREN et al.) beobachtet werden. Auch die Prognose ist ungünstiger, da Todesfälle beschrieben werden (TOBIASCH, TSCHUSCHNER 1954a, CARO-PATON, O'CONNOR, COMAISH et al., KIRCHER, HARA et al.).

Es ist deshalb verständlich, daß die Zugehörigkeit dieser Syndrome zum echten Erythema exsudativum multiforme oft angezweifelt wird, ja STEVENS und JOHNSON lehnen sie in ihrer Originalarbeit ausdrücklich ab. So möchte z.B. MOLINARI-TOSATTI die Ectodermose pluriorificielle vom Erythema exsudativum multiforme abtrennen. Auch STORCK sieht in der Dermatostomatitis ein selbständiges Krankheitsbild, und PROPPE äußert sich dahin, daß die akuten muco-cutaneo-ocularen Syndrome vom idiopathischen Erythema exsudativum multiforme derart verschieden seien, daß sie damit nicht in Zusammenhang gebracht werden dürften, solange die Ätiologie dieser Syndrome unklar sei. Wie schon vorher ausgeführt wurde, nehmen Cerutti, Kumer und Bohnstedt den entgegengesetzten Standpunkt ein, und die von den englischen und amerikanischen Autoren (Ginandes und Thomas) vorgeschlagene Trennung in Erythema exsudativum multiforme minor (Typ Hebra) und Erythema exsudativum multiforme major (Typ Stevens-Johnson) hat sicher eine gewisse Berechtigung, da doch Anhaltspunkte, wie z.B. die Saisongebundenheit (Rodriguez Pascual), für eine Verwandtschaft dieser Affektionen sprechen. Auch Heite und Heite et al. kommen auf Grund statistischer Untersuchungen zum Schluß, daß alle Übergänge vom akuten muco-cutaneo-ocularen Syndrom zum Erythema exsudativum multiforme zu konstatieren sind, so daß es nicht möglich ist, diese Affektionen auf Grund klinischer Kriterien voneinander zu trennen.

Über weitere Fälle, die Übergänge zwischen diesen Syndromen und Erythema exsudativum multiforme zeigen, berichten Gaté et al. (1954), Friedmann und Pathé, Huerkamp. Auch Grignolo beschreibt einen Fall von rezidivierender Hypopyoniritis mit polymorphem Exanthem und Spondylarthritis ankylopoetica.

Es ist offensichtlich, daß die Differentialdiagnose bei einem derart vielfältigen und in seinen Grenzen unbestimmten Krankheitsbild schwierig ist. Schon Tachau hat ausgeführt, daß nicht mit Bestimmtheit ein Krankheitsbild aufgestellt werden kann. Die hauptsächlichsten Affektionen ähnlicher Art sind Maul- und Klauenseuche (Hagemann), Stomatitis aphthosa und Arzneimittelexantheme. Verlauf, Anamnese und epidemiologische Zusammenhänge dürften wohl in der Mehrzahl der Fälle eine Abgrenzung möglich machen (Mletzko, Chevallier et al. 1934).

2. Ätiologie

Überblickt man die reichen Literaturangaben über die Ätiologie des Erythema exsudativum multiforme, so begegnet man den gleichen Schwierigkeiten, wie sie schon in der Einleitung und im Kapitel der klinischen Erscheinungen beschrieben worden sind. Es ist nämlich oft schwer zu beurteilen, welcher Typus des Erythema exsudativum multiforme jeweils beschrieben worden ist. Aus den Literaturangaben, speziell wenn keine Abbildungen vorhanden sind, geht oft nicht hervor, ob es sich wirklich um ein typisches Erythema exsudativum multiforme oder nur um ein multiforme-ähnliches Bild gehandelt hat. Dementsprechend dürfen die Angaben über bestimmte Ursachen auf keinen Fall verallgemeinert werden.

Vorab seien diejenigen Fälle besprochen, bei denen klare Ursachen gefunden wurden und die dementsprechend als symptomatische Form aufgefaßt werden können. Diejenigen Fälle unter ihnen, die im Anschluß an die Verabreichung eines Medikamentes aufgetreten sind, sind am einfachsten zu beurteilen. Als solche werden erwähnt: Phenylbutazon (Vankos et al., Gelber, Cone et al., Steel und Moffatt), Streptomycin (Woringer et al.), Penicillin (Vayre et al.), Jod (Tschuschner 1954b, Kwiatkowski), Sulfomethoxypyridazin (Yaffee, Cohlan), TB 1 (Moore), Phenobarbital (Betron et al.), Sulfonamid (van Vonno et al., Dubois), Optalidon (Strempel). Sujoy sah bei einer Intoxikation mit Kupferarsenit ein dem Erythema exsudativum multiforme ähnliches bullöses Exanthem auftreten. Auf hormonale Zusammenhänge weisen die Beobachtungen von Miller hin, wonach bei einer 22jährigen Frau Erythema exsudativum multiforme-artige, rezidivierende bullöse Erscheinungen mit Methyltestosteron unterdrückt werden konnten, während die Oestrogene keinen Effekt hatten.

Bei internen Krankheiten können ebenfalls Exantheme vom Typus des Erythema exsudativum multiforme auftreten. So sahen HASSELMANN und JOHNE ein typisches idiopathisches Erythema exsudativum multiforme bei einer Paramyeloblastenleukämie, COSTELLO (1953) ein solches bei Hodgkinscher Krankheit im Anschluß an eine Bluttransfusion.

Auch Röntgenbestrahlungen können ein Erythema exsudativum multiforme auslösen. ARNOLD beschreibt drei solcher Fälle, die den klassischen Typus zeigten und nach höheren Dosen (bis zu 12000 r) auftraten. Der Verlauf war gutartig. DAVIS und PACK berichten über fünf eigene Beobachtungen nach Bestrahlung mit Tiefendosen.

Die Zusammenhänge des Erythema exsudativum multiforme mit infektiösen Prozessen standen seit jeher im Vordergrund des Interesses, sind aber wesentlich schwerer zu beurteilen als die bisher besprochenen ätiologischen Faktoren. Zweckmäßigerweise unterscheidet man wohl zwischen denjenigen Fällen von Erythema exsudativum multiforme, die als septische Manifestation aufgefaßt werden können, und denjenigen Fällen von idiopathischem Erythema exsudativum multiforme, die infektiös zu sein scheinen. Bei folgenden Infektionskrankheiten wurde das Auftreten von Erythema exsudativum multiforme beobachtet: Bei Lymphogranuloma inguinale (BOŠNJAKOVIĆ 1933), während einer Massenimpfung gegen Pocken (BOUQUIN et al., HOLTZMAN), nach einer Pertussis-Mischvaccine (KÜLZ), nach Salk-Vaccine (CHERWINSKY), bei Maul- und Klauenseuche (CHEVALLIER et al.), bei Enterokokkensepsis (IZAKI et al.). LANGHOF sah bei elf Frauen, die mit Pocken infizierte Kühe gemolken hatten, ein Erythema exsudativum multiforme. Er beschreibt ferner eine Familieninfektion mit Tularämie, wobei bei allen erkrankten Personen papulo-vesiculöse Exantheme vom Typus des Erythema exsudativum multiforme auftraten. Im Bläscheninhalt konnten Tularämie-Bakterien nachgewiesen werden. GREITHER und LÖHR beschreiben sieben Fälle von typischem Erythema exsudativum multiforme nach intrathorakalen Eingriffen. Medikamentöse Ursachen konnten hierbei ausgeschlossen werden, und die Autoren halten diese Exantheme für septisch bedingt, da eine Reihe von Erregern aus dem Sputum und aus einzelnen inneren Organen gezüchtet werden konnten. Streptokokken hält auch COSTANTINO für ätiologisch bedeutsam, da es in einem Fall von Erythema exsudativum multiforme gelang, aus dem Blut und aus provozierten Blasen einen Streptococcus zu züchten. Die Serumagglutination mit diesen Stämmen war positiv, und auch Intracutanreaktionen mit Streptokokkenvaccine fielen deutlich positiv aus. Die intravenöse Inoculation von Patientenblut bei einem Kaninchen rief eine 2 Wochen lang dauernde Allgemeinstörung hervor, und der Autor konnte eine deutliche dermatotrope Tendenz des zirkulierenden Keimes nachweisen. SELVAAG sah in einem Fall von Erythema exsudativum multiforme mit atypischer Pneumonie einen hohen Antistreptolysintiter. AZIZ EL GAMMAL et al. erzielten bei der Mehrzahl ihrer Fälle von Erythema exsudativum multiforme positive Intracutanteste mit Extrakten aus hämolysierenden Streptokokken. Als Fokalinfekte können vielleicht die Fälle von RICHON et al., BRAUN, BUCHA, SATO, BOŠNJAKOVIĆ (1935) aufgefaßt werden. In allen Fällen wurden Herde in Form von cariösen Zähnen, Zahnabscessen, Tonsillitis oder Mastitis purulenta angetroffen. SATCH et al. fanden bei 65% von 153 Fällen von Erythema exsudativum multiforme chronische Fokalherde.

Demgegenüber fanden RUITER und HAMMINGA in 17 Fällen von idiopathischem Erythema exsudativum multiforme bei genauer Untersuchung auf Zeichen von Streptokokkeninfektion und Tuberkulose keine Anhaltspunkte für eine solche, da Antistreptolysintiter, andere Streptokokkenteste und die Tuberkulin-Cutanreaktion nicht pathologisch waren.

Eigenartig ist der Befund von Lennhoff, der in histologischen Schnitten von Erythema exsudativum multiforme Spirochäten-artige Gebilde nachweisen konnte. Allerdings sind seine Befunde bisher nicht bestätigt worden.

Während die Rolle des Streptobacillus moniliformis (Levaditi et al.) in der Ätiologie des Erythema exsudativum multiforme nicht mehr nachgeprüft worden ist, wird die Diskussion der tuberkulösen Ätiologie des Erythema exsudativum multiforme weitergeführt. Ramel hatte bekanntlich angenommen, daß es sich beim idiopathischen Erythema exsudativum multiforme um ein nicht-follikuläres Tuberkulid handle. Er begründete seine Ansicht mit dem Nachweis von Tuberkelbacillen mittels Ziehl-Neelsen-Färbung im Inhalt von frischen Efflorescenzen bei klinisch nicht tuberkulösen Individuen sowie mit dem positiven Ausfall von Tierversuchen mit diesem Material. Er demonstrierte auch den Fall eines idiopathischen Erythema exsudativum multiforme bei einem 15jährigen Mädchen, wo die Hauterscheinungen innerhalb 4 Wochen von einem Erythema exsudativum multiforme in ein papulonekrotisches Tuberkulid übergingen. Seine experimentellen Angaben wurden mehrfach nachgeprüft und konnten in dieser Form nie bestätigt werden (Kobayashi, Domanski, Hallam et al.). Es werden aber doch klinische Beobachtungen angeführt, die auf einen möglichen Zusammenhang zwischen Erythema exsudativum multiforme und Tuberkulose hinweisen könnten. So beobachteten Tauber und Goldman ein 6jähriges Mädchen, das von Vater und Bruder mit Tuberkulose infiziert wurde. Mit Hilusveränderungen zusammen trat ein ausgedehntes Erythema exsudativum multiforme vom bullösen Typ auf und Tuberkulininjektionen verursachten starke Blasenreaktionen. Auch Mayrhofer vertritt die Ansicht, daß ein Teil der Erythema exsudativum multiforme-Fälle eine tuberkulöse Ätiologie haben könnte, da Tuberkulinkuren Rezidive zu verhindern mögen. Rousset sah eine Frau, bei der im Anschluß an eine Keratitis parenchymatosa tuberkulöser Natur ein Erythema exsudativum multiforme auftrat, das sich kurze Zeit später in ein papulo-nekrotisches Tuberkulid verwandelte. Duvoir et al. beschrieben eine 21jährige Patientin, die 7 Wochen nach einer Geburt gleichzeitig an einer Pneumonie und einem Erythema exsudativum multiforme erkrankte. Nach kurzer Besserung trat ein Rezidiv der Lungen- und Hauterscheinungen auf, wobei sich im Sputum diesmal Tuberkelbacillen nachweisen ließen. Schwer zu interpretieren ist die Beobachtung von Faure-Beaulieu, wonach eine Patientin, die nach Angina und Gelenkentzündung ein Erythema exsudativum multiforme durchmachte, während ihres Spitalaufenthaltes anscheinend eine andere Patientin infizierte, die ihrerseits an einem Erythema nodosum mit stark positiver Tuberkulinreaktion erkrankte.

Man darf somit feststellen, daß der Beweis für einen Zusammenhang zwischen Tuberkulose und Erythema exsudativum multiforme kaum je mit Sicherheit erbracht werden konnte und daß lediglich klinische Beobachtungen auf einen solchen Zusammenhang hinweisen.

Noch weniger erscheint auch klinisch die Beziehung zwischen Lues und Erythema exsudativum multiforme gesichert. Übersichten zeigen, daß an sich schon sehr selten positive Seroreaktionen beim Erythema exsudativum multiforme gefunden werden und daß diese evtl. unspezifisch sind (Saunders). Jedenfalls können die Beobachtungen von Wiedmann und von Gaté et al. (1933) nicht im Sinne eines Zusammenhanges beider Affektionen verwertet werden, da die Möglichkeit besteht, daß es sich in diesen Fällen entweder um eigentliche luische Exantheme oder um eine zufällige Koinzidenz gehandelt hat.

Wichtiger als diese Einzelbeobachtungen erscheinen nun die zahlreichen Beschreibungen von epidemischem Auftreten oder von infektiösen Fällen von Erythema exsudativum multiforme. So sah Koch 20 Fälle von Erythema exsudativum multiforme in einem Konzentrationslager. Die Übertragung erfolgte wahrscheinlich durch den Lagerarzt. KOEHLER beobachtete das Auftreten einer Epidemie von Erythema exsudativum multiforme in einer 186 Mann starken Kompanie. 36 Mann wurden infiziert. GODWIN beschreibt eine Mutter, die zugleich mit ihrem 14 Tage alten Säugling an einem Erythema exsudativum multiforme erkrankte. Der Autor nimmt an, daß die Infektion möglicherweise durch die Muttermilch erfolgte. LEIPNER beschreibt das Auftreten einer Epidemie von Erythema exsudativum multiforme in einem Heim, wo von 56 jugendlichen Insassen 30 an idiopathischem Erythema exsudativum multiforme erkrankten. Die Epidemie wurde offenbar von einem Knaben eingeschleppt, der schon mehrfach Schübe eines Erythema exsudativum multiforme durchgemacht hatte. Interessant ist die Beobachtung von LOZANO. Er sah einen 31jährigen Mann, der lange Jahre an rezidivierenden Aphthen und später an einem rezidivierenden Erythema exsudativum multiforme gelitten hatte. Er war Blutspender, und zweimal traten beim Empfänger seines Blutes schwere Schocks in Form einer generalisierten Dermatitis auf, wenn das Blut kurze Zeit nach einer Attacke eines Erythema exsudativum multiforme entnommen worden war.

Die Natur des infektiösen Agens ist umstritten. Verschiedene Beobachtungen sprechen dafür, daß ein Virus in Frage kommen könnte (STORCK). So gelang BERGAMASCO durch Überimpfung von Blut von drei Patienten mit Erythema exsudativum multiforme auf Hühnereier eine Weiterimpfung des Virus von Ei zu Ei. Aus dem infizierten Ei ließ sich ein Antigen herstellen, das mit dem Blut von Kranken mit Erythema exsudativum multiforme eine deutliche Komplementbildung ergab. Er stellte auch einen Impfstoff aus der Kultur her, der bei acht Kranken zu einem raschen Rückgang der klinischen Erscheinungen führte. SCHMITT, FOERSTER et al. gelang die Züchtung eines Herpesvirus aus Hautblasen eines Patienten mit Stevens-Johnson-Syndrom. YAFFEE konnte bei zwei von vier epidemisch aufgetretenen Fällen Coxsacki B 5-Virus züchten. Auch Ornithose-Virus wird als Ursache vermutet (PAGÈS et al., GJERLOW).

Auch die Tatsache, daß einem Erythema exsudativum multiforme sehr oft ein Herpes vorausgeht, wird im Sinne einer Virusätiologie ausgelegt. Es gelang zwar URBACH und JORDAN et al. im Tierversuch nicht, irgendwelche Übertragungen von Herpesvirus vom Menschen auf das Tier auszuführen, doch ist nach anderen Beobachtungen (MILDER, TRAUB) der Zusammenhang zwischen Herpes und Erythema exsudativum multiforme derart regelmäßig, daß eine ätiologische Bedeutung angenommen werden muß. Neuestens gelang SÖLTZ der Nachweis von Herpesvirus in Efflorescenzen eines Erythema multiforme, das bei einer Patientin aufgetreten war, die wegen eines rezidivierenden Herpes mit virusfreiem S-Antigen geimpft worden war. Auch HRUSZEK nimmt auf Grund von Beobachtungen, nach denen bei Patienten mit Erythema exsudativum multiforme isomorphe Reizeffekte erzielt werden können, eine Virusinfektion an. SIBOULET konnte in fünf Fällen von Ectodermosis pluriorificialis in Abstrichen von der Haut, der Conjunctiva und der Urethra Einschlußkörperchen von der Art der Chlamydozoen finden. Bei der Färbung nach GIEMSA fanden sich in den Hautexcisaten Elementarkörperchen um den Kern in der Form eines Halbmondes. Interessant ist die Beobachtung von ANDERSON et al. Sie sahen das Auftreten eines bullösen Erythema exsudativum multiforme bei einem 6jährigen Knaben, dessen Vater 3 Wochen vorher an einem Herpes simplex gelitten hatte. Es gelang, aus den Blasen des Knaben ein Virus auf Kaninchencornea zu übertragen. Auch JAUSION et al. berichten über Übertragbarkeit eines Virus. Es gelang ihnen, mit Blut und Blaseninhalt einer Patientin mit Erythema exsudativum multiforme zwei Meerschweinchen subcutan zu infizieren. Die Tiere erkrankten unter blutigen

Durchfällen mit Lähmungen und verendeten nach 3 Wochen unter den Erscheinungen einer hämorrhagischen Septicämie. Anschließend erkrankten nacheinander sämtliche 45 Meerschweinchen des Versuchsbestandes unter den gleichen Erscheinungen. Die Autoren nehmen ein filtrierbares Virus als Krankheitserreger an. Verimpfung von Gesamtblut und Plasma der geheilten Patientin hatte keinerlei Effekt.

Vielleicht werden die schon erwähnten Befunde einer Monocytose und von Kälteagglutininen im Blut die Möglichkeit geben, die Virusnatur des infektiösen Agens bei einzelnen Fällen von akutem muco-cutaneo-ocularem Syndrom näher abzuklären.

3. Pathogenese

Aus der Diskussion über die Ätiologie des Erythema exsudativum multiforme lassen sich für seine Pathogenese folgende Schlüsse ziehen: Für eine direkte Infektion der Haut durch irgendeinen Erreger sprechen nur wenige Fälle, nämlich diejenigen, wo sich aus den Hauteffloreszenzen ein übertragbares Virus züchten ließ oder wo ein besonders dermatotroper Streptokokkenstamm gefunden wurde (Costantino). Der Nachweis von Tuberkelbacillen (Ramel) und Spirochäten (Lennhoff) erscheint so wenig gesichert, daß er in diesem Zusammenhang nicht als Basis für eine direkte Infektion der Haut verwertet werden kann. Die Fälle direkter Infektion dürften wohl am ehesten als septische Exantheme aufgefaßt werden.

Viel häufiger läßt sich aber ein solcher Nachweis nicht erbringen, und die Annahme einer fokal-toxischen Reaktion an den Hautgefäßen liegt näher. Damit ist die Möglichkeit gegeben, daß es sich beim Erythema exsudativum multiforme um eine allergische oder hyperergische Manifestation handeln könnte. Diese Annahme wird durch die verschiedenen Befunde erhärtet, bei denen durch Trichophytininjektionen (Hasselmann und Wernsdörfer), Schickreagens (Holtzman), Tuberkulininjektionen (Tauber und Goldman) typische Erythema exsudativum multiforme-Efflorescenzen ausgelöst werden können und wo ein positiver thrombopenischer Index nach Verabreichung der den Schub auslösenden Medikamente gefunden wird (Ström). Auch die später zu besprechenden Effekte der antiallergischen Behandlung könnten dafür sprechen. Zu gleichen Schlußfolgerungen waren schon Gougerot und Hewitt gekommen, die auf Grund klinischer Beobachtungen drei Perioden der Erkrankung unterscheiden: 1. Einige Tage Prodromalstadium ohne Beteiligung der Haut, 2. anfallfreies Intervall von 20—26 Tagen, 3. Ausbruch des Erythema exsudativum multiforme, das 3—6 Wochen dauert. Das zweite Stadium wird als Sensibilisierungszeit für die Haut angesehen.

Auch die Autopsiebefunde können im Sinne einer allergischen Reaktion verwendet werden: Ausgedehnte Arteriolo-Nekrose, verbunden mit fibrinoider Degeneration des Kollagens in Milz und Leber (Alexander und Cope), wurden gefunden.

Neuerdings werden auch Zusammenhänge zwischen Erythema exsudativum multiforme und Kollagenkrankheiten beschrieben. Ito konnte histologisch Ähnlichkeiten finden, Heeres sah bei einer Patientin, die regelmäßig im Frühjahr ein Erythema exsudativum multiforme durchmachte, plötzlich L.E.-Zellen im Blut auftreten. Die Schwester der Patientin litt an einem Libman-Sacksschen Syndrom, ein Bruder war an Erythematodes-Nephritis gestorben. Auch Rallison et al. beschreiben bei drei Kindern, die nach Barbituraten und Hydantoin ein Stevens-Johnson-Syndrom bekamen, L.E.-Zellen im Blut und in der Niere die typischen Erythematodes-Veränderungen. SHORT fand in seinen Fällen von Stevens-Johnson-Syndrom auch eine Periarteriitis nodosa.

In der Pathogenese des Erythema exsudativum multiforme spielen sicher interne und externe Faktoren wohl im Sinne Organ-determinierender Schädigungen mit. So ist bekannt, daß bestimmte Formen des Erythema exsudativum multiforme jahreszeitlich gebunden sind. Schon HEBRA hat den Typus annuus, d.h. den im Frühjahr und Herbst auftretenden Typus, unterschieden. In anderen Fällen wiederum ist eine spezielle Lichtempfindlichkeit beobachtet worden (OPPENHEIM). Diese kann möglicherweise durch Medikamente wie Salvarsan provoziert werden (BUGARSKI). LAUSECKER (1954a) widmet der Klimabedingtheit des Erythema exsudativum multiforme eine Studie. Er beobachtete ein gehäuftes Auftreten schwerer Fälle in einem bestimmten Bergtal Österreichs. Das Klima dieses Tals zeichnet sich durch eine höhere Luftfeuchtigkeit, reichliche Niederschläge und raschen Temperaturwechsel aus. Der Autor glaubt, daß das oft epidemieartige Auftreten des Erythema exsudativum multiforme eher solchen klimatischen Faktoren zuzuschreiben sei als einer Kontagiosität. HÜBNER sah 1935 46 Fälle von Erythema exsudativum multiforme, 15 davon allein im Mai. In acht Fällen wurde eine vermehrte Porphyrinurie festgestellt. Doch kann diese nicht als Erklärung für die Lichtempfindlichkeit dienen, da sie unabhängig davon auftrat. KOEHLER konnte bei einer Epidemie, die in einer militärischen Abteilung auftrat, beobachten, welche externen Faktoren für die Lokalisation der Hauterscheinungen wichtig sind. Sonnenbestrahlung, Capillarstase in den Extremitäten, Kälteeinwirkung und zirkulationsbehindernde Momente bestimmen die Lokalisation des Exanthems.

4. Diagnose

Wie schon TACHAU dargelegt hat und wie aus der ganzen bisherigen Diskussion hervorgeht, dürfte die Diagnose eines Erythema exsudativum multiforme wohl lediglich auf Grund klinisch-morphologischer Kennzeichen vorgenommen werden, da Laboratoriumsuntersuchungen, die für diese Krankheit typische Befunde ergeben würden, noch nicht mit Sicherheit bekannt sind. Nimmt man die Existenz eines idiopathischen Erythema exsudativum multiforme vom Typus Hebra an, so wird man alle diejenigen Fälle nicht in dieses Krankheitsbild einreihen dürfen, die sich in bezug auf die Lokalisation, die Art des Exanthems, den Verlauf und die Schwere des Krankheitsbildes davon unterscheiden. Das Vorhandensein schwerer innerer Erkrankungen und ungünstiger Verlauf sprechen dagegen.

Die toxischen Exantheme vom Typus des Erythema exsudativum multiforme werden dann nicht schwer zu erkennen sein, wenn ein bestimmtes Medikament oder eine bestimmte Noxe bekannt ist. Es dürfte aber noch genügend Fälle geben, die mehr oder weniger typische Erythema exsudativum multiforme-Efflorescenzen bei unbekannter Noxe zeigen. In solchen Fällen muß zunächst an die Möglichkeit infektiöser Exantheme vom Typus des Erythema exsudativum multiforme gedacht werden, speziell wenn Fieber mit Beteiligung anderer Organe usw. bestehen.

Schwierigkeiten dürften sich auch in der Diagnose derjenigen Schleimhauterkrankungen ergeben, die den Typus des muco-cutaneo-ocularen Syndroms zeigen, bei denen aber die Hauterscheinungen minimal oder gar nicht vorhanden sind. In diesen Fällen wird wohl nur eine Beobachtung des Krankheitsverlaufes bzw. der Rezidive eine Abklärung geben können.

Die histologische Untersuchung kann wohl in einzelnen Fällen zu Hilfe gezogen werden, speziell da, wo es sich um die Unterscheidung des Erythema exsudativum multiforme von ähnlichen Prozessen wie Erythematodes, Urticaria in gewissen Stadien usw. handelt. Es ist aber nicht möglich, die verschiedenen Formen des Erythema exsudativum multiforme voneinander zu unterscheiden. Allerdings finden sich auch hier atypische Bilder. LAMBEAU und VAN DER MEIREN sahen in einem Fall von Erythema exsudativum multiforme histologisch ausgedehnte subcorneale und intraepidermale Blasenbildung, die durch Zellnekrosen entstanden waren. Auch GATÉ et al. (1954) beschreiben ähnliche Bilder.

Die Differentialdiagnose zwischen Erythema exsudativum multiforme und der oft ähnlich aussehenden Dermatitis herpetiformis ist nach GOUGEROT et al. mittels Sternalpunktion möglich, da sich bei der Dermatitis herpetiformis im Knochenmark eine Eosinophilie findet, die beim Erythema exsudativum multiforme fehlt. VAN DER MEIREN sieht die wesentlichsten histologischen Unterschiede beider Krankheiten in nekrobiotischen Prozessen in den obersten Epidermisschichten beim Erythema exsudativum multiforme.

Auf Grund der angegebenen Tatsachen läßt sich feststellen (eine Feststellung, die schon TACHAU machen mußte), daß es nicht möglich ist, die Schleimhauteruptionen des Erythema exsudativum multiforme eindeutig differentialdiagnostisch gegen andere Krankheiten abzugrenzen und daß die Diagnose des echten Hebraschen Erythema exsudativum multiforme allein auf Grund der typischen Entwicklung und Metamorphose der Hauterscheinungen gestellt werden kann. Doch wird es genügend Fälle geben, bei denen eine solche Unterscheidung erst nach Beobachtung des Patienten und nach geraumer Zeit möglich sein wird.

5. Therapie

Die leichteren Fälle des Erythema exsudativum multiforme erfordern, da sie nur wenig Allgemeinsymptome machen und den Patienten wenig behelligen, keine besondere Behandlung. Lokal kann mit Puder oder mit desinfizierenden Salben (Antibiotica-haltige Salben, Sterosan usw.) wohl immer ein befriedigendes Resultat erzielt werden.

Wichtig ist die Therapie derjenigen Formen, die mit schweren Schleimhauterscheinungen einhergehen, besonders wenn sie die Augenregion befallen. Hier scheinen nun die Sulfonamide recht gut zu nützen. So berichtet HRUSZEK über sieben Kranke mit Erythema exsudativum multiforme, die täglich eine Prontosiltablette bekamen und in kürzester Frist abheilten. BREGMAN sah einen schnellen Effekt durch Sulfanilamid, SCHREIBER einen solchen mit Prontosil, SZENTKIRÁLYI durch p-Aminobenzolsulfamidal (Deseptyl).

Demgegenüber ist die Wirkung der Antibiotica wesentlich schwerer zu beurteilen. Negative Erfolge, speziell mit Penicillin, beschreibt FRASER in zwei Fällen, MELICK in einem Fall von Stevens-Johnson-Syndrom, die dann auf Aureomycin prompt heilten, VAN DER MEER in einem Fall, der dann auf ACTH ansprach. ROLLIER et al. sahen sogar durch Penicillin eine Verschlimmerung eines Falles von Ectodermosis pluriorificialis erosiva, LAUSECKER (1954b), BUCHA, PEREMANS et al., DOBIN dagegen gute Wirkungen von Penicillin in ihren Fällen. Demgegenüber scheint Aureomycin wirksamer zu sein (JONES, FRASER, GOUGEROT et al. 1950). Auch COSTELLO (1953) sah einen guten Effekt durch Aureomycin in einem Fall, in dem Cortison, ACTH und Terramycin versagt hatten. LOEWENTHAL konnte ebenfalls mit Aureomycin schlagartige Heilung auch der Lungenkomplikationen erzielen. SHALLARD und LAYNG sahen von Aureomycin keinerlei Effekt, doch heilte die Patientin mit Cortison in kürzester Zeit. Ähnliches berichtet SCHERPENHUYSEN, der keinen Effekt durch Antibiotica (Penicillin und Streptomycin) bei einem schweren Fall von Stevens-Johnson-Syndrom sah. ACTH wirkte erst in einer Dosis von 140 mg im Tag. Negative Effekte von Aureomycin sah CHIPPS. LINDQUIST hatte in einem Fall mit Terramycin keinen Erfolg, doch mit 15 E ACTH eine rasche Heilung.

Wirkungsvoller als die Behandlung mit Antibiotica scheint deshalb diejenige mit Cortison und ACTH zu sein. Trotz eines negativen Berichtes von MAURIELLO über ACTH- und Cortison-Therapie in zwei Fällen von Stevens-Johnson-Syndrom gibt die Mehrzahl der Autoren z.T. dramatische Besserungen nach ACTH-Gebrauch an (PERDRUP, REYMANN, WAMMOCK et al., SCHUPBACH et al., WEEKS und LEHMANN, BEHRE, CALDWELL, FERLONI et al., AGOSTAS et al., BLEIER und SCHWARTZ, FRIEDMANN und PATHÉ).

Andere Medikamente, deren Wirksamkeit erwähnt wird, sind: Bismuth (FALK), Elektrargol (DERFL), Quimby (AUDRY), Natriumgentisat (DUVAL und SÉBALD). Dieses letztere Mittel soll imstande sein, speziell die Rezidive zu verhindern. Auch Vitamin C wird empfohlen. So sah LAKAYE von Ascorbinsäure sehr gute Wirkung in 15 von 16 Fällen. Auch HAGEMANN empfiehlt dieses Mittel. Vitamin B_{12}, kombiniert mit Terramycin, wirkte in einem Fall von SCHWARZ günstig.

Besondere Aufmerksamkeit widmen KEINING und OLDACH dem differenten Ansprechen verschiedener Erythema exsudativum multiforme-Formen auf Nicotinsäureamid. Sie unterscheiden diejenige Form, die nicht auf Nicotinsäureamid anspricht — es sind dies die nicht jahreszeitlich gebundenen, mit Angina und Rheuma beginnenden Fälle, die sie Typus rheumatoides oder Typus anginosus bezeichnen —, von derjenigen Form, welche regelmäßig mit Nicotinsäureamid heilt, d.h. den Typus annuus. Diese Fälle treten zur Zeit der größten Ultraviolett-Bestrahlung, d.h. April-Mai, auf und rezidivieren in regelmäßigem Zusammenhang mit den Jahreszeiten. Anginen oder rheumatische Beschwerden sind dabei selten. Auch SAUTER sah einen sehr guten Effekt dieses Mittels bei einem häufig rezidivierenden Fall von Erythema exsudativum multiforme. BRETT und SPRENGER empfehlen das Kombinationspräparat Nicofol (Nicotinsäureamid, Pantothensäure, Folsäure) für die Behandlung der rezidivierenden Fälle von Erythema exsudativum multiforme. Milcheinspritzungen und Bluttransfusionen empfehlen RETT und POTACS. Sehr Günstiges berichten MATANIĆ, NAVARRO-MARTÍN et al. von Irgapyrin.

Literatur

AGOSTAS, W. N., N. REEVES, E. D. SHANKS jr. and V. P. SYDENSTRICKER: Erythema multiforme bullosum (Stevens-Johnson-Syndrome). New Engl. J. Med. **246**, 217 (1952). — ALEXANDER, M. K., and S. COPE: Erythema multiforme exsudativum major (Stevens-Johnson-Syndrome). J. Path. Bact. **68**, 373 (1954). — ANDERSON, J. A., V. BOLIN, W. W. SUTTON u. W. KITTO: Virus als mögliche Ursache eines bullösen Erythema exsudativum multiforme. Arch. Derm. Syph. (Chic.) **59**, 251 (1949). — ARNOLD, H. L.: Erythema exsudativum multiforme nach Röntgenbestrahlung. Arch. Derm. Syph. (Chic.) **60**, 143 (1949). — ASHBY, D. W., and TH. LAZAR: Erythema multiforme exsudativum major (Stevens-Johnson-Syndrome). Lancet **1951I**, 1091. — AUDRY, CH.: Traitement de l'érythème polymorphe par les injections de iodo-bismuthate de quinine. Bull. Soc. franç. Derm. Syph. **40**, 139 (1933). — AZIZ EL GAMMAL, A., AHMED M. ALL and M. FAREE A. ROEYAH: Erythema multiforme, investigation of 26 cases. J. Egypt. med. Ass. **37**, 560 (1954).

BAADER, E.: Dermatostomatitis. Arch. Derm. Syph. (Berl.) **149**, 261—268 (1925). — BAIKOVA, R. A., and Z. L. TSKHOVREBOVA: Affection of the oral mucous membrane in multiforme exsudative erythema. Vestn. Derm. Vener. **34**, 80 (1960). — BANDMANN, H. J., P. KOLB u. H. SACHSE: Erythema exsudativum multiforme mit Beteiligung der Harnblasenschleimhaut. Hautarzt **12**, 379 (1961). — BECKER, S. W.: Fixed eruption of erythema multiforme type, apparently not due to ingestion of a drug. Arch. Derm. Syph. (Chic.) **33**, 1089 (1936). — BEHÇET, HULUSI: Fokalsepsis mit aphthösen Erscheinungen an Mund, Genitalien und Veränderungen an den Augen als wahrscheinliche Folge einer durch Virus bedingten Allgemeininfektion. Derm. Wschr. **105**, 1152 (1937); **107**, 1037 (1938). — BEHRE, R.: Heilung eines Stevens-Johnson-Syndroms mit Bronchiolitis durch Terramycin. Ther. d. Gegenw. **94**, 6

(1955). — BERGAMASCO, A.: Sull'eziologia dell'eritema essudativo polimorfo. Arch. ital. Derm. **23**, 3 (1950). — BERGGREEN: Erythema exsudativum multiforme (mit Schleimhaut- und Zungenbeteiligung). Berliner Dermat. Ges., Sitzg 28. 2. 1939. Ref. in Zbl. Haut- u. Geschl.-Kr. **62**, 337 (1939). — BETSON jr., J. R., and C. D. ALFORD: Stevens-Johnson-Syndrome secondary to phenobarbital administration in the treatment of toxaemia of pregnancy. Obstet. and Gynec. **18**, 195 (1961). — BLEIER, A. H., and E. SCHWARTZ: Cortisone in treating Stevens-Johnson-Syndrome. Report of a case. Amer. J. Ophthal. **34**, 618 (1951). — BØE, J., J. DALGAARD and D. SCOTT: Muco-cutaneous-ocular syndrome with intestinal involvement. A clinical and pathological study of four fatal cases. Amer. J. Med. **25**, 857 (1958). — BOHNSTEDT, R. M.: Das Erythema exsudativum multiforme und verwandte Krankheitsbilder. Z. Haut- u. Geschl.-Kr. **14**, 272 (1953). — BOŠNJAKOVIĆ: Lymphogranuloma inguinale, Erythema exsudativum multiforme. Dermato. ven. Ges. Sektion Zagreb, Sitzg vom 30. 3. 1933. — Erythema exsudativum multiforme. Sitzg vom 31. 5. 1933. Ref. in Zbl. Haut- u. Geschl.-Kr. **49**, 407, 409 (1935). — BOUQUIEN, Y., D. HERVOUET, G. DAUPHIN, R. LHERMITTE et C. ROBIN: Sur un cas de maladie de Stevens-Johnson survenu après une vaccination anti-variolique. Presse méd. **1957**, 956. — BRAUN, H.: Zur Frage des Erythema exsudativum multiforme. Z. Haut- u. Geschl.-Kr. **3**, 341 (1947). — BREGMAN, A.: Treatment of erythema exsudativum multiforme with sulfanilamide. Arch. Derm. Syph. (Chic.) **38**, 623 (1938). — BRETT, R., u. F. SPRENGER: Über Formenkreis und Therapie multiformer Erytheme. Derm. Wschr. **126**, 781 (1952). — BUCHA, G.: Über 3 Fälle der malignen Form des Erythema exsudativum multiforme (Stevens-Johnson-Syndrom). Mschr. Kinderheilk. **103**, 184 (1955). — Beitrag zur Ätiologie des Stevens-Johnson-Syndroms. Mschr. Kinderheilk. **106**, 401 (1958). — BUGARSKI, S.: Der Biotropismus in der Entwicklung derjenigen Fälle von Granuloma anulare und Erythema exsudativum multiforme, bei denen auch eine diffuse Photodermatose bestanden hat. Dermatologica (Basel) **82**, 249 (1940).

CALDWELL, W. G. D.: Stevens-Johnson-Syndrom treated with ACTH. Lancet **1953I**, 1127. — CANTER, H. G., and S. KATZ: Pneumonia in Erythema multiforme exsudativum. Report of a case and a review of the literature. Med. Ann. D. C. **30**, 148 (1961). — CARO-PATON, T.: Syndrome de Stevens-Johnson. Act. dermo-sifiliogr. (Madr.) **44**, 432 (1953). — CARRIÉ: Erythema exsudativum multiforme mit starker Blasenbildung. Vereinig. Düsseldorfer Dermatol. Sitzg 20. 6. 1934. Ref. in Zbl. Haut- u. Geschl.-Kr. **49**, 302 (1935). — CERUTTI, P.: Le sindrome dermato-muco-oculari acute: considerazioni in merito ad alcuni casi. Rass. Derm. Sif. **6**, 107 (1953). — CHERVINSKY, P.: Erythema multiforme following poliomyelitis vaccination. Report of a case. Ann. Allergy **15**, 30 (1957). — CHEVALLIER, P., A. LÉVY-BRUHL, A. FIEHRER et W. SARNOWIEC: Certains érythèmes polymorphes récidivants du type „hydroa vésiculo-bulleux de Bazin" sont-ils dus au virus de la fièvre aphtheuse ou à un virus de la même famille? Rev. Path. comp. **34**, 417 (1934). — CHEVALLIER, P., F. MOUTIER et L. BRUMPT: Magenbefund bei einem Fall von Erythema exsudativum multiforme. Bull. Soc. franç. Derm. Syph. **45**, 1885 (1938). — CHIPPS, J. E.: Erythema multiforme exsudativum (Stevens-Johnson-Syndrome). A review of a case report in which use of aureomycin and pyribenzamine were without apparent benefit. Oral. Surg. **4**, 345 (1951). — COHLAN, S. Q.: Erythema multiforme exsudativum associated with use of sulfamethoxypyridazine. J. Amer. med. Ass. **173**, 799 (1960). — COMAISH, J. S., and D. N. S. KERR: Erythema multiforme and nephritis. Brit. med. J. **1961II**, 84. — CONE, R. B., C. H. HANNIGAN and R. TEICHER: Erythema multiforme bullosum following phenylbutazone treatment for arthritis. Report of a fatal case. Arch. Derm. Syph. (Chic.) **69**, 674 (1954). — COSTANTINO, SAVERIO: Contributo allo studio dell'eziologia dell'eritema essudativo polimorfo. Dermosifiliografo **11**, 92 (1936). — COSTELLO, M. J.: N.Y. St. J. Med. Zit. in W. BURCKHARDT, Erythema exsudativum multiforme. Dermatologica (Basel) **100**, 126 (1950). — Case for diagnosis (an unusual form of erythema multiforme confined to the upper respiratory and possibly the digestive tract?). Arch. Derm. Syph. (Chic.) **68**, 611 (1953). — Keratoconjunctivitis and keratitis with partial and complete blindness as a sequela of Stevens-Johnson-Syndrome (erythema-bullosum malignant). Arch. Derm. Syph. (Chic.) **74**, 444 (1956). — Hodgkin's disease complicated by unusual type of erythema multiforme following blood transfusion. Arch. Derm. Syph. (Chic.) **67**, 225 (1953). — COTTINI, G. B.: Beitrag zur Histopathologie des Erythema exsudativum multiforme der Conjunctiva. Rass. ital. Ottal. 8, 628 (1939). — CROWLEY, R. E.: Erythema multiforme. Report of a case. J. oral. Surg. **9**, 157 (1951).

DAVIS, J., and G. T. PACK: Erythema multiforme following deep X-ray therapy. Arch. Derm. Syph. (Chic.) **66**, 41 (1952). — DERFL, A.: Elektrargol bei Erysipel, Schweinerotlauf und Erythema exsudativum multiforme. Ref. in Zbl. Haut- u. Geschl.-Kr. **48**, 644 (1934). — DOBIN, N. J.: Ein durch Penicillin geheilter Fall von Erythema exsudativum multiforme. Vestn. Vener. Derm. **2**, 87 (1951). — DOMANSKI, M. A.: Résultats des inoculations par passages successifs au cobaye dans les tuberculides, l'acné et les érythèmes polymorphes. Soc. d'Edit. Strasbourgeoise du Rhin 1933, Strasbourg. — DUBOIS, P., L. COLOMB et G. FAYOLLE: Erythème polymorphe par un hypoglycémiant per os. Bull. Soc. franç. Derm. Syph. **64**, 301

(1957). — DUGGAN, J. W., u. S. R. GAINES: Augenkomplikationen bei Erythema exsudativum multiforme. Amer. J. Ophthal. **34**, 189 (1951). — DUVAL, G., et SÉBALD: Action du gentisade de soude dans les érythèmes polymorphes bulleux récidivants. Bull. Soc. franç. Derm. Syph. **57**, 587 (1950). — DUVOIR, M., L. POLLET et A. PICQUART: Erythème polymorphe au cours d'une pneumopathie aiguë à rechute. Streptococcie ou tuberculose? Bull. Soc. méd. Hôp. Paris, III. s. **50**, 1240 (1934).

ELIZADE, F. B., u. O. R. TURRO: Erythema exsudativum multiforme beim Säugling. Ref. in Zbl. Haut- u. Geschl.-Kr. **78**, 356 (1952). — ENKLING, H.: Über Mundschleimhautbeteiligung bei Erythema exsudativum multiforme und nodosum. Diss. Freiburg i. Br. 1933. — EVANS, C. D.: Stevens-Johnson-Syndrome with intestinal symptoms. Brit. J. Derm. **69**, 106 (1957).

FALK, C. A.: The treatment of erythema exsudativum multiforme with bismuth salts and other spirochaeticides. Acta derm.-venereol. (Stockh.) **29**, 516 (1949). — FASAL, P.: Zwei atypische Fälle von Erythema exsudativum multiforme. Wiener Dermat. Ges. Sitzg 4. 12. 1933. Ref. in Zbl. Haut- u. Geschl.-Kr. **48**, 4 (1934). — FAURE-BEAULIEU: Contagion entre érythème polymorphe et érythème noueux; déductions pathogéniques. Bull. Soc. méd. Hôp. Paris, III. s. **52**, 1265 (1936). — FERLONI, A. V. J., y A. F. GIORDANO: Exito de tratamiento con cortisone en un caso de sindrome de Stevens-Johnson. Rev. argent. Dermato-siph. **38**, 58 (1954). — FIESSINGER, N., et R. RENDU: Ectodermose pluriorificielle. Paris méd. **1917**, 54. — FOERSTER, D. W., and L. V. SCOTT: Isolation of herpes simplex virus from a patient with erythema multiforme exsudativum (Stevens-Johnson Syndrome). New Engl. J. Med. **259**, 473 (1958). — FRANÇOIS, J.: Les ectodermoses érosives pluriorificielles. Bull. Soc. franç. Ophtal. **1953**, 169. — FRASER, B. N.: Two cases of Stevens-Johnson-Syndrome. S. Afr. med. J. **1952**, 990. — FRIEDMANN, E., et G. PATHÉ: Le syndrome de Stevens-Johnson n'est qu'une forme grave de l'érythème polymorphe. Ann. Derm. Syph. (Paris) **80**, 132 (1953). — FRÜHWALD: Erythema exsudativum multiforme der Schleimhäute. Demonstrationsabend Chemnitzer Hautärzte, Sitzg 12. 5. 1933. Ref. in Zbl. Haut- u. Geschl.-Kr. **45**, 297 (1933). — FUCHS, E.: Mbl. Augenheilk. **14**, 333 (1876).

GASTINEL, P., et G. SOLENTE: Erythème polymorphe. In: Nouvelle pratique dermatologique von DARIER et al., vol. VII, p. 325. Paris: Masson & Cie. 1936. — GATÉ, J., P.-J. MICHEL et A. CHAPUIS: Erythème polymorphe chez une syphilitique récente sans accident. Bull. Soc. franç. Derm. Syph. **40**, 1085 (1933). — GATÉ, J., J. VAYRE, M. PRUNIERAS et M.-L. POMMIER: Ectodermose pluriorificielle de N. FIESSINGER et R. RENDU. Syndrome de Stevens-Johnson à forme récidivante. Bull. Soc. franç. Derm. Syph. **61**, 225 (1954). — GELBER, A.: Erythema multiforme following phenylbutazone treatment for arthritis. Verh. dtsch. Ges. inn. Med. **1954**, 729. — GINANDES, G. J.: Eruptive fever with stomatitis and ophthalmia. Atypical erythema exsudativum multiforme (Stevens-Johnson). Amer. J. Dis. Child. **49**, 1148 (1935). — GJERLØW, J.: Stevens-Johnson-Syndrome in a case of ornithosis contracted by contact in hospital. Nord. Med. **67**, 349 (1962). — GODWIN, E.: Erythema multiforme simultaneously in mother and child. Case report. Brit. J. Derm. **50**, 33 (1938). — GOUGEROT, H., B. DREYFUS et A. VARAY: Erythème polymorphe et myélogramme. Bull. Soc. franç. Derm. Syph. **44**, 2036 (1937). — GOUGEROT, H., et HEWITT: Erythème polymorphe et allergie. Bull. Soc. franç. Derm. Syph. **55**, 359 (1949). — GOUGEROT, H., J. J. MEYER et RAUFAST: Auréomycine dans deux cas d érythème polymorphe. Bull. Soc. franç. Derm. Syph. **57**, 184 (1950). — GREITHER, A., u. B. LÖHR: Erythema exsudativum multiforme nach thoraxchirurgischen Eingriffen und bei chronischen Infekten der Lunge. Dtsch. med. Wschr. **1954**, 209. — GRIGNOLO, A.: Über einen bisher noch nicht beschriebenen Symptomenkomplex: rezidivierende Hypopyoniritis, polymorphes Erythema exsudativum und Spondylarthritis ankylopoetica. Ophthalmologica (Basel) **118**, 989 (1949). — GRÜTZ: Erythema exsudativum multiforme bullosum faciei, colli et extremitatum. Frühjahrstagg der Vereinig. rheinisch-westfälischer Dermatologen in Wuppertal-Elberfeld. Sitzg vom 27. 5. 1934. Ref. in Zbl. Haut- u. Geschl.-Kr. **49**, 300 (1935).

HAGEMANN, D.: Das Erythema exsudativum multiforme, seine Vitamin-C-Behandlung und Abgrenzung gegen die Maul- und Klauenseuche des Menschen. Med. Welt **1938**, 998. — HALLAM, R., and J. W. EDINGTON: An investigation of the alleged tuberculous aetiology of erythema exsudativum multiforme (Hebra). Brit. J. Derm. **45**, 133 (1933). — HARA, S., and T. KOBAVASHI: On the so-called muco-cutaneous ocular syndrome. An autopsy report of the syndroma muco-cutaneo-oculare acutum Fuchs (Proppe). Jap. J. Derm. **68**, 19 (1958). — HASSELMANN, C. M., u. H. O. JOHNE: Über Erythema exsudativum multiforme (Hebra) als mögliches Initialsymptom der akuten Leukämie. Med. Klin. **1952**, 1626. — HASSELMANN, C. M., u. R. WERNSDÖRFER: Polymorphes, erythematöses Trichophytid bei Trichophytia profunda. Arch. Derm. Syph. (Berl.) **187**, 409 (1949). — HEERES, P. A.: Erythema exsudativum multiforme und Lupus erythematodes disseminatus. Dtsch. med. Wschr. **86**, 349 (1961). — HEITE, H. J.: Zur Abgrenzung des Syndroma muco-cutaneo-oculare acutum Fuchs vom Erythema exsudativum multiforme. Derm. Wschr. **135**, 471 (1957). — HEITE, H. J.,

M. NIHL u. M. WEBER: Zur Abgrenzung des Syndroma muco-cutaneo-oculare acutum Fuchs vom Erythema exsudativum multiforme. Arch. klin. exp. Derm. **207**, 354 (1958). — HÖLSCHER, J. F. M.: Acute viral infections of the lower respiratory tract in children and the Stevens-Johnson-Syndrome. Ned. T. Geneesk. **1958**, 1025. — HOLTZMAN, I. N.: Isoimmune phenomenon in erythema multiforme. Arch. Derm. Syph. (Chic.) **67**, 97 (1953). — HRUSZEK, H.: Sur la signification étiologique des „effets irritatifs" au cours des maladies cutanées, spécialement dans l érythème exsudativum multiforme idiopathicum. Rev. franç. Derm. **12**, 85, 1936. — Behandlung des Erythematodes und Erythema exsudativum multiforme mit Prontosil rubrum. Derm. Wschr. **1939 II**, 162. — HUBER, W.: Zur Kenntnis der Ectodermose érosive pluriorificielle (Stevens-Johnson-Syndrom). Schweiz. med. Wschr. **1949**, 342. — HÜBNER, K. H.: Erythema exsudativum multiforme und Porphyrinurie. Arch. Derm. Syph. (Berl.) **174**, 38 (1936). — HÜLLSTRUNG: Erythema exsudativum multiforme und Porphyrie? Vereinig. Düsseldorfer Dermatologen. Sitzg vom 30. 11. 1936. Ref. in Zbl. Haut- u. Geschl.-Kr. **57**, 84 (1937). — HUERKAMP, B.: Rezidivierendes Hypopyon mit Erythema exsudativum multiforme nach perforierender Eisensplitterverletzung. Klin. Mbl. Augenheilk. **123**, 129 (1953). — HUTSEBAUT, A.: Erythème polymorphe grave: Syndrome de Stevens-Johnson. Arch. belges Derm. **12**, 305 (1956).

ITO, K.: Muco-cutaneo-ocular syndrome. Jap. J. Derm. **69**, 657 (1959). — Vergleichende histopathologische Studien über den akuten und chronischen Typ von muko-cutaneo-okularen Syndromen und Erythema multiforme. Derm. Wschr. **140**, 1053 (1959). — Muco-cutaneo-ocular syndrome, erythema multiforme and „collagenosis". Bull. pharm. Res. Inst. **21**, 19 (1959). — Muco-cutaneo-ocular syndrome. Bull. pharm. Res. Inst. **22**, 1 (1959). — IWAI, T., and T. KOBAYASHI: Histopathological studies of the muco-cutaneous-ocular syndrome. Jap. J. Derm. **69**, Abstr. 78 (1959). Zit. in Zbl. Haut- u. Geschl.-Kr. **105**, 327 (1959/60). — IZAKI, M., S. KUROSAWA and N. TAKASU: Two cases of mucocutaneous ocular syndrome. Zit. in Zbl. Haut- u. Geschl.-Kr. **105**, 327 (1959/60).

JAUSION, H., F. CAILLIAU et S. THÉVENOT: Sur une épizootie massive autour de deux cobayes inoculés d'hydroa vésiculeux. Bull. Soc. franç. Derm. Syph. **45**, 839 (1938). — JONES, J.: Stevens-Johnson syndrome. Lancet **1951 I**, 1280. — JORDAN, P., R. BURKHARDT u. T. NASEMANN: Das Stevens-Johnson-Syndrom. Kasuistik, Versuche zur Klärung der Ätiologie. Beziehungen zu Viruskrankheiten. Arch. klin. exp. Derm. **204**, 624 (1957).

KEIL, H.: Erythema exsudativum multiforme. Eine klinische Einheit mit charakteristischen Merkmalen. Ann. intern. Med. **14**, 194 (1940). — KEINING, E., u. F. A. OLDACH: Behandlungsergebnisse mit Nikotinsäureamiden bei multiformen Erythemen. Derm. Wschr. **112**, 285 (1941). — KIRCHER, W.: Über einen Fall von Ectodermose érosive pluriorificielle (Fiessinger-Rendu). Ein weiterer Beitrag zur Frage des Zusammenhanges dieser Erkrankung mit einer Staphylokokkensepsis. Helv. med. Acta **13**, 239 (1958). — KOBAYASHI, E.: Über die tuberkulöse Natur des Erythema exsudativum multiforme. Jap. J. Derm. **33**, 94 (1933). Ref. in Zbl. Haut- u. Geschl.-Kr. **46**, 58 (1933). — KOCH, F.: Eine Epidemie von Erythema exsudativum multiforme. Sitzg der Südwestdtsch. Dermatologen in Freiburg. 66. Tagg. Ref. in Zbl. Haut- u. Geschl.-Kr. **63**, 480 (1940). — KOEHLER, H.: Epidemisches Auftreten von Erythema exsudativum multiforme. Med. Welt **1938**, 1631. — KORTEN: Erythema exsudativum multiforme. Essener Dermat. Ges. Sitzg vom 17. 6. 1933. Ref. in Zbl. Haut- u. Geschl.-Kr. **46**, 5 (1933). — KRUSPE: Ungewöhnlicher Verlauf eines Erythema exsudativum multiforme. Verein Dresdener Dermatologen. Sitzg vom 10. 1. 1934. Ref. in Zbl. Haut- u. Geschl.-Kr. **48**, 274 (1934). — KÜLZ, J.: Zur pluriorifiziellen Ektodermose Fiessinger-Rendu (Stevens-Johnson-Syndrom). Helv. paediat. Acta **15**, 299 (1960). — KUMER, L.: Ectodermose érosive pluriorificielle und Erythema exsudativum multiforme. Derm. Z. **72**, 62 (1935). — KWIATKOWSKI: Atypisches Erythema exsudativum multiforme. Lemberger Dermat. Ges. Sitzg vom 27. 9. 1934. Ref. in Zbl. Haut- u. Geschl.-Kr. **50**, 274 (1935).

LAKAYE, G., et R. LAKAYE: Vitamine-C et érythème polymorphe. Arch. belges Derm. **4**, 363 (1949). — LAMBEAU, P., et L. VAN DER MEIREN: Erythème polymorphe. Particularités histopathologiques. Arch. belges Derm. **9**, 60 (1953). — LANGHOF, H.: Symptomatische Form des Erythema exsudativum multiforme bei Melkerknoten und Tularämie. Derm. Wschr. **131**, 520 (1955). — LAUSECKER, H.: Zur Geographie des Erythema exsudativum multiforme. Sammelreferat über die Literatur von Ende 1945 bis Anfang 1953. Ref. in Zbl. Haut- u. Geschl.-Kr. **88**, 75 (1954a). — Erythema exsudativum multiforme und Penicillin. Hautarzt **5**, 234 (1954b). — LEIPNER, S.: Beitrag zum epidemischen Auftreten des Erythema exsudativum multiforme. Derm. Wschr. **1935 II**, 1178. — LEMKE, G., u. G. BONSE: Über Lungenveränderungen bei Erythema nodosum und Erythema exsudativum multiforme. Ärztl. Wschr. **1955**, 921. — LENGYEL, N., L. MODRAN u. N. COMSA: Beiträge zur Ätiologie und Pathologie des Erythema exsudativum multiforme im Zusammenhang mit einigen persönlich beobachteten Fällen. Clujul med. **17**, 618 (1936) [Rumänisch]. Ref. in Zbl. Haut- u. Geschl.-Kr. **55**, 357 (1937). — LENNHOFF, C.: Spirochaetes in aetiologically obscure diseases. Acta derm.-venereol. (Stockh.) **28**, 295 (1948). — LEVADITI, NICOLAU et POINCLOUX: Zit. in IVe Congr. des

Dermatologistes et Syphiligraphes de langue française, p. 51, Rapports. Paris: Masson & Cie. 1930. — LINDQUIST, B.: Effect of Corticotropin in erythema exsudativum multiforme (Stevens-Johnson-Syndrome). Nord. Med. **61**, 784 (1959). — LÖFFLER, H., u. E. MARTIN: La monocytose au cours de l érythème polymorphe. Schweiz. med. Wschr. **1947**, 684. — LOEWENTHAL, L. J. A., J. L. B. MARAIS u. H. D. RUSKIN: 2 Fälle von Stevens-Johnson-Syndrom mit Aureomycin behandelt. S. Afr. med. J. **1950**, 686. — LORTAT-JACOB, L.: Les érythèmes polymorphes. IVe Congr. des Dermatologistes et Syphiligraphes de langue française, p. 3, Rapports. Paris: Masson & Cie. 1930. — LOZANO jr., R.: Erythema exsudativum multiforme. Stevens-Johnson-Syndrom. Oral. Surg. **8**, 161 (1955).

MAGNI, S.: Le sindromi muco-cutanee oculari. Riv. oto-neuro-oftal. **27**, 288 (1952). — MANGANOTTI, G.: Osservazioni personali e studio critico sull'eritema essudativo multiforme e sugli eritemi polimorfi sintomatici. Dermosifilografo **13**, 245 (1938). — MATANIĆ, V.: Perorale und parenterale Pyramidon-Pyrazolidin-Therapie bei Erythema exsudativum multiforme, Erythema nodosum contusiforme und Zoster mit Irgapyrin. Z. Haut- u. Geschl.-Kr. **26**, 194 (1959). — MAURIELLO, D. A.: Erythema exsudativum multiforme (Stevens-Johnson-Syndrom). J. Amer. med. Ass. **156**, 1495 (1954). — MAYRHOFER, H.: Bestehen Beziehungen zwischen Erythema exsudativum multiforme und Tuberkulose? Z. Tuberk. **72**, 15 (1935). — MEER, R. VAN DER, D. E. WILSON and J. E. BULTHUIS: Therapeutic effect of ACTH in Stevens-Johnson-Syndrom (erythema exsudativum multiforme). New Engl. J. Med. **248**, 806 (1953). — MEIREN, L. VAN DER: Zur Klinik und Histologie des Erythema exsudativum multiforme. Hautarzt **11**, 246 (1960). — MEIREN, L. VAN DER, C. MESTDAGH, S. ZYLBERSZAC et J. BERNIER: Forme létale de maladie de Stevens-Johnson. Arch. belges Derm. **14**, 209 (1958). — MELICK, R. A.: Stevens-Johnson-Syndrome. Report of a case. Med. J. Aust. **1951**, 194. — MILDER, E.: Post herpetic erythema multiforme. Dermatologica (Basel) **111**, 21 (1955). — MILLER, J. L.: Erythema multiforme (possible endocrine etiology). Arch. Derm. **72**, 186 (1955). — MLETZKO, K.: Das Stevens-Johnson-Syndrom. (Syndroma muco-cutaneo-oculare acutum Fuchs.) Derm. Wschr. **130**, 1151 (1954). — MOLINARI-TOSATTI, P.: Über die Beziehungen zwischen dem Stevens-Johnson-Syndrom, der Ectodermose érosive pluriorificielle und dem Erythema exsudativum multiforme. Med. Parma **1**, 543 (1951). — MOORE, W.: Stevens-Johnson-Syndrom, Erythema multiforme pluriorificialis, in association with the administration of thiosemicarbazone. Tubercle (Lond.) **41**, 448 (1960). — MÜLLER, W. A., u. H. HARTENSTEIN: Die Beteiligung innerer Organe beim Erythema exsudativum multiforme maius. Dtsch. med. Wschr. **85**, 879 (1960).

NADEL: Erythema exsudativum multiforme. Lemberger Dermat. Ges. Sitzg vom 20. 10. 1932. Ref. in Zbl. Haut- u. Geschl.-Kr. **44**, 18 (1933). — NAKAMURA, J., and S. MATSUO: On muco-cutaneous ocular syndrome. Jap. J. Derm. **69**, 77 (1959). — NARÓK, F.: Membranaceous conjunctivitis in E.e.m. Klin. oczna **26**, 395 (1956). — NAVARRO-MARTÍN, A., u. F. MARTÍNEZ-TORRES: Irgapyrin in der Behandlung verschiedener Dermatosen. Act. dermo-sifiliogr. (Madr.) **44**, 628 (1953).

O'CONNOR, F. M.: Erythema multiforme exsudativum (Stevens-Johnson-Syndrom). Report of two cases with post mortem findings and comment. Arch. Derm. **77**, 532 (1958). — OPPENHEIM: Erythema exsudativum multiforme, provoziert durch Besonnung. — Erythema exsudativum multiforme diutinum. Wiener Dermat. Ges. Sitzg vom 22. 6. 1933. Ref. in Zbl. Haut- u. Geschl.-Kr. **46**, 411, 413 (1933). — ORMEA, F.: Erythema exsudativum multiforme von intensiver und fieberhafter Form. Derm. Wschr. **120**, 521 (1949). — OTTOLENGHI-LODIGIANI, F.: „Eritema essudativo multiforme di tipo intenso e pirettico“ (Lortat-Jacob) insorto nel corso di una piodermite subacuta. G. ital. Derm. **83**, 210 (1942). — OWREN, P.: Rezidivierende Haut- und Schleimhautaffektionen mit verschiedenen klinischen Bildern (Behçets Syndrome, Stevens-Johnson disease. Erythema nodosum, erythema multiforme). Nord. Med. **1943**, 698.

PAGÈS, F., et M. BOTREL: Erythème polymorphe grave (Syndrome de Stevens-Johnson) avec pneumopathie. Bull. Soc. franç. Derm. Syph. **63**, 413 (1956). — PERDRUP, A.: Ectodermosis erosiva pluriorificialis (Stevens-Johnson) treated with ACTH, demonstrated to illustrate a report on the same disease in Nordisk medicine, October 24th, 1952. Acta derm.-venereol. (Stockh.) **35**, 230 (1955). — PEREMANS et A. HUTSEBAUT: Erythème polymorphe combiné à un érythème noueux. Arch. belges Derm. **12**, 308 (1956). — PEREYRA, L.: La sindrome di Stevens-Johnson suoi rapporti con l'eritema polimorfo e col pemfigo. Contributo clinico ed istopatologico. G. ital. Oftal. **4**, 132 (1951). — PRAKKEN, J. R.: Leukoderma nach Erythema exsudativum multiforme. Acta derm.-venereol. (Stockh.) **17**, 133 (1936). — PROPPE, A.: Die Baader'sche Dermatostomatitis, die Ectodermosis erosiva pluriorificialis Fiessinger-Rendu, das Stevens-Johnson-Syndrom und die Conjunctivitis et Stomatitis pseudomembranacea (Syndroma muco-cutaneo-oculare Fuchs). Arch. Derm. Syph. (Berl.) **187**, 392 (1949).

RALLISON, M. L., J. W. CARLISLE, R. E. LEE jr., R. L. VERNIER and R. A. GOOD: Lupus erythematosus and Stevens-Johnson-Syndrom. Occurrence as reactions to anticonvulsant medication. Amer. J. Dis. Child. **101**, 725 (1961). — RAMEL, E.: L'érythème exsudatif multiforme. IVe Congr. des Dermatologistes et Syphiligraphes de langue française, p. 59, Rapports. Paris: Masson & Cie. 1930. — L'érythème polymorphe idiopathique, tuberculide non folliculaire. Ref. in Zbl. Haut- u. Geschl.-Kr. **44**, 518 (1933). — RETT, A., u. W. POTACS: Beitrag zur Frage der Beziehung zwischen Erythema exsudativum multiforme und Ectodermose érosive pluriorificielle. Öst. Z. Kinderheilk. **9**, 397 (1954). — REYMANN, F.: Erythema multiforme bullosum treated with ACTH. Acta derm.-venereol. (Stockh.) **35**, 182 (1955). — RICHON, J. GIRARD et D. PICARD: Un cas d érythème polymorphe au cours de la maladie de Bouillaud. Bull. Soc. franç. Derm. Syph. **45**, 1760 (1938). — RODRIGUEZ PASCUAL, L.: Sindrome de Fiessinger-Rendu — Stevens-Johnson. Act. dermo-sifiliogr. (Madr.) **46**, 641 (1955). — ROLLIER, R., P. H. MAURY et MÉRET: Ectodermose pluriorificielle de Fiessinger-Rendu (Syndrome de Stevens-Johnson). Bull. Soc. franç. Derm. Syph. **57**, 357 (1950). — ROUSSET, J.: Tuberculides développées sur des placards d érythèmes polymorphes. Bull. Soc. franç. Derm. Syph. **61**, 59 (1954). — RUITER, M.: Zum gegenwärtigen Stand des Erythema exsudativum multiforme-Problems. Hautarzt **3**, 293 (1952). — RUITER, M., u. H. HAMMINGA: Erythema exsudativum multiforme. (Untersuchungen über die Ätiologie des idiopathischen Typus.) Dermatologica (Basel) **107**, 418 (1953).

SATO, M.: Ein Fall von Erythema exsudativum multiforme und Purpura, die der Mastitis acuta purulenta nachfolgten. Jap. J. Derm. **35**, 23 (1934). Ref. in Zbl. Haut- u. Geschl.-Kr. **48**, 210 (1934). — SATOH, Y., T. ISHII and O. TAKINO: The statistical observation of Erythema exsudativum multiforme. Zit. in Zbl. Haut- u. Geschl.-Kr. **105**, 315 (1959/60). — SAUNDERS jr., H. R.: Erythema multiforme exsudativum. Report of a case with false-positive serology. Yale J. Biol. Med. **21**, 481 (1949). — SAUTER, E. K.: Eine im Kindesalter seltene Form des Erythema exsudativum multiforme und seine Behandlung. Arch. Kinderheilk. **146**, 164 (1953). — SCHERPENHUYSEN, A. A.: Eine Patientin mit Erythema exsudativum multiforme (Syndrom von Stevens-Johnson), behandelt mit Corticotropin (ACTH). Ned. T. Geneesk. **1952**, 1647. — SCHMITT, H.: Isolation of herpes simplex virus from blisters of a patient with Stevens-Johnson-Syndrom. Acta derm.-venereol. (Stockh.) **41**, 53 (1961). — SCHRANK, A.: Lymphoidzellen-Angina mit schwerem septischem Verlauf und Hautveränderungen im Sinne des Erythema exsudativum multiforme. Klin. Wschr. **1942 II**, 794. — SCHREIBER: Behandlung des Erythema exsudativum multiforme mit Prontosil. Verein Dresdener Dermat. Sitzg vom 13. 10. 1937. Ref. in Zbl. Haut- u. Geschl.-Kr. **58**, 508 (1938). — SCHULZE, E.: Stevens-Johnson-Syndrom. Klin. Wschr. **1947**, 721. — SCHUPBACH, H. J., u. B. R. JENDEL: Cortison-Behandlung von rezidivierendem Erythema exsudativum multiforme. Arch. Derm. Syph. (Chic.) **64**, 783 (1951). — SCHWARZ, E.: Über Ectodermosis pluriorificialis erosiva Fiessinger-Rendu (Syndroma muco-cutaneo-oculare acutum Fuchs). Z. Haut- u. Geschl.-Kr. **21**, 167 (1956). — SELVAAG, O.: Erythema exsudativum multiforme und Pneumonie. Acta med. scand. **135**, 34 (1949). — SENRA, J.: Sindrome de Stevens-Johnson. Act. dermo-sifiliogr. (Madr.) **46**, 515 (1955). — SHALLARD, B., and J. M. LAYNG: Cortisone in the treatment of the oculo-mucous membrane (Stevens-Johnson) syndrome. Canad. med. Ass. J. **37**, 560 (1954). — SHORT, J. A.: Stevens-Johnson syndrome. Report of 5 cases and a discussion on aetiology and treatment. Lancet **1957 I**, 290. — SIBOULET, A.: L'ectodermose érosive pluriorificielle. Proc. 10th Internat. Congr. of Derm. London 1952, p. 329, 1953. — SNEDDON, J. B.: Schweres Erythema exsudativum multiforme. Brit. med. J. **1947**, Nr 4512, 925. — SÖLTZ-SZÖTS, J.: Nachweis des Herpes simplex-Virus aus Effloreszenzen eines Falles von Erythema exsudativum multiforme. Z. Haut- u. Geschl.-Kr. **34**, 25 (1963). — SPEKTOROV, R.: Zur Klinik der Komplikationen beim Erythema exsudativum multiforme. Sovet. Vestn. Venerol. i Dermat. **3**, 613 (1934). Ref. in Zbl. Haut- u. Geschl.-Kr. **49**, 512 (1935). — STEEL, S. J., and J. L. MOFFATT: Stevens-Johnson-Syndrom and granulocytopenia after phenylbutazone. Brit. med. J. **1954**, Nr 4865, 795. — STEFANETTI, E.: Rezidivierendes cutan-mycöses exsudatives Syndrom bei intensiver Tuberkulinallergie. Dermosifiliografo **25**, 392 (1950). — STEIGER-KAZAL, D.: Das Verhalten der weißen Blutzellen bei verschiedenen Dermatosen. Arch. Derm. Syph. (Berl.) **154**, 621 (1928). — STEVENS and JOHNSON: A new eruptive fever associated with stomatitis and ophthalmia. Amer. J. Dis. Child. **24**, 526 (1922). — STORCK, H.: Dermatostomatitis (Baader) oder Ectodermose érosive pluriorificielle im Kindesalter. Schweiz. med. Wschr. **1942 II**, 1102. — STREMPEL, R.: Betrachtungen zur Symptomatologie und Pathogenese des Erythema exsudativum multiforme. Hautarzt **10**, 501 (1959). — STRÖM, J.: Erythema multiforme syndrome. Acta derm. venereol. **41**, 501 (1961). — The role of drugs in certain febrile muco-cutaneous manifestations (Syndroma mucocutaneum febrile) as illustrated by provocation of clinical and Thrombocyte reaction. Acta allerg. (Kbh.) **17**, 232 (1962). — SUJOY, E.: Eritema polimorfo ampolloso grave curado con ACTH. Arch. Pediat. Rio de J. **42**, 124 (1954). — SZENTKIRÁLYI, Z.: Behandlung des Erythema exsudativum multiforme und Erythema nodosum mit Para-amino-benzolsulfamidal (Deseptyl). Orv. Hetil. **1937**, 794. Ref. in Zbl. Haut- u. Geschl.-Kr. **57**, 513 (1937).

TACHAU, P.: Erythema exsudativum multiforme. In: Handbuch der Haut- und Geschlechtskrankheiten von JADASSOHN, Bd. VI/2. Berlin: Springer 1928. — TAUBER, E. B., and L. GOLDMAN: Atypical forms of skin tuberculosis in coloured children. 1. Erythema exsudativum multiforme bullosum, probably of tuberculous origin with unusual tuberculine reactions. Arch. Pediat. **53**, 540 (1936). — THIES, O.: Das Auge bei Erythema exsudativum multiforme. Klin. Mbl. Augenheilk. **116**, 44 (1950). — THOMAS, B. A.: The so-called Stevens-Johnson-Syndrom. Brit. med. J. **1950**, Nr 4667, 1393. — TOBIASCH, V.: Über die schwere Verlaufsform des Erythema exsudativum multiforme. Med. Mschr. **7**, 82 (1953). — TRAUB, E. F.: Recurrent herpes simplex, erythema multiforme and stomatitis. Arch. Derm. **80**, 377 (1959). — TRAUTMANN: Zit. in: Handbuch der Haut- und Geschlechtskrankheiten von JADASSOHN, Bd. VI/2, S. 598. Berlin: Springer 1928. — TSCHUSCHNER, A.: Über eine maligne Verlaufsform des Erythema exsudativum multiforme. Kinderärztl. Praxis **22**, 305 (1954). — Jod-Allergie mit tödlichem Ausgang unter dem Bilde eines Erythema exsudativum multiforme. Vereinig. Südwestdtsch. Dermatol. Sitzg 9. u. 10. 10. 1954. Ref. in Zbl. Haut- u. Geschl.-Kr. **92**, 84 (1955). — TSUKADA, S., T. TANIDA and A. AIKAWA: On muco-cutaneous ocular syndrome. Zit. in Zbl. Haut- u. Geschl.-Kr. **105**, 327 (1959/60). — TZANCK, A., et M. CORD: Les érythèmes polymorphes. Maladie infectieuse ou réaction d'intolérance. Ann. Derm. Syph. (Paris) **3**, 1073 (1932).

URBACH: Herpes labialis, Erythema exsudativum multiforme, Stomatitis aphthosa. Wien. Dermat. Ges. Sitzg 22. 6. 1933. Ref. in Zbl. Haut- u. Geschl.-Kr. **46**, 413 (1933). — Gesetzmäßiger Zusammenhang zwischen Herpes labialis und Erythema exsudativum multiforme. Österr. Dermat. Ges. Wien. Sitzg vom 14. 1. 1937. Ref. in Zbl. Haut- u. Geschl.-Kr. **57**, 12 (1958).

VANKOS, J., u. ST. PASTINSZKY: Ein Fall von durch Phenylbutazon hervorgerufenem Stevens-Johnson-Syndrom mit tödlichem Ausgang. Z. Haut- u. Geschl.-Kr. **23**, 54 (1957). — VAYRE, J., et P. COMBEY: Toxidermie géante à type d érythème polymorphe. Bull. Soc. franç. Derm. Syph. **62**, 349 (1955). — VONNO, N. C. VAN, and H. G. S. VAN RAALTE: Erythema exsudativum (macular stage) with marked systemic involvement. Acta derm.-venereol. (Stockh.) **37**, 382 (1957).

WAMMOCK, V. S., A. A. BIEDERMAN u. R. S. VORDAN: Bericht über einen mit ACTH behandelten Fall von Stevens-Johnson-Syndrom. J. Amer. med. Ass. **147**, 637 (1951). — WEEKS, V. T., and W. X. LEHMANN: Erythema exsudativum multiforme treated with Cortisone or ACTH. Report of 4 cases. J. Pediat. **44**, 508 (1954). — WIEDMANN, A.: Erythema exsudativum multiforme bei Lues II. Wiener Dermat. Ges. Sitzg vom 16. 3. 1933. Ref. in Zbl. Haut- u. Geschl.-Kr. **45**, 553 (1933). — WIRZ: Atypisch lokalisiertes Erythema exsudativum multiforme. Münchener Dermat. Ges. Sitzg vom 27. 5. 1932. Ref. in Zbl. Haut- u. Geschl.-Kr. **44**, 259 (1933). — WOLFRAM, G., u. H. STEINHOFF: Zur Frage des E.e.m. Dtsch. Gesundh.-Wes. **11**, 1247 (1956). — WORINGER, F., u. J. G. LÉVY: 2 Fälle von Erythema exsudativum multiforme kombiniert mit Erythema nodosum. Bull. Soc. franç. Derm. Syph. **56**, 536 (1949).

YAFFEE, H. S.: Stevens-Johnson-Syndrom following sulfamethoxy-pyridazine (Kynex), treated successfully with Triamcinolone. U.S. armed Forces med. J. **10**, 1468 (1959). — Erythema multiforme caused by Coxsackie B 5, a possible association with epidemic pustular stomatitis of children. Arch. Derm. **82**, 737 (1960).

Erythema nodosum

Von

Rudolf Schuppli-Basel

Mit 2 Abbildungen

Einleitung

Die ganze Frage des Erythema nodosum wurde in unübertrefflicher Vollständigkeit 1938 an einer Réunion dermatologique in Straßburg diskutiert. Pautrier faßte dabei die wesentlichsten Probleme folgendermaßen zusammen: 1. Während speziell die Pädiater an die tuberkulöse Ätiologie des Erythema nodosum glauben, halten die Dermatologen diese Krankheit für ein Syndrom, dessen Ursache verschiedener Natur sein kann. Möglicherweise beruht dieser Unterschied in der Auffassung darauf, daß das Erythema nodosum bei Erwachsenen und dasjenige bei Jugendlichen verschiedene Krankheiten sind. 2. Es bestehen in 20% der Fälle von Erythema nodosum auch Zeichen von Erythema exsudativum multiforme, so daß der Autor annimmt, daß beide Krankheiten identisch seien und sich nur durch die Beteiligung verschieden tiefer Gefäßgebiete unterscheiden. 3. Sehr wichtig ist die Tatsache, daß das histologische Bild des Erythema nodosum bei allen Fällen unabhängig von ihrer Ätiologie das gleiche ist. Es ließe dies an die Möglichkeit denken, daß das Erythema nodosum eine Krankheit mit eigener Ätiologie sei, doch sei die allergische Natur des Erythema nodosum am wahrscheinlichsten.

Seither hat die Entwicklung der Krankheitsbegriffe des Erythema exsudativum multiforme und des Erythema nodosum derart verschiedene Wege genommen, daß, abgesehen von historischen Gründen, heute wohl keine Notwendigkeit mehr besteht, das Erythema nodosum mit dem Erythema exsudativum multiforme zusammen zu behandeln (Jausion et al.). So wurde auf der einen Seite der Begriff des Erythema exsudativum multiforme durch Einbeziehung verschiedener Haut-Schleimhaut-Syndrome erweitert, auf der anderen Seite haben die neueren Untersuchungen, speziell Mieschers, ergeben, daß das Erythema nodosum eine selbständige Affektion darstellen könnte, so daß sich kaum mehr eine Stütze für die Auffassung des Erythema exsudativum multiforme und des Erythema nodosum als eng zueinander gehörender Krankheiten finden läßt.

Die wenigen neueren Beobachtungen (Touraine et al., Peremans et al., Miura, Nakamura, Sézary et al., Pautrier et al., Faure-Beaulieu, Woringer et al., Lemke und Bonse, Zamfir et al.) sind insofern schwer zu beurteilen, als es sich bei den Hauterscheinungen dieser Fälle um polymorphe Erytheme gehandelt hat, die bei der bekannt schwierigen Abgrenzung dieser Gruppe sehr wohl als septische Manifestationen gedeutet werden könnten.

1. Klinik

In der Regel tritt das Erythema nodosum nach einem prodromalen Stadium mit rapid einsetzendem Fieber und allgemeinen Krankheitserscheinungen akut in

Erscheinung, indem an der Streckseite der Unterschenkel innerhalb weniger Stunden derbe, lebhaft rot gefärbte, druckdolente Knoten auftreten. Ihre Zahl schwankt innerhalb weiter Grenzen. Sie bleiben einige Tage unverändert bestehen werden dann allmählich flacher und weicher, ihre Farbe wechselt vom hellroten in livides blaurot und durchläuft dann die ganze Skala einer sich resorbierenden Kontusion. Zunächst können neue Schübe solcher Knoten auftreten, doch ist die Heilung meist in 3—6 Wochen erreicht. Rezidive sind relativ häufig. So beobachtete LEMMING in über 50% seiner Patienten wiederholtes Auftreten.

Von diesem typischen Verlauf abweichende Fälle werden relativ selten erwähnt. So berichtet LOEWY über typische Herde an den Unterschenkeln, daneben waren auch die Vorderarme, die Ohrmuschelränder und die Nasenwurzel befallen. KERBEL sah Knoten in einer Operationsnarbe auftreten. WOHLSTEIN berichtet über Lokalisation der Knoten an den Fußsohlen. Sie ulcerierten teilweise. Diese Lokalisation wird dadurch erklärt, daß der Patient als Sportler eng zugeschnürte Schuhe trug. Über besonders langdauernde Fälle von Erythema nodosum berichtet MUGGIA: Bei einem 3jährigen Mädchen bestand zunächst ein schweres und wochenlang andauerndes Erythema nodosum an den Unterschenkeln. Während Masern verschwand dieses, trat aber später wieder kurzfristig auf. Leichte Fälle sah PETÉNYI bei mit Tuberkulose infizierten Kindern, bei denen nur ein bis vier kleine Knötchen auftraten, die sich rasch zurückbildeten. BÄFVERSTEDT beschreibt ein atypisches erysipelartiges, aber histologisch typisches Erythema nodosum und das sog. Erythema nodosum migrans. Es unterscheidet sich vom typischen Erythema nodosum durch den chronischen Verlauf und durch die größere Rezidivneigung. Möglicherweise ist dieses Bild mit dem von SHAPOSHNIKOV beschriebenen Erythema nodosum chronicum identisch. GILMAN berichtet über einen Fall, wo zunächst ein Erythema nodosum am Schienbein erschien und nachher rötliche, infiltrierte, quaddelartige Efflorescenzen im Gesicht auftraten. GATÉ et al. sahen bei einem Patienten sehr viele Knötchen an Armen und Beinen auftreten, die z.T. hämorrhagisch waren und teilweise zerfielen. Über einen Fall mit besonders zahlreichen Rezidiven berichtet ROSTENBERG.

Zum typischen Bild des Erythema nodosum gehören Erscheinungen innerer Organe. Hier steht der Respirationstrakt im Vordergrund.

Berichte über Lungenveränderungen sind derart häufig, daß sie kaum vollzählig zitiert werden können. Auf die tuberkulösen Affektionen soll später eingegangen werden. Daneben werden oft Lungen- und Hilusveränderungen nichttuberkulöser Natur beschrieben, die jetzt oft als Löfgren-Syndrom, d.h. als benigne Hiluslymphadenopathie, bezeichnet werden. So berichten VOGT und DÜNNER über lang anhaltende Hilusdrüsenschwellung bei tuberkulinnegativen Patienten mit Erythema nodosum. Auch THOMPSON et al. halten die bei 9 von 100 Patienten beobachteten Hilusdrüsenschwellungen für unspezifisch. PAUL und POHLE beschrieben bei 12 von 20 Kranken mit Erythema nodosum Veränderungen in Mediastinum und Lungen. Drei Patienten zeigten uncharakteristische geringfügige Veränderungen, drei nur Hiluslymphknotenvergrößerungen, ohne daß Zeichen für Tuberkulose bestanden hätten. FAVOUR et al. fanden bei 28 von 65 durchleuchteten Fällen Lungenveränderungen, $^2/_3$ davon waren unspezifisch. GRUPPER und BEAUVOIS sahen einen Patienten an hypertrophischer Bronchitis mit mediastinaler Adenopathie erkranken. Zwei Monate später trat ein Erythema nodosum auf. Die Tuberkulinreaktion war immer negativ. ABRAMSON sah in vier Fällen Erythema nodosum zusammen mit Arthralgie und Hilusdrüsenschwellung bei negativer Tuberkulinreaktion.

Bei Colitis ulcerosa tritt Erythema nodosum in 2,5% der Fälle auf (KELLEY et al.), bei anderen Darmerkrankungen kommt es ebenfalls vor (JACOBS).

Arthralgien und Gelenkschwellungen sind speziell zu Beginn der Krankheit so häufig, daß sie ebenfalls zum typischen Bild des Erythema nodosum gehören. Sie sollen nicht rheumatischer Natur, sondern eher ein allergisches Phänomen sein (DOGRAMACI), da sie an die Gelenkbeteiligung bei Serumkrankheit erinnern (WALLGREN). Über weitere Komplikationen berichtet ESBIERG, der zusammen mit Lungenveränderungen eine Uveoparotitis, und TATÀR, der parallel mit dem Erythema nodosum Veränderungen an der Retina und ebenfalls eine Uveitis beobachten konnte. Auch an der Conjunctiva können Veränderungen in Form von Phlyctaenen (NOBÉCOURT und DUCAS, JACQUET et al.) und Knötchen (GREENE et al., KISIN) auftreten. Histologische Untersuchungen dieser Knötchen zeigten allerdings unspezifische Struktur (BLUEFARB et al.) oder Ähnlichkeit mit Aschoffschen Knötchen (MCCARTHY). KISIN hält diese Knötchen für spezifisch für das Erythema nodosum und möchte sie von phlyctaenischen und episkleritischen Knötchen trennen. Er fand in seinen Fällen negative Tuberkulinreaktionen. Auch KRATKA hält die bei Erythema nodosum auftretenden Augenveränderungen (Episkleritis, Iritis) für allergisch bedingt. Meist sind die Phlyctaenen jedoch tuberkulöser Natur (DICKEY, CERVINI et al., NIKLASSON, W. NEUMANN, PIERRET et al., OROSZ).

JOSEPHSEN beschreibt folgende Komplikationen bei 71 Fällen von Erythema nodosum: dreimal Angina, sechsmal Endokarditis, 27mal rheumatisches Fieber, zweimal Adenitis, dreimal Arthropathia gonorrhoica, einmal Salpingitis, einmal Sepsis. Nur in 26 Fällen traten keine Komplikationen auf. Hie und da wird auch Nephritis beschrieben, die akut hämorrhagisch sein kann, aber eine gute Prognose hat (WALLGREN, COSTE und BERNARD). GOUGEROT und MATHIEU beschreiben das gleichzeitige Auftreten einer Parapsoriasis chronica (Mucha) und eines Erythema nodosum. Diese Autoren glauben, daß beide Affektionen als Abwehrreaktion gegen einen Infekt aufgefaßt werden können.

2. Pathologische Anatomie

Wie schon eingangs erwähnt wurde, zeigen die histologischen Untersuchungen des Erythema nodosum, daß die Gewebsveränderungen unabhängig von der Ätiologie des Erythema nodosum sind. Während seit je stets auf die stark entzündliche Reaktion hingewiesen wurde, die ihren Ausgang vom subcutanen Gefäßnetz nimmt und daher vorwiegend in den tiefen Schichten der Cutis und Subcutis abläuft (GRZYBOWSKI, PAUTRIER und WORINGER, MALLET), hat MIESCHER erstmals spezifische Reaktionsbilder beschrieben. Da seinen Befunden grundlegende Bedeutung für die Auffassung der Pathogenese des Erythema nodosum zukommt, sollen diese in extenso beschrieben werden:

Beim Studium der nodösen Cibazolexantheme stellte der Autor einen oberflächlichen und einen tiefen Typus fest. Der oberflächliche Typus, der in einem Viertel der Fälle angetroffen wurde, zeigte im Bereich der subpapillären Schicht eine massive Infiltration, die ausschließlich aus neutrophilen polynucleären Leukocyten besteht, die Kernzerfall zeigen. Der häufigere tiefe Typus, der klinisch dem Bild des Erythema nodosum entspricht, zeigt eine entzündliche Reaktion im tiefen subcutanen Gewebe. Diese besteht aus einem entzündlichen, vor allem die Bindegewebssepten zwischen den Fettläppchen einnehmenden Ödem und einer von den Gefäßen ausgehenden lockeren Infiltration mit polynucleären Leukocyten. Daneben finden sich in hohem Maße charakteristische granulomatöse Formationen in Gestalt kleinerer und größerer, bald mitten im Fettgewebe, bald im cutanen Grenzgebiet liegender Knötchen (Abb. 1a). Sie sind fast ausschließlich aus kleinen polymorphen Histiocyten aufgebaut, zwischen welchen mehr oder weniger reichlich Leukocytentrümmer liegen. Diese Knötchen lassen bestimmte Strukturen erkennen, indem die Zellen eine nach der Mitte orientierte radiäre Lagerung auf-

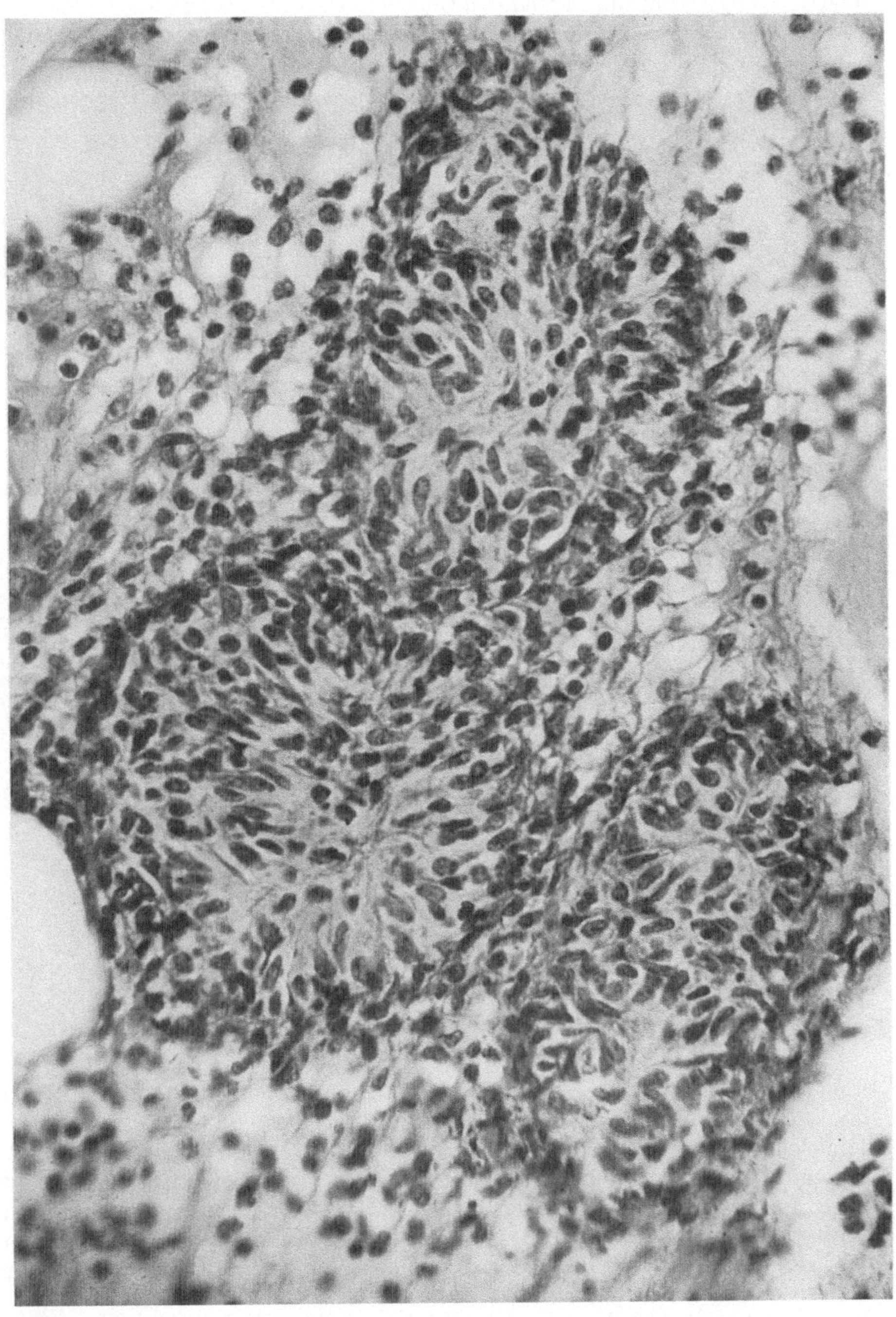

a

Abb. 1a u. b. Knötchen mit Spaltbildung und Palisadenstellung der Zellen. [Aus MIESCHER, G.: Über Cibazolexantheme. Dermatologica (Basel) 86, 66 (1942)]

weisen oder sich, palisadenförmig aneinandergereiht, um ein unregelmäßiges, spaltförmiges Lumen anordnen. Im Zentrum der radiären Knötchen tritt eine Verschmelzung des Protoplasmas der Zellen ein (Abb. 1 b). Diese radiären Formationen fand MIESCHER nicht nur im nodösen Cibazolexanthem, sondern auch in 26 Fällen von genuinem Erythema nodosum, von denen sechs einen typischen tuberkulösen

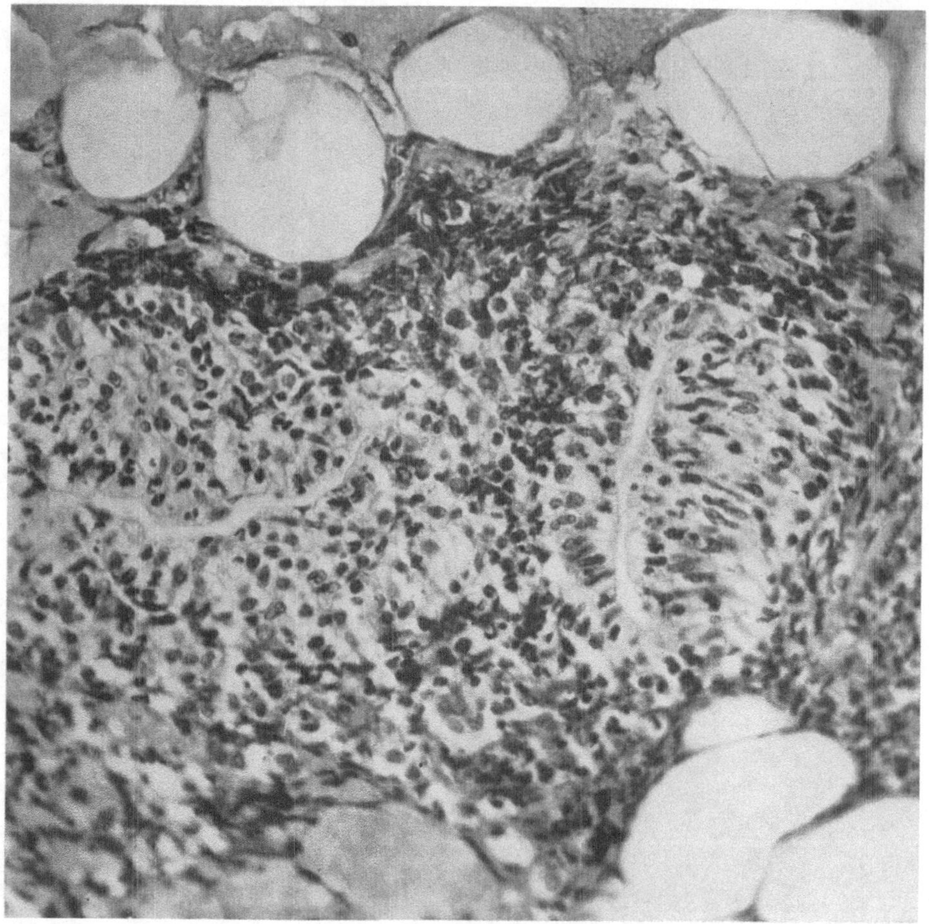

Abb. 1 b

Primärkomplex, neun eine erhöhte Tuberkulinempfindlichkeit, zwei einen Morbus Boeck und acht keine Zeichen von Tuberkulose zeigten. Sämtliche Fälle zeigten die gleichen Veränderungen und stimmten unter sich und mit den Cibazolfällen vollkommen überein. Neben diesen im frischen Stadium gefundenen Veränderungen finden sich später neben den einfachen Knötchen auch größere, die oft eine multizentrische Erweiterung erkennen lassen. Die Gefäße spielen im Reaktionsbild keine hervortretende Rolle. In einem späteren Zeitpunkt gehen Ödem und leukocytäre Infiltration zurück. Das ganze Knötchen geht in einer Anzahl großer Riesenzellen auf, die bald dem Fremdkörper-, bald dem Langhansschen Typus entsprechen. Neben untergehenden bzw. sich riesenzellig umwandelnden Knötchen findet man zerstreut im Gewebe Riesenzellen beider Typen (Abb. 2).

Auf die Deutung, die MIESCHER diesen Vorgängen gibt, soll später eingegangen werden. Die Befunde MIESCHERS wurden in der Folge von REICH, GREITHER,

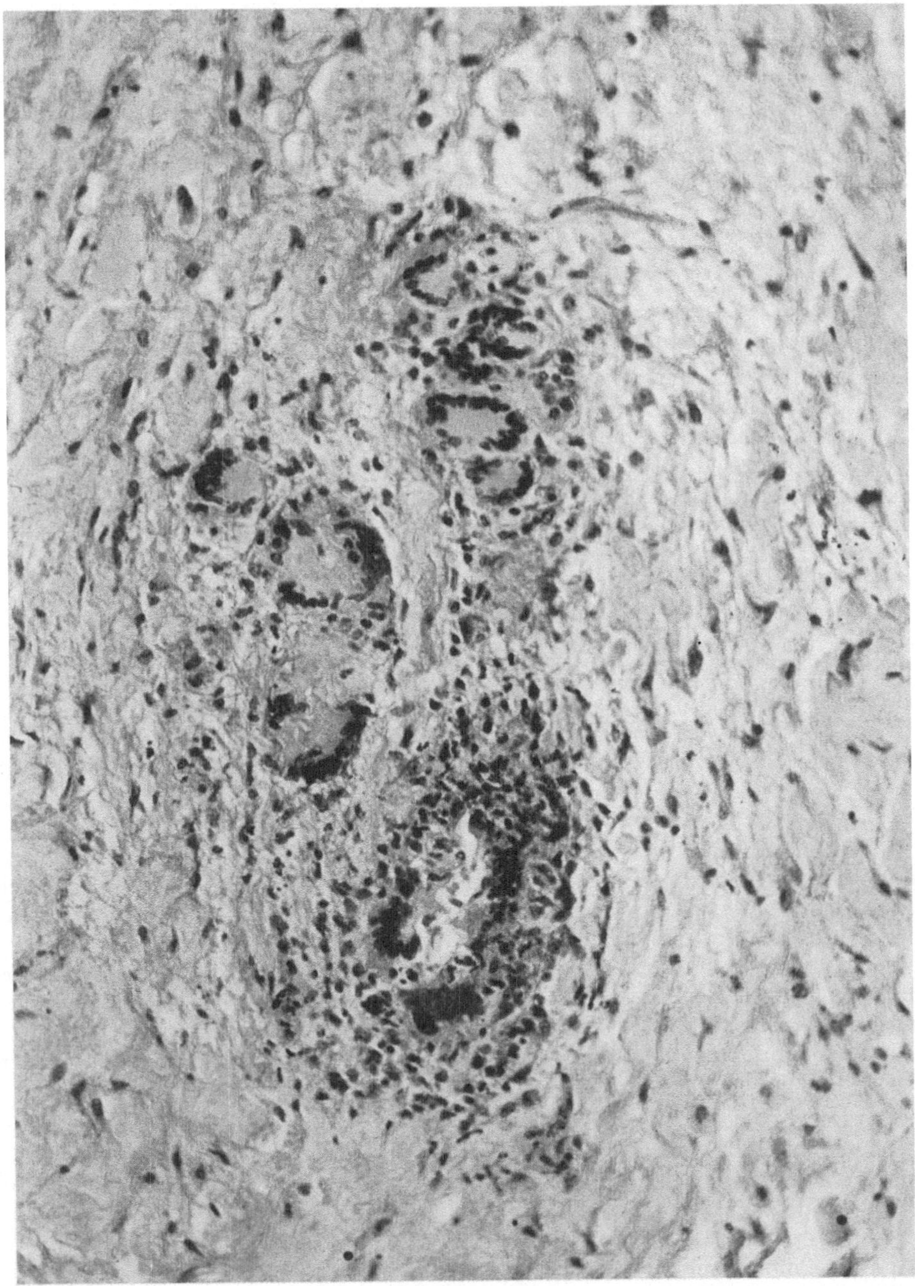

Abb. 2. Riesenzellbildung in einem Fall, bei welchem die Excision in den ersten 24 Std nach Erscheinen des Exanthems gewonnen wurde. [Aus MIESCHER, G.: Über Cibazolexantheme. Dermatologica (Basel) **86**, 67 (1942)]

LÖFGREN und WALLGREN, LEVER, DOXIADIS, NUBÉ bestätigt, wobei allerdings auch der fibrinoiden Degeneration in den Septen des Bindegewebes und der

Wucheratrophie des Fettgewebes Bedeutung zugemessen wird. Es ist sicher, daß die von Miescher beschriebenen Gewebsreaktionen schon früher beobachtet worden sind, daß sie aber möglicherweise falsch interpretiert wurden. So zeigen Bilder in der Arbeit Grzybowskis sehr deutlich ein solches Knötchen, das der Autor als obliterierte Vene auffaßt.

Bergstrand beschreibt demgegenüber in den Knoten des Erythema nodosum ähnliche Veränderungen, wie sie in Hautreaktionen vom anaphylaktischen Typ beschrieben worden sind, nämlich in erster Linie Veränderungen der Gefäße: endotheliale Proliferation, fibrinoide Degeneration, Nekrosen der Gefäßwände und intra- und perivasculäre celluläre Infiltration. Er bestätigt damit weitgehend die Befunde Grzybowskis.

3. Ätiologie und Pathogenese

Wie schon erwähnt, ist die Auffassung des Erythema nodosum als einer tuberkulösen Manifestation bei Internisten und Pädiatern derart verbreitet, daß z.B. Löffler 1947 schreiben konnte, das Erythema nodosum sei in 99% der Fälle tuberkulös bedingt, in 1% gebe es 99 mögliche Ursachen. Die Dermatologen ihrerseits können sich weniger denn je dieser absoluten Meinung anschließen. Auf jeden Fall könnte die Zusammenstellung von Rotnes über die verschiedenen Auffassungen der Ätiologie des Erythema nodosum beliebig durch weitere kontradiktorische Ansichten erweitert werden.

Einen Fortschritt in der Beurteilung des Erythema nodosum brachte nun einerseits die Beobachtung, daß die Cibazolexantheme den Charakter des Erythema nodosum tragen, und andererseits die Feststellung Mieschers über den spezifischen Gewebsaufbau der Erythema nodosum-Knoten. Weiterhin zeigte die Beobachtung, wonach bei Coccidioidomykose regelmäßig ein Erythema nodosum aufzutreten pflegt, daß jedenfalls die unitarische Auffassung des tuberkulösen Ursprungs des Erythema nodosum nicht fundiert ist. Es ist deshalb zweckmäßig, die verschiedenen Ätiologien des Erythema nodosum nacheinander zu diskutieren.

a) Erythema nodosum und Tuberkulose

Beobachtungen über einen engen Zusammenhang zwischen Erythema nodosum und Tuberkulose dominieren in der Literatur derart, daß tatsächlich der Eindruck entstehen könnte, das Erythema nodosum sei eine Form der Hauttuberkulose. Demgegenüber existieren allerdings auch Angaben, daß das gleichzeitige Auftreten beider Krankheiten eher selten sei (Poppel et al., Booth). Eine sorgfältige Überprüfung der für oder gegen die tuberkulöse Ätiologie des Erythema nodosum angeführten Gründe ist deshalb sicher angezeigt.

Als Beweise für die tuberkulöse Ätiologie des Erythema nodosum werden folgende Untersuchungsmethoden herangezogen:

a) Der direkte Bacillennachweis in den Hautknoten oder im strömenden Blut.
b) Feststellung anderer tuberkulöser Organerkrankungen.
c) Das Verhalten des Organismus gegen Tuberkulin.
d) Epidemiologische Feststellungen.
e) Das histologische Gewebsbild.
f) Nachuntersuchungen von Personen, die einmal an einem Erythema nodosum gelitten hatten.

ad a. Am überzeugendsten sind natürlich diejenigen Beobachtungen über direkten Bacillennachweis in den Knoten des Erythema nodosum mittels Färbung, mittels Kultur oder Tierversuch. So konnte Lewkowicz in den Knoten von Erythema nodosum verschiedene Formen des Tuberkelbacillus finden. Dieser

Autor beschreibt Stäbchen, säurefeste Körnchen und im Zellprotoplasma gelöste säurefeste Substanz als Ausdruck außerordentlich gründlicher Vernichtung der Stäbchen, aber auch „Tuberkulosevirus in Kokkenform". Die Beweiskraft dieser Befunde wird dadurch eingeschränkt, daß ähnliche Erscheinungen auch bei tuberkulöser Meningitis, aber auch bei akutem Rheumatismus und in Aschoffschen Granulomen des Herzmuskels gefunden werden konnten. Direkte Nachweise von Tuberkelbacillen in Knoten des Erythema nodosum beschreiben ferner CIBILS AGUIRRE und CERVINI et al. mittels Kultur- und Tierversuch. In einem Fall konnten Bacillen auch im histologischen Schnitt gefunden werden. ARENA fand in einem von 8 Fällen in der Kultur ein positives Resultat. RAMEL nahm von zwölf an Erythema nodosum erkrankten Patienten Überimpfungen von Blut, Urinsediment oder Hautgewebsfiltrat auf Meerschweinchen vor. Acht Patienten zeigten positiven Bacillenbefund. Auch MASSINI konnte aus dem Blut eines Patienten mit Erythema nodosum Tuberkelbacillen züchten. Zwei Monate später erkrankte der Patient an einer Pleuritis exsudativa. DEBRÉ et al. (1935, 1936) fanden zu Beginn der Eruption des Erythema nodosum gleichzeitig im Blut und in Knoten im Tierversuch Tuberkelbacillen vom Typus humanus. SAENZ et al. konnten sowohl mit Blut als auch Gewebsstückchen Bacillen auf Meerschweinchen übertragen, wobei die mit Blut infizierten Tiere viel schneller und massiver erkrankten. Weitere Untersuchungen dieser Autoren sind besonders genau und aufschlußreich. Sie konstatierten, daß es unter Berücksichtigung aller Kautelen gelingt, in Erythema nodosum-Knoten Tuberkelbacillen nachzuweisen, allerdings keineswegs in allen Fällen. Es zeigt sich, daß es bei Kindern in etwa 10%, bei Erwachsenen in 4% möglich ist, Bacillen im Blut oder in den Knoten zu finden. Im Magensaft von Kindern hingegen war der Bacillennachweis bei bestehenden Lungenveränderungen immer positiv. Diese Zahlen entsprechen denjenigen von WALLGREN und GNOSSPELIUS. Diese Autoren konnten selbst nur bei einem von 28 Patienten einen positiven Bacillenbefund in Erythema nodosum-Knoten erheben. Sie stellen 113 Fälle der Weltliteratur zusammen, von denen nur vier ein positives Resultat des direkten Bacillennachweises ergaben. Auf die Tatsache, daß der Bacillennachweis im Blut nur während kurzer Zeit möglich ist, wurde von DEBRÉ et al. hingewiesen. Diese in Frankreich fälschlicherweise Typhobacillose [GATÉ et al. (1937 a), CROSNIER] genannte Tuberkelbacillensepsis konnten auch NÉKÁM, PETROVIČ, BOAS, ARNAUD, NARANJO finden.

Diesen positiven Resultaten stehen auch negative gegenüber. So konnte GRZYBOWSKI weder Tuberkelbacillen noch andere Bakterien in den Knoten von acht Patienten finden. CASTRO FREIRE fand in zwei Fällen von Erythema nodosum weder in Knoten noch im Blut, hingegen aber im Magensaft Bacillen.

ad b. Über Tuberkelbacillennachweis im übrigen Organismus liegen viele Berichte vor: In Lymphdrüsen: GORDON, THOMPSON, NIKLASSON, ITO und ANDO; in pleuritischem Erguß nach Strangdurchtrennung: COSTE und BERNARD; in tuberkulöser Parotis: GATÉ et al. (1937 b); im Sputum: OPITZ in drei von vier Fällen.

Gleichzeitiges Bestehen tuberkulöser Hautmanifestationen erwähnen WHITWELL und FALK. Sie sahen bei ihren Fällen ein Erythema nodosum sich entwickeln und nachher ein Erythema induratum Bazin dazukommen. KOGOJ beschreibt einen Patienten, bei dem das Erythema nodosum von papulo-nekrotischen Tuberkuliden gefolgt war.

Das Zusammentreffen von Lungentuberkulose und Erythema nodosum ist derart häufig, daß hier eine detaillierte Kasuistik unmöglich ist. Im allgemeinen werden die Lungenveränderungen als Frühinfiltrate bezeichnet, die sich in der Regel wieder zurückbilden, sich aber auch in Kavernen umwandeln können. Doch werden auch indurative Prozesse beschrieben. Ebenso werden Pleuraexsudate gefunden, wobei die Prozentzahlen dieser Komplikation ganz verschieden angegeben werden (GIERTSEN). Oft sind die Lungenveränderungen röntgenologisch schwer zu fassen, und nur auf Grund des positiven Tuberkelbacillennachweises läßt sich die richtige Diagnose stellen (LASSEN).

ad c. Die Reaktion des Organismus gegen Tuberkulin wird in ausgedehntem Maße für oder gegen die Auffassung des Erythema nodosum als tuberkulöse Manifestation verwertet. Besonders eindrücklich sind diejenigen Fälle, in denen Positivwerden negativer Tuberkulinreaktionen im Verlauf eines Erythema nodosum beobachtet wurde (LEMAIRE, ONTANEDA et al., JACQUET et al., GAMSTEDT, PUNCH, NOBÉCOURT et al.) oder in denen ein Erythema nodosum durch Tuberkulininjektionen provoziert werden konnte. Solche Fälle beschreiben TINOZZI, LAFOSSE, HUBER, FERRARI, DICKEY, GOUGEROT und DESMOND. ARNAUD gelang es, nach Trennung des Tuberkelbacillus in eine eiweißlösliche und eine fettlösliche Fraktion mittels der eiweißlöslichen Fraktion bei einem an Erythema nodosum erkrankten Individuum Knoten hervorzurufen, die in jeder Hinsicht den spontan aufgetretenen Knoten glichen. Die fettlösliche Fraktion löste keinerlei Reaktion aus.

Die Möglichkeit, das Erythema nodosum mit Tuberkulin provozieren zu können, scheint nicht von langer Dauer zu sein. BINDSCHEDLER beobachtete in vier Fällen zunächst das Auftreten eines Erythema nodosum im Anschluß an Tuberkulininjektionen. Einige Monate später konnte das Erythema nodosum dann nicht mehr provoziert werden, trotzdem die lokale Reaktion auf Tuberkulin sehr stark positiv blieb. Es scheint also, daß die Tuberkulininjektion zu einem bestimmten Zeitpunkt der Tuberkuloseinfektion erfolgen muß, damit ein Erythema nodosum provoziert werden kann. Diese Feststellung kann die Berichte, daß durch Tuberkulininjektionen der Ablauf des Erythema nodosum nicht modifizierbar war (RANTASALO), erklären.

Umgekehrt gelang es PATRIGNANI, durch intradermale Injektion von Tuberkulin Erythema nodosum-Knoten in 1—2 Tagen ganz zum Verschwinden zu bringen.

Besonders heftige, z.T. bullöse Reaktionen nach Tuberkulin als Hinweis auf die tuberkulöse Ätiologie des Erythema nodosum beschreiben RAILLET, STORCK und SPÜHLER, MINAMI und KINGO, STAJIČ, LAURINISCH, CHINI. GOUGEROT und DELORT konstatierten, daß die Tuberkulinreaktion am stärksten im Bereich der Knoten des Erythema nodosum ist und daß ihre Intensität mit zunehmender Entfernung von den Knoten abnimmt. MÓRITZ et al. (1933) untersuchten Erythema nodosum-Knoten mittels eines Hautmikroskops auf das Verhalten der Hautcapillaren und mittels der Methode des „lokalen Blutbildes" (HELMREICH). Mit beiden Reaktionen konnte eine weitgehende Ähnlichkeit des Erythema nodosum mit der Pirquet-Reaktion gefunden werden. Andererseits kann auch eine allgemein erhöhte Reaktivität nachgewiesen werden, da auch Pferdeserum starke Reaktionen geben kann (GOUGEROT und SÉRINGE).

ad d. Besonders eindrücklich sind die Fälle, bei denen Kinder in tuberkulösen Familien angesteckt worden sind und an einem Erythema nodosum erkrankten, wobei z.T. ulceröse Manifestationen auf Haut und Schleimhäuten vorangingen (NORDENSKJÖLD, CIBILS AGUIRRE, GENÉVRIER und BORDET), in anderen Fällen Lungenherde festgestellt werden konnten (HAMBURG-ZETLINA et al., HOFFMANN, BOAS, GÖBEL, KROPATCHEV et al., BROCK). In weiteren Fällen trat nach Kontakt mit Tuberkulösen das Erythema nodosum ohne Zeichen einer internen Tuberkulose auf (BETHOUX et al., CERVINI et al., MÓRITZ, RANTASALO, HOLLANDER, VALLI). Diese Fälle zeigen, daß das epidemische Auftreten von Erythema nodosum wohl meist auf einer tuberkulösen Infektion beruhen dürfte (s. Kapitel 3c).

ad e. Die histologischen Veränderungen des Erythema nodosum sind gar nicht leicht zu beurteilen, wie aus den Ausführungen in Kapitel 2 hervorgeht, und es ist sehr wohl möglich, daß Berichte über typische tuberkulöse Veränderungen beim Erythema nodosum (TANIMURA et al.) auf einer falschen Interpretation des Gewebsbildes beruhen. Zweifellos können die von MIESCHER beschriebenen Granulome in einem gewissen Stadium ihrer Umwandlung, wenn nämlich Riesenzellen vom Langhansschen Typus auftreten, tuberkulösen Veränderungen gleichen.

ad f. Eine ganze Reihe von Arbeiten befassen sich mit dem Schicksal von Patienten, die einmal ein Erythema nodosum durchgemacht hatten. WALLGREN, der wohl die größte Erfahrung auf diesem Gebiet hat, weist auf die Tatsache hin, daß bei Kindern mit Erythema nodosum Tuberkulose weit häufiger sei als bei Kindern ohne Hautmanifestationen. Unter 800 Fällen traf er nur ein Kind an, das an akutem Gelenkrheumatismus erkrankt war, und nimmt an, daß in Schweden etwa 95% der Patienten, die an Erythema nodosum erkrankt seien, tuberkulös infiziert seien. MOGENSEN berichtet über Nachuntersuchungen von 114 meist erwachsenen Patienten mit Erythema nodosum. Fünf davon waren bereits vor dieser Krankheit mit Tuberkulose behaftet. Von den übrigen erkrankten 18% nach einem kürzeren oder längeren Abstand an Tuberkulose. Die Pirquet-Probe war nur bei fünf Patienten negativ. TÖRNELL untersuchte 150 Fälle von Erythema nodosum. Er fand fast immer tuberkulöse Primärinfektion, nur in einem Fall war Tuberkulin-negativ. LORBER sah bei 105 Kindern mit Erythema nodosum in 43% der Fälle eine aktive Tuberkulose, GORDON bei 20% von 66 Fällen. SEVERIN stellte fest, daß unter 3000 Patienten mit Tuberkulose im südlichen Norwegen 511 ein Erythema nodosum hatten (17%). INGEBRIGTSEN fand nördlich des Polarkreises unter 9000 Patienten mit Tuberkulose nur 5% mit Erythema nodosum. Wenn bei einem Erythema nodosum eine Pleuritis auftrat, so wurde dieses Ereignis in $^3/_4$ der Fälle im ersten halben Jahr nach dem Beginn des Erythema nodosum beobachtet, eine komplizierende Phthise in $^2/_3$ der Fälle im Laufe der ersten 3 Jahre. BLANKSMA sah unter 30000 Tuberkulösen 480 Fälle von Erythema nodosum (1,5%). Diese unterschiedliche Häufigkeit des Erythema nodosum ist bemerkenswert. Immerhin ist die niedrigste Zahl von 1,5% höher als die von DOGRAMACI angegebene Zahl von 0,2% und TOMIKAWA et al. von 0,4%, die auf alle poliklinischen Patienten bezogen sind.

Überblickt man nun alle diese Arbeiten, die einen sehr engen Zusammenhang zwischen Tuberkulose und Erythema nodosum anzeigen, so wird der Ausspruch LÖFFLERs verständlich. Es darf aber nicht verschwiegen werden, daß eine ganze Reihe von Arbeiten existieren, aus denen ein viel weniger enger Zusammenhang zwischen Tuberkulose und Erythema nodosum hervorgeht. Die Schwierigkeit besteht eben oft darin, einen ursächlichen Zusammenhang zwischen Tuberkulose und Erythema nodosum sicher festzustellen. Wenn man z.B. nach LÖFFLER alle diejenigen Fälle als tuberkulös betrachtet, bei denen nicht das Gegenteil bewiesen ist, so dürfte es bei sehr vielen Fällen tatsächlich äußerst schwer fallen, einen Zusammenhang dieser beiden Affektionen zu verneinen. Diese Betrachtungsweise dürfte wohl aber doch zu einseitig sein. So geht z.B. aus der statistischen Arbeit von BLOCH und SCHUPPLI hervor, daß lange nicht alle Fälle als tuberkulös bezeichnet werden dürfen, auch wenn man alle ätiologisch unklaren Veränderungen zur Tuberkulose rechnet. Diese Autoren haben festgestellt, daß allerhöchstens 50% ihrer 132 Fälle in irgendeiner Weise mit einer Tuberkulose in Zusammenhang gebracht werden können und daß verschiedene Unterschiede im klinischen Bild zwischen einem Erythema nodosum ohne Tuberkulose und einem solchen mit Tuberkulose bestehen. Im folgenden sollen diejenigen Formen des Erythema nodosum, die in sicherem Zusammenhang mit tuberkulöser Infektion stehen, noch näher in bezug auf ihre Pathogenese besprochen werden.

α) Pathogenese des tuberkulösen Erythema nodosum

Die Tatsache, daß das Erythema nodosum vorwiegend bei tuberkulöser Primoinfektion auftritt, ferner daß es gelingt, in seinen frühen Stadien eine tuberkulöse Bacillämie nachzuweisen und daß ein Positivwerden vorher negativer Tuberkulinreaktionen beobachtet werden kann, hat dazu geführt, das Erythema nodosum mit dem Vorgang der Allergisierung des Organismus in Zusammenhang zu bringen. WALLGREN hält das zu Beginn des Erythema nodosum oft beobachtete Fieber für nichts anderes als tuberkulöses Fieber. Er konnte auch den Infektionstermin verschiedener seiner Fälle feststellen und sah das Erythema nodosum in diesen Fällen 3—8 Wochen nach erfolgter Infektion auftreten, also am Ende der Inkubationsperiode. MÓRITZ und GÖBEL glauben, daß das Inkubationsstadium des Erythema nodosum mit demjenigen der Tuberkulose identisch ist bzw. daß es der vor-allergischen Phase von 4—10 Wochen entsprechen soll. Auch DEBRÉ et al. (1938) kommen bei ihren Fällen auf eine Inkubationsdauer von 4 Wochen bis 4 Monaten.

Die Pathogenese des tuberkulösen Erythema nodosum ist nun umstritten. Während DEBRÉ et al. es als eine kurzdauernde und schnell heilende Tuberkulose auffassen, wird es allgemein eher als eine allergische Manifestation betrachtet (WALLGREN, RYCKEBUSCH, JENSEN, PIERRET et al., FORMAN et al., DOMINGUEZ, KÖNIGSBERGER). Ob die Auffassung, daß es eine tuberkulo-toxische Erscheinung sei (NEUMANN, SIBIRANYI), einen prinzipiellen Unterschied zu dem Begriff einer allergischen Reaktion bedeutet, dürfte wohl eher eine Nomenklaturfrage sein.

Sehr aufschlußreich und im Sinne der Auffassung des Erythema nodosum als einer allergischen Reaktion zu verwerten sind diejenigen Beobachtungen, nach denen im Verlauf einer Tuberkulose im Anschluß an interkurrent auftretende Infekte, die bekanntermaßen die Hautreaktivität verändern, ein Erythema nodosum auftrat (FLANDIN et al.). Hier scheint den Masern eine besonders wichtige Rolle zuzukommen. So berichtet JENSEN, daß von 37 Patienten mit aktiver Lungentuberkulose während einer Masernepidemie zwölf Erwachsene an einem postprimären Erythema nodosum erkrankten. Vier davon starben. NOBÉCOURT et al., KEIZER, COMBY, DEBRÉ et al. erwähnen ebenfalls Masern und Keuchhusten als provozierenden Faktor, TÖRNELL Masern und Lactation. Auch PIERRET et al. beschreiben neue Schübe von Erythema nodosum als Ausdruck von Allergieschwankungen und einer fluktuierenden Immunitätslage.

Für die allergische Genese spricht weiterhin das gleichzeitige Auftreten exsudativer Manifestationen wie Arthritis (STEINBERG), Polyserositis, Endokarditis (TATAFIORE), seröse Meningitis (KAJTÓR, MÓRITZ), Nephritis usw. (WALLGREN).

Nun scheint es sich aber beim Erythema nodosum nicht um eine einfache allergische Reaktion gegen die tuberkulöse Infektion zu handeln. Es existieren Beobachtungen, die zeigen, daß außer der Allergisierung des Organismus gegenüber den Tuberkelbacillen noch zusätzliche Faktoren für die Auslösung eines Erythema nodosum von Bedeutung sind. So beschrieben ITO und ANDO einen Patienten, der seit 12 Jahren an rezidivierendem klassischem Erythema nodosum litt. Es bestand gleichzeitig eine kolliquierende Tuberkulose und eine nicht tuberkulöse, chronische Tonsillitis. Auf Isonicotinsäurehydrazid erfolgte eine starke Exacerbation des Erythema nodosum, das nach Entfernung der tuberkulösen Halslymphknoten besserte. Eine vollkommene Heilung trat aber erst nach Entfernung der nichttuberkulösen, chronisch entzündeten Mandeln ein. BOVENKAMP nimmt an, daß für das Auftreten eines Erythema nodosum neben einer gewissen Disposition noch ein Virus nötig sei. Daß zwei Faktoren für das Entstehen eines Erythema nodosum nötig sind, geht auch aus der Mitteilung von WEBSTER und PASS hervor, wonach bei einem Patienten mit Lungentuberkulose und Erythematodes 9 Tage nach Beginn einer Atebrinbehandlung ein histologisch typisches Erythema nodosum auftrat. GÖBEL et al. sahen ein Erythema nodosum bei einem Knaben, der Lamblien beherbergte, von einer kavernösen Tuberkulose gefolgt werden. Auch SEIDELIN, SCHNOHR u. WESTERGREN halten das Erythema nodosum für eine Affektion mit kombinierter Ätiologie.

Wohl am ehesten im Zusammenhang mit der Tuberkuloseätiologie zu deuten sind die Fälle, bei denen ein Erythema nodosum nach BCG-Impfung auftrat (ITO, STAVROPOULOS). So sahen ROYER et al. bei einem BCG-geimpften Kind nach massiver Ansteckung mit Bacillen das Auftreten eines Erythema nodosum. Seine Schwester, die nicht geimpft war, starb an einer rapid fortschreitenden Tuberkulose. KRISTENSON beobachtete drei tuberkulinnegative Krankenschwestern, die deshalb mit BCG geimpft wurden. Nachdem sie auf einer Tuberkulosestation gearbeitet hatten, trat parallel mit positiv werdender Tuberkulinreaktion ein Schub eines Erythema nodosum auf. Auch die Impfstelle der Vaccine zeigte ein Aufflammen. WALLGREN beschreibt ein 3jähriges Kind, das wegen offener Tuberkulose seiner Eltern mit BCG geimpft wurde. Es erkrankte im Anschluß an eine Angina an einem Erythema nodosum ohne andere tuberkulöse Manifestationen, was wohl im Sinne eines Impfschutzes gedeutet werden kann. Auch DES ROCHETTES et al. erwähnen einen ähnlichen Fall.

β) Die prognostische Bedeutung des Erythema nodosum bei Tuberkulose

Über die prognostische Bedeutung des Erythema nodosum für die gleichzeitig bestehende Tuberkulose gehen die Ansichten auseinander. TISSOT stellte in 20 Fällen fest, daß auf ein Erythema nodosum mit der gleichen Häufigkeit wie bei jeder Primoinfektion eine Lungentuberkulose folgt. OROSZ fand, daß von Kindern mit Erythema nodosum nach einem Jahr 30% vollkommen gesund blieben. 30% zeigten auf latente Tuberkulose verdächtige Erscheinungen, 40% wiesen manifeste tuberkulöse Nacherkrankungen auf. MASCHER untersucht die prognostische Bedeutung des Erythema nodosum bei Erwachsenen im Vergleich zu demjenigen bei Kindern. Er stellt fest, daß in 40% der Fälle eine Pleuritis exsudativa auftrat, $^2/_3$ davon im Zeitraum eines Jahres. In einem Viertel der Fälle entwickelte sich eine Lungenphthise, und zwar schneller als bei Kindern. Auch die primäre Mortalität der sich nach einem Erythema nodosum entwickelnden Tuberkulose ist bei Erwachsenen höher als bei Kindern. USTVEDT et al. sahen, daß von 288 nachkontrollierten Fällen 25% später an Tuberkulose erkrankten. BIRATH konstatierte ähnliche Verhältnisse. Es ist deshalb der Aussage von HEIMBECK zuzustimmen, daß die prognostische Bedeutung des Erythema nodosum umstritten sei. Sie scheint bei Kindern eindeutig besser zu sein als bei Erwachsenen (MONDON) und hier besser bei Frauen als bei Männern (Mortalität bei Erwachsenen nach BIRATH 10%, nach USTVEDT 5%). USTVEDT kommt zum Schluß, daß Personen, die ein Erythema nodosum überstanden haben, mit erheblich größerer Wahrscheinlichkeit an Tuberkulose sterben als der nicht von Erythema nodosum befallene Durchschnitt. Auch BERG kommt zu ähnlichen Schlüssen. Jedenfalls können die Anschauungen über eine abschwächende Wirkung des Erythema nodosum auf die tuberkulöse Infektion (LESNÉ et al., ARAOZ ALVARO) oder über die absolut gute Prognose des Erythema nodosum [CARTAGENOVA et al., NAVARRO et al. (1935)] keineswegs verallgemeinert werden. JOHANNESSEN gibt zwar an, daß die Mortalität im Zeitraum der Jahre 1916—1949 von 5% auf 1% abgefallen sei, und bei Kindern werden Todesfälle relativ selten beschrieben (SLOT et al., OROSZ), andererseits sah BATTISTIG in Bologna bei Kindern mit Erythema nodosum 15% Mortalität an tuberkulösen Komplikationen.

b) Das nodöse Cibazolexanthem

Einen wesentlichen Fortschritt auf dem Gebiet der Erkennung der Ursachen des Erythema nodosum und der Auffassung seiner Pathogenese brachte die Beobachtung, daß typische Erythema nodosum-Eruptionen im Anschluß an gewisse Medikamente, speziell an Sulfathiazol, auftreten. Bereits 1940 beschrieben LOVEMAN und SIMON das Auftreten von Erythema nodosum nach Sulfanilamid. 1943 wurden dann die ersten Sulfathiazolexantheme vom Typus des Erythema nodosum beschrieben (ANTUNES LEAL, JERSILD und IVERSEN, GLASS), z.T. auch bei intravaginaler Applikation von Cibazol (LINDEMAYR). Die Exantheme werden in den meisten Fällen als dem Erythema nodosum sehr ähnlich geschildert, nur in einzelnen Fällen verlaufen sie oberflächlicher. STAFFIERI et al. betonen, daß das Sulfathiazol-Erythema nodosum meist von kürzerer Dauer, nicht symmetrisch, oberflächlicher und weniger schmerzhaft als das typische Erythema nodosum sei. MIESCHER hat die Natur des Cibazolexanthems genauer untersucht. Er kommt zum Schluß, daß es sich dabei wahrscheinlich nicht um eine allergische Manifestation handle, da wesentliche Kriterien der allergischen Reaktion fehlten. So unterscheide es sich vom typischen Arzneimittelexanthem durch die Lokalisation, indem es nicht diffus, sondern auf die Streckseiten der Extremitäten beschränkt sei. Die Gruppenspezifität fehle. Bei Fortsetzung der Behandlung gehe es meistens zurück und kehre bei wiederholter Behandlung meist nicht wieder, eine Feststellung, die auch DIETEL gemacht hat, während GREITHER wiederholt Erythema nodosum durch das gleiche Medikament provozieren konnte.

Wichtig für die Auffassung der Pathogenese des Sulfathiazol-Erythema nodosum ist nun die Feststellung, daß dieses bei verschiedenen mit Sulfathiazol behandelten Krankheiten ganz verschieden häufig auftritt. Aus der aus einer Arbeit von SIMPSON publizierten und ergänzten Tabelle geht hervor, daß es bei Tuberkulose und Lymphogranuloma inguinale weitaus am häufigsten auftritt, während es bei Gonorrhoe und Poliomyelitis praktisch nie beobachtet wird.

Tabelle

Diagnose	Anzahl der mit Sulfathiazol behandelten Fälle	Erythema nodosum	%
Pneumonie (WISSLER)	165	6	3,6
Pneumonie (FRIDERICHSEN)	875	0	0
Pneumonie (JERSILD et al.)	307	9	3,0
Meningitis cerebrospinalis (WISSLER)	26	4	15,0
Tuberkulose (ROLLOF)	231	105	45,0
Nichttuberkulöse Erkrankungen	475	24	5,0
Gonorrhoe (MIESCHER und STRAUSS)	1500	1	0
Lymphogranuloma venereum (SIMPSON et al.) .	504	37	7,5

Aus SIMPSON, R. G.: Erythema nodosum. Dermatologica (Basel) **101**, 94 (1950). Ergänzt durch ROLLOF und MIESCHER.

SIMPSON hat ferner die wichtige Beobachtung gemacht, daß nur bei Kombination von Lymphogranuloma inguinale mit Sulfathiazol ein Erythema nodosum auftrat, während bei anderen Geschlechtskrankheiten, die mit Sulfathiazol behandelt wurden, nur in 0,2% der Fälle und bei Lymphogranuloma inguinale, das mit Sulfanilamid behandelt wurde, überhaupt nie ein Erythema nodosum beobachtet wurde. Ähnliche Verhältnisse sah BRIEGER bei Tuberkulose. Er behandelte tuberkulinpositive und tuberkulinnegative Kinder mit Sulfathiazol. Von 38 tuberkulinpositiven Kindern bekamen 14 ein Erythema nodosum, 10 davon wiesen einen frischen infiltrativen Lungenprozeß und 4 einen verbreiterten dichten Hilus auf. Im Gegensatz hierzu entwickelten sich bei den 31 tuberkulinnegativen Kontrollen nur in zwei Fällen ein Erythema nodosum. Bei beiden ging ein Streptokokkeninfekt voraus. Dieser Autor untersuchte ferner die Blutveränderungen nach Sulfathiazol-Erythema nodosum und stellte fest, daß diese den bei spontanem Erythema nodosum auftretenden Veränderungen vollkommen entsprechen, indem sich eine starke Leukocytose mit typischer Linksverschiebung entwickelt. Er konnte ferner bei Kindern, die spontan ein Erythema nodosum durchmachten, wiederum ein solches durch Sulfathiazol provozieren, wobei klinisch, hämatologisch usw. keine Differenz gefunden werden konnte. Auf Grund dieser Untersuchungen kommt BRIEGER zum Schluß, daß 1. das Erythema nodosum ein charakteristisches Blutbild in bezug auf die Leukocyten aufweist und daß sein Verlauf unabhängig von der Genese ist, und daß 2. das Sulfathiazol imstande ist, als Äquivalent zum Erythema nodosum eine Conjunctivitis phlyctaenulosa zu erzeugen. Auch BAUER sah bei einer frischen Tuberkulose häufig die Auslösung eines Erythema nodosum durch Sulfathiazol.

Wie schon erwähnt, hat die histologische Untersuchung der nach Sulfathiazol auftretenden Fälle von Erythema nodosum keinen Unterschied zwischen den idiopathischen Fällen und den medikamentös ausgelösten Fällen ergeben (MIESCHER). Es kann infolgedessen den Schlüssen MIESCHERs zugestimmt werden, wonach das Sulfathiazol-Erythema nodosum wahrscheinlich kein allergischer Prozeß, sondern am ehesten ein Prozeß mit einheitlicher Pathogenese, nämlich einer Infektallergie oder einer Infektion sui generis, sei.

c) Das kontagiöse Erythema nodosum

Die Tatsache, daß das Erythema nodosum in Form kleiner Endemien auftreten kann, meist im Verband einer Familie, wurde verschieden gedeutet. Während die Familienendemien auf eine besondere Disposition hinweisen, kann damit das Auftreten von Schulepidemien nicht erklärt werden. Jedenfalls könnten Beobachtungen wie diejenige von KOCH, nach der ein Erythema nodosum zu gleicher Zeit bei Drillingen aufgetreten ist, sowohl im Sinne einer besonderen Disposition als im Sinne einer Infektion mit spezifischem Erreger gedeutet werden.

Alle mitgeteilten Beobachtungen lassen nun aber erkennen, daß der tuberkulösen Infektion eine überragende Rolle bei der Entstehung von Epidemien von Erythema nodosum zukommt, indem zum mindesten in einzelnen Fällen eine tuberkulöse Manifestation zu finden war. Solche Endemien von Erythema nodosum in Schulklassen oder Pensionaten beschreiben DEMOLE, DEMURTAS, CHEVALLIER, BROUWER, HAIDVOGL. Familienendemien lassen die tuberkulöse Infektion noch deutlicher erkennen. So berichtet HAROLD über ein Erythema nodosum bei drei Geschwistern, deren Mutter eine offene kavernöse Tuberkulose hatte. PARISOT und SALEUR beobachteten zwei Familien, bei denen mehrere Kinder an Erythema nodosum erkrankten, nachdem ein Familienglied eine offene Tuberkulose zeigte. ROTNES, STOPPELAAR, HELDEMAN et al., CIBILS AGUIRRE, CHABAUD und TOUPANCE, HALBERTSMA, BIEHLER berichten über ähnliche Beobachtungen. Fast überall betrug die Inkubationszeit 4—8 Wochen.

Schwer zu deuten ist die Beobachtung von KESSLER. Dieser Autor beschreibt drei Fälle von Erythema nodosum, die während einer Masernepidemie bei Kindern im Alter von 4—7 Jahren aufgetreten waren. In ganz gesetzmäßiger Weise kam es bei ihnen am 8. Tage der Genesung zu einem erneuten Fieberanstieg und 3 Tage später zu einem typischen Erythema nodosum an den Streckseiten der Extremitäten. Alle acht Kinder hatten längere Zeit vor Ausbruch der Masern täglich Rohmilch aus der gleichen Quelle genossen. Bei Kindern, die die gleiche Milch gekocht genossen hatten, trat nach Masern kein Erythema nodosum auf.

Eine Epidemie von nichttuberkulösem Erythema nodosum wird von NEUMANN beschrieben. Wahrscheinlich war hier eine gastrointestinale Infektion die Ursache.

d) Das Erythema nodosum bei septischen Infektionen

Eine Krankheit, in deren Verlauf das Erythema nodosum häufiger auftritt, ist Scharlach (MORO, MÓRITZ). In diesen Fällen dürften die Streptokokken eine wesentliche Rolle in der Pathogenese des Erythema nodosum spielen, denn es existieren zahlreiche Beobachtungen, nach denen auch andere Streptokokkeninfekte ein Erythema nodosum auslösen können. Neben den zahlreich mitgeteilten Befunden von hämolytischen Streptokokken auf den Tonsillen von Patienten mit Erythema nodosum lassen hauptsächlich eine Reihe von experimentellen Arbeiten auf enge Zusammenhänge zwischen Streptokokkeninfekt und Erythema nodosum schließen:

So gelang es SIMON et al., WOLF mit einer polyvalenten Streptokokkenvaccine bei einem Patienten ein außerordentlich heftiges Erythema nodosum auszulösen. CSERVENKA, KALLNER et al., BJÖRNESJÖ, CARAMANIAN et al. fanden bei verschiedenen Fällen von Erythema nodosum stark erhöhte Antistreptolysintiter. Stark positive Hautteste mit Streptokokkentoxinen konnten CARAMANIAN et al., COLLIS, SASAI, FAVOUR erzielen. Wichtig ist die Mitteilung von SPINK, der durch intradermale Injektion von Bouillonkulturfiltraten von Streptokokken Erythema nodosum-Knoten hervorrufen konnte, die histologisch das gleiche Bild wie die spontan entstandenen Knoten zeigten. Er fand in seinem Krankenmaterial von zehn Patienten mit Erythema nodosum nur einen mit Tuberkulose, die andern zeigten in ihrem Rachenabstrich hämolytische Streptokokken. Auch COBURN u. MOORE beschrieben Experimente, wonach bei 22 Patienten mit Erythema nodosum sehr starke Hautreaktionen mit Nucleoprotein aus Streptococcus haemolyticus ausgelöst werden konnten, während Tuberkulin negativ reagierte. Alle Kranken hatten hohe Antistreptolysintiter. Bei einigen konnten auch neue Schübe von Erythema nodosum nach Injektion des Nucleoproteins ausgelöst werden. LEMAIRE et al. beschreiben Patienten, die einen ansteigenden Antistreptolysintiter im Verlauf eines Erythema nodosum zeigten. NONCLERCQ et al. fanden neben einem hohen Antistreptolysintiter eine γ-Globulin- und Fibrinvermehrung, TRUELOVE einen erhöhten Waaler-Rose-Test. FAVOUR et al. konnten bei 50% ihrer Erythema nodosum-Fälle hämolytische Streptokokken im Rachenabstrich finden. Ein Teil dieser Patienten reagierte auf einen Intracutantest mit einer Vaccine aus diesen Stämmen mit Allgemeinerscheinungen. Auch FORMAN fand ähnliche Verhältnisse. SLOT konnte mit Antistreptokokkenserum in kürzester Zeit vier Fälle von Erythema nodosum zum Verschwinden bringen. Er glaubt, daß in London die Mehrzahl der Erythema nodosum-Fälle durch Streptokokken bedingt seien. Andererseits konnte GARBINI mit Streptokokkenstämmen von Patienten mit Erythema nodosum keinen Dermotropismus im Tierversuch finden. Für eine septische Genese des Erythema nodosum sprechen auch die Beobachtungen von ALMQUIST, wobei bei einem Patienten nach jeder Zahnextraktion ein Erythema nodosum auftrat und nach Extraktion sämtlicher Zähne ausblieb. Auch ELWELL beschrieb den Fall eines Erythema nodosum, das nach Extraktion zweier cariöser Zähne sofort heilte. MEYER glaubt, daß solche septischen Herde in einer latenten Phlebitis der Beine liegen könnten.

e) Das Erythema nodosum bei Lymphogranuloma inguinale Nicolas-Favre

Neben den schon erwähnten Untersuchungen von SIMPSON hat sich speziell HELLERSTRÖM mit der Frage des Erythema nodosum bei Lymphogranuloma inguinale befaßt. Nach seinen Feststellungen tritt das Erythema nodosum dann auf, wenn die Stärke der Freischen Hautreaktion zunimmt und ihren Höhepunkt erreicht. Diese Beobachtung wird durch Carnot et al. bestätigt. Es gelang Hellerström auch, durch wiederholte Injektion des Antigens neue Schübe von Erythema nodosum zu erzeugen. Auch Sézary et al. und Sakurane et al. erwähnen ähnliche Beobachtungen.

f) Erythema nodosum bei Pilzerkrankungen

Über solche Fälle berichten Ballagi, Apffel und Burgun. Walther sah ein typisches, auch histologisch verifiziertes Erythema nodosum bei einer Epidermophytie, Fuhs ebenfalls ein histologisch verifiziertes Erythema nodosum bei einer Trichophytie auftreten. Urbach gelang es, aus den Knoten eines Erythema nodosum bei Trichophytie Trichophyton gypseum zu züchten.

g) Erythema nodosum bei Boeckschem Sarkoid

Es scheint, daß das Boecksche Sarkoid zunehmend häufig im Formenkreis des Erythema nodosum eine Rolle spielt. So berichtet James über 170 Patienten im Alter von 4—70 Jahren, von denen 126 an einer Sarkoidose litten und nur 21 an Tuberkulose. Bock hat mittels Leberpunktion die Diagnose einer Sarkoidose in seinen Fällen histologisch gesichert. James et al. haben den Kveim-Test zur Diagnose verwendet. Er war bei $^2/_3$ ihrer Patienten positiv. Bei den meisten dieser Patienten bestand ebenfalls eine Polyarthritis. Finucane konstatierte bei 37 Patienten mit Lungensarkoidose in 12 Fällen ein Erythema nodosum. Weniger sicher ist der Fall von Boström, bei dem zusammen mit Hilusdrüsenschwellungen ein Erythema nodosum auftrat. Während sich die Lungenveränderungen zurückbildeten, wurden die vorher schwach positiven Tuberkulinreaktionen stark positiv. Auch der von Michel et al. beschriebene Fall von massiven mediastinalen Drüsenschwellungen und Erythema nodosum, der unter Behandlung mit INH rasch zurückging, ist nicht sicher zu beurteilen. Winkler und Leggat machen darauf aufmerksam, daß Erythema nodosum-ähnliche Knoten durch Sarkoidgewebe vorgetäuscht werden können. Parisi beschreibt einen Fall, bei dem nebeneinander Knoten von Boeckschem Sarkoid und Erythema nodosum vorhanden waren.

Diese nichttuberkulöse, deshalb auch benigne Hiluslymphadenopathie (Löfgren-Syndrom) genannte Kombination von Erythema nodosum mit Lungenveränderungen braucht nun nicht unbedingt mit dem Boeckschen Sarkoid identisch zu sein (Waisman et al., Dünner). Sie sind oft so passager, daß kaum ein Boecksches Granulationsgewebe die Ursache der Schwellung sein dürfte. Sicher können auch unspezifische Infekte diese Veränderungen hervorrufen (Stucki). Ob der Name Adénopathies exanthématogènes dieses Krankheitsbild besser charakterisiert (Meyer et al.), sei dahingestellt.

h) Erythema nodosum bei Lues

Ein Zusammentreffen beider Krankheiten wird so selten beobachtet, daß wohl kaum je ein ursächlicher Zusammenhang angenommen worden ist, dies auch deshalb, weil das Erythema nodosum ganz unabhängig vom Stadium der Lues auftreten kann. So wurde die Bildung von Knoten vor der Behandlung (Duvoir et al., Weissenbach et al.), während der Behandlung in der Art einer Herxheimerschen Reaktion [Gougerot et Séringe (1937), Veltman, Mazzanti, Guggenheim] beobachtet oder aber ein Rückgang der Knoten während der Behandlung gesehen.

i) Erythema nodosum bei Coccidioidomykose

Eine wesentliche Bereicherung der Kenntnis der Ursachen des Erythema nodosum haben die Berichte amerikanischer Autoren gebracht, wonach bei der Infektion mit Coccidioides immitis, die in bestimmten Teilen Südkaliforniens endemisch auftritt (San Joaquin valley fever), mit großer Regelmäßigkeit ein Erythema nodosum aufzutreten pflegt. Das klinische Bild dieser Infektion ähnelt zu Beginn einer Bronchopneumonie, an die sich ein Erythema nodosum, dann eine Arthritis oder Conjunctivitis anschließt. Röntgenologisch zeigen sich lokalisierte Lungeninfiltrate. Die Krankheit befällt hauptsächlich Personen im Alter von 10—40 Jahre, und die Prognose ist gut. Nach Berichten von FABER et al., SMITH, THORNER beträgt die Inkubationszeit 1—3 Wochen. Befallen werden vorzugsweise Frauen (75% der Fälle). Die Tuberkulinreaktion ist sehr selten positiv, der Erreger läßt sich manchmal im Sputum nachweisen. Die Hautreaktion mit Coccidioidin wird kurz nach Ausbruch des Erythema nodosum positiv.

k) Erythema nodosum bei Lepra

Es ist bei dieser Krankheit schwer zu entscheiden, ob es sich bei den Knoten um ein echtes Erythema nodosum oder um Leprome handelt. Um solche dürfte es sich dort handeln, wo Virchowsche Zellen und Leprabacillen gefunden werden konnten (PORTUGAL, SALOMÃO). Es wird auch betont, daß die von MIESCHER beschriebenen radiären Knötchen nicht gefunden werden können. VADE faßt deshalb diese nodosumartigen Erscheinungen als Leprareaktion auf. Sie seien seit der Sulfon-Behandlung häufiger geworden. Eine interessante Beobachtung konnten BOLGERT et al. machen. Ein kleines leprakrankes Mädchen zeigte ein echtes kontusiformes Erythema nodosum, das reichlich Bacillen enthielt und nach Behandlung mit Thiosemicarbazon bacillenfrei wurde. Nach BCG-Impfung trat ein neuer Schub auf. Die Knoten waren diesmal oberflächlicher, weniger ausgedehnt, nicht kontusiform und enthielten keine Leprabacillen. Daß auch die Leprareaktion vom Typus des Erythema nodosum irgendwie mit Abwehrphänomenen des Organismus verbunden ist, zeigten SILVA und ANDRADE, die im Serum Lepröser Hämagglutinationen durchführten. Die höchsten Werte fanden sie bei aktiver lepromatöser Lepra, die niedrigsten bei der tuberkuloiden Form. Trat bei Leprösen eine Reaktion vom Typus des Erythema nodosum auf, so fiel der Titer ab. Im ganzen genommen, zeigt aber das Erythema nodosum bei Lepra so wesentliche Unterschiede vom echten Erythema nodosum, daß PEBLER et al. vorgeschlagen haben, den Namen des Erythema nodosum leprosum fallenzulassen und durch akute Panniculitis nodosa leprosa zu ersetzen.

l) Das rheumatische Erythema nodosum

Wie bereits aus der Beschreibung der mit Tuberkulose verbundenen Fälle von Erythema nodosum hervorgeht, sind dabei rheumatoide Erscheinungen in Form von Polyarthritis derart häufig, daß es schwer fällt, ein echtes rheumatisches Erythema nodosum klar abzugrenzen. KEIL betont, daß die Diagnose eines rheumatischen Erythema nodosum nur nach gründlicher und lange dauernder Beobachtung des Patienten gestellt werden könnte. Daß es aber tatsächlich rheumatische Fälle gibt, zeigen diejenigen Statistiken, die über zahlreiche tuberkulinnegative Fälle berichten (ERNBERG et al.), und diejenigen Einzelfälle, die an interkurrenten Krankheiten starben und wo bei der Sektion keine Zeichen von Tuberkulose gefunden werden konnten (STRINGER, ERNBERG et al.). Auch nach den Untersuchungen KAHLMETERs liegt dem Erythema nodosum mit Polyarthritis keineswegs immer Tuberkulose zugrunde.

m) Andere Ursachen des Erythema nodosum

SASLAW et al., LITTLE et al. und NUTTALL-SMITH sahen einen Fall von Erythema nodosum bei einem 13jährigen tuberkulinnegativen Mädchen mit Histoplasmose. THIERS und TIVOLET beobachteten zwei Schübe von Erythema nodosum bei einem 11jährigen tuberkulinnegativen Mädchen, das wegen Katzenkratzkrankheit mit Dihydromycin behandelt worden war. FORD sah zwei Frauen, die nach Leberextraktinjektionen post partum ein Erythema nodosum entwickelten. DITTRICH beschreibt eine 22jährige Patientin, bei der 10% Olobintin wegen einer Pyodermie intramuskulär gegeben wurde. Drei Tage später trat ein typisches Erythema nodosum auf. Die Patientin wies zahlreiche Zahngranulome auf. Nach Zahnextraktion zeigte sich ein neuer Schub des Erythema nodosum. KREMENTCHOUSKY et al. beschrieben das Auftreten eines Erythema nodosum gleichzeitig mit einem ausgedehnten Herpes.

4. Pathogenese

Überblickt man nun die zahlreichen Arbeiten über die Ätiologie des Erythema nodosum, so lassen sich daraus für die Pathogenese folgende Schlüsse ziehen:

1. Das Erythema nodosum beruht auf einer gewissen individuellen Disposition (ROOSVALL). Dafür sprechen die zahlreichen Familieninfektionen mit Tuberkulose, wo gleichzeitig ein Erythema nodosum auftritt, und die Tatsache, daß das weibliche Geschlecht stark bevorzugt ist. Diese Bevorzugung macht sich allerdings im Kindesalter noch nicht so deutlich bemerkbar wie später (SANDRA). So beschreiben PRAG das Auftreten von Erythema nodosum bei Kindern im Verhältnis 1:1, DOXIADIS, NAGI in einem Verhältnis 3 Mädchen : 2 Knaben, während später die Frauen im Verhältnis bis 4:1 (THOMPSON et al., FIERRO, VESEY et al.) überwiegen. Die Ursache dieser Geschlechtsbevorzugung läßt sich vielleicht aus den Beobachtungen vermuten, wonach Stilboestrolinjektionen ein Erythema nodosum auslösen konnten (SONCK) oder dieses immer prämenstruell auftrat (STORCK et al.).

2. Es besteht eine eindeutige Abhängigkeit des Erythema nodosum von der Jahreszeit. So wird übereinstimmend die Häufung der Erythema nodosum-Fälle in den Frühlingsmonaten (NAGY) und ihre Seltenheit im Spätsommer angegeben. Sie entspricht der Erkrankungskurve an Hauttuberkulose (GOLUPZOWA).

3. Bei gewissen Infektionskrankheiten wie Tuberkulose, Streptokokkeninfekten, Coccidioidomykose, Lymphogranuloma inguinale tritt das Erythema nodosum gehäuft auf. Bei diesen Krankheiten kann es auch besonders häufig mittels spezifischer Impfstoffe oder Sulfathiazol provoziert werden. Auch nichthämolysierende Streptokokken in cariösen Zähnen können wahrscheinlich als ätiologischer Faktor eine Rolle spielen (WESTERGREN).

4. Das Erythema nodosum steht in eindeutigem Zusammenhang mit spontanen oder künstlich erzeugten Allergieschwankungen des Organismus. Dies zeigt sich deutlich speziell bei der Tuberkulose, wo diese Allergieschwankungen mittels der Tuberkulinreaktion verfolgt werden können. Möglicherweise spielt hier das vegetative Nervensystem eine Rolle (LOEWENTHAL, SAMAJA).

5. Es besteht kein Unterschied im histologischen Bild des Erythema nodosum bei den verschiedenen Krankheiten.

Für dieses Verhalten können verschiedene Gründe geltend gemacht werden: a) Es kann sich um eine selbständige Krankheit handeln, die auf verschiedene Weise provoziert werden kann und die deshalb unter dem prinzipiell gleichen klinischen und histologischen Bild abläuft (COMBY). b) Es kann sich um eine allergische Reaktion auf verschiedene Toxine und Medikamente handeln.

Es dürfte wohl heute noch zu früh sein, diese Frage definitiv zu entscheiden, da es bisher nicht gelungen ist, einen Erreger zu finden, der für das Erythema nodosum spezifisch wäre. Wohl sprechen die Befunde MIESCHERs über spezifische, sonst nicht beobachtete Granulome für eine selbständige Stellung des Erythema nodosum, doch ist die Auffassung des Erythema nodosum als einer allergischen Reaktion auf verschiedene Noxen durch die verschiedenen Beobachtungen der Bindung an einen bestimmten Reaktionszustand des Organismus, wie er sich bei der Tuberkulose, beim Lymphogranuloma inguinale und bei der Coccidioidomykose experimentell leicht verfolgen läßt, möglicherweise auch auf Grund epidemiologischer Beobachtungen (TRABAUD) derart eindrücklich, daß auch die Befürworter der allergischen Genese des Erythema nodosum (GOUGEROT, PAUTRIER, MOGENSEN, TREPICCIONI, WALLGREN, LANGDORF) sehr zahlreiche Gründe für ihre Anschauung ins Feld führen können.

Eindeutig ist die Auffassung abzulehnen, daß es sich beim Erythema nodosum um eine Hauttuberkulose (ONTANEDA et al.) oder gar um eine autogene Tuberkulinreaktion (ERNBERG) handelt. Wohl spielt die Tuberkulose bei seiner Auslösung in weiten Gebieten der Erde eine wichtige Rolle, so daß in jedem Fall von Erythema nodosum, speziell bei Kindern, auf Tuberkulose als die wichtigste Ursache gefahndet werden muß (CERVINI et al., DOXIADIS, SCHNEIDER, CANTONNET BLANCH, SARROUY et al., MORQUIO, VERGER, HALBRON et al., OPITZ), im Interesse des Patienten darf diese Ätiologie aber auch nicht überwertet werden (BLOCH und SCHUPPLI).

5. Diagnose und Differentialdiagnose

Die Diagnose des typischen Erythema nodosum dürfte wohl kaum Schwierigkeiten machen, da der akute fieberhafte Beginn mit Angina, Gelenkschmerzen und das typische Exanthem mit keiner andern Krankheit verwechselt werden kann. Schwieriger sind diejenigen Fälle zu deuten, bei denen knotenförmige Exantheme ohne Initialsymptome auftreten oder welche einen besonders hartnäckigen und chronischen Verlauf zeigen. Dabei wird ein Erythema induratum Bazin auf Grund des histologischen Bildes und auch der Umwandlung der Knoten in den meisten Fällen abgegrenzt werden können. Schwieriger dürfte die Differentialdiagnose gegenüber den nodösen Vaskulitiden sein, auf die im Kapitel der Periarteriitis nodosa noch näher eingegangen werden soll. CAROL et al. haben der Differentialdiagnose der nodösen Veränderungen eine spezielle Studie gewidmet.

6. Therapie

Daß die alte Salicyltherapie immer noch Gültigkeit hat, zeigen verschiedene Berichte. Außerdem werden empfohlen: Prontosil (SIMON, ENGELHARDT, HÜLLSTRUNG), Sulfathiazol (CIOFFI), Thioharnstoff für alle Formen von Erythema nodosum (THIERS et al.), Deseptyl (SZENTKIRÁLYI), Irgapyrin (NAVARRO-MARTÍN et al.), Penicillin, wenn Streptokokken gefunden werden (MUNTEANU). Quarzlicht kann ebenfalls günstig wirken (MÓRITZ, NIKLASSON). Neuerdings wird Cortison speziell für diejenigen Fälle empfohlen, die auf Salicylate und Antibiotica nicht ansprechen. Die Wirkung setzt sehr rasch ein, wobei Heilungen innerhalb 12 Std (URELES et al.) bis 2 Tagen (FARBER et al., WETZEL, SCHNEIERSON) beschrieben werden.

Literatur

ABRAMSON, L.: Der Komplex Arthralgie, Erythema nodosum, doppelseitige Hilusdrüsenschwellung und Tuberkulinnegativität. Nord. Med. **1943**, 129. — ALMQUIST, A. L.: Erythema nodosum of dental origin. J. oral Surg. **10**, 231 (1952). — ANTUNES LEAL, J.: Erythema nodosum durch Sulfathiazol. Rev. clín. esp. **8**, 116 (1943). — APFFEL, K., u. F. BURGUN: Zur Frage des nicht tuberkulösen Erythema nodosum beim Kinde. Kinderärztl. Prax. **13**, 57 (1942). — ARAOZ ALVARO, G.: Das Erythema nodosum und seine Beziehungen zur Tuberkulose. Rev. argent. Tuberc. **3**, 79 (1937). — ARENA, A.-R.: Existence du Mycobacterium tuberculosis dans les nodules de l'érythème noueux. C. R. Soc. Biol. (Paris) **115**, 340 (1934). — Nachweis von Tuberkelbacillen bei Erythema nodosum. Rev. Inst. bact. (B. Aires) **6**, 170 (1934). — ARNAUD, J.: Bacillémie précédant un érythème noueux apparu au cours d'une granule froide. Rev. Tuberc. (Paris) **5**, 63 (1939). — Reproduction de nodosité d'érythème noueux par des extraits bacillaires chez un malada porteur d'érythème noueux. Rev. Tuberc. (Paris) **5**, 65 (1939).

BÄFVERSTEDT, B.: Erythema nodosum migrans. Acta derm.-venereol. (Stockh.) **34**, 181 (1954). — Zur Kenntnis des atypischen Erythema nodosum. Arch. klin. exp. Derm. **208**, 291 (1959). — BALLAGI, ST.: Ein Fall von Erythema nodosum trichophyticum bei Trichophytia profunda des Kopfes. Ref. in Zbl. Haut- u. Geschl.-Kr. **68**, 361 (1942). — BATTISTIG, A.: L'eritema nodoso e di suoi esiti in un ventegno di clinica pediatrica. Arch. ital. Pediat. **6**, 199 (1938). — BAUER, G.: Erythema nodosum nach Cibazol und Tuberkulose. Schweiz. Z. Tuberk. **6**, 273 (1949). — BERG, G.: Sind früher durchgemachte Pleuritis und Erythema nodosum von Einfluß auf die Prognose der Lungentuberkulose? Ein Beitrag zur Frage über das Vorkommen von erworbener Immunität und über die Bedeutung der Tuberkulinreaktion in prognostischer Hinsicht. Das Gotenburger Material 1910—1934. Beitr. Klin. Tuberk. **98**, 1 (1942). — BERGSTRAND, H.: Is Erythema nodosum a hypersensibility reaction of anaphylactic type? Acta derm.-venereol. (Stockh.) **29**, 539 (1949). — BÉTHOUX, L., et E. BERTHET: Un cas de primo-infection tuberculeuse avec érythème noueux chez une fillette de onze ans. Bull. Soc. méd. Hôp. Paris, III. s. **51**, 508 (1935). — BIEHLER, M. DE: Contribution à l étude de l'érythème noueux. Arch. Méd. Enf. **39**, 817 (1936). — BINDSCHEDLER, J.-J.: L'érythème noueux témoin de l'augmentation de l'allergie à la tuberculine. Son apparition à la suite de réactions tuberculiniques. Bull. Soc. Pédiat. Paris **34**, 545 (1936). — BIRATH, G.: Die Prognose bei Lungentuberkulose, der ein Erythema nodosum vorausgegangen ist. Acta tuberc. scand. **51**, 115 (1941). — BJÖRNESJÖ, K. B.: Erythema nodosum mit Lungenveränderungen nicht tuberkulöser Natur. Svenska Läk.-Tidn. **1949**, 930. — BLANKSMA, P.: Erythema nodosum. Ned. T. Geneesk. **1947**, 2341. — BLOCH, W., u. R. SCHUPPLI: Untersuchungen an 132 Fällen von Erythema nodosum. Dermatologica (Basel) **97**, Suppl. 11 (1948). — BLUEFARB, S. M., S. WALLK and J. LATONI: Erythema nodosum with conjunctival nodules. Arch. Derm. **80**, 107 (1959). — BOAS, E.: Fall von Erythema nodosum mit Tuberkelbacillen im Blute. Hospitalstidende **1933**, 888. — BOCK, H. E.: Zur Allergielage beim Erythema nodosum im Rahmen des Löfgren-Syndroms. Allergie u. Asthma **6**, 121 (1960). — BOLGERT, M., M. L. R. MONTEL et G. LÉVY: Un cas d'érythème noueux d'origine Hansenienne. Rapport de cet érythème avec Erythema nodosum leprosum. Bull. Soc. franç. Derm. Syph. **61**, 528 (1954). — BOOTH, L. E.: Erythema nodosum. Amer. J. Dis. Child. **85**, 648 (1953). — BOSTRÖM, G.: Rückbildung der Lungenveränderungen bei einer gutartigen Lymphogranulomatose im Anschluß an ein Erythema nodosum. Acta derm.-venereol. (Stockh.) **21**, 38 (1940). — BOVENKAMP, G. J. VAN DEN: Erythema nodosum. Ned. T. Geneesk. **1934**, 407. — BRIEGER, H.: Über die allergische Natur des durch Sulfathiazol erzeugten Erythema nodosum. Arch. Kinderheilk. **133**, 161 (1947). — BROCK, J.: Über die klinische und epidemiologische Bedeutung des Erythema nodosum im Kindesalter. Münch. med. Wschr. **1933 II**, 1087. — BROUWER, P.: Einige Beobachtungen über die Bedeutung des Erythema nodosum für die Epidemiologie der Tuberkulose. Ned. T. Geneesk. **1940**, 1501.

CANTONNET BLANCH, P.: Erythema nodosum, Dermatitis contusiforme oder Trousseausche Krankheit. Rev. Tuberc. Urug. **5**, 329 (1936). — CARAMANIAN, M. K., et M. BOUVRY: Erythème noueux streptococcique récidivant. La nature rhumatismale. Bull. Soc. méd. Hôp. Paris **71**, 1129 (1955). — CARNOT, P., R. CACHERA et MALLARMÉ: Maladie de Nicolas-Favre et érythème noueux. Bull. Soc. méd. Hôp. Paris, III. 2. **52**, 1108 (1936). — CAROL, W. L. L., J. R. PRAKKEN and H. A. VAN ZWIJNDREGT: Erythema nodosum and relapsing non-suppurative panniculitis. Arch. Derm. Syph. (Berl.) **182**, 329 (1941). — CARTAGENOVA, L., e M. CAJATI: Ulteriore destino di loro che furono affetti d eritema nodoso. Pediatria (Napoli) **54**, 400 (1956). — CASTRO FREIRE, L. DE, et J. MARQUES PINTO: La bacillémie et l'ultravirus tuberculeux dans l érythème noueux. C. R. Soc. Biol. (Paris) **116**, 165 (1934). — CERVINI, PASCUAL R., u. G. A. BOGANI: Erythema nodosum und Tuberkulose. Arch. argent. Pediat. **4**, 660 (1933). — CHABAUD, H., et TOUPANCE: Epidémie familiale d'érythème noueux. Rev. Tuberc. (Paris) **5**, 1207 (1940). — CHEVALLIER, P.: Une épidémie d'érythème noueux dans un pensionnat de jeunes filles. Bull. Soc. franç. Derm. Syph. **39**, 1236 (1932). — CHINI, V.: Brevi considerazioni intorno al significato di alcune cutireazioni nell'eritema nodoso. Boll. Ist. sieroter. milan. **14**, 163 (1935). — CIBILS AGUIRRE, R.: Tuberkulöse Ätiologie des Erythema nodosum. Arch. argent. Pediat. **4**, 617, 697 (1933). — Vérification expérimentale de l'étiologie tuberculeuse de l'érythème noueux. (Comm. préalable.) Arch. Méd. Enf. **36**, 521

(1933). — Tuberkulöse Primärinfektion mit der Haut als Eintrittspforte und sekundäres Erythema nodosum. Arch. argent. Pediat. **7**, 69, 161 (1936). — Etiologie tuberculeuse de l'érythème noueux. Démonstration bactériologique. Verh. 9. Internat. Kongr. Dermat. **2**, 284 (1936). — Der bakteriologische Beweis der tuberkulösen Ätiologie des Erythema nodosum. Ref. in Zbl. Haut- u. Geschl.-Kr. **56**, 58 (1937). — CIBILS AGUIRRE, R., et A. R. ARENA: Etiologie tuberculeuse de l'érythème noueux, démonstration bactériologique. Arch. Méd. Enf. **39**, 137 (1936). — CIOFFI, E.: I sulfamidi thiazolici nella cura dell'eritema nodoso. Med. trop. **1**, 150 (1941). — COBURN, A. F., and L. V. MOORE: Experimental induction of erythema nodosum. J. clin. Invest. **15**, 509 (1936). — COLLIS, W. R. F.: Erythema nodosum. Brit. med. J. **1933**, Nr 3807, 1162. — COMBY, J.: A propos de l'érythème noueux. Bull. Soc. méd. Hôp. Paris, III. s. **50**, 1740 (1934). — Tuberculose infantile et érythème noueux. Bull. Soc. méd. Hôp. Paris **53**, 975 (1937). — COSTE, F., et J. BERNARD: Erythème noueux et néphrite après section de brides chez une tuberculeuse. Bull. Soc. méd. Hôp. Paris, III. s. **50**, 1680 (1934). — CROSNIER, R.: Erythème noueux et typhobacillose. Actualité de la question. Paris méd. **1942 II**, 388. — CSERVENKA, I.: Antistreptolysinuntersuchungen bei Patienten mit Erythema nodosum. Zit. in Zbl. Haut- u. Geschl.-Kr. **109**, 48 (1961).

DEBRÉ, R.: Erythème noueux et tuberculose. Bull. Soc. franç. Derm. Syph. **45**, 1091 (1938). — DEBRÉ, R., A. SAENZ et R. BROCA: Bacillémie tuberculeuse chez les enfants atteints d'érythème noueux. Arch. Méd. Enf. **39**, 787 (1936). — Bull. Acad. nat. Méd. (Paris) **116**, 26 (1936). — DEBRÉ, R., A. SAENZ, R. BROCA et J. BERNARD: Présence simultanée du bacille de Koch virulent dans les nodosités cutanées et dans le sang d'un enfant au début d'une poussée d'érythème noueux, expression de la primo-infection tuberculeuse. C. R. Soc. Biol. (Paris) **119**, 1290 (1935). — DEBRÉ, R., A. SAENZ, R. BROCA et R. MALLAY: Etude sur l'érythème noueux. Rev. franç. Pédiat. **14**, 433 (1938). — DEMOLE, M.-J.: L'érythème noueux épidémique. Rev. méd. Suisse rom. **53**, 633 (1933). — DEMURTAS, C.: Su un'epidemia di eritema nodoso. Clin. pediat. (Bologna) **17**, 271 (1935). — DES ROCHETTES, M., et P. PAILLAS: Erythème noueux et adénite inguinale tuberculeuse après vaccination de Marbet chez un sujet antérieurement vacciné au BCG. Rev. Tuberc. (Paris) **18**, 929 (1954). — DICKEY, L. B.: Erythema nodosum and tuberculosis in children. Amer. Rev. Tuberc. **26**, 614 (1932). — DIETEL, F.: Erythema nodosum-artiges Exanthem nach Sulfathiazolbehandlung. Derm. Wschr. **119**, 257 (1947). — DITTRICH, O.: Über Olobintin und Herdaktivierung. Ein Beitrag zur Genese des Erythema nodosum. Z. Haut- u. Geschl.-Kr. **7**, 409 (1949). — DOGRAMACI, I.: Erythema nodosum in childhood in Turkey. Ann. paediat. (Basel) **154**, 357 (1940). — DOMINGUEZ LUQUE, J.: Zur Ätiopathogenese des Erythema nodosum. Arch. esp. Pediat. **17**, 298 (1933). — DOXIADIS, S. A.: Ätiologie des Erythema nodosum bei Kindern. Brit. med. J. **1949**, 844. — Erythema nodosum in children. A review. Medicine (Baltimore) **30**, 283 (1951). — DÜNNER, L.: Erythema nodosum und doppelseitige Hilusdrüsenschwellung. Ein klinisches Syndrom. Med. Klin. **1957**, 449. — DUVOIR, M., L. POLLET et J. BERNARD: Erythème noueux et syphilis secondaire. Bull. Soc. méd. Hôp. Paris, III. s. **49**, 42 (1933).

ELWELL, L. B.: Erythema nodosum and focal infection. Brit. med. J. **1935**, 974. — ENGELHARDT: Erythema nodosum. Vereinigung Düsseldorfer Dermat. Sitzung 20. 7. 1936. Ref. in Zbl. Haut- u. Geschl.-Kr. **54**, 488 (1937). — ERNBERG, H.: Erythema nodosum and tuberculosis. Amer. J. Dis. Child. **46**, 1297 (1933). — Das Knotenerythem, ein Warnungssignal. Svenska Nat.-Fören. Tuberk. Kvart. **30**, 1 (1935). — ERNBERG, H., u. O. GABINUS: Häufung von Erythema nodosum-Fällen bei nichttuberkulöser Pathogenese. Nord. med. T. **1938**, 300. — ESBIERG, H. O.: Ein Fall von Uveo-parotitis, begleitet von Erythema nodosum und Lungenveränderungen. Acta ophthal. (Kbh.) **19**, 286 (1941).

FABER, H. K., T. E. SMITH and E. C. DICKSON: Acute coccidioidomycosis with erythema nodosum in children. J. Pediat. **15**, 163 (1939). — FALK, C. A.: Erythema nodosum mit nachfolgendem Erythema induratum. Hygiea (Stockh.) **97**, 572 (1935). — FARBER, S., and H. MANDELBAUM: Use of Cortisone in Erythema nodosum. Arch. intern. Med. **88**, 395 (1951). — FAURE-BEAULIEU: Contagion entre érythème polymorphe et érythème noueux; déductions pathogéniques. Bull. Soc. méd. Hôp. Paris, III. s. **52**, 1265 (1936). — FAVOUR, C. B., and C. M. SOSMAN: Erythema nodosum. Arch. intern. Med. **80**, 435 (1947). — FERRARI, A. V.: Eruzioni a tipo di eritema nodoso dopo applicazione di materiali tubercolinici in individui affetti da tubercolosi cutanea. Boll. Sez. region. Soc. ital. Derm. **3**, 238 (1933). — FIERRO, V. M.: Eritema nuodoso en el joven adulto. Tórax **1**, 105 (1952). — FINUCANE, B.: Erythema nodosum as a manifestation of sarcoidosis. J. Irish med. Ass. **50**, 132 (1962). — FLANDIN, CH., G. POUMEAU-DELILLE et P. AUZEPY: Erythème noueux au cours d'une cortico-pleurite tuberculeuse et d'un abcès bismuthique de la fesse évoluant simultanément. Bull. Soc. méd. Hôp. Paris, III. s. **50**, 1751 (1934). — FORD, F. D. C.: Puerperal erythema nodosum after liver extract injections. Treatment with prednisone. Brit. med. J. **1960 I**, 400. — FORMAN, L.: On the aetiology of erythema nodosum. Brit. J. Derm. **48**, 123 (1936). — FORMAN, L., and G. P. B. WHITWELL: Preliminary observations on erythema nodosum. Guy's Hosp. Rep. **84**, 213 (1934). — FUHS, H.: Ein Fall von Trichophyton gypseum kerium und Erythema nodosum trichophyticum, das histologisch typisch war. Zbl. Haut- u. Geschl.-Kr. **68**, 411 (1942).

GAMSTEDT, E.: Über die Tuberkulinempfindlichkeit bei Erythema nodosum vor der Eruption. Mschr. Kinderheilk. **59**, 111 (1933). — GARBINI, R.: Osservazioni e ricerche sul tropismo degli streptococchi isolati da focolai infettivi di individui con eritema nodoso. Pathologica **27**, 223 (1935). — GATÉ, J., L. GRAVIER, G. CHANIAL et G. BERTRAND: Cellulites nodulaires tuberculeuses caséfiées à type d'érythème noueux. Syndrome fébrile avec arthralgies. Images radiographiques d'ostéite cystoide. Bull. Soc. franç. Derm. Syph. **44**, 738 (1937a). — GATÉ, J., P. J. MICHEL et J. RACOUCHOT: Erythème noueux avec parotite et sous-maxillite chez une jeune fille ayant eu récemment une hémoptysie. Bull. Soc. franç. Derm. Syph. **44**, 173 (1937b). — GENÉVRIER, I., et F. BORDET: Terrain et primo-infection. Rev. Tuberc. (Paris) **6**, 35 (1951). — GIERTSEN, CH.: Four cases of erythema nodosum and „Frühinfiltrat". Acta med. scand. **82**, 55 (1934). — 93 cases of erythema nodosum. Acta med. scand. **82**, 87 (1934). — GILMAN, R. L.: Involuting erythema nodosum followed by an annular eruption of the face. Arch. Derm. Syph. (Chic.) **32**, 536 (1935). — GLASS: Toxisches Exanthem vom Charakter eines Erythema nodosum nach Eleudron. Wiener Dermat. Ges. Sitzg 12. 6. 1943. Ref. in Zbl. Haut- u. Geschl.-Kr. **70**, 499 (1943). — GÖBEL, W.: Eine Schulendemie von Erythema nodosum. Z. Kinderheilk. **55**, 30 (1933). — Über Erythema nodosum. Ther. d. Gegenw. **74**, 496 (1933). — GÖBEL, W., u. E. SCHUHARDT: Beitrag zur Frage des Erythema nodosum. Z. Tuberk. **69**, 260 (1934). — GOLUPZOWA, V. S.: Erythema nodosum in der früheren Kindheit. Pediatr. **11**, 87 (1938). — GORDON, H.: Case of tuberculous infection with erythema nodosum. Brit. J. Derm. **45**, 69 (1933). — Erythema nodosum. A review of 115 cases. Brit. J. Derm. **73**, 393 (1961). — GOUGEROT, H.: Erythème noueux. Syndrome de „réaction de défense par sensibilisation". Arch. derm.-syph. (Paris) 8, 263 (1936). — GOUGEROT, H., et J. DELORT: Erythème noueux et placards érythémato-squameux. Discussion d'une „réaction seconde" tuberculeuse. Bull. Soc. franç. Derm. Syph. **44**, 275 (1937). — GOUGEROT, H., et R. MATHIEU: Parapsoriasis de Mucha chronique. Erythème noueux intercurrent. Bull. Soc. franç. Derm. Syph. **44**, 48 (1937). — Arch. derm.-syph. (Paris) **9**, 509 (1937). — GOUGEROT, H., et PH. SÉRINGE: Erythema haemorrhagicum et necroticum. Arch. dermato-syphlogr. Hôp. St. Louis **9**, 497 (1937). — Anallergie à la tuberculine, à la luétine et à une protéine étrangère au cours d'un érythème noueux classique. Arch. derm.-syph. (Paris) **9**, 501 (1937). — GREENE, L. S., and P. MATTHEW-WHITE: Erythema nodosum with nodules in the conjunctiva. Amer. J. Ophthal. **22**, 389 (1939). — GREITHER, A.: Über das Erythema nodosum, vor allem über die sog. symptomatischen Formen bei Geschlechtskrankheiten und nach Sulfathiazol. Arch. Derm. Syph. (Berl.) **186**, 525 (1948). — GRUPPER, C., et P. BEAUVOIS: Erythème noueux avec adénopathie médiastinale d'origine non-tuberculeuse. Bull. Soc. franç. Derm. Syph. **62**, 140 (1955). — GRZYBOWSKI: Sur l'anatomie pathologique de l érythème noueux. Bull. Soc. franç. Derm. Syph. **45**, 1073 (1938). — GUGGENHEIM, L.: Erythema nodosum bei primärer Syphilis. Dermatologica (Basel) **118**, 311 (1959).

HAIDVOGL, M.: Beobachtungen über die Infektiösität des Erythema nodosum. Beitr. Klin. Tuberk. **60**, 186 (1937). — HALBERTSMA, T.: Erythema nodosum mit negativen Tuberkulinreaktionen. Mschr. Kindergeneesk. **6**, 113 (1936). — HALBRON, P., et H.-P. KLOTZ: L'érythème noueux de l'adulte est-il toujours tuberculeux? Paris méd. **1936 II**, 37. — HALLANDER, H.: Erythema nodosum in a dispensary clientele. Acta tuberc. scand. **23**, 294 (1949). — HAMBURG-ZETLINA, E., u. A. KROPATSCHOV: Über die Ätiologie des Erythema nodosum bei Kindern. [Russisch.] Ref. in Zbl. Haut- u. Geschl.-Kr. **50**, 681 (1935). — HAROLD, J. T.: Familial Erythema nodosum. Tubercle (Lond.) **34**, 279 (1953). — HEIMBECK, J.: The significance of Erythema nodosum tuberculosum. Acta tuberc. scand. **24**, 388 (1950). — HELDENMAN, M. D., and M. SKOLNICK: Erythema nodosum and pulmonary tuberculosis in 2 sisters. Arch. Derm. **84**, 402 (1961). — HELLERSTRÖM, S.: Das Erythema nodosum-Problem im Lichte des Lymphogranuloma inguinale. Acta med. scand. **109**, 1 (1941). — HOFFMANN, M.: Erythema nodosum als Ausdruck einer massiven Infektion mit Tuberkelbacillen. Tuberkulose (Münch.) **14**, 99 (1934). — HUBER, J.: Erythème noueux et tuberculose. Bull. Soc. méd. Hôp. Paris, III. s. **51**, 1118 (1935). — HÜLLSTRUNG, H.: Neuere Anschauungen über die Ätiologie und Pathogenese des Erythema nodosum. Med. Klin. **1939 I**, 805.

INGEBRIGTSEN, G. L.: Erythema nodosum — Intrathoracale Tuberkulose. Acta tuberc. scand. **14**, 158 (1940). — ITO, K.: Skin vasculitis as seen from comparative exanthematology. II. Erythema nodosum following BCG vaccination. Bull. pharm. Res. Inst. **25**, 28 (1960). — ITO, K., and C. ANDO: Erythema nodosum associated with tuberculous cervical lymphadenitis and non-tubercular tonsillitis and its operative treatment. Bull. pharm. Res. Inst. **6**, 40 (1954).

JACOBS, W. H.: Erythema nodosum in inflammatory diseases of the bowel. Gastroenterology **37**, 286 (1959). — JACQUET, P., S. TIEFFRY et A. HAU: Un cas d'érythème noueux avec primo-infection tuberculeuse bénigne chez l'adulte. Bull. Soc. méd. Hôp. Paris, III. s. **51**, 420 (1935). — JAMES, D. G.: Erythema nodosum. Brit. med. J. **1961 I**, 853. — JAMES, G. D.,

A. D. THOMSON and A. WILCOX: Erythema nodosum as a manifestation of sarcoidosis. Lancet 1956 II, 218. — JAUSION, H., et S. TÉVÉNAU: Les vicissitudes de l'expérimentation et matière d'érythème noueux et d'érythème polymorphe. Bull. Soc. franç. Derm. Syph. 45, 1053 (1938). — JENSEN, O.: 12 cases of post primary Erythema nodosum in tuberculosis patients under a Morbilli epidemic. Acta tuberc. scand. 27, 343 (1952). — JERSILD, T., and K. IVERSEN: Erythema nodosum arising from treatment with sulfathiazole. Acta med. scand. 111, 105 (1942). — JOHANNESSEN: Erythema nodosum and subsequent tuberculosis. A follow-up study of 575 cases. Acta tuberc. scand. 26, 138 (1952). — JOSEPHSEN, G.: Erythema nodosum. Ugeskr. Laeg. 1933, 423.

KAHLMETER, G.: Quelques essais de culture, par le procédé de Löwenstein, de bacilles tuberculeux provenant du sang dans les polyarthritis aiguës, dans les endocardites et dans l'érythème noueux. Acta med. scand., Suppl. 50, 90 (1932). — KAJTOR, F.: Über einen Fall von Erythema nodosum im Anschluß an eine benigne abakterielle Meningitis. Wien. Z. Nervenheilk. 2, 291 (1949). — KALLNER, S., u. B. OLHAGEN: Fall von Erythema nodosum rheumaticum, behandelt mit Sulfapyridin. Nord. Med. 1942, 1838. — KEIL, H.: Relation of Erythema nodosum and rheumatic fever. A critical survey. Ann. intern. Med. 10, 1686 (1937). — KEIZER, D. P. R.: Erythema nodosum beim Säugling. Ned. Indie T. Geneesk. 1939, 1503. — KELLEY jr., M. L., and V. W. LOGAN: Erythema nodosum in association with chronic ulcerative colitis. Gastroenterology 31, 285 (1956). — KERBEL, N. C.: An unusual case of erythema nodosum. Canad. med. Ass. J. 83, 820 (1960). — KESSLER, P.: Erythema nodosum nach Masern auf den Genuß von Rohmilch. Münch. med. Wschr. 1937 II, 1209. — KISIN, E. G.: Erythema nodosum mit Beteiligung der Augen. Vestn. Oftal. 16, 506 (1940) [Russisch]. — KOCH, H.: Gleichzeitiges Auftreten eines Erythema nodosum bei Drillingen. Zugleich ein Beitrag zur Frage der Erbbedingtheit des Tuberkulosegeschehens. Klin. Wschr. 1934 II, 1214. — KÖNIGSBERGER, E.: Bemerkungen zur Pathogenese des Erythema nodosum. Acta tuberc. scand. 15, 154 (1941). — KOGOJ: Erythema nodosum et Tuberculosis cutis papulonecrotica. Dermatovenerologische Sektion Zagreb, Sitzg 25. 1. 1934. Ref. in Zbl. Haut- u. Geschl.-Kr. 50, 353 (1935). — KRATKA, W. H.: Episcleritis and Erythema nodosum, a collagen syndrome. Amer. J. Ophthal. 36, 510 (1953). — KREMENTCHOUSKY, BAUER DE LIMOGES et THARAUD: Association d'un érythème noueux et d'un érythème noueux et d'un herpès zostériforme bilatéral. Bull. Soc. franç. Derm. Syph. 42, 801 (1935). — KRISTENSON, A.: Einige Fälle von Erythema nodosum bei BCG-Geimpften. Acta tuberc. scand. 8, 110 (1934). — KROPATCHEV, A. N., u. V. N. VERZNER: Das Erythema nodosum bei kleinen Kindern. [Russisch.] Ref. in Zbl. Haut- u. Geschl.-Kr. 56, 59 (1937).

LAFOSSE, P.: Erythème noueux chez une tuberculeuse après des injections de tuberculine. Revue Tuberc. (Paris) 1, 461 (1935). — LANDORF, N.: Tuberkulinnegatives Erythema nodosum. Acta paediat. 17, Suppl. Nr 1, 180 (1935). — LASSEN, H. C. A.: Erythema nodosum mit Befund von humanen Tuberkelbacillen im Magenspülwasser. Hospitalstidende 1933, 215. — LAURINISCH, A.: Eritema nodoso e tubercolosi. Pediatria (Napoli) 40, 1309 (1932). — LEGGAT, P. O.: Prognosis of sarcoid changes associated with Erythema nodosum. Brit. J. Tuberc. 46, 225 (1952). — LEMAIRE, A., J. DEBRAY et B. HILLEMAND: A propos de deux observations d'érythème noueux survenus parmi des manifestations de type streptococcique. Bull. Soc. méd. Hôp. Paris 72, 942 (1956). — LEMAIRE, R.: Virage de la réaction tuberculinique au cours d'un cas d'érythème noueux. Bull. Soc. méd. Hôp. Paris 52, 1418 (1936). — LEMKE, G., u. G. BONSE: Über Lungenveränderungen bei Erythema nodosum und Erythema exsudativum multiforme. Ärztl. Wschr. 1955, 921. — LEMMING, R.: Über Knotenerythem bei vorher tuberkulösen Menschen, besonders rückfälliges Erythem. Hygiea (Stockh.) 97, 9, 60 (1935). — LESNÉ, E., Y. BOUQUIEN et P. GUILLAIN: Le pronostic éloigné del'érythème noueux. Arch. Méd. Enf. 36, 21 (1933). — LEVER, W. F.: Histopathology of the skin. London: Lippincott 1949. — LEWKOWICZ, K.: Das Erythema nodosum als Prototyp einer tuberkulösen Infektion mit günstigem Ausgang und akutem Beginn. Befund von angedauten Bacillen, säurefesten Granula und Stäubchen oder gelöster säurefester Substanz im Protoplasma von Zellen als Ausdruck der zum Teil völligen Zerstörung der Bacillen und gleichzeitig als Beweis einer sehr starken Immunisierung des Organismus. Ref. in Zbl. Haut- u. Geschl.-Kr. 59, 436 (1938). — Erythema nodosum als Prototyp eines vollen akuten günstigen Verlaufes der Tuberkulose. — In ihm gefundene ausgedehnte Stäbchen, säurefeste Körnchen und Stäubchen oder im Zellprotoplasma gelöste säurefeste Substanz als Ausdruck außerordentlich gründlicher Vernichtung der Keime und damit als Beweis sehr hoher und spezifischer Immunisierung des Organismus. [Polnisch.] Ref. in Zbl. Haut- u. Geschl.-Kr. 59, 511 (1938). — Tuberculococcoidose, érythème noueux, spléno-pneumonie, néphrite haemorrhagique, ictère, rhumatisme. Presse méd. 1939, 558. — LINDEMAYR: Toxisches Exanthem vom Typ des Erythema exsudativum multiforme bzw. Erythema nodosum bei einer mit Radium bestrahlten und mit Cibazolpuder intravaginal behandelten Patientin. Hautarzt 7, 375 (1956). — LITTLE, J. A., and A. J. STEIGMAN: Erythema nodosum in primary histoplasmosis. J. Amer. med. Ass. 173, 875 (1960). — LÖFFLER, W.: Die Bedeutung des Erythema nodosum in der ärztlichen Praxis und in theoretischer Hinsicht. Schweiz. med. Wschr. **1947**, 1152. — LÖFGREN, S., u. F. WALLGREN: Histopathologie des Erythema nodosum. Acta derm.-venereol. (Stockh.) **29**, 1 (1949). — LOEWENTHAL, L. J. A.: Observations on some colinogenic dermatoses including a case of colinogenic Erythema nodosum. Brit. J. Derm. **61**, 403 (1949). — LOEWY, E.: Erythema nodosum tuberculosum. Kölner Dermat. Ges. Sitzg 25. 11. 32. Ref. in Zbl. Haut- u. Geschl.-Kr. **44**, 256 (1933). — LORBER, J.: The changing etiology of erythema nodosum in children. Arch. Dis. Childh. **33**, 137 (1958). — LOVEMAN, A. B., and F. SIMON: Erythema nodosum from Sulfanilamid. Some experimental aspects. J. Allergy **12**, 28 1940).

MALLET, M.: Etude histologique des lésions cutanées de l'érythème noueux. Bull. Soc. franç. Derm. Syph. **45**, 1064—1067 (1938). — MASCHER, W.: Das Erythema nodosum beim Erwachsenen als Symptom der tuberkulösen Primäraffektion und seine Folgezustände. Acta tuberc. scand., Suppl. **10** (1943). — MASSINI, R.: Tuberkelbacillen im Blut bei Erythema nodosum. (Negativer Pirquet bei Tuberkulose und Erythema nodosum.) Verh. schweiz. naturforsch. Ges. 442 (1932). — MAZZANTI, C.: Sindrome di eritema nodoso in una donna con manifestazioni di sifilide recente in atto. Dermosifilografo 8, 505 (1933). — MCCARTHY, J. L.: Episcleral nodules and erythema nodosum. Amer. J. Ophthal., III. s. **51**, 60 (1961). — MEYER, A., M. RAUGEL, J. L. JULLIEN et A. NADOLNY: Adénopathies médiastinales non-tuberculeuses avec érythème noueux (syndrome de Löfgren). Rev. Tuberc. (Paris) **23**, 357 (1959). — MICHEL, P. J., M. TREPPOZ et J. SAINT-PAUL: Un cas de Besnier-Boeck médiastinal avec érythème noueux. Bull. Soc. franç. Derm. Syph. **63**, 261 (1956). — MIESCHER, G.: Über Cibazolexantheme. Dermatologica (Basel) **86**, 64 (1942). — Über Cibazolexantheme und Cibazolfieber. Schweiz. med. Wschr. **73**, 521 (1943). — Zur Histologie des Erythema nodosum. Acta derm.-venereol. (Stockh.) **27**, 448 (1947). — Zur Ätiologie des Erythema nodosum. Schweiz. med. Wschr. **78**, 269 (1948). — Zur Frage der Radiärknötchen beim Erythema nodosum. Arch. Derm. Syph. (Berl.) **193**, 251 (1951). — MINAMI, S., u. KINGO KOGA: 4 Fälle von Erythema nodosum, wahrscheinlich tuberkulöser Natur. [Japanisch.] Ref. in Zbl. Haut- u. Geschl.-Kr. **51**, 130 (1935). — MIURA, OSAMU: Ein Fall von E.n. mit E.e.m. Jap. J. Derm. **45**, 69 (1939). — MOGENSEN, E.: Ätiologie des Erythema nodosum. Ugeskr. Laeg. **1933**, 425. — Reinvestigations in Erythema nodosum. Acta med. scand. **80**, 480 (1933). — MONDON, H.: L'érythème noueux chez l'adolescent et l'adulte. Rev. Tuberc. (Paris) **7**, 225 (1942). — MÓRITZ, DÉNES: Beiträge zur Frage der Inkubationszeit bei Erythema. nodosum. Arch. Kinderheilk. **99**, 177 (1933). — Erythema nodosum und Scharlach. Arch. Kinderheilk. **103**, 227 (1934). — L'influence des rayons ultra-violets sur l'érythème noueux. Arch. Méd. Enf. **37**, 476 (1934). — Meningeale Reaktion bei Erythema nodosum. (Zugleich Beitrag zur Pathogenese der Meningitis tuberculosa.) Mschr. Kinderheilk. **67**, 255 (1936). — MÓRITZ, D., u. S. DÓRA: Das lokale Blutbild des Erythema nodosum. Arch. Kinderheilk. **104**, 65 (1935). — MÓRITZ, D., u. E. v. LEDERER: Die Capillarmikroskopie des Erythema nodosum. Arch. Kinderheilk. **101**, 101 (1934). — MORO, E.: Erythema nodosum bei Scharlach. Z. Kinderheilk. **57**, 321 (1935). — MORQUIO, L.: Erythème noueux et tuberculose. Presse méd. **1934 I**, 409. — MUGGIA, A.: Recidiva di eritema nodoso. Boll. Soc. ital. Pediat. **2**, 330 (1933). — MUNTEANU, M.: Ätiologische Betrachtungen anhand von einigen Fällen von Erythema nodosum. Zit. in Zbl. Haut- u. Geschl.-Kr. **109**, 48 (1962).

NAGY, MARGARETHE: Betrachtungen über das Erythema nodosum bei Kindern. Rev. pédiat. (Cluj) **2**, 83 (1938). — NAKAMURA, MOTOO: Zusammenkommen von Erythema exsudativum multiforme und Erythema nodosum. Jap. J. Derm. **32**, 132 (1932). — NARANJO, F.: Über Tuberkelbacillämie bei Erythema nodosum im Kindesalter. Z. Tuberk. **71**, 11 (1934). — NAVARRO, J. C., u. R. R. SUNDBLAD: Erythema nodosum. Clin. de la Tbc. Méd. Infant. Buenos Aires. Sem. méd. (B. Aires) **1935 I**, 1847. — NAVARRO-MARTÍN, A., u. F. MARTÍNES-TORRES: Das Irgapyrin in der Behandlung des Erythema exsudativum multiforme, des Herpes vulgaris, des Erythema nodosum und anderer Dermatosen. Act. derm.-sifiliogr. (Madr.) **44**, 628 (1953). — NÉKÁM, L.: Ein Fall von Landouzyscher Typhobacillose und Erythema nodosum. Orv. Hetil. **1934**, 98. — Klin. Wschr. **1934 II**, 1464. — NEUMANN, A.: A small endemic of nodous erythema. Contribution to the pathogenesis of Erythema nodosum. Čs. Derm. **34**, 45 (1959). — NEUMANN, W.: Phlyktäne, Erythema nodosum und Poncetscher Rheumatismus. Med. Klin. **1933 II**, 1407. — NIKLASSON, H.: Zur Kenntnis des tuberkulösen Primär-Affektes an der Conjunctiva mit Erythema nodosum. Acta ophthal. (Kbh.) **12**, 244 (1934). — NOBÉCOURT, P., u. BRISCAS: Die negativen Tuberkulin-Cutanproben bei Erythema nodosum. Presse méd. **1941 II**, 713. — NOBÉCOURT, P., et P. DUCAS: Erythème noueux au décours d'un abscès du poumon. Bull. Soc. Pédiat. Paris **32**, 602 (1934). — Erythème noueux et conjunctivite plycténulaire. Presse méd. **1934 II**, 1241. — NONCLERCQ, E., et P. DELLENBACH: Etude biologique d'un cas d'érythème noueux streptococcique. Bull. Soc. franç. Derm. Syph. **63**, 511 (1956). — NORDENSKJÖLD, ANNA: Ein Fall von primärer Scheidentuberkulose mit Erythema nodosum. Acta paediat. (Stockh.) **20**, 257 (1937). — NUBÉ, M. J.: Mieschers Granuloma in Erythema nodosum. Dermatologica (Basel) **101**, 80 (1950). — NUTTALL-SMITH, I.: Pulmonary histoplasmosis accompanied by Erythema nodosum. Canad. med. Ass. J. **74**, 59 (1956).

OHNO, KAZUO: Fall von Erythema nodosum syphiliticum. Jap. J. Derm. **36**, 89 (1934). — ONTANEDA, LUIS E., u. J. MONSERRAT: Pathogenese des tuberkulösen Erythema nodosum. Rev. Asoc. méd. argent. **49**, 923 (1935) [Spanisch]. — ONTANEDA, LUIS E., E. A. ROTTJER u. R. Q. PASQUALINI: Das Erythema nodosum als Erscheinung der ersten tuberkulösen Infektion beim Erwachsenen. Rev. Asoc. méd. argent. **49**, 915 (1935) [Spanisch]. — OPITZ, H.: Zur Infektiösität der an Erythema nodosum leidenden Kinder. Kinderärztl. Prax. **3**, 337 (1932). — OROSZ, D.: Über das Schicksal der Erythema nodosum-Patienten. Wien. med. Wschr. **1933 II**, 869. — Mschr. Kinderheilk. **58**, 180 (1933).

PARISI, P.: Sarcoidi disseminati ed eritema nodoso in rara assoziazione. Arch. ital. Derm. **21**, 39 (1948). — PARISOT, J., et SALEUR: Erythèmes noueux familiaux et contaminations tuberculeuses. Rev. Tuberc. (Paris), IV. s. **1**, 126 (1933). — PATRIGNANI, F.: Contributo allo studio dell'eritema nodoso. L'estinzione dei noduli con iniezione intradermiche di tuberculina. Arch. Sci. med. **73**, 243 (1942). — PAUL, L. W., and L. A. POHLE: Mediastinal and pulmonary changes in Erythema nodosum. Radiology **37**, 131 (1941). — PAUTRIER, L. M.: Comment se pose la question de l'érythème noueux. Bull. Soc. franç. Derm. Syph. **45**, 1046 (1938). Réunion de Strasbourg. — Pathogénie à nature de l'érythème noueux. Bull. Acad. roy. Méd. Belg. **19**, 109 (1954). — PAUTRIER, L.-M., LAUGIER et MERCENIER: Deux cas d'érythème noueux (dont un accompagné d'érythème polymorphe) survenant au cours de l'évolution d'une syphilis secondaire. Bull. Soc. franç. Derm. Syph. **40**, 1092 (1933). — PAUTRIER, L.-M., et F. WORINGER: Contribution à l'étude histologique de l'érythème noueux. Bull. Soc. franç. Derm. Syph **45**, 1068 (1938). — PEBLER, W. J., R. KOOIJ and J. MARSHALL: The histopathology of acute panniculitis nodosa leprosa (erythema nodosum leprosum). Int. J. Leprosy **23**, 53 (1955). — PEREMANS et A. HUTSEBAUT: Erythème polymorphe combiné à un érythème noueux. Arch. belges Derm. **12**, 308 (1956). — PETÉNYI, GÉZA: Über rudimentäre Formen des Erythema nodosum. Ref. in Zbl. Haut- u. Geschl.-Kr. **51**, 101 (1934). — PETROVIĆ, MILAN: Erythema nodosum und tuberkulöse Infektion. Srpski Arkh. tselok. Lek. **35**, 165 (1933). — PIERRET, R., A. BRETON et G. LEFEBVRE: L'érythème noueux, la kératite phlycténulaire, reflets des variations d'allergie tuberculeuse chez l'enfant. Presse méd. **1939**, 255. — POPPEL, M. H., and A. M. MELAMED: Erythema nodosum. New Engl. J. Med. **227**, 325 (1942). — PORTUGAL, H.: Histologie des leprösen Erythema nodosum. Ati 37st Congr. Soc. ital. Dermat. 1951, S. 236. — PRAG, A. R.: Zur Klinik des Erythema nodosum. Hygiea (Stockh.) **94**, 595 (1932). — PUNCH, A. L.: A note on the aetiology of Erythema nodosum. Lancet **1941 I**, 10.

RAILLIET, G.: Erythème noueux à forme rhumatismale avec forte présomption de tuberculose. Bull. Soc. méd. Hôp. Paris, III. s. **51**, 1129 (1935). — RAMEL, E.: De l'étiologie et du traitement de l'érythème noueux idiopathique. Schweiz. med. Wschr. **13**, 715 (1932). — RANTASALO, V.: Ein Fall von Erythema nodosum. Duodecim (Helsinki) **49**, 448 (1933). — Über das Erythema nodosum und seine Beziehung zur Tuberkulose. Duodecim (Helsinki) **49**, 304 (1933). — REICH, H.: Zur Kenntnis der Radiärknötchen (Miescher) beim Erythema nodosum. Hautarzt **3**, 503 (1952). — ROLLOF, S. J.: Erythema nodosum in association with sulfathiazole in thylodone. A clinical investigation with special reference to primary tuberculosis. Acta tuberc. scand. **24**, Suppl. **24** (1950). — ROOSVALL, A.: Endogen factors in the occurrence of erythema nodosum. Acta tuberc. scand. **10**, 351 (1936). — ROSTENBERG, A.: Erythema nodosum of several years' duration. Arch. Derm. Syph. (Chic.) **31**, 762 (1935). — ROTNES, P. L.: Eine Familien-Endemie von Erythema nodosum. Derm. Z. **67**, 259 (1933). — Untersuchungen über Erythema nodosum im Erwachsenenalter. Acta derm.-venereol. (Stockh.) **17**, Suppl. III (1936). — Erythema nodosum im Erwachsenenalter. Nord. med. T. **1937**, 281. — ROYER, J., A. GLOAGUEN et A. PETERS: Erythème noueux 3 ans après une vaccination par le BCG. Rev. Tuberc. (Paris) **18**, 927 (1954). — RYCKEBUSCH: Erythème noueux et tuberculose; deux cas de primo-infection chez l'adulte jeune. Ass. franç. Avancement Sci. **1935**, 428.

SAENZ, A., et R. BROCA: Recherches bactériologiques sur l'érythème noueux. Bull. Soc. franç. Derm. Syph. **1938**, 1100. — SAENZ, A., P. CHEVALLIER, M. LÉVY-BRUHL et L. COSTIL: Sur la présence du bacille de Koch virulent dans les lésions cutanées et dans le sang d'une malade en plein accès d'érythème noueux. C. R. Soc. Biol. (Paris) **112**, 951 (1933). — SAKURANE, Y., u. N. HEIHACHI: Ein Fall von Erythema nodosum kombiniert mit Lymphogranulomatosis inguinalis. Ref. in Zbl. Haut- u. Geschl.-Kr. **55**, 596 (1937). — SALOMÃO, A.: Erythema nodosum leprotischer Ätiologie im Kindesalter. Arch. mineir. Leprol. **11**, 211 (1951). — SAMAJA, M.: L'eritema nodoso nei bambini. Clin. pediat. (Bologna) **15**, 113—164 (1933). — SANDRA, H.: Bemerkungen im Anschluß an 120 Fälle von Erythema nodosum. Ned. T. Geneesk. **1935**, 13. — SARROUY, CH., LE GENISSEL et CH. STORA: Erythème noueux et tuberculose pulmonaire chez l indigène algérien. Arch. Méd. Enf. **39**, 804 (1936). — SASAI, Y.: Supplementary studies on erythema nodosum; especially in relation to nodular vasculitis. Jap. J. Derm. **67**, 627 (1957). — SASLAW, S., and F. M. BEMAN: Erythema nodosum as a manifestation of histoplasmosis. J. Amer. med. Ass. **170**, 1178 (1959). — SCHNEIDER, W.:

Beitrag zur Frage der Ätiologie des Erythema nodosum. Diss. Gießen 1940. — SCHNEIERSON, S. J.: Orally administered cortisone in Erythema nodosum. J. Amer. med. Ass. **150**, 585 (1952). — SEIDELIN SCHNOHR, GERDA: 10 cases of erythema nodosum developing during the course of florid pulmonary phthisis. Acta tuberc. scand. 8, 173 (1934). — SEVERIN, G.: Erythema nodosum und zerstörende Lungentuberkulose. Nord. Med. **1939**, 3048. — SÉZARY, A., R. BERNARD et GOUTNER: Erythème noueux et polymorphe. Bull. Soc. franç. Derm. Syph. **44**, 1048 (1937). — SÉZARY, A., et E. FRIEDMANN: Erythème noueux et maladie de Nicolas-Favre. Bull. Soc. franç. Derm. Syph. **43**, 559 (1936). — SHAPOSHNIKOV, O. K.: Chronic erythema nodosum. Vestn. Derm. Vener. **36**, 21 (1962). — SIBIRANI, M.: Erythema nodosum und seine Beziehung zur Tuberkulose. Arch. ital. Derm. **16**, 501 (1940). — SILVA, C., u. L. ANDRADE: Quantitative Haemagglutination mit Sera Lepröser, die mit durch Tuberkulin BCG sensibilisierten menschlichen roten Blutkörperchen ausgeführt wurde, unter besonderer Berücksichtigung der Fälle vom Typus Erythema nodosum. Mem. 3. Conf. Panamer. Leprol. **1**, 167 (1953). — SIMON, CLÉMENT, DELZANT et VASSAL: Erythème noueux géant fébrile après injection de propidon. Bull. Soc. franç. Derm. Syph. **44**, 1038 (1937). — SIMON, J.: Ein Beitrag zur Behandlung des Erythema nodosum. Ther. d. Gegenw **82**, 142 (1941). — SIMPSON, R. G.: Erythema nodosum. A provocation phenomenon with special reference to lymphogranuloma venereum. Dermatologica (Basel) **101**, 94 (1950). — SLOT, G.: Erythema nodosum treated with antistreptococcal serum. Lancet **1934 II**, 600. — SLOT, G. N. J., and D. MORRIS: Erythema nodosum associated with chorea and tuberculous meningitis. Lancet **1939 I**, 571. — SMITH, C. E.: Epidemiology of acute coccidioidomycosis with Erythema nodosum (San Joaquim valley fever). Amer. J. Publ. Hlth **30**, 600 (1940). — SONCK, C. E.: On the provocative effect of synthetic oestrogen on Erythema nodosum. Preliminary report. Acta allerg. (Kbh.) **2**, 268 (1949). — SPINK, WESLEY W.: Pathogenesis of erythema nodosum with special reference to tuberculosis, streptococcic infection and rheumatic fever. Arch. intern. Med. **59**, 65 (1937). — STAFFIERI, P., e V. ROMEO: Il sulfatiazolo fattore precipitante dell'eritema nodoso. Progr. ter. (Roma) **3**, 133 (1951). — STAJIĆ, S.: Erythema nodosum. Srpski Arkh. tselok. Lek. **35**, 146 (1933). — STAVROPOULOS, J.: Quelques considérations sur un cas d'érythème noueux. Bull. Soc. Pédiat. Paris **33**, 585 (1935). — STEINBERG, L. B.: Zur Ätiologie und Pathogenese des Erythema nodosum bei Kindern. Probl. Tuberk. **9**, 49 (1939). — STOPPELAAR, F. DE: Erythema nodosum bei einem eineiigen Zwilling. Ned. T. Geneesk. **1942**, 772. — STORCK, H., u. O. SPÜHLER: Rezidivierendes Erythema nodosum. Dermatologica (Basel) **112**, 564 (1956). — STRINGER, H. C. W.: Ein Fall von Erythema nodosum und akutem Rheumatismus mit tödlichem Ausgang. Tuberkuloides Gewebsbild in den Lymphknoten. N. Z. med. J. **32**, 35 (1953). — STUCKI, P.: Über das Erythema nodosum und das Löfgren-Syndrom. Praxis (Bern) **50**, 271 (1961). — SZENTKIRÁLYI, Z.: Behandlung des Erythema exsudativum multiforme und Erythema nodosum mit Paraamino-benzol-sulfamidal (Deseptyl). Orv. Hetil **1937**, 794.

TANIMURA, CH., u. S. MORINO: Über Erythema nodosum tuberculosum. Jap. J. Derm. **39**, 94 (1936). — TATAFIORE, E.: Su di un caso di eritema nodoso con complicanza endocarditica. Rinasc. med. **10**, 400 (1933). — TATÁR, J.: Retinitis pseudo-nephritica und Periarteriitis retinae anschließend an Erythema nodosum. Z. Augenheilk. **103**, 84 (1939). — THIERS, H., D. COLOMB et J. FAYOLLE: La sulfathiourée dans le traitement des hypodermites éruptives noueuses ou en placards. Bull. Soc. franç. Derm. Syph. **64**, 140 (1957). — THIERS, H., et TIVOLET: Erythème noueux au cours de l évolution d'une lymphoréticulose bénigne d'inoculation. Bull. Soc. franç. Derm. Syph. **59**, 172 (1952). — THOMPSON, B. C.: Erythema nodosum and cervical gland tuberculosis. Three illustrative cases. Brit. J. Tbc. **30**, 84 (1936). — Erythema nodosum associated with acute tuberculous cervical lymphadenitis. Brit. med. J. **1939**, Nr 4073, 159. — THOMPSON, B. C., M. O. HANSON and C. A. GODD: Erythema nodosum. The possible significance of associated pulmonary hilar adenopathy. Ann. intern. Med. **34**, 983 (1951). — THORNER, J. E.: Erythema nodosum in childhood associated with infection by the oidium coccidioides. Report of 7 cases. Arch. Pediat. **56**, 628 (1939). — TINOZZI, G.: Eritema nodoso e vaccini antitubercolari. Riv. Pat. Appar. resp. **3**, 421 (1934). — TISSOT, F.: Que deviennent les enfants atteints d'érythème noueux? 20 observations. Arch. Méd. Enf. **42**, 627 (1939). — TÖRNELL, E.: Fürsorge bei Fällen von Erythema nodosum und ihrer Umgebung. Nord. med. T. **1933**, 1089. — TOMIKAWA, R., T. NISIWAKI u. A. KAWAGUTI: Über Erythema nodosum. Ref. in Zbl. Haut- u. Geschl.-Kr. **69**, 180 (1943). — TOURAINE, A., et SOULIGNAC: Erythème noueux et érythème polymorphe. Bull. Soc. franç. Derm. Syph. **44**, 458 (1937). — TRABAUD, J.: L'érythème noueux à la lumière d'observations damasquines. Bull. Acad. nat. Méd. (Paris), III. s. **109**, 667 (1933). — TREPICCIONI, E.: La posizione attuale dell eritema nodoso in tisiologia. Lotta c. Tuberc. **4**, 826 (1933). — TRUELOVE, L. H.: Articular manifestations of erythema nodosum. Ann. rheum. Dis. **19**, 174 (1960).

URBACH, E.: Pilznachweis in einem Erythema nodosum trichophyticum. Österreichische Dermatologische Gesellschaft Wien. Sitzung vom 8. 11. 1934. Zbl. Haut- u. Geschl.-Kr. **50**, 552 (1935). — URELES, A. L., and R. B. KALMANSOHN: Oral administration of Cortisone in a case of Erythema nodosum. New Engl. J. Med. **245**, 139 (1951). — USTVEDT, H. J., u. A. S. JOHANNESSEN: Erythema nodosum und darauffolgende Tuberkulose. Norsk. Mag. Laegevidensk. **94**, 532 (1933).

VADE, H. W.: The nature of the Erythema nodosum type of reaction lesions in lepromatous leprosy. A special reference to effects of repeated reactions. Mem. 6. Congr. Internat. Leprol. 1953, p. 725. — VALLI, M.: Contributo clinico allo studio dei rapporti fra i eritemi nodoso e tuberculosi. Riv. Pat. Clin. Tuberc. **13**, 539 (1939). — VELTMAN, G.: Erythema nodosum syphiliticum. Derm. Wschr. **119**, 365 (1947). — VERGER, P.: L'érythème noueux. J. Méd. Bordeaux **119**, 457 (1942). — VESEY, C. M. R., and D. S. WILKINSON: Erythema nodosum. A study of 70 cases. Brit. J. Derm. **71**, 139 (1959). — VOGT, J. H.: Dem Erythema nodosum ähnelndes Exanthem und langanhaltende Hilusdrüsenschwellung beim Tuberkulinnegativen Patienten (Morbus Boeck-Besnier-Schaumann?). Nord. Med. **1939**, 2341.

WAISMAN, N., and M. A. THOMAS: Benign pulmonary hilar lymphadenopathy in erythema nodosum. Arch. Derm. **82**, 754 (1960). — WALLGREN, A.: Erythema nodosum nach Calmette-Impfung. Svenska Läk.-Tidn. **1932**, 1393. — Welche Ätiologie besitzt für das Erythema nodosum die größte Wahrscheinlichkeit? Derm. Wschr. **1934 I**, 624. — Rheumatic erythema nodosum. Amer. J. Dis. Child. **55**, 897 (1938). — Erythema nodosum and pulmonary tuberculosis. Lancet **1938 I**, 359. — Zur Pathogenese des Erythema nodosum. Mschr. Kinderheilk. **80**, 368 (1939). — Nierenreizung bei Erythema nodosum. Acta paediat. (Uppsala) **25**, 331 (1939). — WALLGREN, A., u. A. GNOSSPELIUS: Die Bedeutung der Tuberkelbacillen in den Knoten des Erythema nodosum. Acta med. scand. **103**, 341 (1940). — WALTHER, H.: Beitrag zum Erythema nodosum mycoticum. Z. Haut- u. Geschl.-Kr. **19**, 203 (1955). — WEBSTER, J., u. B. PASS: Erythema nodosum nach Atebrin? Arch. Derm. Syph. (Chic.) **68**, 595 (1953). — WEISSENBACH, R.-J., et H. BROCARD: Erythème noueux et syphilis secondaire cutanéo-muqueuse floride associés. Bull. Soc. franç. Derm. Syph. **43**, 410 (1936). — WESTERGREN, A.: On a complex etiology of Erythema nodosum. Acta derm.-venereol. (Stockh.) **26**, 384 (1946). — WETZEL, U.: Cortisonbehandlung des Erythema nodosum. Ther. d. Gegenw. **95**, 147 (1956). — WHITWELL, G. P. A.: Observations on erythema nodosum and erythema induratum. Guy's Hosp. Rep. **85**, 227 (1935). — WINKLER, M.: Fall von Erythema nodosum-ähnlichen Knoten der Haut oder miliaren Lupoiden mit starken Lungenveränderungen. Schweiz. med. Wschr. **1936 II**, 1923. — WOHLSTEIN, E.: Erythema nodosum exulcerans. Derm. Z. **66**, 335 (1933). — WOLF, M.: Contribution à l'étude des lésions érythématonodulaires. Un cas de nodosités rhumatismales à type d'érythème noueux guéri par les injections intraveineuses de salicylate de soude. Bull. Soc. franç. Derm. Syph. **40**, 516 (1933). — WORINGER, F., et J. G. LÉVY: A propos de 2 cas d'érythème polymorphe associé à l'érythème noueux. Bull. Soc. franç. Derm. Syph. **56**, 536 (1949).

ZAMFIR, D., V. STROESCO u. I. TOMESCO: Über das gleichzeitige Vorkommen eines Erythema multiforme, eines Erythema nodosum und einer Tuberkulose. Bull. méd. (Paris) **1939**, 714.

Periarteriitis nodosa

Von

Rudolf Schuppli-Basel

Einleitung

Obgleich das Krankheitsbild der Periarteriitis nodosa schon seit langer Zeit bekannt ist, ist es im dermatologischen Schrifttum erst seit relativ kurzer Zeit berücksichtigt worden. So fehlt z.B. in der ersten Auflage des Jadassohnschen Handbuches ein entsprechendes Kapitel. Aus verschiedenen Gründen ist nun der Periarteriitis nodosa und ganz allgemein den entzündlichen Gefäßprozessen in den letzten Jahren in zunehmendem Maße Beachtung geschenkt worden, denn einerseits gestattet eine verbesserte klinische Diagnostik auch nichttypische Krankheitsbilder zu Lebzeiten des Patienten zu diagnostizieren, andererseits lassen Statistiken erkennen, daß die entzündlichen Gefäßreaktionen eine deutliche Zunahme erfahren haben, wobei speziell die durch medikamentöse Allergien bedingten Gefäßkrankheiten viel häufiger geworden zu sein scheinen. So berichtete Sandler 1938 erst über 20 Beobachtungen in der Literatur, während wenig später bereits Hunderte von Fällen bekanntgeworden sind. Die Aktualität der Probleme, die sich mit diesen Krankheiten verbinden, geht z.B. daraus hervor, daß verschiedene wissenschaftliche Tagungen der Periarteriitis nodosa gewidmet worden sind (Symposium der Mayo Clinic 1954; Gemeinschaftstagung der Deutschen Gesellschaft für innere Medizin und der Deutschen Gesellschaft für Allergieforschung 1954). Diesen und anderen zusammenfassenden Darstellungen ist es zu verdanken, daß das Krankheitsbild der Periarteriitis nodosa jetzt so weit bekannt ist, daß eine zuverlässige Charakterisierung möglich ist.

Die genauere Erforschung der Pathogenese und der klinischen Bilder der Periarteriitis nodosa hat nun aber zur Folge gehabt, daß Versuche unternommen worden sind, eine Reihe von Krankheitsbildern, die in gewissen Einzelheiten von der klassischen Beschreibung der Periarteriitis nodosa abweichen, von ihr abzutrennen. Es handelt sich hier in erster Linie um die „Vascular Allergy", um die Arteriitis temporalis und um die „Hypersensitive Angitis". Abgesehen davon, daß es schwer fällt, bei der außerordentlichen Mannigfaltigkeit des klinischen Bildes der Periarteriitis nodosa ein „normales Bild" aufzustellen, unterscheiden sich viele dieser Prozesse nur in unbedeutenden quantitativen Einzelheiten vom Bild der Periarteriitis nodosa und haben mit ihr die grundlegende Veränderung der nekrotisierenden Gefäßwandveränderungen gemeinsam. Es wird deshalb der Zukunft überlassen bleiben, ob sich die Sonderstellung dieser Krankheitsbilder rechtfertigt oder ob sie als Spielarten eines gleichartigen Vorganges aufzufassen sind. Daß auch Versuche gemacht worden sind, die Nomenklatur der nodösen Gefäßentzündungen durch Bezeichnungen wie Polyarteriitis, Panarteriitis, „necrotizing arteritis" zu ersetzen, sei hier nur kurz erwähnt, da sie zur eigentlichen Kenntnis des Krankheitsprozesses nichts beigetragen haben.

Da die Periarteriitis nodosa eine den ganzen Organismus befallende Krankheit darstellt, müssen die Veränderungen innerer Organe neben den Hauterscheinungen dem Dermatologen bekannt sein. Sie sollen im folgenden aber nur insoweit genauer beschrieben werden, als sie für die Diagnose wichtig sind, da es sich nicht darum handeln kann, im Rahmen eines dermatologischen Handbuches eine vollständige Übersicht über die Symptomatologie der Periarteriitis nodosa zu geben.

1. Klinisches Bild

Das Leiden befällt nach übereinstimmenden Angaben wesentlich häufiger Männer als Frauen, und zwar in einem Verhältnis von mindestens 3:1. Am häufigsten wird das Alter von 20—45 Jahren bevorzugt, doch werden auch Säuglinge (HENRY et al.), Kinder und Greise nicht verschont. Die Krankheit beginnt nach einem uncharakteristischen prodromalen Stadium von wechselnder Dauer mit einem septischen Krankheitsbild, das durch hohes Fieber, allgemeine Drüsenschwellungen und Splenomegalie beherrscht wird.

Die Prognose wird verschieden angegeben: Während das voll entwickelte Krankheitsbild der Periarteriitis nodosa als infaust gilt (CZICKELI, LOHSE), sind es speziell die oligosymptomatischen Formen (KEMP und ROTH) und hier wiederum die reinen Hautformen, die als gutartig beschrieben werden (SLINGER und STARCK, CROSTI, CAROL, LINDBERG, PORTWICH, BANKE, RUITER). Ob aber tatsächlich die Periarteriitis nodosa dank der Therapie eine „banale Krankheit" geworden ist (SHEDROW), darf bezweifelt werden.

Als Todesursache werden Urämie (BERGER et al.), Verschluß der Coronararterie (RIVES), der schon im Kindesalter beobachtet worden ist (BARNARD et al.), Perforation von Duodenalgeschwüren, Appendicitis mit Peritonitis (DRUSS), Meningitis (KRAHULIK et al.), Perforation der Gallenblase (ROSSNER) angegeben.

a) Interne Veränderungen

Je nach der Lokalisation der Arterienveränderungen wechselt die Symptomatologie außerordentlich stark, so daß es bisher nicht gelungen ist, bestimmte Typen der Periarteriitis nodosa zu charakterisieren. Es ist vielmehr gerade das Uncharakteristische und Diffuse des Organbefalles für die Krankheit typisch. So beherrschen oft selten gesehene Kombinationen von Organerkrankungen das klinische Bild, wie z.B. Neuritis und Nephritis, Pankreatitis und Neuritis, Cholecystitis und Hauterscheinungen usw. Die Häufigkeit der inneren Komplikationen wird wie folgt angegeben: Niere 80%, Herz 70%, Leber 60%, Darm 50%, Pankreas 25%; Nervensystem 58%, davon 35% periphere Nerven allein, 13% zentrales Nervensystem allein, 10% beide zusammen. Im einzelnen manifestieren sich die Organstörungen in folgender Weise:

α) Niere. Meist zeigt sich das Bild einer Glomerulonephritis, die zu Hochdruckkrisen führen kann und in 60% Albuminurie, in 54% Hämaturie verursacht. Hypertonie wird in 57% der Fälle angetroffen (LOHSE).

β) Herz. Es finden sich im EKG Zeichen von Myokarditis; die Coronararterien sind häufig befallen, Zeichen von Angina pectoris dagegen selten (HARRIS et al.). Oft findet sich eine Tachykardie, die zu dem Fieber in keinem Verhältnis steht. Auch Perikarditis wird beobachtet (SCHERF und BOYD).

γ) Leber. Die häufige Gefäßbeteiligung in der Leber verursacht nur in etwa 10% der Fälle klinisch sichtbare Funktionsveränderungen, die sich z.B. als Ikterus manifestieren (KORTING). Porphyria hepatica wurde in einem Fall beschrieben (MULLER et al.). Die Diagnose der Periarteriitis nodosa läßt sich oft auf Grund histologischer Untersuchung der Gallenblase stellen (ROSSNER).

δ) Darm. Die Gefäßveränderungen im Intestinaltrakt führen zu Darmnekrosen, häufiger macht sich die Darmbeteiligung in Form von abdominellen

Schmerzen bei 70% der Kranken, in 17% in Form von Melaena und in 10% als Hämatemesis bemerkbar. Bei Appendektomie kann die histologische Diagnose gestellt werden (DRUSS et al.).

ε) Pankreas. Pankreasbeteiligung zeigt sich in erhöhten Diastasewerten im Urin und kann zu einer fast völligen Nekrose des Pankreas führen.

ζ) Nervenbeteiligung. Besonders genau sind die Veränderungen des Nervensystems untersucht worden (KERNOHAN, STAMMLER, SILLEVIS SMITH, WALTHARD et al.). Es zeigt sich eine durch die Gefäßstörungen bedingte periphere Mononeuritis oder eine segmentale Polyneuritis. In 20—35% ist das periphere Nervensystem befallen, in 8—13% der Fälle das zentrale Nervensystem in Form epileptischer Anfälle oder apoplektischer Insulte. Es kann auch zum Bild der Querschnittsläsion kommen (LOOGEN). Psychische Veränderungen werden ebenfalls beschrieben (JULICH). Klinisch bestehen viele Ähnlichkeiten zwischen der akuten Porphyrie und der Periarteriitis nodosa (BECKER).

η) Muskeln. Eine Polymyositis ist sehr häufig, und die histologischen Veränderungen lassen sich besonders klar in Muskelbiopsien finden.

ϑ) Augen. Augensymptome manifestieren sich als Zentralarterienthrombose (BERNSTEIN), Atrophie des N. opticus (SANNICANDRO). Beteiligung der Chorioidea wird meist zusammen mit Befall der Meningealgefäße angetroffen (KERNOHAN). Retinitis pigmentosa kann ebenfalls durch die Gefäßstörungen verursacht werden (DEJEAN et al.).

ι) Knochen. Seltenere Komplikationen sind Veränderungen in den Schenkelknochen (WEPLER) und in der Schläfenbeinpyramide (DRUSS et al.).

ϰ) Blut. Charakteristisch sind Veränderungen im Blut. Es zeigt sich in 75% eine oft exzessive Leukocytose und eine ebenfalls oft sehr hohe Eosinophilie. Erhöhungen des Antistreptolysintiters auf sonst ungewöhnlich hohe Werte werden beobachtet (LINDGREN). Das Auftreten von Kälteagglutininen (BEUTLER et al.), von unspezifisch positiven Wassermann-Reaktionen, von positivem Coombs-Test (SHEDROW), von L.E.-Zellen (LINCOLN et al.) weist auf ein stark gestörtes Gleichgewicht im Eiweißbild des Serums hin sowie auf das Vorhandensein verschiedener Antikörper. Die Senkung pflegt mäßig bis stark erhöht zu sein. Die γ-Globuline können sehr stark vermehrt sein (MANCKE und PEPER), so daß ein multiples Myelom vorgetäuscht werden kann. Auch die Kombination einer Periarteriitis nodosa mit einem solchen wurde beobachtet (BEST et al.).

λ) Lungen. Lungeninfiltrate im Sinne eines Löfflerschen eosinophilen Infiltrates werden nicht selten beschrieben und haben eine besonders schlechte Prognose (DIVERTIE et al.).

b) Hautsymptome

Eine spezielle Besprechung der Hauterscheinungen bei Periarteriitis nodosa rechtfertigt sich deshalb, weil, wie schon erwähnt, die Prognose der reinen Hautformen der Periarteriitis nodosa ganz wesentlich besser ist als diejenige der Periarteriitis nodosa mit internen Symptomen, so daß CERUTTI et al. diese Form als Polyarteriitis cutis benigna bezeichnen, und weil sich aus den Hauterscheinungen als aus leicht zugänglichen Veränderungen die Diagnose oft ohne Schwierigkeiten stellen läßt.

Hauterscheinungen kommen bei der Periarteriitis nodosa relativ häufig vor. Sie werden von SMITT in etwa 20% der Fälle erwähnt, von CERUTTI in 30%, von LJUBOMUDROV in 47%, von MELCZER und VENKEI in 60%. Verschiedene zusammenfassende Arbeiten sind ihrer Natur gewidmet (MIESCHER, CAROL und PRAKKEN, LINDGREN, MELCZER und VENKEI, KNOTH et al., PUCHOL, LYELL et al.). Es geht aus ihnen hervor, daß es kaum möglich ist, bestimmte Typen aufzustellen.

Auf jeden Fall erscheint die Einteilung von Matras in knötchenförmige, purpuraförmige und gangränöse Erscheinungen zu schematisch, da außerdem hämorrhagische Formen als Apoplexia cutis, papulonekrotische Herde (Mérand), Livedo racemosa (Goldschlag und Chwalibogowski, Arzt), lupusähnliche Knötchen (Kren), Erythema exsudativum multiforme-artige Exantheme (Crosti, Garzón et al.), vesiculöse Eruptionen (Repke), Blasen (v. Cauwenberge, Bureau et al., Joulia et al.) und eine ganze Reihe anderer Morphen beschrieben worden sind. Sie alle können wohl nur auf Grund des histologischen Bildes eindeutig identifiziert werden.

Neben der Haut können auch die Schleimhäute befallen sein (Nobis). Bureau und Barrière beschreiben sie, als den Hauterscheinungen ähnlich, meist als Knötchen, aber auch als Bläschen und Ulcera. Sie sitzen meist an der Mundschleimhaut, seltener an der Nasen- oder Rectalschleimhaut. Eine seltene und atypische Form ist die „Holznase", die von Duperrat und Civatte beschriebene Hypertrophie der Nasenschleimhaut und der ganzen unteren Nasenpartie. Möglicherweise handelt es sich dabei um das gleiche Krankheitsbild, das von Klinger 1931 und von Wegener 1936 als rhinogene Granulomatose beschrieben wurde (Stratton et al., Cambier).

Gleichzeitiges Vorkommen von Periarteriitis nodosa mit anderen Dermatosen scheint selten zu sein. Alkiewicz beschreibt in einem Fall eine Acanthosis nigricans bei typischer Periarteriitis nodosa, Roch et al. Periarteriitis nodosa und M. Recklinghausen zusammen.

2. Histologie

Der für die Periarteriitis nodosa charakteristische Prozeß ist die Nekrose der Gefäßmedia. Sie beginnt als exsudativer Vorgang, der zu fibrinoider Nekrose führt. Dann gehen die elastischen Fasern zugrunde und werden durch ein äußerst zellreiches Granulationsgewebe ersetzt, das zunächst aus polymorphkernigen Leukocyten und manchmal Eosinophilen besteht. Dieses Infiltrat findet sich auch perivasculär, in schweren Formen ist die ganze Gefäßwand davon durchsetzt. Es wird später mehr und mehr monocytär. Intimaveränderungen sind meistens sekundär. Es kann zu Wucherungsvorgängen kommen, die zu mehr oder weniger vollständigem Verschluß des Gefäßlumens führen können. Thrombenbildungen sind verschieden stark ausgeprägt. Sie werden von Miescher als sekundär, von Ketron und Bernstein als zum Prozeß gehörig beschrieben. In einzelnen Fällen treten reichlich Riesenzellen auf, die elastisches Gewebe phagocytieren (Hamperl).

Diese nekrotisierende Gefäßwandentzündung befällt einzelne Abschnitte des Arterienrohres. Es kann in der Folge dort zur Bildung kleiner Aneurysmen kommen (Macaigne und Nicaud, Kazmeier). Sie werden an sämtlichen Gefäßgebieten beschrieben. Für die Periarteriitis nodosa charakteristisch ist, daß in erster Linie die kleinen und mittelgroßen Arterien befallen sind, bei den ausschließlich cutan-subcutanen Formen speziell die tieferen Hautgefäße.

Diese Veränderungen der Gefäßwand zeigen nun oft auch gewisse Modifikationen, auf Grund deren versucht wird, eine Reihe von Krankheitsbildern von der typischen Periarteriitis nodosa abzutrennen. Es handelt sich um die von Harkavy beschriebene „Vascular Allergy", bei der außer den mittelgroßen Arterien auch die Venen Veränderungen vom Typus der nekrotisierenden Entzündung zeigen, wobei außerdem noch fibrinoide Nekrose im angrenzenden Bindegewebe und Endangiitis obliterans beobachtet werden. Auch die von Churg und Strauss als „Allergic granulomatous angitis" beschriebene Krankheit befällt neben sämtlichen Gefäßen das angrenzende Bindegewebe, das fibrinoide Degeneration zeigt und durch Neutrophile und Eosinophile infiltriert ist. Dieses Infiltrat wandelt sich dann in einen Granulationsmantel aus radiär gestellten Makrophagen von Epitheloidzellcharakter um (KRAHULIK et al.). Schließlich zeigt die Arteriitis temporalis ähnliche Veränderungen, wobei aber Fremdkörper-Riesenzellen im Vordergrund stehen und die Zerstörungen der Wand mehr die inneren Schichten betreffen. Riesenzellen können allerdings auch bei der Periarteriitis nodosa in großen Mengen auftreten (ALKIEWICZ).

Für die Periarteriitis nodosa der Haut gibt RUITER an, daß sie zwei Formen zeigen kann. Die erste ist auf die oberflächlichen Hautschichten beschränkt und betrifft vor allem die kleinen oberflächlichen Blutgefäße. Die zweite bevorzugt die mittelkalibrigen Gefäße der Subcutis. SCHOTTE beschreibt eine besondere Gefäßarmut im oberen Cutisdrittel, perivasculäre Infiltrate und eine zwischen Endothel und den anderen Gefäßschichten gelegene homogene strukturlose Masse als Hautamyloidose bei einem Fall, der klinisch als Periarteriitis nodosa imponierte. Auch SZODORAI et al. betonen die Schwierigkeiten der histologischen Unterscheidung der Periarteriitis nodosa cutanea gegenüber dem Erythema nodosum und dem Erythema induratum.

Es ist nach dem Gesagten offensichtlich, daß die histologischen Befunde allein oft nicht zur Differenzierung der einzelnen Fälle ausreichen, daß sie aber interessante Hinweise auf die mögliche Pathogenese der Periarteriitis nodosa geben können.

3. Ätiologie und Pathogenese

Die Beobachtung, daß Periarteriitis nodosa-artige Veränderungen epidemisch bei Tieren vorkommen können, ließ daran denken, daß es sich dabei um ein infektiöses Leiden handeln könnte. Dafür schienen auch einige gelungene Übertragungsversuche zu sprechen, die allerdings in der Folge nie bestätigt werden konnten, so daß die Anschauung, es handle sich bei der Periarteriitis nodosa um eine Krankheit infektiöser Genese, wohl kaum mehr vertreten wird. Nur FEYRTER hält es auf Grund der bei Zoster beobachteten periarteriitischen Gefäßveränderungen in inneren Organen für möglich, daß die Periarteriitis nodosa eine hämatogen ausgelöste Viruskrankheit sei, und KAZMEIER vertritt die Meinung, die Suche nach einem Erreger sei zu Unrecht aufgegeben worden.

Im Vordergrund steht heute vielmehr die Diskussion darüber, inwieweit es sich bei den beschriebenen Gefäßveränderungen um Zeichen eines allergischen Prozesses handeln könne. Dieser Frage sind einige ausgezeichnete Untersuchungen (RANDERATH, KÄMMERER) gewidmet worden, und das Problem kann wie folgt umschrieben werden: Es besteht kein Zweifel, daß bei sensibilisierten Tieren durch wiederholte Injektionen von Antigenen Gefäßveränderungen erzeugt werden können, die weitgehend Ähnlichkeit mit den beim Menschen beobachteten Veränderungen der Periarteriitis nodosa haben (RICH et al., PAGEL). Ob es sich dabei nun tatsächlich um Folgen einer Antigen-Antikörper-Reaktion handelt, ist umstritten, und die Vorstellung, die Periarteriitis nodosa komme durch eine chronische Urticaria der Blutgefäße zustande (SHEDROW), dürfte wohl zu einfach sein. Zahlreiche Befunde weisen nämlich darauf hin, daß auch toxische, hämodynamische und nervöse Einflüsse, die unabhängig von Antikörperbildungen die Gefäße treffen, histologisch faßbare Veränderungen vom Typus einer entzündlichen Arteriitis zur Folge haben können. So haben speziell die Versuche zur Erzeugung künstlichen Hochdruckes ergeben, daß Injektionen von DCA Gefäßwandveränderungen zur Folge haben können. Auch bei künstlich erzeugter Perinephritis lassen sich typische Gefäßveränderungen in der Niere erkennen, sobald nach Entfernung der andern Niere eine Hypertonie auftritt, so daß Smith und Zeek z. B. der Ansicht sind, daß die Periarteriitis nodosa eher einem rapid einsetzenden Hochdruck als dem Einfluß irgendeines Antigens zuzuschreiben sei. Die Hypertonie scheint auch beim Menschen eine wichtige Rolle in der Genese der Periarteriitis nodosa zu spielen, da von Selzer et al. ein ausschließliches Befallensein der Gefäße des Lungenkreislaufs bei Hypertonie im kleinen Kreislauf infolge Mitralstenose gefunden worden ist. Auch Meessen erwähnt eine Reihe von Experimenten, die dagegen sprechen, daß die Periarteriitis nodosa ausschließlich die Folge eines allergischen Prozesses sei. Auf jeden Fall kann die Ansicht von Albertini, daß heute einzig die allergische Genese der Periarteriitis nodosa gesichert erscheint, noch nicht ohne weiteres angenommen werden, da bisher nur in wenigen Fällen ein eindeutiger Allergennachweis geglückt ist. Ein solcher war bisher nur dort möglich, wo die Periarteriitis nodosa im Anschluß an eine medikamentöse Allergie aufgetreten war. Rasmussen stellt an Hand einer eigenen Beobachtung die bisher als Ursache der Periarteriitis nodosa beschriebenen Allergene zusammen. Es besteht danach kein Zweifel, daß tatsächlich Medikamente, speziell Serum, Jod, dann Sulfonamide, Penicillin, Arsen, Thiouracil, Phenylbutazon u. a., imstande sind, Veränderungen im Organismus hervorzurufen, die weder klinisch noch histologisch von spontan entstandenen Fällen von Periarteriitis nodosa zu unterscheiden sind.

Immerhin muß festgestellt werden, daß sich wesentliche Unterschiede zwischen dieser Form der Periarteriitis nodosa und einer anaphylaktischen Reaktion, der sie den Gewebsveränderungen nach am ehesten entsprechen würde, finden. Der wesentlichste Unterschied besteht darin, daß die durch Medikamente ausgelöste Periarteriitis nodosa weiterzugehen pflegt, auch wenn das Medikament abgesetzt wird (Barnum et al.). Ob man berechtigt ist, diese Fälle unter dem Begriff der „Hypersensitiven Angitis" (Zeek et al.) zusammenzufassen, erscheint fraglich. Denn die als Unterscheidungsmerkmale gegenüber der klassischen Periarteriitis nodosa angegebenen Unterschiede, nämlich daß die Teilungszonen der Gefäße nicht besonders bevorzugt werden, daß sowohl Venen als Arterien fibrinoide Nekrose zeigen, daß die Milzarterien ausgedehnt befallen sind, daß alle histologischen Veränderungen das gleiche Stadium zeigen, daß die Gewebsveränderungen der „Hypersensitiven Angitis" auch in den Lungen zu finden sind, daß ihr Beginn akuter, ihr Verlauf kürzer ist, sind wohl mehr quantitative als prinzipielle Abweichungen von den spontan entstehenden Formen der Periarteriitis nodosa. Auch die Abgrenzung der „Allergic Granulomatosis" (Strauss et al.) und die Unterscheidung von primärer Periarteriitis nodosa und von sekundärer Periarteriitis nodosa als Endstadium von hypertonischen Zuständen (Blankenhorn et al.) erscheint zunächst von geringem heuristischem Wert. Jedenfalls ist die Tendenz zur Unterteilung der Periarteriitis nodosa in weitere Krankheitsbilder (s. Schema bei Randerath, Bock, Reich, Stüttgen) vorläufig noch problematisch, da es Übergangsformen und Kombinationen z. B. von Periarteriitis nodosa und Arteriitis temporalis gibt (Touraine et al.) und da damit weder für die Erkenntnis der Pathogenese noch in bezug auf die Beurteilung der Prognose viel gewonnen ist.

Neben den einigermaßen abgeklärten medikamentösen Ursachen der Periarteriitis nodosa sind es nun hauptsächlich die bakteriellen Allergene, die für das Zustandekommen der Gefäßveränderungen verantwortlich gemacht werden. So hat Harkavy in seinen Fällen durchwegs Sinusitiden angetroffen. Dietrich sah Periarteriitis nodosa nach Erysipel auftreten. Die Beobachtungen über das Auftreten nekrotisierender Arteriitiden nach Impfungen dürften wohl auch in dieses Kapitel gehören (Barner). Auch wird die Anwesenheit eines Corynebacteriums in den Hautknoten (THIERS et al.), von Staphylokokken, Streptokokken, Pneumokokken oder Tuberkelbacillen in Organen (TISELL), Organ-Preßsäften (WEIDMAN) oder Urin (ARZT) erwähnt. Im Blut konnten OLINER et al. Streptokokken, VRÁNOVÁ Tuberkelbacillen nachweisen, während PIERINI dieser Nachweis nicht gelang. Es ist daher die Möglichkeit erwogen worden, daß durch die Wirkung dieser Bakterien im menschlichen Gewebe ein Auto-Antigen entstehen könne (HARKAVY, SARRE) und damit die Periarteriitis nodosa ins Gebiet der Kollagenkrankheiten gehöre (BUREAU et al. 1956) oder aber daß es sich um eine Herxheimersche Reaktion handeln könne (STÜTTGEN).

Einer Erwähnung bedürfen noch die Beziehungen der Periarteriitis nodosa zum rheumatischen Formenkreis. KLINGE et al. führen beide Erkrankungen als Beispiele typisch allergischer Gefäßschäden an. Nach RÖSSLE finden sich Übergänge zwischen den klassischen Formen rheumatischer Gewebsveränderungen und der Periarteriitis nodosa. Es gelang auch, in einem Fall von Periarteriitis nodosa im Herzmuskel Aschoffsche Knötchen festzustellen (UNVERRICHT). Auch klinisch wird der Zusammenhang beider Affektionen immer wieder erwähnt (FROBOESE, PIERINI). Es dürfte sich bei sehr vielen Auseinandersetzungen über dieses Thema wohl mehr um Nomenklaturfragen als um wirkliche Unterschiede handeln, da weder das rheumatische Reaktionsbild noch die hyperergischen Veränderungen der Periarteriitis nodosa in ihren Grenzen scharf umrissen werden können.

Als Stütze für die Auffassung der Periarteriitis nodosa als allergischer Manifestation wird schließlich oft die allergische Disposition der Kranken herangezogen (KLEIN, COHEN et al., BERGER et al.) bzw. das oft beobachtete Zusammentreffen von Asthma bronchiale (TRASOFF et al., FAHRLÄNDER), urticariellen Hauterscheinungen (SAWYER) und Periarteriitis nodosa. Nun fehlen aber in den meisten Publikationen Angaben darüber, ob es sich beim Asthma bronchiale wirklich um eine allergische Form oder um ein symptomatisches Asthma bei anderen Lungenveränderungen gehandelt hat (WILSON und ALEXANDER). Das gleiche gilt für die Urticaria, die ebenfalls nicht immer allergischen Ursprungs sein muß. Lediglich in dem von MIALE et al. beschriebenen Fall ließ sich ein eindeutiger Zusammenhang zwischen einem Nahrungsmittelantigen und Periarteriitis nodosa klinisch und in dem von MCLETCHIE et al. beschriebenen Fall zwischen einer Antibiotica-Allergie und den Gefäßveränderungen auch histologisch an passiv übertragenen Hautreaktionen feststellen, während der von LEJTES beschriebene Fall von Periarteriitis nodosa bei einem mit Penicillin behandelten Luetiker in dieser Beziehung schwer zu beurteilen ist.

Schließlich wird noch die familiäre Disposition für Gefäßkrankheiten erwähnt (ANHEGGER).

Zusammenfassend kann der heutige Stand der Kenntnis der Pathogenese der Periarteriitis nodosa so definiert werden, daß es sich bei der Periarteriitis nodosa theoretisch wohl um eine echte Antigen-Antikörper-Reaktion handeln kann, daß aber in den allermeisten Fällen der schlüssige Beweis für eine solche Auffassung bisher nicht erbracht werden konnte und daß diejenigen Fälle, bei denen die Periarteriitis nodosa als Arzneimittelallergie aufgefaßt wird, streng nachgeprüft werden sollten. Denn da es sich dabei oft um chronisch Kranke handelt, bei denen alle möglichen Medikamente im Verlauf ihrer Krankheit angewendet worden sind, ist auf einen sicheren Nachweis besonders Gewicht zu legen, damit nicht falsche Vorstellungen über die Schädlichkeit gewisser Medikamente entstehen können. Es bedarf jedenfalls einer besonderen immunbiologischen und endokrinologischen Konstellation, damit die Gefäßläsionen entstehen können (STÜTTGEN).

4. Diagnose und Differentialdiagnose

Es ist klar, daß bei der Vielfältigkeit der Symptomatologie der Periarteriitis nodosa die Diagnose, speziell derjenigen Formen, die ohne Hautbeteiligung verlaufen, sehr schwer sein kann. Außer den histologisch faßbaren Veränderungen gibt es eben kein für die Periarteriitis nodosa typisches Krankheitsbild. Am ehesten wird aus dem Syndrom eines septischen Zustandes verbunden mit hoher Senkung, Leukocytose, Eosinophilie und Lymphopenie, einem nephritischen Urinbefund und einer passageren Hypertonie die Diagnose zu stellen sein. Beim Bestehen von Hautveränderungen dürften die typischen Knötchen wohl ohne weiteres eine eindeutige Diagnose ermöglichen. Wesentlich schwieriger ist die Diagnose derjenigen Hautformen, die ohne die typischen internen Befunde verlaufen und bei denen das histologische Bild außer der Beteiligung der Arterien auch eine solche der Venen und der Capillaren zeigt. Hier kommen in erster Linie differentialdiagnostisch die von Storck beschriebenen Mikrobide hämorrhagischen Charakters in Frage sowie die Schönlein-Henochsche Purpura. Daß Zusammenhänge zwischen beiden Affektionen bestehen, zeigt die Angabe von Spiegel, daß bei 12 von 17 Patienten Purpura zu Beginn der Periarteriitis nodosa auftrat, und die Beobachtung von Gadermann et al., wonach bei Periarteriitis nodosa das Auftreten der Purpura möglicherweise durch chronischen Alkoholismus ausgelöst werden kann. Berardinelli beobachtete ebenfalls das Auftreten einer Periarteriitis nodosa nach Alkoholabusus. Auch Übergänge von Periarteriitis nodosa zu Erythematodes werden beschrieben (Neuss), doch läßt sich eine klare Unterscheidung der Periarteriitis nodosa von ähnlich verlaufenden „Kollagenkrankheiten“ wohl meist treffen (Habib). Die von Degos beschriebene Papulosis atrophicans maligna kann im Anfangsstadium der Periarteriitis nodosa gleichen. In verschiedenen Fällen wird es nicht möglich sein, eine definitive Diagnose zu stellen, sondern der Verlauf der Krankheit dürfte Aufschluß über die Natur der Erkrankung geben.

So gibt McCombs an, daß es möglich sei, die „allergische“ Vaskulitis von der Periarteriitis nodosa klinisch zu differenzieren. Die allergische Gefäßentzündung ist gekennzeichnet durch Gelenkschmerzen, Purpura, Ödem, gastrointestinale Blutungen und Nierenschäden. Sie heilt oft spontan und spricht gut auf Cortison an. Demgegenüber ist die Periarteriitis nodosa eine progrediente Krankheit, die mit Fieber, Gewichtsabnahme, peripherer Neuritis, Asthma und Hypertonie verläuft und Eosinophilie und Hämaturie hervorruft.

Es empfiehlt sich deshalb, den Begriff der Periarteriitis nodosa nicht zu weit zu fassen, sondern ihn auf die Fälle mit ausschließlicher Arterienbeteiligung nekrotisierenden Charakters zu beschränken. In diesem Krankheitsbild hätten dann die „Vascular Allergy“ und die „Hypersensitive Angitis“ ihren Platz. Alle anderen Prozesse wären dann unter dem Begriff der vasculären Allergide abzugrenzen oder als Arteriolitis allergica zu bezeichnen (Ruiter et al.).

5. Therapie

Daß alle als Allergene in Frage kommenden Medikamente abzusetzen sind, ist klar (v. Rijssel et al.). Während früher Bismuth und Salvarsan speziell in den reinen Hautfällen von Nutzen befunden wurden (Goldschlag, Goldschlag und Chwalibogowski), während sie bei interner Organbeteiligung versagten (Curtis et al.), wird neuerdings den Antibiotica, Sulfonamiden und Cortison-Derivaten der Vorzug gegeben. Tatsächlich gelingt es, mit ACTH und Cortison Heilung oder doch wenigstens vorübergehende Besserungen zu erreichen (Lit. bei Malkinson und Wells, Nobis), wobei Prednison speziell günstig wirken soll

(Lit. in „*CIBA*", Therapie mit Ultracorten). Auch durch Antibiotica (Stüttgen, Reynaers, v. Cauwenberge, Holmes) und Sulfonamide (Venkei) sind Heilungen erzielt worden (Lit. bei Bock). Baggenstoss et al. und Siegenthaler et al. sahen unter Cortison histologisch Heilungen der Periarteriitis nodosa, allerdings konnte der Tod an Urämie nicht verhindert werden. Yonis, Winkelmann et al. und Lincoln et al. sahen vollständige Heilung mit hohen Dosen Cortison, de Rose et al. mit ACTH. Schwangerschaft kann günstig wirken (Fornara). Gaté et al. sahen bei einer Patientin mit gangränöser Form der Periarteriitis nodosa und starken rheumatischen Schmerzen, bei der ACTH und Cortison versagt hatten, mit Nivaquin eine rasche Heilung der Haut und völliges Verschwinden der Schmerzen. Carrick et al. konnten einen Fall mit ausschließlicher Hautbeteiligung mit 12 g PAS täglich während Monaten heilen, Bessière et al. konnten bei einem Kind mittels Jodölinjektionen neue Schübe verhindern. Jørgensen empfiehlt Fiebertherapie, die in einem Fall Heilung gebracht hatte, nachdem Sulfonamide und Antibiotica versagt hatten. Hill konnte in einem Fall ausgedehnte gangränöse Hautdefekte plastisch decken, nachdem durch massive Dosen Cortison der pathologische Prozeß zur Heilung gebracht worden war.

Literatur

Albertini, A. v.: Bedeutung der Allergielehre für die Pathologie. Schweiz. Z. allg. Path. **17**, 1 (1954). — Alkiewicz, Jan: Die subcutanen Veränderungen bei einem Fall von Periarteriitis nodosa. Przegl. Derm. Wener. **28**, 630 (1933). — Multiple nekrotisierende Periarteriitis nodosa der Haut in Gemeinschaft mit Acanthosis nigricans. Arch. Derm. Syph. (Berl.) **168**, 522 (1933). — Anhegger, E.: Beobachtungen zur Periarteriitis nodosa. Z. ärztl. Fortbild. **45**, 407 (1951). — Arzt, L.: Zu Nekrose und Ulceration führende Purpura. (Periarteriitis nodosa ?) Österr. Dermat. Ges. Wien, Sitzg vom 10. 12. 1936. Ref. in Zbl. Haut- u. Geschl.-Kr. **56**, 87 (1937).

Baggenstoss, A. H., R. M. Shick and H. F. Polley: The effect of cortisone on the lesions of periarteriitis nodosa. Amer. J. Path. **27**, 537 (1951). — Banke, S.: Periarteriitis nodosa. Ugeskr. Laeg. **1941**, 532. — Barnard, W. G., and W. M. Burbury: Gangrene of the fingers and toes in a case of polyarteritis nodosa. J. Path. Bact. **39**, 285 (1934). — Barner, F. R.: Über nekrotisierende Arteriitis nach Impfungen und ihre Deutung im Rahmen der heutigen Allergielehre. Schweiz. Z. allg. Path. **19**, 411 (1956). — Barnum, D. R., G. de Takats and R. E. Dolkart: Periarteriitis nodosa following thiouracil therapy of hyperthyroidism: resultant hypertension benefited by sympathectomy. Report of a case. Angiology **2**, 256 (1951). — Becker, J.: Akute Porphyrie und Periarteriitis nodosa in der Neurologie. Monogr. aus dem Gesamtgebiet der Neurologie und Psychiatrie. Hrsg. von M. Müller, H. Spatz u. P. Vogel. H. 92. Berlin-Göttingen-Heidelberg: Springer 1961. — Berardinelli, W.: Le premier cas de péri-artérite noueuse ou maladie de Kussmaul-Maier observé au Brésil. Presse méd. **1933I**, 280. — Berger, S. S., and M. A. Weitz: Periarteriitis nodosa. J. Allergy **9**, 489 (1938). — Bernstein, A.: Periarteriitis nodosa without peripheral nodules diagnosed ante mortem. Amer. J. med. Sci. **190**, 317 (1935). — Bessière, L., et Massoulier: Périartérite noueuse. Amélioration des signes cliniques et biologiques coincidents avec un traitement par l'huile iodée. Bull. Soc. franç. Derm. Syph. **65**, 651 (1958). — Best, W. R., and G. Fine: Periarteriitis nodosa and multiple myeloma. Report of simultaneous occurence in a patient receiving Stilbamidine. Ann. intern. Med. **34**, 1472 (1951). — Blankenhorn, M. A., and H. C. Knowles jr.: Periarteritis nodosa: Recognition and clinical symptoms. Ann. intern. Med. **41**, 887 (1954). — Bock, H. E.: Allergische Erkrankung des Herzens und des Gefäßsystems. In: Hansen, Allergie, 3. Aufl., S. 532. Stuttgart: Georg Thieme 1957. — Die Bedeutung der allergischen Pathogenese bei der Arteriitis. Kongr.-Zbl. ges. inn. Med. **60**, 391 (1954). — Bureau, Y., et H. Barrière: Les manifestations cutanéo-muqueuses de la périartérite noueuse (Maladie de Kussmaul). Ann. Derm. Syph. (Paris) **1954**, 601. — Bureau, Y., H. Barrière, Jarry et Coignard: Périartérite noueuse avec manifestation cutanée necrotique et érythémato-squameuse. Bull. Soc. franç. Derm. Syph. **60**, 434 (1953).. — Bureau, Y., A. Jarry et H. Barrière: Maladie du collagène. Périartériite noueuse. Bull. Soc. franç. Derm. Syph. **63**, 516 (1956). — Butler, K. R., and J. A. Palmer: Cryoglobulinaemia in polyarteritis nodosa with gangrene of extremities. Canad. med. Ass. J. **72**, 686 (1955).

Cambier, J.: Le syndrome de Wegener et les formes „respiratoires" de la périartérite noueuse. Presse méd. **1955**, 821. — Carol, W. L. L.: Die cutane Form der Periarteriitis nodosa. Ned. T. Geneesk. **1936**, 358. — Carol, W. L. L., u. J. R. Prakken: Die cutane Form der Periarteriitis nodosa. Acta derm.-venereol. (Stockh.) **18**, 102 (1937). — CARRICK, L., and E. C. VON DER HEIDE: Periarteriiti nodosa. Report on a case treated with Paraaminosalicylic acid. Arch. Derm. Syph. (Chic.) **64**, 359 (1951). — CAUWENBERGE, VAN, et VAN CAUWENBERGE: Aspects cliniques et histologiques de la périartérite noueuse, sa pathogénie et son traitement. Arch. belges Derm. **7**, 191 (1951). — Panvascularite nodulaire chronique. Arch. belges Derm. **7**, 152 (1951). — Périartérite noueuse ou maladie de Kussmaul-Maier. Arch. belges Derm. **7**, 152 (1951). — CERUTTI, P.: Periarterite nodosa cutanea. Minerva derm. **36**, 187 (1961). — CERUTTI, P., u. G. SANTOJANNI: Über die Polyarteriitis cutanea benigna. Hautarzt **8**, 109 (1957). — CHURG,. J, and L. STRAUSS: Allergic granulomatosis, allergic angitis and periarteritis nodosa. Amer. J. Path. **27**, 277 (1951). — CHWALIBOGOWSKI, A., u. F. GOLDSCHLAG: Ein Fall von Periarteriitis nodosa bei einem 5jährigen Kind. Arch. Derm. Syph. (Berl.) **171**, 622 (1935). — *CIBA*: Zur Therapie mit Ultracorten. Basel: Ciba 1958. — COHEN, M. B., B. S. KLINE and A. M. YOUNG: The clinical diagnosis of periarteriitis nodosa. J. Amer. med. Ass. **107**, 1555 (1936). — CROSTI, A.: Contributo alla conoscenza dei quadri clinici e dermatologici della periarterite nodosa degli eventuali loro rapporti con l'infezione reumatica. G. ital. Derm. **76**, 15 (1935). — CURTIS, A. C., and R. M. COFFEY: Periarteriitis nodosa. A brief review of the literature and a report of one case. Ann. intern. Med. **7**, 1345 (1934). — CZICKELI, H.: Das Krankheitsbild der neuritischen Form der Periarteriitis nodosa. Wien. med. Wschr. **1954**, 801.

DEGOS, R.: Papulose atrophi ante maligne (Syndrome cutaneo-intestinal mortel). In: Dermatologie. Paris: Editions Médicales Flammarion 1956. — DEJEAN, VIALLEFONT et CHAMPION: Périartérite noueuse et rétinite pigmentaire. Bull. Soc. Ophtal. France **1953**, 252. — DIETRICH, K.: Periarteriitis nodosa in der Haut des Vorderarmes nach Erysipel derselben. Z. Kreisl.-Forsch. **25**, 305 (1933). — DIVERTIE, M. B., and A. M. OLSEN: Pulmonary infiltration associated with blood eosinophilia: a clinical study of Löffler's syndrome and of periarteriitis nodosa. Dis. Chest **37**, 340 (1960). — DRUSS, J. G., and J. L. MAYBAUM: Periarteriitis nodosa of the temporal bone. Arch. Otolaryng. **19**, 502 (1934). — DUPERRAT, B., et J. CIVATTE: Gros nez ligneux. Zit. bei Y. BUREAU et H. BARRIÈRE.

FAHRLÄNDER, H.: Über Periarteriitis nodosa. Schweiz. med. Wschr. **1953**, 575. — FEYRTER, F.: Über die Pathogenese der Periarteriitis nodosa, insbesondere der Periarteriitis nodosa zosterica. Dtsch. Arch. klin. Med. **201**, 377 (1954). — Über die Periarteriitis nodosa zosterica. Verh. dtsch. Ges. inn. Med. **1954**, 694. — FORNARA, P.: Consulto di un pediatra su di un caso di periarterite nodosa seguito dall'età infantile a quelle adulta. Minerva med. **1955 II**, 1793. — FROBOESE, C.: Beitrag zur Stütze der rheumatologischen Ätiologie der Periarteriitis nodosa und zum subtotalen Pankreasinfarkt. Virchows Arch. path. Anat. **317**, 430 (1949).

GADERMANN, E., u. K. FOIGT: Die Schönlein-Hennoch'sche Purpura und ihre Beziehungen zur Periarteriitis nodosa. Frankfurt. Z. Path. **62**, 255 (1955). — GARZÓN, R., R. A. ARGÜELLO, L. J. FERRARIS y R. CRESPO: Periarteriitis nodosa. Dos observaciones. Arch. argent. Derm. Syph. **3**, 453 (1953). — GATÉ, J., J. CONDERT et J. VAYRE: Périartérite noueuse ulcérée actuellement guérie par la nivaquine. Bull. Soc. franç. Derm. Syph. **1955**, 174. — GOLDSCHLAG, F.: Periarteriitis nodosa. Öster. Dermat. Ges. Wien, Sitzg v. 14. 1. 1937. Ref. in Zbl. Haut- u. Geschl.-Kr. **57**, 19 (1938). — GOLDSCHLAG, F., u. A. CHWALIBOGOWSKI: Periarteriitis nodosa. Lemberger Dermat. Ges. Sitzg v. 26. 4. 1934. Zbl. Haut- u. Geschl.-Kr. **49**, 1, 3 (1935).

HABIB, R.: Rapports entre la périartérite noueuse, les autres artérites nodulaires et les maladies du collagène. Ann. Méd. **56**, 496 (1955). — HAMPERL, N.: Elastische Fasern als Fremdkörper. Virchows Arch. path. Anat. **323**, 591 (1953). — HARKAVY, J.: Vascular allergy. Arch. intern. Med. **67**, 709 (1941). — J. Allergy **14**, 507 (1943). — HARRIS, A. W., G. W. LYNCH and J. P. O'HARE: Periarteriitis nodosa. Arch. intern. Med. **63**, 1163 (1939). — HENRY, M. J., H. G. E. STOECKLE and H. C. HOPPS: Periarteriitis in a 4-month-old infant unresponsive to penicillinase. Amer. Heart J. **60**, 817—835 (1960). — HILL, E. J.: Skin grafting in periarteritis nodosa. Plast. Reconstr. Surgery **15**, 186 (1955). — HOLMES, J. G.: Die Hauterscheinungen der Periarteriitis nodosa unter besonderer Berücksichtigung hämorrhagischer Veränderungen. Hautarzt **4**, 180 (1953).

JØRGENSEN, J.: On the treatment of Periarteritis nodosa. Acta derm.-venereol. (Stockh.) **31**, 167 (1951). — JOULIA, P., P. LECOULANT, L. TEXIER, J. MALEVILLE et GAGGINI: Un cas de périartérite noueuse à manifestation cutanée et pluriviscérale. Confirmation anatomique du diagnostique. Bull. Soc. franç. Derm. Syph. **66**, 779 (1959). — JULICH, H.: Beitrag zur Klinik der Periarteriitis nodosa. Dtsch. Gesundh.-Wes. **1950**, 134.

KÄMMERER, H.: Zur allergischen Genese der Arthritis. Verh. dtsch. Ges. inn. Med. **60**, 417 (1954). — KAZMEIER, F.: Symptomatologie und Differentialdiagnose der Periarteriitis nodosa. Med. Welt **1951**, 774. — KEMP, G., u. F. ROTH: Zur Periarteriitis nodosa im Kindesalter. Zbl. Kinderheilk. **75**, 60 (1954). — KERNOHAN, J., and H. W. WOLTMAN: Periarteriitis nodosa. A clinico-pathologic study with special reference to the nervous system. Arch. Neur. Psychiat. (Chic.) **39**, 655 (1938). — KETRON, L. W., and J. C. BERNSTEIN: Cutaneous manifestations of periarteritis nodosa. Arch. Derm. Syph. (Chic.) **40**, 929 (1939). — KLEIN, P. S.: Periarteriitis nodosa. Study of chronicity and recovery with report of 2 cases. Arch. intern. Med. **84**, 983 (1949). — KLINGE, F., u. H. G. FASSBENDER: Pathologische Anatomie der experimentellen Grundlagen. In HANSEN, Allergie, 3. Aufl. Stuttgart: Georg Thieme 1957. — KLINGER: Zit. bei STRATTON et al. — KNOTH, W., u. W. MEYHÖFER: Beitrag zum Formenkreis der Periarteriitis nodosa und zur Bewertung der Riesenzellen bei Gefäßerkrankungen. Dermatologica (Basel) **119**, 1 (1959). — KORTING, G. W.: Über cutane Periarteriitis nodosa unter besonderer Berücksichtigung begleitender Leberstörungen und der sog. Thrombophlebitis migrans. Arch. Derm. Syph. (Berl.) **199**, 333 (1955). — KRAHULIK, L., M. ROSENTHAL and E. H. LOUGHLIN: Periarteriitis nodosa (necrotizing panarteriitis) in childhood with meningeal involvement. Report of a case with study of pathologic findings. Amer. J. med. Sci. **190**, 308 (1935). — KREN: Periarteriitis nodosa cutis. Wiener Dermat. Ges. Sitzg vom 4. 12. 1933. Ref. in Zbl. Haut- u. Geschl.-Kr. **48**, 1 (1934).

LEJTES, F. L.: Bei der Syphilistherapie entstandene Periarteriitis nodosa. Vestn. Vener. Derm. **30**, 49 (1956). — LINCOLN, M., and W. A. RICKER: A case of periarteriitis nodosa with L.E. cells; apparent complete remission with cortisone therapy. Ann. intern. Med. **41**, 639 (1954). — LINDBERG, KAJ: Über eine subcutane Form der Periarteriitis nodosa mit langwierigem Verlauf. Arb. path. Inst. Helsingfors (Jena), N.F. **7**, 159 (1933). — LINDGREN, J., and C. LUNDMARK: Periarteritis nodosa as a skin disease. Acta derm.-venereol. (Stockh.) **36**, 343 (1956). — LJUBOMUDROV, V. E.: Affection of the skin in periarteritis nodosa. Vestn. Derm. Vener. **35**, 15 (1961). — LOHSE, R.: Zur klinischen Diagnose der Periarteriitis nodosa. Ärztl. Forsch. **6**, (I) 270 (1952). — LOOGEN, F.: Über die Periarteriitis nodosa. Z. klin. Med. **150**, 182 (1952). — LYELL, A., and R. CHURCH: The cutaneous manifestations of polyarteritis nodosa. Brit. J. Derm. **66**, 335 (1954).

MACAIGNE, et P. NICAUD: Les lésions de la périartérite noueuse à forme chronique. (Maladie de Kussmaul). Ann. Anat. path. **11**, 235 (1934). — MALKINSON, F. D., and C. G. WELLS: Adrenal steroids in Periarteriitis nodosa. Arch. Derm. Syph. (Chic.) **71**, 492 (1955). — MANCKE, R., u. R. PEPER: Zur Problematik der Periarteriitis nodosa. Schweiz. med. Wschr. **87**, 918 (1957). — MATRAS, A.: Zur cutanen Form der Periarteriitis nodosa. Wien. klin. Wschr. **1938 II**, 991. — MCCOMBS, R. P.: The clinical differenciation of "allergic" vasculitis from periarteriitis nodosa. Int. Arch. Allergy **12**, 98 (1958). — MCLETCHIE, N. G. B., R. M. MACDONALD and J. H. CUTTS: Polyarteritis nodosa. Report of a case with proof of drug allergy. Canad. med. Ass. J. **76**, 213 (1957). — MEESSEN, H.: Über allergisch bedingte Arteriitis Verh. dtsch. Ges. inn. Med. **60**, 385 (1954). — MELCZER, N., u. T. VENKEI: Über die Hautformen der Periarteriitis nodosa. Arch. Derm. Syph. (Berl.) **186**, 107 (1944). — Dermatologica (Basel) **94**, 214 (1947). — MÉRAND: Periarteriitis nodosa papulosa. Ver.igg Südwestdtsch. Dermat. Sitzg 7./8. 5. 1955 Freiburg i. Br. Ref. in Zbl. Haut- u. Geschl.-Kr. **92**, 400 (1955). — MIALE, J. B., K. H. DOEGE and M. PIEHL: Acute panarteritis in allergic persons. Arch. intern. Med. **80**, 791 (1947). — MIESCHER, G.: Über kutane Formen der Periarteriitis nodosa. Dermatologica (Basel) **92**, 225 (1946). — Akut entzündliche Gefäßkrankheiten und deren Auswirkung auf die Haut (vaskuläre Allergide). Arch. Derm. Syph. (Berl.) **206**, 135 (1957). — Vascular allergids. Excerpta med. (Amst.), Sect. XIII **11**, H. 11 (1957). — MULLER, S. E., R. C. FRAVEL and W. ESMOND: Porphyria hepatica associated with panarteritis. Ann. intern. Med. **45**, 288 (1956).

NEUSS, O.: Über 2 Fälle von generalisiertem „collagen disease", Periarteriitis nodosa und Lupus erythematodes disseminatus. Medizinische **1953**, 328. — NOBIS, L.: Ein Fall von kutaner Periarteriitis nodosa. Z. Haut- u. Geschl.-Kr. **11**, 469 (1951).

OLINER, L., M. TAUBENHAUS, T. M. SHAPIRA and N. LESHIN: Non-syphilitic interstitial keratitis and bilateral deafness (Cogan's syndrome) associated with essential polyangitis (periarteriitis nodosa). A review of the syndrome with consideration of a possible pathogenic mechanism. New Engl. J. Med. **248**, 1001 (1953).

PAGEL, W.: Pathologie und Histologie der allergischen Erscheinungen. In: Fortschritte der Allergielehre, Bd. I. Basel: S. Karger 1939. — PIERINI, L. E., u. J. C. LASCANO GONZALEZ: Periarteriitis nodosa oder Kussmaul-Maiersche Krankheit. Rev. argent. Dermatosif. **20**, 302 (1936). — PORTWICH, F.: Periarteritis nodosa (Kussmaul'sche Krankheit). Ergebn. inn. Med. Kinderheilk., N.F. **12**, 428 (1959). — PUCHOL, J. R.: Histopatología de las angeítis cutáneas. C S.I C. Madrid 1962.

RANDERATH, E.: Die Bedeutung der allergischen Pathogenese bei der Arthritis. Verh. dtsch. Ges. inn. Med. **60**, 359 (1954). — RASMUSSEN, H.: Iodide hypersensitivity in the etiology of Periarteriitis nodosa. J. Allergy **26**, 394 (1955). — REICH, H.: Allergische granulomatöse Angiitiden. Arch. Derm. Syph. (Berl.) **206**, 229 (1957). — REPKE, K.: Zur Klinik der Periarteriitis nodosa. Z. ärztl. Fortbild. **44**, 191 (1950). — REYNAERS, H.: Périartérite noueuse. Arch. belges Derm. **10**, 45 (1954). — RICH, A. R.: Hypersensitivity in disease with a special reference to periarteritis nodosa, rheumatic fever, disseminated lupus erythematosus and rheumatoid arthritis. Harvey Lect. **42**, 106 (1947). — RICH, A. R., and J. E. GREGORY: Bull. Johns Hopk. Hosp. **72**, 65 (1943). — Zit. in C. W. BOYD, Fundamentals of immunology, 3rd edit. London: Interscience Publishers 1956. — RIJSSEL, TH. VAN, u. L. MEYLER: Arteriitis generalisata necroticans nach Gebrauch von Sulfonamiden. Ned. T. Geneesk. **1947**, 2649. — RIVES, J.: Ein Fall von klinisch festgestellter Periarteriitis nodosa. Fol. neuropath. eston. **13**, 44 (1934). — ROCH, M., et E. MARTIN: Neurofibromatose. Périartérite noueuse. Hypertension. Helv. med. Acta **5**, 661 (1938). — RÖSSLE, R.: Zum Formenkreis der rheumatischen Gewebsveränderungen, mit besonderer Berücksichtigung der rheumatischen Gefäßveränderungen. Virchows Arch. path. Anat. **288**, 780 (1933). — ROSA, M. A. DE, y M. N. PIEGARI: Periarteriitis nodosa. Forma cutánea. Pren. méd. argent. **1954**, 2436. Ref. in Zbl. Haut- u. Geschl.-Kr. **92**, 155 (1955). — ROSSNER, H.: Über die Periarteriitis nodosa. Dtsch. Mil.-Arzt **3**, 308 (1938). — RUITER, M.: Die cutane Form der Periarteriitis nodosa. Ned. T. Geneesk. **1952**, 794. — The so-called cutaneous type of periarteriitis nodosa. Brit. J. Derm. **70**, 102 (1958). — RUITER, M., u. C. H. BRANDSMA: Arteriolitis allergica. Dermatologica (Basel) **97**, 265 (1948).

SANDLER, B. P.: Periarteriitis nodosa. Report of a case diagnosed clinically and confirmed by necropsy. Amer. J. med. Sci. **195**, 651 (1938). — SANNICANDRO, G.: Periarterite nodosa a localizzazione cutaneo-ghiandolare col quadro clinico di una elefantiasi ed eruzione nodulare dell'arto inferiore sinistro. Arch. ital. Derm. **9**, 70 (1933). — SARRE, H.: Die Bedeutung der allergischen Genese bei der Arteriitis. Kongr.-Zbl. ges. inn. Med. **60**, 413 (1954). — SAWYER, C. F.: Necrotizing arteriitis (periarteriitis nodosa). Surgery **6**, 717 (1939). — SCHERF, D., u. L. J. BOYD: Herzkrankheiten und Gefäßerkrankungen, 5. Aufl. Wien: Springer 1951. — SCHOTTE: Periarteriitis nodosa cutanea. Derm. Wschr. **141**, 326 (1960). — SELZER, G., and M. HORWITZ: Polyarteritis nodosa. Pathological and clinical features. With a report on seven cases. S. Afr. med. J. **23**, 8 (1949). — SHEDROW, A.: Etude clinique de la périartérite noueuse. Sem. Hôp. Paris **1953**, 170. — SIEGENTHALER, W., u. U. ISTER: Klinische und pathologisch-anatomische Beobachtungen bei einem Fall von Periarteriitis nodosa. Schweiz. med. Wschr. **1956**, 355. — SILLEVIS SMITT, W. G.: Der neurologische Aspekt der Periarteriitis nodosa. Ned. T. Geneesk. **1952**, 2851. — SLINGER, W. N., and V. STARCK: Cutaneous form of polyarteritis nodosa. Arch. Derm. Syph. (Chic.) **63**, 461 (1951). — SMITH, C. C., and P. M. ZEEK: Studies on periarteriitis nodosa. II. The role of various factors in the etiology of periarteriitis nodosa in experimental animals. Amer. J. Path. **23**, 147 (1947). — SPIEGEL, R.: Clinical aspects of Periarteriitis nodosa. Arch. intern. Med. **58**, 993 (1936). — STAMMLER, A.: Neurologische Syndrome bei der Periarteriitis nodosa. Fortschr. Neurol. Psychiat. **18**, 606 (1950). — STORCK, H.: Über haemorrhagische Phänomene in der Dermatologie. Dermatologica (Basel) **102**, 197 (1951). — STRATTON, H. J. M., T. M. L. PRICE and M. O. SKELTON: Granuloma of the nose and periarteriitis nodosa. Brit. med. J. **1953**, Nr 4802, 127. — STRAUSS, L., J. CHURG and F. G. ZAK: Cutaneous lesions of allergic granulomatosis. J. invest. Derm. **17**, 349 (1951). — STÜTTGEN, G.: Zum Begriff der Periarteriitis nodosa cutanea. Arch. Derm. Syph. (Berl.) **206**, 231 (1957). — Periarteriitis nodosa. Ver.igg Düsseldorfer Dermatologen. Sitzg v. 6. 7. 1955. Ref. in Zbl. Haut- u. Geschl.-Kr. **93**, 64 (1955/56). — Arteriitis und Gangrän der Haut. Ein Beitrag zur Abgrenzung der Periarteriitis nodosa cutanea. Hautarzt **7**, 353 (1956). — SZODORAI, L., u. K. N. VEZEKÉNYI: Über die an den Unterschenkeln junger Frauen auftretende Periarteriitis nodosa cutanea. Seu Vaskulitis nodularis. Hautarzt **10**, 263 (1959).

THIERS, H., H. PELLOUX, D. COLOMB, J. FAYOLLE et R. TRUCHOT: Syndrome de périartérite noueuse avec présence d'un corynebactérium dans les nodules cutanés. Bull. Soc. franç. Derm. Syph. **67**, 141 (1960). — TISELL, F.: Periarteriitis nodosa und Allergie. Nord. Med. **1939**, 3629. — Periarteriitis nodosa und ihre Beziehung zu allergischen Zuständen. Acta med. scand., Suppl. **123**, 284 (1941). — TOURAINE, A., BOLTANSKI et L. VISSIAN: Périartérite noueuse avec artérite temporale. Bull. Soc. franç. Derm. Syph. **1950**, 303. — TRASOFF, A., and MAXWELL SCARF: Periarteriitis nodosa and asthma. Case report. J. Allergy **11**, 277 (1940).

UNVERRICHT, W.: Zur Periarteriitis nodosa. Ther. d. Gegenw. **1949**, 152.

VENKEI, T.: Periarteriitis nodosa (Kussmaul-Maier). Tagg der Ungar. Dermat. Ges. Budapest. Sitzg vom 12./13. 6. 1942. Ref. in Zbl. Haut- u. Geschl.-Kr. **70**, 334 (1943). — VRÁNOVÁ: Ein Fall von Periarteriitis nodosa mutilans. Ref. in Zbl. Haut- u. Geschl.-Kr. **54**, 512 (1937).

WALTHARD, B., u. K. M. WALTHARD: Periarteriitis nodosa. In: Handbuch der speziellen pathologischen Anatomie und Histologie. Hrsg. von O. LUBARSCH, F. HENKE u. R. RÖSSLE, Bd. 13, Teil 1, Bandteil B. Berlin-Göttingen-Heidelberg: Springer 1957. — WEGENER, F.: Zit. in H. REICH. — WEIDMAN, F. D.: Periarteriitis nodosa. Arch. Derm. Syph. (Chic.) **27**, 717 (1933). — WEPLER, W.: Über Skelettveränderungen bei Periarteriitis nodosa. Verh. dtsch. ges. Path. **1950**, 153. — WILSON, u. ALEXANDER: Zit. in J. HARKAVY. — WINKELMANN, R. K., u. H. MONTGOMERY: Über die kutane Periarteriitis nodosa. Hautarzt **11**, 82 (1960).

YONIS, I. Z.: Periarteriitis nodosa. Report of 3 cases successfully treated by cortisone and ACTH. Ann. paediat. (Basel) **192**, 65 (1959).

ZEEK, P. M., C. C. SMITH and J. C. WEETER: Studies on periarteritis nodosa. III. The differentiation between the vascular lesions of periarteritis nodosa and of hypersensitivity. Amer. J. Path. **24**, 889 (1948).

Phlebitis saltans (migrans)

Von

Rudolf Schuppli-Basel

Mit 2 Abbildungen

Einleitung

Das 1890 von ERLENMAYER erstmals als selbständige Krankheit beschriebene Leiden bietet im Rahmen der Gefäßkrankheiten ein gut charakterisiertes Bild. Verschiedene Probleme, die bereits bei der Besprechung der Periarteriitis nodosa erörtert worden sind, stellen sich hier wieder. Der Klarheit des Krankheitsbildes ist es zuzuschreiben, daß es seit der ersten Beschreibung kaum eine Erweiterung erfahren hat. Lediglich die von FAVRE beschriebene Phlébite fil de fer und die sog. Mondorsche Erkrankung müssen in bezug auf ihre Zugehörigkeit zum klassischen Bild der Phlebitis saltans diskutiert werden.

1. Klinisches Bild

Die Krankheit befällt vorwiegend Männer in jüngeren Jahren, wohl ausschließlich starke Raucher. Sie beginnt — hie und da nach Trauma — meist ohne stärkere Störungen des Allgemeinbefindens mit einer Hautschwellung an den Extremitäten entlang den Venen. Diese lassen sich nach einer gewissen Zeit als bleistiftdicker Strang palpieren. Diese Verhärtungen finden sich auf eine Strecke von einigen Zentimetern und verschwinden nach kürzerer oder längerer Zeit unter Hinterlassung einer braunen Pigmentierung wieder, um unvermittelt wieder an anderen Venenpartien aufzutreten. Befallen sind vorwiegend die subcutanen Venen der Streck- und Außenseiten der unteren Extremität, seltener der oberen Extremität und der Rumpfhaut. In einem Fall waren die Analgefäße beteiligt (SAKURANE). Als Zeichen der venösen Zirkulationsstörung kann eine Erythrocyanose der peripheren Extremitätenteile bestehen (DAHLENBURG). Das schwere Krankheitsbild der Phlegmasia caerulea dolens kann ebenfalls mit einer Phlebitis saltans kombiniert sein (OECHSLIN). In einem allerdings nicht restlos klaren Fall beschreibt FUJINAMI Phlebitiden auch im Gesicht.

Dieses sprungweise Auftreten ist für die Phlebitis saltans absolut charakteristisch, weshalb die Krankheit besser mit „saltans" als mit „migrans" bezeichnet wird, indem ein lokales Fortschreiten des Venenbefalles seltener als neues Auftreten fern vom ersten Herd beobachtet wird. Die befallenen Venen können schmerzhaft sein, doch ist dieses Merkmal nicht obligat.

Das Allgemeinbefinden der Patienten ist wenig verändert. KONRADS erwähnt eine starke Schlaflosigkeit. Fieberschübe können einen neuen Schub der Venenerkrankung einleiten, doch kann die Temperatur dauernd normal sein. Das Blutbild zeigt keine charakteristischen Veränderungen. Die von einigen Autoren beschriebene Leukopenie und relative Lymphocytose gehört nicht zum Bild der Phlebitis saltans. Die Blutsenkung ist mäßig beschleunigt, der Blutdruck wenig verändert. Komplikationen innerer Organe werden selten erwähnt. Häufiger sind Gelenkschwellungen. Im Falle von KEIBL und KÖBERLE fand sich eine rheumatische Myokarditis, die wohl unabhängig von der Phlebitis saltans bestand. HARTFALL et al. erwähnen Befall der Pulmonal-, Coronar- und Mesenterialgefäße außer den Extremitätenvenen. Der Verlauf der Krankheit ist ausgesprochen chronisch. Im Falle GOUGEROTS et al. ließen sich die Erscheinungen über 20 Jahre hin verfolgen.

Äußerst wichtig sind die Beziehungen der Phlebitis saltans zur Endarteriitis obliterans. Obwohl BUERGER schon im Jahre 1910 auf die Beziehungen zwischen beiden Krankheiten aufmerksam gemacht hatte, wurde diese erst in neuerer Zeit (ELSCHNER) wieder stärker beachtet, während lange Zeit beide Affektionen nur selten im Zusammenhang genannt worden sind (HENSCHEN). Tatsächlich findet sich in einem großen Prozentsatz der kasuistischen Mitteilungen die Erwähnung arterieller Durchblutungsstörungen als Claudicatio intermittens (LINDNER und SCHEFFLER, WAGNER und LINDNER, NOGUER-MORÉ), als Gangrän des Fußes (BUSCHKE und JOSEPH) oder der Zehenspitzen (FUJINAMI). LINDNER und SCHEFFLER gelang der Nachweis eines völligen Verschlusses der Femoralarterie mittels Arteriographie. Diese Feststellungen führten ELSCHNER dazu, zu fordern, daß bei allen Patienten, die an einer Phlebitis saltans erkranken, unbedingt nach einer Arterienerkrankung im Sinne einer Endangiitis obliterans gefahndet werden muß.

2. Histologie

Befallen sind meist mittelgroße Venen in der Subcutis. Die Veränderung betrifft die ganze Venenwand. Sie scheint im Bereich der Vasa vasorum zu beginnen, wo sich ein Infiltrat aus Histiocyten, Fibroblasten und Lymphzellen bildet, das die Muskelbündel der Media auseinanderdrängt. Polynucleäre Leukocyten sind ebenfalls in wechselnder Anzahl vorhanden. Die elastischen Fasern werden nicht zerstört, sondern aufgesplittert. Das Endothel ist geschwollen und kann massive Zellwucherungen zeigen, die zur Bildung eines Granuloms führen können. Dieses ins Lumen reichende Granulationsgewebe wird von EDWARDS als sehr charakteristisch für die Phlebitis saltans angesehen. Es kann dadurch zu einem völligen Verschluß des Venenlumens kommen. In diesen Fällen dürfte die histologische Unterscheidung der Phlebitis saltans vom Erythema nodosum nicht immer leicht sein (GANS). FRIEDLÄNDER et al. sahen allerdings diese Intimabeteiligung selten; doch dürfte es sich wohl eher um den Zeitpunkt der Untersuchung handeln, welche Teile der Venen besonders beteiligt sind. Die Bildung eines Thrombus gehört zum Bild der Phlebitis saltans. Er wird unter Riesenzellbeteiligung organisiert. Die Riesenzellen haben den Charakter von Fremdkörperriesenzellen (Abb. 1 und 2).

3. Ätiologie

Während früher der Lues eine wesentliche Rolle in der Entstehung der Phlebitis saltans zugeschrieben wurde (NEISSER), lassen jetzt die nahen Beziehungen der Phlebitis saltans zur Endangiitis obliterans die Frage der durch Tabak bedingten Schädigung besonders aktuell erscheinen. Andererseits weisen die Erkenntnisse auf dem Gebiete der allergischen Gefäßschädigung auf eine mögliche Rolle allergischer Vorgänge in der Entstehung der Phlebitis saltans hin.

HARKAVY konnte bei Rauchern, die Gefäßschäden zeigten, in 78% positive Hautreaktionen mittels Tabakextrakten auslösen, während bei gesunden Rauchern dies nur in 9% möglich war. Kontrollteste mit anderen Antigenen waren demgegenüber bei den gefäßgeschädigten Personen seltener positiv als bei den normalen. Es gelang ihm auch, in einem Fall durch Injektion von Tabak-Antigen bei einem starken Raucher, der an Phlebitis saltans und Endangiitis obliterans litt, neue Schübe von Phlebitis auszulösen. Damit dürfte die tatsächliche Rolle des Tabaks in der Genese der Phlebitis saltans sichergestellt sein und auch die Bevorzugung des männlichen Geschlechts und der starken Raucher darunter eine Erklärung finden.

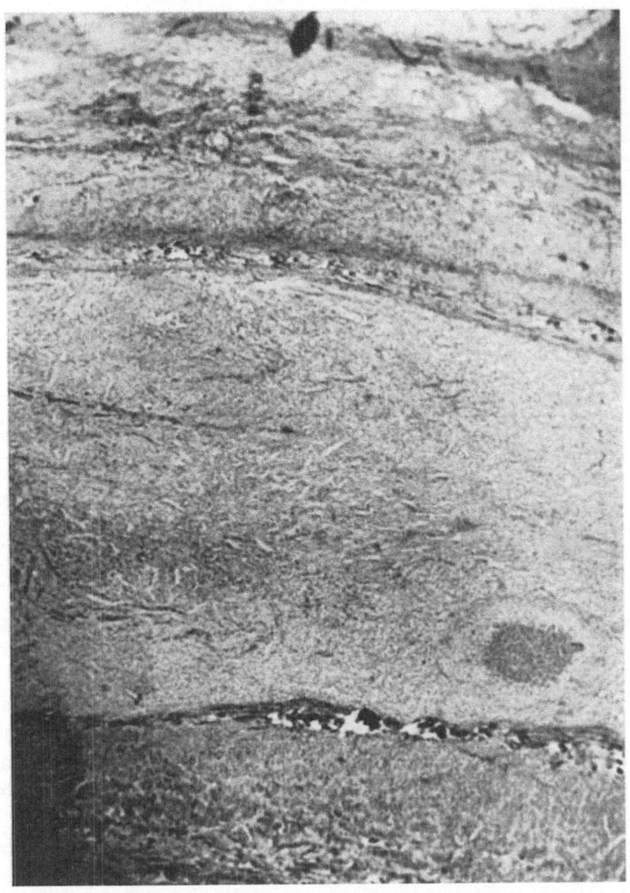

Abb. 1. Längsschnitt durch thrombosierte oberflächliche Armvene. Starke Verbreiterung und Aufsplitterung der Venenwand. Wucherung der Intima

Andererseits spielen sicher noch andere Antigene eine wichtige Rolle, so im Fall von HANEKE Hundehaare, in anderen Fällen (zit. bei HARKAVY) Fisch und Citrusfrüchte. SCHUPPLI beobachtete in einem Fall eine Allergie gegenüber Pilzallergenen in Form von Trichophytin und pilz- und schimmelhaltigen Nahrungsmitteln. Bakterielle Allergene können auch eine Rolle spielen, da Fälle nach Erysipel (NASTASE et al.) oder bei Streptokokkensepsis (FLORIAN) beobachtet wurden und da nach Sanierung eines Focus die Phlebitis saltans zum Stillstand kommen kann (HENSCHEN, GOUGEROT et al.). Dieser Focus kann tuberkulöser Natur sein (ITO et al.).

Alle diese Befunde sprechen dafür, daß die Pathogenese der Phlebitis saltans in einer allergisch-hyperergischen Entzündung zu suchen ist, die dem von KLINGE beschriebenen Reaktionstypus entspricht. Der Befund von Diplokokken direkt im Endothel der Gefäße (GOUGEROT et al.) widerspricht dieser Auffassung nicht, da im betreffenden Fall die negativen Blutkulturen und die negativen Übertragungsversuche eine septische Erkrankung ausschließen ließen.

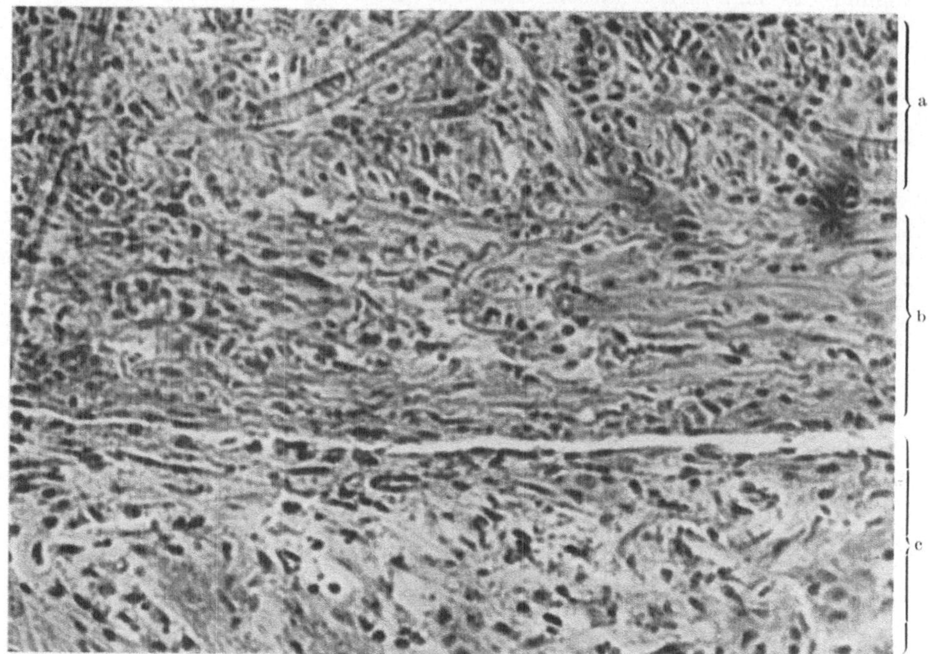

Abb. 2. Infiltrat in der Intima und im anliegenden Thrombus. a Media, b Intima, c Thrombus

4. Diagnose und Differentialdiagnose

Die Diagnose ist nicht schwer, da das Bild der Phlebitis saltans wohl mit keiner andern Krankheit verwechselt werden kann. Subcutane knotenförmige Schwellungen wie das Erythema nodosum, Erythema induratum Bazin usw., die zu Beginn des Leidens ähnlich aussehen können, lassen sich durch ihren Verlauf und das nicht strangförmige Befallensein zum mindesten nach einer gewissen Zeit sicher erkennen. Schwieriger ist die Frage zu entscheiden, wie weit die von FAVRE beschriebene Phlébite „fil de fer" und die von MONDOR beschriebene Thrombose der Rumpfhautvenen in das gleiche Bild gehören. Sowohl klinisch wie histologisch fehlen bei beiden Krankheiten stärkere Entzündungserscheinungen, obwohl sich eine Endophlebitis nachweisen läßt (RAUHS). Nach BRAUN-FALCO können diese oberflächlichen Phlebitiden jedoch schubweise verschiedene Venengebiete befallen, so daß eine sichere Entscheidung, ob diese nicht-entzündlichen, oberflächlichen, strangförmigen Venenthrombosen in das gleiche Kapitel wie die klassische Phlebitis saltans gehören, zur Zeit noch nicht getroffen werden kann.

5. Therapie

Während früher mit Quecksilber-Schmierkuren Erfolge erzielt wurden (BUSCHKE et al.), wird man heute viel eher neueren Mitteln wie Cortison-Derivaten, ACTH und Nivaquin den Vorzug geben. Nähere Angaben über die Wirkung dieser Mittel fehlen allerdings. WAGNER und LINDNER erzielten mit Penicillin einmal eine völlige Heilung. KEIBL und KÖBERLE beschrieben einen Erfolg mit

Alttuberkulin-Injektionen. NEUMANN erwähnt die gute Wirkung eines speziell Kastanienextrakt enthaltenden Präparates, WENTHOLT Besserung durch Fieberkur. NOBL empfiehlt, die Patienten möglichst wenig liegen zu lassen, damit die Thrombosierung vermieden werde. Nach KRIEG soll das Präparat Venostasin am besten wirken, während TOURNAY sich ganz auf Lokalbehandlung beschränkt.

Literatur

BRAUN-FALCO, O.: Über strangförmige, oberflächliche Phlebitiden. Derm. Wschr. **127**, 506 (1953). — BUERGER, L.: Zit. in ELSCHNER, H. — BUSCHKE, A., u. A. JOSEPH: Zur Kenntnis der wandernden Venenentzündung (Phlebitis migrans) und deren Behandlung. Klin. Wschr. **1933 II**, 1483.

DAHLENBURG: Phlebitis migrans. Schlesische Dermat. Ges. Sitzg. v. 2. 7. 1938. Ref. in Zbl. Haut- u. Geschl.-Kr. **60**, 379 (1938).

EDWARDS, A. E.: Phlebitis and the diagnosis of thromboangitis obliterans. Ann. intern. Med. **31**, 1019 (1949). — ELSCHNER, H.: Die Phlebitis saltans und das Krankheitsbild der Endangiitis obliterans. Derm. Wschr. **127**, 534 (1953). — ERLENMAYER, A.: Zit. in H. ELSCHNER.

FAVRE, W.: La phlébite „fil de fer". Presse méd. **61**, 579 (1953). — FLORIAN, J.: Les thromboses veineuses récidivantes (phlébite migrante) en pathologie générale. Phlébologie **11**, 99 (1958). — FRIEDLÄNDER, E., u. M. SGALITZER: Die Phlebitis migrans und ihre Behandlung. Med. Klin. **1938 I**, 223. — FUJINAMI, T.: Fall von Phlebitis migrans. Jap. J. Derm. **35**, 85 (1934).

GANS, O., u. G. K. STEIGLEDER: Histologie der Hautkrankheiten, 2. Aufl., Bd. I. Berlin-Göttingen-Heidelberg: Springer 1955. — GOUGEROT, H., et PHAN HUN CHI: Phlébite migrante. Bull. Soc. franç. Derm. Syph. **4**, 596 (1935). — Phlébite migrante; septicémie veineuse subaigüe (Rôle possible d'un streptocoque anaérobie). Arch. derm.-syph. (Paris) **7**, 359 (1935). — GOUGEROT, H., P. FRUMUSAN et O. ELIASCHEFF: Histobactériologie de la phlébite migrante. Bull. Soc. franç. Derm. Syph. **43**, 708 (1936).

HANEKE, H.: Ein Beitrag zur allergischen Genese der Phlebitis saltans. Hautarzt **8**, 75 (1957). — HARKAVY, J.: Cardio-vascular allergy. In: Progress in allergy, vol. III. Basel: Karger 1952. — HARTFALL, S. J., and G. ARMITAGE: Thrombo-phlebitis migrans. A report of two cases. Guy's Hosp. Rep. **82**, 424 (1932). — HENSCHEN, C.: Venopathia saltans (sog. Thrombophlebitis migrans) als Folgekrankheit eines chronischen Gallenblasenempyems. Schweiz. med. Wschr. **1936**, 38.

ITŌ, MINOR, u. SABURŌ, SATO: Ein Fall von Phlebitis nodosa cutanea migrans. Jap. J. Derm. **45**, 100 (1939).

KEIBL, E., u. F. KÖBERLE: Über Thrombophlebitis migrans. Wien. klin. Wschr. **1939 II**, 648. — KLINGE, F., u. H. G. FASSBENDER: Pathologische Anatomie der experimentellen Grundlagen. In: HANSEN, Allergie. Stuttgart: Georg Thieme 1957. — KONRADS, J.: Ein Beitrag zum seltenen Krankheitsbild der Thrombophlebitis migrans. Dtsch. med. Wschr. **1949**, 552. — KRIEG, E.: Phlébite migrante. Phlébologie **9**, 99 (1956).

LINDNER, B., u. H. S. F. SCHEFFLER: Ist die Thrombophlebitis migrans eine Schwestererkrankung der Endangiitis obliterans von Winniwarter-Buerger? Derm. Wschr. **125**, 341 (1952).

MONDOR, H., et J. BERTRAND: Thrombophlébitides et périphlébitides de la paroi thoracique antérieure. Presse méd. **1951**, 1533.

NASTASE, G., M. MUNTEANU, A. ALEXANDRESCU-PURICE u. M. TRANDAFIRESCU: Phlebitis migrans. Zit. in Zbl. Haut- u. Geschl.-Kr. **112**, 188 (1962). — NEISSER, E.: Zit. bei H. ELSCHNER. — NEUMANN, W.: Eine Therapie der Phlebitis migrans. Wien. med. Wschr. **1933 I**, 740. — NOBL, G.: Bemerkungen zur Phlebitis migrans. Med. Klin. **1933 II**, 972. — NOGUER-MORÉ, S.: Ischämische Gangrän der Finger und Phlebitis migrans. Act. dermo-sifiliogr. (Madr.) **42**, 484 (1951).

OECHSLIN, R.: Phlegmasia caerulea dolens. Schweiz. med. Wschr. **93**, 27 (1963).

RAUHS, R.: Der Morbus Mondor. Klin. Med. **11**, 500 (1956).

SAKURANE, K.: Weiterer Verlauf von Phlebitis migrans. Jap. J. Derm. **41**, 139 (1937). — SCHUPPLI, R.: Zur Ätiologie der Phlebitis saltans. Hautarzt **10**, 466 (1959).

TOURNAY, R.: A propos de phlébite migrante. Phlébologie **9**, 105 (1956).

WAGNER, H., u. B. LINDNER: Ein Beitrag zur Kasuistik der Thrombophlebitis migrans. Z. Haut- u. Geschl.-Kr. **10**, 259 (1951). — WENTHOLT, H. M. M.: Thrombophlebitis migrans. Dermatologica (Basel) **110**, 177 (1955).

Panniculitis

Von

Rudolf Schuppli-Basel

Einleitung

Die Pathologie und Pathophysiologie des Unterhautfettgewebes ist im großen und ganzen bisher wenig studiert worden, und die meisten Ergebnisse dieser Studien sind Nicht-Dermatologen zu verdanken (Blanc, Pfuhl). Baumgartner und Riva weisen in ihrer ausgezeichneten Monographie über die Panniculitis auf die Tatsache hin, daß sich im Fettgewebe unter dem Einfluß der verschiedensten nervösen und hormonalen Faktoren intensivste Stoffwechselvorgänge abspielten. Trotz des relativ einfach aufgebauten Gewebes, in dem diese vor sich gingen, seien die Funktionen des Fettgewebes aber auffallend wenig bekannt.

Es ist deshalb nicht verwunderlich, daß auf dem Gebiete der krankhaften Erscheinungen, die das Fettgewebe und speziell das Unterhautfettgewebe betreffen, keine einheitliche Auffassung herrscht und daß die verschiedenen Krankheitsbilder z.T. mit widersprechenden, oft die persönliche Auffassung des Autors wiederspiegelnden Bezeichnungen belegt werden. So sind die Bezeichnungen Lipogranulomatose, Liponekrose, mikrocystische disseminierte Steatonekrose (Gans), cutane Dyslipoidosen (Fleck), Panniculitis, die auf den ersten Blick verwirrend vielfältig erscheinen, im Grunde genommen nur Umschreibungen verschiedener Stadien eines ähnlichen Phänomens, nämlich einer entzündlichen Reaktion und eines Abbaues des Fettgewebes. Schon Rothmann hat 1894 auf die höchst auffällige Tatsache hingewiesen, daß dieselben Veränderungen der Fettzelle, die sich bei der Atrophie herausbilden, auch bei der Entzündung des Fettgewebes zu konstatieren sind. Es kann deshalb schwierig sein, im einzelnen Falle zu entscheiden, welches Phänomen primäre und welches sekundäre Bedeutung hat. So kann es einerseits durch infektiöse Prozesse zu Schädigung der Fettzelle kommen, andererseits kann eine primär traumatisch entstandene Nekrose im Fettgewebe zu Entzündungserscheinungen und zu Granulombildung Anlaß geben. Es ist also von vornherein zu erwarten, daß aus einer einmaligen histologischen Untersuchung erkrankten Fettgewebes nicht immer ein bindender Schluß gezogen werden kann. Dementsprechend sind für die verschiedenen Formen der Fettgewebsentzündung, die im folgenden mit Panniculitis als dem einfachsten Begriff bezeichnet werden sollen, verschiedene Einteilungsversuche gemacht worden. Baumgartner und Riva, ergänzt durch Kooij, schlagen folgende Einteilung vor:

a) Panniculitis als sekundäre Reaktion auf Prozesse in der Umgebung, z.B. Entzündungen und maligne Tumoren.

b) Artifizielle Panniculitis durch äußere Faktoren (Traumen, Injektionen).

c) Spontan auftretende, umschriebene Panniculitis.

d) Panniculitis, die durch Medikamente (z.B. Brom und Jod) hervorgerufen wird.

e) Panniculitis als Folge infektiöser Prozesse, z.B. Tuberkulose, Lues, Lepra usw.

Keil unterscheidet primäre Panniculitis von febrilem und afebrilem Typus, und sekundäre Panniculitis, wie sie als ständige Begleiterscheinung bei Erythema induratum Bazin, Darier-Roussyschem Sarkoid und anderen nodulären Erythemen angetroffen wird.

Röckl und Thies wiederum teilen die herdförmigen chronisch rezidivierenden Krankheitszustände des subcutanen Fettgewebes in drei Gruppen ein:

1. Panniculitis als Nachbarschaftsreaktion.
2. Panniculitis nach Traumen.
3. Spontane Panniculitis: a) Typ Pfeifer-Weber-Christian, b) Typ Rothmann-Makai.

Abweichend davon betrachten Faninger et al. die spontanen Panniculitiden als eine einzige Krankheitsgruppe, da Übergänge zwischen den verschiedenen Formen bestehen.

Im folgenden sollen nun diejenigen Formen der Panniculitis, die nach Trauma, Injektionen usw. auftreten, und die sekundären Panniculitiden als Begleitsymptome anderer Krankheiten nur so weit erwähnt werden, als sie für die Differentialdiagnose wichtig sind. Besprochen werden die spontan auftretenden Formen, also die primäre idiopathische Panniculitis, die ein einigermaßen gut abgegrenztes Krankheitsbild darstellt, was speziell für die von Pfeifer 1892, Parkes Weber 1925 und Christian 1928 beschriebene Panniculitis nodularis febrilis non-suppurativa zutrifft, die im französischen Schrifttum als Panniculite atrophiante fébrile bezeichnet wird. Demgegenüber erscheinen die von Rothmann und Makai beschriebenen Formen der Panniculitis zu wenig einheitlich, als daß sie als Krankheit sui generis aufgefaßt werden könnten. Auch die Sonderstellung der von Vilanova et al. beschriebenen Hypodermite nodulaire subaigüe migratrice und der von Carpentier erwähnten Hypodermite nodulaire bénigne récidivante de la femme muß noch weiter abgeklärt werden.

I. Panniculitis nodularis febrilis non-suppurativa (Pfeifer-Weber-Christian)

1. Klinik

Das Leiden scheint die weiße Rasse zu bevorzugen, indem erst zwei Fälle bei Negern beschrieben worden sind (Samitz und Coletti). Auch scheint es in südlichen Gegenden seltener als in nördlichen zu sein (Gay Prieto et al.). Es sind davon bisher etwa 120 Fälle bekannt geworden. Frauen sind 3—4mal häufiger befallen als Männer. Bevorzugt werden die mittleren Lebensjahre, doch sind auch Fälle bei kleinen Kindern und Säuglingen beschrieben worden (Brain, Urbas et al.). Die Krankheit ist charakterisiert durch Fieberschübe, wobei die Temperatur bis 40° steigen kann. Parallel dazu treten subcutane Knoten auf, die von Erbsen- bis Faustgröße variieren. Sie können einzeln oder herdweise auftreten. Bevorzugt sind die Extremitäten, speziell die Oberschenkel, doch können auch Abdomen, Rücken, Handrücken und Gesicht (Sweitzer, Pfeifer) befallen sein. In einem Fall wird auch Lokalisation auf der Lippen- und Mundschleimhaut beschrieben (Sosa Bens et al.). Ihre Oberfläche ist oft gerötet und über das Niveau der normalen Haut erhaben. Die Schmerzhaftigkeit variiert stark. Die Knoten können sich nach kurzer Zeit ohne Narben wieder zurückbilden, in der Regel verschwinden sie aber erst nach längerer Zeit unter Hinterlassung einer eingedellten atrophischen Hautpartie. In verschiedenen Fällen (Grupper et al. 1955, Peterkin, Samitz und Coletti, Sheffer, Tolman und Cox) wurde eine zentrale Erweichung der Knoten beschrieben, wobei sich spontan eine ölig-gelbliche Flüssigkeit entleerte, deren Menge bis zu 120 cm³ betrug. Diese Flüssigkeit kann auch eitrig werden, so daß BENDEL den Ausdruck non-suppurativa in der Bezeichnung der Krankheit wegzulassen empfiehlt. Das Leiden verläuft ausgesprochen chronisch. Rückfälle werden in kürzeren oder längeren Intervallen beschrieben, die Jahre betragen können.

Die Prognose der Pfeifer-Weber-Christianschen Krankheit ist nicht durchwegs gut, da bisher sieben Todesfälle beschrieben worden sind. Als Todesursache werden folgende Affektionen erwähnt: MILLER und KRITZLER fanden Fettembolien in den Lungen, Verfettung und Fettnekrosen in der Leber, Splenomegalie, hydropische Degeneration der Nebennierenrinde und Phagocytose der Erythrocyten im reticulo-endothelialen System. In anderen Fällen wurden Tuberkulose (TILDEN), Glomerulonephritis (SPAIN und TOBY), Sepsis (FRIEDMANN, UNGAR) beschrieben. Es ist also in den meisten Fällen zweifelhaft, ob die erwähnten Todesursachen mit der Panniculitis in direktem Zusammenhang stehen. Meist scheint die Prognose allerdings gut zu sein, auch völlige Heilungen werden beschrieben (ROTHMAN et al.).

Interne Symptome werden nur selten beschrieben. DORFMAN sah Verbreiterung des Hilusschattens, die er einer Affektion des mediastinalen Fettgewebes zuschreibt, da sie parallel mit den Hautknoten zurückging. DOSTROVSKY et al. konnten ein Magencarcinom finden. CACCIALANZA et al. sahen die Kombination mit akutem Gelenkrheumatismus und Polyserositis, ARNER mit Asthma und Heuschnupfen. In zwei Fällen wurde ein Erythematodes beobachtet (ROTHMAN et al., CAROL). Im Blut können keine charakteristischen Befunde erhoben werden. Die Senkungsreaktion kann normal und erhöht sein. Die Leukocytenzahlen können erhöht sein. In der Hälfte der Fälle findet sich allerdings eine ausgesprochene Leukopenie (SPIER, HERING). WIGLEY beobachtete in einem Fall eine makrocytäre Anämie und Steatorrhoe, ORAM et al. Leberverfettung und hypochrome Anämie. ARNER sah stark erhöhten Antistreptolysintiter bei normalem Antistaphylolysintiter. Die Blutkulturen waren außer in den von PUENTE und von BERNDT et al. beschriebenen Fällen steril.

2. Histologie

Die Erkrankung ist ausschließlich in der Subcutis lokalisiert, während die Epidermis normal ist und sich in den oberen Schichten der Cutis höchstens ein leichtes perivasculäres Infiltrat findet. Es lassen sich nach LEVER und UNGAR drei Stadien unterscheiden: Innerhalb der ersten 24 Std werden die subcutanen Fettzellen durch Einwanderung segmentkerniger Leukocyten voneinander getrennt. An den Rändern der Fettzellen tauchen dann Histiocyten auf, die die Fettzelle rosettenartig ausfüllen, so daß sich das Bild der Wucheratrophie ausbildet. Das Fett wird phagocytiert, und nach etwa 3 Wochen finden sich im Gewebe nur noch wenige Fettzellen, es besteht in der Hauptsache aus Histiocyten und Makrophagen mit schaumigem Cytoplasma und gelegentlich mehreren Kernen. Zuletzt wird der Herd mit Strängen von kollagenen Fasern durchzogen, so daß eine Fibrose zurückbleibt. Die Gefäße sind verschieden stark beteiligt. Während von einzelnen Autoren nur geringe Verbreiterung und Infiltration der Arteriolenwand und Schwellung der Endothelien gefunden wurden, beschrieben CUMMINS et al. schwere Gefäßveränderungen mit subendothelialem Ödem und Lamellisation der Gefäßwände, die zum Verschluß der Gefäße führen kann. Außer diesen Veränderungen finden sich hie und da noch Granulome aus palisadenförmig angeordneten Epitheloidzellen (REYNAERS), so daß manchmal die Differentialdiagnose gegenüber tuberkulösen Prozessen schwer zu stellen ist.

3. Ätiologie und Pathogenese

Die Ätiologie der Pfeifer-Weber-Christianschen Krankheit ist unbekannt. Der klinische Verlauf mit den Fieberschüben macht den Eindruck eines infektiösen Geschehens, um so mehr, als Fälle infektiöser Panniculitis bei Tieren beschrieben worden sind, die ähnliche Veränderungen im Gewebe zeigen (DURAN-REYNALS). Weiter sprechen die Beobachtungen über Auftreten von Panniculitis nach Flecktyphus (ABRIKOSSOFF) dafür, daß bekannte Infekte eine Panniculitis auslösen können. Auch in den meisten Fällen der Pfeifer-Weber-Christianschen Krankheit werden neben erhöhtem Antistreptolysintiter fokale Infekte erwähnt (PIERINI et al., NETHERTON, MIEDZINSKY, TILDEN et al., SMITH et al., DUBOIS et al.). PUENTE konnte in seinem Fall stark positive Hautreaktionen mit Tuberkulin und Staphylokokkentoxin auslösen. Direktere Beweise konnte KORTING erbringen, der mit Injektion einer aus Keimen aus Duodenalgalle hergestellten Streptokokkenvaccine neue Herde hervorrufen konnte. ANDRUP sah das gleiche nach Staphylokokkenvaccine. Auch VILANOVA et al. konnten bei einigen Fällen, bei denen eine Panniculitis mit Aphthosis zusammen auftrat, mit Speichelantigen neue Knoten provozieren.

Auf einen anderen Entstehungsmechanismus weisen diejenigen Fälle hin, in denen Medikamente, speziell Halogene (PARKES WEBER 1935, MILLER) eine typische Pfeifer-Weber-Christiansche Erkrankung verursachen.

Die Ähnlichkeit schließlich, die manche Fälle von Panniculitis mit dem Erythema induratum Bazin zeigen, hat Anlaß zur Erörterung der tuberkulösen Ätiologie gegeben (CAROL, CAROL et al.), ohne daß es allerdings bisher gelungen wäre, einen Beweis für diese Arbeitshypothese zu finden.

Die Pathogenese der Panniculitis läßt sich aus experimentellen Befunden ableiten, wonach Injektionen öliger Substanzen, lokale mechanische Traumen, thermische Einflüsse zu Veränderungen führen können, die einer Panniculitis entsprechen. Daß auch bei der Pfeifer-Weber-Christianschen Krankheit mechanische Momente für die Lokalisation neuer Knoten von Bedeutung sind, zeigt die Beobachtung von ARNER, der durch subcutane Injektionen Knoten von Panniculitis hervorrufen konnte. Auch STUHLERT sah das Auftreten eines Panniculitis-Knotens nach Trauma. Auch Störungen in der Gefäßversorgung, z.B. im Gefolge thrombosierender Prozesse oder venöser Stauungen, können Entzündungen im Unterhautfettgewebe zur Folge haben, so daß wohl die Aussage erlaubt ist, daß dem zirkulatorischen Faktor in der Genese der Panniculitis eine wesentliche Rolle zufällt. Dieser Faktor könnte möglicherweise analog den bei der Periarteriitis nodosa und Phlebitis saltans beschriebenen Verhältnissen auf einer bakteriell bedingten Antigen-Antikörper-Reaktion beruhen (MEYER), so daß das Bild der Pfeifer-Weber-Christianschen Krankheit in den Bereich der hyperergischen Gewebsreaktionen einzureihen wäre. Am klarsten hat wohl KELLNER das Problem charakterisiert, wonach nach Zerstörung von Fettzellen durch Trauma, aber auch durch Infektion und wohl auch durch Ernährungsstörungen das aus den Zellen ausgetretene körpereigene Fett zum Fremdkörper werde und Anlaß zu einer resorptiven Entzündung, zum lipophagen Granulom geben kann. Die Pfeifer-Weber-Christiansche Krankheit wäre demnach durch ihren Verlauf, durch die rezidivierenden Fieberschübe von anderen lipophage Granulome verursachenden Leiden zu unterscheiden und als selbständige Krankheit charakterisiert.

4. Diagnose und Differentialdiagnose

Zu differentialdiagnostischen Schwierigkeiten geben naturgemäß sämtliche nodösen Exantheme Anlaß, so daß die Diagnose der Pfeifer-Weber-Christianschen

Krankheit nur aus dem klinischen und histologischen Bild gemeinsam gestellt werden kann. Wohl selten wird man sich der Grenzen der histologischen Beweisführung so recht bewußt wie hier (GANS). Die Schwierigkeiten ergeben sich speziell deshalb, weil Fettgewebsveränderungen sich sekundär bei einer ganzen Reihe von Krankheiten finden, die wie das Erythema induratum Bazin, das Sarkoid Darier-Roussy, das Boecksche Sarkoid Wucherungen im Fettgewebe zeigen, die der Panniculitis sehr ähnlich sind. Typisch ist das histologische Bild der Panniculitis ja nur in den ersten 24 Std, später kann es starke Angleichungen an andere nodöse Prozesse zeigen. Die Schwierigkeiten werden dadurch noch vermehrt, daß offenbar Übergangsformen bestehen, die z.B. von CAROL et al. unter dem Namen Erythema nodosum lipogranulomatosum beschrieben wurden, und daß Fälle, die klinisch unter dem Bilde des Sarkoides Darier-Roussy verliefen, sich histologisch als Panniculitis erwiesen. Der Vergleich der Panniculitis mit dem Sarkoid Darier-Roussy erhöht die Verwirrung noch mehr, da die Existenzberechtigung des Sarkoids Darier-Roussy in den letzten Jahren bestritten wird und ein Teil dieser Formen als zum Morbus Boeck, ein anderer als zum Erythema induratum Bazin gehörig erkannt wurde. Verschiedene Autoren (KOOIJ, KELLNER) treten dafür ein, daß auf die Bezeichnung Sarkoid Darier-Roussy wegen Begriffsverwirrung verzichtet werde. Die Auffassung von CAROL et al., daß die Panniculitis eine akute Form des Sarkoides Darier-Roussy wäre, würde damit hinfällig.

Zur Verwechslung Anlaß können auch die von MONTGOMERY et al., WINER, WOODBURNE et al. als „Nodular vasculitis“ beschriebenen Krankheiten geben. Es handelt sich dabei um histologisch dem Erythema induratum Bazin sehr nah verwandte Zustände, die sich ausschließlich bei Frauen an den Unterschenkeln finden. Diese Patienten lassen aber zum Unterschied vom Erythema induratum Bazin keinerlei Zeichen einer tuberkulösen Affektion erkennen (RIST et al.). Auch ein Teil der von DEGOS als Dermo-hypodermite à cocci pyogènes beschriebenen Fälle dürfte wohl hier zu klassieren sein. Schließlich sei noch der Versuch von VILANOVA et al. erwähnt, die Hypodermite nodulaire subaigüe migratrice als selbständiges Krankheitsbild abzugrenzen. Diese Affektion, die er ausschließlich bei Frauen beobachten konnte, unterscheidet sich von der Panniculitis, abgesehen vom afebrilen Verlauf dadurch, daß die entzündlichen Infiltrate in den Bindegewebssepten des Unterhautzellgewebes im Vordergrund stehen und das Fettgewebe nur sekundär verändert ist. Diese Krankheit dürfte mit dem von BÄFVERSTEDT beschriebenen Erythema nodosum migrans identisch sein. Schließlich muß in tropischen Gegenden die unter dem Bild eines Erythema nodosum leprosum von PEBLER et al. beschriebene Panniculitis nodosa leprosa differential-diagnostisch beachtet werden.

Die Frage, ob die bei Säuglingen beschriebene Panniculitis wirklich der Panniculitis der Erwachsenen entspricht, ist noch keineswegs abgeklärt, da histologisches und klinisches Bild oft uncharakteristisch sind (MITCHELL et al.) und die verschiedenen Formen der Adiponecrosis neonatorum ähnliche Bilder machen können (CAROL et al.). Auch die Identität der Panniculitis granulomatosa (FISCHER) mit der Pfeifer-Weber-Christianschen Erkrankung ist unabgeklärt.

Auf Grund des Genannten würde es sich zur Zeit sicher verantworten lassen, die nicht typischen Formen der Panniculitis in eine der Gruppe der von GOUGEROT als Hypodermite zusammengefaßten Krankheiten einzureihen, da sonst die Gefahr besteht, daß das Krankheitsbild der Pfeifer-Weber-Christianschen Krankheit ungebührlich erweitert wird.

5. Therapie

Die Berichte über die Beeinflußbarkeit der Panniculitis sind schwer zu beurteilen, da die Krankheit nach Entfernung eines Focus (STUHLERT, MIEDZINSKY,

PIERINI et al.) heilen oder wenigstens jahrelange Remissionen zeigen kann. ARNOLD sah einen günstigen Effekt von Sulfapyridin. Seine Angaben konnten von WIGLEY et al. nicht bestätigt werden, Sulfapyridin verschlechterte im Gegenteil das Krankheitsbild. MOE konnte die Entwicklung neuer Knoten in einem Fall mit Phenergan aufhalten. Antibiotica scheinen sicherer zu wirken, speziell Chloramphenicol (SCHWARTZ, WIGLEY et al.) und Penicillin (MESTDAGH, KOOIJ, ZEE). Erfolglos erwiesen sich Sulfonamide und Antibiotica bei DUBOIS et al., MÉNARD, DEGOS et al. GRUPPER et al. berichten über einen sehr guten Effekt von Cortison, POMERANTZ et al. sahen mit diesem Mittel dagegen einen Mißerfolg.

II. Die Panniculitis Typus Rothmann-Makai

Die von ROTHMANN 1894 und von MAKAI 1928 beschriebenen Formen der Panniculitis unterscheiden sich durch den afebrilen Verlauf von der Pfeifer-Weber-Christianschen Form der Panniculitis. GOTTRON et al. halten zum mindesten die von MAKAI beschriebene Form für eine selbständige Affektion, während BAUMGARTNER und RIVA beide Formen mit anderen nicht zum Pfeifer-Weber-Christianschen Syndrom gehörigen Formen in einer provisorischen Gruppe zusammenfassen, in der eine Anzahl heterogener Krankheitsbilder mangels besserer Kriterien untergebracht werden müßten und von der in Zukunft wohl einzelne Krankheiten als einheitliche Affektion abgetrennt werden könnten. Es ist klar, daß eine auf vorwiegend negativen Kriterien aufgebaute Einteilung die bei den Panniculitiden schon bestehenden Schwierigkeiten diagnostischer Art nur vergrößern kann, so daß in diesem Rahmen nicht näher auf eine genauere Beschreibung der Klinik dieser Formen eingegangen werden soll, da sich im Schrifttum die widersprechendsten Angaben finden. So beschreibt z.B. RINALDI einen Fall von chronischer progressiver Panniculitis vom Typ Rothmann-Makai mit chronisch kontinuierlichem Verlauf seit 5 Jahren, der unter Vitamin D_2 vollkommen abheilte. KONOPIK beschreibt einen Fall von Rothmann-Makaischer Panniculitis, wo es gelang, aus den Infiltraten Tuberkelbacillen zu züchten und wo die Differentialdiagnose zum Erythema induratum Bazin und Erythema nodosum schwer zu stellen war. Er glaubt, daß die Pathogenese der Panniculitiden in einer Herabsetzung der Resistenz des mesenchymalen Gewebes zu suchen sei, wobei Staphylokokken den Typus Pfeifer-Weber-Christian, Tuberkelbacillen den Typus Rothmann-Makai verursachen. Auch Würmer sollen in der Genese dieser Panniculitisform eine Rolle spielen (DUPERRAT).

Da in diesem Kapitel nur Hypothesen zu diskutieren wären, soll es der Zukunft überlassen bleiben, in dieses Dunkel Licht zu bringen.

Literatur

ABRIKOSSOFF, A.: Zit. in W. BAUMGARTNER u. G. RIVA. — ANDRUP, O.: Panniculitis. Acta derm.-venereol. (Stockh.) **37**, 396 (1957). — ARNER, S.: Spontaneous circumscribed panniculitis (Weber-Christian disease). Acta derm.-venereol. (Stockh.) **34**, 194 (1954). — ARNOLD, H. L.: Nodular non-suppurative Panniculitis (Weber-Christian's disease). Arch. Derm. Syph. (Chic.) **61**, 94 (1945).

BÄFVERSTEDT, B.: Erythema nodosum migrans. Acta derm.-venereol. **34**, 181 (1954). — BAUMGARTNER, W., u. G. RIVA: Panniculitis, die herdförmige Fettgewebsentzündung. Helv. med. Acta, Suppl. **14**, Ser. A (1945). — BENDEL jr., W. L.: Relapsing febrile nodular panniculitis (Weber-Christian disease). Review of the literature and report of a case. Arch. Derm. Syph. (Chic.) **160**, 570 (1949). — BERNDT, H., u. W. FRIEDRICHS: Beitrag zur Klinik der Panniculitis Weber-Christian. Z. ges. inn. Med. **15**, 67 (1960). — BLANC: Syndromes nouveaux de pathologie adipeux. Paris: Masson & Cie. 1951. — BRAIN, R. T.: Relapsing panniculitis. Brit. J. Derm. **70**, 260 (1928).

CACCIALANZA, P., e R. CAZZOLA: Pannicolite nodulare recidivante febbrile non suppurativa. (Sindrome di Weber-Christian). Contributo alla conoscenza della sindrome con illustrazione di un caso clinico. G. ital. Derm. **89**, 1137 (1949). — CAROL, W. L. L.: Über akute und auch subakute nodöse Panniculitis. Ned. T. Geneesk. **1941**, 134. — CAROL, W. L. L., J. R. PRAKKEN and H. A. VAN ZWIJNDREGT: Erythema nodosum and relapsing febrile non-suppurative panniculitis. Arch. Derm. Syph. (Berl.) **182**, 329 (1941). — CARPENTIER, E.: Les hypodermites nodulaires bénignes récidivantes de la femmes. Excerpta med. (Amst.), Sect. XIII **6**, 346 (1952). — CHRISTIAN, H. A.: Relapsing febrile nodular non-suppurative panniculitis. Arch. intern. Med. **42**, 338 (1928). — CUMMINS, L. J., and W. F. LEVER: Relapsing nodular febrile non-suppurative panniculitis. (Weber-Christian disease). Report of two cases. Arch. Derm. Syph. (Chic.) **38**, 415 (1938).

DEGOS, R.: Erythème induré de Bazin ayant cédé très rapidement au traitement sulfamidé (Dermo-hypodermite à cocci pyogènes ?). Bull. Soc. franç. Derm. Syph. **1942**, 150. — DEGOS, R., et J. HEWITT: Panniculite atrophiante fébrile et récidivante (Weber-Christian). Bull. Soc. franç. Derm. Syph. **1954**, 341. — DORFMAN, M.: Pulmonary hilar enlargement associated with Weber-Christian disease. Arch. Derm. Syph. (Chic.) **68**, 693 (1953). — DOSTROVSKY, A., D. KOPEL and J. TAS: A case of Weber-Christian disease. (Coincident with a gastric carcinoma and characterized by liquefying lesions). Dermatologica (Basel) **114**, 39 (1957). — DUBOIS, P., A. BEAUDOING et L. COLOMB: Un cas de panniculite nodulaire fébrile récidivante de Weber-Christian. Bull. Soc. franç. Derm. Syph. **1957**, 57. — DUPERRAT, B.: Panniculite de Rothman-Makai. Med. Infant. **67**, 5 (1960). — DURAN-REYNALS, F.: Necrotizing disease in rabbits affecting fatty acid muscular tissues. Analogies with Weber-Christian disease of humans. Yale J. Biol. Med. **18**, 583 (1946).

FANINGER, A., u. M. ISVANESKI: Ein Beitrag zur Kenntnis der spontanen chronisch-rezidivierenden Panniculitis. Hautarzt **9**, 372 (1958). — FISCHER, E.: Panniculitis granulomatosa. Dermatologica (Basel) **112**, 545 (1956). — FLECK, F.: Über cutane Dyslipoidosen, Steatonekrosen und verschiedene Einzelformen abnorm-regionaler Fettverteilung. Z. Haut- u. Geschl.-Kr. **24**, 1 (1958). — FRIEDMAN, N. B.: Fatal panniculitis (including autopsy). Arch. Path. **39**, 42 (1945).

GANS, O., u. G. K. STEIGLEDER: Histologie der Hautkrankheiten, 2. Aufl., Bd. 1. Berlin-Göttingen-Heidelberg: Springer 1955. — GAY-PRIETO, J., M. ALVAREZ-CASCO y F. VEGA-DIAZ: Paniculitis nodular recidivante febril. Enfermedad de Weber-Christian. Act. dermo-sifiliogr. (Madr.) **42**, 835 (1951). — GOTTRON, H. A., u. W. NIKOLOWSKI: Pfeifer-Christian-Weber'sche Krankheit in ihrer Nosologie und Pathogenese. Hautarzt **3**, 530 (1952). — GOUGEROT, H.: La nosologie des hypodermites. Ann. Derm. Syph. (Paris) **1946**, 369. — GRUPPER, CH., et M. HERBERT: Panniculite atrophiante fébrile de Weber-Christian. Lésions ramollies précédant l'atrophie (2e présentation). Bull. Soc. franç. Derm. Syph. **1955**, 14. — GRUPPER, CH., M. HERBERT et J. HEWITT: Panniculite atrophiante fébrile de Weber-Christian. Bull. Soc. franç. Derm. Syph. **1954**, 344.

HERING, H.: Pfeifer-Weber-Christian-Syndrom. Med. Wiss. Ges. Derm. Dresden. Sitzg 6./7. 2. 1954. Derm. Wschr. **129**, 593 (1954).

KEIL, H.: Panniculitis: Its place in nosology. Brit. J. Derm. **47**, 512 (1935). — KELLNER, H.: Zur Frage der Zusammenhänge zwischen lipophager Granulombildung und Erythema induratum, Sarkoid Darier-Roussy und Panniculitis non-suppurativa nodularis recidivans. Hautarzt **2**, 299 (1951). — KONOPIK, J.: On the pathogenesis and aetiology of panniculitis. Čs. Derm. **30**, 259 (1955). — KOOIJ, R.: Weber-Christian's disease, a form of spontaneous panniculitis. Dermatologica (Basel) **101**, 332 (1950). — KORTING, G. W.: Afebrile suppurative Pfeifer-Weber-Christian'sche Erkrankung mit Herdprovozierbarkeit durch Schlag und körpereigene Streptokokkenvakzine. Derm. Wschr. **133**, 521 (1956).

LEVER, W. F.: Histopathology of the skin. Lippincott London 1949. — Nodular non-suppurative panniculitis. (Weber-Christian disease.) Report of a case in which an infiltrate of polymorphonuclear leukocytes represented the earliest lesion. Arch. Derm. Syph. (Chic.) **59**, 31 (1949).

MAKAI, E.: Über Lipogranulomatosis subcutanea. Klin. Wschr. **1928 II**, 2343. — MÉNARD, E.: Deux cas de maladie de Weber-Christian. Bull. Soc. franç. Derm. Syph. **1957**, 108. — MESTDAGH, C.: Panniculite nodulaire subfébrile non suppurante. Arch. belges Derm. **4**, 75 (1948). — MEYER, A.: Die herdförmige unspezifische Entzündung der Subcutis (Panniculitis). Praxis (Bern) **1955**, 201. — MIEDZINSKI, F.: Some remarks about Weber-Christian disease. Acta derm.-venereol. (Stockh.) **37**, 88 (1957). — MILLER, J. L.: Panniculitis (Lipogranulomatosis). Arch. Derm. Syph. (Chic.) **43**, 725 (1941). — MILLER, L. J., and R. A. KRITZLER: Nodular non-suppurative panniculitis. Arch. Derm. Syph. (Chic.) **47**, 82 (1943). — MITCHELL, J. H., and H. SANFORD: Panniculitis (Weber-Christian disease ?). Chicago Dermat. Society. April 18, 1951. Arch. Derm. Syph. (Chic.) **65**, 732 (1952). — MOE, P. J.: Weber-Christian disease. T. norske Laegeforen. **76**, 919 (1956). — MONTGOMERY, A., P. A. O'HEARY and N. W. BARKER: Nodular vascular diseases of the legs. J. Amer. med. Ass. **128**, 335 (1945).

NETHERTON, E. W.: Relapsing nodular non-suppurative panniculitis. Arch. Derm. Syph. (Chic.) **28**, 258 (1933).

ORAM, S., and G. M. COCHRANE: Weber-Christian disease with visceral involvement. An example with hepatic enlargement. Brit. med. J. **1958**, Nr 5091, 281.

PARKES WEBER, F.: A case of relapsing nonsuppurative panniculitis, showing phagocytosis of subcutaneous fat cells by macrophages. Brit. J. Derm. **37**, 301 (1925). — A further note on relapsing febrile nodular non suppurative panniculitis. Brit. J. Derm. **47**, 230 (1935).— PEBLER, W. J., R. KOOIJ and J. MARSHALL: The histopathology of acute panniculitis nodosa leprosa (erythema nodosum leprosum). Int. J. Leprosy **23**, 53 (1955). — PETERKIN, G. A.: Relapsing febrile non-suppurative panniculitis (Weber-Christian disease). Brit. J. Derm. **65**, 288 (1953). — PFEIFER, V.: Über einen Fall von herdweiser Atrophie des subkutanen Fettgewebes. Dtsch. Arch. klin. Med. **50**, 438 (1892). — PFUHL, W.: Zit. in O. GANS. — PIERINI, D. O., e I. M. POMPOSIELLO: Paniculitis nodular recidivante no supurativa febril. (Sindrome de Weber-Christian). Rev. argent. Dermatosif. **33**, 128 (1949). — POMERANTZ, H. Z., and M. A. SIMON: An unusual case of Weber-Christian-Syndrom. Ann. intern. Med. **47**, 1251 (1957). — PUENTE, J. J.: Panniculitis nodularis recidivans febrilis durch Staphylokokken. Ein Fall von Granuloma lipophagicum der Brust. Ref. in Zbl. Haut- u. Geschl.-Kr. **63**, 672 (1940).

REYNAERS, H.: Panniculite nodulaire chronique. Arch. belges Derm. **8**, 78 (1952). — RINALDI, V. G.: Pannicolite nodulare cronica progressiva tipo Rothmann-Makai. Ann. ital. Derm. Sif. **10**, 44 (1955). — RIST, E., et M. RENAUD: Erythème induré de Bazin à poussées récidivantes à caractère prémenstruel. Relations avec la maladie de Weber-Christian. Presse méd. **1947**, 437. — RÖCKL, H., u. W. THIES: Herdförmige chronisch rezidivierende Krankheitszustände des subkutanen Fettgewebes. Zur Histopathogenese der Lipogranulomatosis. Hautarzt 8, 58 (1957). — ROTHMAN, ST., and A. L. LORINCZ: Recovery from relapsing febrile non-suppurative panniculitis (Weber-Christian disease). Arch. Derm. Syph. (Chic.) **70**, 535 (1954). — ROTHMANN, M.: Über Entzündung und Atrophie des subcutanen Fettgewebes. Virchows Arch. path. Anat. **136**, 159 (1894).

SAMITZ, M. H., and J. M. COLETTI: Weber-Christian disease occurring in a Negro Woman. Arch. Derm. Syph. (Chic.) **65**, 487 (1952). — SCHWARTZ, B.: Liquefying nodular panniculitis. Brit. J. Derm. **64**, 291 (1952). — SHAFFER, B.: Liquefying nodular panniculitis. Report of a case. Arch. Derm. Syph. (Chic.) **38**, 535 (1938). — SMITH, P. A. J., and B. RUSSELL: Nodular panniculitis with atrophy. Brit. J. Derm. **69**, 101 (1957). — SOSA BENS, D., A. HERNÁNDEZ y F. SALAS PANISELLO: Paniculitis nodular no supurativa recidivante y febril (enfermedad de Weber-Christian) en un niño de tres años. Rev. cuba. Pediat. **27**, 531 (1955). Ref. in Zbl. Haut- u. Geschl.-Kr. **95**, 345 (1956). — SPAIN, D. M., and I. M. TOBY: Non-suppurative nodular panniculitis (Weber-Christian disease). Amer. J. Path. **20**, 783 (1944). — SPIER, H.: Panniculitis non suppurativa chronica Typ Weber-Christian. Dermatologen-Tagg in Hamburg, 24.—26. 9. 1948. Ref. in Zbl. Haut- u. Geschl.-Kr. **73**, 178 (1949). — STUHLERT, H.: Pfeifer-Christian-Weber'sche Krankheit und Panniculitis traumatica. Z. Haut- u. Geschl.-Kr. **16**, 321 (1954). — SWEITZER, S. E.: Panniculitis. Arch. Derm. Syph. (Chic.) **39**, 1096 (1939).

TILDEN, I. L., H. C. GOTSHALK and E. V. AVAKIAN: RELAPSING febrile non-suppurative panniculitis. Report of a case. Arch. Derm. Syph. (Chic.) **41**, 681 (1940). — TOLMAN, M. M., and J. H. COX: Nodular non-suppurative panniculitis. Arch. Derm. Syph. (Chic.) **70**, 693 (1954).

UNGAR, H.: Relapsing febrile nodular inflammation of adipose tissue (Weber-Christian syndrome): Case with autopsy. J. Path. Bact. **58**, 175 (1946). — URBAS, N., et A. GOSPODNETIC: Panniculitis non-suppurativa nodularis recidivans febrilis Parkes-Weber-Christian chez l'enfant à l'issue mortelle. Zit. in Zbl. Haut- u. Geschl.-Kr. **106**, 319 (1960).

VILANOVA, X., et J. PINOL AGUADÉ: Hypodermite nodulaire subaiguë migratrice. Ann. Derm. Syph. (Paris) **1956**, 369. — VILANOVA, X., u. J. P. AGUADÉ: Noduläre Aphthose, Aphthose en plaques und Pfeifer-Weber-Christian'sche Panniculitis. Experimentelle Reproduktion der nodulären Läsionen bei Aphthose. Hautarzt **9**, 389 (1958).

WIGLEY, J. E. M., and O. L. S. SCOTT: Febrile relapsing nodular non-suppurative panniculitis (Weber-Christian disease). Brit. J. Derm. **64**, 460 (1952). — WINER, L. H.: Histopathology of the nodose lesions of the lower extremities. Arch. Derm. Syph. (Chic.) **63**, 347 (1951). — WOODBURN, A. R., and O. S. PHILPOTT: Nodular vasculitis. Arch. Derm. Syph. (Chic.) **60**, 294 (1949).

ZEE, M. L.: Nodular non suppurative panniculitis treated with penicillin. J. Amer. med. Ass. **130**, 1219 (1946).

Cheilitis granulomatosa und Melkersson-Rosenthal-Syndrom

Von

Rudolf Schuppli-Basel

Mit 4 Abbildungen

Einleitung

Das Gebiet der persistierenden Lippenschwellungen, der Makrocheilie, ist als typisches Grenzgebiet zwischen Dermatologie, Otologie und Chirurgie lange Zeit wenig beachtet worden. Erst seit MIESCHER im Jahre 1945 das Krankheitsbild der essentiellen granulomatösen Makrocheilie (Cheilitis granulomatosa) aufgestellt hatte, wandte sich die Aufmerksamkeit der Dermatologen diesen Veränderungen zu. MIESCHER fand bei mehreren in der Zürcher Klinik beobachteten Fällen von Makrocheilie histologische Veränderungen, die weitgehend gemeinsame Merkmale aufwiesen, so daß es ihm berechtigt schien, eine besondere Krankheitsgruppe zu bilden. 1949 wies dann LÜSCHER anhand eigener Beobachtungen auf das von MELKERSSON 1928 beschriebene Syndrom von rezidivierenden Gesichtsschwellungen und Facialisparese hin, das ROSENTHAL 1931 dahin ergänzt hatte, daß er das Vorhandensein einer Lingua plicata bei diesem Syndrom konstatierte. Über dieses Syndrom hatten 1942 schon in Skandinavien EKBOM und WAHLSTRÖM berichtet, während es in der deutschsprachigen Literatur kaum erwähnt worden war. Seither sind eine ganze Reihe von Arbeiten erschienen, die sich mit diesen beiden Krankheitsbildern befassen. Merkwürdigerweise stammen sie beinahe ausschließlich aus dem skandinavischen und deutschen Beobachtungsgebiet. Dabei gewinnt man den Eindruck, daß beide Krankheitsbilder zunehmend häufig auftreten und nicht etwa nur jetzt besser erfaßt werden können. Dagegen sollen sie in Amerika viel seltener sein (LAYMON).

Einen weiteren Fortschritt in der Erkenntnis dieser Krankheitsbilder brachten die Beobachtungen von GAHLEN und BRÜCKNER und von RICHTER und JOHNE, daß die von MIESCHER beschriebenen histologischen Veränderungen bei klinisch typischen Fällen von Melkersson-Rosenthal-Syndrom vorhanden sein können. Seither sind noch wesentlich mehr solcher Fälle beschrieben worden, so daß es nach MIESCHER (1956) berechtigt erscheint, das Melkersson-Rosenthal-Syndrom und die Cheilitis granulomatosa zusammenzufassen.

Weiter gelang der Nachweis, daß die histologischen Veränderungen, die für das Melkersson-Rosenthal-Syndrom typisch sind, sich nicht nur in der Lippe finden, sondern daß sie auch in der Wangenschleimhaut, der Zunge, in Nervengewebe (SCHUERMANN), Lymphknoten und Gesichtshaut (HORNSTEIN 1954) anzutreffen sind, so daß neben der Bezeichnung Cheilitis granulomatosa auch diejenige einer Pareiitis und Glossitis granulomatosa aufgestellt worden ist. Es rechtfertigt sich deshalb, die histologischen Veränderungen als das eigentliche Wesen der Krankheit anzusehen und alle Fälle, die diese aufweisen, unabhängig von ihrem klinischen Aussehen der gleichen Krankheitsgruppe zuzuordnen. Es sollen deshalb die Cheilitis granulomatosa, die Pareiitis granulomatosa und das Melkersson-Rosenthal-Syndrom gemeinsam besprochen werden, obwohl PIERARD und MAGE der Auffassung sind, daß es sich um voneinander unabhängige Prozesse handelt. Zur Nomenklatur sei bemerkt, daß es wohl am zweckmäßigsten ist, die Krankheitsbilder nach ihrem wichtigsten Symptom zu benennen, also nach wie vor eine Cheilitis, Glossitis, Pareiitis zu unterscheiden und den Namen des Melkersson-Rosenthal-Syndroms dem kompletten Trisymptomenkomplex zu reservieren. Da es möglicherweise ein Melkersson-Rosenthal-Syndrom verschiedener Genese gibt (HAMMINGA et al., LANDES und HERGER), wären dann die das histologisch charakteristische Bild aufweisenden Fälle als Miescher-Melkersson-Rosenthal-Syndrom zu bezeichnen (HERING und SCHEID).

1. Klinisches Bild

In den letzten 10 Jahren sind mehrere hundert Fälle beschrieben worden, die in das genannte Krankheitsbild gehören und z.T. außerordentlich genau untersucht worden sind. Da die Beschreibung der meisten Fälle nur in Einzelheiten differiert, läßt sich ein recht zuverlässiges klinisches Bild aufstellen.

a) Krankheitsverlauf

Der Krankheitsprozeß setzt unvermittelt, d.h. ohne äußeren Grund oft über Nacht ein, indem Schwellungen im Bereiche des Gesichts auftreten, die in seltenen Fällen dieses in seiner Gesamtheit, meist aber nur eine oder beide Lippen und die angrenzenden Wangenpartien betreffen. Prodrome fehlen meist völlig. Nur gelegentlich wird eine Störung des Allgemeinbefindens mit Temperaturerhöhung angegeben (KUSKE). Vorausgehende infektiöse Prozesse im Bereiche des Gesichtes, wie Pyodermien oder Erysipel, werden nie beobachtet. Nur gelegentlich treten wenige Stunden vor Beginn der Schwellung kleine Bläschen auf der Lippe auf, die als Herpes recidivans gedeutet worden sind (RACOUCHOT).

Der Verlauf der Erkrankung ist ausgesprochen schubweise, indem es zunächst zur Schwellung einer bestimmten Gesichtspartie, später dann zu einer solchen benachbarter Gebiete kommt, bis schließlich eine mehr oder weniger konstante Verdickung des Gewebes resultiert. Diese betrifft meist beide Lippen oder eine allein, wobei nach MIESCHER die Unterlippe, nach HORNSTEIN die Oberlippe häufiger befallen ist.

Leichte Remissionen können vorkommen, doch ist die Dauer des Leidens außerordentlich chronisch. Sie kann Jahrzehnte betragen (MORDANT). Gelegentlich allerdings wird spontaner Rückgang der Schwellung beobachtet.

Die Altersverteilung der Patienten ist uncharakteristisch. Die Erkrankung wird vom Kindes- bis zum Greisenalter beobachtet. Bei Frauen scheint allerdings das jugendliche Erwachsenenalter bevorzugt zu sein. Frauen überwiegen im Verhältnis 3:2.

Außer an den Lippen werden ähnliche Schwellungen an der Zunge, am Zahnfleisch (SATO, BAZEX et al.), an der Nase und am Kinn beschrieben.

Die Veränderungen der Zunge sind speziell beachtet worden, da sie ein Teilsymptom des Melkersson-Rosenthal-Syndroms darstellen. Nach SCHUERMANN (1952) kommt die Lingua plicata durch eine ausgeprägte Makroglossie zustande, die zu einer Starre und Trägheit der Zunge führen kann. Die Schleimhaut wird glasig, an Rändern und Spitze sind Zahnabdrücke markiert, was auf ein Ödem schließen läßt. Die stark ausgeprägte Furchung teilt die Oberfläche in zahlreiche Lappen ein, hie und da finden sich leukoplakische Epitheltrübungen. In seltenen Fällen findet sich auch das Bild der Exfoliatio areolaris linguae (KUSKE). Diese

Zungenveränderungen werden in etwa $^1/_3$ der Fälle gefunden. Für ihr Zustandekommen wird oft eine erbliche Disposition angenommen (Hambraeus).

Die Schwellungen im Bereiche des Gesichtes können die verschiedenen Partien betreffen und zum Bild der Blepharochalasis und in extremen Fällen zu einer Facies leonina führen. Sie können auch isoliert die Gesichtshaut betreffen und die Lippen verschonen (Musger 1953).

Neben den Haut- und Schleimhautschwellungen werden in verschiedenen Fällen auch Schwellungen der regionären Lymphdrüsen beobachtet, die sich speziell vor oder während neuen Schüben finden lassen. Hornstein sah in mehr als der Hälfte seiner Fälle Lymphknotenvergrößerung. Sie werden auch von Hering und Scheid beschrieben.

b) Nervenbeteiligung

Während von Melkersson nur eine Facialisparese beobachtet worden ist, ist seither auch das Befallensein anderer Nerven beschrieben worden. Nach der Zusammenstellung von Hornstein fanden sich bei 25 Fällen siebenmal Zeichen einer bestehenden kompletten peripheren Facialisparese. Einmal fand sich eine Ptose der Oberlider, dreimal waren Geschmacksstörungen vorhanden, vereinzelt ließ sich eine Hyperakusis feststellen. In drei Fällen bestanden Druckschmerzhaftigkeit der Trigeminus- und Occipitalnerven-Austrittspunkte, einmal eine Hyperästhesie im Wangenbereich. Broser et al. sahen außer Facialisparese eine Neuritis retrobulbaris, Befall des Trigeminus und zentralnervöse Syndrome mit Befallensein des Hirnstamms und mit Hemiparese. Auch Schimpf et al. sahen Bewußtseinsstörungen, Hemiparese und Reflexdifferenzen bei einer 29jährigen Frau mit Melkersson-Rosenthal-Syndrom. Schuermann beschreibt bei einem Kranken mit histologisch gesicherter Cheilitis granulomatosa wiederholt gleichzeitig mit rezidivierender Facialisparese und Lippenschwellung Geschmacksstörungen und häufige Schluckkrisen. Lüscher sah in seinem Fall Facialislähmung, Störung des N. statoacusticus und leichte Hyperalgesie im Bereich der zweiten und dritten Cervicalnerven. Damit zeigt sich, daß außer dem Facialis auch Oculomotorius, Trigeminus, Statoacusticus, Glossopharyngicus, Vagus und möglicherweise auch Hypoglossus betroffen sein können. Darüber hinaus können auch pathologische Befunde im Liquor (Kettel) und im Elektroencephalogramm erhoben werden (Pierard et al., Hornstein, Midana et al.). Von neurologischer Seite werden ferner speziell Schmerzhaftigkeit im Trigeminusgebiet (Massmann et al., Günther und Meinertz, Hamminga et al.) angegeben, und Hornstein hat schließlich den sehr interessanten Befund erhoben, daß eine Patientin 4 Monate nach dem Auftreten eines Melkersson-Rosenthal-Syndroms an einer zentralnervösen, caudal-spinalen Affektion erkrankte.

c) Interne Symptome

Naturgemäß können bei Patienten, die an einer jahrelang bestehenden chronischen Krankheit wie dem Melkersson-Rosenthal-Syndrom leiden, interne Störungen auftreten. Wieweit diese in Zusammenhang mit diesem Leiden gebracht werden können, ist fraglich. Auf jeden Fall ist bisher keine Veränderung bekannt geworden, die mit größerer Regelmäßigkeit zu konstatieren wäre. Höchstens verschiedene Augensymptome wie Conjunctivitis, Exophthalmus, Corneatrübungen scheinen häufiger zu sein (Gassler et al.). Beschrieben werden Angina (Hornstein) in 4 von 25 Fällen, Gelenkrheumatismus in 5 von 25 Fällen, Herzvitium (Tappeiner), Hypertonie (Kuske, Hornstein, Duperrat und Goetschel). Das Blutbild zeigt meist normale Werte, abgesehen von einer leichten Leukocytose im

Schub. HORNSTEIN fand in 6 von 25 Fällen erhöhte Eosinophilenzahlen. Die Senkungsreaktion ergibt normale oder schwach erhöhte Werte.

Kombinationen mit anderen Hautkrankheiten werden nur sehr selten erwähnt. So beschreibt KLÜKEN einen Fall von Melkersson-Rosenthal-Syndrom bei einem Patienten, der gleichzeitig eine Epidermodysplasie (LEWANDOWSKI-LUTZ) aufwies. HORNSTEIN beschreibt einen Patienten mit Melkersson-Rosenthal-Syndrom und Akrodermatitis.

2. Histologie

Charakterisiert ist die Cheilitis granulomatosa durch einheitliche Veränderungen, die in ihrer Intensität und in gewissen Einzelheiten differieren können, die

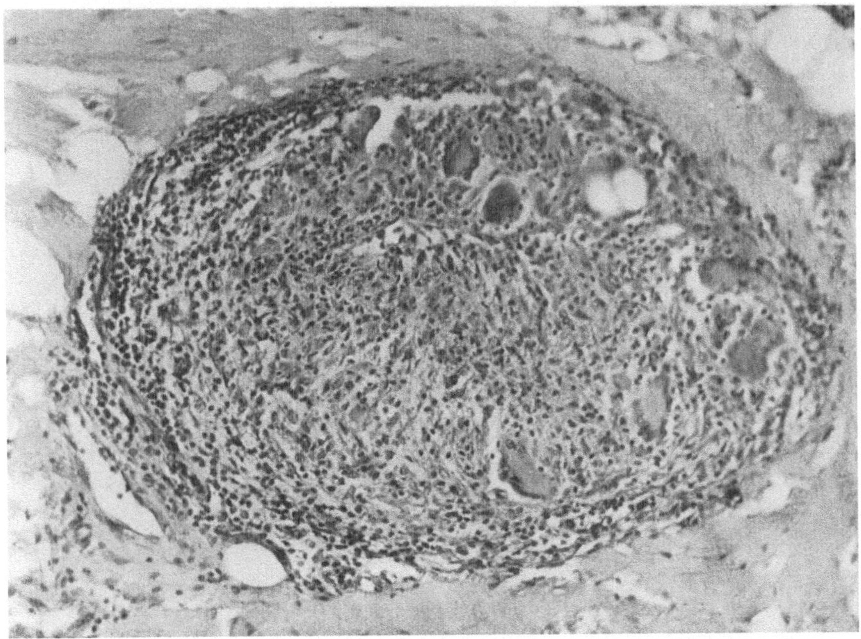

Abb. 1. Scharf begrenztes Knötchen, aus Epitheloidzellen und Riesenzellen bestehend. [Aus MIESCHER, G.: Über essentielle granulomatöse Makrocheilie (Cheilitis granulomatosa). Dermatologica (Basel) **91**, 66 (1945)]

aber im Prinzip die gleichen sind. Aus dem histologischen Bild geht hervor, daß es sich um eine diffuse Entzündung handelt, welche zur Infiltration und zu einem Ödem des ganzen mukösen und submukösen Gewebes führt. Es fehlen dabei auch bei mehrjährigem Verlauf ausgesprochene Zeichen von fibröser und bindegewebiger Hyperplasie. MIESCHER gibt folgende Beschreibung: Die entzündlichen Infiltrate sind ausgesprochen peri- und paravasculär orientiert, selten vermißt man eine direkte Beziehung zum Gefäß. Sie haben bald diffusen, bald ausgesprochen knötchenförmigen Charakter, wobei das Gefäß sowohl im Innern des Knötchens als auch an seinem Rande gelegen ist. Die Mehrzahl der Infiltrate besteht aus Lymphocyten und einigen Histiocyten und enthält dadurch ein ganz uncharakteristisches Gepräge. Im Gegensatz dazu finden sich in allen Fällen auch granulomatöse Formationen, welche mehr oder weniger ausgesprochen tuberkuloiden Charakter aufweisen (Abb. 1). Es handelt sich um kleinere oder größere knötchenförmige Haufen epitheloider Zellen, welche von Lymphocyten durchsetzt und eingerahmt sind. Zuweilen begegnet man Riesenzellen vom Langhansschen Typus. Das lymphocytäre Element kann sowohl prävalieren als auch vollständig zurücktreten, so daß Bilder entstehen, die an das Sarkoid von Besnier-Boeck erinnern, und das um so mehr, als die Knötchen dann meist scharf gegen das umgebende Gewebe abgesetzt sind. Elastische Fasern fehlen im Innern der Knötchen. Die Knötchen sind bald rundlich, bald walzenförmig, wobei sie das Gefäß oft eine längere Strecke weit mantelförmig umschließen (Abb. 2). Bei den Gefäßen handelt es sich meist um kleinere Venen und Subcapillaren, in deren adventitieller Scheide der granulomatöse Prozeß sich entwickelt. Intima und Media sind in der Regel unverändert. Die

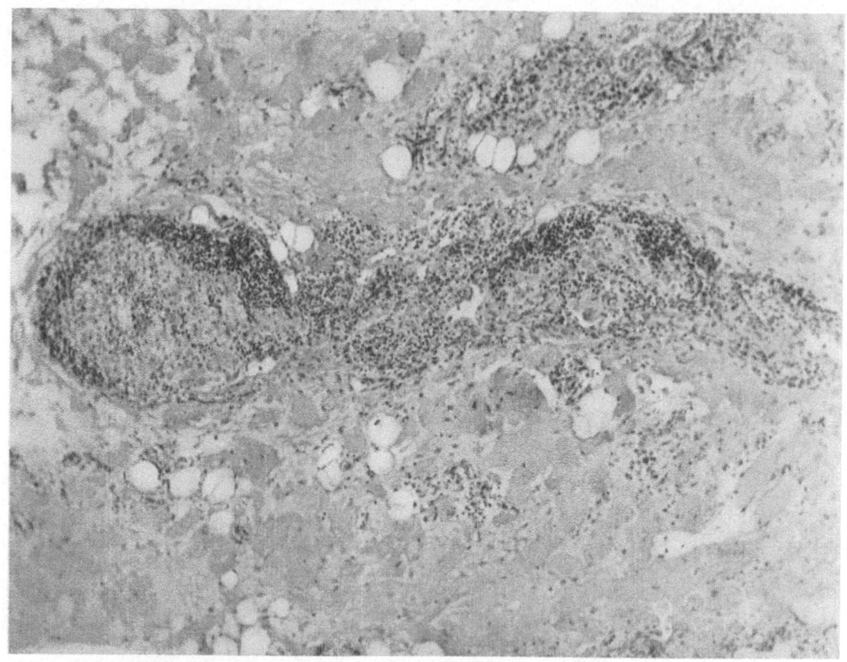

Abb. 2. Perivasculäres Knötchen. [Aus MIESCHER, G.: Über essentielle granulomatöse Makrocheilie (Cheilitis granulomatosa). Dermatologica (Basel) **91**, 64 (1945)]

Entzündung geht einher mit einer ödematösen Auflockerung des gesamten Gewebes, so daß dadurch die Lamina propria der Schleimhaut um das Doppelte bis Dreifache verbreitert wird. Das Ödem kann auch die Granulationsknoten erfassen, so daß dieselben vollkommen in ihre Elemente dissoziiert werden. Dasselbe kann mit Muskelbündeln geschehen, die sich ebenfalls in ihre einzelnen Fasern auflösen.

Die Lippenspeicheldrüsen zeigen keine pathologischen Veränderungen, oder es finden sich bloß interstitielle Lymphocyteninfiltrate in dem dem Entzündungsherd zugewandten Teil der Drüse. Einzig in einem Fall wurden auch mitten im Drüsenparenchym tuberkuloide Bildungen angetroffen (Abb. 3). Die Größe der Drüsen überschreitet nicht die üblichen Maße, welche zwischen Hirsekorn- und Erbsgröße schwanken. Die Intensität der Veränderungen und ihre Differenzierung kann von Fall zu Fall schwanken, da bei einem so chronischen Leiden die Excisionen naturgemäß nicht im gleichen Zeitpunkt gemacht werden können, doch sind sie im Prinzip einheitlich.

Diese histologischen Befunde werden von allen Untersuchern bestätigt. SCHUERMANN hat darüber hinaus noch Excisionen aus der geschwollenen Wangenschleimhaut (Makropareiie), aus der verdickten Zunge und aus Schwellungen der Gesichtshaut untersucht. Er konstatiert, daß die histologischen Befunde zwar

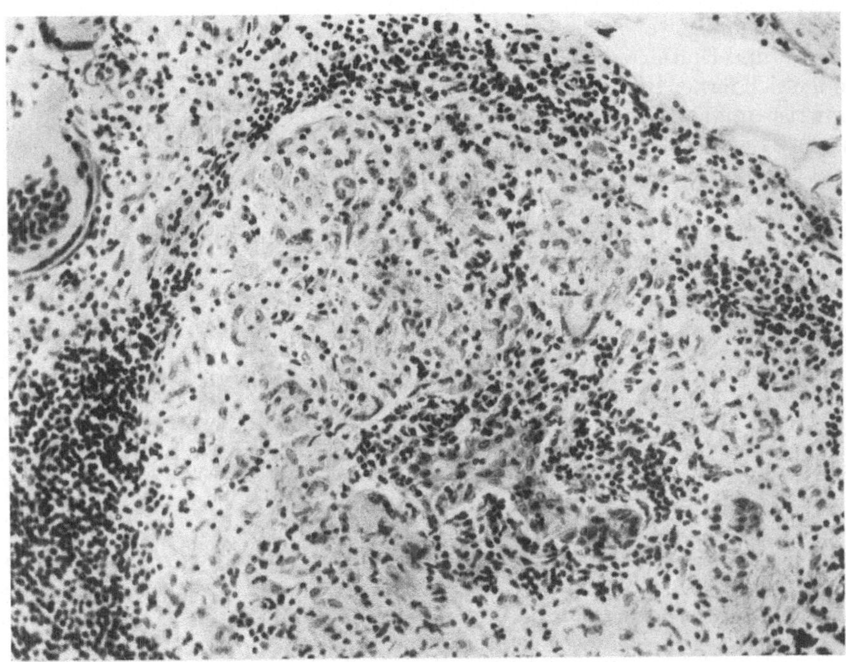

Abb. 3. Zwischen Drüsen gelegenes Knötchen. [Aus MIESCHER, G.: Über essentielle granulomatöse Makrocheilie (Cheilitis granulomatosa). Dermatologica (Basel) **91**, 69 (1945)]

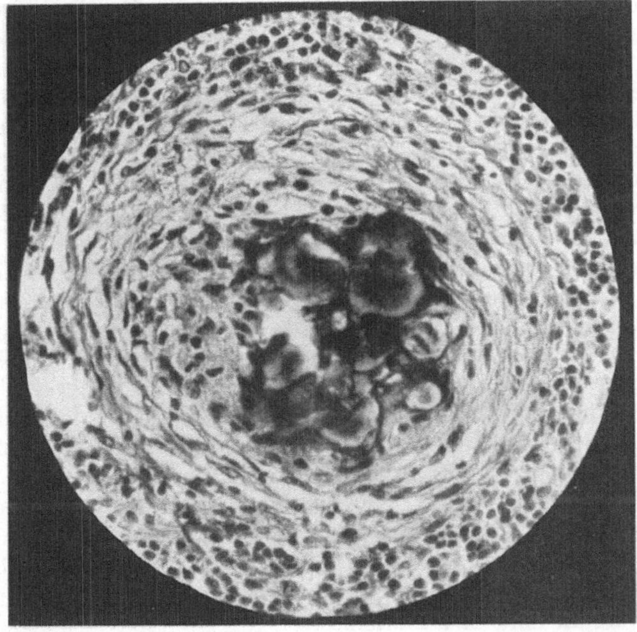

Abb. 4. Halslymphknoten: Reticulumknötchen mit konzentrischer Schichtung außen und großen verkalkten Einschlußkörperchen im Zentrum. [Aus HERING, H., u. P. SCHEID: Kritische Bemerkungen zum Melkersson-Rosenthal-Syndrom als Teilbild des Morbus Besnier-Boeck-Schaumann. Arch. Derm. Syph. (Berl.) **197**, 355 (1954)]

untereinander gewisse Abweichungen zeigen, aber jeweils ihrem Wesen nach zusammengehörig sind. Er fand in einem hyperämischen und ödematösen

Schleimhautbindegewebe Granulationsgewebe, das aus wechselnd zahlreichen Reticulum- und Epitheloidzellen und verschieden zahlreichen Leukocyten bestand. Es fanden sich ferner Riesenzellen vom Langhansschen Typus in wechselnder Zahl. Stellenweise fanden sich Plasmazellen in größerer Zahl, sowie abweichend von Mieschers Befunden in der Zunge ein beträchtlicher Reichtum an zelligen und faserigen Bindegewebselementen, der die Derbheit der Zunge und ihre Starre erklärt.

Interessant sind die Befunde, die Hering und Scheid an excidierten Halslymphknoten erheben konnten. Sie fanden eine teils diffuse, teils knötchenförmige Retikulose und epitheloidzellige Granulomatose, oft mit konzentrischer Schichtung peripherer Knötchen, teils mit kalkhaltigen konzentrisch geschichteten Einschlußkörperchen (Abb. 4).

Auch in der Muskulatur von Lippe und Wange fanden sie eine epitheloidzellige Granulomatose, einen Befund, den auch Musger (1953) und Santler erheben konnten. Auch Hornstein fand in Lymphknoten riesenzellhaltige Epitheloidzellknötchen.

3. Ätiologie und Pathogenese

Es liegt auf der Hand, daß bei den erwähnten einheitlichen histologischen Befunden einer epitheloidzelligen Granulomatose in erster Linie Zusammenhänge mit tuberkulösen Prozessen auf der einen Seite und dem Boeckschen Sarkoid auf der anderen Seite gesucht wurden. Bisher haben weder direkte Überimpfung von Gewebsstückchen, noch Kulturen den Nachweis einer tuberkulösen Ätiologie erbringen können. Auch die Tuberkulinempfindlichkeit der Patienten kann für die ätiologische Abklärung nicht verwendet werden, da sie innerhalb weiter Grenzen schwankt und wohl den Verhältnissen der Durchschnittsbevölkerung entspricht. In einem einzigen Fall (Klüken) konnte eine verkäsende Tuberkulose der Hilus- und Bifurkationslymphknoten gefunden werden. Als Beweis der Identität des Krankheitsbildes der Cheilitis granulomatosa mit dem Boeckschen Sarkoid führen Hering und Scheid die histologischen Befunde an, die in allen Einzelheiten einem Boeckschen Sarkoid entsprechen sollen. Ob diese Auffassung stimmt, wird sich erst bei Beobachtung weiterer Fälle ergeben. Es muß immerhin festgestellt werden, daß bisher in keinem Fall andere für Morbus Boeck typische Lokalisationen gefunden werden konnten, so daß jetzt mehrheitlich eine Identität beider Affektionen abgelehnt wird (Schuppener, Hornstein et al.).

Auf eine ganz andere Pathogenese weisen nun die Angaben von Tappeiner hin. Er beschreibt eine 56jährige Frau, die an einem schubweise verlaufenden, histologisch verifizierten Melkersson-Rosenthal-Syndrom litt. Nach Entfernung einer Kunstharzprothese trat bei der Patientin in kürzester Zeit eine völlige Heilung ein. Auch Röckl beschreibt einen Fall, in dem 2 Jahre nach Einlegen einer Zahnprothese eine Cheilitis granulomatosa auftrat, und Pezzarossa sah Heilung nach Gebißsanierung. Andere Autoren erwähnen eine allergische Konstitution bei ihren Patienten (Massmann und Schilf, Meyer, Andrup), während Miescher in seinen Fällen keine solche fand. Schuppener sah wiederum eine abortive Form bei durch Bohnenkaffee auslösbarer Urticaria, Machacek ein typisches Syndrom bei einer polyvalenten Allergikerin, die zudem noch eine Retentionscyste im Sinus maxillaris zeigte.

Auf andere Möglichkeiten der Erklärung weist das Bestehen septischer Herde hin. So hat schon Miescher darauf hingewiesen, daß in der Vorgeschichte häufig Furunkel angegeben werden. Auch in der Zusammenstellung von Hering und Scheid fanden sich in 6 von 24 Fällen eitrige Prozesse im Körper erwähnt. Musger beobachtete in einem Fall eine Salpingitis kurz vor dem Auftreten eines

Melkersson-Rosenthal-Syndroms. Direkter Nachweis von Streptokokken in Schwellungsherden gelang MACHACEK, STEVENS, SATO. GAHLEN und GILLMANN sahen ein histologisch typisches Melkersson-Rosenthal-Syndrom bei einer Patientin mit Filariasis und glauben an eine infekt-allergische Genese dieses Syndroms. Dafür sprechen auch die Beobachtungen von KOCHS, der unter 1600 Fällen von Hautleishmaniose 26 Fälle von histologisch typischer Cheilitis granulomatosa fand, und die sehr interessanten Feststellungen von DAHM et al. über einen positiven Sabin-Feldman-Test für Toxoplasmose bei sechs Patienten mit Melkersson-Rosenthal-Syndrom.

Nach diesen sehr differenten Befunden ist wohl die Feststellung TAPPEINERs und HORNSTEINs, daß es sich um ein polyätiologisches Krankheitsbild handeln könnte, die zur Zeit beste Umschreibung unserer Unkenntnis der eigentlichen Ätiologie.

Eine völlig andere Pathogenese diskutiert DÖRING mit der Frage der Beziehung des Nervensystems zu lokalen Gewebsveränderungen. Er stellte fest, daß sich die Lingua plicata auf die vorderen $^2/_3$ der Zunge beschränkt, die durch den Trigeminus innerviert wird, dem über die Chorda tympani ein parasympathischer Anteil zugeordnet ist. Parasympathische Erregung könnte auch andere beim Melkersson-Rosenthal-Syndrom beobachtete Symptome wie den Tränenfluß, die Atrophie der Nasenschleimhaut, rezidivierende Ödeme erklären. Das Melkersson-Rosenthal-Syndrom sei also eine Funktionsstörung der parasympathischen Innervation, die vom Ganglion geniculi ausgeht und mit der Störung des Facialis verbunden ist. Allerdings sind damit die Granulationsbildungen nicht erklärt. Auch WALLK et al. messen nervösen Störungen speziell des vegetativen Nervensystems große Bedeutung bei, ADERHOLD et al. außerdem noch erblicher Anlage. Schließlich werden auch noch Lichteinflüsse und Kälte (JORDAN und REICHEL; Berliner Demonstrationen) für das Entstehen der Facialisparese verantwortlich gemacht.

4. Diagnose und Differentialdiagnose

MIESCHER hat in seiner ersten Publikation die Differentialdiagnose der Cheilitis granulomatosa ausführlich besprochen und auf folgende Krankheitsbilder hingewiesen, die dabei in Frage kommen können:

1. kann es sich um eine primäre Makrocheilie als Ausdruck chronisch entzündlicher Vorgänge in der Lippe handeln.

2. gibt es eine primäre Makrocheilie als Ausdruck der geschwulstartigen Hyperplasie einzelner Gewebselemente. Die Lymphangiome, Hämangiome lassen sich ohne weiteres unterscheiden, während diejenigen Fälle, die auf Hyperplasie der Lippenspeicheldrüsen beruhen, schwieriger abzugrenzen sind. Es sind verschiedene solcher Fälle beschrieben worden, wobei meistens die Oberlippe befallen war. Die vergrößerten Speicheldrüsen lassen sich durch die Schleimhaut hindurch palpieren. In diese Gruppe von Lippenveränderungen gehört das Aschersche Syndrom (durch Drüsenhypertrophie bedingte Doppellippe, Blepharochalasis und Struma). FINDLAY beschreibt fünf Fälle von idiopathischer Lippenverdickung, wovon drei zum Ascherschen Syndrom gehörten.

3. Von diesen primären Makrocheilien lassen sich die entzündlichen Cheilitiden, die z.T. infolge Schwellung der Schleimdrüsen zu einer Lippenverdickung führen können, ohne weiteres abgrenzen (Cheilitis glandularis apostematosa), da sie mit starken Entzündungserscheinungen einhergehen.

4. Weitere differentialdiagnostisch wichtige Lippenvergrößerungen lassen sich anamnestisch, klinisch und histologisch unterscheiden, indem diesen auf chronischer Entzündung beruhenden Prozessen (Lupus, Erysipelas recidivans, Lepra

usw.) typische Erscheinungen vorausgehen. Speziell auch die tertiärluische Lippenverdickung muß ausgeschlossen werden (Hauser).

Schwierigkeiten werden sich speziell im Beginn der Erkrankung ergeben, bevor die Schwellung dauerhaft geworden ist und die typischen histologischen Veränderungen sich finden. Hier sind hauptsächlich vasoneurotische Ödeme auszuschließen.

Die Diagnose wird hingegen nicht schwer zu stellen sein, wenn die typischen histologischen Veränderungen angetroffen werden, wobei die Einschränkung gemacht werden muß, daß diese nicht in allen Stadien gleich ausgebildet sein können, so daß bei negativem Ausfall der histologischen Untersuchung das Vorliegen eines Miescher-Melkersson-Rosenthalschen Syndroms nicht ausgeschlossen werden kann. So existieren Berichte über typische Fälle dieses Syndroms, bei denen die histologische Untersuchung ein vollkommen negatives Resultat ergeben hat (Landes und Herger).

Schwierig einzuordnen sind auch diejenigen Fälle, bei denen die Schwellung unter Fieber auftritt (Kuske) und wo dementsprechend an das Bestehen eines Erysipels gedacht werden muß, speziell wenn die Facialisparese nicht von Anfang vorhanden ist. Auch Monilia-Infektionen (Bazex et al.) können eine Makrocheilie hervorrufen, die histologisch Entzündungsgranulome aufweist.

5. Therapie

Die meisten Berichte über therapeutische Effekte sind negativ. So sah Hamminga keinen Erfolg bei Röntgenstrahlen, Penicillin, Sulfadiazin, Calciferol. Kuske brauchte ebenfalls Röntgenstrahlen ohne Erfolg. Hering und Scheid sahen keinen Erfolg von Vitamin D_2 in einer Gesamtdosis von 150 mg; Tebethion, ein Antihistaminicum, brachte ausgesprochene Verschlechterung. Gipperich erzielte weder mit Röntgenstrahlen, noch mit Dijodthyroxin, noch mit antiallergischer Medikation einen Erfolg. Penicillin verschlechterte einen Fall von Gahlen und Brückner und nützte in einem andern Fall (Berliner Demonstrationen) nichts. Gumpesberger erzielte mit Penicillin dagegen wenigstens einen gewissen Rückgang der Induration und Rötung. Positive Berichte stammen von Tappeiner, der durch Entfernung einer Kunstharzprothese und durch Sanierung von Zahnherden in einem andern Fall einen raschen Rückgang der Symptome sah, während Gahlen und Brückner durch Focussanierung keinen Erfolg erzielen konnten. Antistin wirkte bei einem Fall von Hamminga wenigstens subjektiv günstig, während Hornstein und Schuppener Cortison und ACTH empfehlen. Einen raschen Erfolg erzielten Hering und Scheid in einem Fall mit Isonicotinsäurehydrazid, bei dem alle übrigen Therapien versagt hatten, während Wagner von dem gleichen Mittel keine Wirkung sah. Berger erwähnt günstige therapeutische Resultate mit Tuberculostatica und Cortison, Sales et al. solche mit Streptomycin und Cortison, während andere Tuberculostatica und Cortison lokal versagt hatten; Braun-Falco et al. erzielten mit Neoteben und massiven Dosen von Nicofol in einem von drei Fällen einen Erfolg. Meist jedoch wird chirurgisches Vorgehen im Sinne einer Cheiloplastik (Thomsen, Stava et al.) oder Schleimhautabtragung (Faninger et al.) empfohlen.

Literatur

Aderhold, K., E. Krönke u. H. Pawlik: Melkersson-Rosenthal-Syndrom mit Megacolon congenitum — Ein selbständiges Krankheitsbild. Dtsch. Gesundh.-Wes. **1957**, 513. — Andrup, O.: Melkerssons Syndrom auf allergischer Basis. T. norske Laegeforen. **73**, 9 (1953).

Bazex, Dupré et Parant: Moniliase bucco-pharyngée avec granulome et macrochéilite glandulaire datant de l'enfance (Discussion avec le syndrome d'Ascher). Bull. Soc. franç.

Derm. Syph. **63**, 527 (1956). — Makrochéilites parenchymateuses. Bull. Soc. franç. Derm. Syph. **64**, 114 (1957). — BERGER, J.: Beitrag zum Problem Cheilitis granulomatosa Miescher, Melkersson-Rosenthal-Syndrom, mit atypischen Fällen. Wien. med. Wschr. **1956**, 441. — *Berliner Demonstrationen* aus der Universitäts-Hautklinik der Charité, sowie aus der ihr angeschlossenen Haut-Abteilung des Städt. Krankenhauses Berlin-Buch. Cheilitis granulomatosa. Ref. in Zbl. Haut- u. Geschl.-Kr. **89**, 364 (1954). — Cheilitis et Pareiitis granulomatosa. Ref. in Zbl. Haut- u. Geschl.-Kr. **89**, 364 (1954). — Melkersson-Rosenthal'sches Syndrom. Ref. in Zbl. Haut- u. Geschl.-Kr. **89**, 364 (1954). — BRAUN-FALCO, O.: Cheilitis granulomatosa Miescher. Arch. Derm. Syph. (Berl.) **200**, 589 (1955). — BRAUN-FALCO, O., u. B. RATHJENS: Zum Bild der Pareiitis granulomatosa. Derm. Wschr. **128**, 1073 (1953). — BROSER, F., u. R. M. BENDER: Über zentralnervöse Symptome bei Cheilitis granulomatosa Miescher, bzw. Melkersson-Rosenthal-Syndrom. Nervenarzt **29**, 21 (1958).

DAHM, G., u. H. SCHINKO: Zur Genese der Cheilitis granulomatosa bzw. des Melkersson-Rosenthal-Syndroms. Arch. klin. exp. Derm. **212**, 616 (1961). — DÖRING: Diskussionsbemerkung zum Melkersson-Rosenthal-Syndrom. 4. Tagg Hamburger Derm. Ges. 28./29. 1. 1950. Hautarzt **1**, 279 (1950). — DUPERRAT, B., et M. G. GOETSCHEL: Macrochéilite de Miescher. Bull. Soc. franç. Derm. Syph. **62**, 140 (1955).

EKBOM, K. A., u. ANNIE WAHLSTRÖM: Melkerssons Syndrom. Chronische Gesichtsschwellung mit rezidivierender Gesichtslähmung. Nord. Med. **1942**, 2373.

FANINGER, A., u. M. ISVANESKI: Cheilitis granulomatosa Miescher. Med. Pregl. **7**, 147 (1954). — FINDLAY, G. H.: Idiopathic enlargements of the lips: Cheilitis granulomatosa, Ascher's syndrome and double lip. Brit. J. Derm. **66**, 129 (1954).

GAHLEN, W., u. B. BRÜCKNER: Beitrag zur Pathogenese des Melkersson-Rosenthal-Syndroms. Arch. Derm. Syph. (Berl.) **192**, 468 (1951). — GAHLEN, W., u. H. GILLMANN: Melkersson-Rosenthal-Syndrom bei Filariasis. Münch. med. Wschr. **1954**, 189. — GASSLER, H., u. H. BERTHOLD: Ein Beitrag zum Melkersson-Rosenthal-Syndrom aus ophthalmologischer Sicht. Klin. Mbl. Augenheilk. **139**, 44 (1961). — GIPPERICH, L.: Sindrome di Melkersson e Rosenthal. G. Clin. med. **32**, 519 (1951). — GÜNTHER, H., u. F. MEINERTZ: Das Melkersson-Rosenthal'sche Syndrom. Nervenarzt **23**, 22 (1952). — GUMPESBERGER: Cheilitis granulomatosa (Miescher). Österr. Derm. Ges. Wissenschaftl. Sitzg 13. 10. 56. Hautarzt **7**, 285 (1956).

HAMBRAEUS, L.: Rezidivierende Facialisparese mit Lingua plicata und Gesichtsschwellung (Melkersson-Syndrom). Nord. Med. **48**, 1342 (1952). — HAMMINGA, H.: Cheilitis granulomatosa. Dermatologica (Basel) **110**, 177 (1955). — HAMMINGA, H., u. T. A. J. VAN DOORMAAL: Das Syndrom von Melkersson-Rosenthal. Ned. T. Geneesk. **1953**, 27. — HAUSER, W.: Das Melkersson-Rosenthal-Syndrom und die Cheilitis granulomatosa. Dtsch. zahnärztl. Z. 8, 986 (1953). — HERING, H., u. P. SCHEID: Kritische Bemerkungen zum Melkersson-Rosenthal-Syndrom als Teilbild des Morbus Besnier-Boeck-Schaumann. Arch. Derm. Syph. (Berl.) **197**, 344 (1954). — HORNSTEIN, O.: Beteiligung des lymphatischen Systems am Komplex der „Cheilitis" (Pareiitis etc.) granulomatosa. Arch. Derm. Syph. (Berl.) **198**, 396 (1954). — Klinische und histologische Untersuchungen über „Cheilitis granulomatosa" (Miescher) bzw. Melkersson-Rosenthal-Syndrom. Hautarzt **6**, 433 (1955). — Über die Pathogenese des sog. Melkersson-Rosenthal-Syndroms (einschließlich der „Cheilitis granulomatosa" Miescher). Arch. klin. exp. Derm. **212**, 570 (1961). — HORNSTEIN, O., u. H. SCHUERMANN: Das sog. Melkersson-Rosenthal-Syndrom (einschließlich „Cheilitis granulomatosa" Miescher). Ergebn. inn. Med. Kinderheilk. **17**, 191 (1962).

JORDAN, P., u. K. REICHEL: Das Melkersson-Rosenthal-Syndrom. Hautarzt **1**, 37 (1950).

KETTEL, K.: Zit. in E. LÜSCHER. — KLÜKEN, N.: Epidermodysplasia verruciformis mit Cheilitis granulomatosa. Hautarzt **3**, 405 (1952). — KOCHS, A. G.: Die spezifisch proliferative Cheilitis bei Hautleishmaniose als Modellfall granulomatöser Makrocheilie. Derm. Wschr. **1956**, 553. — KUSKE, H.: Granulomatöse Makrocheilie (Cheilitis granulomatosa) mit rezidivierender Facialislähmung rechts (Melkersson-Rosenthal-Syndrom). Dermatologica (Basel) **110**, 392 (1955). — Cheilitis granulomatosa. Dermatologica (Basel) **110**, 394 (1955). — Makrocheilie bei chronisch rezidivierendem Erysipel der Oberlippe. Dermatologica (Basel) **110**, 395 (1955).

LANDES, E., u. R. HERGER: Melkersson-Rosenthal-Syndrom. Hautarzt **4**, 440 (1953). — LAYMON, C. W.: Cheilitis granulomatosa and Melkersson-Rosenthal syndrome. Arch. Derm. **83**, 112 (1961). — LÜSCHER, E.: Syndrom von Melkersson-Rosenthal. Schweiz. med. Wschr. **79**, 1 (1949).

MACHACEK, G. F.: Melkersson-Rosenthal-Syndrom. N.Y. Derm. Soc. Sitzg v. 25. 10. 1955. Arch. Derm. **74**, 440 (1955). — Melkersson-Rosenthal syndrome. Arch. Derm. **74**, 440 (1956). — MASSMANN, W., u. E. SCHILF: Experimenteller Beitrag zum Melkersson-Rosenthal'schen Syndrom. Psychiat. Neurol. med. Psychol. (Lpz.) **5**, 294 (1953). — MELKERSSON: Zit. in E. LÜSCHER. — MEYER, K.: Das Syndrom von Melkersson-Rosenthal. Ann. paediat. (Basel) **180**, 111 (1953). — MIDANA, A., e G. BONU: Considerazioni sulla sindrome di Melkersson e

Rosenthal. Minerva derm. **33**, 323 (1958). — Miescher, G.: Über essentielle granulomatöse Makrocheilie (Cheilitis granulomatosa). Dermatologica (Basel) **91**, 57 (1945). — Cheilitis et Pareiitis granulomatosa ohne Facialisparese bei Vorhandensein einer Lingua scrotalis. Dermatologica (Basel) **112**, 536 (1956). — Mordant, H.: Syndrome de Melkersson-Rosenthal. Arch. belges Derm. **13**, 87 (1957). — Musger, A.: Chronisch-entzündliche, ohne Beteiligung der Lippen einhergehende Schwellung der Gesichtshaut mit dem histologischen Bild der Cheilitis granulomatosa Miescher. Ein Beitrag zur Cheilitis granulomatosa Miescher bzw. zum Melkersson- Rosenthal-Syndrom. Wien. klin. Wschr. **1953**, 796. — Drei Fälle zum Problem der Cheilitis granulomatosa Miescher. Österr. Dermat. Ges. Sitzgsber. 1953. Ref. in Zbl. Haut- u. Geschl.-Kr. **85**, 262 (1953).

Pezzarossa, G.: Ulteriori osservazioni sulla macrocheilite granulomatosa (con particolare riferimento ai suoi rapporti con la sindrome di Melkersson-Rosenthal). G. ital. Derm. **98**, 545 (1957). — Pierard, J., et J. Mage: Le syndrome de Melkersson-Rosenthal. Arch. belges Derm. **10**, 1 (1954). — Pierard, J., J. Mage et R. Baes: Syndrome de Melkersson-Rosenthal. Arch. belges Derm. **10**, 278 (1954).

Racouchot, J., et G. Leger: Syndrome de Melkersson-Rosenthal avec herpes récidivant. Bull. Soc. franç. Derm. Syph. **65**, 590 (1958). — Richter, R., u. H. O. Johne: Über Beziehungen des Melkersson-Rosenthal-Syndroms zur Cheilitis granulomatosa (Miescher). Arch. Derm. Syph. (Berl.) **190**, 486 (1950). — Röckl: Cheilitis granulomatosa Miescher. Vereinigung Südwestdeutscher Dermatologen, Sitzung vom 9./10. 10. 1954. Ref. in Zbl. Haut- u. Geschl.-Kr. **91**, 222 (1955). — Rosenthal: Zit. in E. Lüscher.

Sales, Gadel et Masson: Macrochéilite de Miescher. Bull. Soc. franç. Derm. Syph. **64**, 115 (1957). — Santler, R.: Cheilitis granulomatosa. Österr. Dermat. Ges. Sitzg v. 23. 4. 53. Ref. in Zbl. Haut- u. Geschl.-Kr. **85**, 254 (1953). — Sato, Y.: Ein Fall von Cheilitis granulomatosa. Jap. J. Derm. **66**, 193 (1956). — Schimpf, A., u. J. Suckow: Cerebrale Störungen beim Melkersson-Rosenthal-Syndrom. Arch. Psychiat. Nervenkr. **196**, 27 (1957). — Schuermann, H.: Glossitis und Pareiitis granulomatosa. Hautarzt **3**, 538 (1952). — Spezifische Veränderungen am lymphatischen System bei „Cheilitis" („Pareiitis" usw.) granulomatosa. Hautarzt **5**, 174 (1954). — Schuppener, H. J.: Zum Melkersson-Rosenthal-Syndrom. Erhebungen an einer Gruppe von 21 Patienten. Dtsch. Gesundh.-Wes. **1956**, 1598. — Abortives Melkersson-Rosenthal-Syndrom bei durch Bohnenkaffee auslösbarer Urticaria mit Horner-Symptomen-Komplex. Zit. in Zbl. Haut- u. Geschl.-Kr. **98**, 313 (1957). — Štavá, Z., and T. Bielický: Melkersson-Rosenthal's syndrome and its problems. Čs. Derm. **28**, 283 (1953). — Stevens, F. A.: Streptococcic infection of the „fibroedema" of Melkersson's syndrome. J. Amer. med. Ass. **156**, 223 (1954).

Tappeiner, S.: Cheilitis granulomatosa Miescher. Österr. Dermat. Ges. Sitzg vom 20. 11. 1952. Ref. in Zbl. Haut- u. Geschl.-Kr. **85**, 241 (1953). — Zur Klinik und Pathogenese der Cheilitis granulomatosa (Miescher). Hautarzt **4**, 130 (1953). — Thomsen, K. A.: Cheiloplasty and ACTH in Melkersson's syndrome. Nord. Med. **49**, 718 (1953).

Wagner: Zwei Fälle von Cheilitis granulomatosa Miescher. Ver.igg Schleswig-Holstein. Dermatologen, Sitzg vom 14. 2. 1954. Ref. in Zbl. Haut- u. Geschl.-Kr. **87**, 296 (1954). — Wallk, S., and S. Bluefarb: Melkersson-Rosenthal syndrome. Arch. Derm. **84**, 798 (1961).

Granuloma anulare — Necrobiosis lipoidica diabeticorum — Granulomatosis disciformis — Necrobiosis maculosa

Von

Rudolf Schuppli-Basel

Mit 1 Abbildung

Einleitung

Auf dem Gebiet der granulomatösen Reaktionen der Haut sind, abgesehen von den gut charakterisierten Formen des Besnier-Boeckschen Sarkoides, der tuberkulösen, luischen, lepromatösen Granulome usw. eine ganze Reihe von Krankheitsbildern beschrieben worden, die auf Grund klinischer oder histologischer Merkmale einigermaßen gegen ähnliche Prozesse abgegrenzt werden können. Daneben existieren aber zahlreiche Beobachtungen, die sich in keines der bekannteren Bilder einordnen lassen und für die deshalb zunächst neue Bezeichnungen geschaffen werden müssen. Da die Ätiologie dieser Granulomatosen meist vollkommen unklar ist, lassen sich zunächst nur typische Fälle der einzelnen Krankheitsgruppen klar voneinander abgrenzen, während andere Fälle nach dem klinischen Bild der einen, nach dem histologischen Bild der andern Gruppe zugeordnet werden müssen. Dabei zeigt sich, daß das Hauptgewicht bei der Beurteilung der Granulomatosen unbekannter Ätiologie auf die histologischen Veränderungen zu legen ist, da das klinische Bild oft irreführend ist. Es sollen deshalb zunächst die histologischen Merkmale folgender Krankheitsbilder beschrieben werden:

1. Granuloma anulare.
2. Necrobiosis lipoidica (Urbach-Oppenheim).
3. Granulomatosis disciformis (Miescher).
4. Necrobiosis maculosa (Miescher).

I. Histologie

1. Granuloma anulare

Der für das Granuloma anulare charakteristische Prozeß läuft in der Cutis ab. Es finden sich dort herdförmige Veränderungen, die deutlich verschiedene Zonen unterscheiden lassen: Es hebt sich ein zentraler, mehr oder weniger nekrotischer Bezirk von einem peripheren, zellig infiltrierten ab, der die zentrale Nekrose umschließt. Das Infiltrat wird aus zwei Zellarten gebildet. Einmal finden sich gewucherte Bindegewebszellen mit breitem Protoplasmasaum und runden, ovalen oder spindelförmigen Kernen, gegen die Peripherie dieser Herde häufen sich dagegen Lymphocyten, zwischen denen vereinzelte polynucleäre Leukocyten und selten Plasmazellen anzutreffen sind. Die Gefäße in der Umgebung des Herdes zeigen ein leichtes perivasculäres Infiltrat. Die Venen können durch eine deutliche

Intimawucherung in wechselndem Grade verschlossen sein, während die Arterien unverändert sind. Zahlreich sind Gefäßsprossen, die ebenfalls geschwollene Endothelien und Intimawucherungen zeigen (GANS und STEIGLEDER).

Die zentrale Nekrose zeigt je nach dem Zeitpunkt der Untersuchung ein verschiedenes Bild. In frischeren Fällen ist das Bindegewebe im nekrotischen Herd nur schlecht oder gar nicht mehr erkennbar. Vom nekrotischen Zentrum aus ziehen sich radiär angeordnete Bindegewebssepten in das umgebende Infiltrat, die ebenfalls nekrotisch verändert sind. Das nekrotische kollagene Gewebe färbt sich nach VAN GIESON schmutzig-gelb. Es finden sich in ihm Einlagerungen von Mucin und von homogenen, leuchtend rot gefärbten, in kleinen Haufen zusammenliegenden Kugeln (Russell-Körper) hyalin umgewandelten Bindegewebes. In länger bestehenden Krankheitsherden dagegen tritt die Nekrose gegenüber einer reichlichen Neubildung von Bindegewebszellen und Bindegewebsfasern zurück, und das periphere Zellinfiltrat wird lockerer. Veränderungen der Epidermis fehlen in den meisten Fällen und sind nur sekundärer Art.

MEZZADRA betont, daß das histologische Bild stark von der Phase der Krankheit abhängt und bemerkenswert polymorph sein kann.

2. Necrobiosis lipoidica

Auch hier zeigt die Epidermis ausschließlich sekundäre Veränderungen. Der eigentliche Sitz der Krankheit findet sich in der mittleren Cutis in Form einer Nekrobiose mit homogenisierten Bindegewebsschollen. Das Gewebe ist hier sehr kernarm oder kernlos und färbt sich unregelmäßig mit Eosin. Totale Nekrose wird niemals beobachtet. Die elastischen Fasern fehlen fast vollkommen. Zwischen den nekrotischen Massen finden sich extracelluläre Fettablagerungen in wechselnder Menge. Es scheint sich dabei vorwiegend um Neutralfett, Fettsäuren und Lipoide zu handeln, ferner um Mucin, Hämosiderin und eine Diastaseresistente PAS-positive Substanz (WOOD et al.). Intracelluläre Fettphagocytose tritt demgegenüber stark in den Hintergrund. Das die Nekrose umgebende Granulationsgewebe ist verschieden stark ausgebildet. Bei älteren Herden kann es sehr gering sein. Es ist sowohl schalenförmig um die Nekrose als auch perivasculär angeordnet und besteht aus Lymphocyten, Histiocyten und Fibroblasten. Gelegentlich werden reichlich Eosinophile gefunden. Riesenzellen von uncharakteristischem Typus kommen häufig vor. Sie können Asteroidkörperchen enthalten (SMITH et al.). Wichtig sind die Veränderungen der Gefäße, die sich hauptsächlich an der Grenze zwischen Cutis und Subcutis finden. Sie sind erweitert, ihre Wand ist verdickt, wobei speziell die Intima gewuchert ist, so daß es manchmal zu völligem Gefäßverschluß kommen kann. Die enge Beziehung zu Gefäßveränderungen zeigte der von STÜTTGEN publizierte Fall, wo eine Necrobiosis lipoidica bei einem Patienten auftrat, der während 5 Jahren an einer Purpura Schönlein gelitten hatte.

3. Granulomatosis disciformis chronica et progressiva (MIESCHER)

In frischen Herden ist die Epidermis ziemlich breit und normal zusammengesetzt. Die Veränderungen finden sich ausschließlich in der Cutis, an der Grenze zwischen Cutis und Subcutis, vor allem im Bereich der Gefäße, und steigen von hier aus den Gefäßen folgend bis in die Nähe der subpapillären Schicht. An der Grenze gegen die Subcutis bildet sich ein kontinuierlicher Infiltrationsstreifen. Dieses Infiltrat setzt sich aus Fibroblasten, die teilweise den Aspekt von Epitheloiden annehmen können und regellos gelagert sind, zusammen. Es finden sich im Infiltrat mehrkernige Zellen, die dem Fremdkörpertypus entsprechen, z.T. aber auch Langhansschen Zellen ähnlich sind. Das Bindegewebe zeigt keine Veränderungen. Es ist durch ein wechselnd dichtes lymphocytäres und plasmocytäres Infiltrat durchsetzt. Die Gefäße zeigen ausgesprochene Wucherung der Endothelien, z.T. auch einen breiten granulomatösen Mantel aus Fibroblasten, Epitheloiden und Langhansschen Riesenzellen. Nekrosen fehlen.

4. Necrobiosis maculosa (Miescher)

Die Epidermis ist normal. In den mittleren Partien der Cutis finden sich nekrobiotische Zonen, die unregelmäßig gelagert sind. Sie besitzen bei frischen Herden nur geringe Ausdehnung, in älteren Herden nehmen sie die ganze Breite der Cutis bis an die Subcutis ein. Sie sind vollkommen kernlos, während das kollagene Gewebe sich nach van Gieson z.T. noch rot anfärbt. In jüngeren Herden ist die nekrobiotische Zone von einem ziemlich dichten Granulationsgewebe umschlossen, das reichlich längliche, hellkernige und Protoplasma-reiche, nach der Mitte ausgerichtete Elemente und daneben Lymphocyten und vereinzelt auch mehrkernige Zellen enthält. Im umgebenden Gewebe sind die Fibroblasten vermehrt, und es findet sich eine Anhäufung fibrocytärer Elemente. Leukocyten fehlen dort vollständig. Ausgesprochene Gefäßveränderungen, abgesehen von perivasculären Infiltraten, sind nicht anzutreffen. Das elastische Gewebe ist im Innern der Herde untergegangen. Fettfärbungen ergeben keine Anwesenheit lipoider Substanzen.

II. Differentialdiagnose

Die Granulomatosis disciformis nimmt innerhalb der vier erwähnten Affektionen dadurch eine Sonderstellung ein, daß nie nekrobiotische Prozesse beobachtet werden. Nach Miescher ist hauptsächlich die Abgrenzung gegen Tuberkulose wichtig. Dagegen spricht das vollständige Fehlen typischer Tuberkel, auch in den frischen Efflorescenzen, gegen den Morbus Boeck die wenig scharfe Begrenzung der Infiltrate, gegen ein knotiges Tuberkulid vom Typus Bazin oder Darier-Roussy, an welches die Mitbeteiligung der großen Gefäße denken läßt, die Lokalisation vorwiegend in der Cutis sowie die herabgesetzte Tuberkulinempfindlichkeit, gegen tertiäre Lues die negative Wassermann-Reaktion und der Mißerfolg einer Salvarsankur. Immerhin haben mehrere Autoren (Gertler, Ringrose, Heite et al.) auf Grund statistischer und histologischer Studien die Ansicht ausgesprochen, daß die Granulomatosis disciformis nur ein Stadium der Necrobiosis lipoidica sei, das bei Nichtdiabetikern und auch Rauchern auftrete. Auch zum Granuloma anulare bestehen Übergänge (Frenken).

Die drei mit nekrobiotischen Prozessen verlaufenden Affektionen gegeneinander abzugrenzen, ist nun nicht in allen Fällen leicht. Nach Miescher schafft die Necrobiosis maculosa Beziehungen zwischen Necrobiosis lipoidica, dem Granuloma anulare und den Noduli rheumatici, was auf eine einheitliche Pathogenese aller dieser Affektionen hindeutet. Nach Gans und Steigleder ist histologisch die Necrobiosis maculosa nach Aufbau des granulomatösen Randwalles und in bezug auf die Nekrobiose mit dem Granuloma anulare völlig identisch. Es ist deshalb schwer festzustellen, ob ihr eine selbständige Stellung zukommt oder ob sie nur ein Stadium einer der andern Granulomatosen darstellt.

Die Differentialdiagnose zwischen Granuloma anulare und Necrobiosis lipoidica ist deshalb von Wichtigkeit, weil beide Affektionen relativ häufig vorkommen und weil es sich bei beiden Affektionen um klinisch recht gut charakterisierte Krankheitsbilder handelt. Folgende Kriterien sind für die Differentialdiagnose beider Krankheiten aufgestellt worden. Nach ELLIS und KIRBY-SMITH lassen sich typische Fälle von Granuloma anulare und Necrobiosis lipoidica histologisch dadurch unterscheiden, daß beim Granuloma anulare das Infiltrat um die nekrotische Zone herum besser differenziert und schärfer abgegrenzt sei als bei der Necrobiosis lipoidica. Auch die Nekrose sei beim Granuloma anulare schärfer begrenzt. Bei der Necrobiosis lipoidica hingegen sind die kollagenen Fasern weniger fragmentiert und nicht gequollen wie beim Granuloma anulare. Die Zellen des Infiltrats sind beim Granuloma anulare palisadenförmig angeordnet und ausgerichtet, was bei der Necrobiosis lipoidica weniger der Fall ist. Wichtig ist das Alter der Läsion; nur die länger bestehenden Herde der Necrobiosis lipoidica sind histologisch typisch, die jüngeren gleichen einem Granuloma anulare (WORINGER, WORINGER et al.).

Besonderes Interesse verdient nun die Frage der Lipoideinlagerungen; wurde doch von URBACH angenommen, daß dies für die Necrobiosis lipoidica typisch sei. Nun zeigen aber Untersuchungen von älteren Fällen von Granuloma anulare, daß auch bei dieser Affektion Lipoideinlagerungen möglich sind (LAYMON und FISHER), so daß dieses Kriterium kaum für die Differentialdiagnose verwendet werden kann.

Am ehesten können wohl die Gefäßveränderungen verwertet werden. Es wurde längere Zeit angenommen, daß die Störungen der Gefäßdurchgängigkeit die Ursache der Necrobiosis lipoidica seien, indem diese zu der Bionekrose des Gewebes führten, die nachher mit Lipoid imbibiert würde. Zwar können auch beim Granuloma anulare Gefäßveränderungen vorkommen wie bei der Necrobiosis lipoidica, doch nehmen sie nie das gleiche Ausmaß an. Besonderes Gewicht messen BAZEX et al. dabei den Veränderungen der Arteriolen bei. Diese sind bei der Necrobiosis lipoidica wesentlich schwerer als beim Granuloma anulare.

Einen neuen Gesichtspunkt haben nun die Befunde von HARE gebracht, der in neun Fällen von Necrobiosis lipoidica Glykogenablagerungen fand. Dies liegt frei und in Histiocyten phagocytiert in den peripheren Partien der nekrobiotischen Herde und im unmittelbar anschließenden Corium. Das Vorhandensein des Glykogens ist unabhängig von Fettablagerungen. Zwar wurde es auch in zwei Fällen von Granulomatosis disciformis und in zehn von zwölf Fällen von Granuloma anulare gefunden, aber in wesentlich geringerer Quantität als bei der Necrobiosis lipoidica. In anderen Fällen war es nur in Spuren vorhanden, so z.B. in Knoten bei rheumatoider Arthritis. Es wurde weder im Gewebe bei rheumatischem Fieber gefunden, noch in Fällen von Hautveränderungen, die auf Gefäßstörungen beruhten, noch bei Xanthomen oder Fettnekrosen. Die Menge des Glykogens war unabhängig davon, ob es sich um diabetische oder nicht-diabetische Individuen handelte. Obgleich die Bedeutung der Glykogenablagerung bei der Necrobiosis lipoidica bisher nicht völlig abgeklärt ist, so kann doch gesagt werden, daß sie in quantitativer Hinsicht für die Diagnose verwertet werden kann. Es scheint, daß die Necrobiosis maculosa in dieser Beziehung engste Verwandtschaften mit der Necrobiosis lipoidica hat und daß sie möglicherweise nur ein Vorstadium der echten Necrobiosis lipoidica ist.

Die Beziehungen des Granuloma anulare zu nekrobiotischen Knoten bei der rheumatischen Arthritis sind von BOWERS, JAEGER, BOLGERT untersucht worden. Alle Autoren kommen zum Schluß, daß enge histologische Beziehungen zwischen beiden Krankheiten bestehen, doch zeigten sich gewisse Unterschiede, die es gestatten, die beiden Affektionen zu unterscheiden. 1. sind in arthritischen Knoten die degenerierten Herde gewöhnlich breiter als in einem Granuloma anulare. 2. ist in arthritischen Knötchen das degenerierte Material (wahrscheinlich Kollagen) homogener. Das Bindegewebe ist ohne Unterbrechung von Epitheloiden infiltriert, im Gegensatz zum Granuloma anulare, wo eine weniger regelmäßige Anordnung besteht. 3. Gefäßneubildungen sind in rheumatischen Knoten weniger häufig als beim Granuloma anulare. 4. Die Zellreaktion bei den rheumatischen Knoten ist einförmiger: es handelt sich meist um Histiocyten vom endotheloiden Typus, oft mit Fibroblasten, während beim Granuloma anulare gewöhnlich Eosinophile, viele Lymphocyten und gelegentlich Plasmazellen gesehen werden, zusätzlich zu den fibroblastischen Zellen in den umgebenden Granulationswällen.

Auch zu den juxtaartikulären Knoten bestehen Beziehungen (PFLEGER-SCHWARZ, DUPERRAT et al.).

Schließlich ist die Beziehung des Granuloma anulare zu tuberkulösen Granulationsformen immer wieder diskutiert worden. Speziell die Abgrenzung des Granuloma anulare von den papulonekrotischen Tuberkuliden kann schwer sein (PINKUS).

Zusammenfassend läßt sich wohl feststellen, daß sich in verschiedenen Fällen von Granulomatosen mit den heute zur Verfügung stehenden Methoden keine klaren Unterscheidungsmerkmale finden lassen, so daß eine klinische Differenzierung der Fälle nach wie vor unumgänglich ist. Jedenfalls ist es oft nicht möglich, die besprochenen Krankheitsbilder nur auf Grund histologischer Kriterien voneinander trennen zu wollen.

III. Klinik

1. Granuloma anulare

Die Literatur über Einzelbeobachtungen von Granuloma anulare ist recht reichhaltig, wobei neben typischen Fällen auch zahlreiche atypische beschrieben worden sind, die sich in bezug auf Ausdehnung, Zahl der Herde, Sitz der Herde, Dauer der Erkrankung usw. vom typischen Verlauf unterscheiden. Es soll im folgenden bewußt auf Mitteilung dieser Einzelfälle verzichtet werden, da sie meist keinen neuen Beitrag für die Erkenntnis des Krankheitsprozesses des Granuloma anulare liefern. Wichtiger sind die zusammenfassenden Arbeiten über das Granuloma anulare.

So versuchen GLEITZ und HEITE mit Hilfe des sog. häufigkeits-analytischen Verfahrens an Hand von 490 in der Literatur beschriebenen Krankheitsfällen einen Normbegriff des klinischen Bildes des Granuloma anulare herauszufinden. Es ergibt sich, daß die Frauen mit etwa 60% häufiger betroffen sind, in 40% aller Fälle beginnt die Krankheit im ersten Dezennium, aber auch in den höchsten Altersstufen kann das Granuloma anulare auftreten. In 42% der Fälle besteht ein einziger Herd, doch sind bis zu 30 Herde beschrieben worden. Die Lokalisation des Granuloma anulare wird wie folgt angegeben: Hand und Handgelenk ist in 78% betroffen, Arme und Beine 19%, Fuß 14%, Kopf 12%, Stamm 11%. Dabei zeigt sich, daß die Hand bei Kindern weniger häufig befallen ist als bei Erwachsenen. Die Dauer der Erkrankung schwankt zwischen 3 Monaten und 29 Jahren, wobei in 80% der Fälle eine solche von 5 Monaten bis 6 Jahren angegeben wird, was einem Mittelwert von $1^1/_2$ Jahren entspricht. Rezidive treten in 13% der Fälle auf. Sie sind bei Frauen häufiger als bei Männern. Auch MEYER bestätigt die Bevorzugung des frühen Kindesalters durch das Granuloma anulare. Es tritt am häufigsten in den ersten 5 Lebensjahren auf. In England scheint das Granuloma anulare häufiger zu werden (ROOK et al.).

a) Ätiologie

LEINBROCK diskutiert in einer Arbeit die Ätiologie des Granuloma anulare. Er stellt fest, daß zur Zeit zwei unterschiedliche Auffassungen vertreten werden:

1. es sei eine tuberkulöse Affektion und 2. es sei nicht als spezifische Erkrankung zu betrachten, sondern als polyätiologisches Syndrom, bei dem die Tuberkulose, Fokalinfekte, Rheumatismus, Autointoxikationen und andere Ursachen eine Rolle spielen können. Für die tuberkulöse Ätiologie sprechen neben den tuberkuloiden Strukturen, die in einzelnen Herden von Granuloma anulare angetroffen werden können, diejenigen Fälle, bei denen es mit tuberkulösen Veränderungen innerer Organe zusammen auftritt. Beweisender sind natürlich diejenigen Fälle über positiven Tuberkelbacillennachweis aus Herden von Granuloma anulare. Ferner wurde beobachtet, daß Granuloma anulare-ähnliche Erscheinungen an Stellen positiver Tuberkulinreaktionen auftreten konnten. Sehr interessant, aber schwer zu beurteilen, sind diejenigen Fälle, bei denen ein Granuloma anulare nach Vigantolgaben (JORDAN und WULF, DEPAOLI) und Rimifon (TAPPEINER) sich generalisierte. Auch wird der Übergang eines generalisierten Granuloma anulare während einer Vitamin D-Therapie in ein papulonekrotisches Tuberkulid beschrieben. Gegen eine tuberkulöse Ätiologie spricht der meist negative Ausfall der Tuberkulinreaktionen bei Kindern mit Granuloma anulare sowie wohl am ehesten die Tatsache, daß das Granuloma anulare nach Probeexcisionen spontan abheilen kann, was bei einer Hauttuberkulose und einem Tuberkulid wohl nie beobachtet wird. Als Resultat dieser Untersuchungen kann festgestellt werden, daß der Beweis der tuberkulösen Herkunft des Granuloma anulare mit den derzeit zu fordernden Mitteln (Bacillennachweis, Tierversuch) bis heute in überzeugender Weise nicht erbracht ist (BOLDT).

BRAUN diskutiert an Hand eines Falles von Granuloma anulare, der insofern atypisch war, als sich neben typischen ringförmigen Herden auch tuberöse Efflorescenzen von histologisch tuberkuloidem Bau zeigten, die Ätiologie des Granuloma anulare. Er hält es für wahrscheinlich, daß das Granuloma anulare in den Formenkreis der Hauttuberkulose bei gesteigerter Allergie zugeordnet werden müsse.

Daß Beziehungen auch zum Rheumatismus bestehen können, zeigt die Beobachtung von ROLLIERS et al. Familiäres Auftreten wird auch beobachtet (SPITZER).

Die Beziehungen des Granuloma anulare zu internen Störungen interessieren hauptsächlich im Hinblick auf die nahe histologische Verwandtschaft des Granuloma anulare mit der Necrobiosis lipoidica, und da auch Fälle, bei denen beide Dermatosen nebeneinander auftraten, beschrieben sind (RÉLIAS et al., FRAIN-BELL, TRUFFI). BOLDT hat deshalb der Beziehung des Granuloma anulare zu Diabetes eine Studie gewidmet und festgestellt, daß verschiedene Fälle von sog. Granuloma anulare, die in der Literatur als mit Diabetes kombiniert beschrieben worden sind, in das Krankheitsbild der Necrobiosis lipoidica hineingehören. Immerhin konnte der Autor in der Literatur 20 Beobachtungen von sicherem Granuloma anulare bei Diabetes ausfindig machen. Dabei sollen sich verschiedene, als atypisches Granuloma anulare bezeichnete Fälle in dieser Gruppe befinden (BOLGERT et al.), doch kann diese Stoffwechselstörung nicht mit größerer Regelmäßigkeit beim Granuloma anulare angetroffen werden. Interessant ist die Beobachtung von OLIVIER et al., wonach sich bei einem tuberkulösen Diabetiker unter der Behandlung mit Tuberculostatica aus einem Lupus vulgaris zuerst ein Granuloma anulare und dann eine Necrobiosis lipoidica entwickelte.

Die Theorie, daß das Granuloma anulare eine hyperergische Reaktion auf verschiedene Ursachen sei, wird hauptsächlich von der französischen Schule vertreten. BOLGERT kommt auf Grund histologischer Studien und des Vergleiches dieser Veränderungen bei Granuloma anulare und subcutanen rheumatischen Knoten zum Schluß, daß es sich beim Granuloma anulare um eine hyperergische Reaktion auf verschiedene infektiöse Agentien handelt: Syphilis, Lepra, Tuberkulose, aber auch auf verschiedene banale Infekte. Die fibrinoide Nekrose sei dabei das fundamentale Geschehen, die entzündlichen Reaktionen seien sekundär. Gougerot geht in einer sehr genauen Studie auf die Schwierigkeiten ein, die sich oft daraus ergeben, daß das klinische Bild nicht mit dem histologischen übereinstimme und daß es eine ganze Reihe atypischer Formen von Granuloma anulare gebe. Er hält das Granuloma anulare für ein Syndrom einheitlicher allergischer Genese auf verschiedene Ursachen. Dies dürfte auch die Meinung von Grupper et al. sein, die das Granuloma anulare zu den Kollagenosen rechnen, d.h. zu allergischen Reaktionen, die eine Veränderung des kollagenen Bindegewebes zur Folge haben.

Schließlich weist Leinbrock an Hand eines selbst beobachteten Falles darauf hin, daß möglicherweise nervöse Einflüsse für die Lokalisation der Herde des Granuloma anulare verantwortlich seien und Othaz et al. diskutieren die Möglichkeit einer infektiösen Genese durch ein filtrierbares Virus.

b) Differentialdiagnose

Es ist nach den vorausgegangenen Ausführungen klar, daß die Unterscheidung des Granuloma anulare von der Necrobiosis lipoidica in verschiedenen Fällen nicht leicht ist, speziell wenn die Herde atypisch aussehen, flächenhaft angeordnet sind und die granulomatösen Einzelherde vermissen lassen oder wo sie tief subcutan gelegen sind. Degos et al. (1949) beschreiben auch eine Diabetikerin, bei der klinisch ein Granuloma anulare neben einem Herd einer Necrobiosis lipoidica vorlag. Daß auch das histologische Bild in solchen Fällen im Stiche lassen kann, wurde ebenfalls ausgeführt.

Es darf also festgestellt werden, daß verschiedene Fälle von Granuloma anulare bisher weder auf Grund klinischer noch histologischer Kriterien eindeutig klassiert werden können und daß oft nur die Kombination von klinischem und histologischem Bild zur Diagnose führen kann (Woringer 1950).

Schwierig ist auch die Frage zu beurteilen, ob das als Erythema elevatum et diutinum beschriebene Krankheitsbild eine Krankheit sui generis darstellt oder nur ein abgewandeltes Granuloma anulare. Nach Baccaredda und Jacobi handelt es sich um die gleiche Affektion und die Bezeichnung Erythema elevatum et diutinum sollte vollkommen fallen gelassen werden, während Combes und Bluefarb beide Krankheitsbilder auf Grund histologischer und klinischer Unterschiede trennen wollen.

c) Therapie

Die Tatsache, daß Granuloma anulare-Herde oft nach einer nicht totalen Probeexcision oder nach Vereisung mit CO_2-Schnee (Kuske et al.) oder mit Chloräthyl (Földvári) abzuheilen pflegen, ist allgemein bekannt. Hämel hält diese Tatsache für einen möglichen Hinweis darauf, daß nervöse Einflüsse im Sinne der Dystrophielehre Speranskis für dieses Verschwinden verantwortlich gemacht werden könnten. Cochrane empfiehlt Vitamin E zur Behandlung von Granuloma anulare und sah in 9 von 13 Fällen ein rasches Verschwinden der Herde nach Gaben von Vitamin E in täglichen Dosen von 150—600 mg. Meist waren die Herde in 5—9 Wochen verschwunden. May und Couperus behandelten sieben Fälle von disseminiertem Granuloma anulare mit Plaques-Bildung an den Beinen auf Grund der Theorie, daß auch Streptokokken die granulomatösen Bildungen verursachen könnten, mit Penicillin und erreichten in kurzer Zeit ein völliges Verschwinden der Hauterscheinungen. Senigagliesi et al. injizierten in fünf Fällen Streptomycin in die Herde und erzielten stets völlige Heilung. Tolbach sah bei einem Tuberkulösen rasche Heilung des Granuloma anulare mit Rimifon,

Beltram bei einem luischen Tuberkulösen mit INH, Magnin et al. bei einem Patienten mit Darmparasiten und sehr vielen Granulomen mit Emetin. Auch Cortison ist wirksam (Daubresse).

2. Die Necrobiosis lipoidica

Dieses 1932 von Urbach und vorher von Oppenheim beschriebene Krankheitsbild wurde zunächst nur bei Diabetikern angetroffen und als für Diabetes typische Lipoidose angesehen. In der Folge mehrten sich die Mitteilungen über typische Fälle von Necrobiosis lipoidica ohne Diabetes (Degos et al. 1948). Neben Einzelbeobachtungen sind es hauptsächlich die zusammenfassenden Arbeiten von Boldt und Knoth und Füller, die sich mit diesem Krankheitsbild besonders eingehend befaßten. Die letzteren Autoren berichten über 113 auswertbare Fälle aus der Literatur, die sie bezüglich Alters- und Geschlechtsverteilung, Diabetes, Kreislaufverhältnisse, Lokalisation der Hauterscheinungen usw. untersuchten. Sie kommen zu folgenden Ergebnissen:

Die Altersverteilung reicht vom 10. bis zum 73. Lebensjahr, wobei die Krankheit am häufigsten zwischen 30 und 65 Jahren auftritt. Das weibliche Geschlecht überwiegt mit 75% deutlich. Der Blutdruck ist bei mehr als der Hälfte der Patienten abnorm, d.h. entweder erhöht oder besonders labil. Die Dermatose ist in den meisten Fällen an den unteren Extremitäten lokalisiert, doch sind in einem Zehntel der Fälle auch der Stamm und in einem Fünftel der Fälle auch die obere Extremität befallen. Miescher und Storck beschreiben eine disseminierte kleinfleckige Form der Necrobiosis lipoidica mit Infiltraten am Stamm und an den Extremitäten. Das Bild der Einzelefflorescenz hat seit der Beschreibung durch Urbach keine Änderung erfahren. Es handelt sich um lividrote, ziemlich scharf begrenzte Herde, die bei der Diaphanoskopie einen dunkelgelben Farbton ergeben. Die Affektion beginnt mit einer intensiv roten, derben, linsengroßen, peripher wachsenden Papel, die über das Niveau der Haut erhaben ist. Bei längerem Bestand sinkt das Zentrum ein, nimmt eine Sklerodermie-artige Konsistenz an und wird schwefelgelb. An der Peripherie etabliert sich ein 2—3 mm breiter, violett-roter Ring. Die gelbe Farbe des Herdes ist nicht gleichmäßig, sondern etwas durch dunklere Fleckchen unterbrochen und von zahlreichen Telangiektasien durchzogen. Die Herde können konfluieren und dadurch zu einer unregelmäßigen Konturierung führen. Gleichzeitig wird das Zentrum atrophisch, blaß und eingesunken. Auch eine kolliquierende Form wurde beschrieben (Corti et al.). In einem Fall bestand beim gleichen Patienten ein Sarkoid der Kopfhaut (Williams).

a) Ätiologie und Pathogenese

Während Urbach die Necrobiosis lipoidica als direkte und obligate diabetische Stoffwechseldermatose bezeichnete, wurde sehr rasch die unbedingte Verquickung von Diabetes und Necrobiosis lipoidica als unzutreffend erkannt. Boldt hat sich in einer ausgedehnten Studie näher mit der Frage des Zusammenhanges zwischen Diabetes und Necrobiosis lipoidica befaßt. Er stellt fest, daß in einem Krankengut von 51 sicheren Fällen von Necrobiosis lipoidica in sieben Fällen, d.h. in 15%, ein Diabetes fehlte. Ellis und Kirby-Smith sahen in ihrem Material sogar 40%, Chernosky 60% der Fälle ohne Diabetes verlaufen. Rollins et al. sahen $^1/_3$ Nichtdiabetiker, beinahe alles Frauen. McKenzie fand nur bei 17% seiner Fälle Diabetes, Gertler et al. dagegen in 109 von 137 Fällen, während unter 1000 Diabetikern nur einer eine Necrobiosis zeigte, doch kommt sie auch bei Bronzediabetes vor (Hewitt et al.). Wahrscheinlich liegt aber der Prozentsatz in Wirklichkeit noch höher, da vielfach angenommen wird, daß zur Diagnose der Necrobiosis lipoidica Diabetes gehört und die entsprechenden Fälle ohne Diabetes deshalb unter anderer Diagnose beschrieben werden. Ist die Necrobiosis lipoidica mit Diabetes kombiniert, so findet sich diese Kombination vorwiegend bei mittelschweren und schweren Fällen von Diabetes. Ferner disponiert der schwere konstitutionelle Diabetes der jugendlichen und mittleren Lebensjahre stärker zur Necrobiosis lipoidica als der leichtere arteriosklerotische Altersdiabetes. In einem Fall trat nach Kopftrauma ein Hypercorticismus mit erhöhtem Blutzucker und Necrobiosis lipoidica auf (ROTHMAN et al.). Die Gesamtfettsäuren und Gesamtlipoide sind in etwa 50% der Fälle erhöht, allerdings nur in engen Grenzen. Die Mehrzahl der Cholesterinwerte liegt im Bereich normaler Werte. Es läßt sich also feststellen, daß bei der Necrobiosis lipoidica keine konstanten Stoffwechselstörungen angetroffen werden. Diese Schlußfolgerungen finden sich praktisch auch in sämtlichen Einzelbeobachtungen über Necrobiosis lipoidica mit oder ohne Diabetes, so daß in der Pathogenese Stoffwechselstörungen allein keine Rolle spielen können.

In dieser Beziehung kommt den Gefäßveränderungen eine besondere Bedeutung zu. Schon die klinische Untersuchung zeigt, daß es sich bei Patienten mit Necrobiosis lipoidica um vegetativ stigmatisierte Individuen mit Neigung zu Vasolabilität handelt, und auch die histologischen Untersuchungen zeigen, daß bei der Necrobiosis lipoidica Gefäßveränderungen obligat vorhanden sind. Sie lassen sich auch im Röntgenbild nachweisen (BONSE). So hält LEVER die Necrobiosis des Kollagens für eine Folge der Gefäßveränderungen. Dies ist auch die Meinung der meisten Forscher, die sich mit dieser Frage befaßt haben. Umstritten ist nur, wie die Lipoidablagerung in der Necrobiosis lipoidica zu bewerten, d.h. ob sie primärer oder sekundärer Natur sei. Während URBACH die Lipoidablagerungen für das sekundäre Phänomen hält, glauben LAYMON und FISHER, es sei unmöglich zu entscheiden, welches das primäre und welches das sekundäre Geschehen sei. Sie halten die Ansicht von GOTTRON und von BOLDT, daß die Zirkulationsstörung in der Cutis die primäre Störung sei, für zu einseitig. Auch SENDRAIL et al. halten die Möglichkeit einer lokalen Stoffwechselstörung für wahrscheinlicher als eine primäre Gefäßkrankheit. Tatsache ist jedenfalls, daß Lipoidablagerung unabhängig vom Lipoidspiegel im Blut auch bei andern nekrobiotischen Prozessen wie Gummen, Hautgangrän usw. gefunden werden kann. Jedenfalls ist die Necrobiosis lipoidica keine Lipoidose (GANS). Nach ENGEL et al. muß daran gedacht werden, daß außer den Lipoiden andere Blutfaktoren für die Entstehung der Nekrobiosis verantwortlich sind. Sie fanden eine erhöhte Serumviscosität, Erhöhung der α-Globuline und der proteingebundenen Hexose. Auch PEZZAROSSA sah im Serum von Patienten mit Necrobiosis lipoidica eine verminderte Emulgierfähigkeit für Cholesterin.

Eine von den bisherigen Fällen abweichende Beobachtung von SCHEFFLER und HAGEN könnte darauf hinweisen, daß auch allergische Prozesse beim Entstehen der Necrobiosis lipoidica mitspielen, indem als Reaktion auf antigenes Insulin histologisch typische Herde von Necrobiosis lipoidica auftraten, die nach Wechsel des Präparates wieder verschwanden.

APLAS stellt die Theorie auf, daß die Necrobiosis lipoidica nur ein Teilsymptom eines durch eine gemeinsame Ursache ausgelösten generalisierten Krankheitsprozesses sei.

b) Therapie

Die verschiedenen therapeutischen Maßnahmen werden von KNOTH und FÜLLER diskutiert. Insulintherapie dürfte naturgemäß nur bei den diabetischen Fällen eine Berechtigung haben. Ihr Wert ist aber sehr umstritten (THIERS und

Colomb), speziell auch die lokale Applikation von Insulin mit Injektionen (Rasmussen) oder mittels Umschlag. Ist der Diabetes aber mit Insulin eingestellt, so können die Herde ohne Rezidiv chirurgisch entfernt werden (Nylén et al., Dougherty). Lokale Cortisonbehandlung wird von Dejenariu et al., Chernosky, Smith, Marten et al., Feldman, Newman als wirksam bezeichnet, von Cordero et al. speziell in Verbindung mit Hyaluronidase. Gertler sah einen partiellen Erfolg durch Unterspritzung der Herde mit $^1/_4$% Novocain. Eine eindeutige Besserung mit Chloräthylvereisung sahen Rasiewicz et al., mit dem Zirkulationshormon Padutin Clevinghaus. Eine Verbesserung der Zirkulation dürfte nach dem Vorhergesagten überhaupt das Wesentliche sein, und die Fälle von spontanem Zurückgehen von Necrobiosis lipoidica, die z.B. bei Auftreten eines Ekzems in der Region der Herde beobachtet werden, dürften wohl auf die Verbesserung der Zirkulation zurückzuführen sein.

3. Granulomatosis disciformis chronica et progressiva

Miescher und Leder beschrieben 1948 eine Patientin, die wahrscheinlich aus Psoriasisefflorescenzen heraus eigenartige, große, scheibenförmige Herde an den Unterschenkeln entwickelte, die bei der histologischen Untersuchung als eine Granulomatose der Cutis von ganz ungewöhnlichem Aspekt erschien. Klinisch waren die Herde gekennzeichnet durch düster-braunrote Farbe, durch scharfe, mehr oder weniger polycyclische Konturen und durch einen ausgesprochen gelblich-lupoiden Farbton unter Glasdruck. Die Oberfläche zeigte eine unbedeutende Schuppung, und durch die verdünnte Epidermis schimmerten stellenweise die Gefäße durch (Abb. 1).

In einem zweiten Fall zeigte eine Patientin am Unterschenkel über der Tibiakante linsengroße rote Flecken, die sich zentrifugal in der Art von Öltropfen ausdehnten und konfluierten. Die Herde zeigten große, stellenweise polycyclische, unregelmäßig begrenzte Plaques mit scharfen Konturen von düsterroter Farbe, untermischt mit gelblichen Farbtönen. Zwischen Peripherie und Zentrum bestanden deutliche Unterschiede. Der periphere Teil der Herde stellte einen flach-tuberösen, breiten Randstreifen dar, der nach außen von einem 2—3 mm breiten roten Saum umgeben war. Ähnliche Herde fanden sich an der Stirn-Haargrenze. In der Folge wurden dann noch von Walter, Wells und Goldsmith, Santler, Pinetti, Tappeiner, Machacek, Cairns, Fleck, Kogoj et al., Arzt, Šabatová, Ullmo et al., Woringer et al., Götz weitere Fälle beschrieben. Nach diesen Berichten sitzen die Herde meist an den Unterschenkeln, doch sind auch solche an der Stirn, den Handrücken, den Vorderarmen beschrieben worden. Traumen scheinen ein wichtiger Faktor für die Entstehung und Lokalisation der Herde zu sein. Interne Befunde, die mit einiger Regelmäßigkeit bei der Granulomatosis disciformis beobachtet werden könnten, sind bisher nicht bekannt geworden.

a) Ätiologie und Pathogenese

Nach Miescher ist die Natur der Affektion ungeklärt. Das Granulom erinnert an Bilder der Tuberkulose, der tertiären Lues und des Morbus Besnier-Boeck, ohne aber mit ihnen identisch zu sein. Pinetti hält die Affektion für tuberkulös bedingt. Auch Knoth, Curth, Degos et al. diskutieren eher im Sinne einer Zusammengehörigkeit von Tuberkulose und Granulomatosis disciformis. Keining et al. glauben an eine sehr nahe Verwandtschaft zwischen Granulomatosis disciformis und Morbus Boeck, da sie beim gleichen Patienten typische Herde von Morbus Boeck und solche einer Granulomatosis disciformis sahen. Die Tuberkulinreaktion war negativ. Neotebenbehandlung hatte einen gewissen Erfolg. Auch

KOGOJ et al. halten die Granulomatosis disciformis auf Grund des histologischen Bildes und des Verhaltens gegenüber Tuberkulin für ein dem Boeckschen Sarkoid nahe verwandtes Geschehen, betonen aber als großen Unterschied dazu, daß bisher bei der Granulomatosis disciformis noch nie interne Veränderungen, die für Morbus

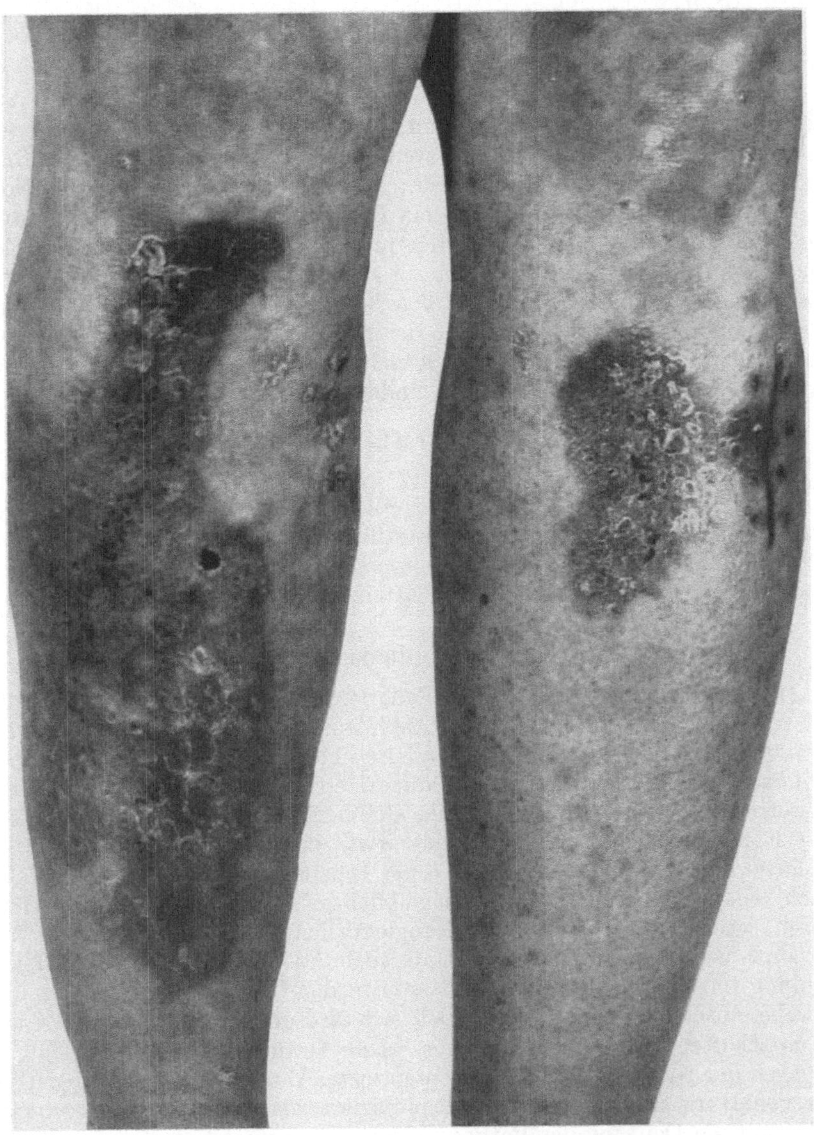

Abb. 1

Boeck charakteristisch wären, beobachtet worden sind. Sie schlagen vor, die Bezeichnung Granulomatosis disciformis durch „sarkoides" zu ergänzen. WORINGER hält auf Grund einer umfassenden Betrachtung die Granulomatosis disciformis für ein Vorstadium der Necrobiosis lipoidica, da die Nekrobiose sekundär durch Gefäßveränderungen zustande kommt, und solche Gefäßveränderungen bei der Granulomatosis disciformis bereits vorhanden seien. GÖTZ hält ebenfalls die Angiopathie für das beide Krankheitsbilder verbindende ursächliche Geschehen. Er macht darauf aufmerksam, daß bisher kein sicherer Fall von Diabetes bei Granulomatosis disciformis angetroffen worden ist. Auch SANTLER hält die Granulomatosis disciformis für eine Gefäßerkrankung. Den Übergang eines von KROEPFLI als Granulomatosis disciformis demonstrierten Falles in eine tödliche Kollagenkrankheit beschreibt ZISWILER.

b) Differentialdiagnose

Die beschriebenen Herde der Granulomatosis disciformis sehen denen der Necrobiosis lipoidica sehr ähnlich, und die Differentialdiagnose kann nur auf Grund des histologischen Bildes gestellt werden. Bei der Granulomatosis disciformis fehlen Nekrobiosen vollständig, während sie bei der Necrobiosis lipoidica vorhanden sind. Klinisch ähnlich sah ein Fall von Mycosis fungoides (BORDA et al.) aus, doch konnte auch hier die Differentialdiagnose auf Grund des histologischen Bildes einwandfrei gestellt werden. ARZT diskutiert ebenfalls die Differentialdiagnose granulomatöser Prozesse und betont die Schwierigkeit der Abgrenzung der Granulomatosis disciformis von der Necrobiosis lipoidica und von atypischen Tuberkulosegranulomen. Es wird in vielen Fällen wohl nur auf Grund des histologischen und klinischen Bildes ein eindeutiger Entscheid gefällt werden können.

c) Therapie

FLECK sah im Gegensatz zu PINETTI keinen Erfolg weder von Tuberculostatica noch von ACTH, hingegen konnte er mit CO_2-Schnee und Phenolätzungen einen befriedigenden Erfolg erzielen. WORINGER sah eine schnelle Heilung eines Falles mit Natriumsalicylat bei Gelenkrheumatismus. GOETZ et al. empfehlen Antimalariamittel. TEODORESCU et al. hatten einen Versager mit INH.

4. Necrobiosis maculosa

1949 beschrieb MIESCHER einen Fall, der klinisch mit der Necrobiosis lipoidica den klinischen Aspekt gemeinsam hat, histologisch dagegen an die Vorgänge bei Granuloma anulare erinnert. Es handelte sich um eine 70jährige Frau, die an den Unterschenkeln und an der Brust einige Herde aufwies, die scharf begrenzt, von düsterroter Farbe mit einem Stich ins Gelblich-Braune sind. Der Rand der Herde war leicht prominent, das Zentrum etwas eingesunken, die Oberfläche glatt. Kleinere Herde fanden sich auch an der Innenseite des Kniegelenkes. Sie waren flach erhaben, ziemlich derb, von gelblich-roter Farbe und glatter Oberfläche, durch welche bereits einige Teleangiektasien durchschimmerten. Wie oben erwähnt, zeigte die histologische Untersuchung eine ausgebreitete Affektion mit Bildung torpider nekrobiotischer Herde in der Cutis, welche von Granulationsgewebe umschlossen sind. Es handelt sich also um einen Prozeß, der engste Verwandtschaften mit den Vorgängen beim Granuloma anulare zeigt, klinisch dagegen der Necrobiosis lipoidica entspricht. Ähnliche Beobachtungen sind seither von HARE u. TAPPEINER et al. publiziert worden. MIESCHER geht zunächst nicht auf die Deutung der Pathogenese ein, er erwähnt einzig, daß Beziehungen bestehen zwischen der Necrobiosis maculosa, dem Granuloma anulare, der Necrobiosis lipoidica und den Noduli rheumatici, was möglicherweise auf eine einheitliche Pathogenese aller dieser Affektionen hindeutet.

Literatur

APLAS, V.: Über das Wesen der sog. Necrobiosis lipoidica diabeticorum. Z. Haut- u. Geschl.-Kr. 28, 84 (1960). — ARZT, L.: Zur Differentialdiagnose granulomatöser Prozesse (Granulomatosis disciformis chronica et progressiva, Necrobiosis lipoidica diabeticorum, atypisches Tuberkulosegranulom). Hautarzt **3**, 488 (1952). — Granulomatosis disciformis chronica et progressiva Miescher? Granuloma anulare? (Demonstration.) Zbl. Haut- u. Geschl.-Kr. **88**, 358 (1954).

BACCAREDDA, A.: Granuloma anulare atipico (Erythema elevatum et diutinum). Minerva derm. **30**, 1 (1955). — BAZEX, A., A. DUPRÉ, M. PARANT et CHRISTOL: Etude critique sur le diagnostic différential anatomo-pathologique entre le granuloma anulaire et la nécrobiose lipoidique. Bull. Soc. franç. Derm. Syph. **67**, 598 (1960). — BELTRANI, G.: Considerazioni sopra un caso anomale di granuloma anulare. Dermatologia (Napoli) **11**, 70 (1960). — BOLDT, A.: Zur Kenntnis der Necrobiosis lipoidica („diabeticorum"). Arch. Derm. Syph. (Berl.) **179**, 74 (1939). — Beitrag zur Klinik und Ätiologie des Granuloma anulare. Arch. Derm. Syph. (Berl.) **179**, 603 (1939). — BOLGERT, M.: A propos de la pathogénie du Granulome annulaire. Ann. Derm. Syph. (Paris) **4**, 136 (1944). — BOLGERT, M., et L. LAFOURCADE: Granulomes annulaires multiples chez un diabétique ignoré. Bull. Soc. franç. Derm. Syph. **1949**, 280. — BONSE, G.: Weichstrahl-Röntgenbefunde bei Necrobiosis lipoidica („diabeticorum"). Arch. Derm. Syph. (Berl.) **192**, 509 (1951). — BORDA, J. M., y J. ABULAFIA: Micosis fungoide con carácter de granulomatosis disciforme crónica de Miescher. Arch. argent. Derm. **4**, 173 (1954). — BOWERS, R. E.: The histology of Granuloma anulare compared with that of the necrobiotic nodules of rheumatoid arthritis. Brit. J. Derm. **61**, 247 (1949). — BRAUN, O.: Über einen atypischen Fall von Granuloma anulare. Arch. Derm. Syph. (Berl.) **190**, 438 (1950).

CAIRNS, R. J.: Miescher's granulomatosis with mediastinal gland enlargement. Proc. roy. Soc. Med. **48**, 173 (1955). — CHERNOSKY, M. E.: Current concepts of necrobiosis lipoidica. Sth med. J. (Bgham, Ala.) **54**, 25 (1961). — CLEVINGHAUS, A.: Ein Fall von Necrobiosis lipoidica. Med. Welt **1941 II**, 825. — COCHRANE, T.: Granuloma anulare: treatment with Vitamine E. Brit. J. Derm. **62**, 316 (1950). — COMBES, F. C., and S. M. BLUEFARB: Erythema elevatum diutinum. Arch. Derm. Syph. (Chic.) **42**, 441 (1940). — CORDERO, A. A., y R. N. CORTI: Necrobiosis lipoidica. Pren. méd. argent. **1957**, 787. — CORTI, R. N., y A. A. CORDERO: Necrobiosis lipoidica diabetica (Forme abscedada). Rev. argent. Dermatosif. **39**, 208 (1955). — CURTH, W.: Granulomatosis disciformis (Miescher). Arch. Derm. **74**, 685 (1956).

DAUBRESSE, E., et J. L. DAUBRESSE: Granulome anulaire extensive. Arch. belges Derm. **13**, 103 (1957). — DEGOS, R. R., J. DELORT, E. HOUSSET et P. DEVEMY: Dermatite lipoidique des diabétiques d'Oppenheim-Urbach, à type de granulome anulaire. Bull. Soc. franç. Derm. Syph. **56**, 48 (1949). — DEGOS, R., O. DELZANT et J. CIVATTE: Tuberculose cutanée pauci-bacillaire faisant discuter une granulomatose disciforme de Miescher. Bull. Soc. franç. Derm. Syph. **67**, 427 (1960). — DEGOS, R., et E. LORTAT-JACOB: Dermatitis atrophicans lipoides diabetica. (Necrobiosis lipoidica diabeticorum Urbach.) Bull. Soc. franç. Derm. Syph. **1948**, 215. — DEJENARIU, I., A. SZENTMIKLOSYA u. T. DAVID: Über einen Fall von diabetischer lipoidischer Nekrobiose (Oppenheim-Urbach). Derm.-Vener. (Buc.) **3**, 171 (1958). — DEPAOLI, A.: Un caso non commune di granuloma anulare. Minerva derm. **26**, 107 (1951). — DOUGHERTY, J. W.: Necrobiosis lipoidica diabeticorum treated by skin grafting. Arch. Derm. **76**, 803 (1957). — DUPERRAT, B., et G. E. GOETSCHEL: Nodules juxta-articulaires du granulome anulaire. Bull. Soc. franç. Derm. Syph. **64**, 158 (1957).

ELLIS, F. A., and H. KIRBY-SMITH: Necrobiosis lipoidica and Granuloma anulare. Arch. Derm. Syph. (Chic.) **45**, 40 (1942). — ENGEL, M. F., and W. J. HAMMACK: Necrobiosis lipoidica diabeticorum. A biochemical, histochemical and electrophoretic study. Arch. Derm. **78**, 73 (1958).

FELDMAN, F. F.: Diskussionsbemerkung zu H. PRICE, Necrobiosis lipoidica diabeticorum. Arch. Derm. Syph. (Chic.) **67**, 638 (1953). — FLECK, F.: Zum Problem der Granulomatosis disciformis chronica et progressiva. Derm. Wschr. **127**, 541 (1953). — FÖLDVÁRI, F.: Granuloma anulare. Ungarische Dermat. Ges. Sitzg vom 12. 10. 1934. Ref. in Zbl. Haut- u. Geschl.-Kr. **50**, 358 (1935). — FRAIN-BELL, W.: Necrobiosis lipoidica diabeticorum and Granuloma anulare. Proc. roy. Soc. Med. **50**, 1020 (1957). — FRENKEN, J. H.: Granuloma anular y Granuloma de Miescher. Son aspectos diferentes del mismo padecimiento? Comentarios a propósito de dos casos. Dermatologia (Méx.) **3**, 301 (1959).

GANS, O., u. G. K. STEIGLEDER: Histologie der Hautkrankheiten, Bd. I, S. 163, 592. Berlin-Göttingen-Heidelberg: Springer 1955. — GERTLER, W.: Necrobiosis lipoidica bei Hyperlipämie. Derm. Wschr. **137**, 522 (1958). — Die nosologische Stellung der Granulomatosis (tuberculoides) pseudosclerodermiformis symmetrica chronica (Gottron). [Granulomatosis disciformis chronica et progressiva (Miescher).] Derm. Wschr. **141**, 241 (1960). — GERTLER u. SCHIECK: Zur Häufigkeit der Necrobiosis lipoidica bei Diabetikern. Derm. Wschr. **141**, 456 (1960). — GLEITZ, T., u. H.-J. HEITE: Das Krankheitsbild des Granuloma annulare in häufigkeitsanalytischer Betrachtungsweise. Arch. Derm. Syph. (Berl.) **199**, 92 (1954). — GÖTZ, H.: Zur Frage der Beziehungen zwischen der Granulomatosis disciformis chronica et progressiva (Miescher) und der Necrobiosis lipoidica diabeticorum. Hautarzt **7**, 156 (1956). — GÖTZ, H., u. M. GARRETTS: Klinische und experimentelle Beobachtungen zur

Frage der Wirkung von Antimalariamitteln bei Hautkrankheiten (Granulomatosis disciformis chronica et progressiva). Hautarzt **11**, 155 (1960). — GOLDSMITH, W. N.: Granulomatosis disciformis chronica et progressiva (Miescher). Proc. 10th Internat. Congr. of Dermatol. London 1952, S. 459 (1953). — GOTTRON, A.: Zur Kenntnis und Pathogenese der Dermatitis atrophicans lipoides diabetica. Med. Klin. **34**, 145 (1938). — GOUGEROT, A.: Révision de la nosologie du granulome annulaire. Bull. Soc. franç. Derm. Syph. **1949**, 153. — GRUPPER, CH., et G. PLAS: Granulome annulaire et maladies du collagène. Bull. Soc. franç. Derm. Syph. **1950**, 178.

HÄMEL, J.: Zur Behandlung der Verrucae, des Molluscum contagiosum und des Granuloma anulare. Derm. Wschr. **120**, 678 (1949). — HARE, P. J.: Necrobiosis lipoidica. Brit. J. Derm. **67**, 365 (1955). — HEITE, H. J., u. H. X. SCHARWENKA: Erythema elevatum diutinum, Granuloma anulare, Necrobiosis lipoidica und Granulomatosis disciformis Gottron-Miescher. Eine vergleichende häufigkeitsanalytische Studie. Arch. klin. exp. Derm. **208**, 260 (1959). — HEWITT, J., P. DESVIGNES et C. SCHOTT: Nécrobiose lipoidique au cours d'un diabète bronzé. Bull. Soc. franç. Derm. Syph. **65**, 282 (1958).

JACOBI, F.: Granuloma anulare. In: Handbuch v. JADASSOHN. Berlin: Springer 1931. — JAEGER, H.: Granulome annulaire (Lésions histologiques identiques à celles des nodules souscutanés rhumatismaux). Dermatologica (Basel) **92**, 325 (1946). — JORDAN, P., u. K. WULF: Vitamin-D-Tuberkulid (papulo-nekrotisches Tuberkulid, Granuloma anulare) bei Lupuspatientin. Verh. der wissenschaftl. Dermat.-Tagg in Hamburg. Sitzg vom 26. 9. 1948. Demonstrationen. Arch. Derm. Syph. (Berl.) **189**, 440 (1949).

KEINING, E., u. O. BRAUN-FALCO: Zur Ätiologie der Granulomatosis disciformis chronica et progressiva (Miescher). Derm. Wschr. **131**, 1 (1955). — KNOTH, W.: Die Begutachtung eines Granulomatosis disciformis chronica et progressiva-Kranken mit abgeheilter Tuberculosis cutis fistulosa. Berufsdermatosen **7**, 136 (1959). — KNOTH, W., u. H. FÜLLER: Zur Patho- und Histogenese der Necrobiosis lipoidica „diabeticorum". Arch. Derm. Syph. (Berl.) **199**, 109 (1954). — KOGOJ, F., u. S. PURETIĆ: Zur Frage der Granulomatosis disciformis chronica et progressiva Miescher. Hautarzt **4**, 305 (1953). — KROEPFLI, P.: Granulomatosis disciformis chronica et progressiva. Dermatologica (Basel) **112**, 499 (1956). — KUSKE, H., u. W. SOLTERMANN: Granuloma anulare, erfolgreiche Behandlung mit CO_2-Schnee. Dermatologica (Basel) **115**, 732 (1957).

LAYMON, C. W., and J. FISHER: Necrobiosis lipoidica (diabeticorum). Arch. Derm. Syph. (Chic.) **59**, 150 (1949). — LEINBROCK, A.: Granuloma anulare giganteum. Hautarzt **6**, 447 (1955). — LEVER, W. F.: Histopathology of the Skin. London: J. B. Lippincott Company 1949.

MACHACEK, G. F.: Granulomatosis disciformis chronica et progressiva. Arch. Derm. **72**, 485 (1955). — MAGNIN, P. H., y A. A. CORDERO: Granuloma anulare diseminado y Parasitosis intestinal. Rev. argent. Dermatosif. **41**, 54 (1957). — MARTEN, R. H., u. M. DULAKE: Hydrocortison in necrobiosis lipoidica diabeticorum. Brit. J. Derm. **69**, 395 (1957). — MAY, S. B., and M. COUPERUS: An unusual case of disseminated Granuloma anulare with plaque formation on the legs. Arch. Derm. **74**, 324 (1956). — MCKENZIE, A. W.: Carbohydrate studies in necrobiosis lipoidica. Brit. J. Derm. **74**, 191 (1962). — MEYER, K.: Granuloma anulare. Arch. Kinderheilk. **145**, 161 (1952). — MEZZADRA, G.: Sull'etiopatogenesi del granuloma anulare. Contributo clinico istologico. Arch. ital. Derm. 18, 201 (1942). — MIESCHER, G.: Necrobiosis maculosa. Dermatologica (Basel) **98**, 199 (1949). — MIESCHER, G., u. M. LEDER: Granulomatosis disciformis chronica et progressiva. Schweiz. med. Wschr. **1948**, 1182. — Granulomatosis disciformis chronica et progressiva (atypische Tuberkulose). Dermatologica (Basel) **97**, 25 (1948). — MIESCHER, G., u. H. STORCK: Disseminierte kleinfleckige Necrobiosis lipoidica bei Diabetikern. Dermatologica (Basel) **102**, 382 (1951).

NEWMAN, B. A., and F. F. FELDMAN: Effects of topical cortisone on chronic discoid lupus erythematosus and necrobiosis lipoidica diabeticorum. J. invest. Derm. **17**, 3 (1951). — NYLÉN, B. O., and T. SKOOG: Surgical treatment of necrobiosis lipoidica. Acta derm.-venereol. (Stockh.) **38**, 366 (1958).

OLIVER, L., et E. REBOUL: Dyslipoidose Oppenheim-Urbach à type de granulome annulaire chez un diabétique tuberculeux. Bull. Soc. franç. Derm. Syph. **63**, 250 (1956). — OTHAZ, E. L., SANTIAGE PONCE DE LÉON y DERMIDIO PALAU: Granuloma anulare. Rev. Asoc. méd. argent. **49**, 2099 (1936).

PEZZAROSSA, G.: Sulla necrobiosi lipidica e sui rapporti con il granuloma anulare. G. ital. Derm. **98**, 129 (1957). — PFLEGER-SCHWARZ, L.: Zur Ätiologie der juxtaartikulären Knoten und des Granuloma anulare. Wien. klin. Wschr. **1949**, 913. — PINETTI, P.: Sulla granulomatosi disciforme cronica et progressiva (Miescher). G. ital. Derm. **93**, 105 (1952). — PINKUS, H.: Über atypische Tuberkulide, zugleich ein Beitrag zur Ätiologie des Granuloma anulare. Arch. Derm. Syph. (Berl.) **170**, 194 (1934).

RASIEWICZ, W., and T. KOCHANOWICZ: A case of necrobiosis lipoidica of the skin, treated by ethyl chloride freezing. Przegl. Derm. **46**, 169 (1959). — RASMUSSEN, K. A.: Necrobiosis lipoidica diabeticorum. Transactions of the Danish Dermatological Society. Oct. 4, 1950. Acta derm.-venereol. (Stockh.) **33**, 255 (1953). — Rélias, A., et S. Maissa: Nécrobiose lipoidique à type de granulome anulaire géant. Bull. Soc. franç. Derm. Syph. **65**, 40 (1958). — Ringrose, E. J.: Smoking, Necrobiosis lipoidica, Granulomatosis disciformis progressiva. Arch. Derm. **79**, 635 (1959). — Rolliers, M., R. Rollier et A. Zniber: Purpura rhumatoide et granulome anulaire. Maroc. méd. **35**, 500 (1956). — Rollins, T. G., and R. K. Winkelmann: Necrobiosis lipoidica — Granulomatosis. Necrobiosis lipoidica diabeticorum in the non-diabetic. Arch. Derm. **82**, 537 (1960). — Rook, A., R. Davies and D. Stevanovic: Familial granuloma anulare, Report of two cases with observations on the incidence of the disease in Britain. Acta derm.-venereol. (Stockh.) **37**, 160 (1957). — Rothman, S., and Y. Lynfield: Acanthosis nigricans, juvenile type, combined with necrobiosis lipoidica diabeticorum. Arch. Derm. **79**, 113 (1959).

Šabatová, Marie: Granulomatosis disciformis chronica et progressiva Miescher. Ref. in Zbl. Haut- u. Geschl.-Kr. **95**, 21 (1956). — Santler, R.: Granulomatosis disciformis chronica et progressiva. Österr. Dermat. Ges. Sitzg vom 26. 6. 1952. Ref. in Zbl. Haut- u. Geschl.-Kr. **81**, 399 (1952). — Zwei Fälle von Granulomatosis disciformis chronica et progressiva (Miescher). Hautarzt **5**, 14 (1954). — Granulomatosis disciformis chronica et progressiva. Demonstration. Ref. in Zbl. Haut- u. Geschl.-Kr. **88**, 372 (1954). — Granulomatosis disciformis chronica et progressiva. Österr. Dermat. Ges. Sitzg vom 28. 10. 1954. Ref. in Zbl. Haut- u. Geschl.-Kr. **90**, 166 (1954/55). — Scheffler, H., u. H. Hagen: Allergische Hautreaktion nach Insulin in Form der Necrobiosis lipoidica. Med. Klin. **1956**, 2128. — Sendrail, M., et A. Bazex: Les lipoidoses cutanées. Ann. Derm. Syph. (Paris) **1941**, 259. — Senigagliesi, S., e M. Gentilli: Ulteriore contributo alla parigione del granuloma anulare con streptomicina topica. Minerva derm. **30**, 153 (1955). — Smith jr., J. G.: Necrobiosis lipoidica. A disease of changing concepts. Arch. Derm. **74**, 280 (1956). — Smith jr., J. G., and B. A. Wansker: Asteroid bodies in necrobiosis lipoidica. Arch. Derm. **74**, 276 (1956). — Spitzer, R.: Granuloma anulare familiare. Dermatologica (Basel) **123**, 38 (1961). — Stüttgen, G.: Panangiitis haemorrhagica lipoidica. Derm. Wschr. **134**, 1149 (1956).

Tappeiner, J., u. P. Wodniansky: Necrobiosis maculosa. Derm. Wschr. **146**, 569 (1962). — Tappeiner, S.: Zur Klinik und Histologie der Granulomatosis disciformis chronica et progressiva (Miescher). (Atypisches Sarkoid.) Arch. Derm. Syph. (Berl.) **194**, 341 (1952). — Granuloma anulare der Ohrmuschelränder (nach Rimifon?). Hautarzt **7**, 374 (1956). — Teodorescu, St., u. P. Vulcan: Chronische und progressive diskoide Granulomatose Miescher. Derm.-Vener. (Buc.) **2**, 537 (1957). — Thiers, H., et D. Colomb: Nécrose lipidique des diabétiques simulant l'érythème noueux. Bull. Soc. franç. Derm. Syph. **1953**, 98. — Tolmach, J. A.: Coincidence of micropapular tuberculid and granuloma anulare. Arch. Derm. **75**, 912 (1957). — Truffi, M.: Granuloma anulare di Crocker. Boll. Sez. region. Soc. ital. Derm. 1, 76 (1937).

Ullmo, A., et F. Woringer: Granulomatosis disciformis chronica et progressiva Miescher. Bull. Soc. franç. Derm. Syph. **1956**, 62. — Urbach, E.: Lipoidstoffwechselerkrankungen der Haut. In: Handbuch von Jadassohn, Bd. XII/2. Berlin: Springer 1932.

Walter: Granulomatosis disciformis chronica et progressiva (Miescher). Österr. Dermat. Ges. Sitzg vom 10. 5. 1951. Ref. in Zbl. Haut- u. Geschl.-Kr. **78**, 408 (1952). — Wells, G. C., and W. N. Goldsmith: Granulomatosis disciformis chronica et progressiva (Miescher). Proc. roy. Soc. Med. **44**, 360 (1951). — Williams, R. M.: Necrobiosis lipoidica diabeticorum with alopecia showing sarcoid-like reaction. Arch. Derm. **79**, 366 (1959). — Wood, M. G., and H. Beerman: Necrobiosis lipoidica, Granuloma anulare and rheumatoid nodule. J. invest. Derm. **34**, 139 (1960). — Woringer, F.: A propos du granulome anulaire. Bull. Soc. franç. Derm. Syph. **1950**, 144. — Relations entre la granulomatose disciforme et la nécrobiose lipoidique. Bull. Soc. franç. Derm. Syph. **1956**, 394. — Granulomatose disciforme chronique et progressive de Miescher. Bull. Soc. franç. Derm. Syph. **63**, 282 (1956). — A propos d'une confusion de termes: la nécrobiose lipoidique. Bull. Soc. franç. Derm. Syph. **68**, 680 (1961). — Woringer, F., et A. Ullmo: Granulomatosis disciformis chronica et progressiva Miescher. Ann. Derm. Syph. (Paris) **84**, 22 (1957). — Woringer, F., et J.-P. Weill: Comparaison d'une lésion jeune et d'une lésion adulte de nécrobiose lipoidique diabétique. Bull. Soc. franç. Derm. Syph. **66**, 226 (1959).

Ziswiler, H.: Über die Prognose und den Verlauf des generalisierten Lupus erythematodes. Dtsch. med. Wschr. **86**, 1302 (1961).

Hautmanifestationen rheumatischer Krankheiten

Von

Otto Hornstein-Düsseldorf

Mit 24 Abbildungen

I. Einleitung (mit Nomenklatur)

Bei nur wenigen Krankheiten haben sich in den letzten Jahrzehnten die pathogenetischen Vorstellungen so gewandelt wie bei den seit alters her „rheumatisch" genannten. Bei nur wenigen Krankheiten dürfte aber auch die nosologische Begriffsbestimmung ähnlich schwierig und problematisch sein. Dies macht beispielsweise die seit KLEMPERER nicht mehr zur Ruhe gekommene Diskussion um den Begriff der „Kollagenkrankheiten" bzw. der „pararheumatischen Krankheiten" (HEILMEYER; ROST u.a.) deutlich. Andererseits hat man schon früher verschiedene para- oder postinfektiöse Gelenksyndrome als „Rheumatoide" (GERHARDT) zusammengefaßt, ohne über das Wesen des „echten" Rheumatismus Klarheit erzielt zu haben. Der „fließende" Gliederschmerz, dem dieser den Namen verdankt, ist zwar klinisches Leitsymptom, zur nosologischen Klassifizierung aber unbrauchbar. Wie so häufig, ist für den fachkundigen Rheumatologen eine Definition des rheumatischen Formenkreises weit schwieriger als für den schmerzgeplagten Rheumatiker, dem die Art seiner Gelenkbeschwerden Beweis genug ist. Dem Arzt hingegen erschwert das Fehlen eines gemeinsamen oder überhaupt ausreichend fundierten *ätiologischen* Prinzips alle Bemühungen um eine exakte nosologische Begriffsbestimmung.

Dennoch hat die klinische Rheumatologie durch fortschreitende Grundlagenforschung und sorgfältige Auswahl diagnostischer Kriterien — also letztlich durch Übereinkunft der Experten — eine gewisse Umgrenzung der rheumatischen Krankheiten im engeren Sinne erreicht. Es zählen hierzu einerseits das *Rheumatische Fieber* einschließlich seiner zentralnervösen Sondermanifestation als Chorea minor, andererseits die *Primär-chronische Polyarthritis,* zu der auch das Felty-Syndrom, die Stillsche Krankheit und wohl auch das — nur im kontinentaleuropäischen Schrifttum anerkannte — Wissler-Fanconi-Syndrom gehören. Nur auf diese beiden Krankheitsgruppen soll sich unser Beitrag beziehen. Dagegen können die „pararheumatischen" Krankheiten (Lupus erythematodes integumentalis et visceralis, Dermatomyositis, Progressive Sklerodermie, Peri- oder Polyarteriitis nodosa, Gougerot-Sjögren-Syndrom), zu denen vielfach auch das Erythema nodosum und das Erythema exsudativum multiforme, die Purpura Schönlein-Henoch und teilweise sogar die Endangiitis obliterans v. Winiwarter-Buerger und der Morbus Boeck gerechnet werden (ROST 1960), nicht oder höchstens am Rande erwähnt werden. Das gleiche gilt für den Formenkreis der „Rheumatoide" mit der häufig dort eingeordneten Reiterschen Krankheit.

Verschiedene Kriterien der Grenzziehung um die sog. „rheumatischen" Krankheiten haben zweifellos etwas Künstliches an sich; denn einerseits werden immer mehr nosologische Berührungspunkte oder Überschneidungen zwischen „rheumatischen" und „pararheumatischen" Krankheitsformen entdeckt (vgl. etwa einzelne Beobachtungen von Felty-Syndrom und visceralem Lupus erythematodes), andererseits bestehen zwischen dem Rheumatischen Fieber und der Primär-chronischen Polyarthritis doch zahlreiche Unterschiede, die vielleicht sogar die Gemeinsamkeiten überwiegen. Im angelsächsischen und skandinavischen Schrifttum wird dieser Tatsache schon lange Rechnung getragen, indem hier statt von Primär-chronischer von „Rheumatoider" Arthritis gesprochen wird. Es ist also wichtig, sich des terminologischen Provisoriums, das die verschiedenen Klassifikationsschemata für den Rheumatismus bis heute errichtet haben, bewußt zu bleiben[1]. Alle diese Ordnungsprinzipien haben sicherlich ihren heuristischen Wert — das mag in gewisser Hinsicht auch für den Begriff der „Kollagenkrankheiten" gelten —, sie dürften aber mit dem Fortschreiten der Grundlagenforschung, besonders auf dem Gebiet der Immunopathologie, wohl noch manche Korrektur und Neuorientierung erfahren.

Zur *Nomenklatur* einige kurze Hinweise: Der in den ersten Jahrzehnten dieses Jahrhunderts im angelsächsischen und skandinavischen Schrifttum aufgekommene Terminus „*Rheumatisches Fieber*" hat sich fast allgemein durchgesetzt, da er im Gegensatz zu den Bezeichnungen Polyarthritis rheumatica acuta bzw. akuter Gelenkrheumatismus die Vielfalt der möglichen Organmanifestationen begrifflich nicht einschränkt. Als Synonyma werden (besonders im schweizerischen Schrifttum) „Rheumatismus verus" (NAEGELI; v. NEERGAARD), „Rheumatismus acutus", „Rheumatische Infektion" (LEICHTENTRITT; GLANZMANN) oder einfach Morbus rheumaticus gebraucht. Bei französischen Autoren (aber z.B. auch bei RICKER) ist daneben der historisch gerechtfertigte Name Bouillaudsche Krankheit, bei russischen Autoren Bouillaud-Sokolskische Krankheit in Übung. FAHR prägte die (heute meist verlassene) Bezeichnung „Granulomatosis rheumatica", womit er die rheumatische Krankheitsgruppe als spezifische Infektionskrankheit deklarieren und gewissermaßen der Tuberkulose, Lues usw. an die Seite stellen wollte.

Der Begriff der *Primär-chronischen Polyarthritis* ist zwar seit langem in der deutschsprachigen Fachliteratur eingebürgert, in der fremdsprachigen, besonders in der angelsächsischen Medizin, aber nur wenig geläufig. Hier dominiert die Bezeichnung „*Rheumatoid Arthritis*", die bei uns wegen der Verwechslungsmöglichkeit mit dem para- oder postinfektiösen Komplex der „Rheumatoide" nur zögernd gebraucht wird. Neuerdings sprechen manche Autoren auch von „Rheumatoid Disease", um den nosologischen Wesenszug als Systemkrankheit stärker zum Ausdruck zu bringen. Im gleichen Sinne kann man auch von „Primärchronischem Rheumatismus" oder — in historischer Sicht — von der Charcotschen Krankheit sprechen.

In den deutschsprachigen Handbüchern der Dermatologie sind die zum Rheumatismus im engeren Sinne gehörigen Hautveränderungen bisher nur im Handbuch GOTTRON-SCHÖNFELD dargestellt worden (HORNSTEIN u. SCHUERMANN 1958). Im Jadassohnschen Handbuchwerk der Dreißigerjahre fehlt ein dermatologisches Kapitel zum Rheumatismusproblem. Aber auch in den meisten Lehrbüchern der

---

[1] Die in verschiedenen Ländern geltenden Klassifikationen der rheumatischen Krankheiten weichen mehr oder minder wesentlich voneinander ab. Auch das 1954 von der Weltgesundheitsorganisation aufgestellte Einteilungsschema ist in mancher Hinsicht noch problematisch; hier werden als „Diseases commonly accepted as rheumatic" aufgeführt:

A. With articular localization:

1. Inflammatory.

a) Rheumatic fever.

b) Rheumatoid arthritis. (Special forms: Psoriatic arthritis, STILLs disease, FELTYs syndrome, SJÖGRENs syndrome.)

c) Ankylosing spondylitis or rheumatoid spondylitis.

d) Arthritis due to specific infection.

e) REITERs syndrome.

f) Articular hypersensitivity against drugs, protein etc.

g) Palindromic rheumatism and intermittent hydrarthrosis. (Die unter d—f genannten Arthritiden entsprechen teilweise dem „Rheumatoid"-Begriff der deutschen Literatur.)

2. Degenerative.

(Die hier genannten arthropathischen Zustände, ferner solche „with non-articular localization", z.B. Tendosynovitis, Periarthritis, Fibrositis, Bursitis, außerdem die zweite Hauptgruppe der „*para-rheumatic*", *collagen, and other diseases presenting rheumatic features* brauchen in unserem Zusammenhang nicht aufgezählt zu werden.)

Rheumatologie ist zugehörigen Dermatosen kein oder nur ein unbedeutender Platz eingeräumt. So findet sich z.B. in der 1. Auflage der von HOCHREIN herausgegebenen „Rheumatischen Krankheiten“ (1942) zwar noch ein kurzes dermatologisches Kapitel von SPIETHOFF; in der 2. Auflage (1952) hat man aber auf einen entsprechenden Beitrag gänzlich verzichtet. Bezeichnend für den in den letzten 20 Jahren auch in der Dermatologie eingetretenen Umschwung der nosologischen Klassifikationen mag sein, was SPIETHOFF 1942 noch unter „Rheuma und Hauterkrankungen“ abhandelte: das Erythema exsudativum multiforme, das Erythema nodosum und die Purpura rheumatica als „klassische Vertreter der Rheumadermatosen“[1], Nagelveränderungen beim Rheumatismus, Herpes zoster, Morphaea und progressive Sklerodermie, Acrodermatitis chronica atrophicans, Psoriasis arthropathica und Rheumatismusknötchen. Nur die letzteren würden wir heute zum rheumatischen Formenkreis sensu strictiori rechnen.

Dem verhältnismäßig kargen Interesse in der Dermatologie an Problemen des engeren Rheumatismus steht eine um so intensivere Beschäftigung mit „pararheumatischen“ Krankheiten — bereits lange vor der inneren Medizin — gegenüber. Der historischen Objektivität wegen muß man aber feststellen, daß in der zweiten Hälfte des vorigen Jahrhunderts auch von dermatologischer Seite sehr wesentliche Beiträge zur Klinik des Rheumatismus geleistet worden sind (vgl. BAZIN als Schöpfer des lange Zeit nachwirkenden „Arthritismus“-Begriffs, BESNIER, BROCQ, BOURDILLON u.a.). Später mag die Spezialisierung des Schrifttums das ihrige dazu getan haben, daß rheumatologische Probleme für die Dermatologie scheinbar an Aktualität verloren haben. Die Rheumatologie ist freilich bereits zum Range einer eigenen medizinischen Fachdisziplin aufgerückt und als solche teilweise verselbständigt. Es bestehen aber zu den verschiedensten Fachgebieten und — wie beispielsweise der dermatologische Anteil an der Erforschung der „pararheumatischen“ Krankheiten lehrt — auch zur Dermatologie eine ganze Reihe von Wechselbeziehungen, auf die in neuerer Zeit besonders GOTTRON, SCHUERMANN, ROST u.a. aufmerksam gemacht haben. Es leuchtet ohne weiteres ein, daß die Dermatologen bei der Miterforschung der großen „*pararheumatischen*“ Mesenchymkrankheiten auch den „*rheumatischen*“ ihre Aufmerksamkeit nicht versagen können, auch wenn sich ihr Beitrag nur auf einen Teilsektor beschränkt.

Unter diesem Gesichtspunkt sollen nachstehend die Hautmanifestationen folgender Krankheiten behandelt werden:

I. Febris rheumatica.
  1. Vorwiegend unspezifische integumentale Begleiterscheinungen.
  2. Erythema anulare Lehndorff-Leiner.
  3. Nodi (sive Noduli) rheumatici.

II. Primär-chronische bzw. Rheumatoide Polyarthritis des Kindesalters.
  1. Wissler-Fanconi-Syndrom.
  2. Chronische Polyarthritis sensu strictiori.
  3. Stillsche Krankheit.

III. Primär-chronische bzw. Rheumatoide Polyarthritis des Erwachsenenalters.
  1. Chronische Polyarthritis sensu strictiori.
  2. Felty-Syndrom.
  3. Monosymptomatischer „Rheumatismus nodosus“ (und das Problem des Granuloma anulare).

---

[1] So hat bereits 1926 ROST in seinen „Hautkrankheiten“ die verschiedenen Purpuraformen, das Erythema nodosum und das Erythema exsudativum multiforme als „rheumatoide“ Erkrankungen zusammengefaßt und dieser Gruppe 1948 auch den Lupus erythematodes zugerechnet.

Außer den schon erwähnten Beziehungen zu verschiedenen „pararheumatischen" Systemkrankheiten weist die Primär-chronische Polyarthritis auch mehrere Analogien zur Psoriasis arthropathica auf, die besonders im angelsächsischen Schrifttum zu der Tendenz geführt haben, diese Extremvariante der Schuppenflechte (TIEDEMANN) der „Rheumatoiden Arthritis" als Sonderform einzugliedern (vgl. auch das Klassifikationsschema der Weltgesundheitsorganisation).

Nach unserer Auffassung ist jedoch die *nosologische Sonderstellung der Psoriasis arthropathica* — jedenfalls in ihrer „klassischen" Form — *voll gerechtfertigt*, so daß keine Notwendigkeit besteht, dieses Krankheitsbild in die unmittelbare Thematik unseres Handbuchbeitrags einzubeziehen. Wir werden lediglich an Hand einer kurzen tabellarischen Übersicht der wichtigsten Unterscheidungskriterien zwischen Psoriasis arthropathica und Primär-chronischer Polyarthritis eine kurze kritische Stellungnahme beziehen und verweisen im übrigen auf das Psoriasis-Kapitel in diesem Handbuchwerk sowie auf eine 1962 erschienene eigene Arbeit über die nosologische Stellung der Psoriasis arthropathica.

Wahrscheinlich hat auch das Krankheitsbild der „multiplen cutanen Reticulo-Histiocytome" trotz seiner häufigen arthropathischen Komponente keine rheumatische Basis. Die Problematik der nosologischen Deutung und Klassifikation spiegelt sich in Termini wie „paraxanthomatöse (thesaurotische) System-Histiocytose" (BACCAREDDA-BOY), „Lipoid Dermato-Arthritis" (WARIN) oder „Reticulo-Histiocytic Granulomas of the Skin" — entweder „simulating Rheumatoid Arthritis" (GRAHAM und STANSFIELD) oder „associated with Arthritis mutilans" (JOHNSON und TILDEN) — wider. Wir verwenden im folgenden die möglichst wenig präjudizierende Bezeichnung „*Reticulo-Histiocytosis disseminata partim arthropathica*", da die Frage einer echten Speicherkrankheit oder einer primär entzündlichen Granulomatose noch offen ist. Höchstwahrscheinlich kann man aber das klinisch ähnliche Krankheitsbild der sog. xanthomatösen Arthritis (LAYANI) in die Gruppe der Lipoidstoffwechselkrankheiten einordnen.

Auch das Gougerot-Sjögren-Syndrom als vorwiegend „pararheumatisches" Krankheitsbild, das zweifellos verschiedene klinische und immunpathologische Beziehungen zum Formenkreis der Primär-chronischen Polyarthritis aufweist, kann angesichts der notwendigen Beschränkung auf obligat rheumatische Krankheitsbilder nicht näher dargelegt werden. Das gleiche gilt für das Problem des Morbus Reiter, der zwar viele symptomatologische Beziehungen zum Rheumatismus aufweist, nosologisch aber am ehesten bei der Krankheitsgruppe der „Rheumatoide" einzuordnen ist.

Zum Verständnis des Folgenden erscheint es uns unumgänglich, in ganz knappen Zügen wenigstens einen kurzen Überblick über den heutigen Wissensstand zur Ätiologie und Pathogenese der rheumatischen Krankheiten zu geben. Im Rahmen dieses Handbuchbeitrags mag dabei die Wiedergabe einiger wichtiger Ergebnisse genügen. Hinsichtlich näherer Einzelheiten sei auf die im Literaturverzeichnis unter „Einleitung" aufgeführten Arbeiten verwiesen.

Überblick über den heutigen Wissensstand zur Ätiologie und Pathogenese der rheumatischen Krankheiten

a) Rheumatisches Fieber

Die alte Kontroverse zwischen den Verfechtern der „spezifischen" Infektionstheorie (ASCHOFF, SCHOTTMÜLLER, GRÄFF, FAHR u.a.) und der Allergietheorie (KLINGE, RÖSSLE, COBURN, SWIFT u.a.) des Rheumatismus hat für das Rheumatische Fieber gewissermaßen mit einem „Kompromiß" geendet. Es wird zwar in der Regel durch initiale Infekte der oberen

Luftwege mit β-hämolysierenden A-Streptokokken (meist als Tonsillitis oder Pharyngitis) vorbereitet und ausgelöst, doch führen diese Infekte zu einer zunehmenden Sensibilisierung gegen Streptokokken-Antigene mit dem schließlichen Resultat einer infektionsallergischen Reaktion, die zur rheumatischen Gewebsläsion führt. So hat bereits COBURN (1931) zwischen einer *Sensibilisierungsphase* durch den prodromalen Streptokokkeninfekt, einer *Latenzphase* mit Antikörperbildung und einer hyperergischen *Reaktionsphase* — dem Rheumatischen Fieber — unterschieden. Nach VORLAENDER ist der initiale Streptokokkeninfekt in 90—95% aller Fälle beweisbar. Da es allein innerhalb der A-Streptokokken (LANCEFIELD) über 40 serologisch differenzierbare Typen mit typenspezifischem Antigenmuster gibt, ist es verständlich, daß zahlreiche Streptokokken-Erkrankungen in den ersten Lebensjahren durchgemacht werden können, bevor der Organismus gegen die meisten A-Streptokokken immunisiert ist. Anscheinend kann der das Rheumatische Fieber auslösende Infekt von allen Typen hervorgerufen werden (EHRICH; RAMMELKAMP). Für den Krankheitsausbruch hat wahrscheinlich die rasche Aufeinanderfolge solcher Streptokokkeninfekte — darunter die Reinfektion mit dem gleichen Erregertyp (COBURN; GOLDBERGER) — und eine konstitutionelle, teilweise vererbbare Disposition zur rheumatischen Reaktionsbereitschaft erhebliche Bedeutung. Die höhere Morbiditätsquote in feuchtkalten Klimaregionen und der jahreszeitliche Häufigkeitsgipfel im Winter und Frühjahr hängen wahrscheinlich von epidemiologischen Faktoren der humanpathogenen Streptokokkenbesiedlung ab.

Die kollektive Altersverteilung des Rheumatischen Fiebers erreicht ihren *Gipfel etwa um das 10. Lebensjahr* (FANCONI u. WISSLER; LEIBER; EWERBECK u.a.), was vielleicht damit erklärt werden kann, daß einerseits bereits eine ausreichende infektionsallergische Umstimmung, andererseits noch keine vollständige Immunität erreicht ist (F. SCHMID). Während die Krankheit früher kaum vor dem 4. Lebensjahr beobachtet wurde, ist in den letzten Jahrzehnten, wahrscheinlich unter dem Einfluß der allgemeinen Acceleration (BENNHOLDT-THOMSEN), eine Vorverlegung des Beginns und gleichzeitig eine Zunahme der frühkindlichen kardialen Erkrankungsformen, also eine *Präzession* und eine *Akzentuation* eingetreten (LEIBER; EWERBECK; KÖTTGEN u. CALLENSEE u.a.). Andererseits ist die Gesamtmorbidität an Rheumatischem Fieber geringer geworden (HALL), was wahrscheinlich auf ihre verbesserte Prophylaxe — durch Behandlung der A-Streptokokkeninfekte mit Penicillin — zurückzuführen ist (CATANZARO; DENNY; STOLLERMANN; WANNAMAKER u.a.).

Zwar gelingt der Streptokokkennachweis im Rachen bei Ausbruch des Rheumatischen Fiebers nur in etwa 50—60% der Fälle (KLEIN; CHRIST), da oft ein 2—3wöchiges Intervall zwischen auslösendem Infekt und rheumatischer Manifestation besteht; doch führt in den übrigen, bakteriologisch „stummen" Fällen der Antikörpernachweis weiter, da sowohl gegen celluläre als auch gegen extracelluläre Streptokokkenantigene (Streptokinase, Hyaluronidase, Streptolysin O und S) Antikörper mit charakteristischem Titeranstieg gebildet werden. Weiter wird die Streptokokkenätiologie gestützt durch epidemiologische Beobachtungen [vermehrter Ausbruch des Rheumatischen Fiebers nach epidemischen Streptokokkenanginen (WINBLAD)], durch die Erfolge der Prophylaxe und Rezidivverhütung mit Penicillin sowie durch experimentelle Erzeugung von generalisierten hyperergischen Granulomen nach wiederholten subcutanen Streptokokkeninjektionen (MURPHY u. SWIFT). Allerdings ist es bis heute nicht gelungen, auf experimentellem Wege entzündliche, dem Bild des menschlichen Rheumatismus völlig identische Gewebsveränderungen am Endomyokard und an den Gelenken zu erzeugen (GRAM u. BÖHMIG; VORLAENDER).

Als Folge der infektionsallergischen Antigen-Antikörperreaktion werden entzündungsfördernde Substanzen („H-Substanzen", „Menkin-Stoffe") freigesetzt, die ihrerseits durch Permeabilitätserhöhung der Gefäße, seröse und fibrinöse Exsudation sowie wahrscheinlich durch Aktivierung körpereigener Fermente (Serokinase, Fibrinolysin) erst die eigentliche rheumatische Gewebsschädigung verursachen (BÖHMIG; LETTERER; EHRICH u.a.). Diese pathogenetische Kettenreaktion läuft weitgehend eigengesetzlich und unabhängig vom auslösenden Streptokokkeninfekt ab, sie kann durch Penicillinbehandlung nicht mehr beeinflußt werden. Dabei werden die mesenchymalen Gewebe der Gelenksynovia, der serösen Häute und des Endokards — die „Resonanzmembranen" nach KÜSTER — bevorzugt befallen. Mit der Gewebsschädigung geht eine proliferative Entzündung einher, die wahrscheinlich nicht nur auf resorptiven, sondern auch auf spezifisch hyperergischen Zelleistungen beruht (LETTERER). Anscheinend rufen die Gewebsläsionen (unter zusätzlicher Komplexbindung von Streptokokken-Antigenen?) auch die Bildung von organspezifischen Auto-Antikörpern hervor (STEFFEN; VORLAENDER u.a.), die sich immuno-elektrophoretisch nachweisen lassen. Diese Auto-Antikörper bzw. serologischen Zusatzfaktoren, die bisher bei der rheumatischen Karditis und bei Endokarditisrezidiven nach Mitralstenoseoperationen („Postcommissurotomie-Syndrom") am besten bekannt sind, spielen möglicherweise für die vorherrschende *Lokalisation* der rheumatischen Entzündungsherde eine determinierende Rolle. So konnte VORLAENDER tierexperimentell zeigen, daß sich mit niedrig dosierten (einmaligen oder wiederholten) Streptokokken-Injektionen nur dann endomyokarditische Veränderungen erzeugen ließen, wenn gleichzeitig intravenös ein homologes Antiserum gegen Endomyokard verabreicht wurde. (Dagegen blieb die alleinige Einwirkung der Erreger oder des Antiserums ohne nachweisbaren gewebspathogenen Effekt.)

Zusammenfassend ist festzustellen, daß es ohne Streptokokken offenbar kein Rheumatisches Fieber gibt und daß die überwältigende Mehrheit aller epidemiologischen, klinischen und bakteriologisch-serologischen Befunde für eine infektionsallergische Genese der Krankheit spricht. Dabei wird die primäre Antigen-Antikörperreaktion rasch in die mesenchymalen Gewebe „abgelenkt", wo degenerative Bindegewebsläsionen mit herdförmiger granulomatös-hyperergischer Entzündung entstehen. Im Zuge dieser „rheumatischen" Entzündung werden auch autoimmunologische Sekundärreaktionen in Gang gesetzt, die möglicherweise für die jeweiligen Prädilektionen der rheumatischen Organmanifestationen von entscheidender Bedeutung sind.

b) Primär-chronische Polyarthritis („Rheumatoid Arthritis")

„Rheumatoid arthritis is a chronic inflammatory disease of unknown etiology and pathogenesis which is systemic in nature and characterized by the manner in which it involves joints." Zu dieser lapidaren Feststellung kommen SHORT, BAUER u. REYNOLDS am Ende ihrer Monographie über diese Krankheit (1957). Im Gegensatz zum Rheumatischen Fieber ist die kausal-genetische Rolle infektiöser Faktoren für die Mehrzahl der Fälle, jedenfalls für die *symmetrische* progressive Form der Primär-chronischen Polyarthritis, nicht bewiesen. Therapeutische „Fokalsanierungen" bleiben meist ohne Erfolg, allenfalls kann die allgemeine Resistenzlage des Organismus verbessert werden (MIEHLKE; VOIT u. GAMP u.a.). Dennoch legen verschiedene klinische und serologische Befunde die Mitwirkung infektiöser Prozesse nahe, die sich aber „gewissermaßen im Hintergrund abspielen" (SCHOEN u. TISCHENDORF).

In letzter Zeit hat diese Auffassung einen gewissen Auftrieb erhalten durch die Abgrenzung einer *asymmetrischen*, in Schüben verlaufenden *Sonderform* der chronischen Polyarthritis (VOIT; TICHY), die hohe Antistreptolysin O-Titer, aber niedrige oder negative rheumaserologische Hämagglutinationsteste aufweist und daher auch als „*Antistreptolysin-Typ*" (im Gegensatz zum häufigeren „Agglutinations-Typ") bezeichnet wird (VOIT; v. KRESS; TICHY; VORLAENDER). Zu dieser infektabhängigen Sonderform sollen rund 25% der ganzen Krankheitsgruppe gehören (TICHY). Nach VORLAENDER kommt entzündliche Herzbeteiligung nur bei dieser nosologischen Untergruppe vor, was im Hinblick auf die streptokokkeninduzierte Karditis des Rheumatischen Fiebers Beachtung verdient[1]. Andererseits fehlt das der akuten Polyarthritis eigentümliche „Springen" von einem Gelenk zum anderen, vielmehr setzt sich die Entzündung an den einmal ergriffenen Gelenken hartnäckig fest, so daß sekundär-entzündliche Zerstörungen entstehen können.

Ob außerdem der besonders in der französischen Rheumatologie anerkannte Begriff einer meist gutartigen „*Primär-subakuten Polyarthritis*" (mit initialem Befall großer Gelenke) im Sinne von RAVAULT, VIGNON und BERTHIER zu Recht besteht — dieses Krankheitsbild wäre klinisch und serologisch sowohl von der Primär-chronischen Polyarthritis als auch vom Rheumatischen Fieber abzugrenzen —, wird von TICHY bejaht, von SCHOEN, MIEHLKE und BARGON bezweifelt[2]. Zwar werden mit zunehmender Verfeinerung der serologischen Diagnostik immer mehr Patienten meist mittleren Alters beobachtet, die auch nach langer Nachbeobachtungszeit weder hohe Antistreptolysin O-Titer noch positive rheumaserologische Reaktionen noch Karditis aufweisen, doch bleibt immer noch die Möglichkeit einer atypischen Spielart der Primär-chronischen Polyarthritis oder einer mitigierten Verlaufsform des Rheumatischen Fiebers offen, zumal das letztere nach dem 40. Lebensjahr praktisch ohne Herzbeteiligung verläuft (SCHOEN).

Ein kurzer Hinweis zur „*Sekundär-chronischen Polyarthritis*" („Rhumatisme fibreux" von JACCOUD): Diese Diagnose ist nach SCHOEN in der deutschen Medizin früher zu oft gestellt worden. Sie setzt eine Erkrankung an Rheumatischem Fieber voraus, die in ein destruierend-arthropathisches Stadium übergeht. Bei Anlegung strenger klinisch-katamnestischer und serodiagnostischer Maßstäbe läßt sich nur in Ausnahmefällen ein solcher nosologischer Zusammenhang aufrechterhalten (MOLL). Bei der großen Mehrzahl dürfte es sich dagegen um Fälle von Stillscher Krankheit, Wissler-Fanconi-Syndrom, atypischer Primär-chronischer Polyarthritis vom „Antistreptolysin-Typ" u.ä. handeln.

---

[1] Vielleicht erklären sich nunmehr auch die recht unterschiedlichen Angaben über das Vorkommen kardialer Manifestationen (Klappensklerose, diffuse interstitielle und granulomatöse Myokarditis, adhäsive Perikarditis) auch bei der Primär-chronischen Polyarthritis (COATES; KAHLMETER; BAGGENSTOSS u. ROSENBERG; CRUICKSHANK; SOKOLOFF; GOEHRS u.a.).

[2] Wahrscheinlich steht dieser Polyarthritis-Typ dem „postanginösen Rheumatismus" von LAYANI und CHAOUAT nahe, der als mono- bis oligoartikuläre Entzündung bei Männern, seltener Frauen im 3. und 4. Lebensjahrzehnt vorkommt.

Bei der Krankheitsgruppe der Primär-chronischen Polyarthritis tritt nicht selten ein *konstitutionelles, teilweise hereditär-familiäres Fundament* deutlich hervor (HANGARTER; STECHER u. Mitarb.), und zwar noch mehr als beim Rheumatischen Fieber (SHORT; BAUER u. REYNOLDS). Vererbt wird aber nicht die Krankheit als solche, sondern die krankhafte Reaktionsbereitschaft, zu deren Manifestation es einer ganzen Reihe von Realisationsfaktoren bedarf. Nach DE BLÉCOURT u. Mitarb. folgt die Primär-chronische Polyarthritis (und die ankylosierende Spondylarthritis) wahrscheinlich einem nicht-geschlechtsgebundenen dominanten Erbmechanismus, wobei zwischen Männern und Frauen jedoch Unterschiede hinsichtlich der Penetranz der Erbanlage bestehen.

Auf welche Weise der in verschiedenem Grade konstitutionell vorgezeichnete Reaktionsmechanismus in Gang gesetzt wird, hängt wahrscheinlich von der *Konstellation zusätzlicher exo- und endogener Krankheitsfaktoren* ab. Unter den letzteren werden Adaptationsstörungen des endokrinen Gleichgewichts — besonders im Hypophysen-Nebennierenrindensystem —, pathologische Regulationsmechanismen übergeordneter diencephaler Zentren, psychische Traumen u.ä. genannt. Viele Befunde sprechen zwar für eine tiefgreifende Alteration der neurohormonalen Regulationssysteme, doch erfaßt das von SELYE inaugurierte Stadienschema des „Allgemeinen Adaptationssyndroms" nicht die ganze Reaktionsbreite des Krankheitsbildes, da sich beim gleichen Patienten Symptome des „Resistenzstadiums" und (während subakuter Schübe) der „Alarmreaktion" vermischen (JUNG u. BÖNI). Nach SCHOEN und TISCHENDORF stehen dysproteinämische Vorgänge mit Hyper-γ-Globulinämie im Mittelpunkt des Krankheitsgeschehens („humorales Rheumasyndrom")[1]. Der günstige therapeutische Einfluß von ACTH und Corticosteroiden spricht ebenfalls gegen direkte infektiöse Einflüsse und mehr für einen *gleichsam verselbständigten entzündlichen Reaktionsprozeß*, der mit dem Rheumatischen Fieber das ähnliche histomorphe Substrat, die systematisierte Ausbreitung und die bevorzugte Lokalisation um die Gelenke teilt.

Im Mittelpunkt der nosologischen Erörterungen steht heute das Problem des sog. „*Rheumafaktors*", der mit serologischen Methoden in einem hohen Prozentsatz der Fälle nachweisbar ist und wahrscheinlich die Bedeutung eines Auto-Antikörpers hat. Dieser Serumfaktor, der im Sinne eines klinisch brauchbaren Testes zuerst durch das von WAALER (1940) und ROSE mit Mitarbeitern (1948) entwickelte Hämagglutinationsverfahren mit sensibilisierten, d.h. mit Wa.R.-Amboceptor vorbehandelten Hammel-Erythrocyten nachgewiesen wurde, ist zwar nicht spezifisch, aber doch *hochcharakteristisch für die Primär-chronische Polyarthritis*[2]. Seine differentialdiagnostische Bedeutung ist unbestritten, besonders wenn er hohe Titerwerte (1:512 und darüber) erreicht. Allerdings erfolgt der Titeranstieg meist ganz allmählich, so daß der serologische Nachweis mitunter überhaupt erst nach 10—15jähriger Dauer der Krankheit gelingt (DIXON). Dieser Umstand sowie die Tatsache, daß mit den meisten Hämagglutinationsverfahren bei der juvenilen Form der Primär-chronischen Polyarthritis (bzw. bei der Stillschen Krankheit) nur in etwa einem Drittel der Fälle ein positiver serologischer Befund besteht, ziehen die ätiologische Bedeutung des „Rheumafaktors" erheblich in Zweifel.

Biologisch „*falsch positive*" Resultate des „Rheumafaktors" — oft aber mit niedrigen Titerwerten — kommen, abgesehen vom Lupus erythematodes visceralis, vereinzelt bei chronischen Leber- und Nierenkrankheiten, Lues, verschiedenen Virusinfekten, Morbus Waldenström und bei den Plasmocytomen vor, also bei Krankheiten, die vielfach mit erheblicher Dys- und Paraproteinämie und Hyper-γ-Globulinämie einhergehen (VAUGHAN; SCHEIFFARTH u. Mitarb. u.a.).

Nach eigenen Erfahrungen, die mit denen anderer Autoren übereinstimmen, werden auch bei der *Psoriasis arthropathica* positive Hämagglutinationsteste nur ausnahmsweise — und

---

[1] Wiederholt ist aber auch Primär-chronische Polyarthritis bei Patienten mit *Agammaglobulinämie* beobachtet worden (VAUGHAN u. GOOD; GOOD u. ROTSTEIN).

[2] In den letzten 10 Jahren ist eine ganze Reihe von technischen Variationen und Verbesserungen entwickelt worden, die die serologischen Reaktionen teils in ihrer Empfindlichkeit gesteigert, teils exakter standardisiert und vereinfacht haben: Vorabsorption der gewöhnlich im Humanserum vorhandenen Heteroagglutinine für normale Hammelblutkörperchen (HELLER u. Mitarb. 1949), Kältepräcipitation des Patientenserums (SVARTZ u. SCHLOSSMANN 1954), Beladung bzw. Sensibilisierung der mittels Tannin vorbehandelten Erythrocyten mit humanem γ-Globulin bzw. mit der Cohnschen γ-Globulinfraktion II (JACOBSON u. Mitarb. 1956), Verwendung menschlicher, mit einem inkompletten Antikörper des Rh-Systems sensibilisierter Erythrocyten (JACQUELINE u. Mitarb. 1957), Verwendung künstlicher Polymere (z.B. Latexpartikel) an Stelle von Erythrocyten zur Sichtbarmachung der agglutinierenden Fähigkeit des Rheumafaktors (SINGER u. PLOTZ 1956), Entwicklung eines Hämagglutinations-Inhibitionstests, der auf dem indirekten Nachweis eines agglutinations*hemmenden*, bei Primär-chronischer Polyarthritis fehlenden zweiten Serumfaktors beruht und eine besonders hohe Empfindlichkeit aufweist (ZIFF u. Mitarb. 1957), aber auch relativ viele „falsch positive" Resultate ergibt (DRESNER u. TROMBLY).

dann mit niedrigen Titerwerten unterhalb des für die Primär-chronische Polyarthritis pathognomonischen Grenzbereichs — beobachtet (vgl. unter „Psoriasis arthropathica").

Die *klinische Bedeutung* des „Rheumafaktors" beruht einerseits auf der hohen statistischen Signifikanz seines Auftretens im Rahmen der Primär-chronischen Polyarthritis, andererseits auf der Regelmäßigkeit, mit der er die gesteigerte Aktivität des Krankheitsprozesses mit hohen Titerwerten anzeigt. (Eine ähnliche Indicatorfunktion für entzündlich-rheumatische Aktivität hat auch der Nachweis des zur β_1-Globulin-Fraktion gehörenden C-reaktiven Proteins (CRP), das aber im Gegensatz zum „Rheumafaktor" diagnostisch völlig unspezifisch ist.) Zwar werden positive serologische Rheumateste bei fortgeschrittenen Fällen mit röntgenologisch nachweisbaren Gelenkveränderungen häufiger als bei Frühformen gefunden (VORLAENDER u. a.), doch erlaubt der serologische Befund keine eindeutigen prognostischen Schlüsse (JESSAR), da Titerhöhe und Schwere des klinischen Krankheitsverlaufs nicht immer übereinstimmen.

Antirheumatische Therapie hat meist keinen direkten Einfluß auf den Agglutinationstiter, in Einzelfällen wird aber mit dem Rückgang der klinischen Krankheitsaktivität auch ein Absinken der Titerhöhe beobachtet (SVARTZ; SCHLEGEL; VORLAENDER).

Über die *pathophysiologische Natur des „Rheumafaktors"* besteht noch keine völlige Klarheit. Er bleibt innerhalb eines p_H-Bereichs von p_H 4—11 stabil und wird bei 56° nicht zerstört, ist also nicht identisch mit Serumkomplement (VORLAENDER). Bei chromatographischen Untersuchungen an Cellulosesäulen hat man ihn in der γ-Globulin-Fraktion (s. bei MÜLLER-EBERHARD), bei zweidimensionaler Elektrophorese jedoch im Bereich der β-Globuline angereichert gefunden (BRAUNSTEINER u. Mitarb.). Beobachtungen von klinisch eindeutiger, aber rheumaserologisch negativer Primär-chronischer Polyarthritis bei Patienten mit *Agammaglobulinämie* sprechen indirekt wieder für die Zugehörigkeit des Faktors zur γ-Globulin-Fraktion.

Ultrazentrifugen-Untersuchungen haben nun gezeigt, daß der Faktor als *Makroglobulin* mit der Sedimentationskonstante 22 S (Svedberg-Einheiten) auftritt (FRANKLIN u. Mitarb.; SVARTZ u. a.). Er besteht aus einem dissoziierbaren Komplex von 19 S- und 7 S-γ-Globulinen, die in einem molekularen Mengenverhältnis von etwa 1:7 verbunden sind (KUNKEL; MÜLLER-EBERHARD u. a.). Beide Globuline kommen getrennt auch bei Gesunden vor, aber nicht in Komplexverbindung. Wahrscheinlich gibt es mehrere, dem „Rheumafaktor" ähnliche Makroglobuline, die auch für „falsch positive" Hämagglutinationsbefunde verantwortlich sein können (CHRIST). Auch konnte SVARTZ im Tierexperiment mit pleomorphen, aus dem Nasopharynx von Patienten mit Primär-chronischer Polyarthritis gezüchteten Streptokokken der Gruppe B einen kältepräcipitierbaren, dem menschlichen Rheumafaktor anscheinend nahe verwandten Eiweißkörper erzeugen.

Diese und andere experimentelle Untersuchungen fördern die Vermutung, daß der „Rheumafaktor" seinem Wesen nach eine Art von Auto-Antikörper darstellt, zumal er an Immunpräcipitate und auch an lösliche AgAk-Komplexe adsorbiert werden kann (VAUGHAN; EDELMANN u. Mitarb.; RAGAN u. a.). Vielleicht fungieren dabei die 7 S-γ-Globuline als Antigen, das 19 S-γ-Globulin als Antikörper[1]. Jedenfalls fallen die Hämagglutinationsproben sowohl mit S 19- als auch mit S 22-γ-Globulin positiv aus. ROST äußerte auch die Vermutung, daß der „Rheumafaktor" analog zum (gegen DNS gerichteten) L.E.-Zellfaktor durch Autosensibilisierung gegen cytoplasmatische *Ribo*nucleinsäuren von gelenknahen Bindegewebszellen und gegen interfibrilläre Grundsubstanzen zustande kommt. Nach SVARTZ sind an der Entstehung des „Rheumafaktors" abnorme, vielleicht durch Mikroorganismen verursachte enzymatische Prozesse beteiligt.

Zieht man das Resumé einer Unsumme an bisher geleisteter immunopathologischer Arbeit, so muß man feststellen, daß die echte Antikörpernatur des „Rheumafaktors" trotz aller Ansätze in dieser Richtung bislang *nicht sicher bewiesen* ist. In pathogenetischer Hinsicht hat er vielleicht nur sekundäre, untergeordnete Bedeutung, da er nicht sofort bei Krankheitsbeginn nachweisbar ist. Aus der Tatsache, daß typische Primär-chronische Polyarthritis auch bei Agammaglobulinämie vorkommen kann, wird man mit VAUGHAN, GOOD und ROTSTEIN sogar den Schluß ziehen dürfen, daß γ-Globulin und Rheumafaktor für das klinische Krankheitsbild nicht unbedingt als Conditio sine qua non zu gelten haben.

c) Psoriasis arthropathica

Wie bereits einleitend ausgeführt, würde eine nähere Besprechung der Psoriasis arthropathica den Rahmen des vorliegenden Handbuchbeitrags sprengen, da dieses Krankheitsbild in nosologischer Hinsicht außerhalb der Gruppe der rheumatischen Krankheiten im engeren Sinne steht. Wir haben diese Auffassung kürzlich in einer größeren Arbeit begründet [Arch. klin. exp. Derm. **214**, 622—651 (1962)]

[1] Neuerdings gibt SVARTZ den genauen Sedimentationskoeffizienten dieses Makroglobulins mit S 18,7—18,8 an (1960/61).

Tabelle 1

	Psoriasis arthropathica	Primär-chronische Polyarthritis
Häufigkeitsmaximum des Krankheitsbeginns	3. und 4. Lebensjahrzehnt	bei Männern 4. Lebensjahrzehnt, bei Frauen 4. und frühes 6. Lebensjahrzehnt
Geschlechtsverteilung	fast gleich (analog zur Psoriasis vulgaris)	mehr Frauen als Männer (♀:♂ = 3:1)
Symmetrie der Polyarthritis	meist erst in Spätstadien	meist schon in Frühstadien (70%)
Interphalangeale Prädilektionsgelenke	häufiger distal als proximal	meist proximal, nur selten distal
Beteiligung der Wirbelsäule oder der Sakro-Iliacalgelenke	relativ häufig (zusammen etwa 30%)	selten (Ausnahme Stillsche Krankheit)
Subcutane Knoten	fehlend	relativ häufig vorhanden (15—25%)
Psoriatische Hautveränderungen	fast stets vorhanden, oft atypisch, sehr häufig mit Nagelbeteiligung	in Einzelfällen (gemäß statistischer Erwartung)
Serologischer Nachweis der „Rheumafaktoren“	negativ (selten mit niedrigem Titer positiv)	meist mit hohem Titer positiv (70—95%)

und müssen es uns hier versagen, nochmals auf Einzelheiten einzugehen. Die wichtigsten nosologischen Unterschiede sind aus Tabelle 1 ersichtlich. Im übrigen sei auch auf die neueren Arbeiten von Wright, Coste, Reed und Krebs verwiesen.

d) Reticulo-Histiocytosis disseminata partim arthropathica

Die bisherigen klinischen Erfahrungen über diese seltene Krankheitsform sprechen gegen eine Zugehörigkeit zum Rheumatismus im engeren Sinne. Das klinische und histologische Bild ähnelt in vieler Hinsicht einer Speicherkrankheit, wobei auf Grund histochemischer Befunde an eine Störung des intermediären Lipoid- bzw. Glykolipoid-Stoffwechsels gedacht werden kann. Meist treten die Gelenkerscheinungen erst lange nach dem Aufschießen der cutanen Knötchen auf. Bemerkenswert erscheinen gewisse symptomatologische Analogien zur Psoriasis arthropathica (Einbeziehung der distalen Interphalangealgelenke, Häufung von „Arthritis mutilans“, mitunter Beteiligung der Wirbelsäule). Vollends fragwürdig wird die Beziehung zum Rheumatismus durch die Beobachtung einzelner Fälle *ohne arthropathische Zweiterkrankung* (vgl. Cramer) und durch die Erfolglosigkeit antirheumatischer Therapie mit Corticosteroiden.

Zum gegenwärtigen Zeitpunkt ist die nosologische Stellung des Krankheitsbildes — primäre Stoffwechselstörung oder primäre Entzündung — noch umstritten. Zur Klärung fehlt eine Reihe von diagnostischen Voraussetzungen. Die Einbeziehung spezieller rheumatologischer Untersuchungen — nicht nur lipoidchemischer Serum- und Gewebeanalysen — erscheint in jedem Falle geboten. Bezüglich näherer Literaturangaben verweisen wir auf Graham und Stansfield, Johnson und Tilden, Montgomery u. Mitarb., D. Walther, Lyell und Carr, Baccaredda-Boy und Cramer.

II. Rheumatisches Fieber

Nach den von der American Heart Association angegebenen Kriterien für die Diagnose des Rheumatischen Fiebers[1] zählen zu den *Symptomen I. Ordnung:* Poly-

[1] Diese Kriterien sind niedergelegt in: Circulation **13**, 617—620 (1956) unter dem Titel „Jones' Criteria (modified) for guidance in the diagnosis of rheumatic fever. (Report of the Committee on Standards and Criteria for Programs of Care.)“

arthritis, Karditis, *Erythema anulare, subcutane Knötchen* und Chorea minor. Alle Laboratoriumsbefunde sind dagegen zu den minder pathognomonischen Symptomen II. Ordnung verwiesen. Den Hauterscheinungen des Rheumatischen Fiebers kommt also im Rahmen der übrigen Symptomatologie eine eminente *diagnostische* — und im Hinblick auf rechtzeitige und gezielte Behandlung indirekt auch eine prognostische — *Bedeutung* zu. Dies gilt um so mehr, als die genannten rheumatischen Hautsymptome (und die Chorea minor) wesentlich häufiger bei Kindern als bei (jungen) Erwachsenen vorkommen und somit gerade in diesem Lebensalter eine frühzeitige Einleitung der Therapie zur Vermeidung bleibender, die Lebenserwartung verringernder Schäden äußerst wichtig ist.

Außer dem Erythema anulare Lehndorff-Leiner und den rheumatischen Knötchen, die jeweils eine fast spezifische Bedeutung haben, gibt es noch eine Reihe von Dermatosen, deren Häufung beim Rheumatischen Fieber — oder aber deren eigenständige „rheumatoide" Symptomatologie! — immer wieder dazu geführt hat, ihre echte rheumatische Genese zu postulieren. Hierzu rechnen die Schönlein-Henochsche Purpura („rheumatica"), Fälle von Urticaria („rheumatica"), von Erythema nodosum und von Erythema exsudativum multiforme, um nur die bekanntesten zu nennen. Ihnen allen ist eine *hyperergisch-anaphylaktoide Pathogenese* und ein offenbar polyätiologisches Ursachenspektrum — darunter auch mit *streptogenen* Infekten — gemeinsam, so daß eine relative oder absolute Zunahme beim Rheumatischen Fieber nicht überrascht. Wir fassen im folgenden diese verschiedenartigen entzündlichen Eruptionen als *vorwiegend unspezifische Begleitreaktionen* des Rheumatischen Fiebers zusammen und gehen daher nicht näher auf sie ein. Nur muß man sich darüber im klaren sein, daß in manchen Fällen doch eine spezifisch-rheumatische Basis anzunehmen ist. Dafür sprechen dann vor allem das gemeinsame Auftreten mit typischen rheumatischen Krankheitsmanifestationen, verstärkte allgemeine Aktivitätszeichen der Grundkrankheit, zeitliche Unabhängigkeit von sonstigen, erfahrungsgemäß häufig auslösenden Ursachen (z.B. Medikamenteneinnahme).

1. Vorwiegend unspezifische Begleitreaktionen

a) Allgemeiner Hautstatus beim Rheumatischen Fieber

Auffällig ist zunächst die universelle *Blässe* der Haut, die nur zum geringeren Teil auf einer echten Anämie beruht, wie die Inspektion der Schleimhäute zeigt. An den Extremitätenenden wird oft — als Ausdruck einer latenten peripheren Kreislaufinsuffizienz — eine gewisse livid-cyanotische Verfärbung sichtbar. Bei Myokarditis oder beginnender Herzinsuffizienz pflegen sich diese Kreislaufsymptome noch zu verstärken. Die Hände sind schweißfeucht, im Thenar-Hypothenarbereich manchmal fleckig gerötet. Über den geschwollenen Gelenken erscheint die Haut glänzend und blaß, dabei heißer als in der Umgebung.

Als charakteristisch gilt der eigentümlich säuerliche *Geruch des Schweißes*, der sich allerdings bei Erwachsenen deutlicher als bei Kindern bemerkbar macht (Feer). Diese profusen Schweiße kommen auch unabhängig von der Salicylatbehandlung vor. Nicht selten sind sie von einer überwiegend an Brust und Oberarminnenseiten lokalisierten Miliaria cristallina gefolgt. Bei Kindern kann die Schweißneigung auch fehlen, manchmal ist die Haut in subakuten Krankheitsstadien sogar auffallend rauh und trocken (Fanconi und Wissler).

Mitunter werden akute Schübe von einem *Herpes simplex* (labialis) eingeleitet (Schoen und Tischendorf).

b) Urticaria (rheumatica)

Abgesehen von der gering urticariellen Variante des Erythema anulare Lehndorff-Leiner, die deshalb von manchen Autoren auch „Erythema marginatum" genannt wird, kommt auch eine echte Urticaria („Urticaria gyrata rheumatica" nach Traub) nicht selten vor, besonders in Frühstadien (Canizares). Urticarielle und erythematös-anuläre Schübe können alternierend auftreten; dies soll auf nahe Beziehungen zum eigentlichen Erythema anulare hinweisen (Grenet; Traub;

Keil; Fanconi und Wissler). Campbell, Griffith und Leake fanden auf Grund von Beobachtungen in einem amerikanischen Marinelazarett Urticaria beim Rheumatischen Fieber ungleich häufiger als beim übrigen Krankengut. Dagegen beobachtete Canizares — ebenfalls in einem amerikanischen Militärlazarett des letzten Weltkrieges — nur bei 4 von 233 Rheumatikern (1,7%) urticarielle Schübe. Diese begleiteten die polyarthritischen und sonstigen Krankheitsexacerbationen unter gleichzeitigem Anstieg der BSG und klangen zusammen mit den akuten Symptomen wieder ab.

c) Purpura

Purpurische Eruptionen — oft klinisch ähnlich, aber nur selten pathogenetisch identisch mit der Schönlein-Henochschen Purpura — können auch beim Rheumatischen Fieber aufschießen (Griffith u. Mitchell; Campbell u. Mitarb.) Sie sind ein Ausdruck abnormer vasomotorischer Irritabilität und erhöhter Gefäßdurchlässigkeit, also vasculärer und nicht thrombopathischer Natur. Daß sie beim Rheumatischen Fieber überhaupt nicht vorkommen sollen (Naegeli), wird von Fanconi und Wissler bestritten. Keil sah hämorrhagische Hauterscheinungen sogar bei 10% seiner Patienten. Andere Autoren fanden sie dagegen viel seltener (Swift; Wright; Küster; Canizares). Sie sind subjektiv symptomlos und müssen wegen ihrer Geringfügigkeit gesucht werden. Am ehesten findet man sie in Form von Petechien und kleinen Sugillationen an den Knöcheln und um die Knie, doch gibt es anscheinend keine besondere Vorzugslokalisation. Paunescu-Podeanu und Baltaceanu unterscheiden innerhalb verschiedener „rheumapurpurischer Zustände" beim echten Gelenkrheumatismus eine spezifische und eine unspezifische Purpura.

Unabhängig von purpurischen Efflorescenzen äußert sich eine latente *hämorrhagische Diathese* des Rheumatikers nicht selten in einem positiven Rumpel-Leede-Zeichen, in Epistaxis (wichtiges Frühsymptom!), gelegentlich auch in Mikrohämaturie.

Im allgemeinen klingen die purpurischen Erscheinungen erst nach 3—5 Wochen, oft parallel zum Rückgang des übrigen rheumatischen Schubes ab. Vereinzelt sind sie bereits vor dem Ausbruch anderer rheumatischer Symptome nachweisbar (Canizares). Vielleicht spielen für das zeitweilig gehäufte Auftreten von kleinen Hautblutungen auch epidemiologische Besonderheiten eine Rolle (Chester u. Schwartz). Bei Choreatikern findet man öfters zahlreiche kleine Sugillationen, die auf banale Traumatisierungen infolge der ataktischen Hyperkinese bei vermehrter Gefäßfragilität zurückzuführen sind. Wright weist außerdem auf die zusätzliche Bedeutung einer K-Hypovitaminose hin. Nach seiner Ansicht sind viele hämorrhagische Phänomene beim Rheumatischen Fieber nur die Folge einer toxischen Gefäßschädigung durch Salicylate. Ausgedehnte Sugillationen pflegen auch bei schweren Rheumatismusformen zu fehlen (Fanconi u. Wissler).

Eine prognostische Bedeutung soll purpurischen Eruptionen nach Campbell u. Mitarb. nicht zukommen.

d) Papulöse Erytheme

Unter den dermalen Begleiterscheinungen des Rheumatischen Fiebers ist von manchen Autoren auf eigentümliche papulöse Veränderungen hingewiesen worden. Bei diesen als „simple papular form" bzw. „Erythema papulatum rheumaticum" (Keil), „Erythema papulosum urticatum" (Vilanova, Piñol und Rotés Querol) oder „papular erythema multiforme" (Canizares) bezeichneten Efflorescenzen dürfte es sich jeweils um die gleichen Hautveränderungen handeln. Sie finden sich in symmetrischer und diskreter, mitunter gruppierter Anordnung an den Hand- und Fußrücken, in der Umgebung der Fußknöchel, der Knie- und Ellbogengelenke, bevorzugen also die *Streckseiten* der Extremitäten. Weit seltener treten die Veränderungen an den Beugeseiten oder am Stamm auf (KEIL). Die einzelnen Knötchen sind tiefrot und stecknadelkopf- bis linsengroß. Mitunter besteht zu Beginn ein leichtes Brennen (CANIZARES) oder ein mäßiger Juckreiz. Die papulösen Eruptionen entstehen schubweise und bilden sich binnen weniger Tage bis zu 3—4 Wochen wieder zurück, manchmal unter vorübergehender Hinterlassung einer geringen Pigmentierung. Nach KEIL, der über 14 eigene Beobachtungen (unter 523 Fällen von Rheumatischem Fieber) berichtete, können die Efflorescenzen auch bereits nach wenigen Stunden wieder verschwinden. Anscheinend variiert also die Dauer der Schübe von Fall zu Fall beträchtlich.

Im allgemeinen treten papulöse Erytheme während aktiver Krankheitsphasen auf bzw. sind ein Aktivitätszeichen des Rheumatischen Fiebers (KEIL). Sichere Rückschlüsse auf die Gesamtprognose des Krankheitsprozesses sind aber nicht möglich, auch wenn gelegentlich auf den relativ milden Krankheitsverlauf hingewiesen worden ist (KEIL u.a.). In der Regel sind Kinder und Adoleszente betroffen, nur ausnahmsweise auch Erwachsene (BARLOW).

Differentialdiagnostisch kann die Abgrenzung von fixen Arzneiexanthemen schwierig oder unmöglich sein; doch hält ein so erfahrener Autor wie VILANOVA diese papulösen Efflorescenzen für echte rheumatische Manifestationen. Dafür sprechen auch gelegentliche Beobachtungen von kombiniertem oder alternierendem Auftreten mit „Erythema marginatum" (SEVESTRE; GARROD; KEIL — vgl. unter „*Erythema anulare*").

e) Erythema nodosum

Dieses anscheinend polyätiologische und pathogenetisch vielschichtige Krankheitsbild gesellt sich manchmal einem Rheumatischen Fieber zu. Ein spezifischer Zusammenhang mit dem letzteren ist aber nur selten hinreichend beweisbar (vgl. etwa Fall WALLGREN 1938) und wohl auch nur selten eindeutig gegeben. Immerhin weisen die häufig — auch unabhängig vom Rheumatischen Fieber — deutlich erhöhten Antistreptolysin-O-Titer gegebenenfalls auf *streptogene* Einflüsse und somit auf enge pathogenetische Beziehungen zum rheumatisch-infektiösen Formenkreis hin. Erwähnt sei in diesem Zusammenhang auch das mit „rheumatoiden" Gelenkerscheinungen einhergehende *Löffgren-Syndrom,* ein infektionsallergisches (gelegentlich auch mit dem Morbus Boeck in Verbindung gebrachtes) Krankheitsbild mit bilateraler Schwellung der Hiluslymphknoten, Erythema nodosum und polyarthritischen Erscheinungen.

Hinsichtlich des beim Rheumatischen Fieber gleichfalls häufig auftretenden *Erythema exsudativum multiforme* gelten ähnliche Überlegungen wie beim Erythema nodosum. Ein direkter Zusammenhang mit der Grundkrankheit ist im allgemeinen abzulehnen. Ätiologisch sind meist toxische oder allergisierende Vorgänge beteiligt (Arzneimittelsensibilisierung u.ä.), die auf dem Boden der rheumatisch-hyperergischen Reaktionslage besonders leicht zum Ausbruch kommen. So ist das Erythema exsudativum multiforme meist nur als Komplikation und nicht als Teilmanifestation des Rheumatischen Fiebers anzusehen.

Wahrscheinlich ist auch das von A. MEYER beschriebene „Erythema pustulosum" nichts anderes als eine z.T. ungewöhnliche (Unterarmstreckseiten) lokalisierte und pustulöse Variante eines Erythema exsudativum multiforme, bei dem ja vesiculo-pustulöse Morphen vorkommen können. Von MEYER waren die Efflorescenzen als eine besondere Sepsisform im Rahmen der „rheumatischen Infektion" aufgefaßt worden.

f) Sonstige Hauterscheinungen

Mit den genannten, in der Mehrzahl unspezifischen Begleitphänomenen des Rheumatischen Fiebers ist sicherlich noch keine vollständige Übersicht über das ganze Panorama exanthematischer Veränderungen erreicht. So gibt es z.B. „angioneurotische Ödeme" (SCHLOSS) und morbilliforme oder scarlatiniforme „*rashs*", die sich einer klaren nosologischen Klassifizierung entziehen. Teilweise dürfte es sich nur um flüchtige Arzneiexantheme handeln.

Als Folgeerscheinung des Rheumatischen Fiebers kann u. U. an den Extremitäten eine Livedo racemosa-artige bläuliche Netzzeichnung zurückbleiben, wie sie von GRINSPAN und ZURITA als „*Livedo postrheumatica*" beschrieben worden ist. Im Gegensatz zur echten Livedo racemosa soll dabei ein Reflexerythem fehlen, da die Durchblutungsstörung sowohl auf allgemeine klimatische als auch auf örtliche thermische Reize hin nicht zur Verstärkung, sondern zur Abschwächung tendiert und auch von statischen Lageveränderungen abhängig ist. GRINSPAN und ZURITA schließen daraus auf die Möglichkeit einer bleibenden postrheumatischen Funktionsstörung der vasomotorischen Nerven des betroffenen Gebiets.

2. Erythema anulare Lehndorff-Leiner[1]

[Synonyma: *Erythema anulare rheumaticum* (LEICHTENTRITT). In der angelsächsischen Literatur: *Erythema marginatum (rheumaticum)* (BARLOW u. WARNER), *rheumatic erythema multiforme, flat anular erythema, anular erythema multiforme* (KEIL)]

a) Historischer Rückblick

Sieht man davon ab, die Fülle der seit der antiken Medizin bei „rheumatischen" Beschwerden beschriebenen Hautveränderungen auf ihre in heutiger Sicht *mögliche* Zugehörigkeit zum echten Rheumatismus zu überprüfen (vgl. *Einleitung*), so findet man die ersten, nosologisch klar definierbaren Beschreibungen rheumatischer Erytheme in der ersten Hälfte des 19. Jahrhunderts. So berichtete 1831 R. BRIGHT über ringförmige, als „Roseola annulata" bezeichnete Erytheme im Verlaufe von Sydenhamscher Chorea[2]. Vier Jahre später beschrieb PIERRE FRANÇOIS RAYER in seinem „Traité théorique et pratique des maladies de la peau", im Kapitel über die exanthematischen Entzündungen, eine bei akutem Gelenkrheumatismus vorkommende „*éruption érythémateuse roséolée, fugace*", lokalisiert an Brust und Bauch, gekennzeichnet durch „plaques arrondies ou réunies en placards, à contours festonnés, rougeâtres à la périphérie, sans desquamation, sans prurite". 1862 wies FERRAND im Rahmen seiner Dissertation über rheumatische Exantheme bereits auf die besondere Häufung bei Herzkomplikationen hin. RAYER grenzte das Exanthem auch ausdrücklich von einer Urticaria ab. 1876 — 3 Jahre nach einer weiteren Veröffentlichung im französischen Schrifttum über „Érythème marginé et rhumatisme" von SEVESTRE — griff ERNEST BESNIER in einer umfassenden Arbeit über rheumatische Hautveränderungen auch dieses Thema wieder auf, wobei er bei den akut-rheumatischen Erythemen unter anderem zwischen einer „forme papuleuse" und „formes marginées, en plaques discoides" unterschied (letztere „en lignes sinueuses festonées, généralement de coloration intense à la périphérie")[3]. Dagegen dürften sich unter den von PERROUD (1873) beschriebenen Fällen von „Erysipèle rhumatismal" auch ätiologisch heterogene Exantheme befunden haben.

1881 beschrieben BARLOW und WARNER bei mehreren rheumakranken Kindern und jungen Erwachsenen außer typischen rheumatischen Knötchen ein „*Erythema marginatum* (sive papulatum)", und CHEADLE (1889) sowie GARROD (1890) führten weitere Beobachtungen an, bereits mit dem Hinweis auf das „nicht seltene" Zusammentreffen „... mit Endokarditis und Perikarditis in den schwersten Fällen" (CHEADLE). Noch recht ungenau sind im deutschen Schrifttum die von SINGER (1897) und RIEBOLD (1905) gegebenen Beschreibungen: Beide Autoren schildern zwar „gyrierte, figurierte und urticarielle" Erytheme, grenzen sie aber offensichtlich vom E. exsudativum multiforme und E. nodosum nicht scharf ab. 1913 erwähnte STAMM bei einem kasuistischen Bericht zwar ein „Erythema marginatum", ging aber nicht näher darauf ein.

Erst 1922 beschrieben die Wiener Pädiater HEINRICH LEHNDORFF und CARL LEINER in allen Einzelheiten „*ein typisches Exanthem bei Endokarditis*" unter der Bezeichnung „*Erythema annulare*". Die seither vielfach übliche Benennung nach diesen beiden Autoren ist um so berechtigter, als sie als erste den „pathognomonischen" Zusammenhang mit einer rheumatischen Endokarditis ganz klar erkannten. Ihre Schilderung des Exanthems ist unübertroffen.

In der pädiatrischen Literatur hat sich das E. a. seit den Dreißigerjahren durch Arbeiten von LEHNDORFF, LEICHTENTRITT, RIETSCHEL, WALLGREN, ABT, TRAUB, GRENET, DEBRÉ, PERRY, FANCONI u. WISSLER u. a. einen festen Platz erobert, während es in der Dermatologie

[1] Sprachlich unrichtig ist das Adjectivum a*nn*ulare!

[2] Nach KEIL (1936) geht eine noch frühere Beschreibung auf W. C. WELLS zurück.

[3] Außerdem nannte BESNIER noch die Urticaria, das Erythema exsudativum multiforme, scarlatiniforme und morbilliforme Exantheme sowie das Erythema nodosum. Selbst der Hinweis auf einen dem Pocken-Vorexanthem vergleichbaren „*rash*" fehlte nicht (Einbeziehung des späteren Morbus Still?).

nur wenig beachtet und beinahe sogar vergessen wurde. Einzelne Mitteilungen von CAROL und VAN KRIEKEN, BINDSCHEDLER, URBACH und BLEIER, selbst eine so umfassende Arbeit wie die von KEIL (aus dem Mount Sinai Hospital New York), blieben lange Zeit ungehobene Schätze.

b) Klinisches Erscheinungsbild

So diskret, unscheinbar und flüchtig das E.a. sich auch zeigt, so charakteristisch — geradezu unverwechselbar — ist sein klinischer Aspekt. „Die Schwierigkeit liegt nicht im Erkennen des Exanthems als vielmehr im Finden und im Darandenken" (FANCONI u. WISSLER). Man muß bei Patienten mit Rheumatischem Fieber immer wieder den Stamm absuchen, um schließlich bei manchen dieses sehr eigentümliche Exanthem zu entdecken. Es besteht teilweise nur aus linsen- bis kleinfingernagelgroßen, selten größeren maculösen Erythemen, überwiegend aber aus schmalen, meist nur 2—3 mm breiten Erythemstreifen, die in buntem Wechsel von kreisförmigen oder ovalären *Ringen*, verschieden großen *Kreissegmenten*, polycyclischen und *girlandenförmigen Figuren* auf der Haut ausgebreitet sind. Das Kolorit dieser wie spielerisch, manchmal fast arabesk gezeichneten Erythemmuster entspricht einem zarten, hie und da etwas intensiveren Rot oder Rosa, manchmal mit einem lividen Unterton, der sich bis zu einem leichten Blaugrau verstärken kann. Der Untergrund der Haut ist auffallend blaß. Meist liegt das Exanthem im Hautniveau, läßt sich leicht wegdrücken und ist frei von jeglicher Infiltration. Gelegentlich besteht aber eine angedeutet papulöse oder urticarielle Note, so an einzelnen Rändern[1]. Sehr typisch ist die *Tendenz zu peripherer, ringförmiger „Wanderung"* der Einzelmorphen, wobei sie sich an gegenseitigen Berührungsstellen teilweise auslöschen und so in gyrierte, vielbogig zusammengesetzte Kreisfiguren von Münzen- bis beinahe Kleinhandtellergröße übergehen können. Die von ihnen umschlossenen Hautbezirke erscheinen blaß, manchmal mit einem Stich ins Bräunliche („like chamois skin" — KEIL), aber frei von Schuppung, eigentlicher Pigmentierung oder Atrophie. Juckreiz oder sonstige lokale Mißempfindungen fehlen.

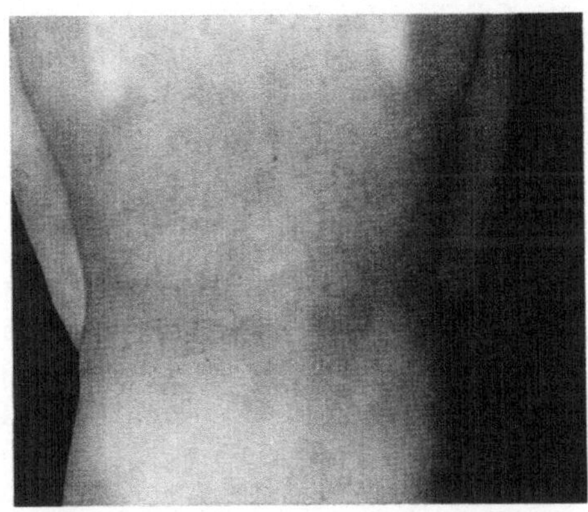

Abb. 1. Erythema anulare Lehndorff-Leiner. Typisch *diskretes* Erscheinungsbild am Stamm mit zartroten, wie mit feinstem Pastell auf den bräunlich-blassen Untergrund der Haut gemalten polycyclischen Kreisbögen und Ringfiguren von wechselnd großem Durchmesser. (Patient der Univ.-Kinderklinik Bonn, Abbildung von Herrn Prof. Dr. HUNGERLAND freundlicherweise zur Verfügung gestellt)

Nicht nur die geometrische Polymorphie, auch die *Flüchtigkeit* und *Variabilität* dieses „kapriziösen" Exanthems (DEBRÉ) ist äußerst charakteristisch. Es pflegt

[1] Die Unterscheidung eines (leicht erhabenen) Erythema marginatum und eines (flachen) Erythema anulare (z.B. bei KEIL) erscheint uns etwas künstlich, da beide Varianten fließende Übergänge aufweisen. („Erythema marginatum" wird allerdings in der angelsächsischen Literatur vielfach synonym für „Erythema anulare" gebraucht.) Auch KEIL, der unter 523 Fällen von Rheumatischem Fieber 15mal „Erythema marginatum rheumaticum" und 24mal „Flat erythema annulare rheumaticum (LEHNDORFF and LEINER)" beobachtete, erwähnt morphologisch ununterscheidbare Zwischenformen, so etwa dann, wenn sich ein Erythema marginatum unter Abflachung zurückbildet. Wahrscheinlich beruht auch die von manchen Autoren betonte, manchmal leicht pruriginöse (KEIL) *urticarielle Erscheinungsform* („Urticaria gyrata rheumatica" nach TRAUB) nur auf einer graduellen Steigerung des E. a. infolge stärkerer entzündlicher Exsudation, abgesehen von den mit stärkerem Juckreiz verbundenen Fällen echter Urticaria beim akuten Rheumatismus.

rasch, oft unbemerkt aufzutreten, dauert nur wenige Stunden bis ein oder zwei Tage (selten länger) und klingt meist etwas langsamer als gekommen wieder ab, manchmal unter kurzdauernder Hinterlassung einzelner kleinmaculöser Erytheme. Die Rezidivneigung ist erheblich, mit Intervallen zwischen Tagen, Monaten, selbst Jahren. Auch der Gesamtverlauf kann mehrere Jahre (COBURN; im Falle URBACHs 12 Jahre) dauern („Dauerexanthem" LEHNDORFFs). Während der einzelnen Schübe ändert sich das Erscheinungsbild oft innerhalb weniger Stunden; kleinfleckige Erytheme breiten sich zu zierlichen Ringen aus, neue Kreisbögen entstehen, andere blassen ab. Manchmal kommt es nur zu flüchtigen roseolären Efflorescenzen; nach FANCONI u. WISSLER handelt es sich vielleicht um Abortivformen des E.a.

Hinsichtlich der *Lokalisation* ist der *Stamm* deutlich bevorzugt (Brust, Bauch, Flanken, Rücken). Manchmal sind auch noch die proximalen Extremitätenanteile (besonders die Oberschenkelinnenseiten) einbezogen, nur selten der Hals oder die Beugeseiten der Unterarme (z.B. bei BINDSCHEDLER, GRENET, DEBRÉ, FANCONI u. WISSLER, HADLEY).

Alleiniges Auftreten an den Armen oder Beinen ist atypisch (MENOZZI; WORINGER u. LUTZ). *Gesicht und Mundschleimhaut bleiben fast stets frei*, nach LEHNDORFF auch die Streckseiten der Extremitäten. Die einzige uns bekannte Ausnahme stammt von MACKENZIE, der bei einem Kind mit tödlichem Krankheitsverlauf vorübergehend auch im Gesicht Hauterscheinungen beobachtete.

Häufig besteht zur Zeit des Exanthems Fieber. Mitunter überdauern die Hauterscheinungen aber dessen Rückgang um Stunden bis Tage und können in seltenen Fällen auch während fieberfreier klinischer Ruhephasen beobachtet werden (FANCONI u. WISSLER; CAMPBELL u. Mitarb.; BURKE). In akuten Krankheitsstadien genügen oft schon psychische Aufregungen, ängstliche Erwartungsspannungen, der Wärmereiz eines heißen Bades, selbst die Menstruation (WALLGREN) zur Verstärkung oder Auslösung neuer Erytheme. Auch in fieberfreien Latenzstadien sind infolge interkurrenter Infekte, Operationen (Tonsillektomie!) oder banaler Traumen wiederholt Rezidive beobachtet worden — ein Hinweis auf das Weiterbestehen der rheumatischen Reaktionslage (LEICHTENTRITT). UV-Bestrahlungen können u.U. die Erytheme zunächst, unter Juckreiz, urticariell umwandeln, dann aber (vorübergehend?) zum Verschwinden bringen (URBACH u. BLEIER).

c) Klinische und prognostische Bedeutung

Für sich allein betrachtet wäre dem Erythema anulare ob seiner spielerischen Flüchtigkeit und subjektiven Beschwerdefreiheit keine wesentliche Krankheitsbedeutung beizumessen. Und doch ist es so charakteristisch, daß es FANCONI und WISSLER geradezu als die „*Visitenkarte*" des echten Rheumatismus bezeichnet haben: „Leider gibt er sie nur in verhältnismäßig wenigen Fällen ab und auch da meist nicht zu Beginn, sondern erst, wenn er sich schon festgesetzt hat." So hat dieses unscheinbare Exanthem in zweifacher Hinsicht Bedeutung: Es gilt als *diagnostisches* Specificum des rheumatischen Grundprozesses (LEICHTENTRITT; WALLGREN; ABT; TRAUB; GRENET; DEBRÉ u. Mitarb.; FANCONI u. WISSLER; PERRY u.a.), und es weist mit fast *pathognomonischer* Sicherheit (LEHNDORFF u. LEINER; SHELDON; RIETSCHEL; WALLGREN; TRAUB; KEIL; FANCONI u. WISSLER u.a.) auf das *gleichzeitige Bestehen einer rheumatischen Herzaffektion* (meist Endokarditis, seltener Myo-, Peri- oder Pankarditis) hin. So fand NATTENHEIMER bei katamnestischen Untersuchungen von 23 Kindern mit E.a. jedesmal eine durchgemachte rheumatische Herzbeteiligung. Das gleiche konstante Zusammentreffen war schon LEHNDORFF u. LEINER, LEICHTENTRITT, GRENET sowie DEBRÉ aufgefallen. Dabei zeigte sich eine eigentümliche Prävalenz des Exanthems für schwere, auch tödlich endende Verlaufsformen, wodurch es die Bedeutung eines Signum mali ominis gewann (LEICHTENTRITT; GRENET; DEBRÉ; KRAMÁR; TRAUB). In FANCONIs Krankengut war innerhalb einer durchschnittlichen Nachbeobachtungszeit von knapp 7 Jahren etwa jeder dritte Patient mit früherem E.a. gestorben. GRENET hatte 4 seiner 8 Patienten mit E.a. verloren. Allerdings stellt die Koinzidenz mit rheumatischer (Endo-)Karditis keine „Conditio sine qua non" dar; so fanden WALLGREN unter 18, TRAUB unter 10 Patienten mit E.a. jeweils einen, BURKE unter 19 fünf, CAMPBELL u. Mitarb. unter 35 neun ohne nachweisliche Herzerkrankung. Nach TARANTA können Chorea minor und E.a. gelegentlich die einzige Manifestation eines Rheumatischen Fiebers sein. Dennoch muß die *Prognose in jedem Falle mit Vorsicht* gestellt werden, da das Endokard doch nur ausnahmsweise verschont bleibt und häufig Herzklappenfehler resultieren. In den letzten Jahren werden die prognostischen Chancen allgemein etwas optimistischer beurteilt; so konnte BURKE (1955) unter 14 Kindern mit früher durchgemachter rheumatischer Karditis und „Erythema marginatum" sechsmal einen normalen Herzbefund erheben. Wahrscheinlich haben die therapeutischen Fortschritte des letzten Jahrzehnts (Rezidivprophylaxe durch Penicillin, Behandlung mit Corticosteroiden und ACTH) entscheidend zu dieser Verbesserung beigetragen.

Häufig stellt sich ein E.a. *erst im Verlaufe* des rheumatischen Krankheitsprozesses ein, oft sogar erst nach dem Höhepunkt eines Schubes. Den Erfahrenen zwingt es dennoch — trotz echter oder nur vorgetäuschter klinischer Besserung — zu erhöhter Vorsicht und laufender Herzkontrolle. Seltener macht sich das E.a. zum Vorläufer des rheumatischen Krankheitsprozesses. Solche Fälle mit Ausbruch kurz vor oder zu Beginn des ersten polyarthritischen Schubes (SWIFT; WALLGREN; KEIL; WORINGER u. LUTZ; BURKE), einer Chorea minor (WALLGREN; TRAUB) oder einer Endokarditis (LEHNDORFF u. LEINER; SCHMIDEK; BARCAGLIA; FANCONI u. WISSLER; BURKE; HORNSTEIN) sind mehrfach beobachtet worden. Im allgemeinen ist das E.a. aber kein initiales, sondern ein sekundäres Symptom des rheumatischen Grundprozesses, freilich von hoher diagnostischer und prognostischer Bedeutung: Es ist ganz allgemein ein Ausdruck unverminderter Akuität und Rezidivneigung des Krankheitsprozesses und muß in jedem Falle nach einer Herzbeteiligung fahnden lassen.

Umgekehrt, d.h. von der Gesamtheit rheumatischer (Endo-)Karditiden aus betrachtet, muß man allerdings feststellen, daß nur der weitaus kleinere Teil von diesem flüchtig-rezidivierenden Erythem begleitet ist. Jedoch ist eine *Zunahme bei schweren kardialen Verlaufsformen* unverkennbar (LEICHTENTRITT; TRAUB; WALLGREN; FANCONI u. WISSLER). So fand WALLGREN in einem großen Krankengut bei leichten Formen der Endokarditis nur in etwa 8%, bei schweren Formen dagegen in etwa 30% ein E.a., was einem 3—4fachen Anstieg bei den letzteren entspricht. Unter TRAUBs Patienten betrug diese Zunahme sogar fast das Sechsfache. Bei der Chorea minor — einer rheumatischen Encephalitis des extrapyramidalen Systems mit vorwiegend günstiger Gesamtprognose — kommt es dagegen nur relativ selten zu E.a. (nach NATTENHEIMER innerhalb 20 Jahren unter 47 „reinen" Chorea minor-Fällen der Zürcher Kinderklinik nur 3mal, unter 116 „reinen" Polyarthritis-Fällen dagegen 18mal, unter 34 Fällen mit alternierenden Rezidiven von Chorea minor und Polyarthritis wieder nur 2mal; jedesmal aber war das E.a. von einer Herzaffektion begleitet!).

Zusammenfassend muß betont werden, daß auch heute noch — trotz aller therapeutischen Fortschritte — *die Prognose eines Rheumatischen Fiebers mit E.a. quoad sanationem (et vitam) generell vorsichtiger gestellt werden sollte als ohne dieses Exanthem.* Doch wußten schon LEHNDORFF u. LEINER, daß es „auch bei ganz leichten Fällen" vorkommen kann und „gerade bei den schwersten vermißt" wird.

Über seine *Häufigkeit im Rahmen der Gesamtmorbidität an Febris rheumatica* ist nicht leicht ein Urteil zu gewinnen, da die verschiedenen Angaben teilweise erheblich divergieren (FINDLAY 0,57%, CANIZARES 1,7%, GRENET 3%, TRAUB

6%, Keil 7,5%[1], Wallgren 12%, Fanconi u. Wissler 15%, Leichtentritt sogar über 60% — allerdings durchwegs bei schweren Karditisformen!). Sicherlich spielen die Altersverteilung des Krankenguts (bei Kindern häufiger, bei Erwachsenen seltener), die Beobachtungsdauer, die Häufigkeit schwerer Fälle in manchen Kliniken, vielleicht auch klimatische und regionale Einflüsse (Traub), Aufmerksamkeit des Pflegepersonals u.ä. eine Rolle. Denn das E.a. drängt sich der Beobachtung nicht auf, es muß gesucht werden. Wahrscheinlich liegt die durchschnittliche Häufigkeit *etwa bei 10%* (Lehndorff; Feer; Wallgren; Dyer).

Die *Altersverteilung* des Exanthems stimmt mit der des Rheumatischen Fiebers grundsätzlich überein, dürfte also ihren Gipfel etwa um die Wende des 1. zum 2. Lebensjahrzehnt erreichen (vgl. Einleitung). Ein E.a. im 4. Lebensjahr (Schmidek) oder noch früher (Burke) ist daher als große Ausnahme anzusehen. Dagegen kommt es auch bei jugendlichen Erwachsenen vor (Keil; Urbach u. Bleier; Woringer u. Lutz; Canizares u.a.), wie auch die militärmedizinischen Erfahrungen des letzten Weltkriegs, besonders in den USA, gezeigt haben. Eine Geschlechts- oder Konstitutionsgebundenheit besteht offenbar nicht.

d) Nosologische Stellung

Ist das Erythema anulare Lehndorff-Leiner ein spezifisches Exanthem des Rheumatischen Fiebers? Diese Frage ist zunächst allgemein bejaht worden. Allerdings sind inzwischen einige Beobachtungen bekannt geworden, wonach ein typisches E.a. das einzige „rheumaverdächtige" Symptom war und blieb. Bei einem 9jährigen Patienten von Fanconi und Wissler (Fall 53), ebenso bei einem gleichaltrigen Patienten von Winkler, bestand nicht einmal eine Senkungsbeschleunigung, im letzteren Falle lediglich eine chronische Tonsillitis; Burke konnte unter 19 Fällen von „Erythema marginatum" 5mal überhaupt keine rheumatischen Organmanifestationen feststellen: Bei einem 9jährigen mit Bronchiektasien trat es nach zwei Penicillininjektionen(!) auf, bei einem 5jährigen während einer Glomerulonephritis, bei einem 7wöchigen Säugling während einer Dyspepsie (ohne Medikamente), bei einem 7jährigen zur Zeit einer Ascaridiasis, bei einer 3jährigen nach einer Tonsillitis. Fanconi und Wissler sahen mehrfach in der Rekonvaleszenz eines Scharlachs (mit und ohne sog. Scharlachrheumatoid) ein typisches E.a., so einmal am 35. Krankheitstag ohne Temperaturerhöhung, Gelenk- oder Herzsymptome. In einem anderen Falle wechselte ein anuläres Erythem zeitweilig mit charakteristischen Efflorescenzen einer Stillschen Krankheit. Solche Beobachtungen sind im ganzen zwar Ausnahmen geblieben, *schränken aber zweifellos die Spezifität des Exanthems ein.*

e) Differentialdiagnose

α) Erythema infectiosum. Diese (auch mäßig kontagiöse) wahrscheinlich durch ein Virus hervorgerufene Krankheit weist dem E.a. sehr ähnliche, polycyclisch-variabel konfigurierte, etwa eine Woche lang bestehende Erytheme auf („Ringelröteln"). Der Hauptunterschied betrifft die Lokalisation: Schmetterlingsförmiger Beginn im Gesicht (Glanzmann: „Diagnose ins Gesicht geschrieben"), dann Ausbreitung auf die Streckseiten der Glieder (besonders Unterarme), dagegen nur selten auf den Stamm. Das Exanthem kann leicht infiltriert sein. Das Allgemeinbefinden ist nur gering beeinträchtigt, selbst Temperaturerhöhung kann fehlen.

β) Erythema anulare centrifugum Darier. Die großbogige und leicht erhabene Konturierung der Kreisfiguren, die bräunlich-livide, wie vergilbt aussehende Verfärbung und gelegentliche feinlamellöse Schuppung der davon umschlossenen Hautbezirke, die protrahiertere Ausbreitung ermöglichen eine rasche klinische Unterscheidung. Auch bleibt das Allgemeinbefinden fast unverändert. Das mittlere Lebensalter ist bevorzugt.

[1] „Erythema marginatum" und „Flat erythema annulare" zusammengerechnet (39 von 523 Patienten). Die Gesamtzahl aller „rheumatischen Erytheme" beläuft sich im Krankengut von Keil auf 53 (10%). Nicht einbezogen sind in diese Zahl verschiedenartige hämorrhagische Eruptionen (53), scarlatiniforme Eruptionen (8), echte Urticaria (7) und Erythema nodosum (5).

γ) **Erythema chronicum migrans.** Die Chronizität des Fortschreitens, der große, gelegentlich den ganzen Rücken einnehmende Durchmesser der leicht infiltrierten Erytheme, gegebenenfalls eine Zeckenbißanamnese sind diagnostisch wegweisend.

δ) **Anuläres sekundärsyphilitisches Rezidivexanthem.** Vor einer Verwechslung schützen die Gleichmäßigkeit der Einzelmorphen, ihr etwas kleinerer Durchmesser und bräunlich-erythematöser Unterton, die häufige Beteiligung der Handteller und Fußsohlen sowie weitere klinische Symptome einer Lues II (die aber mit Temperaturerhöhung und ausgesprochen „rheumatoiden" Beschwerden einhergehen kann).

ε) **Cutis marmorata.** Sie bevorzugt die Extremitäten und weist eine gleichbleibende netzförmige, nicht anuläre Zeichnung auf. Noch deutlicher zeigt ein *Erythema caloricum*, das bei antirheumatischer Lokalbehandlung mit heißen Kataplasmen beobachtet werden kann, ein grobbalkiges und weitmaschiges, die tiefcutanen Gefäßplexus nachzeichnendes bräunlich-erythematöses Netzwerk.

ζ) **Urticaria gyrata.** Der vorhandene heftige Juckreiz bietet meist eine Unterscheidungsmöglichkeit gegenüber dem E. a., das gelegentlich ein leicht urticarielles Aussehen annehmen kann.

η) **Toxische oder allergische Exantheme.** Bei anulärer Konfiguration und flüchtigem Verlauf können sie erhebliche differentialdiagnostische Schwierigkeiten bereiten; so sah BURKE bereits bei einem 7 Wochen alten Säugling mit Dyspepsie (ohne Medikamenteneinnahme!) ein 5 Tage dauerndes typisches E. a. an Stamm und Beinen, bei einem 7jährigen Jungen mit Ascaridiasis ebenfalls ein solches seit 2 Jahren intermittierend auftretendes Exanthem (unabhängig von Medikamenteneinnahme!). Im allgemeinen lassen sich aber arzneibedingte u. ä. Exantheme durch stärkere Polymorphie und Rötung der Efflorescenzen, durch Bevorzugung der Acren und distalen Extremitätenabschnitte, durch ein häufig vorhandenes Enanthem, gegebenenfalls auch mit Hilfe eines Expositionsversuchs, erkennen.

ϑ) **Trypanosomiasis („Schlafkrankheit").** Bei dieser durch Trypanosoma gambiense (oder rhodesiense) hervorgerufenen, besonders in West-Afrika endemischen Protozoenkrankheit können eigentümlich *circinäre Erytheme* auftreten („Érythème en placards", „Érythème circiné" nach DARRÉ), die in verschiedener Hinsicht dem Erythema anulare, besonders seiner leicht erhabenen Variante, ähneln, zumal sie meist auf den Stamm beschränkt sind, morphologisch ähnliche Kreisfiguren beschreiben, meist kurzlebig oder doch variabel sind und keine subjektiven Beschwerden verursachen (DARRÉ). Auch gilt das Exanthem als ein Frühsymptom der Krankheit, wenngleich es auch in späteren, von schweren Alterationen des ZNS beherrschten Krankheitsstadien vorkommen kann. Die Beachtung der übrigen klinischen Symptome (unter anderem variable Ödeme, nuchale Lymphknotenschwellungen, furunkelartige Schwellungen an der Stelle von Insektenstichen), der mikroskopische Nachweis der Flagellaten im dicken Tropfen und natürlich auch die spezielle geographisch-epidemiologische Situation sind für die Diagnose maßgebend.

ι) **Exantheme des Morbus Still und des Wissler-Fanconi-Syndroms.** Hierzu sei auf die entsprechenden Kapitel (jeweils unter „Differentialdiagnose") verwiesen.

f) Histopathologie

Der erste histologische Befund eines E. a. wurde 1935 von CAROL u. VAN KRIEKEN aus der Amsterdamer Hautklinik mitgeteilt. Auch KEIL (1938) und CAMPBELL (1946) gehen kurz auf das Gewebsbild ein. In den letzten Jahren haben GREITHER (1957), HORNSTEIN (1958, 1961) und GRIMMER (1961) weitere Untersuchungen veröffentlicht. Ein kurzer histopathologischer Hinweis — als Vergleich zum Exanthem der Stillschen Krankheit — findet sich auch bei ISDALE und BYWATERS (1956) sowie bei ALLEN (1954).

Der Vergleich der einzelnen Befunde lehrt, daß es zur richtigen histologischen Interpretation des wechselhaften klinischen Bildes besonders auf den Zeitpunkt und die Entnahmestelle der Excision ankommt; so erklären sich einige Detailunterschiede in den jeweiligen Beschreibungen. Man kann aber auch im gleichen Excisat, sofern es groß genug ist und *quer zur Ausbreitungsrichtung der erythematösen Ringe* verläuft, alle histomorphen Phasen des Entzündungsablaufs nebeneinander finden (HORNSTEIN), so daß sich etwa folgender zeitlicher „Längsschnitt" ergibt:

Hauptsächlicher Reaktionsort ist der subpapilläre Gefäßplexus bis zu den anschließenden „Venolengabeln", also der postcapillare Schenkel der Endstrombahn im oberen Corium. Hier kommt es — wahrscheinlich nach einer flüchtigen

Hyperämie der vorgeschalteten Arteriolen und Capillaren — zu einer anfänglichen Vasodilatation, die (offenbar im Zusammenwirken mit arteriolärer Konstriktion) zu verlangsamter Blutströmung führt und so eine *Diapedese von neutro- und*

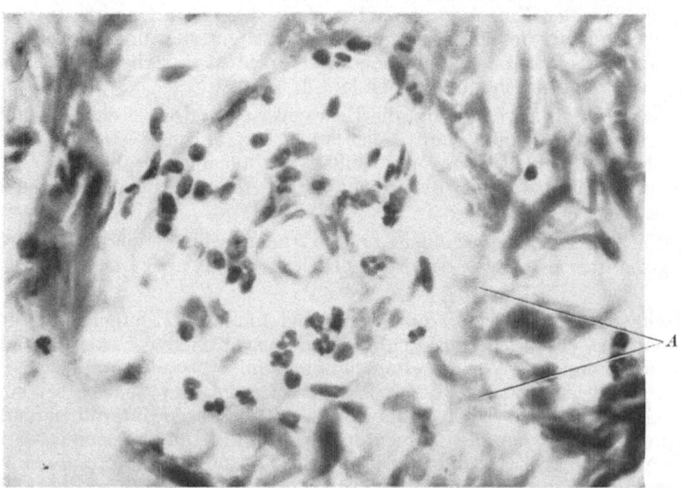

Abb. 2. Erythema anulare Lehndorff-Leiner. Gewebsschnitt, van Gieson, 600mal vergr. — Frühphase der Entzündung im subpapillaren Gefäßplexus: noch relativ weites Gefäß mit Endothelschwellung; im circumvasalen Lymphraum Ödem und emigrierte neutrophile Granulocyten. *A* verquollenes kollagenes Bindegewebe in Gefäßnähe, im Schnitt gelb-orange angefärbt. [Aus O. Hornstein: Hautarzt **9**, 120—125 (1958)]

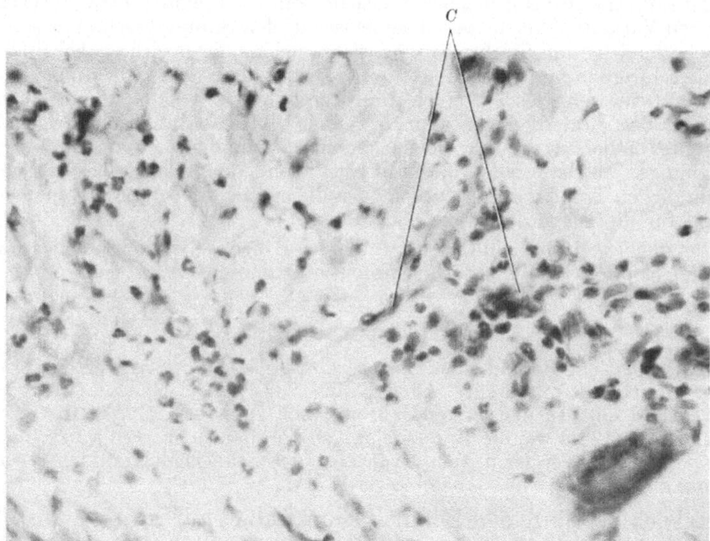

Abb. 3. Erythema anulare Lehndorff-Leiner. Gewebsschnitt, HE, 360mal vergr. — Höhepunkt der exsudativen Entzündung: deutliches Gewebsödem mit granulocytärer Infiltration auch in der entfernteren Gefäßumgebung. *C* durch Endothelschwellung scheinbar verschlossene Capillarlumina. Rechts unten ein schräg getroffener Schweißdrüsenausführungsgang. [Aus O. Hornstein: Hautarzt **9**, 120—125 (1958)]

einzelnen eosinophilen Granulocyten aus der Blutbahn in die Umgebung ermöglicht. Die Plasmaexsudation bleibt relativ gering und führt nur zu leichter „*Verquellung*“ *des gefäßnahen Bindegewebes* (Abb. 2), keineswegs aber zu „fibrinoider Nekrose“. Es folgt eine lockere *granulocytäre Infiltration* des circumvasalen Bindegewebes, während die Gefäße selbst jetzt *Engstellung und Endothelschwellung* zeigen

(Abb. 3). Die am weitesten emigrierten Granulocyten weisen zuerst *Kernzerfall* auf, der dann auch bei den übrigen einsetzt. Es kommt also nicht sofort zur Leukocytoklasie, auch fehlen Hämorrhagien vollständig. Vergleicht man mit den bisherigen Entzündungsphasen nun Gewebsbezirke *innerhalb* der erythematösen Kreisbögen, über die also das Exanthem teilweise schon „gewandert" ist, so ergibt sich eine Wandlung des Befundes: die Gefäßlumina sind wieder deutlich sichtbar oder leicht erweitert, die Granulocyten samt Kerntrümmern sind verschwunden, es besteht lediglich noch eine *geringe lympho-monocytoide uncharakteristische Proliferation* des circumvasalen Mesenchyms (Abb. 4). Wahrscheinlich handelt es sich dabei um Resorptionsvorgänge. Auch die oberflächlichen Lymphgefäße sind etwas

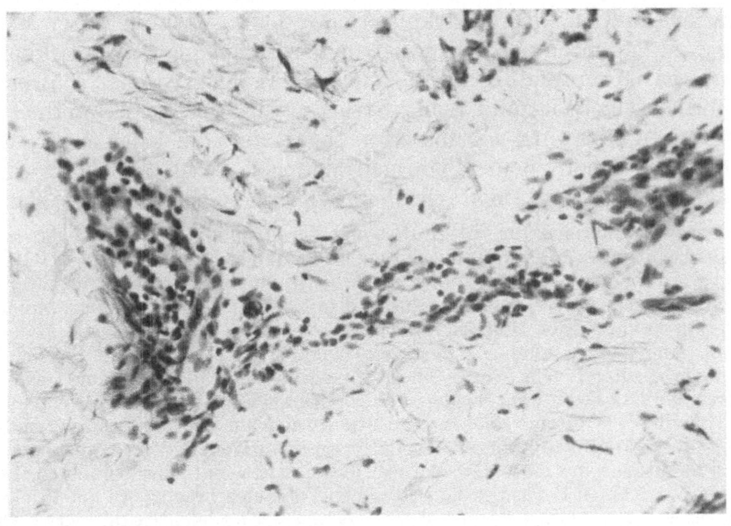

Abb. 4. Erythema anulare Lehndorff-Leiner. Gewebsschnitt, HE, 210mal vergr. — Rückbildungsphase der Entzündung: geringe lympho-histiocytoide Proliferation des circumvasalen Mesenchyms; keine Granulocyten mehr nachweisbar; Gefäßlumina teilweise wieder offen. [Aus O. Hornstein: Hautarzt 9, 120—125 (1958)]

erweitert, sonst aber unverändert. Auffällig ist dagegen eine gewisse Vermehrung von Gewebsmastzellen im Corium. Die Epidermis bleibt fast unbeteiligt, kann aber stellenweise (Greither) etwas Acanthose und Parakeratose aufweisen.

Dieser aus histologischen Einzelphasen „rekonstruierbare" Entzündungsablauf zeigt, daß das E.a. ein *„unspezifisches" gewebliches Substrat* aufweist. Ansätze zur Granulombildung fehlen, sie wären bei der Flüchtigkeit des Exanthems auch gar nicht zu erwarten. Einige Unterschiede in den histologischen Befunden dürften sicher, wie schon erwähnt, von der Bestehensdauer des gerade excidierten Herdes und von graduellen Schwankungen der entzündlichen Exsudation abhängen; so fand Greither nur eine lympho-histiocytäre Entzündung ohne Granulocyten, also das Bild der Sekundärphase. Isdale u. Bywaters verglichen dagegen das entzündliche Substrat sogar mit dem der Schönlein-Henochschen Purpura, nur ohne Erythrocytenaustritte. Carol und van Krieken beschrieben zwar gleichfalls die granulocytäre Infiltration, aber nicht die (manchmal nur geringe) Karyorrhexis der Infiltratzellen. Auf diesen Kernzerfall der Entzündungszellen wies zuerst Keil hin. Grimmer fand bezirksweise eine außerordentlich starke Erweiterung der Gefäße mit verstärkter Blutfülle und — abweichend von allen sonstigen Befunden — eine geringe Erythrodiapedese in circumvasale Lymphräume.

g) Pathogenese

Der Schwerpunkt der ersten Arbeiten über das E.a. (LEHNDORFF u. LEINER; LEICHTENTRITT; LEHNDORFF) lag mehr auf diagnostischem und prognostischem als auf pathogenetischem Gebiet. Doch hatten bereits LEHNDORFF und LEINER eine mikrobiell-metastatische Genese des Exanthems — entgegen einer damals noch weit verbreiteten Auffassung vom Wesen „septischer“ Hautveränderungen — bezweifelt. Einen wesentlichen pathogenetischen Gesichtspunkt brachte WALLGREN (1935), indem er das E.a. als „*Angioneurose auf rheumatisch-allergischer Basis bei bestimmten hochempfindlichen Individuen*“ ansah. Einen ähnlichen Standpunkt vertrat BINDSCHEDLER TRAUB zog außerdem hinsichtlich der rheumatisch-allergischen Reaktionsbasis des Exanthems Vergleiche mit dem Generalisationsstadium der Tuberkulose oder Lues. DEBRÉ, LAMY u. JAMMET gelang bei zwei Patienten der Nachweis von vergrünenden Streptokokken aus der Blutkultur, was sie veranlaßte, auf fließende Übergänge zwischen schweren Rheumatismusformen einerseits und Lenta-Sepsis sowie Stillscher Krankheit andererseits hinzuweisen. IACCHIA sah das E.a. sogar als Vorzeichen einer drohenden Sepsis an, da er es bei einem 12jährigen Mädchen — im Anschluß an mehrere Zahnextraktionen — vor Ausbruch einer septischen Endokarditis beobachtete.

Besonders aufschlußreich für die Aufklärung der Ätiologie und Pathogenese des E.a. waren die Beobachtungen, die WINKLER an einem 9jährigen Jungen mit seit 3 Jahren rezidivierendem E.a., aber ohne (sonstige) rheumatische Organmanifestationen machte. Das Kind bot lediglich einen reduzierten Allgemeinzustand mit chronischer Tonsillitis, ohne Beschleunigung der Blutsenkung oder Blutbildveränderungen. Nach Tonsillektomie klang das E.a. zunächst ab. Aus hämolysierenden und vergrünenden Streptokokken, die sich aus dem Tonsillengewebe züchten ließen, wurde eine Autovaccine hergestellt. Bereits nach der ersten Injektion erschien das Exanthem wieder und konnte auch später in gleicher Weise beliebig reproduziert werden. Während solcher Rezidive wurden im Rachenabstrich wiederholt die gleichen Streptokokken nachgewiesen (wiederum mit antigener, d.h. exanthemauslösender Wirkung nach Autovaccination). Der Beweis, daß das E.a. auf einer echten *AgAk-Reaktion* beruht, wurde durch einen Prausnitz-Küstnerschen Versuch erbracht: An der Injektionsstelle entstand sofort ein akuter Entzündungsherd, der am 6. Tag leicht rezidivierte, am 12. Tag nach einer zweiten Injektion sich in ursprünglicher Stärke wiederholte und sich dann in ein derbes indolentes Knötchen umwandelte. Histologisch ließ sich eine schwere Entzündung mit starkem Ödem und vermehrter granulocytärer Infiltration nachweisen.

Wenn auch durch WINKLERs Experiment bewiesen wurde, daß eine *AgAk-Reaktion* beim E.a. von entscheidender Bedeutung ist, so erklärt sie doch noch nicht die anuläre Konfiguration der Morphen. Diese und der flüchtige Verlauf des Exanthems weisen auf *zusätzliche Faktoren von seiten der terminalen Strombahn bzw. deren Gefäßnervensystem* hin. Auch die Verstärkung durch psychische, thermische, neurovegetative und hormonale Einflüsse deutet in die gleiche Richtung. WALLGREN hatte dementsprechend von einer „Angioneurose“ gesprochen.

Auf der Grundlage der bisherigen klinischen, histologischen und immunbiologischen Beobachtungen läßt sich daher etwa folgende Vorstellung über die Pathogenese des E.a. formulieren (HORNSTEIN 1958):

Das E.a., fast stets im Rahmen des akuten Rheumatismus auftretend, beruht auf einer *flüchtigen AgAk-Reaktion im Bereich der cutanen terminalen Strombahn*. Das histologische Abbild dieser spezifischen Reaktion(en) erscheint zwar — wie immer beim geweblichen Substrat allergisch-hyperergischer Entzündungen — relativ „unspezifisch“, entspricht im wesentlichen aber dem frühen anaphylaktoiden Reaktionstyp einer hyperergischen Entzündung im Sinne LETTERERs, wenn auch in verhältnismäßig blander Form. Da im Prausnitz-Küstnerschen Versuch eine (auch histologisch) schwere Entzündung nachzuweisen ist (WINKLER), muß das relativ geringe Ausmaß des Exanthems von *modifizierenden Faktoren* abhängen. Hierzu rechnen wir — gerade auch im Hinblick auf das flüchtigerythematöse, anulär wandernde Erscheinungsbild — überwiegend constrictorische Tonusschwankungen und passagere Spasmen der präterminalen kleinen Arterien und Arteriolen, wodurch die Blutgefäße gedrosselt werden, die reagible Menge des hämatogen herangeführten Antigens mit den (z.T. zellständigen?) Antikörpern im Bereich der Endstrombahn reguliert und so das Ausmaß der örtlichen AgAk-Reaktion verringert wird („gelenkte Allergie“ nach KLINGE u. Mitarb.). Bekanntlich ermöglicht gerade die anatomische Architektur der cutanen arteriellen Gefäßplexus (mit anastomosierenden „Candelaber-Arterien“) über vasomotorische Tonusschwankungen rasche funktionelle Verschiebungen der peripheren Blutverteilung. Möglicherweise werden beim E.a. die vasoconstrictorischen Impulse selbst bereits initial, zu Beginn der AgAk-Reaktion, ausgelöst, wobei die hyperämisch-entzündliche Reaktionsphase gewissermaßen nach dem Rand der sich rasch vergrößernden ischämischen Zone „abgelenkt“ wird. Jedenfalls vermag die Vorstellung einer derart „dosierten“ und vom örtlichen Gefäßnervensystem gesteuerten hyperergischen Reaktion die klinischen Phänomene pathophysiologisch gut zu erklären. Im übrigen weist auch die Tatsache, daß nur der kleinere Teil der rheumatischen Herzpatienten vom E.a. befallen wird, auf besondere individual-pathologische Einflüsse — so von seiten des vegetativen Nervensystems — hin.

Nach unserer Ansicht beruht also das E.a. auf einer *flüchtig-exsudativen AgAk-Reaktion im subpapillaren Gefäßplexus*, die hinsichtlich ihrer Quantität und klinischen Ausbreitung anscheinend *vom Gefäßnervensystem der vorgeschalteten Strombahn in charakteristischer Weise modifiziert* wird.

h) Therapie

Eine separate Behandlung des E.a. wäre unsinnig — und im übrigen kaum erfolgversprechend, da meist weder Corticosteroide oder ACTH, noch Salicylate oder Antihistaminica eine *direkte* Wirkung auf das Exanthem erkennen lassen (BURKE). Die Therapie hat nur dem rheumatischen Grundprozeß als solchem zu gelten, mit dessen Rückgang meist auch die Hauterscheinungen abklingen. Im Hinblick auf die fast stets vorhandene Herzbeteiligung — auch bei trügerischem Wohlbefinden — ist es sehr wichtig, auf die Einhaltung strikter Bettruhe zu achten.

3. Nodi (sive Noduli) rheumatici

[Synonyma: *Nodi rheumatosi*, *Nodosis rheumatica* (STRAUSS), *Meynetsche Knötchen* (besonders im französischen Schrifttum), *Rheumatismus nodosus* (REHN), *rheumatische Sehnenknötchen*, *parartikuläre (subcutane) Knötchen* u.a.]

a) Historischer Rückblick

Obwohl die subcutanen rheumatischen Knötchen eigentlich die sinnfälligste, weil makroskopisch wahrnehmbare Form des Rheumagranuloms sind, gehören sie zu den klinischen Manifestationen des Rheumatischen Fiebers, die erst relativ spät die Aufmerksamkeit der Ärzte auf sich gelenkt haben. Vielfach gilt P. MEYNET als Erstbeschreiber, nachdem er 1875 der Medizinischen Gesellschaft von Lyon einen 14jährigen Knaben mit akuten polyarthritischen Schüben, Endokarditis und multiplen periartikulären und periostalen, rapid aufschießenden und wieder verschwindenden Knötchen vorstellte. Aber schon 1868 gab der amerikanische Pädiater HILLIER in seinem Lehrbuch der Kinderkrankheiten eine Beschreibung solcher Knötchen[1]. Wenn dennoch die besonders im französischen Schrifttum geläufige Benennung nach MEYNET für die Knötchen des Rheumatischen Fiebers zu Recht besteht, so wegen der ihm zu verdankenden klaren Zuordnung zum akuten Rheumatismus. Die später viel gebrauchte

[1] Zum Teil gehören hierher wohl auch die sog. „*rheumatischen Schwielen*“ des Unterhautzellgewebes, wie sie der Berliner Arzt ROBERT FRORIEP 1843 im Rahmen seiner „Beobachtungen über die Heilwirkung der Electricität“ beschrieben hat.

Bezeichnung „Rheumatismus nodosus“ geht auf den deutschen Pädiater H. REHN zurück, der sie in seinem Rheumatismusbeitrag zum Handbuch der Kinderheilkunde von GERHARDT (1878) wählte. Die erste histologische Beschreibung stammt von BANG (1876), dann von BARLOW und WARNER (1881); eine erneute histologische Darstellung gab BANG im Anschluß an eine klinische Abhandlung von HIRSCHSPRUNG (vier Beobachtungen). Übrigens diagnostizierten auch BARLOW und WARNER schon 1875 bei einem Kind rheumatische Knötchen; 1881 konnten sie auf dem internationalen medizinischen Kongreß in London bereits über 27 Patienten zwischen $4^1/_2$ und 18 Jahren berichten.

Die erste Beschreibung bei einem Erwachsenen gaben die beiden Dermatologen E. TROISIER u. L. BROCQ (1881), die über einen 45jährigen Mann berichteten, bei dem sich nach einem akuten polyarthritischen Schub mit Endokarditis und Pleuritis multiple erbsen- bis haselnußgroße, sehr schmerzhafte Knötchen an Stirn, Hinterhaupt und beiden Ohrmuscheln entwickelten.

Bezeichnend für das damals in der französischen Medizin (insbesondere in der Dermatologie) außerordentlich rege Interesse an Problemen des Rheumatismus sind Veröffentlichungen von DAVAINE („Contribution à l'Histoire du Rhumatisme; Oedème rhumatismal; Nodosités éphémères rhumatismales du tissu céllulaire sous-cutané“, 1879), FÉRÉOL (1879, 1883), TROISIER (1881) und BROCQ (1884), in denen sehr eingehend die klinische Phänomenologie der subcutanen Rheumaknötchen erörtert wird. So trennt BROCQ unter diesen „nicht-erythematösen“ Rheumaknoten scharf zwischen einem „ephemeren cutanen“ und einem „subcutanen“ Typ. Die Exaktheit der klinischen Beschreibung macht auch heute noch die Lektüre dieser Arbeiten interessant.

Diese und andere Untersuchungen gaben den Anstoß, daß sich in den folgenden Jahrzehnten — noch vor der 1904 durch ASCHOFF und GEIPEL erfolgten histologischen Entdeckung der rheumatischen Granulome im Herzmuskel — eine rege Kasuistik und Diskussion über die Rheumaknötchen und ihre prognostische Bedeutung entwickelte. Dabei ergab sich die eigenartige Feststellung, daß diese Knötchen von englischen Ärzten sehr häufig gefunden wurden, während sie in den USA — auch in den Nordstaaten — lange Zeit als ausgesprochene Rarität galten. Erst in den letzten 25—30 Jahren ist diese Ansicht unter dem Einfluß der Arbeiten von BRENNEMANN, WALLACE, MERRITT, ANDERSON u.a. grundlegend revidiert worden.

Im *dermatologischen* Schrifttum ist den Nodi rheumatici verhältnismäßig wenig Beachtung geschenkt worden. Zwischen den Veröffentlichungen von BROCQ und der Beschreibung einer rein cutanen Aussaat von rheumatischen Knötchen durch ROSENBERG (1934) besteht eine erstaunlich große Lücke. Um so mehr konzentrierte sich das Interesse auf die „juxtaartikulären Knoten“ luischer und anderer Genese. Auch seither sind klinische und histologische Beiträge zum Thema (einschließlich der Knoten der Primär-chronischen Polyarthritis) nur relativ selten von dermatologischer Seite erfolgt (KUMER u. LANG; MATRAS; GRAUER; SUTTON-SUTTON; HAMPEL; MOHRMANN; GOTTRON; HOLTZ; HORNSTEIN u. SCHUERMANN; RUITER u.a.).

b) Klinischer Lokalbefund

Um Nodi rheumatici (N.rh.) zu finden, muß man daran denken, ihre Prädilektionsstellen kennen und systematisch — nach ihnen suchen. Manchmal springen sie sichtbar etwas über die Haut vor, oft sind sie aber nur bei sorgfältiger Palpation zu erfassen. Meist handelt es sich um *multiple, reiskorn- bis kirschkerngroße Knötchen,* die sich kugelig, ovoid oder kegelförmig anfühlen und entweder lose in der *Subcutis* liegen oder einer (osteo-periostalen) Unterlage breitbasig oder nur stielartig (z.B. an Sehnenscheiden, Gelenkkapseln) aufsitzen. Gelegentlich kommen auch größere (bis über kirschgroße) oder kleinere, kaum noch fühlbare (hanfkorn- oder stecknadelkopfgroße) Gebilde vor. Die Konsistenz ist meist gleichmäßig *derb,* bisweilen bei größeren Knoten infolge partieller Erweichung etwas fluktuierend, umgekehrt bei (seltener) sekundärer Verkalkung steinhart. Häufig besteht nur geringe oder gar keine Schmerzhaftigkeit, was die Auffindung erschweren kann. Seltener wird über heftigen Spontan- oder Druckschmerz geklagt.

Topographisch bevorzugt sind ganz allgemein solche Körperregionen, die ein relativ spärliches Fettpolster aufweisen und mechanischen Insulten leichter ausgesetzt sind, so die *Umgebung von Sehnenscheiden, Gelenken, Knochenvorsprüngen und größeren Periostflächen.* Dementsprechend findet man N.rh. besonders an den *Streckseiten* der großen und kleinen Extremitätengelenke *(Ellenbogen, Knie,*

Knöchel, Hand- und Fußrücken), seltener entlang der vertebralen Dornfortsätze, des Darmbein- und Schulterblattkamms, der Tibia, im Bereich der Galea aponeurotica (occipital, retroauricular, frontal) oder des Sternums. Gelegentlich kommen sie auch im medialen Sulcus bicipitalis, über dem M. trapezius, selbst an Palmar- und Plantaraponeurosen vor und können dann zu Verwechslungen mit cubitalen Lymphknoten, Myogelosen, rachitischen Exostosen, Hygromen usw. führen. Auffällig ist die Tendenz zu *bilateral-symmetrischer* Verteilung.

Da während polyarthritischer Schübe die Gelenke in semiflektierter Schonstellung gehalten werden und die paraartikulären Gewebe kollateral entzündlich geschwollen sind, lassen sich die Knötchen manchmal erst bei *forcierter Flexion* nachweisen. Durch diesen Kunstgriff kann man gegebenenfalls auch noch schrotkorngroße Noduli tasten.

Meist treten die Knötchen *schubweise* und *rezidivierend* zu mehreren auf, über den Gelenken manchmal gruppiert, über der Wirbelsäule einzeln oder perlschnurartig aufgereiht. Sie pflegen rasch, oft „über Nacht" aufzuschießen und ebenso schnell oder etwas langsamer wieder zu verschwinden. So können sie Tage, Wochen, manchmal Monate in wechselnder Größe und Konsistenz nachweisbar sein. Persistenz über mehr als ein Jahr beobachteten FINDLAY sowie CAMPBELL u. a. Die Zahl der Knötchen variiert von Fall zu Fall und auch während der verschiedenen Schübe beträchtlich. Manchmal sind nur einzelne (z. B. an den Ellenbogen und Fußknöcheln), dann wieder eine Vielzahl vorhanden. In Einzelfällen sind mehr als 60 gefunden worden (FRENCH: 150!). Im allgemeinen liegen sie voneinander getrennt, können bei längerem Bestehen aber zu schrotbeutelartigen Konglomeraten verbacken und (sehr selten) unter Entleerung kreidig-krümeliger Massen nach außen durchbrechen (GOTTRON). Infolge reaktiver verruköser Mitwucherung der Epidermis ergeben sich dann u. U. diagnostische Schwierigkeiten. Meist verschwinden die Knötchen aber spurlos, ohne klinisch nachweisbare Sklerosierungen oder Narben zu hinterlassen.

Gewöhnlich bleibt die Haut über den N.rh. gut verschieblich und verändert ihre Farbe nicht wesentlich. Bei oberflächlichem Sitz können die Knötchen u. U. mit dem Corium verschmelzen. Das ist besonders bei den „ephemeren" Noduli im Sinne von TROISIER, FÉRÉOL und BROCQ der Fall.

c) Allgemeine nosologische Hinweise

α) Häufigkeit. Generell läßt sich sagen, daß rheumatische Knötchen häufiger beim Rheumatischen Fieber als bei der Primär-chronischen Polyarthritis und innerhalb des ersteren wiederum häufiger bei Kindern als bei Erwachsenen vorkommen. Dennoch stellen sie ein zumindest sehr inkonstantes, nach manchen Autoren sogar ein relativ seltenes Symptom dar. Den größten Prozentsatz gab DAWSON mit 50—60%, dann STILL mit 27,5% an. ANDERSON sah Knötchen bei etwa 15% aller klinisch behandelten Kinder unter 14 Jahren, MERRITT bei 11,5%, INGERMAN und WILSON bei 11%, FINDLAY bei 10%. Hingegen fanden CERKOVNAJA und ŠKRUDNEVA unter 530 kindlichen Rheumatikern nur 34 (6,4%), CAMPBELL, GRIFFITH u. LEAKE (in einem US-Marinelazarett) unter 835 Patienten nur 46 (5,5%), EDSTRÖM (in einem internistischen Krankengut) unter 850 Patienten wiederum 92 (10,8%) betroffen. Nach MOLL differiert die Häufigkeitsskala zwischen 2 und 37%. Ebenso stimmen die Ansichten darüber nicht überein, ob N.rh. beim Rheumatischen Fieber seltener oder häufiger als das Erythema anulare vorkommen.

Mehrere Faktoren dürften für diese statistischen Divergenzen von besonderer Bedeutung sein: Vor allem die Dauer der Beobachtungszeit und die Altersverteilung des Krankenguts. So wies bereits STILL darauf hin, daß bei fast der Hälfte seiner unter 12 Jahre alten *klinisch* behandelten Patienten N.rh. gefunden wurden, gegenüber 30% sämtlicher Fälle mit choreatischen, kardialen und polyarthritischen Manifestationen und gegenüber nur 10% der ambulant betreuten Fälle. Andererseits konnte CANIZARES bei jungen, an Rheumatischem Fieber erkrankten Soldaten in einem amerikanischen Lazarett des letzten Weltkrieges nur in 1,2% subcutane Knötchen feststellen.

Außer altersbiologischen Unterschieden ist es aber auch wichtig, ob die Patienten von Anfang an oder erst im weiteren Verlauf des Krankheitsprozesses in klinische Beobachtung kommen. So machte HANSEN besonders darauf aufmerksam, daß N.rh. als Frühsymptom nur in 2,5%, als späteres Symptom aber in 20% seiner Fälle vorkamen (ähnlich, aber weniger groß ist auch die Differenz zwischen früh und spät auftretenden Exanthemen). Außerdem gibt es auch eigentümliche, vielleicht von besonderen epidemiologischen Bedingungen abhängende Jahresschwankungen im Auftreten rheumatischer Knötchen, worauf früher besonders angelsächsische Autoren hingewiesen haben.

β) Disposition. Eine Konstitutions- oder Geschlechtsprävalenz für das Auftreten von N.rh. beim Rheumatischen Fieber besteht anscheinend nicht. Wahrscheinlich leisten aber alle resistenzmindernden *äußeren* Einflüsse (ungünstiges soziales Milieu, Unterernährung, Verspätung der Behandlung usw.) infolge ihrer ungünstigen allgemeinen Auswirkung auf den Verlauf aller rheumatischen Krankheiten indirekt auch dem Auftreten von N.rh. Vorschub. Die Altersdisposition deckt sich mit der des rheumatischen Grundprozesses, der seinen Gipfel zwischen dem 8. und 14. Lebensjahr erreicht, neuerdings aber auch schon vor dem 4. Lebensjahr beobachtet wird (KÖTTGEN u. CALLENSEE; EWERBECK u.a.). Ganz außergewöhnlich dürfte allerdings der von THALHAMMER mitgeteilte Fall eines 7 Monate alten Säuglings sein, der neben einem auf Endokarditis verdächtigen Herzbefund lediglich zahlreiche (zeitweilig bis 64) N.rh. aufwies.

d) Diagnostische Bedeutung

Wie schon erwähnt, zählen die subcutanen Knötchen zu den *Kardinalsymptomen* des Rheumatischen Fiebers. Nach den Richtlinien der American Heart Association verleiht bereits der Nachweis dieses und eines weiteren diagnostisch gleichrangigen Symptom (Polyarthritis, Karditis, Chorea minor, Erythema anulare) der Diagnose Rheumatisches Fieber hohe Wahrscheinlichkeit. Vielfach treten die pathognomonischen Knötchen aber erst *im Verlauf der rheumatischen Schübe* auf und lassen dann den klinischen Verdacht zur Gewißheit werden. Dabei ist der klinische Höhepunkt der Exacerbation oft schon überschritten (FANCONI u. WISSLER). Weit seltener setzen sich die Knötchen an den Krankheitsbeginn oder treten bereits im Intervall zwischen dem auslösenden Streptokokkeninfekt und dem typischen Ausbruch des Rheumatischen Fiebers in Erscheinung.

In seltenen Fällen können subcutane Knoten die *einzige akut-rheumatische Manifestation* im Kindesalter bleiben („Rheumatismus nodosus“)[1] (BERKOWITZ; COATES u. COOMBS; NAVARRO; KEIL; ZIEGLER; TIZARD; THALHAMMER; TARANTA; DRAHEIM u. Mitarb.). Häufig bestehen in solchen Fällen aber gewisse Hinweise auf die unterschwellige rheumatische Reaktionslage (vorausgehende Strepto-

[1] GOTTRON wendet sich gegen den Terminus „Rheumatismus nodosus“, der die nosologische Verselbständigung eines Krankheitssymptoms vortäusche, und möchte ihn lieber durch „Nodi rheumatosi“ o.ä. ersetzt wissen. Auch FANCONI und WISSLER kritisieren die Bezeichnung aus ähnlichen Gründen. Was den Rahmen des akuten Rheumatismus betrifft, so ist diesen Einwänden völlig beizustimmen. Allerdings gibt es beim chronisch-rheumatischen Formenkreis mitunter klinisch und anatomisch monosymptomatisch bleibende „Rheumaknoten“, für die der besonders von FAHR, KLINGE und WEHSARG begründete Begriff „Rheumatismus nodosus“ noch Gültigkeit beanspruchen kann.

kokkeninfekte, beschleunigte BSG, flüchtige Gelenkschmerzen usw.). Da es bislang noch keinen rheuma-*spezifischen* Labortest gibt, muß sich die Diagnose auf derartige Indizien und vor allem auf den histologischen Befund stützen.

In einer Arbeit über „rheumatic-like nodules" bei 9 nicht-rheumatischen Kindern berichtet BEATTY, daß diese Knötchen hinsichtlich Lokalisation (Sehnenscheiden der Hand, Tibiakante, Fascia temporalis, Galea aponeurotica, Fußknöchel) und Gewebsbild von eindeutigen N.rh. nicht zu unterscheiden waren. Als Ursache werden ungewöhnliche Reaktionen auf Traumen diskutiert. Wahrscheinlich handelt es sich hier um monosymptomatische „Rheumatismus nodosus"-Formen im Sinne der älteren Literatur.

e) Prognostische Bedeutung

Seit den Untersuchungen von BARLOW und WARNER (1881), CHEADLE (1887) und besonders von BERKOWITZ (1913) aus der v. Pfaundlerschen Klinik (München), die unter 78 Kindern mit N.rh. 69mal entzündliche Herzbeteiligung feststellte, weiß man um die ernste prognostische Bedeutung der N.rh. Sie signalisieren noch regelmäßiger als das Erythema anulare Lehndorff-Leiner das Bestehen einer *rheumatischen Karditis*, von deren Ausgang ja meist die Prognose quoad sanationem et vitam abhängt. Das Auftreten dieser ominösen Knötchen *deutet fast stets auf eine Verschlechterung des Krankheitsgeschehens hin.* Hauptsächlich sind sie bei schweren und *langen* Krankheitsverläufen, dagegen weit seltener bei kürzeren oder foudroyant-deletär verlaufenden Formen des Rheumatischen Fiebers zu beobachten (BRENNEMANN; BRONSON; MERRITT; GIBSON u.a.). Dabei besteht eine gewisse Affinität zu *schweren* Herzerkrankungen (meist als Endo- oder Pankarditis, nur selten als alleinige Myokarditis), während bei milden Formen selten Knötchen vorkommen (GRENET; NATTENHEIMER; FANCONI u. WISSLER; KEIL; GIBSON; BALDWIN u. Mitarb. u.a.). So werden die — an sich banalen — Knötchen gewissermaßen zum *kardiopathischen Stigma.*

Die Häufigkeit des gleichzeitigen Bestehens einer rheumatischen Herzaffektion liegt nach den Angaben der Literatur zwischen 88—100%. So fand BERKOWITZ eine Herzbeteiligung bei 69 von 78 Kindern mit N.rh., MERRITT bei 24 von 25, HAYES und GIBSON bei 167 von 173, CERKOVNAJA und ŠKRUDNEVA ohne Ausnahme bei 34 Kindern. Ebenso lückenlosen Herzbefall, z.T. als Pankarditis mit episodischem Vorkommen von N.rh., beobachteten andere Autoren, allerdings bei zahlenmäßig kleinerem Krankengut (WALLACE 15, ZWEIG 8, LEICHTENTRITT 16, FANCONI u. WISSLER 15 Fälle).

Bei Erwachsenen kommt die Syntropie mit rheumatischen Kardiopathien anscheinend weniger gesetzmäßig vor. So fanden CAMPBELL u. Mitarb. unter 835 an Rheumatischem Fieber erkrankten Marinesoldaten zwar 46mal N.rh., doch bestand nur bei knapp $^{2}/_{3}$ dieser Fälle eine Herzaffektion; sie war allerdings meist schwer.

Die *Mortalität* — meist infolge akuter oder chronischer Herzinsuffizienz — ist bei Kindern *erschreckend hoch.* Von 167 Patienten verloren HAYES und GIBSON 52 (31%), von 90 SCHLESINGER 36 (40%), von 34 CERKOVNAJA und ŠKRUDNEVA 13 (etwa 38%), von 15 FANCONI und WISSLER 8 (über 50%), letztere innerhalb einer Nachbeobachtungszeit von 7 Jahren. Dabei scheint das Zusammentreffen von N.rh. und Erythema anulare besonders ungünstig zu sein (NATTENHEIMER). HAYES und GIBSON fanden bei zusätzlichen N.rh. eine Verdoppelung der Mortalitätsquote gegenüber der Gesamtheit aller Kinder mit rheumatischer Kardiopathie. Sie betonen auch, daß die Prognose eines Rheumatischen Fiebers mit Erythema anulare allein noch wesentlich besser sei als mit N.rh.

Rheumatische Knötchen sind natürlich nicht nur mit Karditis, sondern mindestens ebenso oft auch mit gleichzeitigen polyarthritischen Schüben kombiniert. Dagegen finden sie sich weit seltener bei Chorea minor und anderen rheumatischen Organmanifestationen. BERKOWITZ stellte zwar in der früheren Literatur die Kombination N.rh./Chorea minor bei

39% der Patienten fest, doch wurde dies von späteren Autoren in dieser Höhe nicht mehr bestätigt. So fand Nattenheimer N.rh. in 10% der polyarthritischen Verlaufsformen (gegenüber 16% Erythema anulare) und nur in 2% der choreatischen Erkrankungen (gegenüber 6% Erythema anulare). Anscheinend wird die Prognose der Chorea minor auch beim Hinzutreten von rheumatischen Knötchen nicht wesentlich verschlechtert (Nattenheimer). Entscheidend bleibt im allgemeinen die Schwere der Herzbeteiligung.

Da seit Einführung der modernen antirheumatischen Prophylaxe und Therapie mit Penicillin und Corticosteroiden die *schweren* Karditiden eindeutig seltener geworden sind (Köttgen u. Callensee; Graser; Hall u.a.) — während die Beteiligung des Herzens am rheumatischen Grundprozeß im ganzen nicht abgenommen hat (Köttgen u. Callensee) —, erhebt sich die Frage, ob sich auch die düstere kardiale Prognose der Noduli aufgehellt hat. Zwar sieht man heute rheumatische Knötchen (und Erythema anulare) seltener als früher (Graser), was gleichfalls für den Rückgang der malignen Verläufe spricht, doch ist damit die Frage nach ihrer *individuellen* Prognose noch nicht beantwortet. Wahrscheinlich wird das Problem dadurch noch kompliziert, daß mit der Präzession des Rheumatischen Fiebers in den letzten Jahrzehnten gerade im frühen Kindesalter die kardialen Manifestationen zugenommen haben (Ewerbeck u.a.). Eine genaue Klärung steht wohl noch aus, auch wenn man weiß, daß die Frühprognose des Rheumatischen Fiebers (mit weniger als 2% Mortalität) heute wesentlich besser als noch vor 10 Jahren ist (Hall) und auch die Spätprognose mit dem Risiko der rheumatischen Herzkrankheit durch ausreichende Prophylaxe der Rezidive mit Penicillin weiter gebessert werden kann[1].

f) Differentialdiagnose

Im Grunde ist das Auftreten von N.rh. *im Rahmen des Rheumatischen Fiebers* so pathognomonisch, daß differentialdiagnostisch nicht viel in Betracht kommt. Daher beschränken wir uns darauf, einige Verwechslungsmöglichkeiten nur zu erwähnen: cartilaginäre Exostosen, Heberdensche Knötchen, verkalkte Atherome, traumatische Epithelcysten, Granuloma anulare, subcutane Knoten einer Periarteriitis, sog. Sehnenscheidenganglien, Sehnenscheidenfibrome, nodöse oder noduläre Herde von Calcinosis universalis, sog. Glomustumoren, subcutane Neurinome, Leiomyome usw. Von allen diesen Veränderungen bzw. Teilmanifestationen verschiedenartiger Grundkrankheiten lassen sich auf Grund der übrigen klinischen Kriterien die N.rh. meist klar abgrenzen. Im Zweifelsfall dürfte das charakteristische histologische Bild der Knoten den Ausschlag geben.

Nur das *Granuloma anulare* bedarf einer kurzen differentialdiagnostischen Erörterung, und zwar einerseits im Hinblick auf abortive Rheumatismusformen mit *monosymptomatischen* N.rh., andererseits wegen des außerordentlich *ähnlichen Gewebsbildes*. Vom letzteren her ist eine sichere Unterscheidung gar nicht möglich; wenn man beim Granuloma anulare die schärfere Trennung von fibrinoider Nekrosezone und umgebendem Granulationswall als Unterscheidungsmerkmal ansehen will, so ist dem entgegenzuhalten, daß es sich wahrscheinlich nur um die Folge eines längeren Bestehens handelt. Wir haben wiederholt frisch aufgetretene Granuloma anulare-Herde untersucht, die von N.rh. ähnlicher Bestehensdauer rein histomorph und auch histochemisch nicht eindeutig zu unterscheiden waren.

[1] Sicherlich dürfte der Pessimismus Kissels, der in den ersten Jahrzehnten dieses Jahrhunderts 40 Kinder mit zeitweiligen N.rh. sämtlich ad exitum kommen sah, unter heutigen medizinisch-sozialen Verhältnissen nicht mehr begründet sein. Es wäre aber ebenso ungerechtfertigt, auf Grund verschiedener Beobachtungen von monosymptomatisch-nodulären „formes frustes" die prognostische Bedeutung rheumatischer Knötchen zu verharmlosen (Navarro, Argentinien). Bei diesem Problem sind auch wohl geographische und klimatische Einflüsse zu berücksichtigen, da Streptokokkeninfekte (und damit das Rheumatische Fieber als Streptokokken-Allergie) in den tropischen und subtropischen Zonen relativ selten vorkommen.

Lediglich der schichtmäßig meist (nicht immer) höhere, cutane Sitz der Herde ermöglicht gegebenenfalls eine Abgrenzung.

So ist die Differentialdiagnose des Granuloma anulare rein klinisch noch leichter als histologisch, da das noduläre bis kleintuberöse, perlfarben-grau schimmernde Erscheinungsbild der Einzelmorphen, die Tendenz zu ringförmiger Gruppierung und die lange Persistenz meist genügende Anhaltspunkte geben. Hinsichtlich der Lebensaltersverteilung, der Prädilektionsstellen, der Symmetrie und der Schmerzlosigkeit bestehen aber auffällige Parallelen mit den rheumatischen Knötchen.

Aus differentialdiagnostischen (und nosologischen) Gründen erscheint auch ein vergleichender Hinweis auf die subcutanen Knoten der *Primär-chronischen bzw. „Rheumatoiden" Polyarthritis* angebracht. Bei dieser Krankheit sind die Knoten meist größer (bis walnußgroß) und weniger zahlreich vorhanden (mitunter nur in der Einzahl); auch persistieren sie bei klinisch inaktiven, stationären Krankheitsverläufen manchmal jahrelang. Die Prädilektionsstellen beschränken sich meist auf die oberen Extremitäten (Ellenbogen, Ulnarkanten!); die beim Rheumatischen Fieber ebenfalls häufige Lokalisation an den Knöcheln und am Hinterhaupt fehlt meist. Im übrigen haben die Knoten nicht die prognostische Bedeutung wie beim Rheumatischen Fieber.

g) Histologie

Das histomorphe Substrat der N.rh. weist die wesentlichen Kriterien des rheumatischen Granuloms auf, wie sie einleitend beschrieben worden sind und daher hier keiner Wiederholung mehr bedürfen. Je nachdem, wie lange die Knötchen vor der Excision bestanden haben, kann der Grad der granulomatösen Proliferation verschieden sein. Meist bilden sich in ihnen nur kleinere, sero-fibrinös durchtränkte Verquellungsnekrosen des Bindegewebes aus, wobei nur ein Teil der kollagenen Fasern zerstört erscheint. Das zellig-entzündliche Moment kann im ganzen etwas zurücktreten, dann finden sich lediglich lockere großzellig-histiocytäre Proliferate an den Rändern und relativ spärliche lympho-monocytoide Ansammlungen um stehengebliebene „Gefäßinseln" (Abb. 5). Dieser letztere Befund gilt sogar als besonders typisch (Collins, Bennett, Zeller u. Bauer u.a.). Die ausgeprägte und großflächige Koagulationsnekrose, wie sie in den größeren Knoten der Primär-chronischen Polyarthritis und manchmal auch in lange bestehenden Granuloma anulare-Herden vorzukommen pflegt, wird in den Knötchen des Rheumatischen Fiebers oft vermißt. So erklärt sich auch ihr bisweilen verblüffend schnelles Verschwinden, das offenbar auf rascher Resorption bei noch wenig fortgeschrittener Gewebszerstörung beruht.

Man muß sich hüten, die subcutanen akuten Rheumaknötchen mit den eigentlichen Aschoff-Geipelschen Granulomen, wie sie im Herzmuskel und subendo-perikardial gefunden werden, gleichzusetzen. Bei diesen bewirkt die resorptive Begleitreaktion auf mitzerstörte Muskelfasern gewisse Besonderheiten im Granulomaufbau mit organspezifischem Auftreten von sog. Kardiohistiocyten bzw. Anitschkow-Zellen (v. Albertini). Auf diese Unterschiede hat schon Symmers aufmerksam gemacht.

h) Pathogenese

Entsprechend dem Wandel der pathogenetischen Auffassungen über das Rheumatische Fieber haben sich auch die Vorstellungen über die formale und kausale Genese der N.rh. geändert. Brocq dachte als Ursache noch an eine temporäre Überfüllung der örtlichen Lymphgefäße, da ein von ihm beobachteter Patient zur gleichen Zeit am Hals einen dicken Lymphstrang aufwies. Barlow dagegen sah die Knötchen für identisch mit den rheumatischen Vegetationen auf den Herzklappen an und hielt ihre Pathogenese durch Embolie von kardialen Fibrinthromben für geklärt, sofern die gleichen Mikroben hier wie dort gefunden würden. (Bekanntlich hat sich dieses Postulat bis heute nicht beweisen lassen; die ganz vereinzelt von Leichtentritt u.a. gezüchteten Viridansstreptokokken sind Ausnahmefälle geblieben.) Lange Zeit wurde eine teils bakteriell-embolische, teils toxisch-reaktive Genese vertreten (Roy; Berkowitz u.a.), bis schließlich vor etwa 30 Jahren — hauptsächlich unter dem Einfluß der Arbeiten Klinges und seiner Schule — die Lehre von der hyperergisch-allergischen Entstehung aller rheumatischen Organmanifestationen sich Bahn gebrochen hat.

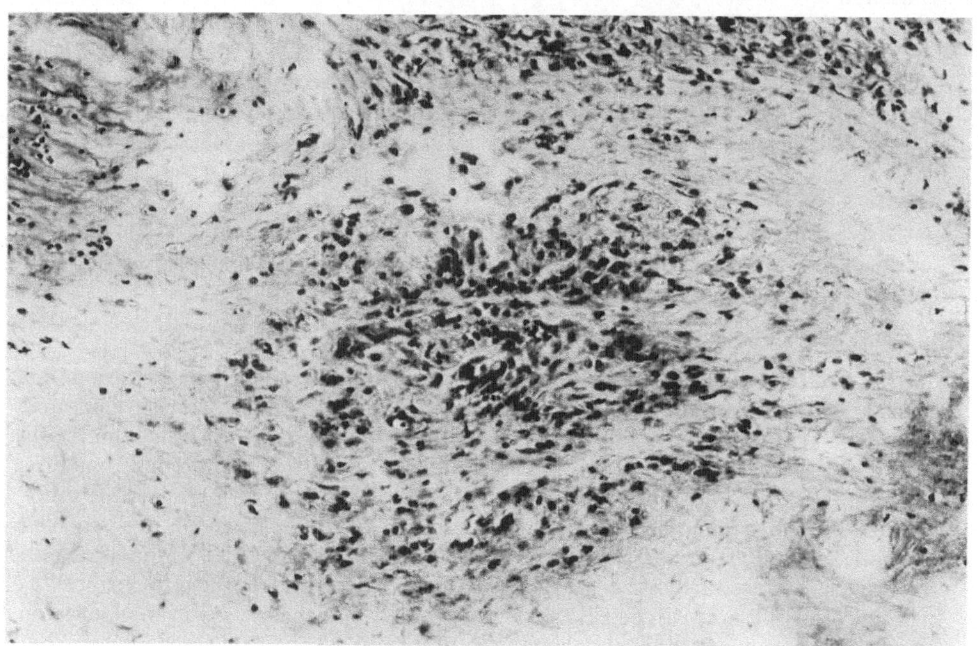

Abb. 5. Nodulus rheumaticus bei Rheumatischem Fieber. Gewebsschnitt, HE, 135mal vergr. — „Gefäßinseln" mit umgebender lympho-histiocytärer Entzündung inmitten zell- und strukturarmer fibrinoider Bindegewebsnekrose. Am oberen Bildrand Granulationsgewebe vom Rand der Nekrosezone erkennbar. Keine typische palisadenförmige Anordnung des Granulationsgewebssaumes

Wenn damit auch der Fundamentalprozeß der rheumatischen „Reaktionskrankheit" geklärt ist (vgl. Einleitung), so bleibt doch noch die Frage zu beantworten, wie sich gerade die cutan-subcutane Lokalisation der Rheumaknötchen erklärt. Die Art der Prädilektionsstellen (Akrolokalisation! Symmetrie!) läßt einerseits an traumatogene Faktoren, andererseits auch an Einflüsse der regionalen Durchblutung und ihrer zentralnervösen Steuerung denken. So hat besonders Ricker im Rahmen seiner relationspathologischen Betrachtungsweise zentralnervösen, vasomotorisch-vegetativen Impulsen eine entscheidende Bedeutung für die Entstehung der N.rh. — und darüber hinaus der ganzen Bouillaudschen Krankheit — beigemessen. In interessanten Versuchen haben Massell, Coen und Jones zeigen können, daß es durch subcutane Injektionen von Blut rheumatischer Patienten in einem großen Prozentsatz gelingt, rheumatische Knötchen bei den Patienten zu induzieren, und zwar in Abhängigkeit von der Aktivität des Rheumatischen Fiebers[1]. Auch mit Hyaluronidase-Injektionen ließen sich z. T. Knötchen erzeugen.

[1] Im übrigen hat Küster (1954/57) in ähnlichen Versuchen einen „Nekrosefaktor" im Serum von Patienten mit Rheumatischem Fieber nachgewiesen.

Nach GOTTRON soll für das Auftreten der rheumatischen Knötchen auch eine gewisse familiäre Disposition bzw. eine „genmäßige Voraussetzung" von Bedeutung sein. Auch LEICHTENTRITT wies auf eine hereditäre Belastung in Einzelfällen hin. Es erscheint uns aber fraglich, ob die in erster Linie für die Primär-chronische Polyarthritis erwiesene erbliche Basis auch auf spezielle Teilmanifestationen des chronischen und akuten Rheumatismus ausgedehnt werden kann.

i) Therapie

N.rh. bedürfen im allgemeinen keiner lokalen Behandlung, da sie mit dem Rückgang der rheumatischen Krankheitsaktivität meist von selbst verschwinden. Ausnahmsweise persistierende, örtlich störende Knoten können exstirpiert werden.

III. Chronische Polyarthritis des Kindesalters

[Synonyma: *Juvenile or childhood rheumatoid arthritis* (MORSE), *Rheumatoid disease* (ELLMANN-BALL), *Rheumatoid arthritis, juvenile type* (New York Rheumatism Association), *Stills disease, Poliartrite cronica anchilosante giovanile* u.a.m.]

Vorbemerkung

In etwa 4—5% der Fälle tritt der chronische Rheumatismus bereits im Kindesalter auf (COSS u. BOOTS; FANCONI; KLINKE u.a.)[1]. Bei rund zwei Dritteln der Fälle entwickelt er sich ähnlich torpid und reaktionsträge wie meist im Erwachsenenalter, *bei einem Drittel aber verläuft er unter subakuten bis akuten, oft schweren Allgemeinerscheinungen.* Diese letztere Variante wird nach dem eigentlichen Erstbeschreiber auch als Stillsche Krankheit bzw. als Stillsches Syndrom (SACREZ u. JUIF; SCANO; SPODICK u.a.) bezeichnet. Im kontinental-europäischen Schrifttum wird neuerdings noch das sog. Wissler-Fanconi-Syndrom abgegrenzt (s. unten), während in den angelsächsischen Ländern eine solche Unterscheidung nicht gemacht wird und vielfach sogar die ursprüngliche Abgrenzung des Morbus Still von der „juvenilen rheumatoiden Arthritis" wieder aufgegeben worden ist.

Hinsichtlich familiärer Belastung (COSS u. BOOTS; JOHNSON u. DODD; KELLEY; KLINKE; TOUMBIS, ANSELL, BYWATERS u. LAWRENCE), überwiegend negativer Streptokokkenätiologie und uncharakteristischer Vorgeschichte bestehen *Analogien zur adulten Primär-chronischen Polyarthritis.* Auch die Bevorzugung der Mädchen ist deutlich, zumindest bei der schleichenden Verlaufsform. Bei der Stillschen Krankheit im engeren Sinne ist das Geschlechtsverhältnis ausgeglichener (KLINKE). Im Gegensatz zur akuten Febris rheumatica treten beide Krankheitsformen häufig *schon in früher Kindheit*, gelegentlich bereits in der Säuglingsperiode auf (VERDURA; FANCONI; KLINKE u.a.) und sinken bis zur Präpubertät nur leicht, dann aber jäh ab (KÖTTGEN u. CALLENSEE). (Postpuberal erfolgt wieder ein allmählicher Anstieg der Morbidität.) SCHLESINGER u. Mitarb. (1961) fanden ausgesprochene Häufigkeitsgipfel des Krankheitsbeginns im 2. und 4. Lebensjahr, COSS und BOOTS bei den Mädchen im 2. und 3., bei den Knaben sogar im 1. Lebensjahr.

Hinsichtlich des allgemeinen klinischen Bildes, dessen Darlegung den Rahmen dieses Handbuchbeitrags überschreiten würde, sei auf die entsprechende pädiatrische Literatur verwiesen (vgl. Schrifttum). Nur auf eine erst in jüngster Zeit bekanntgewordene und uns

[1] Nach den Untersuchungen von GAUCHAT und MAY werden in den USA jährlich etwa 1200 Neuerkrankungen bei Kindern unter 15 Jahren festgestellt, was umgerechnet einer Morbidität von 3 auf 100000 Kindern entspricht. Diese Zahl ist etwa die gleiche wie beim kindlichen Diabetes mellitus und bei der kindlichen (Lipoid-)Nephrose.

wichtig erscheinende Feststellung darf am Rande hingewiesen werden: Eine *ankylosierende Spondylitis* und *Sacro-Iliitis* kommt im Kindesalter nicht so selten vor, wie bisher angenommen wurde. Nicht weniger als 48 der 202 von CARTER untersuchten Kinder (23,7%) zeigten eine Sacro-Iliitis, davon 21 in schwerem Ausmaß. Das typische Erscheinungsbild der Spondylarthritis ankylopoetica ist im Kindesalter jedoch extrem rar (DEBRÉ-LELONG). Solche und andere, schon seit langem bekannte Beobachtungen unterstreichen die besonders von pädiatrischer Seite verfochtene Forderung, den chronischen Rheumatismus der Kindheitsperiode — trotz mancher Übergänge in das Erwachsenenalter und mancher Spätrezidive (vgl. ZIFF, CONTRERAS u. MCEWEN) — als einen Rheumatismus eigener Prägung zu betrachten.

1. Wissler-Fanconi-Syndrom

[Synonyma: *„Subsepsis hyperergica“* (WISSLERs ursprüngliche Bezeichnung), *„Subsepsis allergica“* (FANCONI, WISSLER), *„Pseudosepsis allergica“* (DENYS), *Wissler-Fanconische Krankheit, Wisslersche Krankheit*]

Vorbemerkung

1943 wurde das Krankheitsbild von WISSLER als besondere Verlaufsform des kindlichen chronischen Rheumatismus beschrieben. Der Zahl der bis Ende 1961 veröffentlichten europäischen Beobachtungen — über 70 — nach zu schließen, ist es ziemlich selten (oder selten diagnostiziert). Im angelsächsischen Schrifttum hat es sich bisher nicht eingebürgert; entsprechende Fälle werden dort wahrscheinlich dem Rheumatischen Fieber zugerechnet (FERRIER u. MÉGEVAND). Beide Geschlechter sind etwa gleich häufig beteiligt, das erste Lebensjahrzehnt (abgesehen von dem fast nie betroffenen Säuglingsalter) ist bevorzugt.

a) Allgemeines klinisches Bild

Es ist durch die *Trias von „septischen“ intermittierenden Fieberschüben, flüchtigen Exanthemen und* (meist später folgenden) *variablen Gelenkerscheinungen* charakterisiert, außerdem durch eine erhebliche *Leukocytose* mit Linksverschiebung, aber meist *ohne Eosinopenie.* Blutkulturen sind praktisch immer steril. Die BSG ist stets deutlich beschleunigt. Erhöhungen des Antistreptolysin-O-Titers über die obere Normgrenze kommen — im Gegensatz zum Rheumatischen Fieber — nur in Einzelfällen vor. Peri- und Myokard sind manchmal (relativ benigne) beteiligt, dagegen nie das Endokard. Obwohl die Krankheit *rezidivierend* über Wochen bis mehrere Monate geht, bleibt das Allgemeinbefinden der Patienten meist relativ gut. Jahrelange, ständig remittierende Verläufe sind selten (DENYS; GARBY; GRISLAIN; KLINKE). Meist endet die Krankheit mit vollständiger Ausheilung; Todesfälle sind nur ganz selten beschrieben worden; Übergänge in schwere chronische Polyarthritis kommen aber zu etwa 10% vor (WISSLER 1958; KLINKE u.a.).

b) Ätiologie und Pathogenese

Hierüber bestehen noch erhebliche Unklarheiten. WISSLER hat seine ursprüngliche Vermutung einer oligobakteriellen hämatogenen Streuung („Subsepsis“) mit hyperergischer Reaktion inzwischen etwas korrigiert zugunsten der Annahme einer *überschießenden infektionsallergischen Reaktionsform* auf uneinheitlicher ätiologischer Basis. Streptokokkenantigene, eine Primärtuberkulose (im Falle von BALLOWITZ, FLEISCHHAUER und LOESCHKE mit außerordentlich hoher Tuberkulinempfindlichkeit), Vaccinationen (GRISLAIN u. Mitarb.), selbst vermeintliche „Fokalsanierungen“ können das Krankheitsbild auslösen oder neu entfachen. Eine krankheitsspezifische AgAk-Reaktion konnte bisher nicht nachgewiesen werden. KÜSTER u. POTHMANN diskutieren die Möglichkeit autoimmunologischer Vorgänge, ausgelöst durch verschiedene Vorkrankheiten, z.B. Tuberkulose. Auch Viruskrankheiten (im Falle von ONYSZKIEWICZ-BIELEWICZOWA z.B. Varicellen), aber auch polyvalente nutritive und andere Antigene (NOWAK) können den Pathomechanismus in Gang setzen. Nach Transfusionen sind mehrfach schwere hämolytische Krisen beschrieben worden. Indirekt wird die hyperergisch-allergische und *nicht*-septische Genese auch ex juvantibus bestätigt: Antibiotica und Sulfonamide sind ohne Effekt, Corticosteroide dagegen hochwirksam.

c) Nosologische Stellung

In dieser Hinsicht nimmt das Krankheitsbild, das mit dem von Denys vorgeschlagenen Terminus „Pseudosepsis allergica" wohl am besten umschrieben wird, eine eigentümliche Zwischenstellung zwischen dem akuten Rheumatischen Fieber und der chronischen Polyarthritis des Kindesalters ein (Fanconi). Symptomatologisch gleicht es zwar in mancher Hinsicht dem ersteren, prognostisch (fehlende Endokarditis, aber gelegentlicher Übergang in chronische Polyarthritis) und vom Verlauf her (zeitweilige Milz- und Lymphknotenschwellungen ähnlich der Stillschen Krankheit) ist es aber doch dem *chronisch-rheumatoiden Formenkreis* im Sinne einer Extremvariante zuzurechnen (Wissler; Janbon; Fischer; Küster; Denys; Spartà; Klinke). Dominierend im Vordergrund des teils an eine Sepsis, teils an eine Serumkrankheit erinnernden Krankheitsgeschehens steht gewissermaßen eine anaphylaktoide „Initialzündung" (Wissler), die nur selten vom chronischen Stadium gefolgt ist[1]. Wir haben es hier mit einer ausgesprochenen „*Reaktionskrankheit*" zu tun, gekennzeichnet durch minimale Ursache und maximale, perakute Wirkung.

d) Die Hauterscheinungen des Wissler-Fanconi-Syndroms

Die *klinische Bedeutung* des Exanthems erhellt bereits aus der Feststellung Wisslers, *daß ohne Fieber und Exanthem die Diagnose nicht gestellt werden kann.* Dabei bieten die Einzelefflorescenzen ein weit weniger pathognomonisches Erscheinungsbild als etwa diejenigen des Erythema anulare Lehndorff-Leiner oder auch der Stillschen Krankheit. Das Hauptcharakteristikum des Exanthems ist gerade seine *enorme Polymorphie*, daneben die *Sprunghaftigkeit* und *Flüchtigkeit.* Meist finden sich die Hauterscheinungen vom Krankheitsbeginn an, pflegen fast gleichzeitig mit den kurzen hektischen Fieberstößen aufzutauchen und zu verschwinden, können aber um Stunden (bis wenige Tage) länger dauern und gelegentlich sogar in fieberfreien Intervallen rezidivieren. Polyarthritische Symptome der großen und kleineren Gelenke können hinzutreten, kommen ohne Exanthem aber fast nie vor.

Die *morphologische und topographische Variabilität des Exanthems* — beim gleichen Patienten, oft sogar im gleichen Schub — kann nicht genug betont werden. Das wechselhafte Spiel der Hauterscheinungen reicht von roseolären, kleinpapulösen, unregelmäßig circinären und urticariellen Efflorescenzen bis zu landkartenförmigen Figurationen (Abb. 6). Scarlatiniforme, rubeoliforme, auch morbilliforme Eruptionen können das Bild vollends verwirren. Selbst einzelne Bläschen (Bourel u. Mitarb.), Petechien (Wissler; Denys; Onyszkiewicz-Bielewiczowa), Erythema exsudativum multiforme-artige Morphen (Küster u. Pothmann), Scrotumschwellungen (Kölbl) und Ödeme der Wangen und Lider (Bourel u. Mitarb.) ähnlich Quincke-Ödemen sind vereinzelt beobachtet worden. Ferrier und Mégevand sahen unmittelbar nach einer Bluttransfusion die schlagartige Entwicklung einer Erythrodermie, die 3 Std. später nach Behandlung mit einem Calcium-Antihistaminicum (Calcium-Sandosten) wieder ebenso abrupt verschwand. Dabei bestanden weder Schocksymptome noch Temperaturerhöhung! Der exsudativanaphylaktoide Grundzug der Krankheit spiegelt sich gleichsam im jähen Aufflackern und in der raschen Wechselhaftigkeit des Hautbildes wider. Manchmal besteht mäßiger Juckreiz.

[1] Sekundär-chronische Polyarthritis nach echter Febris rheumatica kommt im Kindesalter wahrscheinlich überhaupt nicht vor; bei entsprechenden Fällen dürfte es sich meist um Spätstadien des Wissler-Fanconi-Syndroms handeln (Klinke).

In lokalisatorischer Hinsicht tritt das Exanthem scheinbar wahllos *an den Extremitäten, am Stamm oder im Gesicht (bisweilen solitär)* auf. Nur ein Enanthem fehlt nach den bisherigen Erfahrungen regelmäßig (Wissler).

Eine besondere — und hinsichtlich der Hauterscheinungen und des klinischen Gesamtverlaufs sicher auch atypische — Beobachtung teilten Caussade, Neimann, Pierson und Lascombes mit. Ein $6^1/_2$jähriger Junge erkrankte nach einer heftigen Angina zunächst unter dem Bild einer vermeintlichen Septikämie mit Arthralgien, in deren Verlauf an Stamm und Extremitäten sehr polymorphe Veränderungen auftraten: fleckförmige Erytheme, linsen- bis

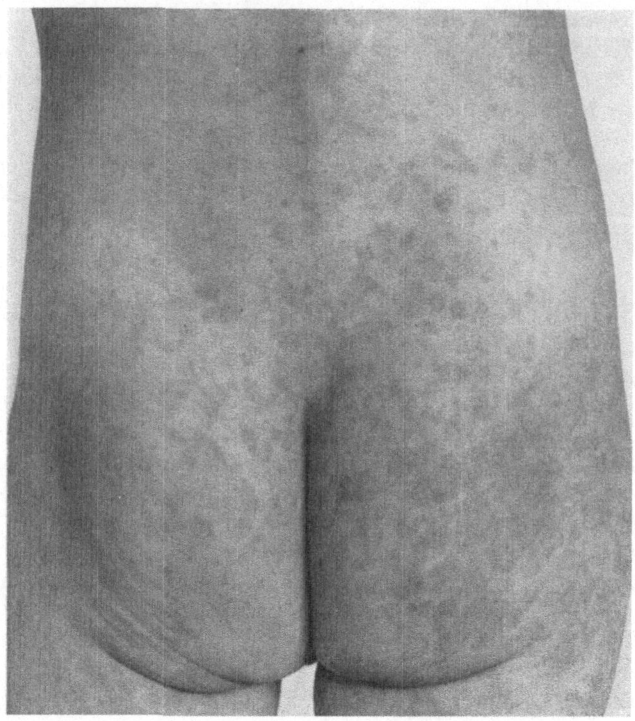

Abb. 6. Wissler-Fanconi-Syndrom. — Maculöses, aus unterschiedlich großen und unregelmäßig begrenzten Einzelmorphen bestehendes Exanthem über den unteren Rücken- und Gesäßpartien eines 10jährigen Mädchens. Teils roseoläre bis angedeutet anuläre, teils konfluierende Ausbreitung. [Abbildung von H. Wissler freundlicherweise zur Verfügung gestellt]

haselnußgroße derbe *Knoten, Petechien* und *kleinere Ekchymosen, Teleangiektasien.* Nach vorübergehender Entfieberung und Rückbildung des Exanthems durch Antibiotica und Cortison erneuter febriler Schub mit profuser Aussaat von maculösen, papulösen, nodösen Efflorescenzen und Ekchymosen an Stamm und Extremitätenstreckseiten. Am unteren Thorax Confluenz zu teilweise *hämorrhagischen Plaques.* Nach zeitweiliger Besserung durch Cortison zweites fieberhaftes Rezidiv eines nodulär-purpurischen Exanthems. Therapeutischer Versuch mit Na-Salicylat wegen Acidose vorzeitig abgebrochen. Rapide Entwicklung von *Hautnekrosen* an Knien, Knöcheln und Unterarmstreckseiten, gleichzeitig schwerstkranker Allgemeinzustand mit Somnolenz und körperlichem Verfall. ACTH ohne Erfolg. Auf Butazolidin Entstehung eines *Raynaud-Syndroms* mit beginnenden Fingernekrosen. Dann dramatische Besserung auf Na-Gentisat, Rückbildung der Hauterscheinungen (teilweise unter Vernarbung), klinische Heilung nach insgesamt 10monatiger Dauer.

Das Ungewöhnliche dieser Beobachtung besteht — abgesehen von den auffallend langen Fieberschüben — in den Hauterscheinungen, die von dem sonst beim Wissler-Fanconi-Syndrom beschriebenen Exanthem *verschieden* sind. Die französischen Autoren halten die nodösen, hämorrhagischen und teilweise nekrotisierenden Elemente zwar für nosologisch zugehörig zum Wissler-Fanconi-Syndrom, da der histologische Befund auf eine „cutane Allergie" (?) hinweise und da sich die sonstigen klinischen Symptome gut in den Rahmen des Syndroms einfügen würden. Die Beschreibung des Exanthems läßt u.E. aber mit der Möglichkeit *zusätzlicher* dermaler Komplikationen im Sinne infektiös bedingter „vasculärer Allergide“ (Antistreptolysin-O-Titer zeitweilig 1:800—1:1600!) oder auch eines Sanarelli-Shwartzman-Phänomens rechnen.

Eine *Lymphknotenschwellung* gehört nicht regelmäßig zum Krankheitsbild, kann interkurrent aber in meist *diskreter* Form auftreten. Übergänge zur Stillschen Krankheit (?) sind vereinzelt beschrieben worden (DENYS u. PROVIS; SPARTÀ u. DISERTORI u.a.).

e) Differentialdiagnose

1. *Sepsis.* Ausschlaggebend sind die bakteriologischen Blutkulturen, indirekt der zunehmend schlechtere Allgemeinzustand, die häufige Eosinopenie des Blutbildes sowie nicht zuletzt die therapeutische Beeinflussung durch Antibiotica.

2. *Serumkrankheit.* Die exanthematischen Phänomene können verblüffend ähnlich sein, doch besteht meist stärkerer Juckreiz. Das Fieber pflegt niedriger zu sein. Meist deckt die Anamnese den ursächlichen Zusammenhang auf.

3. *Arzneiexanthem.* Das klinische Bild entscheidet, auf die Anamnese ist oft weniger Verlaß. Längere Dauer der Morphen, stärkere Ausprägung (gerade bei hochfieberhaftem Krankheitsverlauf), häufige Lokalisation an den Körperöffnungen und der Mundschleimhaut erleichtern die Diagnose. Übrigens sind auch beim Wissler-Fanconi-Syndrom gelegentlich zusätzliche Arzneiexantheme beobachtet worden.

4. *Erythema anulare (Lehndorff-Leiner).* Die Ähnlichkeit mit diesem Exanthem kann tatsächlich beträchtlich sein, sofern man — z.B. bei einer konsiliarischen Untersuchung — nur eine momentane Phase und nicht den weiteren Verlauf der Krankheit zu sehen bekommt. Bei längerer Beobachtung fällt aber die größere Vielfalt und ausgedehntere Lokalisation der Efflorescenzen des Wissler-Fanconi-Syndroms (häufig auch Gesicht und Acren!) auf. Auch ein Blick auf die „septisch“ anmutende Fieberkurve kann aufschlußreich sein. Eine Endokarditis fehlt! So entscheidet manchmal erst die Epikrise über die nosologische Einstufung in den akuten Rheumatismus oder in das Wissler-Fanconi-Syndrom.

5. *Exanthem beim Morbus Still.* Auch hier hat der Quer- und Längsschnitt *aller* Symptome entscheidende differentialdiagnostische Bedeutung. WISSLER ist so vorsichtig, nur solche klinische Verlaufsformen, bei denen zwischen den stürmischen Erscheinungen einer „Subsepsis allergica“ und einem polyarthritisch-deformierenden Spätstadium ein erscheinungsfreies Intervall liegt, als nosologisch zusammengehörig aufzufassen. Bestehen dagegen fließende Übergänge, so ist er mehr zur Annahme einer primären Stillschen Krankheit mit akutem Beginn geneigt.

Das Exanthem des Morbus Still ist zwar gleichfalls pleomorph und flüchtig, neigt aber doch im Vergleich zum Wisslerschen Exanthem zu einer etwas größeren Konstanz im Erscheinungsbild der Einzelefflorescenzen.

6. *Chronische Form (sog. Lenta-Form) der Meningokokkensepsis.* Dieses früher häufiger diskutierte, auch als „Febris maculosa intermittens“ (DECASTELLO u. WELTMANN) bezeichnete Krankheitsbild wird heute kaum noch beobachtet; vielleicht verbarg sich in ihm in Wirklichkeit die eine oder andere „Subsepsis allergica“ (WISSLER). Die Diagnose hängt vom bakteriologischen Meningokokkennachweis im Blut, vom klinischen Verlauf, der die Gefahr einer eitrigen Meningitis birgt, schließlich auch von der Wirksamkeit einer antibiotischen Therapie ab. Das Exanthem dieses Krankheitsbildes soll vielfach stärker infiltriert (Erythema nodosum-ähnlich) und nur selten rein maculös sein (WISSLER). Erwähnt sei, daß bei dieser nosologisch etwas unklaren (und uneinheitlichen?) „Sepsis“ auch Zusammenhänge mit Gonorrhoe diskutiert worden sind (DECASTELLO u. WELTMANN).

f) Histopathologie des Exanthems

Es ist uns nur eine einzige Veröffentlichung bekannt, in der unter anderem über das Gewebsbild von Hauterscheinungen beim Wissler-Fanconi-Syndrom berichtet wird (CAUSSADE, NEIMANN, PIERSON u. LASCOMBES). Allerdings erscheint gerade dieser Krankheitsfall atypisch (vgl. oben). Histologisch fanden sich im Bereich einer auf dem Höhepunkt des dritten Schubes excidierten hämorrhagischen Papel zwar Ödem, Hämorrhagien und herdförmige fibrinoide Bindegewebsnekrosen mit Zellzerfall im oberen Corium, aber keine Gefäßwandveränderungen oder entzündlichen Infiltrate. Dagegen ließ sich während der Rückbildungsphase in der Subcutis eine lympho-plasmocytäre Entzündung um die erweiterten, sonst unauffälligen Gefäße nachweisen. Die Reste des subcutanen Bindegewebes zeigten ebenfalls lympho-plasmocytäre Infiltrate mit einigen Histiocyten sowie neutro- und eosinophilen Granulocyten.

Wissler erwähnt bei einem seiner Patienten den histologischen Befund zweier hämorrhagischer Knötchen, in dem von einer pericapillaren akuten fibrinös-leukocytären Entzündung gesprochen wird, ähnlich derjenigen in Hautherden der Lenta-Sepsis sowie mit „Anklängen" an die Periarteriitis nodosa (v. Albertini). Allerdings bestand in diesem Fall eine „anaphylaktoide Purpura", also wiederum ein atypischer Krankheitsverlauf. Die Flüchtigkeit des typischen Exanthems und das Fehlen narbiger Residuen gibt eben im allgemeinen zu histologischen Untersuchungen keine besondere Veranlassung.

Im Zusammenhang mit der häufig bestehenden relativen Eosinophilie des Blutbildes trotz gehäufter Fieberschübe erscheint es bemerkenswert, daß auch in histologischen Befunden von Tonsillen (Künstler) und Lymphknoten (Musso) eine Vermehrung der eosinophilen Granulocyten beschrieben wurde.

g) Therapie

Sie besteht heute im allgemeinen in der Anwendung von *Corticosteroiden* (oder ACTH), worauf meist schlagartig die Entfieberung und Symptomfreiheit folgt. Allerdings können bei vorzeitigem Absetzen der Therapie Rezidive auftreten

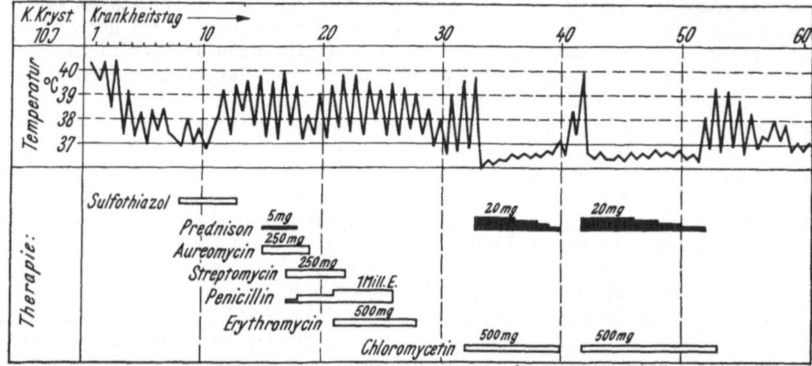

Abb. 7. Typischer Verlauf der Temperaturkurve bei einem Kind mit Wissler-Fanconi-Syndrom. Sulfonamide und Antibiotica ohne Einfluß auf die „septischen" Fieberzacken, nach ausreichender Prednison-Therapie (unter Chloromycetinschutz) dagegen sofortiger Temperaturabfall. Rezidiv nach Absetzen und Remission nach Wiederbeginn der Therapie. [Aus H. Wissler: Helv. Paed. Acta **13**, 405—425 (1958)]

(Abb. 7). Antibiotica und Sulfonamide sind durchwegs ohne Einfluß; vermeintliche Erfolge müssen vielmehr der Spontanheilungstendenz der Krankheit zugeschrieben werden.

Die verschiedenartigen ätiologischen Voraussetzungen des Krankheitsbildes machen u. U. ein individuelles therapeutisches Vorgehen erforderlich; z. B. gelang es Ballowitz u. Mitarb., bei einem offenbar tuberkulogenen Wissler-Fanconi-Syndrom durch Desensibilisierung mit kleinsten Tuberkulininjektionen Abheilung zu erzielen. Obwohl *infektions*allergische Einflüsse sicher von wesentlicher Bedeutung sind — nicht selten tritt das Wissler-Fanconi-Syndrom nach infektiösen (katarrhalischen oder eitrigen) Vorkrankheiten auf —, führt eigentümlicherweise die Beseitigung (vermuteter) Fokalinfekte fast nie zum Ziel oder löst im Gegenteil neue Schübe aus (Wissler).

2. Chronische Polyarthritis sensu strictiori

Der klinische Verlauf ähnelt in vieler Hinsicht dem bei den meisten Erwachsenen: uncharakteristische Prodromi, schleichender Beginn, wechselnde, aber meist symmetrische Gelenkschmerzen und Kapselschwellungen mit distaler Primärlokalisation und Tendenz zu zentripetalem Fortschreiten, Muskelatrophien, afebrile Temperatur.

Dagegen pflegen die üblichen rheumaserologischen Nachweisverfahren nur selten (oder schwach) positiv auszufallen, und zwar um so seltener, je jünger das Kind ist (Bywaters,

Carter u. Scott; Kelsey; Dahl u.a.). Mit besonders empfindlichen Methoden (Hämagglutinations-Hemmungstest) gelingt aber meist doch ein positiver serologischer Nachweis (Ziff; McEwen; Toumbis u.a.). Eine sichere Korrelation zwischen Krankheitsdauer und positivem Waaler-Rose-Test besteht nicht, vielleicht aber eine gewisse Abhängigkeit von der allgemeinen Aktivität des Krankheitsprozesses (Bywaters, Carter u. Scott). Relativ spät sind Veränderungen im Röntgenbild zu sehen. Sind die Handgelenke an der Entzündung beteiligt, so resultiert meist eine beschleunigte Entwicklung der karpalen Knochenkerne. Manchmal kommt es zu vorzeitigem Schluß der Epiphysenfugen mit Wachstumshemmung. Bei etwa jedem dritten Kind entwickelt sich eine Peri- und Myokarditis (Klinke u.a.).

Die *Prognose* quoad vitam ist bei rechtzeitiger und ausreichender Behandlung in neun von zehn Fällen heutzutage gut, quoad restitutionem aber immer noch dubiös (Köttgen; Sacrez, Debré u.a.). Nach Sury (1961) erfolgt zu je einem Drittel völlige Heilung, partielle Defektheilung oder schwere Verkrüppelung. Tödliche Gefahren drohen vor allem bei Mitbeteiligung der Nieren, der Lungen, des Herzens. Auch allgemeine Amyloidose kann vereinzelt bereits im Kindesalter eintreten.

An *Hauterscheinungen* sieht man gelegentlich *flüchtige variable Exantheme*, ähnlich denen der Stillschen Krankheit (Klinke). Auch *Noduli rheumatici* können vorkommen, aber seltener als bei der adulten Verlaufsform. Mitunter besteht eine gewisse *Xerostomie* infolge Verminderung der Speichelsekretion, während ein voll ausgebildetes Sjögren-Syndrom bei Kindern sehr selten ist (Klinke).

3. Stillsche Krankheit

a) Klinische Vorbemerkungen

Das Wesen dieser besonderen Verlaufsform des kindlichen chronischen Rheumatismus liegt in einer *deutlich verstärkten allgemeinen Reaktionsbereitschaft des Organismus, wobei Krankheitsmanifestationen des RHS vorherrschen.* Die klassischen *Kardinalsymptome* bestehen in chronisch-progredienter Polyarthritis mit (sub-)akuten fieberhaften Schüben, generalisierter Lymphknoten- und Milzschwellung, toxisch-infektiöser Anämie und mäßiger bis hoher Leukocytose mit relativer Lymphopenie. Herzbeteiligung, meist als *Perikarditis*, ist relativ häufig (etwa 30%) und für die Vitalprognose gravierend. Kleine *und* große Extremitätengelenke werden bevorzugt ergriffen, nicht selten aber auch die *Halswirbelsäule* (Coss u. Boots; Ansell u. Bywaters; Potter u. Mitarb.) und die *Iliosacralgelenke* (Carter). *Augenbeteiligung* kommt relativ häufig vor (Franceschetti; Schlesinger; Bonnet; v. Wolffersdorff; François; Edström u.a.), nach Sury sogar in 20% (Conjunctivitis, Skleritis, Iridocyclitis mit Cataracta complicata, bandförmige Keratitis). In den letzten Jahren, wohl unter dem Einfluß der Corticosteroid-Behandlung, sind zwar die letalen Krankheitsverläufe seltener geworden — nach Sury (1961) noch 10% —, nicht aber die deformierenden oder ankylosierenden Endstadien der Polyarthritis, die bis zu völliger Kachexie reichen können.

Die obige Feststellung, daß der chronische Rheumatismus des Kindesalters in verschiedener Hinsicht von dem der Erwachsenen abweicht, gilt in besonderem Maße für die Stillsche Krankheit, auch wenn dieser das Felty-Syndrom teilweise an die Seite gestellt werden kann. Darum seien kurz einige *Besonderheiten* der Stillschen Krankheit angeführt, für die teils nur altersabhängige, teils aber auch spezielle krankheitsbedingte Faktoren maßgeblich sein dürften:

Im weißen Blutbild herrscht eine *Leukocytose* vor, zumindest während der Fieberstadien. Selbst Werte über 50000 mit myeloischen Reaktionen kommen gelegentlich vor. Unter Kelleys Patienten wiesen nur 15% eine Leukopenie auf (dabei Grenze bereits bei 6000/mm^3 angesetzt). Nach Schlesinger und Cathie finden sich leukopenische Reaktionen, verbunden mit relativer Leukocytose und Anämie, meist erst in fieberfreien Spätperioden.

Eine Hepatomegalie ist selten (bei Lockie u. Norcross z.B. bei 3 von 28 Kindern); ebenso entwickelt sich im juvenilen Alter nur selten bereits eine Amyloidose (Trasoff u. Mitarb.; Pickard; James u. Bolton u.a.).

Die Polyarthritis kann bereits in Frühstadien *auch die größeren Gelenke* mitergreifen, desgleichen die *Sacro-Iliacalfugen* und die *Halswirbelsäule*, die beiden letzteren allerdings mehr im späteren Kindesalter. Lokale Wachstumshemmungen können zur *Brachydaktylie* einzelner Finger oder Zehen führen, besonders bei Krankheitsausbruch in den ersten 3 Lebensjahren oder vor der zweiten Dentition (Coss u. Boots). Auch die allgemeine körperliche Entwicklung bleibt häufig auffällig zurück (vgl. unter Entwicklungsmerkmale).

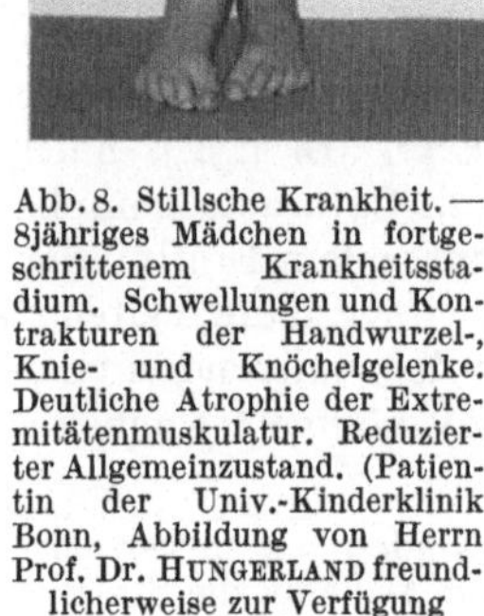

Abb. 8. Stillsche Krankheit. — 8jähriges Mädchen in fortgeschrittenem Krankheitsstadium. Schwellungen und Kontrakturen der Handwurzel-, Knie- und Knöchelgelenke. Deutliche Atrophie der Extremitätenmuskulatur. Reduzierter Allgemeinzustand. (Patientin der Univ.-Kinderklinik Bonn, Abbildung von Herrn Prof. Dr. Hungerland freundlicherweise zur Verfügung gestellt)

Eine bisher nur bei der juvenilen, nicht dagegen bei der adulten chronischen Polyarthritis beobachtete Sonderform von rheumatoider Corneabeteiligung äußert sich in einer *bandförmig* horizontal verlaufenden *Keratitis* (Edström 1961 u.a.).

Die üblichen rheumaserologischen Agglutinationsteste bleiben, wie schon erwähnt, im Kindesalter *meist negativ*. Dieser Unterschied gegenüber dem Erwachsenenalter hängt möglicherweise aber nur von der Gesamtdauer des Krankheitsprozesses ab, da auch bei der adulten, Primär-chronischen Polyarthritis die entsprechenden Rheumateste bisweilen erst nach 10—15 Jahren positiv werden (Dixon).

Von Bedeutung ist schließlich auch das häufige Auftreten von „*rheumatoiden*“ *Exanthemen*, die geradezu ein Charakteristikum der Stillschen Krankheit (bzw. der chronischen kindlichen Polyarthritis überhaupt) darstellen und wahrscheinlich mit der systematisierten Reaktionsbereitschaft des RHS und der erhöhten Gefäßirritabilität dieser Lebensperiode zusammenhängen.

b) Spezielle Hauterscheinungen der Stillschen Krankheit

Sie haben große *diagnostische Bedeutung*, werden aber wegen ihrer Flüchtigkeit und relativen Beschwerdefreiheit häufig übersehen. Auch Still hatte sie noch nicht erwähnt. Genauere Beschreibungen sind erst relativ spät erfolgt (Gauchat u. May; Sacrez u. Juif; Kelley u.a.), besonders eingehend von Isdale und Bywaters. Nach Gauchat und May sind die Exantheme so typisch, daß ihre Kenntnis weitere komplizierte Laboratoriumsuntersuchungen zur Klärung der Diagnose erübrigt.

Die meisten Autoren begnügen sich mit dem Hinweis auf *morbilliforme oder scarlatiniforme Exantheme* („*rashs*“), die „wie angeflogen“ an Stamm, Gesicht und Extremitäten entstehen und wieder abklingen. Bisweilen ist eine urticarielle Note angedeutet. In der Regel begleiten diese flüchtigen, meist nur Stunden währenden Hauterscheinungen fieberhafte Exacerbationen des Krankheitsprozesses, können aber auch monosymptomatisch bereits während Phasen von erhöhter Senkungsbeschleunigung auftreten.

α) Erythema multiforme rheumatoides

Mit diesem Terminus ist von Gauchat und May ein Exanthem bezeichnet worden, das ein durchaus pathognomonisches Erscheinungsbild aufweist. Andere angelsächsische Autoren sprechen von „*rheumatoid rash*“ (Abb. 9a—f). Es handelt sich meist um kleinfleckige, etwas unregelmäßig begrenzte *maculöse Erytheme* von 3 mm oder weniger Durchmesser, manchmal (besonders beim Erstausbruch) angedeutet papulös erhaben (Isdale u. Bywaters). Seltener — nach Isdale und Bywaters in etwa 20% — finden sich größere, über 5 mm messende Einzelherde, oft mit zentraler Abblassung. Auf diese Weise und gelegentlich durch leichte Anhebung des Randes kann eine ringförmige Konfiguration entstehen (Abb. 9e). Im Gegensatz zum Erythema anulare Lehndorff-Leiner fehlt aber die bogige, periphere Randausbreitung der einzelnen Efflorescenzen. Wenn flächenhaft, unregelmäßig-landkartenförmig begrenzte Erytheme auftreten (z.B. an Gesäß, Flanken und Unterbauch), so kommen sie in erster Linie durch *Konfluenz dichtstehender Einzelherde* zustande (Abb. 9f). Das Kolorit entspricht einem zarten Lachsrot oder hellen Rosa, das häufig durch einen schmalen anämischen Hof um die Erythemflecke noch deutlicher hervortritt. Entsprechende Beobachtungen wurden von FAHR und KLEINSCHMIDT, BOLDERS, LANGMEAD, BAILEY, KEIL u.a., am eingehendsten von ISDALE und BYWATERS mitgeteilt.

Hinsichtlich der *Lokalisation* sind die Streckseiten der Extremitäten, der Stamm und das Gesicht in fallender Häufigkeit betroffen; so fanden ISDALE und BYWATERS unter 46 Patienten mit rheumatoidem „rash“ die Arme und Beine in 97%, den Stamm in 82%, das Gesicht und den Nacken in 59% intermittierend befallen.

Eigentümlicherweise lassen sich die Efflorescenzen durch leichtere Druck- und Kratzreize provozieren (ISDALE u. BYWATERS), ein Verhalten, das an Köbnersche *isomorphe Reizeffekte* erinnert (Abb. 9a). So können sich die erythematösen Morphen an Druckstellen von Falten des Bettzeugs oder des Schlafanzugs streifenförmig aneinanderreihen. Auch experimentell ist das Phänomen *in gewisser Abhängigkeit von der Reizquantität auslösbar:* Während eines „rash“ können einfache Kratzstriche mit Reflexerythem binnen weniger Stunden von neuen, linear angeordneten Erythemen an der Einwirkungsstelle gefolgt sein, während starkes Kratzen mit striemenartiger Reaktion die anschließende Entstehung dieser Efflorescenzen häufig verzögert oder sogar unterdrückt (ISDALE u. BYWATERS).

Typischerweise ist das Exanthem *flüchtig, rezidiviert aber häufig*; oft dauert es nur wenige Stunden, bevorzugt dabei die zweite Tageshälfte (abendlicher Temperaturanstieg!) und überschreitet selten 24 Std. Endo- und exogene Wärmeeinflüsse (Fieberschübe, Sonnenbestrahlung, heiße Bäder usw.) können es provozieren oder steigern. GAUCHAT und MAY beobachteten sogar nur für die Dauer einiger Minuten — z.B. während der klinischen Untersuchung — das plötzliche Aufschießen und Verschwinden typischer „rashs“. Meist erscheinen die Efflorescenzen der Rezidive nicht mehr an genau den gleichen Stellen, ändern aber während der Einzelschübe ihre Größe nur unwesentlich.

Im allgemeinen fehlen Diapedeseblutungen; ausnahmsweise können sie aber streifenförmig umschrieben in Erscheinung treten. SCHLESINGER u. Mitarb. (1961) beobachteten bei einem 10jährigen Mädchen sogar eine Noma-ähnliche Gangrän der Nasenspitze, die später ohne wesentliche Residuen abheilte.

Die Angaben über *die Häufigkeit* des bei der Stillschen Krankheit auftretenden „rheumatoiden Rash“ wechseln, möglicherweise bedingt durch die unterschiedliche Beachtung dieses Symptoms oder durch verschieden lange klinische Beobachtungszeit der Patienten. TOUMBIS fand entsprechende Hauterscheinungen bei 6 von 50 Kindern (12%), ISDALE und BYWATERS bei 46 von 166 Kindern (27,7%); SCHLESINGER (1961) gibt eine Häufigkeit von ungefähr 40%, GAUCHAT und MAY sogar von 75—80% an. Bei Knaben soll das Exanthem etwas häufiger als bei Mädchen vorkommen, besonders im ersten Lebensjahrzehnt (ISDALE u. BYWATERS). Bei späterem Krankheitsbeginn wird es zunehmend seltener beobachtet; im Krankengut von BYWATERS, CARTER und SCOTT bestand eine fallende Häufigkeit von etwa 30—18—10% vom ersten bis zum dritten Dezennium.

Ganz allgemein sind die Exanthemschübe ein *Ausdruck erhöhter Krankheitsaktivität.* Vor allem die intermittierenden Fieberperioden, aber auch generalisierte Lymphknotenschwellungen und Splenomegalie treten zusammen mit ihnen signifikant gehäuft auf (ISDALE u. BYWATERS). Nicht selten aber eilt das Exanthem den sonstigen klinischen Symptomen um Wochen bis Monate, gelegentlich um Jahre voraus oder tritt innerhalb der ersten beiden Wochen nach Ausbruch des typischen Krankheitsbildes auf. Gelenkschwellungen, selbst Gelenkschmerzen können in diesem Stadium noch fehlen (KELSEY; SCHLESINGER u. Mitarb. 1961).

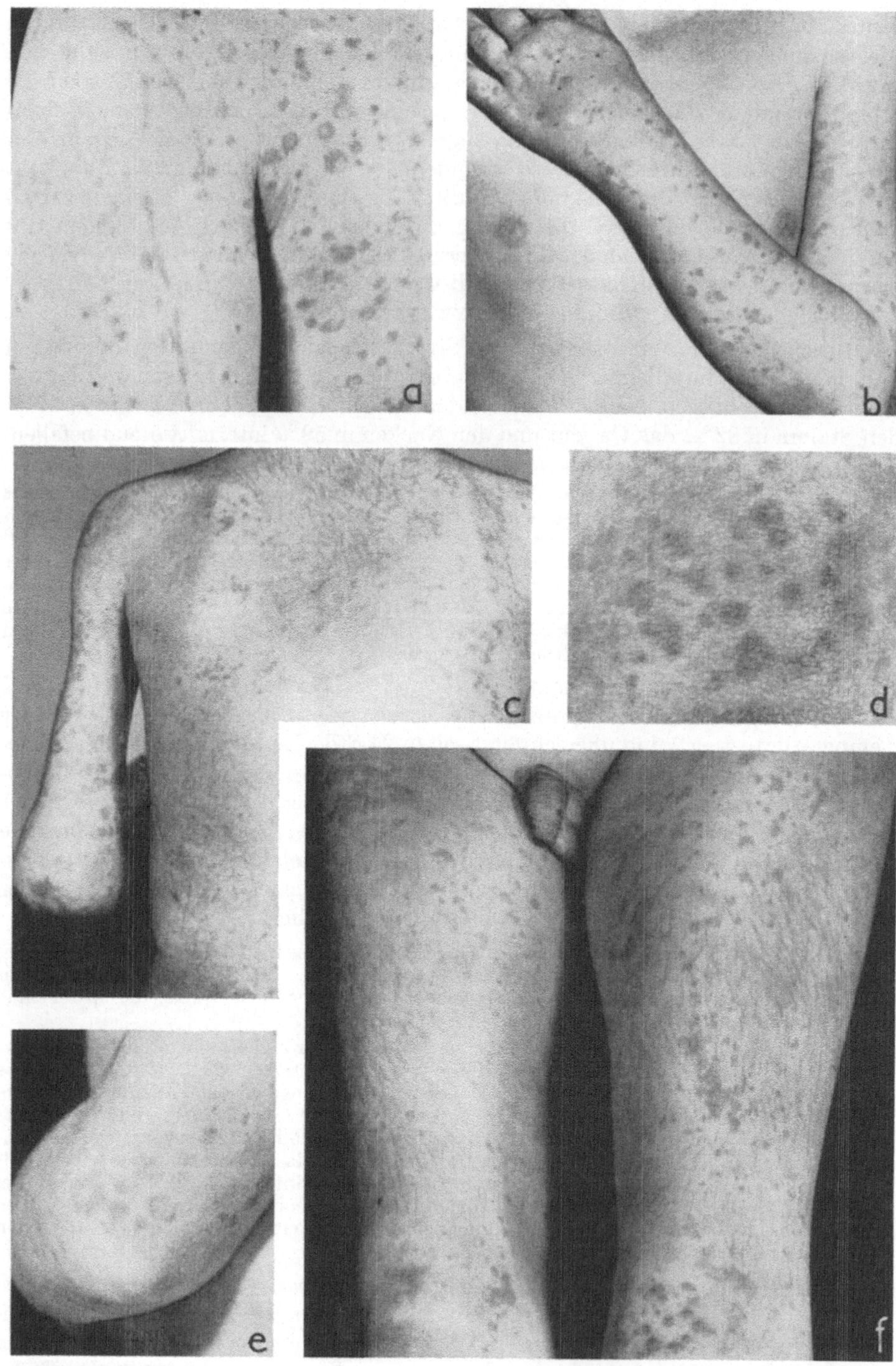

Abb. 9 a—f. Charakteristische Erscheinungsformen des „Rash“ der Stillschen Krankheit. — a Streifenförmige Erytheme nach Kratzstrichen ähnlich Köbner-Effekten. b Typische Ausbreitung an den Armen. c Gruppierte Erytheme am Rücken und an den Armen. d Einzelerytheme über der Streckseite des Knies. e Typische Erytheme mit pseudo-anulärem Erscheinungsbild infolge Abblassung der Zentren. f Verstärkte Hautblässe um gruppierte und teilweise konfluierte Erytheme. [Aus J. C. ISDALE and E. G. L. BYWATERS: Quart. J. Med. N.S. **25**, 377—587 (1956)]

Nur die BSG pflegt regelmäßig beschleunigt zu sein. Das Exanthem ist also ein *Frühsymptom.* Erstausbruch in der Spätphase der Stillschen Krankheit ist selten. Die Gesamtdauer — ungeachtet des unregelmäßig rezidivierenden Auftretens — variiert zwischen wenigen Tagen und mehreren Jahren. ISDALE und BYWATERS errechneten bei ihren Patienten eine mittlere Dauer von 13 Monaten, die sich bei Fällen mit weit vorauseilenden Hauterscheinungen noch wesentlich verlängerte. Je frühzeitiger das Exanthem vor der eigentlichen Polyarthritis auftritt, desto ausgedehnter, höher fieberhaft und rezidivbereiter bleibt es nach ihren Erfahrungen. Eine *prognostische* Aussage für die Gesamtkrankheit ist aber *nicht möglich* (KELSEY; SCHLESINGER, FORSYTH, WHITE, SMELLIE u. STROUD). Beim Vergleich von Krankheitsgruppen mit und ohne Exanthem fanden ISDALE und BYWATERS 5 Jahre nach Beginn keine eindeutigen Unterschiede im klinischen Status. Auch zeigten die rheumaserologischen Hämagglutinationsteste, soweit überhaupt positiv, keine signifikante Bevorzugung einer der beiden Gruppen.

Nicht nur für die Frühdiagnose der Stillschen Krankheit, auch zur Erkennung atypischer Verläufe und zur Abgrenzung vom Rheumatischen Fieber hat das Exanthem eine besondere Bedeutung. Insofern kann seine rechtzeitige Erkennung gegebenenfalls doch etwas die Gesamtprognose beeinflussen: je weniger Zeit bis zur Einleitung einer gezielten Therapie verloren wird, desto günstiger sind die Spätergebnisse.

αα) Differentialdiagnose

1. Erythema anulare rheumaticum (Lehndorff-Leiner). Die Efflorescenzen sind gleichfalls flüchtig, häufig rezidivierend, maculös bis angedeutet urticariell und von blaßroter Farbe, neigen aber zum peripheren Fortschreiten in bogen- und kreisförmigen Figuren. Schon zu Beginn sind die maculösen Einzelherde meist größer als beim Morbus Still. Auch bleiben im Gegensatz zu diesem das Gesicht und meist auch die Streckseiten der Extremitäten frei. Desgleichen fehlen isomorphe Reizeffekte. Schon FAHR und KLEINSCHMIDT betonten die Verschiedenheit gegenüber dem Exanthem der Stillschen Krankheit.

Im übrigen besteht beim E.a. fast regelmäßig eine Endokarditis (beim Morbus Still dagegen seltener eine Herzbeteiligung, vorwiegend als Peri- oder Myokarditis), ist der Anti-O-Streptolysin-Titer fast stets erhöht, die Grundkrankheit durch Salicylate gut beeinflußbar, und das Fieber etwas geringeren Schwankungen unterworfen als bei der Stillschen Krankheit (MCMINN u. BYWATERS).

2. Arzneiexantheme. Sie neigen zwar gleichfalls zur bevorzugten Manifestation an den Acren und distalen Extremitätenanteilen, pflegen aber mehr polymorph zu sein und — auch noch nach Absetzen der Noxe — länger zu dauern als der flüchtige „rash“ der Stillschen Krankheit.

3. Masernexanthem. Es kann dem Beginn eines Still-Exanthems zunächst ähneln, ist aber durch die gleichzeitigen katarrhalischen Erscheinungen, die initialen Koplikschen Flecken und den weiteren Verlauf leicht abgrenzbar.

4. Rötelnexanthem. Da Rubeolen mit Lymphknotenschwellungen einhergehen und gelegentlich von einer passageren, 3—21 Tage dauernden Polyarthritis begleitet sind (KANTOR), können sie differentialdiagnostische Schwierigkeiten bereiten. Die charakteristische Ausbreitung des Exanthems, der cervico-nuchale Beginn der Polylymphadenitis, die meist geringeren Allgemeinerscheinungen, das charakteristische Blutbild mit Vermehrung plasmazellartiger Elemente, gegebenenfalls noch epidemiologische Hinweise sind diagnostisch ausschlaggebend.

5. Pfeiffersches Drüsenfieber. Bei etwa 30% der Erkrankten können zu Beginn flüchtige morbilli- oder scarlatiniforme Exantheme bestehen (SEITZ u. BALLOWITZ). Der Befall des lymphatischen Systems mit generalisierter Lymphknoten- und Milzschwellung vermag eine Stillsche Krankheit vorzutäuschen. Differentialdiagnostisch ist daher auf gleichzeitige Angina, ulcerös-pseudomembranöse Veränderungen der Mundschleimhaut, Monocytose des Blutbildes zu achten. Das Exanthem allein ist uncharakteristisch und auf den Krankheitsbeginn beschränkt.

6. Purpura Schönleini. Differentialdiagnostische Schwierigkeiten können nur im präpurpurischen Stadium des Exanthems auftreten. Nur in seltenen Ausnahmen kommen purpurische Efflorescenzen auch bei der Stillschen Krankheit vor.

ββ) Histopathologie

Nach ISDALE und BYWATERS finden sich im oberen Corium, besonders um den subpapillaren Gefäßplexus, lockere Ansammlungen von rund- und segmentkernigen Leukocyten. Die letzteren weisen im Zentrum der Einzelherde Zerfallsneigung auf, doch bleiben die entzündlichen und regressiven Veränderungen erheblich hinter denen des Erythema anulare rheumaticum zurück (Abb. 10). Nach SCHLESINGER u. Mitarb. (1961) handelt es sich bei den rundkernigen Zellen um Lympho-, Histio- und Plasmocyten. Das begleitende Gewebsödem bleibt relativ geringfügig, auch färberisch bestehen keine stärker degenerativen Veränderungen des Bindegewebes.

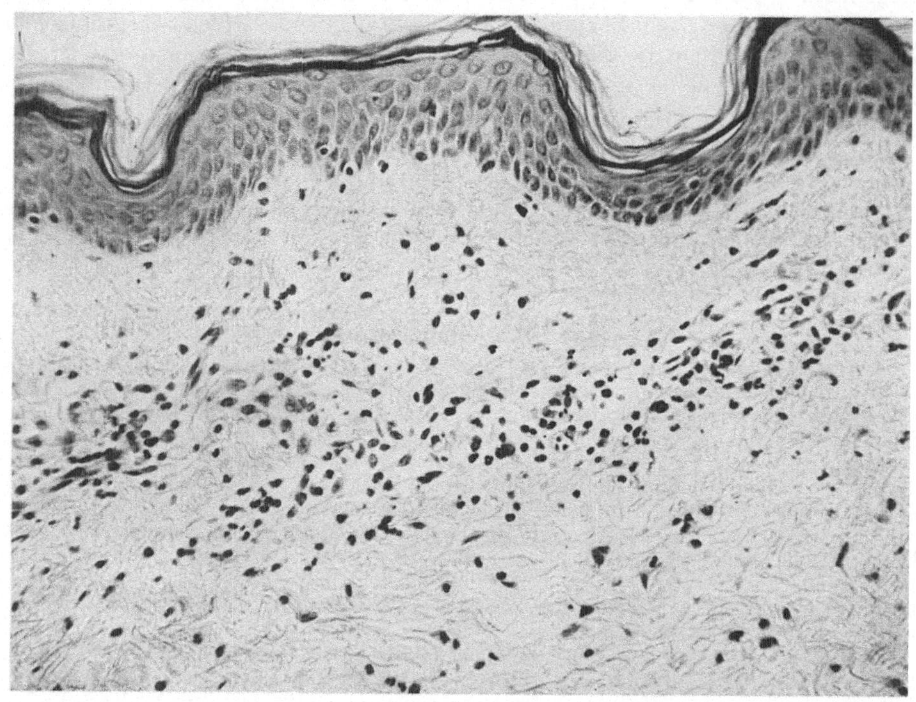

Abb. 10. Histologischer Befund des „Rash" der Stillschen Krankheit. — HE, 220mal vergr. Vorwiegend lymphomonocytoide Entzündung um Gefäße des subpapillaren Strombahnplexus. Keine granulocytäre Komponente. [Aus J. C. ISDALE and E. G. L. BYWATERS: Quart. J. Med. N.S. **25**, 377—587 (1956)]

γγ) Pathogenese

Der klinische Verlauf und die histologischen Befunde des Exanthems sprechen für eine flüchtige exsudative Entzündung, die auch von der lebhaften neurovegetativen Reagibilität der terminalen Strombahngefäße wesentlich mitbestimmt sein dürfte. Außerdem ist wahrscheinlich noch eine klinisch nicht unmittelbar faßbare Schädigung des cutanen Bindegewebes von Bedeutung. So läßt sich nach Untersuchungen von ISDALE und BYWATERS durch Einspritzung von Hoden-Hyaluronidase ein vorübergehendes „Auslöschphänomen" des Exanthems für 2—3 Tage erzielen. Dagegen haben Injektionen von physiologischer Kochsalzlösung oder percutane Applikationen von Hydrocortison-haltigen Salben keinen Einfluß auf die Efflorescenzen. Offenbar stehen also die Hauterscheinungen auch mit Veränderungen der mesenchymalen Grundsubstanz in Zusammenhang und sind somit nicht nur vasculäres Begleitphänomen, sondern auch echter Ausdruck des „rheumatoiden" Grundprozesses.

δδ) Therapie

Corticosteroide und ACTH, aber auch Salicylate und Antihistaminica haben auf das Exanthem keine spezifische Wirkung. Seine Beeinflussung hängt vorwiegend von der Bekämpfung der allgemeinen Krankheitsaktivität durch Corticosteroide oder ACTH ab. Gelegentlich bleiben auch nach therapeutischer Remission der übrigen Krankheitszeichen noch rezidivierende „rashs" bestehen, sie kündigen dann erneute Exacerbationen an. Von der Therapie her gesehen beansprucht also das Exanthem eine gewisse Sonderstellung innerhalb der klinischen Manifestationen der Stillschen Krankheit, wie überhaupt seine vasomotorisch-vegetative Komponente einen empfindlichen und schwer beeinflußbaren (konstitutionell bedingten?) pathogenetischen Faktor darstellt.

β) Subcutane Knoten

Vom klinisch-palpatorischen Befund und von der topographischen Prädilektion her unterscheiden sich die Nodi und Noduli der Stillschen Krankheit nicht von denen des Rheumatischen Fiebers. Sie liegen gleichfalls bevorzugt an den Streckseiten der großen und kleinen Extremitätengelenke, manchmal auch entlang der Wirbelsäule, im Bereich der Galea aponeurotica oder größeren Sehnenscheiden. Im ganzen treten sie aber *seltener als beim Rheumatischen Fieber* und sogar *wesentlich seltener als bei der Primär-chronischen Polyarthritis der Erwachsenen* auf (Edström u. Gedda; Kelley; Schlesinger u. Mitarb. 1961; Toumbis u. Mitarb.; Fanconi; Debré u.a.). Die unterschiedliche Häufigkeitsverteilung in Abhängigkeit von Lebensalter und Krankheitsbeginn kommt z.B. in Untersuchungen von Bywaters, Carter und Scott zum Ausdruck, die eine allmähliche Zunahme vom 1. bis zum 6. Lebensjahrzehnt konstatierten (auf die einzelnen Dezennien verteilt: 5—10—25—40—25—40%).

In *prognostischer* Hinsicht haben die Knoten wohl nicht die gleiche gefährliche Bedeutung wie beim Rheumatischen Fieber, wenngleich sie ebenfalls auf die noch bestehende Aktivität des Krankheitsprozesses hinweisen. Allerdings können sie gelegentlich auch in fieberfreien Ruhephasen der Krankheit (u.U. sogar jahrelang) persistieren. Bei langer Dauer und ungünstiger Lokalisation, z.B. bei subperiostalem Sitz im Schädelbereich (Schlesinger u. Mitarb. 1961), sind Usurierungen des benachbarten Knochens möglich.

Anscheinend besteht eine gewisse *Beziehung zwischen dem Vorkommen subcutaner Knötchen und dem rheumaserologischen Verhalten* beim kindlichen chronischen Rheumatismus; so fanden Bywaters, Carter und Scott gerade unter den Patienten mit Rheumaknötchen auffällig häufig positive serologische Agglutinationsteste. Dagegen ließ sich zu den übrigen klinischen Symptomen (Splenomegalie, Lymphknotenschwellungen, Polyarthritis, Rash) keine entsprechende Relation herstellen.

αα) Histopathologie

Das Gewebsbild der subcutanen Knoten beim kindlichen chronischen Rheumatismus weist alle Kennzeichen des „rheumatischen" oder „rheumatoiden" Gewebsschadens in Verbindung mit einer entzündlich-granulomatösen Reaktion auf. Insofern ist der histologische Befund recht charakteristisch und erlaubt wohl stets die Diagnose „rheumatisches Granulom". Früher nahm man an, daß zwischen den Knoten der juvenilen und der adulten rheumatoiden Arthritis kein wesentlicher histologischer Unterschied bestehe. Neuere systematische Untersuchungen von Bywaters, Glynn und Zeldis haben hier aber ein überraschendes Ergebnis gebracht.

Diese Autoren verglichen rein histologisch — ohne Berücksichtigung der klinischen Diagnosen — die subcutanen Knoten von 91 Patienten, davon 57 mit Rheumatischem Fieber, 12 mit Stillscher Krankheit und 22 mit adulter rheumatoider Arthritis. Dabei ergab sich weitgehende Übereinstimmung der Gewebsbefunde bei der Stillschen Krankheit und beim Rheumatischen Fieber, abgesehen von einer beim Morbus Still häufigeren und deutlicheren Fibrose. Dagegen bestanden zwischen den Knoten der juvenilen und adulten Rheumatoiden Arthritis verschiedene histologische Unterschiede: Bei den letzteren waren fibrinoide Nekrosen, palisadenförmige Ausrichtung des umsäumenden Granulationsgewebes und periphere Fibrosierung wesentlich ausgeprägter. Demgegenüber fehlte bei der Stillschen Krankheit meist der charakteristische dreizonale Aufbau der Granulome.

Das fibrinoid-nekrotisierende Material im Zentrum der juvenilen Rheumaknötchen ist oft ödematös aufgelockert, zwischen dissoziierten Bindegewebsbälkchen verteilt und von intakten „Gefäßinseln" durchsetzt. Vorwiegend diese vasculären Bezirke sind die Zentren einer geringen lympho-histiocytären Entzündung, während ausgesprochen granulomatöse, die Nekroseherde umsäumende Gewebsformationen fehlen oder nur angedeutet sind. Nur selten ist die Fibrosierung der Knoten so ausgeprägt wie bei den Erwachsenen, jedoch oft etwas stärker als beim Rheumatischen Fieber (Bywaters, Carter u. Scott).

Die genannten Vergleichsuntersuchungen sind insofern bemerkenswert, als sie zeigen, daß die *histomorphen Unterschiede der beiden nosologisch so nahe verwandten, aber altersbiologisch getrennten Formen der „Rheumatoiden" Arthritis wesentlich größer sind als diejenigen der ätiologisch zwar verschiedenen, aber der gleichen Altersstufe angehörenden Krankheitsprozesse des Rheumatischen Fiebers und der Stillschen Krankheit.* Sie führen außerdem erneut vor Augen, daß das Gewebsbild der rheumatischen Entzündung ätiologisch uneinheitlich bzw. unspezifisch ist, aber von einer besonderen morphologischen Reaktionsweise des Organismus — eben der „rheumatisch" genannten — geprägt wird. Für Art und Ausmaß dieser Reaktionsweise ist anscheinend auch die Altersdisposition von wesentlicher Bedeutung, wofür gerade die histomorphen Parallelen der Knoten beim Rheumatischen Fieber und bei der Stillschen Krankheit sprechen.

c) Atypische Hauterscheinungen

Hierzu ist u.E. das ganz selten erwähnte Vorkommen eines Erythema anulare vom Typ Lehndorff-Leiner zu rechnen. Solche Fälle sollten stets eine Überprüfung der Diagnose veranlassen, was übrigens auch für die vermeintlichen seltenen Übergänge zwischen dem Rheumatischen Fieber und der Stillschen Krankheit gilt.

Über eine ungewöhnliche Beobachtung von Stillscher Krankheit berichteten Sacrez und Juif: 10jähriges Mädchen, Krankheitsbeginn nach Angina und Stomatitis unter fieberhaftem rezidivierenden Aufschießen mehrerer tiefroter, transitorischer Papeln an Beinen, Rücken und Bauch. Später Ulcerationen an den Ellenbogen. Dann über den entzündlich geschwollenen Kniegelenken einzelne rot-violette, infolge Atrophie radiär gefältelte Striae distensae, histologisch mit Verlust der elastischen Fasern im mittleren Corium. Deshalb zunächst *Verdacht auf Dermatomyositis.* Dann erneutes Auftreten kleinpapulöser, binnen 1—2 Tagen plaqueförmig ausgedehnter, kleinfingernagel- bis halbhandtellergroßer indurierter, spontan- und druckschmerzhafter Efflorescenzen. Wechselnd rasche Rückbildung unter bräunlicher Pigmentierung, teilweise nach Suppuration. Insgesamt jetzt *Ähnlichkeit mit hochsitzendem Erythema nodosum.* Histologisch degenerativ-entzündliche Gefäßveränderungen mit Verdacht auf Periarteriitis nodosa (Befund von F. Woringer). Zeitweiliges Zurücktreten der Symptome der Stillschen Krankheit. Später zunehmende Ausdehnung und Neuentstehung von Striae distensae an den Knien. Dann erneuter Schub von papulo-tuberösen bis plaqueförmigen Efflorescenzen mit Persistenz und Induration. Histologisch jetzt einem *Morbus Osler ähnliche,* teilweise von Entzündung begleitete Gefäßveränderungen.

Dieser Krankheitsprozeß, in dessen Verlauf zeitweilig eine Dermatomyositis, eine Periarteriitis nodosa und eine Oslersche Krankheit erwogen wurde, ist ein Beispiel dafür, daß bei der Stillschen Krankheit auch atypische, nosologisch schwierig einzuordnende Hauterscheinungen vorkommen. Der geschilderte Fall erinnert u.E. in mancher Hinsicht an sog. vasculäre Allergide.

d) Unterschenkelgeschwüre

Offenbar nur sehr selten treten bereits bei der juvenilen Rheumatoiden Arthritis Ulcera an den Unterschenkeln auf. Über eine solche Beobachtung berichtete RIDLEY: 14jähriges Mädchen, Beginn der Krankheit mit 6 Jahren unter polyarthritischen Erscheinungen, bereits ein Jahr später ständig rezidivierende Unterschenkelgeschwüre. Die Gelenkdeformitäten der Beine waren in diesem Falle sehr ausgeprägt, so daß das Mädchen völlig an das Bett bzw. den Lehnstuhl gefesselt war.

Die pathogenetischen Faktoren dürften ähnlicher Art sein wie bei den Ulcera des Felty-Syndroms. Schwere Störungen der Haut- und Muskeltrophik, zunehmende Inaktivitätsatrophie, degenerative Veränderungen des Gefäß-Bindegewebes, zusätzliche banale Traumatisierungen wirken hier wahrscheinlich ursächlich zusammen.

e) Muskelveränderungen

Besonders in Spätstadien pflegt hochgradige, durch Inaktivität und interstitielle Myositis bedingte *Atrophie* vieler Extremitätenmuskeln zu bestehen, wodurch dann die kugelig verdickten großen Extremitätengelenke (besonders Knie und Ellenbogen) geradezu grotesk hervortreten können.

Eine gleichzeitige *Dermatomyositis* bei Stillscher Krankheit fanden SCHLESINGER u. Mitarb. (1961) bei 3 von 100 Kindern. Diese Patienten wiesen außerdem histologisch gesicherte Rheumaknötchen auf. Bei einem weiteren Kind entstanden bakteriologisch sterile *Muskelabscesse*, als deren Ausgangspunkt erweichende intramuskuläre Rheumaknoten in Betracht gezogen wurden.

f) Entwicklungsstörungen

Zu den Spätfolgen der Stillschen Krankheit gehört auch eine nicht selten zu beobachtende Retardierung des allgemeinen Körperwachstums und der Entwicklung der sekundären Geschlechtsmerkmale. Solche *Reifungshemmungen* treten offenbar besonders bei schweren Verlaufsformen der Krankheit auf (COSS u. BOOTS; ANSELL u. BYWATERS; FANCONI u.a.), erreichen aber nur bei kachektisierenden Prozessen ein schweres Ausmaß. Gelegentlich kommt auch eine ausgeprägte *Hypertrichose* vor (DEBRÉ-LELONG).

Bei manchen Kindern entwickelt sich durch vorzeitigen Wachstumsstillstand der Unterkiefer *(Brachygnathie)* eine eigenartig „spitze" Physiognomie mit fliehender Kinnpartie, die bereits von STILL erwähnt und als „Vogelgesicht" bezeichnet wurde[1]. COSS und BOOTS fanden unter 56 Patienten mit juveniler Rheumatoider Arthritis bei jedem Vierten eine deutliche solche Brachygnathie.

IV. Primär-chronische Polyarthritis (bzw. „Rheumatoide Arthritis") des Erwachsenenalters

1. Chronische Polyarthritis sensu strictiori

Diese Hauptgruppe des chronischen Gelenkrheumatismus erscheint trotz ihrer symptomatologischen Vielfalt klinisch und serologisch recht gut charakterisiert. Die Kardinalsymptome betreffen den Bewegungsapparat, insbesondere Gelenke und Muskulatur, können sich aber auch mit visceralen Manifestationen verschiedenster Art verbinden, so daß oft das Vollbild einer schweren, gleichsam *systematisiert-progredienten Allgemeinkrankheit* vorliegt.

Auffällig ist die *Bevorzugung des weiblichen Geschlechts* und die Altersverteilung: Frauen sind etwa dreimal so oft wie Männer betroffen und erkranken am häufigsten im 4. und um die Wende zum 6. Lebensjahrzehnt (SCLATER; LEWIS-FANING;

[1] Ganz ähnliche Verkürzungen des Gesichtsschädels mit hypoplastisch wirkendem Kinn haben wir übrigens auch bei Patienten mit sehr frühzeitiger, bereits in den ersten Lebensjahren beginnender *Psoriasis arthropathica* beobachtet.

Short u. Mitarb. u.a.). Bei den Männern ist kein so akzentuierter Häufigkeitsgipfel festzustellen; allenfalls ist bei ihnen das vierte Dezennium leicht bevorzugt (Clemmesen u. Arnsø). Im Kindesalter und besonders jenseits 60 Jahren, wo die Morbidität stark abnimmt, nähert sich das Geschlechtsverhältnis etwa 1:1. Diese statistischen Resultate weisen ebenso wie die klinisch-empirische Erfahrung auf besondere Beziehungen zur geschlechtsreifen Lebensphase der Frau hin; häufige Besserungen in der Gravidität (Stimulation der Nebennierenrinde!), Verschlimmerung oder Erstausbruch post partum, besonders aber während des Klimakteriums sprechen für eine tiefgreifende Abhängigkeit von neurohormonalen Regulationen.

Das gehäufte Auftreten der Krankheit in den gemäßigten Zonen (besonders in feuchtkalten Regionen mit ozeanischem Einfluß) und ihre Seltenheit in tropischen Ländern macht den Einfluß *klimabiologischer* peristatischer Faktoren deutlich, der im Verein mit anderen, noch weniger bekannten Ursachen (Konstitution, Heredität u.a.) in einigen Ländern der nördlichen Erdhemisphäre die Gesamtmorbidität auf über 1% ansteigen läßt. Da am Ende des Krankheitsprozesses oft chronisches Siechtum und Hilflosigkeit infolge vollständiger Gelenkversteifung stehen, bedeutet die Krankheit auch in sozialmedizinischer und volkswirtschaftlicher Hinsicht ein enormes Problem. Die Ausgabenstatistiken der Versicherungsträger für langfristige Behandlungs- und Kurmaßnahmen sprechen für sich.

Die Langwierigkeit und schleichende Progression des sich am drastischsten an den Gelenken abspielenden Krankheitsgeschehens hat dazu geführt, ein *Frühstadium*, ein *Stadium der vollen Entwicklung* und ein *Endstadium* zu unterscheiden. In jeder dieser Phasen kann der Prozeß zum Stillstand kommen und ausheilen, aber auch nach jahrelanger trügerischer Remission weiter um sich greifen. Mit zunehmender Dauer sind irreversible Gelenkläsionen meist unvermeidlich.

Das Frühstadium beginnt oft zögernd mit uncharakteristischen Allgemeinbeschwerden (Müdigkeit, Appetitlosigkeit, Gewichtsverlust, subfebrile Temperaturen, Parästhesien), bis sich morgendliche Steifigkeit der Finger und (meist symmetrische) Gelenkschmerzen, besonders an den kleinen Extremitätengelenken, hinzugesellen. Der „Rheumafaktor" ist um diese Zeit im Serum meist noch nicht nachweisbar. Wesentlich seltener beginnt die Krankheit sofort unter subakuten oligo- oder polyarthritischen Erscheinungen; am seltensten ist monartikulärer Beginn. Beim „Antistreptolysin-Typ" der Primär-chronischen Polyarthritis (vgl. Einleitung), der nach einleitenden Infekten der oberen Luftwege aufzutreten pflegt, werden oligo- bis monartikuläre Anfangsstadien häufiger beobachtet. Dabei besteht charakteristischerweise ein *asymmetrischer* Gelenkbefall mit Rezidivattacken im gleichen Bereich (etwa 25% aller Fälle nach Tichy).

Im weiteren Verlauf werden allmählich, zentripetal fortschreitend, auch die größeren Gelenke ergriffen und langsam zerstört, so daß nach einigen Jahren vollständige fibröse und knöcherne Ankylosierung — oft in funktionell ungünstigen Stellungen — eintreten kann. Die chronisch entzündeten Gelenke bleiben meist relativ „trocken", entzündliche Ergüsse treten hinter fibröser Kapselverdickung und bindegewebiger Knorpel-Knochendestruktion zurück. Die kugel- oder spindelförmig geschwollenen Gelenke kontrastieren mit der abgemagerten Muskulatur, deren Schwund auf Schonung und entzündlicher Infiltration beruht. Relativ häufig werden auch die Sternoclavicular- und Kiefergelenke in Mitleidenschaft gezogen, nur selten dagegen die Iliosacral- und Wirbelgelenke (am ehesten noch im Cervicalbereich). Auch die distalen Interphalangealgelenke bleiben — ein wichtiger Unterschied zur Psoriasis arthropathica — vielfach verschont.

Entsprechend ihrem Charakter als generalisierte „Mesenchymkrankheit" pflegt die Primär-chronische Polyarthritis auch den ganzen Organismus mehr oder minder stark in Mitleidenschaft zu ziehen. *Es gibt kein Organsystem, das nicht alteriert sein kann.* Dazu gehören z.B. entzündliche Hepato-Splenomegalien und generalisierte Lymphknotenschwellungen, die in ausgeprägter Form das sog. Felty-Syndrom kennzeichnen, aber auch monosymptomatisch bei den gewöhnlichen Verlaufsformen auftreten können. Entgegen früheren Ansichten ist auch das Herz gar nicht selten in recht verschiedener, offenbar krankheitseigener Weise mitbeteiligt. Auch das interstitielle Lungenmesenchym, das Zentralnervensystem, die Augen (Iridocyclitis u.a.), der Magen-Darmtrakt, die Blutbildungsstätten des Knochenmarks können entzündliche und bindegewebig-degenerative Veränderungen aufweisen, die nicht allein auf der

Entstehung von Rheumagranulomen, sondern auch auf funktionell und anatomisch faßbaren Durchblutungsstörungen beruhen. Gerade die *Beteiligung des Gefäßsystems* fehlt bei der Primär-chronischen Polyarthritis so gut wie nie, wenn sie auch nur gelegentlich im klinischen Bild stärker hervortritt. Die Schädigung des Knochenmarks äußert sich meist in normochromer Anämie, während die Granulocytopoese seltener gestört ist. Die Blutsenkung ist mäßig bis hochgradig beschleunigt, das Serumeisen als Folge des erhöhten entzündlichen Verbrauchs im Gewebe meist stark erniedrigt, das Serumkupfer dagegen erhöht. Temperaturerhöhungen, meist von subfebrilem protrahierten Charakter, können mit afebrilen Phasen abwechseln; häufig begleiten sie schubweise Steigerungen der Krankheitsaktivität. Die empfindlichsten Aktivitätszeichen liegen jedoch auf serologischem Gebiet (Nachweis des CRP und des „Rheumafaktors" mit hohen Titerwerten).

In fortgeschrittenen Endstadien erschöpft sich die erhöhte entzündliche Krankheitsaktivität, dann stehen die degenerativ-arthropathischen Defektzustände im Vordergrund, die Krankheit ist gewissermaßen „ausgebrannt" und nimmt immer mehr den Charakter eines irreversiblen Leidens an. In anderen Fällen setzen sekundäre, unaufhaltsame Komplikationen wie Amyloidose, Lebercirrhose, Agranulocytose und allgemeine Kachexie dem Leben ein Ende. Freilich kann die Primär-chronische Polyarthritis auch in jedem früheren Stadium zum Stillstand kommen und ausheilen. Somit läßt sich der Verlauf nie voraussagen, die *Prognose quoad sanationem* und auch *quoad vitam* bleibt *dubiös.*

a) Allgemeiner Hautstatus

Im klinischen Gesamtbild der Primär-chronischen Polyarthritis haben die Hauterscheinungen eine relativ untergeordnete Bedeutung, obwohl sie in der einen oder anderen Form bei ausgeprägten Fällen nur selten vermißt werden. In nosologischer Hinsicht dokumentieren sie den systematisierten, potentiell das ganze Mesenchym einbeziehenden Krankheitscharakter, in diagnostischer Hinsicht sind sie dagegen weniger eindrucksvoll, etwa verglichen mit den charakteristischen dermalen Morphen des Lupus erythematodes (visceralis). Im großen und ganzen gilt die Regel, daß dermale Manifestationen der Primär-chronischen Polyarthritis vorwiegend bei schweren und langwierigen Krankheitsverläufen vorkommen (SHORT, BAUER u. REYNOLDS). Dennoch müßte das diagnostische Augenmerk allgemein noch mehr auf die Vielfalt der vorkommenden Hautveränderungen gerichtet werden; so kommt es, daß beispielsweise über ihre — mögliche — frühdiagnostische Bedeutung kaum etwas bekannt ist. Nur die Psoriasis, die bei Patienten mit chronischem Gelenkrheumatismus wesentlich häufiger als bei der Durchschnittsbevölkerung vorkommt, erfährt größere Beachtung (vgl. den einleitenden Abschnitt „Psoriasis arthropathica").

Die *Hand des Kranken* — an klinischem Ausdrucksgehalt vielleicht ebenso aufschlußreich wie das Gesicht, zumal sie der willkürlichen Beherrschung stärker entzogen ist (MAX BÜRGER) — bietet gerade in fortgeschrittenen Stadien der Primär-chronischen Polyarthritis einen sehr charakteristischen Aspekt. Die Fingergrund- und proximalen Fingergelenke sind verdickt, die Mittelhand weicht ulnarwärts ab, der 2.—5. Finger ist unter Semiflexion und lateraler Abduktion im Metacarpo-Phalangealbereich versteift, ein Bild, das CHARCOT treffend als „main en coup de vent" bezeichnet hat. Andererseits können die Interphalangealgelenke — vorwiegend proximal, selten distal — in Hyperextension ankylosiert sein. Diese *meist symmetrischen* Kontrakturen und Deviationen resultieren aus dem Kräftespiel zwischen entzündlicher Kapselschrumpfung der Gelenke und Zugwirkung der atrophierenden Unterarmflexoren und Mittelhandmuskeln. Tritt die Kapsel- und Weichteilverdickung über den Fingergrundgelenken zusammen mit einer kollateralen Schwellung über dem Handgelenk auf, so entsteht eine muldenförmige Einsenkung des mittleren Handrückens, die von französischen Autoren als „dos de chameau" charakterisiert worden ist.

Die Haut über den geschwollenen Handgelenken erscheint glatt-atrophisch, glänzend und über die Gelenke gespannt („glossy skin"), im ganzen leicht bräunlich-cyanotisch. Die Querrunzeln über den Fingerstreckseiten sind verstrichen, manchmal unter derber Verhärtung nach Art einer Sklerodaktylie. Dabei sind die Fingerenden aber meist nicht verschmächtigt, im Gegenteil manchmal sogar trommelschlegelartig verbreitert, was nach SCHOEN und TISCHENDORF ein Ausdruck der allgemeinen Dysproteinämie ist, aber auch auf chronische rheumatische Affektionen im kardio-pulmonalen Bereich hinweisen kann. Die Fingerrücken weisen eine schmutzig-bräunliche *Pigmentierung* auf, die besonders über den proximalen Interphalangealgelenken verstärkt ist (LUCHERINI u. CERVINI). Die Hände, seltener die Füße fühlen sich im ganzen oft feucht und kühl, manchmal aber auch besonders warm an.

Auch die *Nägel* der Finger (und Zehen) zeigen bisweilen *trophische Störungen* (uhrglasartig verstärkte Krümmung, Brüchigkeit, Glanzlosigkeit, Längsauffaserung, Onycholysis, Querfurchen). Gelegentlich findet man in der Literatur (wohl fälschlicherweise) auch punktförmige Nagelgrübchen als „Rosenausches Zeichen" hinzugerechnet, die in Wirklichkeit meist ein psoriatisches Merkmal (manchmal das einzige!) darstellen und als solches besondere differentialdiagnostische Bedeutung haben (vgl. Abschnitt „Psoriasis arthropathica"). SHORT, BAUER und REYNOLDS fanden trophische Nagelstörungen bei rund einem Siebtel ihrer Patienten, besonders in höherem Alter und bei langwierigem, schwerem Krankheitsverlauf. Nach ihren Beobachtungen sind Nagelveränderungen und verstärkte Neigung zur Hautatrophie im Rahmen des Krankheitsbildes häufig kombiniert.

Gelegentlich findet man im Bereich des Thenar und Hypothenar fleckige, netzförmig konfluierende Erytheme von rosa bis kräftig rotem Farbton (DAWSON; LUCHERINI u. CERVINI u.a.), wie sie ähnlich auch bei schweren Leberparenchymschäden als „*liver palms*" vorkommen. In diesem Zusammenhang sei daran erinnert, daß auch bei der Primär-chronischen Polyarthritis die Leber häufig in Mitleidenschaft gezogen ist und bei histologisch-bioptischen Untersuchungen sogar auffällig häufig chronisch-entzündliche Veränderungen erkennen läßt (LÖVGREN; MOVITT u. DAVIS u.a.).

Die geschilderten Hautveränderungen treten zwar an den Händen besonders augenscheinlich hervor, können aber auch das übrige Integument betreffen. Manchmal nimmt die Haut, besonders am Stamm, ein verwaschen grau-bräunliches Kolorit an, das sogar an einen Morbus Addison erinnern kann (SHORT, BAUER u. REYNOLDS). Auf die Pigmentverschiebungen haben schon ältere Autoren aufmerksam gemacht (R. L. JONES; MCCRAE; DOUTHWAITE u.a.). Beim Felty-Syndrom tritt die großflächig-bräunliche Hautverfärbung sogar mit einer gewissen Regelmäßigkeit auf. Andererseits ist wiederholt auf das Bestehen einer Vitiligo bei Primär-chronischer Polyarthritis hingewiesen worden, so daß entsprechende Herde nach DAWSON sogar eine besondere Teilmanifestation der Krankheit darstellen sollen. Dieser Ansicht wird jedoch von anderen Autoren widersprochen. So fanden SHORT u. Mitarb. unter 293 Patienten 3, unter 300 Kontrollprobanden 2 mit Vitiligo, was also die Annahme einer Prävalenz bei der Primär-chronischen Polyarthritis nicht stützt.

Im äußeren Erscheinungsbild bleiben die entzündlich-degenerativen Alterationen des äußeren Integuments oft klinisch unterschwellig, wie die Untersuchungen von CURTIS und POLLARD zeigen. Diese Autoren fanden bei einer größeren Zahl von Patienten in makroskopisch unauffälligen Haut- und Muskelbiopsien vom Wadenbereich deutliche Atrophie der Epidermis sowie entzündliche Zellansammlungen im Corium und in der Muskulatur, wobei die Gefäßumgebung betont und bindegewebige Sklerosierung mit teilweiser Aufbrauchung des subcutanen Fettgewebes mitvorhanden war. Überhaupt gehören *entzündliche Veränderungen der Extremitätenmuskulatur* — besonders in Gelenknähe — zu den häufigsten extraartikulären Gewebsveränderungen der Primär-chronischen Polyarthritis (MORRISON u. Mitarb.; BUNIM u. Mitarb.; STEINER u. Mitarb.; MORITZ u.a.). Diese myositischen Veränderungen bestehen meist in locker disseminierten lympho-monocytoiden knötchenförmigen Proliferaten im Interstitium bzw. um die kleinen Gefäße, während ausgesprochene Rheumagranulome mit nekrotischem Zentrum nur ausnahmsweise vorkommen. So fanden MORRISON u. Mitarb. myositische Veränderungen in 60—75%, perineurale Entzündungsherde ähnlicher Art in 70% ihrer Fälle. Die Muskelfasern können in verschiedenem Grade atrophieren, ohne daß die Atrophie immer circumfokal an granulomatöse Entzündungsherde gebunden ist. Nach MORRISON ist der muskuläre und perineurale Entzündungstyp des visceralen Lupus erythematodes von dem der Primär-chronischen Polyarthritis morphologisch nicht zu unterscheiden. Ähnliche differentialdiagnostische Schwierigkeiten können bei den Muskelveränderungen der übrigen „pararheumatischen" Krankheiten Dermatomyositis, Progressive Sklerodermie, u.U. sogar Polyarteriitis nodosa und Sklerödem Buschke entstehen (SCHUERMANN; LE COULANT u. TEXIER u.a.).

Bei *elektromyographischen* Untersuchungen fand MORITZ pathologische Potentialschwankungen bei Ableitung von den kleinen Handmuskeln in ungefähr 60%, bei Ableitung vom M. biceps in 25%. In der Handmuskulatur konnten die Veränderungen bereits wenige Monate nach Beginn der Gelenkbeschwerden beobachtet werden; in den größeren, gelenkfernen Muskeln waren sie erst wesentlich später nachzuweisen. Im allgemeinen verläuft das Ausmaß der elektromyographischen Veränderungen etwa parallel zur allgemeinen Krankheitsaktivität; in klinischen Ruhephasen kann sich die Potentialkurve trotz bleibender Muskelatrophie weitgehend normalisieren (MORITZ).

Die *Pathogenese* der die Primär-chronische Polyarthritis begleitenden Hautveränderungen ist noch ungenügend bekannt und wahrscheinlich komplexer Natur. An den Hyperpigmentierungen ist möglicherweise eine neuro-hormonale Gleichgewichtsstörung im Hypophysen-Nebennierenrinden-System beteiligt, wenngleich die Pigmentverschiebungen nicht als Ausdruck eines echten Hormonmangels, etwa analog zur Addisonschen Nebennierenrindeninsuffizienz anzusehen sind. Auch die häufig mitvorhandene Leberparenchymschädigung kann die Pigmentverschiebungen mit-verursachen.

Die sonstigen degenerativ-atrophischen Haut- und Nagelveränderungen hängen wohl nur z.T. mit primär-entzündlichen Einflüssen zusammen. Eine nicht minder große Rolle dürften vasomotorische Störungen spielen, wie überhaupt die peripheren Durchblutungsverhältnisse für die Entstehung sekundärer rheumatischer Gewebsläsionen große Bedeutung haben. So zeigen periphere Kreislauffunktionsproben und capillarmikroskopische Untersuchungen vom Nagelfalz schon in den Frühstadien der Erkrankung eine auffällig träge vasomotorische Reaktion mit deutlich verzögerter Anpassung an funktionelle Belastungen. Auf diesem vasomotorischen Stigma beruht eine ganze Reihe von diagnostischen Kreislauftesten.

Der pathogenetische Einfluß übergeordneter Zentren im Stammhirn liegt zwar auf Grund verschiedener klinischer Indizien nahe, läßt sich aber nicht leicht beweisen[1]. Eine interessante, an neuralpathologische Gedankengänge von VEIL und STURM anknüpfende Ansicht, die auch die Hautveränderungen dem pathogenetischen Verständnis näherbringen kann, äußert MOLL im Hinblick auf die häufig im Gewebsbild vorhandenen perineuralen Entzündungserscheinungen. Nach seiner Meinung bedingen die engen topischen und trophischen Beziehungen des peripheren Nervensystems zu den rheumatisch alterierten Gelenkmembranen einen dauernden Reizzustand receptorischer und zentripetaler Nervenfasern und damit eine Störung im Gleichgewicht der den Stoffwechsel regulierenden neurotrophischen Reflexe. Diese örtliche Dysreflexie irritiert übergeordnete Zentren,

[1] So sprechen psychische Wesensänderungen, die auffällige Symmetrie der Polyarthriti- und anderer Krankheitsmanifestationen, Störungen des vegetativen Gleichgewichts mit Vasomotorenlabilität und vermehrter Schweißsekretion, Veränderungen der Mimik (Maskent gesicht) und gewisse klinische Parallelen im Erscheinungsbild der Hände (Ulnardeviation) mi) der Handstellung bei degenerativen Stammganglienerkrankungen (SCHOEN u. TISCHENDORF- für eine Beeinflussung von seiten des Zentralnervensystems, insbesondere der vegetativautonomen und extrapyramidalen Anteile (HILLER; MOLL u.a.). Desgleichen kann der pathologische Ausfall verschiedener Funktionsproben des Hypophysenvorder- und -hinterlappens auf Funktionsstörungen des diencephal-hypophysären Systems hinweisen.

die ihrerseits möglicherweise mit abnormen efferenten Impulsen reagieren und so eine Art von Circulus vitiosus herbeiführen[1].

b) Rheumatoide Erytheme

Im Gegensatz zur Stillschen Krankheit bzw. zur Primär-chronischen Polyarthritis des Kindesalters werden rheumatoide Exantheme bei Erwachsenen nur sehr selten beobachtet. Short, Bauer und Reynolds fanden unter 293 erwachsenen Patienten überhaupt keinen mit entsprechenden Hauterscheinungen. So bedeutet es eher eine Ausnahme, daß Isdale und Bywaters unter mehr als 500 adoleszenten und adulten Patienten 7 mit Erythemen vom Typ des „Rash" der Stillschen Krankheit beobachteten.

Bei zwei ihrer Patienten trat das Exanthem zugleich mit dem Krankheitsbeginn im 17. Lebensjahr auf. Bei den übrigen Patienten, durchwegs Frauen zwischen 20 und 49 Jahren, kam es teils ebenfalls zu Beginn, teils erst im weiteren Krankheitsverlauf zum Ausbruch. Bei einer 49jährigen Patientin, die seit dem 19. Lebensjahr eine rezidivierende Colitis ulcerosa, seit dem 25. Lebensjahr eine Primär-chronische Polyarthritis mit Milztumor aufwies, bestanden seit fast drei Jahrzehnten flüchtig-intermittierende Erytheme, gingen also dem Ausbruch der Gelenkerscheinungen um mehrere Jahre voraus. Während Phasen gesteigerter Krankheitsaktivität stellte sich das Exanthem fast regelmäßig ein, oft nur in den Abendstunden während des Temperaturanstiegs. Bei einer anderen Patientin sistierten die Hauterscheinungen ebenso wie die fieberhaften polyarthritischen Beschwerden während einer Gravidität, um anschließend wieder gehäuft aufzutreten. Bemerkenswerterweise war bei allen Patienten trotz jahre- bis jahrzehntelanger Krankheitsdauer weder der Rheuma- noch der L.E.-Faktor im Serum nachzuweisen.

Das klinische Erscheinungsbild der rheumatoiden Erytheme zeigt nach Isdale und Bywaters praktisch das gleiche Aussehen wie im Kindesalter, so daß auf seine Besprechung im Rahmen der Stillschen Krankheit verwiesen sei. Immer pflegt das Exanthem flüchtig, oft nur stundenweise, aufzutreten, so daß es leicht übersehen werden kann. Daß es die Abendstunden bevorzugt, hängt wahrscheinlich mit dem häufigen Vorkommen abendlicher Temperaturerhöhungen zusammen. Auch in topographischer Hinsicht stimmen der adulte und der juvenile Exanthemtyp überein, da sowohl die Arme und Beine als auch der Stamm und das Gesicht befallen sein können.

In seltenen Fällen können bei der Primär-chronischen Polyarthritis auch *Purpura*-Schübe auftreten. Short u. Mitarb. fanden solche zwar nie bei der ersten Hospitalisation der Patienten, vereinzelt aber doch im späteren Verlauf. Umgekehrt stellte Davis unter 500 Patienten mit nicht-thrombopenischer Purpura eine Primär-chronische Polyarthritis in 4% als Ursache fest.

c) Ulcera crurum

In den letzten Jahren ist mehrfach, besonders im angelsächsischen Schrifttum, auf das Vorkommen ungewöhnlich torpider und therapieresistenter Unterschenkelgeschwüre bei der Primär-chronischen Polyarthritis hingewiesen worden (Granirer; Kirpilä; Beninson u. Ensign). Verhältnismäßig häufig besteht in diesen Fällen die klinische Sonderform eines Felty-Syndroms. Es darf daher auf das entsprechende Kapitel verwiesen werden, in dem auch die Pathogenese der Geschwürsbildungen erörtert wird.

[1] Während die meisten Autoren (ebenso wie Moll) das neurodystrophische Element nur als pathogenetische Teilkomponente bewerten, messen Veil und Sturm dem „neuralen Störungsfeld" schlechthin die Führungsrolle bei, das auch nach Wegfall der auslösenden ätiologischen Faktoren das Krankheitsgeschehen eigenrhythmisch weiter unterhalte. Diese nosologische (Über-)Bewertung der neurogenen Pathodynamik wird heute allerdings nur noch von sehr wenigen Autoren akzeptiert.

Unterschenkelgeschwüre sind zu häufig die Folge einer Varicosis, als daß im allgemeinen ihrer Entstehung im Rahmen einer Primär-chronischen Polyarthritis besondere Bedeutung beigemessen würde. SHORT, BAUER und REYNOLDS haben aber bei umfangreichen Vergleichsuntersuchungen an chronisch Rheumakranken und Kontrollpersonen festgestellt, daß die letzteren fast doppelt so häufig eine Varicosis aufwiesen (14,7% gegenüber 8,2%). Nach ihrer Ansicht erklärt sich dies vielleicht durch die zwangsläufig größere statische Schonung der Beine bei chronischer Polyarthritis. Im übrigen ließen sich *Unterschenkelödeme*, die die genannten Autoren in der Patientengruppe bei 9,6%, in der Kontrollgruppe bei 5,5% fanden, durch venöse Stase allein meist nicht erklären, zumal sie vielfach parartikulär bestanden. Möglicherweise sind sie analog zu den Gelenkergüssen der Ausdruck einer krankheitsspezifischen Gewebsinsudation (KULKA u. Mitarb.; SHORT u. Mitarb.).

Insgesamt sind Unterschenkelgeschwüre, ihrer spärlichen Erwähnung nach zu schließen, bei der Primär-chronischen Polyarthritis doch relativ selten. Nach BENINSON und ENSIGN lassen sich zwei pathogenetisch verschiedene Geschwürstypen unterscheiden, ein *unspezifischer* (banal-traumatischer) und ein *rheumatoider Typ*. Der letztere entsteht durch Erweichung und Ulceration von Rheumaknoten, wobei im Gewebsbild noch die charakteristische dreizonale Struktur erhalten sein kann: schwielig-fibröse Außenzone mit zahlreichen entzündlich veränderten Blutgefäßen, granulierende Mittelzone mit palisadenförmig aufgereihten Histiocyten, zerfallendes Zentrum (Ulcusgrund) mit fibrinoider Bindegewebsdegeneration. Demgegenüber erscheint der andere Ulcustyp histologisch uncharakteristisch.

Die Therapie dieser Ulcerationen besteht einerseits in der Bekämpfung der Grundkrankheit (vgl. unter Felty-Syndrom), andererseits in gezielten Lokalmaßnahmen. So berichtet KIRPILÄ über die Totalexcision und plastische Deckung der Geschwüre bei 21 Patienten, ohne jedoch die Spätresultate zu erwähnen. GRANIRER wandte Antibiotica und Corticosteroide, örtlich proteolytische Fermente, unterstützt durch prolongierte Bettruhe, mit unterschiedlichem Erfolg an. BENINSON und ENSIGN empfehlen eine Behandlungsmethode, mit der sie die bisher therapieresistenten Unterschenkelgeschwüre von neun chronischen Polyarthritikern relativ rasch und dauerhaft zur Abheilung brachten. Ihr Verfahren besteht in der kombinierten örtlichen Anwendung eines durch Gaze abgedeckten, Sekret-absorbierenden Gelatinepuders mit elastischer Wicklung des Beines unter stufenweise erhöhter Zugspannung, begünstigt durch eine sehr eiweißreiche Diät und mediko-mechanische sowie orthopädische Maßnahmen gegen die Gelenkversteifungen.

d) Sichtbare Schleimhäute

Eine ausgeprägte entzündlich-atrophische Alteration der Conjunctiva, der Nasen- und Mundschleimhaut (sowie der Speicheldrüsen, des Gastro-Intestinaltraktes und der Bronchialschleimhaut) liegt beim Gougerot-Sjögren-Syndrom vor, das zwar nosologisch anscheinend uneinheitlich ist, aber relativ häufig Beziehungen zur Primär-chronischen Polyarthritis aufweist. In abortiver Form kann sich in der Mundschleimhaut aber auch nur eine fleckige entzündliche Rötung einstellen, die an das Erscheinungsbild einer Ariboflavinose bzw. B_2-Avitaminose erinnert (BAYLES u. Mitarb.; LUCHERINI; SHORT u. Mitarb.). Gelegentlich zeigen die Zungenränder eine diffuse Rötung mit Schwellung der fungiformen Papillen, was v. NEERGAARD als „Glossitis papillaris" bezeichnet hat. Auch kann die Zungenschleimhaut von filiformen Papillen entblößt und glatt werden und zunehmend atrophieren.

e) Ischämische Finger- und Zehennekrosen

Nach Scott u. Mitarb. (1961) lassen sich *drei Typen von entzündlicher Gefäßbeteiligung* bei Rheumatoider Arthritis unterscheiden: 1. Subakute Gefäßveränderungen in der Muskulatur (Steiner; Bunim; Morrison u. a.) und in anderen Organen (Cruickshank u. a.). 2. Fälle von Rheumatoider Arthritis mit schwerer generalisierter und nekrotisierender Arteriitis der großen Gefäße vom Typ der Polyarteriitis nodosa (Levin u. Mitarb.; Ball; Nyström; Ogryzlo; F. R. Schmid u. a.). 3. Fälle von obliterierender Endarteriitis der Hände und Finger, wie sie Bywaters beschrieben hat. Im Rahmen dieses Handbuchbeitrags soll nur die letztere Gruppe näher besprochen werden, da sie ein typisches klinisches Korrelat aufweist, während die anderen Gefäßprozesse mehr von allgemeiner

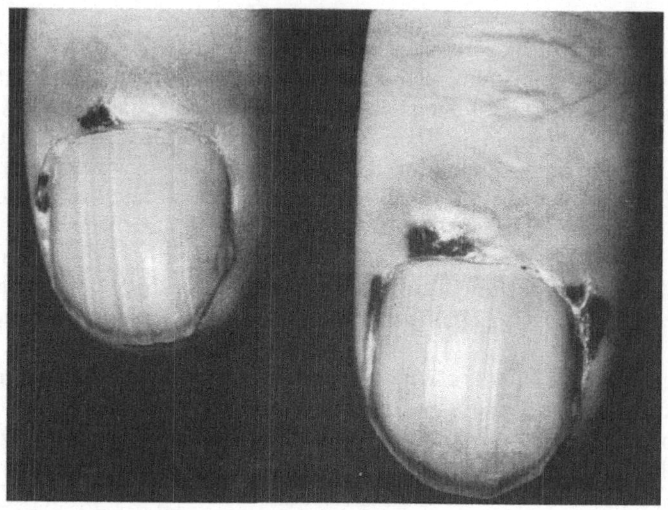

Abb. 11. Paronychiale kleine ischämische Nekrosen bei Primär-chronischer Polyarthritis. [Aus E. G. L. Bywaters: Ann. rheum. Dis. **16**, 84—103 (1957)]

nosologischer Bedeutung sind (hinsichtlich der 1. Gruppe vgl. auch unter „Allgemeiner Hautstatus“ im vorigen Abschnitt).

Bywaters berichtete 1957 über 10 Patienten mit Rheumatoider Arthritis (6 Frauen, 4 Männer), die obstruierende arterielle Gefäßprozesse an den Fingerarterien, teilweise auch im Bereich der inneren Organe aufwiesen. Die klinischen Symptome reichten von umschriebenen bräunlich-hämorrhagischen *„Paronychie“-artigen Mikroinfarkten* an den Nagelfalzen (Abb. 11), Fingerkuppen und übrigen Endphalangen (Abb. 12) bis zu vollständiger Gangrän der Finger oder der ganzen Hand. Bei zwei Patienten, die mit 31 und 41 Jahren unter Periarteriitis nodosa-artigen Generalisationserscheinungen ad finem kamen, waren auch die Nieren, das Pankreas, der Darm, die Milz, das Herz und die Lungen ergriffen. Ein Zusammenhang mit vorangegangener Cortisontherapie konnte in der Mehrzahl der Fälle ausgeschlossen werden.

Teilweise gingen dem Auftreten der remittierenden Mikroinfarkte akroasphyktische Zustände vom Raynaud-Typ voraus, manchmal entwickelten sich auch umschriebene hämorrhagische Blasen an den Fingerenden. Nach Abheilung der Veränderungen blieben feine narbige Einziehungen und Abflachungen der Fingerkuppen zurück. Bei allen Fällen waren auch tendinöse, cutane und subcutane Noduli an den Fingern (und z. T. auch an den Ellenbogen) nachweisbar. Vereinzelt entstanden aus solchen Knötchen ausgestanzte, schlecht heilende Ulcera.

Pathologisch-anatomisch fanden sich konzentrische Einengungen oder Obliterationen der kleinen Arterien durch subintimale histio-reticuläre Zellwucherungen bei meist intakter Elastica interna und Lamina media (Abb. 13). Die akuten gangränösen Erscheinungen waren durch zusätzliche thrombotische Verschlüsse hervorgerufen, die bei mitigierteren Verlaufsformen bindegewebig organisiert und teilweise rekanalisiert wurden.

In nosologischer Hinsicht rechnet BYWATERS seine Beobachtungen auf Grund der übrigen klinischen Symptomatologie, des Krankheitsverlaufes und der pathologisch-anatomischen Befunde zur Primär-chronischen Polyarthritis, wenngleich er nahe Beziehungen zur Endangiitis obliterans v. Winiwarter-Buerger, zum visceralen Lupus erythematodes und zur Progressiven Sklerodermie hervorhebt. Nach seiner Ansicht sind die Gefäßläsionen als eine idiopathische rheumatoide Krankheitsmanifestation analog zu den subcutanen Knötchen anzusehen. Gegen einen visceralen Lupus erythematodes, der ähnliche Gefäßveränderungen hervorrufen kann, sollen der relativ günstige Verlauf bei der Mehrzahl der Fälle und das fehlende L.E.-Zellphänomen

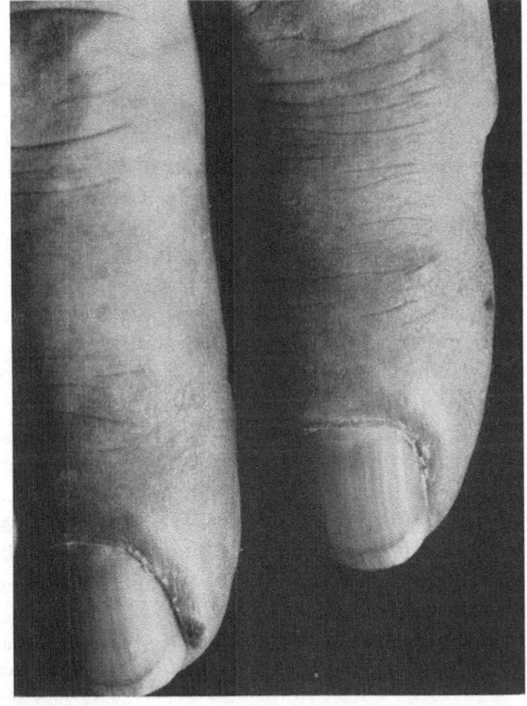

Abb. 12. 48jähriger Patient mit Primär-chronischer Polyarthritis. 2 Jahre nach Krankheitsbeginn erstmals kleinste bräunliche Nekroseherde am rechten Zeigefinger und Nagelfalz des 3. Finger. [Aus E. G. L. BYWATERS: Ann. rheum. Dis. **16**, 84—103 (1957)]

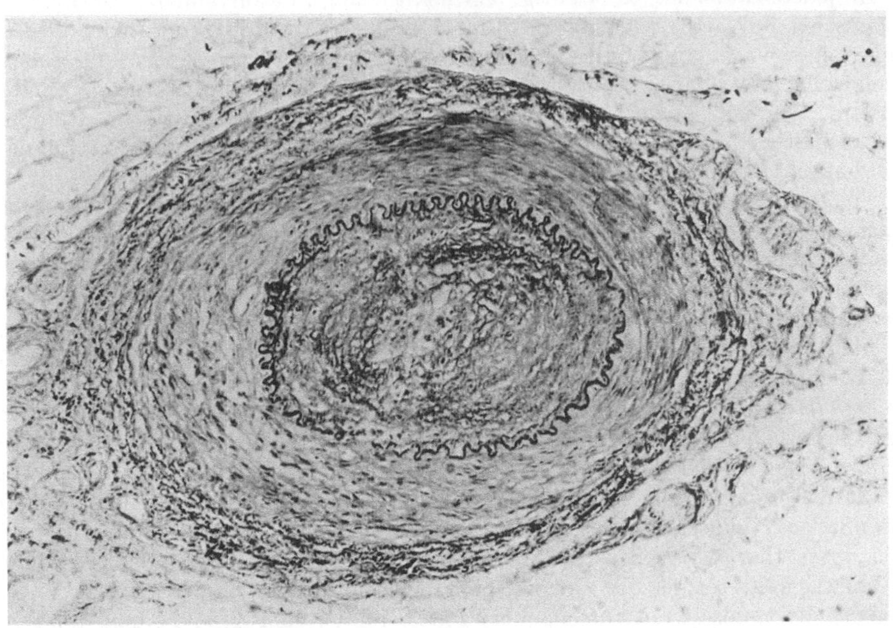

Abb. 13. Gewebsbild zu Abb. 11. Histologische Veränderungen im Bereich einer kleinen Fingerarterie. Elastica-Färbung, 300mal vergr. — Subintimale Zellproliferation mit Obliteration des Gefäßlumens. Elastica interna rechts und unten aufgesplittert, sonst noch weitgehend erhalten. Lockere histiocytäre Proliferation und granulocytäre Infiltration in der Gefäßumgebung. [Aus E. G. L. BYWATERS: Ann. rheum. Dis. **16**, 84—103 (1957)].

sprechen, zumal der „Rheumafaktor" (schwach) positiv nachweisbar war. Das Freibleiben der Venen und größeren Arterien war differential-diagnostisch gegen eine Endangiitis obliterans, das Intaktbleiben der mittleren und äußeren Arterienschichten gegen eine Periarteriitis nodosa anzuführen. Zur Diagnose einer Progressiven Sklerodermie, mit der die Gefäßveränderungen sehr viel Ähnlichkeit hatten, fehlten sonstige pathognomonische Symptome. Kryoglobuline konnten nie nachgewiesen werden. In der Mehrzahl der Fälle bestand auch keine Abhängigkeit von vorangegangener Cortisonbehandlung, während umgekehrt diese Therapie die Gefäßalterationen nicht zu bessern vermochte.

Die unmittelbare pathologisch-anatomische Beteiligung des Gefäßsystems am Krankheitsprozeß, schon früher von KLINGE u. a. hervorgehoben, hat im rheumatologischen Schrifttum der letzten Jahre erhöhte Beachtung gefunden. Nach BÖNI fehlen periphere Durchblutungsstörungen bei der Primär-chronischen Polyarthritis fast nie. RATSCHOW fand zwar keine zahlenmäßige Koinzidenz von Rheumatismus und peripheren Kreislaufstörungen, hält es jedoch für sicher, daß sich die „Endangiitis obliterans" der 20—35jährigen als *Polyangiitis rheumatica* — mit oder ohne polyarthritische oder polymyositische Begleiterscheinungen — entwickeln kann. Zu ähnlichen Schlußfolgerungen kommt FEYRTER, der bei rheumatischen Angitiiden den gleichen histomorphen 3-Phasenablauf wie bei der Endangiitis obliterans fand. Außerdem wies er beim Gougerot-Sjögren-Syndrom und beim Felty-Syndrom arteriitische Veränderungen ähnlich der Periarteriitis nodosa nach. Im übrigen können rheumatische Gefäßprozesse — ähnlich wie beim visceralen Lupus erythematodes — auch osteolytische Einschmelzungsvorgänge verursachen.

Auch mit Hilfe arteriographischer Röntgenuntersuchungen gelingt es relativ oft, arterielle Gefäßverschlüsse im Bereich der Hände und Füße nachzuweisen (SCOTT u. Mitarb.; SOILA u. BERGLUND; BARCELÓ, ALEGRE-MARCET u. VALLS SERRA).

In jedem Falle ist es wichtig, vermeintlichen „Paronychien" bei Primär-chronischer Polyarthritis erhöhte Aufmerksamkeit zu widmen, um nicht die Anfänge einer vasculären Generalisation des Krankheitsprozesses zu übersehen. Auch sollte stets nach etwa vorhandenen Kryoglobulinen im Serum gefahndet werden, da solche auch bei der Primär-chronischen Polyarthritis im Rahmen des vielfältigen immunopathologischen Reaktionsspektrums auftreten können (FELDAKER, PERRY u. HANLON).

Noch häufiger als anatomische Läsionen weisen die peripheren Gefäße *funktionelle Störungen* auf, die sich mit verschiedenen Untersuchungsmethoden (Capillarmikroskopie am Nagelfalz, Plethysmographie bzw. Verschlußdruckplethysmographie der Finger, elektro-oscillographische Messungen, Wärmedurchgangsmessungen der Handinnenfläche usw.) nachweisen lassen. So konnte RATSCHOW bei über der Hälfte seiner Patienten mit Primär-chronischer Polyarthritis (oder mit Rheumatischem Fieber) eine *abnorm gesteigerte angiospastische Reaktionsbereitschaft* in der Kreislaufperipherie feststellen. Nach BETZ und MAULER fehlen dem chronischen Rheumatiker die spontanen vasomotorischen Schwankungen und fein angepaßten Gefäßreaktionen des Gesunden auf thermische Reize. Die Capillarresistenz ist meist herabgesetzt, zeigt aber keine sichere Abhängigkeit von mittleren peristatischen Temperaturschwankungen (POTTER und DUTHIE). Erst unter therapeutischen Bedingungen mit Corticosteroiden pflegt sich die Durchlässigkeitsstörung der Gefäße mehr oder minder zu normalisieren.

Auch der venöse Kreislaufschenkel ist nicht immer vom Krankheitsprozeß verschont. Entsprechende Beobachtungen von *rheumatischer bzw. „rheumatoider" Phlebitis* sind z. B. von TANASESCU u. Mitarb. sowie von LUCHERINI und CECCHI publiziert worden. Diese Venenentzündungen sind nach LUCHERINI und CECCHI vorwiegend in den subcutanen Unterschenkelplexus lokalisiert, begleiten Phasen erhöhter Krankheitsaktivität und sprechen auf antirheumatische Therapie an (was allerdings auch bei unspezifischen Thrombophlebitiden der Fall ist). TANASESCU beobachtete in zwei Fällen nach Tonsillektomie sofortige Abheilung. Die entzündlichen Veränderungen sind fast ausschließlich auf den adventitiellen Bereich beschränkt, während die Lamina interna meist intakt ist und dementsprechend die Gefäßdurchlässigkeit nach Abheilung der Phlebitis erhalten bleibt.

f) Subcutane Knoten (Rheumaknoten)

[Synonyma: *Rheumatische Knoten, rheumatoid nodules* (ALLEN u.a.), *nodosités juxta-articulaires* (JEANSELME), *nodules de Lutz-Jeanselme* (FURTADO u.a.), *subcutaneous nodules of juxta-articular type* (HOPKINS); im übrigen vgl. unter „Nodi rheumatici" im Kapitel über das Rheumatische Fieber]

Ähnlich wie beim Rheumatischen Fieber sind die subcutanen bzw. parartikulären und -ossalen Nodi und Noduli ein sehr charakteristisches Stigma der Grundkrankheit, die ob ihres geweblichen Substrats ja auch als rheumatische Granulomatose (FAHR) bezeichnet worden ist. Aber erst gegen Ausgang des 19. Jahrhunderts zogen diese Knotenbildungen ein regeres ärztliches Interesse auf sich (FAGGE u. PAYE-SMITH; BANNATYNE; HAWTHORNE; WICK). Lange Zeit galt gerade das Vorkommen subcutaner Knoten beim Rheumatischen Fieber und bei der Primär-chronischen Polyarthritis als eines der wesentlichsten Beweismittel für die nosologische Zusammengehörigkeit beider Krankheiten, die dementsprechend nur als verschiedene Phasen ein und derselben pathogenetischen Entwicklung gedeutet wurden (RÖSSLE; KLINGE; FAHR; WEHSARG u.a.). Auch die histomorphe Analogie und vielfache Übereinstimmung der Knoten schien in die gleiche Richtung zu weisen. Erst relativ spät — mit zunehmender Aufdeckung wichtiger klinischer und immunbiologischer Unterschiede zwischen Rheumatischem Fieber und „Rheumatoider" Arthritis — hat man auch feinere Unterschiede im Gewebsbild der Knoten höher bewertet (DAWSON u. BOOTS; COLLINS; BENNETT u. Mitarb.).

In der Dermatologie ist eine Zeitlang die rheumatische Genese „juxtaartikulärer Knoten" zugunsten ihrer (gleichfalls möglichen) tertiär-*luischen* Bedingtheit vernachlässigt worden (vgl. H. HOFFMANN). Wiederholt hat sogar in Zweifelsfällen allein das Vorhandensein solcher juxtaartikulärer Knoten den Ausschlag zugunsten der Diagnose Lues gegeben. In histologischen Vergleichsstudien haben dann KUMER und LANG gezeigt, daß der rheumatische und der luische Knoten ein durchaus unterscheidbares Gewebsbild aufweisen. Wesentlich schwieriger kann dagegen die Abgrenzung von einem *Granuloma anulare (giganteum)* sein, auf dessen „rheumatoides" Gewebssubstrat man erst relativ spät aufmerksam geworden ist. Daneben kommt eine ganze Reihe von klinisch ähnlich imponierenden subcutanen Knoten anderer Ätiologie in Betracht, worauf wir im Abschnitt über die Differentialdiagnose noch eingehen werden.

Die *Häufigkeit* der subcutanen Knoten wird in der Literatur recht unterschiedlich angegeben. SHORT, BAUER und REYNOLDS fanden sie unter 293 Patienten bei der Klinikaufnahme 34mal (11,6%) gegenüber nur 2mal unter 300 Kontrollpersonen (0,7%). Allerdings stieg die Häufigkeit der Rheumaknoten auf 21,3% an, sobald auch der spätere klinische Verlauf berücksichtigt wurde. Einen ähnlich hohen Wert (20%) fanden DAWSON und BOOTS, die allerdings selbst einräumen, daß ihr spezielles Interesse an Rheumaknoten zu einer Selektion entsprechender Klinikeinweisungen geführt haben kann. Nach anderen Autoren variiert die Häufigkeit zwischen 3 und 12,2% (BENNETT; LEWIS-FANING; McCRAE; COATES u. DELICATI), nach MOLL sogar zwischen 5 und 25%. Eine statistisch gesicherte Bevorzugung bestimmter Altersstufen oder eine Abhängigkeit von der Krankheitsdauer besteht anscheinend nicht (SHORT u. Mitarb.). Auch die Geschlechtsverteilung entspricht etwa der allgemeinen Relation bei der Grundkrankheit.

α) Klinischer Befund

In vieler Hinsicht bestehen Analogien zu den subcutanen Knoten des Rheumatischen Fiebers. Meist treten die Gebilde in *Mehrzahl* auf, aber nur selten so zahlreich wie beim Rheumatischen Fieber. Auch solitäres Vorkommen ist möglich.

Die Größe der Knoten differiert zwischen kaum wahrnehmbaren, stecknadelkopfgroßen und kirsch- bis walnußgroßen Ausmaßen. An den *Ellenbogen*, die eine ausgesprochene Prädilektionsstelle darstellen, sowie an den Knien können noch

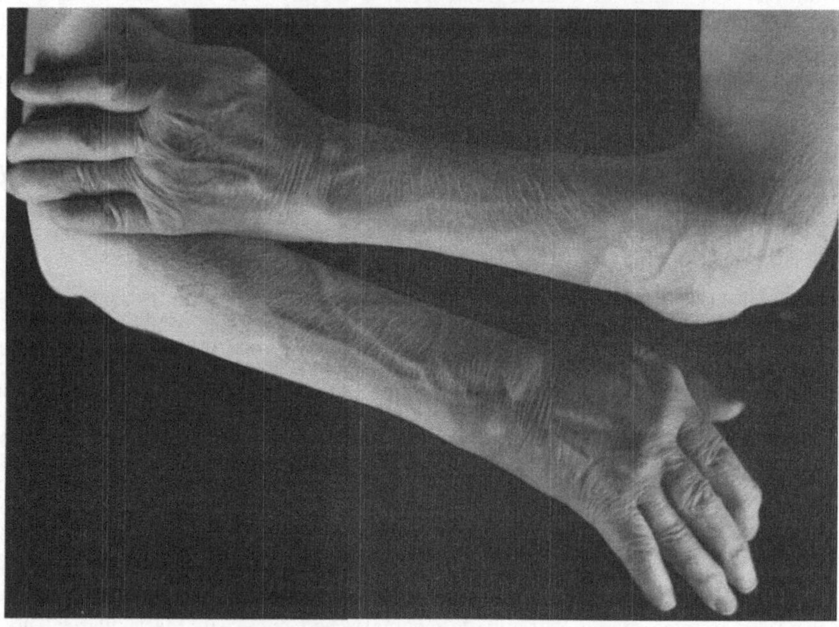

Abb. 14. 64jährige Patientin mit fortgeschrittener Primär-chronischer Polyarthritis. Beidseits in Höhe des Olecranons sowie an der Dorsalseite der Handgelenke unterschiedlich große subcutane Knoten. Typische ulnare Abduktion der Finger besonders der rechten Hand

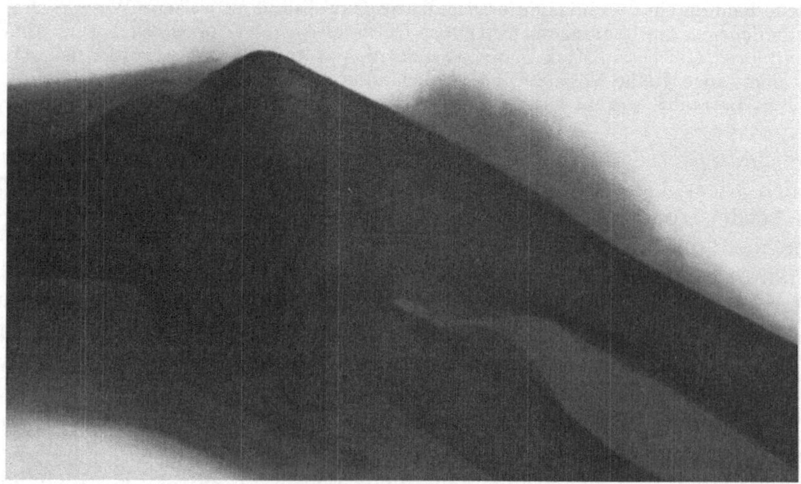

Abb. 15. Röntgen-Weichteilaufnahme eines in Olecranon-Nähe gelegenen subcutanen Knotens der Patientin von Abb. 14. Fast homogene, anscheinend aus mehreren Knoten konglomerierte schattengebende Struktur. [Aus O. HORNSTEIN u. H. SCHUERMANN: In GOTTRON-SCHÖNFELD, Dermat. u. Venerol. II/1, S. 639 (1958)]

größere, u. U. konfluierende Exemplare vorkommen. Im übrigen sind die Finger- und Handrücken, die Streckseiten der distalen Extremitätenanteile (besonders Unterarme), die Kreuzbein- und Trochantergegend, die Umgebung der Wirbelsäulendornfortsätze, der Scapula usw. topographisch bevorzugt, also *gelenk- und knochennahe Regionen* mit relativ spärlichem Fettpolster und erhöhter mechanisch-traumatischer Exposition (Abb. 14). Auch die Beugeseiten der Finger können befallen sein. Charakteristisch ist die Neigung zu *symmetrischer* Ausbreitung, wie sie im übrigen auch die nodösen Manifestationen des Rheumatischen Fiebers kennzeichnet.

Palpatorisch sind die Knoten meist scharf begrenzt, manchmal schmerzhaft, seltener indolent, auf der Unterlage stielartig verschieblich oder breitbasig angeheftet (Abb. 15). Die Konsistenz ist derb-elastisch, sie kann ebenso wie die Größe während des Bestehens der Knoten wechseln. Sekundäre Veränderungen (zentrale Erweichungen oder Verkalkungen) können sich reaktionslos abkapseln, in seltenen Fällen aber auch zur spontanen Perforation mit Entleerung des nekrotischen Materials führen. Die mikroskopische und chemische Untersuchung des Gewebedetritus (negative Murexid-Probe) ermöglicht eine Abgrenzung von Gichtknoten, die *typischerweise* zu Zerfall, Fistelbildung und Ulceration neigen.

Im allgemeinen bestehen die Knoten der Primär-chronischen Polyarthritis *länger* als beim Rheumatischen Fieber. Monatelange Persistenz, selbst jahrelanges Verharren trotz Rückgang der allgemeinen Krankheitsaktivität ist nicht selten. In solchen inveterierten Knoten, die zu „erratischen Findlingen" einer früheren Aktivitätsperiode der Krankheit geworden sind, läßt sich oft ausgeprägte Hyalinisation und Kalkinkrustation des geschädigten Bindegewebes nachweisen. Da sie ihren Trägern meist keine Beschwerden mehr verursachen, werden sie bei der klinischen Untersuchung oft nur zufällig entdeckt.

β) Klinische und prognostische Bedeutung

Grundsätzlich kann man feststellen, daß die Knotenbildungen der Primär-chronischen Polyarthritis *nicht die gleiche ominöse Bedeutung wie beim Rheumatischen Fieber* haben. Zwar besitzen sie eine gewisse Affinität zu schweren und gesteigert entzündlichen Verlaufsformen (DAWSON u. BOOTS; WEHSARG; MOLL u.a.), kommen auch nach den Erfahrungen von SHORT u. Mitarb. etwas häufiger bei Krankheitsfällen mit akutem Beginn vor, sind aber anscheinend kein für rheumatoide Herzbeteiligung signifikantes Warnsymptom. Ihre prognostische Bedeutung ist daher relativ gering. Auch gehören sie *nicht* zu den Früh-Symptomen der Primär-chronischen Polyarthritis, da sie nur ausnahmsweise — sofern man vom monosymptomatischen „Rheumatismus nodosus" absieht — schon in den ersten Krankheitsmonaten nachweisbar sind. Bei einseitiger Polyarthritis pflegen sie zu fehlen, sind also nur für die bilateral-symmetrische Form der Primär-chronischen Polyarthritis charakteristisch. Im übrigen sind adäquate Nodi auch in den verschiedensten inneren Organen, z.B. im Herzen, in der Dura mater, in Skeletmuskeln, peripheren Nerven, Lungen, Oesophagus, serösen Häuten, Gelenkkapseln, Skleren (BENNETT u. Mitarb.; BEVANS u. Mitarb.; VERHOEFF u. KING; MAHER u.a.) autoptisch gefunden worden, was daran denken lassen muß, daß die cutan-subcutanen Rheumaknoten immer nur ein ins makroskopisch Wahrnehmbare gesteigertes Teilsymptom der Grundkrankheit sind, das in der Haut auch dann fehlen kann, wenn innere Organe beteiligt sind.

γ) Histopathologie

Da das Gewebsbild der subcutanen Knoten die Grundzüge des „rheumatischen" bzw. „rheumatoiden" Granuloms aufweist, sei hier an den entsprechenden Abschnitt der Einleitung angeknüpft. Der histologische Befund ist in ausgeprägten Fällen so charakteristisch, daß er früher oft als „spezifisch" angesehen wurde. Im Zentrum der Knoten bestehen mehr oder minder ausgedehnte, landkartenförmig verteilte „fibrinoide“ Nekrosen, die mit Verquellung und scholliger

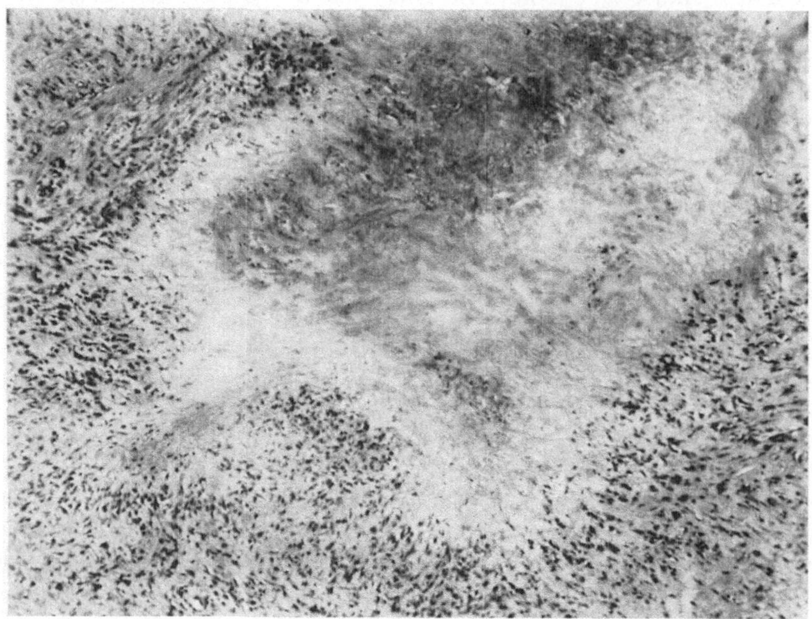

Abb. 16. Subcutaner Knoten bei Primär-chronischer Polyarthritis. Gewebsschnitt, HE, 75mal vergr. — Randbezirk einer ausgedehnten, landkartenförmig-unregelmäßig begrenzten Nekrosezone. Die Zellproliferation des umgebenden Granulationsgewebes ist charakteristischerweise bürsten- bzw. palisadenförmig radiär gestellt

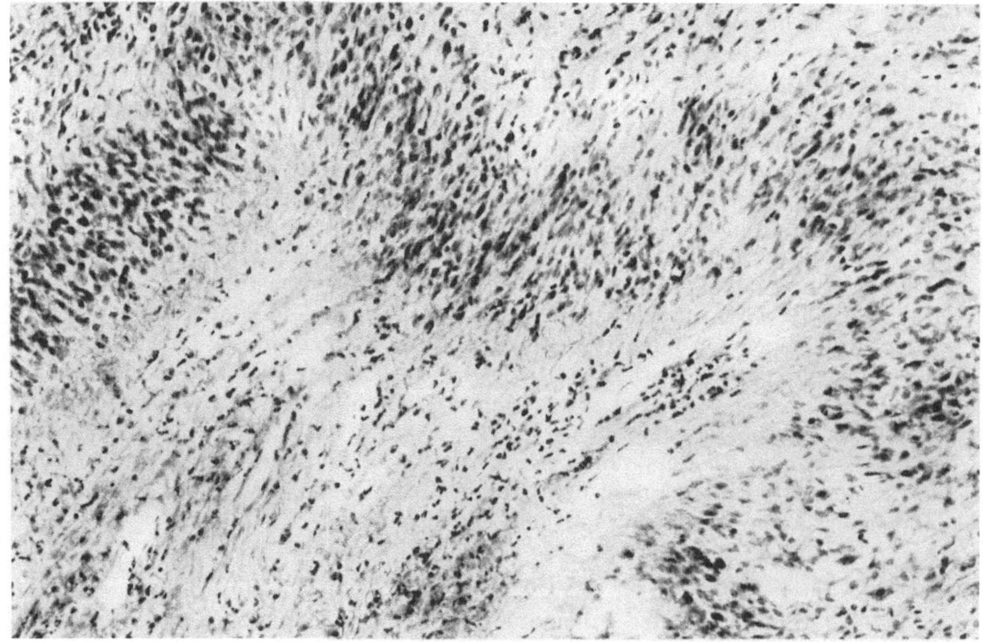

Abb. 17. Subcutaner Knoten bei Primär-chronischer Polyarthritis. Gewebsschnitt, HE, 135mal vergr. — Randanteil einer fibrinoiden Bindegewebsnekrose mit reichlichem Zell- und Kernzerfall (teilweise ähnlich, aber nicht identisch mit zerfallenden Granulocyten). Daran anschließend ein mehrreihiger Granulationsgewebswall, in dem großzellige, radiär gestellte Histiocyten vorherrschen

basophiler Degeneration des präexistenten Bindegewebes einhergehen. Bei stärkerem Ausmaß erinnert der Befund an eine Koagulationsnekrose (Abb. 16). Dieses Zentrum wird im typischen Fall von radiär stehenden, großzellig-langgestreckten, basophilen Histiocyten umsäumt, denen sich noch Lymphocyten, Plasmazellen und vereinzelte mehrkernige Riesenzellen zugesellen können (Abb. 17). In dieser Zone sowie in der sich anschließenden schwielig-bindegewebigen Peripherie der Knoten fallen häufig entzündliche Gefäßveränderungen mit Einengung des Lumens durch subintimale Granulome auf (Abb. 18 und 19). Besonders ausgeprägte Gefäßläsionen, z. T. in Form umschriebener fibrinoider Wandver-

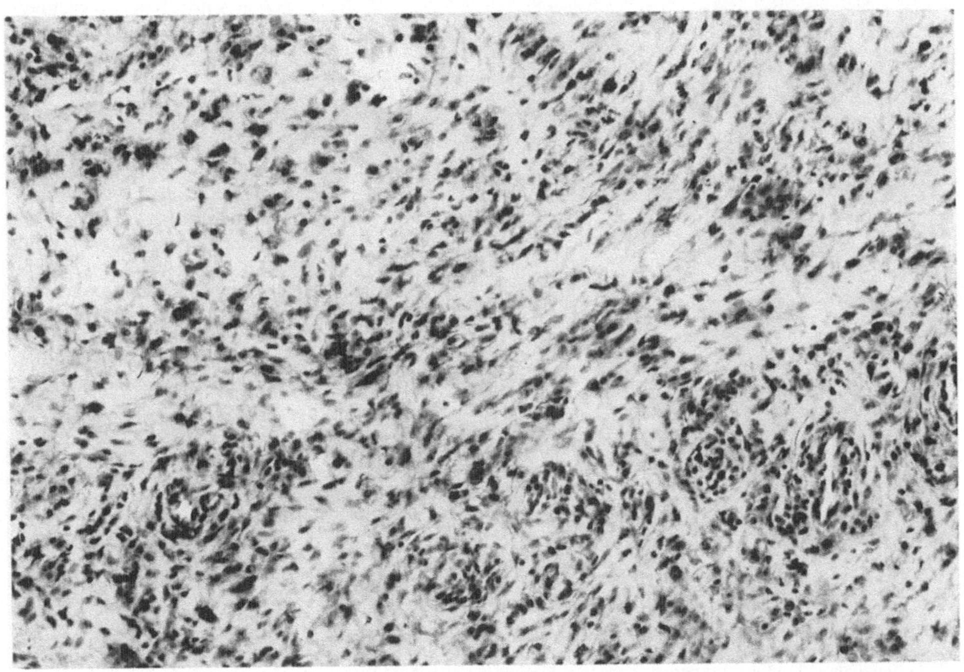

Abb. 18. Gleiches Präparat wie Abb. 17, 135mal vergr. — Peripherie des subcutanen Knotens mit granulierenden Gefäßwucherungen, entzündlichen Gefäßverschlüssen und begleitender histio-monocytoider und lymphocytärer Entzündung. Außerdem Tendenz zu hyaliner Fibrosierung des Interstitiums

quellungen, hat z. B. Ruiter in mehreren subcutanen Knoten eines Patienten mit Primär-chronischer Polyarthritis beschrieben.

Nicht immer weisen chronische Rheumaknoten einen „klassischen" trizonalen Gewebsaufbau auf. Zu Beginn der Knotenbildung sieht man oft nur entzündliche lympho-monocytoide und granulocytäre Infiltrate um die Gefäße mit Ödem und kleinknotiger fibrinoider Verquellung des Bindegewebes (Kersley u. Gibson; Ruiter u. a.), während in fortgeschrittenen Stadien durch Colliquationsnekrose im Zentrum der Knoten cystoide Hohlräume entstehen können. Im subcutanen Fettgewebe entwickeln sich die Knoten meist im Bereich interlobulärer Bindegewebssepten. Synovia-nahe Knoten weisen häufig Lymphknötchen mit und ohne „Keimzentren" sowie Plasmazellansammlungen in der Peripherie auf (Allen).

Ruiter untersuchte bei einem 63jährigen chronisch-rheumatischen Patienten eine Reihe von cutan-subcutanen Knoten in verschiedenen Entwicklungsstadien. In frischen Knötchen fand er um die kleinen Gefäße entzündliche Infiltrate mit Kernzerfall, teilweise mit fibrinoiden Veränderungen der Gefäßwände und mit Ödem des umgebenden Bindegewebes, stellenweise also das Bild einer nekrotisierenden Vasculitis im oberen Corium. Kleine Arterien zeigten ein mucinöses, deutlich metachromatisches Intimaödem. Erst in älteren Knötchen waren außer den vorwiegend vasculären Entzündungszeichen auch degenerative Bindegewebsveränderungen mit basophilen Feulgen-positiven Fibrinoidsäumen um verquollene, kernhaltige Bindegewebsherde nachzuweisen. Ruiters Fall demonstriert den entscheidenden Einfluß entzündlicher Gefäßveränderungen auf das Zustandekommen der Knoten, wobei allerdings die vasculären Läsionen über das gewohnte Maß hinausgingen und den Typ nekrotisierender Vasculitiden boten. Ähnliche Gefäßveränderungen, allerdings an inneren Organen, beschrieben Ball, Cruickshank und Bywaters. Davon abzugrenzen sind vorwiegend proliferative und obliterierende Gefäßveränderungen, wie sie als subintimale und intramurale Zellknötchen fast regelmäßig im Randbereich rheumatischer Knoten zu sehen sind. Ruiter rechnet seine Beobachtung — trotz einer mitvorhandenen Nierenstörung, eines positiven L.E.-Zell-Phänomens und der histologisch dominierenden Gefäßveränderungen — nicht zum visceralen Lupus erythematodes, sondern— angesichts des prognostisch günstigen Verlaufs — zum sog. atypischen primär-chronischen Rheumatismus im Sinne von Bywaters, wobei allerdings nahe Beziehungen zwischen beiden Krankheitsformen bestehen.

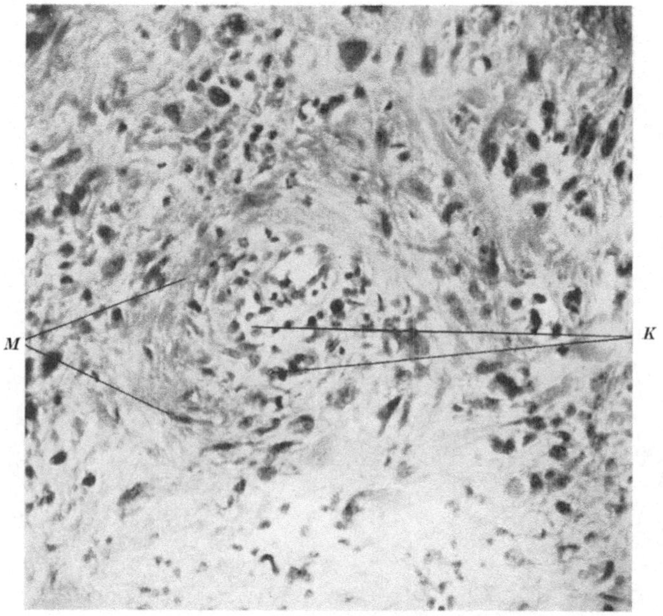

Abb. 19. Subcutaner Knoten bei Primär-chronischer Polyarthritis. Gewebsschnitt, HE, 220mal vergr. — Degenerative und proliferativ-entzündliche Gefäßveränderung im rheumatoiden Granulationsgewebe. Subintimal und intramural gelegenes, etwas ödematös aufgelockertes histiocytäres Zellknötchen mit exzentrischer Einengung des Gefäßlumens. In der Umgebung große basophile Histiocyten. *M* hyaline Verquellung der Tunica media. *K* endovasales Granulom. [Aus O. Hornstein u. H. Schuermann: In Gottron-Schönfeld, Dermat. u. Venerol. II/1, 636 (1958)]

In histochemischer und histoenzymatischer Hinsicht ist die Natur des ,,Fibrinoids" im Zentrum der Knoten noch nicht völlig aufgeklärt. Nach Fawns und Landells besteht das nekrotische Granulomzentrum teils aus zerfallenen kollagenen Fasern, teils aus einer körnigen, färberisch wie Fibrin reagierenden, stets PAS-positiven Substanz. Beide Bestandteile können histoenzymatisch unterschieden werden, da das Kollagen durch Kollagenase, das körnige Material durch Trypsin verdaut wird. Bei dem letzteren handelt es sich um Fibrinoid, das nach Meyer, Böhmig, Movat u.a. aus Exsudatfibrin im Rahmen der primären interstitiell-fibrinösen Entzündung entsteht. Als Beweis für die exsudative Herkunft des Fibrinoids sehen Movat u.a. den histochemischen Nachweis der freien Aminosäuren Tyrosin, Tryptophan, Cystein und Cystin an. Offenbar sind am Zustandekommen der fibrinoiden Gewebsnekrose exsudative proteolytische und desmolytisch-mesenchymale Komponenten beteiligt. Die granulomatöse Reaktion als solche ist dagegen ein Sekundärphänomen. Im übrigen hat man neuerdings mit immunohistologischen Fluorescenzmethoden in subcutanen Knoten (sowie in der Gelenksynovia und in Lymphknoten) den ,,Rheumafaktor" mit selektiver Bindung an Plasmazellen spezifisch nachweisen können (Mellors, Heimer, Corcos und Korngold).

δ) Differentialdiagnose

Nimmt man die „juxtaartikulären Knoten“ als Ganzes, so stellen die „rheumatisch“ bzw. „rheumatoid“ bedingten nur einen kleinen Teil dar. Da der tiefe, meist subcutane Sitz einen relativ nuancenarmen klinischen Befund — oft sogar nur einen Palpationsbefund — ergibt, muß sich die Differentialdiagnose in erster Linie auf den Zusammenhang mit den übrigen klinischen Symptomen stützen. Daher soll an dieser Stelle nur andeutungsweise auf die verschiedenen möglichen Ursachen juxtaartikulärer Knotenbildungen eingegangen werden.

1. Treponematosen. Sowohl bei der *Lues im Stadium III* als auch bei der *Frambösie* („Pian“ bzw. „Yaws“) und bei der *Pinta* (Mal del Pinto bzw. Carate) kommen subcutane („juxtaartikuläre“) Knoten (A. LUTZ 1891; E. JEANSELME 1904) in wechselnder Häufigkeit vor. Nach BURNIER war in Europa um die Dreißigerjahre dieses Jahrhunderts die Lues zu 98% die Ursache solcher treponematös bedingter Knoten. In den letzten Jahrzehnten ist es — infolge zeitweiligen Rückgangs der Morbidität an Lues oder infolge zunehmend exakterer Diagnostik? — um die juxtaartikulären Luesknoten bei uns recht still geworden. Im südamerikanischen Schrifttum wird dagegen noch recht häufig von entsprechenden Beobachtungen berichtet (Literatur s. bei FURTADO). Die innere Zugehörigkeit zur Lues kann sich aus der Anamnese und dem klinischen Gesamtrahmen, aus serologischen Indizien, aus dem Erregernachweis im Gewebe (nach HASSELMANN u.a. mit großen Fehlerquellen behaftet!) oder „ex juvantibus“ (z.B. mittels antiluischer Therapie) ergeben, wobei allerdings inveterierte Knoten manchmal resistent bleiben. Der „Rheumafaktor“ kann gelegentlich auch bei älterer Lues — ebenso wie umgekehrt die Wa.R. bei chronischer Polyarthritis — „falsch positiv“ sein, ist für sich allein also kein sicheres Unterscheidungskriterium.

Wichtig ist der histologische Befund, da das Gewebsbild trotz dreizonaler Struktur vom typischen Befund rheumatischer Knoten etwas abweicht (KUMER u. LANG): So besteht im Zentrum eine zellfreie, vom histomorphen Gepräge der „fibrinoiden“ Nekrose abweichende hyalin-fibröse Bindegewebszone mit cystoiden, von amorphen Massen erfüllten Hohlräumen, während die beiden anderen Schichten größere Ähnlichkeit mit dem Rheumagranulom aufweisen.

Die Knoten der vorwiegend tropischen Treponematosen Frambösie und Pinta sind zwar histopathologisch nicht von luisch bedingten zu unterscheiden (FURTADO), lassen sich aber klinisch und epidemiologisch meist abgrenzen. Bei der Frambösie können sie gelegentlich ein monströses Ausmaß annehmen (Apfelgröße und darüber).

2. Tuberkulose, Sarkoid Darier-Roussy und Lepra. Bei diesen drei Krankheitsgruppen können vereinzelt gelenknahe Knoten auftreten, so bei Knochen- und Gelenktuberkulose als Folge der tuberkulösen Ausbreitung in das benachbarte Gewebe, häufig mit anschließender Fistelbildung. Auch bei der tuberkuloiden Lepra können subcutane Knoten auftreten. WISE demonstrierte einen solchen Patienten mit subcutanen Knoten an Knien und Ellenbogen, wobei histologisch kein Unterschied zu den juxtaartikulären Knoten syphilitischen oder frambösischen Ursprungs bestand (H.FOX). Über juxtaartikuläre Knoten beim Sarkoid Darier-Roussy berichtete SILVA. Hier dürften der klinische Gesamtrahmen und der histologische Befund die diagnostische Zuordnung der Knoten ermöglichen.

3. Acrodermatitis chronica atrophicans. Das häufige Auftreten von juxtaartikulären („fibroiden“) Knoten und tiefen Plaques („Ulnarstreifen“ usw.) bei dieser wahrscheinlich infektiös bedingten dermatotropen Allgemeinkrankheit kann diagnostische Irrtümer hervorrufen, wenn die charakteristischen livid-atrophischen Erytheme übersehen werden (vgl. Handbuchbeitrag HAUSER). Meist sind die Knoten am einen oder an beiden Ellenbogen und über der proximalen Ulnarkante, seltener über den Knien und Schienbeinen lokalisiert. So gut wie immer sind ihnen typische atrophische Akrodermatitisherde zugeordnet, teils distal davon, teils über den Knoten selbst. Die Diagnose kann bei Kenntnis der Krankheit leicht gestellt werden, wobei zu berücksichtigen ist, daß schlaffe Atrophie (als Charakteristikum der Akrodermatitis) bei der Primär-chronischen Polyarthritis meist fehlt. Bei dieser weisen die Hände eine mehr hautfarbene straffe Atrophie auf. Im histologischen Bild der fibroiden Knoten fehlt die für Rheumagranulome charakteristische Zonenbildung, es findet sich nur ein schwielig-fibröses, teilweise hyalinisiertes Zentrum mit zunehmender Plasmazellproliferation in den Randbezirken.

4. Granuloma anulare. Gelegentlich können die typischen cutanen Herde auch subcutan, perichondral (Ohr) oder parartikulär auftreten (CIVATTE, BOLGERT und POISSON; DUPERRAT, GOETSCHEL u.a.). Die histologische Unterscheidung von echten Rheumaknoten kann dann praktisch unmöglich sein (ALLEN u.a.). Hinsichtlich der „rheumatoiden“ Note des Granuloma anulare und seiner nosologischen Problematik vgl. im Kapitel „Rheumatismus nodosus“.

5. *Progressive Sklerodermie.* Nach Crocker, Gray u.a. kommen subcutane Knötchen bei Progressiver Sklerodermie gar nicht so selten vor, besonders im Rahmen des Thibièrge-Weissenbach-Syndroms. Dabei sind die subcutanen Knötchen meist verkalkt und lassen sich dadurch auch röntgenologisch leicht darstellen. Gray fand bei einer 26jährigen Patientin subcutane Knötchen in großer Zahl an den Hand- und Fußrücken, an den patellaren Sehnenansätzen, in der Nachbarschaft der Darmbeinkämme, der vertebralen Dornfortsätze und der Schulterblätter, also in ganz ähnlicher Lokalisation wie bei rheumatischen Prozessen. Jedoch waren röntgenologisch und histologisch keine Verkalkungen nachweisbar, lediglich eine hyaline Bindegewebsdegeneration mit fleckförmigen circumvasalen Rundzellinfiltraten an der Knötchenperipherie. Auch an den Fingerstreckseiten können in Verbindung mit einer Sklerodaktylie kleine subcutane Knötchen auftreten (Lipschütz; Fletcher). Histologisch findet sich dabei hyaline Umwandlung des Bindegewebes mit Elasticaschwund und circumvasalen Lymphocyteninfiltraten in der Peripherie.

6. *Juxtaartikuläre Knoten bei Stoffwechselkrankheiten.* In erster Linie ist hier die *Gicht* zu nennen, die im chronischen Stadium häufig durch knotige Uratablagerungen besonders in der Umgebung der Fußgelenke (sog. Tophi) charakterisiert ist. Diese Knoten sind oft sehr schmerzhaft und neigen zur Fistelbildung, wobei sie krümelig-schmierige Massen mit reichlichen Uratkristallen (positive Murexid-Probe!) entleeren. Histologisch besteht eine ausgeprägt verschwielende, in Verbindung mit den Uratdepots sehr kennzeichnende Entzündung vom Fremdkörpertyp. Die Anamnese mit den typischen Gichtanfällen, die Prädilektion der distalen Fußgelenke („Podagra") und der Ohrmuscheln („Ohrtophi"), das bevorzugte Auftreten bei Männern von pyknischem Habitus im mittleren und höheren Alter, eine hereditäre Disposition zur gleichen und zu sonstigen Stoffwechselkrankheiten (Diabetes mellitus, Lipoidosen usw.), der charakteristische Röntgenbefund mit umschriebenen Usuren an den Gelenkflächen sind diagnostisch wegweisend.

Der Vollständigkeit halber seien auch tiefcutane knotige Hautherde *systematisierter Lipoidosen* (mit und ohne Blutfetterhöhung) erwähnt, ferner knoten- und plattenförmige Kalkablagerungen bei universeller Calcinosis, die aber nur bei atypischem Krankheitsverlauf das Bild eines Rheumatismus nodosus vortäuschen können (Uhlmann).

7. *Heberdensche Knoten.* Bei diesen langsam entstehenden, schmerzlosen, bilateral-symmetrisch verteilten Knoten handelt es sich um flachkugelige, fibröse Verdickungen an den Lateralseiten der distalen Interphalangealgelenke, wovon hauptsächlich der 2.—5. Finger, selten der Daumen oder die Zehen betroffen sind. Meist ist in benachbarten oder in entfernteren Gelenken eine blande Osteoarthritis röntgenologisch nachweisbar. Die Fingerendglieder können subluxiert und in ihrer Beweglichkeit behindert sein. Es besteht eine hereditäre Belastung für das Leiden mit deutlicher Bevorzugung von Frauen im mittleren Lebensalter. Dennoch dürfte die Diagnose angesichts der stereotypen Lokalisation, der Chronizität und des Fehlens eindeutiger rheumatischer Veränderungen im allgemeinen keine Schwierigkeiten bereiten.

8. *Sonstige Knotenbildungen.* Der Erwähnung bedürfen noch die gutartigen, häufig xanthomatösen *Riesenzellfibrome der Sehnenscheiden*, die meist an den Fingern im Bereich der Streckseiten lokalisiert sind, ferner die sog. *Fingerknöchelpolster* (knuckle pads), die eine Art von walzenförmig plattgedrückter Bindegewebsschwiele über den proximalen Interphalangealgelenken bilden, ferner *chronische Bursitiden* mit fibröser Verödung und Verkalkung, cartilaginäre und periostale *Exostosen, gutartige mesenchymale Geschwülste*, sog. *traumatische Epithelcysten* u.a. Bei allen diesen Gebilden ermöglicht, sofern der klinische Befund keine eindeutige Aussage zuläßt, die histologische Untersuchung eine klare Diagnose.

ε) Pathogenese

Als typische, geradezu pathognomonische Manifestation des entzündlich-rheumatischen Grundprozesses haben die subcutanen Knoten die gleiche Pathogenese wie alle anderen im Organismus entstehenden rheumatischen Granulome. Die Grundprinzipien der formalen Genese sind praktisch identisch, basierend auf der initialen Gewebsschädigung durch eine (wahrscheinlich immunologisch ausgelöste) fibrinös-interstitielle Entzündung und auf der nachfolgenden granulomatösen Reaktion mit schließlicher fibröser Umwandlung (vgl. Einleitung).

Für die spezielle Pathogenese bedürfen nur folgende Faktoren einer besonderen Hervorhebung: *Dysregulationen der örtlichen Durchblutung* und *traumatische Insulte.* Für die Annahme örtlicher Durchblutungsstörungen lassen sich die Vorzugslokalisation der Knoten an den Acren, therapeutische Erfolge mit physikalisch-balneologischen, im wesentlichen durchblutungsfördernden Maßnahmen, die klinischen Symptome peripherer Kreislauffunktionsstörungen und nicht zuletzt der histologische Befund der Knoten selbst anführen. Hier besteht besonders in den Anfangsstadien eine erhebliche Gefäßneubildung in der Umgebung der fibrinoiden Bindegewebsnekrose, oft noch vor Ausbildung des eigentlichen granulomatösen Randwalls. In den Spätstadien nimmt die Gefäßsprossung wieder deutlich ab, so daß alte hyalin-fibröse Knoten nur noch eine spärliche Vascularisation zeigen und sich daher häufig nicht mehr vollständig zurückbilden.

Die Acrolokalisation der Knoten, vor allem der Sitz im Ellenbogenbereich, weist aber auch auf exogene *mechanische* Einflüsse hin. So ist es bekannt, daß *professionelle Alltagstraumen* auch banaler Art (ständige Druckbeanspruchung durch Knien, Aufstützen usw.) die Entstehung von Rheumaknoten begünstigen (KOELSCH; FRANÇON u. Mitarb.). Für die Pathogenese hat das Moment des Traumas hauptsächlich die Bedeutung eines Realisationsfaktors, der neben anderen, teilweise noch unbekannten äußeren Einflüssen bei gegebener Erkrankungsdisposition die Entstehung von Rheumaknoten provoziert.

ζ) Therapie

Eine örtliche Behandlung der Rheumaknoten erscheint nur dann sinnvoll, wenn sich diese gegenüber der Allgemeintherapie des rheumatischen Grundprozesses resistent verhalten und durch Schmerzhaftigkeit, örtliche Verunstaltung, Funktionsbehinderung oder Ulceration Beschwerden verursachen. In solchen Fällen kommt Exstirpation der Knoten in Betracht, während intra- und perifokale Injektionen von Hyaluronidase oder von Corticosteroiden in kristalliner Depotform wegen der geringeren Erfolgschance weniger zu empfehlen sind.

g) Pseudo-sklerodermische Begleiterscheinungen

Im Verlaufe einer Primär-chronischen Polyarthritis können sklerodermiforme Veränderungen an den Händen, seltener auch an den Füßen entstehen, die dem ungeübten Untersucher das Bild einer Sklerodaktylie bei progressiver Sklerodermie (pr. Skl.) vortäuschen — zumal auch bei der letzteren manchmal degenerativ-atrophische Gelenkveränderungen vorkommen. *Derartigen pseudo-sklerodermischen Zuständen fehlt aber die Progressivität*; ihre differentialdiagnostische Abgrenzung von der pr. Skl. hat also nicht nur therapeutische, sondern auch prognostische Bedeutung.

Folgende diagnostische Kriterien erleichtern nach JABLONSKA und BUBNOW die Unterscheidung:

1. Die Sklerosierung der Hand erreicht nie die Ausdehnung und Einförmigkeit der echten Sklerodaktylie. Eine gewisse Verschieblichkeit der Cutis auf der Unterlage bleibt meist erhalten.
2. Die Gelenkveränderungen sind primärer Natur, *die dermale Sklerose ist sekundäre Begleiterscheinung*. Bei der pr. Skl. vom Sklerodaktylie-Typ sind dagegen die artikulären Läsionen eine Folge des primären benachbarten Sklerosierungsprozesses, der außer dem Corium und der Subcutis auch die Ligamente und Schleimbeutel einbezieht.
3. Die Handinnenflächen fühlen sich *zart und schweißfeucht* an, während sie bei pr. Skl. eine mumienhaft derbe und trockene Beschaffenheit mit verminderter Schweißsekretion aufweisen.
4. Die Physiognomie mancher Patienten erfährt zwar eine eigentümliche Änderung durch Verschmälerung der Nasenflügel und des Saumgebietes der Lippen (mitunter mit angedeuteter Mikrostomie und perioraler radiärer Furchenbildung), doch fehlen in solchen Fällen makulöse teleangiektatische Erytheme (als Frühsymptom der pr. Skl.!) und diagnostisch gleichrangige Indizien in der Mundhöhle (z. B. ein sehnig verkürztes Zungenbändchen).
5. Die Histologie pseudo-sklerodermischer Zustände ist durch degenerative Homogenisierung des kollagenen Bindegewebes sowie durch Fragmentierung und scholligen Zerfall der elastischen Fasern gekennzeichnet, während bei der pr. Skl. eine noch stärkere Sklerosierung des Bindegewebes mit besser erhaltenen, oft parallel zur Hautoberfläche verlaufenden elastischen Fibrillen kontrastiert.
6. Die *sensible Chronaxie* pflegt bei Primär-chronischer Polyarthritis *nur über den sklerosierten Hautbezirken etwas verlängert* zu sein, während sie *über den unveränderten Anteilen normal* bleibt. Demgegenüber besteht bei der pr. Skl. — und zwar bereits im Frühstadium — eine

Verlängerung der sensiblen Chronaxie am *gesamten* Hautorgan. Diese sehr zielsichere diagnostische Unterscheidung ist von Jablonska und ihren Mitarbeitern klar herausgearbeitet worden.

Differentialdiagnostischen Wert besitzt auch die *Capillarmikroskopie* am Nagelfalz: Während bei der Primär-chronischen Polyarthritis nur relativ uncharakteristische Verdünnungen und Erweiterungen der subepidermalen Capillarschlingen zu sehen sind, ist der pr. Skl. ein recht charakteristischer capillarmikroskopischer Befund mit abnormer Deformation und Verminderung der Capillarschlingen sowie mit verzögerter und intermittierend stockender Durchströmung eigentümlich (Jablonska).

Raynaud-Phänomene gehören zu den seltenen, *atypischen* Begleitsymptomen einer Primär-chronischen Polyarthritis. Im capillarmikroskopischen Bild sind einzelne Gefäßschlingen maximal erweitert. Eine nosologische Zuordnung zur Primär-chronischen Polyarthritis kann erst dann erfolgen, wenn die bekannten, teilweise genannten differentialdiagnostischen Kriterien eine pr. Skl. auszuschließen erlauben. Auf die Wichtigkeit der Bestimmung der sensiblen Chronaxie sei hier nochmals hingewiesen.

Einer kurzen differentialdiagnostischen Erwähnung bedarf noch der *Morbus P. Marie-Bamberger* („Osteoarthropathie hypertrophiante pneumique"), neuerdings von Uehlinger auch *Osteopathia hypertrophicans toxica* genannt. Dieses vorwiegend die Diaphysen der Röhrenknochen, gelegentlich aber auch das übrige Skelet im Sinne einer ossifizierenden Periostitis, Osteoporose und generellen Osteophytose befallende Krankheitsbild stellt eine *pathognomonische, jedoch fakultative Begleiterscheinung verschiedenartiger kardio-pulmonaler Krankheitsprozesse* (Pneumokoniosen, chronische Bronchiektasien, Bronchialcarcinome, kongenitale Herz- und Gefäßvitien etc.) dar. Die pathogenetischen Voraussetzungen sind noch unklar (peripheres Sauerstoffdefizit? Toxische Kachexiewirkung? Hypophysär-diencephale Funktionsstörung?).

Während leichtere Fälle — unabhängig von Schwere und Prognose der kardialen oder broncho-pulmonalen Primärkrankheit — nur durch schmerzhafte Steifigkeit und Schwellung der Finger mit trommelschlägelartiger Umbildung der Endglieder und uhrglasförmiger Verkrümmung der Nägel charakterisiert sind, *kann bei ausgedehnter Osteopathie ein der Primär-chronischen Polyarthritis ähnlicher Zustand mit pseudo-sklerodermischen Veränderungen resultieren.* Hierzu eine eigene Beobachtung:

60jährige Patientin, wegen „atypischer progr. Sklerodermie oder Pseudo-Sklerodermie bei atypischer Primär-chronischer Polyarthritis" in die Klinik aufgenommen. Krankheitsdauer bis zum Tod 11 Monate. *Beginn mit bläulicher Anschwellung der Finger und Handrücken, zum Teil mit Raynaud-artigen Symptomen.* Plumpe Hände, Trommelschlägelfinger, Uhrglasnägel. BSG 57/95 mm n.W. Dysproteinämie mit starkem Anstieg der α_2-Globulin-Fraktion, CRP +, Rheuma-Serologie negativ. *Zunehmend schmerzhafte Schwellung der Unterarme und Unterschenkel,* verstärktes Schwitzen, Verschlechterung des Allgemeinbefindens. Röntgenologische Feststellung einer parahilären, zunächst als Tuberkulose verkannten Lungenverschattung. Bei späterer Kontrolle als bereits inoperables *Bronchialcarcinom* diagnostiziert. *Typischer Röntgenbefund einer Osteopathia hypertrophicans toxica an beiden Händen, Unter- und Oberarmen mit Einbeziehung des Schultergelenks und der Clavicula.* Rapider Verfall erst 2 Monate ante finem. Autoptische Bestätigung eines Bronchialcarcinoms.

2. Felty-Syndrom

[Synonyma: *(Still-) Chauffard-Felty-Syndrom, Chauffard-Ramond-Syndrom, Poliartrite cronica primaria adenosplenomegalica* (Gigante u.a.)]

Vorbemerkung

1924 beschrieb A. R. Felty (Baltimore) bei fünf Patienten eine besondere Form der chronischen Polyarthritis, gekennzeichnet durch zusätzliche Splenomegalie und Leukopenie, ferner (inkonstant) durch generalisierte Lymphknotenschwellungen, mäßige Anämie, zeitweilige Temperaturerhöhungen, Gewichtsverlust, subcutane (rheumatoide) Knoten und bräunliche Hautpigmentierungen. Zunächst war man auf Grund verschiedener klinischer Parallelen mit der Stillschen Krankheit des Kindesalters geneigt, beide Krankheitsformen grundsätzlich zusammenzufassen. Diese Ansicht vernachlässigte jedoch eine ganze Reihe von echten Unterschieden, die nicht nur in der verschiedenen Altersdisposition, sondern anscheinend auch in bestimmten pathophysiologischen Besonderheiten begründet sind, weshalb sie neuerdings von vielen Autoren zugunsten einer schärferen Abgrenzung beider „Syndrome" wieder verlassen wurde. So gilt heute fast allgemein das Felty-Syndrom ebenso als eine besondere Verlaufsweise des adulten primär-chronischen Rheumatismus, wie es für die Stillsche Krankheit im Rahmen der juvenilen chronischen Polyarthritis schon lange anerkannt ist.

Ohne FELTYs Verdienst um die nosologische Präzisierung des Syndroms zu schmälern, sei darauf hingewiesen, daß einige vergleichbare Beobachtungen schon früher publiziert wurden. So berichteten POLLITZER (1914) und STRAUSS (1915) über Krankheitsfälle, die mit dem heutigen Felty-Syndrom identisch sein dürften. Damals hatte man aber zu sehr die Ähnlichkeit mit der Stillschen Krankheit im Auge, um das Neuartige genügend herauszustellen. Auch hatten bereits 1896 CHAUFFARD und RAMOND über generalisierte Lymphknotenschwellungen (aber nicht über Splenomegalie) beim chronischen Rheumatismus der Erwachsenen berichtet, so daß POLLITZER bei seinen Beobachtungen noch von einem „Typus Still-Chauffard" sprach.

Die erste ausdrückliche Beschreibung des „Felty-Syndroms" im deutschsprachigen Schrifttum stammt von BREU und FLEISCHHACKER (1938). Seither ist eine größere Zahl von kasuistischen Veröffentlichungen erfolgt, die aber meist nur einzelne Beobachtungen umfassen, da das typische Krankheitsbild innerhalb des primär-chronischen Rheumatismus doch ziemlich selten vorkommt. So fand es PETRY unter 8000 Rheumakranken nur ein einziges Mal. H. MÜLLER schätzte die Zahl der bis 1960 veröffentlichten Fälle auf nicht mehr als etwa 125. Zweifellos sind aber in dieser Zeit die abortiven Erscheinungsformen nicht enthalten; weiß man doch, daß besonders Anämien, aber auch Milzschwellungen und Leukopenien bei der Primär-chronischen Polyarthritis in wechselnder Häufigkeit, gewissermaßen monosymptomatisch, auftreten können.

Noch wenig bekannt ist, daß das Krankheitsbild nicht nur rheumatologische und hämatologische, sondern auch interessante *dermatologische* Aspekte aufweist. Beiträge hierzu stammen von SCHOCH, HJORTH, KORTING u. HOLZMANN, STOLTE u.a.

a) Klinische Hauptkennzeichen

Das Felty-Syndrom stellt einen besonderen, *durch enorme Aktivierung des RHS gekennzeichneten Reaktionstyp der Primär-chronischen Polyarthritis* dar und beginnt meist im mittleren bis höheren Lebensalter, im allgemeinen erst *lange nach dem Beginn der Polyarthritis*. Bei Kindern tritt es fast nie auf (Ausnahme: 7jähriges Mädchen bei LOUYOT, VINCENT u. MATHIEU). Vielleicht lassen sich solche Fälle auch einer atypischen Stillschen Krankheit zuordnen. Ebenso wie bei der „einfachen" Primär-chronischen Polyarthritis überwiegt das weibliche Geschlecht. Der Krankheitsverlauf erstreckt sich langsam progredient, von subakuten Schüben unterbrochen, über Jahre bis Jahrzehnte. Mehrfach ist tödlicher Ausgang infolge Panmyelopathie, Amyloidose oder Lebercirrhose beschrieben worden.

Zu den *obligaten Symptomen* des Krankheitsbildes gehört die um Jahre bis Jahrzehnte vorausgehende, in Schüben verlaufende *chronische Polyarthritis*, eine deutliche *Milzschwellung* und eine *Leukopenie des Blutbildes*, meist mit relativer Lymphocytose. Die Leukocytenzahlen liegen häufig zwischen 1000—3000/mm^3, manchmal noch darunter. Als *fakultative Symptome* können hinzutreten *generalisierte Lymphknotenschwellungen*, *Hepatomegalie*, *Nodi rheumatici*, leichte *Fieberschübe*, eine *Anämie*, die nur selten stärkere Grade erreicht, *Achylie der Magenschleimhaut*, *verschiedenartige Hauterscheinungen*. Agranulocytotisch bedingte Komplikationen können vorkommen. Auf Übergänge in Lebercirrhose oder allgemeine Amyloidose, auf Beziehungen zur Periarteriitis nodosa (NYSTRÖM), zum Sjögren-Syndrom (GEILER), zum Plummer-Vinson-Syndrom (LINDEBOOM) sowie auch zum visceralen Lupus erythematodes (HASERICK; STOLTE[1]) ist besonders hingewiesen worden. BUSER beschrieb die Umwandlung einer Stillschen Krankheit in ein typisches Felty-Syndrom mit gleichzeitiger autoptisch gesicherter Endokarditis vom Typ Libman-Sacks bei einer 20jährigen Frau. In den Fällen von SCHMENGLER und PETRIDES sowie H. MÜLLER traten im Krankheitsverlauf schwere hämolytische Anämien auf.

Alle diese Beobachtungen deuten auf *autoimmunisatorische* Vorgänge hin, wie sie gerade beim rheumatischen Formenkreis (einschließlich der pararheumatischen sog. „Kollagenosen") gehäuft vorkommen. Ebensowenig wie beim sonstigen primär-chronischen Gelenkrheumatismus hat sich beim Felty-Syndrom eine wesentliche ursächliche Rolle spezifischer Erreger nachweisen lassen, wenngleich infektiösen Noxen letzten Endes doch ein mitbestimmender Einfluß zuerkannt wird. Der pathogenetische Schwerpunkt liegt aber auf der *hyperergischen Reaktionsweise eines chronisch stimulierten RHS*, dessen Hyperaktivität wahrscheinlich durch (infektiös ausgelöste) autoallergische Prozesse auf dem Boden der rheumatischen Gewebsschädigung hervorgerufen wird. Morphologisch äußern sich diese abnormen Reaktionen in erheblicher reticulo-plasmocytärer Proliferation der sog. lymphatischen Organe (vor allem Milz und Lymphknoten), humoral in einer Dys- und Paraproteinämie, die gelegentlich — wie schon erwähnt — in Amyloidose oder Lebercirrhose einmündet.

Die *Ursache der Leukopenie* — als wesentlichster Unterschied zur Stillschen Krankheit, die mit Normo- oder Hyperleukocytose einhergeht — wird heute eher in einer *autoimmunologisch bedingten Knochenmarksschädigung* (vorzugsweise der *Granulocytopoese* im Sinne eines myelotropen „Schockfragments") als in einer „splenogenen Markhemmung" erblickt (SCHMENGLER u. PETRIDES, SCHOEN u. TISCHENDORF u. a.). Bei der letzteren kommt es mehr zu einer generellen Knochenmarkshemmung mit Pancytopenie, die beim Felty-Syndrom nur manchmal beobachtet wird. Gesteigerte Phagocytosebereitschaft, z. B. als Erythrophagocytose im peripheren Blut nach einem L.E.-Induktionsversuch (KORTING u. HOLZMANN), systematisierte reticuläre Proliferation des engeren RHS einschließlich des Knochenmarks, Hyper-γ-Globulinämie, positiver Latex-Test u. a. unterstützen diese Auffassung. Auch führt die Splenektomie nur in einem Teil der Fälle zur bleibenden Beseitigung der hämopoetischen Störung.

In *therapeutischer* Hinsicht war das Felty-Syndrom früher eine Indikation zur Splenektomie, während es heute — basierend auf den veränderten pathogenetischen Vorstellungen — mehr und mehr zu einer Domäne der Behandlung mit Corticosteroidhormonen geworden ist. Daneben werden roborierende Maßnahmen und Bluttransfusionen empfohlen.

b) Hauterscheinungen beim Felty-Syndrom

Im wesentlichen kann man drei Typen von dermatologischen Veränderungen unterscheiden, die beim Felty-Syndrom in mehr oder minder charakteristischer Weise vorkommen: 1. Abnorme Pigmentierungen, 2. Unterschenkelgeschwüre von auffälliger Therapieresistenz, 3. fleckförmige Erytheme. Außerdem sind vereinzelt nekrotisierende Ulcera der Mundschleimhaut und der Gaumentonsillen (Leukopenie bis Agranulocytose!), Xerostomie, Atrophie der Zungenschleimhaut, Glossodynie und Dysphagie beobachtet worden, die im Verein mit Achylie des Magens und entzündlichen Speicheldrüsenveränderungen auf eine Kombination mit dem Sjögren-Syndrom hinweisen (vgl. GEILER) und daher hier unberücksichtigt bleiben können.

α) Pigmentierungen

Sie wurden bereits von FELTY beschrieben und kehren auch in der Mehrzahl der Kasuistiken wieder. Es handelt sich um *schmutzig-bräunliche Verfärbungen*

[1] Auch SCHOCH fand bei einem seiner Felty-Patienten im Knochenmark L.E.-Zellen, sonst jedoch keinerlei Anzeichen für einen integumentalen oder visceralen Lupus erythematodes.

der Haut von *meist fleckförmiger* Anordnung und verwaschen-unscharfer Begrenzung. Meist sind die frei getragenen Partien, vor allem das Gesicht betroffen, wo manchmal eine Chloasma-artige oder auch bandförmig-pellagroide Färbung an Stirn und Wangen, manchmal eine mehr schmetterlingsförmige Zeichnung in den mittleren Gesichtspartien besteht. Hände, Unterschenkel und Füße können mitbeteiligt sein. Mitunter weist außerdem das *gesamte* Integument ein fahles, schiefrig-bräunliches Kolorit, ähnlich dem eines beginnenden Bronze-Diabetes oder einer Lebercirrhose, auf.

Die meisten Pigmentierungen sind *durch die allgemeine Corticosteroidtherapie günstig zu beeinflussen.* Solche therapeutischen Beobachtungen lassen den vorsichtigen Schluß zu, daß am Zustandekommen der Pigmentierungsstörung — ähnlich wie beim Morbus Addison — ein Unterfunktionszustand der Nebennierenrinde einen wesentlichen Anteil hat[1].

β) Geschwüre

Wiederholt sind beim Felty-Syndrom Ulcera an den Unterschenkeln erwähnt oder ausdrücklich beschrieben worden (Rogers u. Langley; Peden; Sutton u. Sutton; Schoch; Hjorth; Lutz; Lodin u. Gentele; Granirer; Stolte; Beninson u. Ensign u.a.). Diese Geschwüre waren meist großflächig, tief nekrotisierend und gegenüber den üblichen Therapiemaßnahmen *ungewöhnlich resistent.* Teilweise waren die für Ulcera varicosa typischen supramalleolaren Prädilektionsstellen betroffen, teilweise aber auch die Streck- und Beugeseiten der Unterschenkel. Mehrfach wurden Hinweise auf venöse oder arterio-venöse Durchblutungsstörungen ausdrücklich verneint. Überraschenderweise bewirkten Splenektomien (Rogers u. Langley; Peden) oder neuerdings Corticosteroid- und ACTH-Behandlung (Hjorth; Stolte), also *am Grundprozeß angreifende Maßnahmen,* trotz vorheriger hartnäckiger Therapieresistenz baldige narbige *Abheilungen!*

Angesichts der Häufigkeit des Ulcus cruris varicosum bei Frauen mittleren und höheren Lebensalters — also angesichts der gleichen Geschlechts- und Altersdisposition wie beim Felty-Syndrom — ist naturgemäß besondere Zurückhaltung hinsichtlich einer nosologischen Zuordnung der Geschwüre zu diesem Syndrom geboten. Histologische Untersuchungen (Schoch; Hjorth; Lodin u. Gentele) führten in dieser Frage nicht weiter, da die Gewebsbefunde unspezifisch waren. Dagegen sprechen die durch Corticosteroid-Behandlung „ex iuvantibus" erzielten Erfolge in gewisser Weise doch für eine ursächliche (indirekte) Abhängigkeit der Geschwürsbildungen von der Grundkrankheit.

Bei einer 58jährigen Patientin von Lodin und Gentele traten rezidivierende Ulcera außer an den Unterschenkeln auch an den Ellenbogen, einigen Fingerknöcheln und an der distalen Fußsohle auf (ähnlich einem sog. trophoneurotischen Ulcus).

Über den *Pathomechanismus der Ulcusentstehung* beim Felty-Syndrom ist noch wenig bekannt. Wahrscheinlich wirken chronische Störungen der dermalen Trophik, entzündliche und inaktivitätsbedingte Muskelatrophie[2] sowie mangelhafte, durch die allgemeine Granulocytopenie bedingte Abwehrreaktionen auf banale Schädigungen ursächlich zusammen. In diesem Zusammenhang sei daran

[1] Im übrigen ist das Felty-Syndrom mehrfach mit dem „allgemeinen Adaptationssyndrom" Selyes — im Sinne einer chronischen Erschöpfungsphase des Hypophysen-Nebennierenrinden-Systems — in Verbindung gebracht worden (Aslan u.a.).

[2] Curtis und Pollard fanden bei histologischen Untersuchungen von Haut-Muskelexcisionen der Wadenregion Atrophie der Epidermis, Fibrose des Coriums und geringe interstitielle Entzündung der Muskulatur vom Typ der bei Rheumatoider Arthritis von Steiner u. Mitarb. beschriebenen myositischen Veränderungen.

erinnert, daß torpide Ulcera cruris (häufig mit hämosiderotischer Randpigmentierung) auch bei der Sichelzellanämie, der Thalassaemia major (Cooley-Anämie), T. minor et „minima", beim familiären hämolytischen Ikterus, bei der echten Polycytämie, beim Morbus Werlhof sowie beim Banti-Syndrom vorkommen und teilweise ebenfalls durch Splenektomie geheilt werden können.

γ) Erythematöse, purpurische und andere Hautveränderungen

Sie sind vereinzelt bei typischen Felty-Patienten beschrieben worden und anscheinend ebenso „unspezifischer" Natur wie die Pigmentverschiebungen und Unterschenkelgeschwüre. So berichtet MacCormac über fleckförmige, unter Atrophie und Pigmentierung abheilende Erytheme an beiden Fußknöcheln. Eine

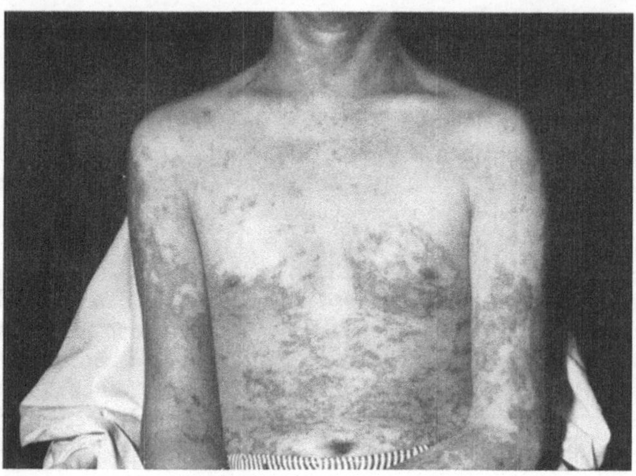

Abb. 20. Patient mit Felty-Syndrom. — Hauptsächlich im Brust- und oberen Bauchbereich lokalisiertes, aus unregelmäßig begrenzten, zentrifugal wandernden anulär-squamösen Erythemen bestehendes Exanthem. [Aus G. W. Korting u. H. Holzmann: Arch. klin. exp. Derm. **210**, 472—484 (1960)]

von Hjorth demonstrierte Patientin zeigte außer Unterschenkelgeschwüren und flächenhaften, besonders die Beugefalten betonenden Pigmentvermehrungen dunkelrote *Striae distensae* an Bauch, Hüften und Brüsten sowie fleckige, aus Teleangiektasien, Purpura und rötlich-brauner Pigmentierung gemischte Erytheme. Außerdem wies die Patientin Palmarerytheme auf (Leberschädigung?). Purpurische Schübe werden auch von Schoch, Lodin und Gentele, Korting und Holzmann erwähnt.

Über ein ungewöhnliches, an Brust, Oberbauch, Armen und Beinen lokalisiertes braun- bis bläulich-rotes Exanthem bei einem 40jährigen Felty-Patienten berichteten Korting und Holzmann (Abb. 20). Es handelte sich dabei um dichtstehende bis *grobnetzig konfluierende*, teilweise *polycyclisch begrenzte* und mäßig erhabene, zentral meist abgeblaßte und eingesunkene, dadurch *anulär imponierende Erytheme* (Abb. 21), die stellenweise pseudoatrophische Runzelung und kleinlamellöse Schuppung oder Colerette-artige Schuppensäume aufwiesen. An den Unterschenkeln trat eine petechial-hämorrhagische Note hinzu und bei der Kneifprobe an unveränderter Haut entstanden Punktblutungen. Im Laufe der klinischen Behandlung griffen die Herde auch auf den Rücken über, zeigten *allmähliche zentrifugale Ausbreitung*, hie und da kleinfingernagelgroße Erosionen und Schuppenkrusten, an den Unterschenkeln flächenhaft konfluierende *hämorrhagische* Erytheme. Histologisch fand sich eine lockere lymphohistiocytäre und von einzelnen Eosinophilen durchsetzte Aktivierung des subpapillären Gefäßbindegewebes sowie eine herdförmige geringe lymphocytäre Infiltration des epidermalen Rete Malpighi (Abb. 22). Außerdem waren epidermale Zellveränderungen im Sinne der „altération cavitaire" mit acidophiler Zelldegeneration und Corps rond-artigen, McManus- und Feulgen-negativen Einschlußkörperchen sowie geringe ortho- und parakeratotische Verbreiterungen der Hornschicht nachweisbar. Unter einer kombinierten *Dexamethason*-Antibiotica-Behandlung kam es zu fortschreitender, lediglich verwaschene Braunpigmentierungen hinterlassender *Abheilung* der Hautveränderungen und zu erheblicher allgemeiner Besserung, teilweise sogar mit Normalisierung verschiedener klinischer Befunde.

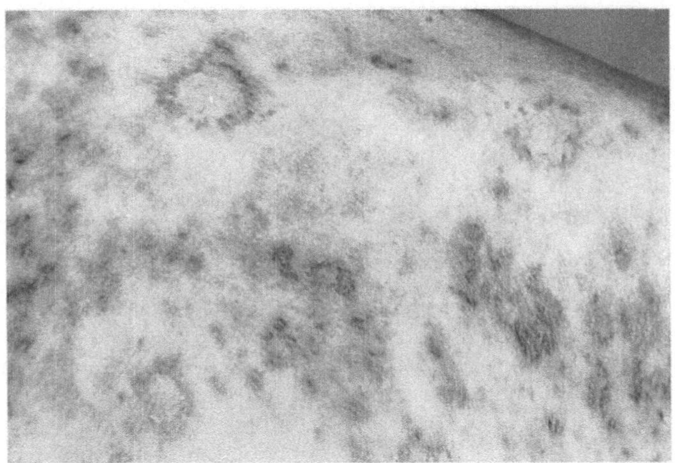

Abb. 21. Gleicher Patient wie Abb. 20. Teilvergrößerung des Exanthembefundes. [Aus G. W. KORTING u. H. HOLZMANN: Arch. klin. exp. Derm. **210**, 472—484 (1960)]

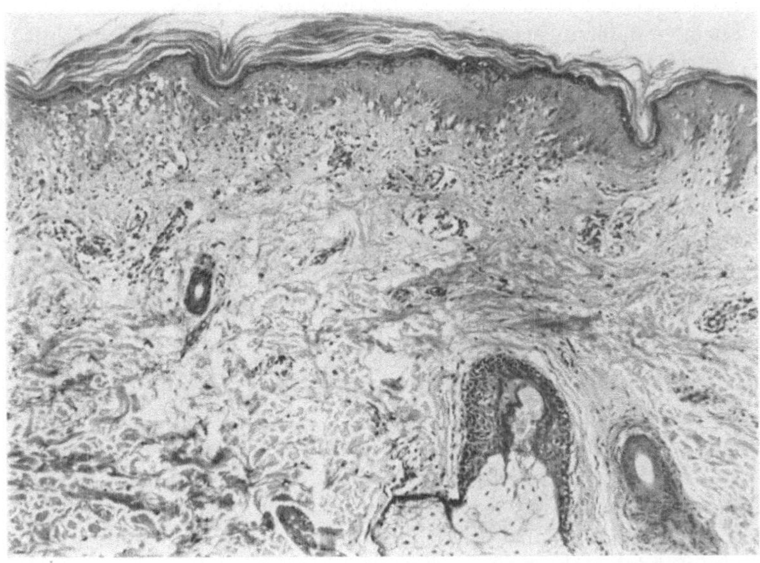

Abb. 22. Gleicher Patient wie Abb. 20 und 21. Histologische Übersicht einer Gewebsexcision aus dem Exanthembereich. HE, 100mal vergr. — Nur geringfügige lympho-histiocytäre Entzündung im Bereich des subpapillaren Gefäßplexus. Keine Granulomstrukturen. [Aus G. W. KORTING u. H. HOLZMANN: Arch. klin. exp. Derm. **210**, 472—484 (1960)]

Mit Recht stellen KORTING und HOLZMANN die Frage, ob nicht manche der immer wieder in der Kasuistik beschriebenen Pigmentierungen ein derartiges erythemato-squamöses Vorstadium durchlaufen, das nur nicht genügend beachtet oder bewertet wird. Gewisse Hinweise für diese Möglichkeit finden sich in den Arbeiten von KEIL sowie von ARONSON und MONTGOMERY.

3. Monosymptomatischer „Rheumatismus nodosus" und das Problem des Granuloma anulare

Wie schon oben ausgeführt, können subcutane bzw. parartikuläre Knoten die einzige klinisch nachweisbare Manifestation einer chronisch-rheumatischen Reaktionslage sein. Klinge hat solche abortive Krankheitsformen als „Rheumatismus nodosus ohne Gelenkrheumatismus" bezeichnet, und Fahr prägte sogar den Begriff des „chronisch-spezifischen Rheumatismus nodosus", was besagen soll, daß auch diese monosymptomatische Rheumatismusform „spezifisch" zur chronisch-rheumatischen Krankheitsgruppe gehört. Wie wir schon früher (gemeinsam mit Schuermann) ausgeführt haben, dürfte das Krankheitsbild als *relativ selbständige und blande Erscheinungsform eines chronischen Rheumatismus* nicht allzu selten sein. Genaue Zahlenangaben stehen uns allerdings nicht zur Verfügung.

In dem Maße, in dem die nosologische Differenzierung zwischen Rheumatischem Fieber und Primär-chronischer Polyarthritis auf Grund klinischer, immunopathologischer, bakteriologischer und anderer Kriterien an Umfang gewonnen hat, hat das rheumatische Granulom als histomorphes Bindeglied zwischen beiden Krankheitsgruppen an spezifischer Bedeutung eingebüßt. Auch der Begriff des Rheumatismus nodosus, ursprünglich im pathologisch-anatomischen *und* im klinischen Sprachgebrauch sehr geläufig, ist heute vielfach im Schwinden begriffen. Ihn ganz auszumerzen, wie es Gottron aus terminologischen und allgemein-pathologischen Erwägungen vorschlägt, erscheint nur für die Fälle gerechtfertigt, bei denen doch noch andere rheumatische Organmanifestationen — und sei es nur in abortiver Form — nachzuweisen sind. Die Diagnose darf also nur gestellt werden, *wenn die Beteiligung anderer Organsysteme weitgehend ausgeschlossen ist,* was besonders strenge diagnostische Maßstäbe erfordert.

Die Berechtigung, von einem „Rheumatismus nodosus" zu sprechen, gilt nicht für solche Fälle, in denen subcutane Knoten nach Remission der übrigen rheumatischen Krankheitssymptome persistieren (vgl. auch vorigen Abschnitt). Ausschlaggebend ist hier die Anamnese, weniger der rheumaserologische Befund, da nach Rückgang der allgemeinen Krankheitsaktivität auch die Titerhöhe der immuno-serologischen Agglutinationsteste wieder unter den pathognomonischen Grenzwert absinken, also den Verhältnissen beim eigentlichen Rheumatismus nodosus ähnlich werden kann.

Hinsichtlich ihrer klinischen und histologischen Erscheinungsform unterscheiden sich die Knoten des „Rheumatismus nodosus" praktisch nicht von subcutanen Knoten als Teilmanifestation einer Primär-chronischen Polyarthritis. Eine nochmalige Besprechung erübrigt sich daher unter Hinweis auf das vorangehende Kapitel. So gut wie immer handelt es sich um eine *relativ inaktive Verlaufsform des chronischen Rheumatismus,* was unter anderem in dem guten Allgemeinzustand, in der kaum beschleunigten Blutsenkung und in den meist *negativen oder nur schwach positiven rheumaserologischen Befunden* zum Ausdruck kommt. Negative Agglutinationsteste (sowie Antistreptolysintiter unter der Signifikanzgrenze) schließen also die Diagnose keineswegs aus. Wahrscheinlich entgehen die meisten Fälle schon deshalb der klinischen Beobachtung, weil Ärzte und Patienten meist eine ambulante Behandlung für ausreichend ansehen.

Bezüglich der *Differentialdiagnose* sei an die im vorigen Abschnitt (unter „Subcutane Knoten") aufgeführten Verwechslungsmöglichkeiten erinnert. Hier sind zusätzlich noch die häufigen knotigen *Myogelosen* („Hartspann") bei Arthrosis deformans, Osteochondrosen und Haltungsschäden der Wirbelsäule zu nennen, ferner der Sammelbegriff des sog. „*Muskel*"- oder „*Weichteilrheumatis-*

mus“, der im angloamerikanischen Schrifttum unter der Bezeichnung „Fibrositis“ bzw. „Fibrositis-Syndrom“ läuft und neuerdings erhöhte Beachtung bei Rheumatologen und Orthopäden erfährt. Es handelt sich hierbei nicht nur um funktionelle Störungen mit reversibler Änderung des physikalisch-chemischen Aggregatzustandes der mesenchymalen Grundsubstanzen, sondern um echte degenerative und entzündliche Läsionen des muskulären Bewegungsapparats mit mehr oder minder deutlichen entzündlichen Erscheinungen im Endo- und Perimysium (vgl. MIEHLKE u. SCHULZE; TICHY u. Mitarb. u.a.).

Auf eine Gefahr, die bei der regen heutigen Diskussion über neue Probleme des „Weichteilrheumatismus“ auftaucht, muß gerade von dermatologischer Seite hingewiesen werden: daß relativ gut definierte, wenn auch ätiologisch ungenügend geklärte Krankheitsbilder (z.B. die Panniculitis non-suppurativa Pfeiffer-Weber-Christian), ferner Neuritiden, Bursitiden usw. dieser im Entstehen begriffenen Krankheitsgruppe allzu voreilig zugezählt werden. Die Erfahrungen mit dem Begriff der „Kollagenkrankheiten“, der 1957 auf einem französischen Internisten-Kongreß „bis zur Unkenntlichkeit zerpflückt worden ist“ (HARTMANN), sollten eigentlich zu besonderer Zurückhaltung mahnen.

Für den Dermatologen enthält der Fragenkomplex des monosymptomatischen „Rheumatismus nodosus“ noch ein besonderes Problem, das bisher noch der genaueren Erforschung harrt: das Problem der *„rheumatoiden“ histomorphen Analogie des Granuloma anulare zu den Rheumaknoten* (BOLGERT; HORNSTEIN u. SCHUERMANN; VAN CANEGHEM u. FIEVEZ; DANNENBERG, YOUNG u. TUNCALI u.a.). Auch von pathologisch-anatomischer Seite haben sich kürzlich v. ALBERTINI und VOGEL zu dieser Frage geäußert und in elektronenoptischen Untersuchungen auf die weitgehende Identität der degenerativen Primärläsion des kollagenen Bindegewebes bei beiden Krankheitsformen hingewiesen.

Die Frage lautet also, ob das Granuloma anulare auf Grund seines histomorphen Aspekts mit den subcutanen Knoten des chronischen Rheumatismus gleichgesetzt werden kann oder ob es überhaupt eine nosologische Variante des „Rheumatismus nodosus“ darstellt.

Vom histologischen Substrat aus gesehen, könnten diese Fragen durchaus bejaht werden. Wie wir schon vor Jahren ausgeführt haben, ist der gewebliche Aufbau der Granulome mit ihrem fibrinoid-nekrotischen Zentrum, dem palisadenartig angeordneten Demarkationswall aus Fibroblasten und großen basophilen Histiocyten sowie den entzündlichen Gefäßveränderungen in den Randanteilen und der Umgebung einem typischen Rheumagranulom so ähnlich, daß ohne Kenntnis des klinischen Bildes die histologische Differentialdiagnose unmöglich sein kann, wenn die Granulome subcutan gelegen sind, was gelegentlich vorkommt (JACOBI; GRAY; GOLDSCHMIDT; GRAUER; DANNENBERG). Zwar pflegen die Einzelherde kleiner, der entzündliche Granulationswall lockerer und der Gehalt an metachromatischen (Mucin-ähnlichen) Substanzen im Nekrosebereich manchmal etwas deutlicher als in Rheumaknoten ausgeprägt zu sein (WOOD u. BEERMAN; GOTTRON u.a.), doch sind diese Vergleichskriterien im Einzelfall höchst unzuverlässig. Da auch beim Granuloma anulare die Alteration des Bindegewebes am Anfang steht und erst sekundär durch die zellige Reaktion zum Granulom wird (CIVATTE; v. ALBERTINI u. VOGEL u.a.), ist die Übereinstimmung mit echten Rheumaknoten so groß, daß man eigentlich erstaunt sein muß, wie ausgerechnet der Gewebsbefund so lange Zeit als Kronzeuge für die tuberkulöse Ätiologie des Granuloma anulare angeführt werden konnte, während die histomorphen Parallelen zum Rheumatismus früher übersehen wurden.

Es kann an dieser Stelle nicht unsere Aufgabe sein, auf die klinischen, ätiologischen und pathogenetischen Aspekte des Granuloma anulare näher einzugehen. Nur im Hinblick auf die „rheumatoide“ Problematik des Krankheitsbildes seien einige allgemeine nosologische Gesichtspunkte kurz angeführt.

Die aus mehreren papulösen bis kleintuberösen Einzelgranulomen ringförmig zusammengesetzten Krankheitsherde bevorzugen die *Acren* der Extremitäten und hier besonders — in fallender Häufigkeit — die Handrücken, Fingerstreckseiten, Handgelenke, Ellenbogen, Knie, Knöchel und Fußrücken. Ihre Ausbreitung kann zwar annähernd symmetrisch, nicht selten aber auch einseitig oder doch asymmetrisch erfolgen. Prinzipiell können die gleichen Regionen wie bei rheumatischen Knoten befallen sein, jedoch mit besonders starker Betonung der *distalen Abschnitte der oberen Extremitäten.*

Die *Altersverteilung* zeigt bei beiden Geschlechtern ein Maximum im ersten Lebensjahrzehnt — speziell um das 5. und um das 10. Lebensjahr —, eine *relative Abnahme während der Pubertät* und einen deutlichen Wiederanstieg — besonders beim weiblichen Geschlecht — im dritten Lebensjahrzehnt (Gleitz u. Heite u.a.). In späteren Lebensabschnitten nimmt die Morbidität bei beiden Geschlechtern ab. In jeder Lebensperiode, auch in der Kindheit, ist jedoch *das weibliche Geschlecht gegenüber dem männlichen deutlich bevorzugt,* insgesamt etwa im Verhältnis 2:1.

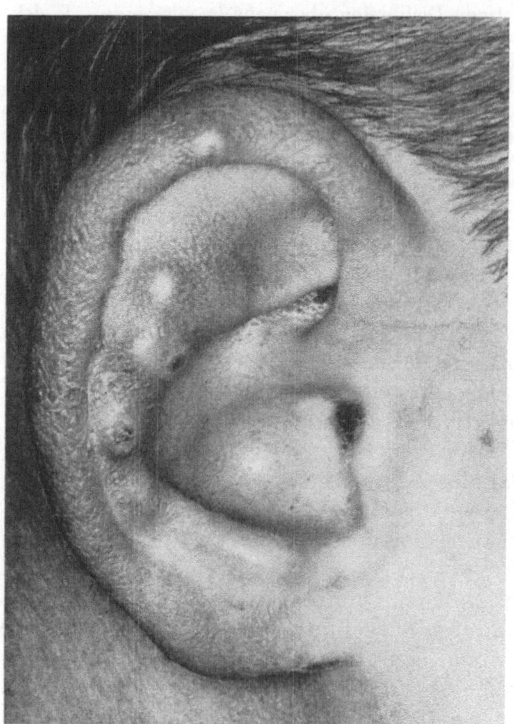

Abb. 23. 14jähriger Patient. Mehrere Granuloma anulare-Knötchen unter dem Bild eines monosymptomatischen „Rheumatismus nodosus" im Bereich beider Ohrmuscheln. Seit 5 Jahren typische Granuloma anulare-Herde an den Hand- und Fingerrücken, seit mehreren Monaten auch an den Ohrmuscheln. Histologischer Aufbau von Rheumagranulomen nicht sicher unterscheidbar. Rheumaserologie negativ. Nosologische Zuordnung zum Granuloma anulare nur wegen der zeitlichen Koinzidenz und histomorphen Analogie mit klinisch und lokalisatorisch typischen Granuloma anulare-Herden

Die *Zahl* der ringförmig gruppierten Einzelherde ist meist gering (am häufigsten 1—3), kann aber auch unter schubweiser Generalisation erheblich zunehmen (40 und mehr Herde). Die einzelnen Morphen entstehen binnen einiger Tage — über ein nur selten zu beobachtendes erythematöses Vorstadium —, pflegen dann aber mehrere Monate bis Jahre vorhanden zu sein. Nach Heite folgt die Häufigkeitsverteilung der Krankheitsdauer einer logarithmischen Normalverteilung mit einem Medianwert von etwa 1,5 Jahren. Als Schwankungsbreite fand er 3 Monate bis 29 Jahre, wobei eine Verlaufsdauer von 5—6 Jahren am häufigsten, kürzere und längere Zeiträume weit seltener vorkamen.

Im allgemeinen sind die Granulomata anularia durch symptomenarme, beschwerdefreie Chronizität bei guter allgemeiner Gesundheitsverfassung der Patienten charakterisiert. Soweit in kasuistischen Mitteilungen überhaupt Vor- und Begleitkrankheiten erwähnt werden, geschieht es oft als Beleg für eine ätiologische Hypothese. In diesem Sinne wird mehrfach auf eine Tuberkulose in der Anamnese, auf Diabetes mellitus (auch im Hinblick auf die vermeintliche Verwandtschaft des Granuloma anulare zur Necrobiosis lipoidica), auf eine traumatische oder postinfektiöse Genese hingewiesen. Häufig besteht *Akrocyanose.* Relativ selten wird über die Kombination mit arthritischen oder arthrotischen Veränderungen berichtet, so im Falle von Leinbrock. Ob es sich auch in anderen Fällen (z.B. Menard) wirklich um Granulomata anularia gehandelt hat, erscheint fraglich; so berichtete Menard über das Auftreten multipler kleiner Knoten an den Ohrmuscheln bei einem 11jährigen Knaben mit polyarthritischen Beschwerden, wobei die nodösen Herde unter Salicyltherapie abheilten, anschließend aber rezidivierten. Wahrscheinlich hat es sich in diesem Falle um echte Nodi rheumatici bei Rheumatischem Fieber gehandelt. Wir selbst sahen bei einem 14jährigen Patienten gleichfalls an den Ohrmuscheln multiple, seit 5 Jahren bestehende Knötchen, die wir nur deshalb als Granuloma anulare-Herde auffaßten, weil entsprechende cutane Herde in typischer anulärer Konfiguration an den Handrücken bestanden. Rein histologisch und histochemisch war uns dagegen eine sichere Unterscheidung von Rheumaknötchen nicht möglich.

Unter den mannigfachen „*Ursachen*“, die für das Granuloma anulare diskutiert werden, wird vor allem Traumen jeglicher Art, Lichteinflüssen, infektions-allergischen Reaktionen, endokrinen und neurovegetativen Regulationsstörungen eine erhöhte Bedeutung beigemessen. Rätselhaft bleibt, daß die gleichen Faktoren (z. B. Traumen, interkurrente Infekte, Vigantolinjektionen) teils provozierend, teils restituierend wirken können. So neigen viele Autoren, die sich nicht auf eine bestimmte ätiologische Hypothese festgelegt haben, zu einer polyätiologischen Deutung des Krankheitsbildes.

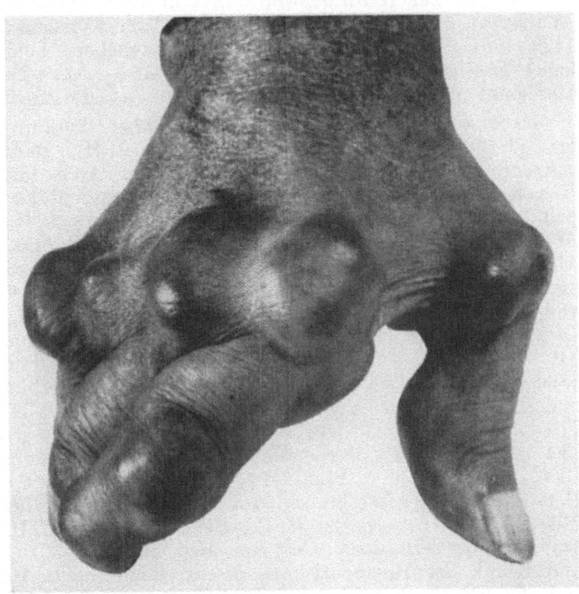

Abb. 24. Multiple juxta-articuläre Knoten bei Primär-chronischer Polyarthritis (57jähriger Patient von Prof. GAHLEN, Hautklinik Düsseldorf). Weitere Knoten an Ellenbogen, Knien und Fußgelenken. Histologisch typische Rheumagranulome. Gichttophi ausschließbar

Eigenartigerweise spielt bisher die Idee einer „*rheumatoiden*“ *Genese* eine ganz untergeordnete Rolle, obwohl sie nach dem Gewebsbefund noch am besten fundiert wäre. Auch viele der erwähnten allgemeinen nosologischen Hinweise — der Erkrankungsgipfel im Kindesalter, die relative Abnahme um die Pubertät, die Bevorzugung des weiblichen Geschlechts, die gelenknahe Akrolokalisation der Herde, das häufige Mitvorhandensein einer Akrocyanose, der günstige Einfluß der Gravidität usw. — zeigen auffällige Parallelen zu rheumatischen Krankheitsformen. Im übrigen rechnen v. ALBERTINI und VOGEL auf Grund ihrer licht- und elektronenoptischen Untersuchungen das Granuloma anulare (sowie die Aschoffschen Rheumaknötchen im Herzmuskel, die parartikulären Knoten des Rheumatismus nodosus und die sog. Senile Elastose der Haut) sogar zu den „*echten Kollagenosen*“, da hier neben der Grundsubstanz auch die Kollagenfibrille nachweislich primär geschädigt sei, was bekanntlich bei den „collagen diseases“ im Sinne von KLEMPERER nicht der Fall ist.

Wenn auch eine ganze Reihe gewichtiger Kriterien die Annahme einer *engen Verwandtschaft des Granuloma anulare zur rheumatischen Krankheitsgruppe* stützen, so erscheint uns doch eine Gleichsetzung in Anbetracht der bisher ungenügenden pathogenetischen und ätiologischen Forschungen noch nicht statthaft, zumindest verfrüht. Solange die Ätiologie noch ungeklärt ist, sollte auch die nosologische Selbständigkeit des Granuloma anulare unangetastet bleiben, wenn auch mit besonderem Nachdruck auf seine klinischen und vor allem histomorphen Überschneidungen mit dem „Rheumatismus nodosus" hinzuweisen ist.

Literatur *

I. Einleitung

ALBERTINI, A. v.: Zur Pathogenese des rheumatischen Granuloms. Schweiz. med. Wschr. **83**, 772—776 (1953). — Zur Morphologie und Pathogenese des fibrinoiden Gewebsschadens im rheumatischen Granulom. (Vortrag.) Z. Rheumaforsch. **20**, 1—16 (1961). — ALBERTINI, A. v., u. A. GRUMBACH: Die experimentelle Streptokokkeninfektion des Kaninchens in ihren Beziehungen zur Herdinfektion. Ergebn. allg. Path. path. Anat. **33**, 314—423 (1937). — ALBERTINI, A. v., u. A. VOGEL: Über wirkliche Kollagenosen. Dtsch. med. Wschr. **86**, 1421—1426 (1961). — ASCHOFF, L.: Die „rheumatischen" Leiden im Lichte der deutschen Pathologie. Dtsch. med. Wschr. **60**, 7—11 (1934). — AZUA DOCHAO, L. DE: Etiopatogenia de las afecciones cutaneas reumatoides (A.C.R.). Act. dermo-sifiliogr. (Madr.) **45**, 683—718 (1954).

BACCAREDDA-BOY, A.: Paraxanthomatöse (thesaurotische) System-Histiocytose. Hautarzt **11**, 58—63 (1960). — BAGGENSTOSS, A. H., and E. F. ROSENBERG: Cardiac lesions associated with chronic infectious arthritis. Arch. intern. Med. **67**, 241—258 (1941). — BAKER, D. M.: Changes in the corium and subcutaneous tissues as a cause of rheumatic pain. Ann. rheum. Dis. **14**, 385—391 (1955). — BAKER, H., D. N. GOLDING and M. THOMPSON: Arthritis and psoriasis. Atti X. Congr. Lega Internaz. contro il Reumatismo, vol. II, p. 341—342, Roma 1961. — BALL, J., and J. S. LAWRENCE: Epidemiology of the sheep cell agglutination test. Ann. rheum. Dis. **20**, 235—243 (1961). — BATEMAN, M., J. M. MALINS and M. J. MEYNELL: Rheumatic arthritis and systematic lupus erythematodes. Ann. rheum. Dis. **17**, 114—118 (1958). — BAYER, F.: Rheumatismus und Lues. Z. Rheumaforsch. **15**, 140—151 (1956). — BAZIN, E.: Affections cutanées d'origine arthritique et nerveuse. Paris 1860. — BESNIER, E.: Étude sur les dermopathies rhumatismales ou arthritides rhumatismales. Ann. Derm. Syph. (Paris) 8, 254—268, 320—337 (1876/77). — BLAND, E. F., and T. D. JONES: Rheumatic fever and rheumatic heart diseases. Circulation **4**, 836—843 (1951).— The natural history of rheumatic fever in a 20 year perspective. Ann. intern. Med. **37**, 1006—1026 (1952). — BLÉCOURT, J. J. DE, A. POLMAN and T. DE BLÉCOURT-MEINDERSMA: Hereditary factors in rheumatoid arthritis and ankylosing spondylitis. Ann. rheum. Dis. **20**, 215—223 (1961). — BOCK, H. E.: Der Stand der ACTH-Cortison-Therapie allergischer Erkrankungen. Verh. dtsch. Ges. inn. Med. **62**, 288—301 (1956). — BÖHMIG, R.: Pathogenese und Klinik des Rheumatismus. Mschr. Kinderheilk. **103**, 97—103 (1955). — BÖHMIG, R., u. P. KLEIN: Pathologie und Bakteriologie der Endocarditis. Berlin-Göttingen-Heidelberg: Springer 1953. — BONOMO, L.: Il quadro umorale dell'artrite reumatoide. Acta rheumat. (Documenta Geigy) S. 64—75. Basel 1961. — BOUILLAUD, J. B.: Traité clinique du rhumatisme articulaire. Paris: J. B. Baillière 1840. — BOUISSOU, M.: Les lésions du conjonctif dermique cliniquement sain au cours de la maladie de Bouillaud (Essai pathogénique). Arch. franç. Pédiat. **14**, 241—260 (1957). — BOURDILLON, C.: Psoriasis et arthropathies. Thèse pour le doctorat en médecine, No. 328. Paris: A. Davy 1888. — BRAUNSTEINER, H., F. EGGHART, H. PUXKANDL, F. REINHARDT u. G. WIEDERMANN: Untersuchungen zur Charakterisierung des Rheumafaktors. Wien. Z. inn. Med. **39**, 97—105 (1958). — BROCQ, L.: Nonerythematous nodes in rheumatic subjects. J. cutan. vener. Dis. **2**, 281—283 (1884). — BRUGSCH, H. G.: Rheumatic diseases, rheumatism and arthritis. Philadelphia and Montreal: J. B. Lippincott Company 1957. — BÜRGER, M.: Altern und Krankheit. Leipzig: Georg Thieme 1949. — Altern und Rheuma. Z. Rheumaforsch. **11**, 314—331 (1952). — BUSANNY-CASPARI, W.: Pathologische Anatomie der rheumatischen Herz- und Gefäßerkrankungen. Medizinische **1959**, 2021—2026. — BYWATERS, E. G. L.: Preventive use of antibiotics in medicine. Brit. med. Bull. **16**, 47—50 (1960).

CATANZARO, F. J., CH. R. RAMMELKAMP and R. CHAMOVITZ: Prevention of rheumatic fever by treatment of streptococcal infections. New Engl. J. Med. **259**, 51—57 (1958). — CATANZARO, F. J., CH. A. STETSON, A. J. MORRIS, R. CHAMOVITZ, CH. R. RAMMELKAMP, B. L. STOLZER and W. D. PERRY: Symposium on rheumatic fever and rheumatic heart disease; role of Streptococcus in pathogenesis of rheumatic fever. Amer. J. Med. **17**, 749—756 (1954). — CAVELTI, PH. A.: Experimentelle Studien über die Pathogenese des fieberhaften Rheumatismus (Polyarthritis acuta rheumatica). Schweiz. med. Wschr. **78**, 83—85 (1948). — Sensitization with tissue antigens. In: Rheumatic Diseases, Proc. 7th Intern. Congr. Rheum. Philadelphia: W. B. Saunders Company 1952. — CHARCOT, J. M.: Maladies des vieillards. Paris: Delahaye 1867. — CHIARI, H.: Die pathologische Anatomie

* Abgeschlossen am 31. 12. 1961.

des akuten Rheumatismus. Dresden u. Leipzig: Theodor Steinkopff 1938. — CHRAPOWICKI, T., and T. PATZEROWA: Some criteria of the condition of the peripheral vascular system in children suffering from rheumatic fever. Pediat. pol. **33**, 1145—1156 (1958). — A trial of estimation of morphologic changes of the peripheral vascular system in children suffering from rheumatic fever. Pediat. pol. **33**, 1157—1162 (1958). — CHRIST, P.: Untersuchungen mit der Antistreptokinase-Antihyaluronidase und der Antistreptolysinreaktion. Z. Rheumaforsch. **12**, 141—156 (1953). — Über die Bedeutung von Streptokokkeninfektionen in der Pathogenese der akuten Polyarthritis und der akuten Nephritis. Ergebn. inn. Med. Kinderheilk. **11**, 379—465 (1959). — CHRIST, P., E. VANEK, R. SCHIESSL, K. H. KRACHUDEL u. HJ. BECKER: Zur Serologie rheumatischer Erkrankungen. Z. Rheumaforsch. **20**, 81—98 (1961). — CIHULA, J., u. J. POLÁK: Die Kapillarpermeabilität beim akuten Rheumatismus. Z. ges. inn. Med. **15**, 396—399 (1960). — CLEVE, H., u. F. HARTMANN: Immunelektrophoretische Serumuntersuchung beim Gelenkrheumatismus. Verh. Dtsch. Ges. Inn. Med., 63. Kongr. 1957, S. 637—641. — CLEVE, HARTWIG: Neuere immunelektrophoretische Untersuchungen im Serum Rheumakranker. Z. Rheumaforsch. **17**, 350—361 (1958). — COATES, V. M., and J. L. DELICATI: Rheumatoid arthritis and its treatment. Lewis: London 1931. — COBURN, A. F.: The factor of infection in the rheumatic state. Baltimore: Williams & Wilkins Company 1931. — Some basic insolved problems in the prevention of rheumatic fever. Ann. intern. Med. **47**, 402—517 (1957). — COBURN, A. F., and R. H. PAULY: Studies with immune response of the rheumatic subject and its relationship to activity of the rheumatic process. J. clin. Invest. **14**, 769—781 (1935). — COLLINS, D. H.: Fibrositis and infektion. Ann. rheum. Dis. **2**, 114—126 (1940). — *Committee on Prevention of Rheumatic Fever and Bacterial Endocarditis of the American Heart Association*, „Control of streptococcal infections". Circulation **15**, 154—158 (1957). — COPE, S., G. SANDERSON, C. A. ST. HILL and E. N. CHAMBERLAIN: Prophylactic use of oral penicillin in rheumatic fever, chorea and carditis. Brit. med. J. **1960** I, No 5177, 913—917. — CROSS, R. J. (Edit.): Current views on pathogenesis and therapy of rheumatic fever. Amer. J. Med. **22**, 422—436 (1957). — CRAMER, H.-J.: Multiple Reticulohistiocytome der Haut ohne nachweisbare Zweiterkrankung. Hautarzt **14**, 297—302 (1963).

DEICHER, H.: Mechanismus und Anwendung des Latex-Hemmungstests zur Diagnostik der Primär-chronischen Polyarthritis. I. Mitt.: Über die Natur der Serum-Inhibitoren. Klin. Wschr. **39**, 612—618 (1961). — DENNY, F. W., L. W. WANNAMAKER, W. R. BRINK, C. H. RAMMELKAMP and E. A. CUSTER: Prevention of rheumatic fever. J. Amer. med. Ass. **143**, 151—153 (1950). — DIAMOND, E. F.: Is there a rheumatic constitution? J. Pediat. **54**, 341—347 (1959). — DIXON, A. ST. J.: „Rheumatoid arthritis" with negative serological reactions. Ann. rheum. Dis. **19**, 209—228 (1960). — DORTMANN, A., u. F. KÜSTER: Die Antistreptolysinreaktion als Differentialdiagnosticum beim rheumatischen Fieber. Kinderärztl. Prax. **25**, 515—521 (1957). — DRESNER, E.: Some current concepts of the etiology of rheumatoid arthritis. J. chron. Dis. **5**, 612—629 (1957).

EDELMANN, G. M., H. G. KUNKEL and E. C. FRANKLIN: Interaction of the rheumatoid factor with antigen-antibody complexes and aggregated gamma-globulin. J. exp. Med. **108**, 105—120 (1958). — EDSTRÖM, G.: Die Klinik des rheumatischen Fiebers. Ergebn. inn. Med. Kinderheilk. **52**, 439—503 (1937). — Rheumatic fever, its symptoms, prevention and treatment. Acta rheum. scand. **1**, 145 (1953). — EHRICH, W. E.: Die Entzündung. In: Handbuch der allgemeinen Pathologie, Bd. VII/1, S. 1—324. Berlin-Göttingen-Heidelberg: Springer 1956. — ELGHAMMER, H. W.: Rheumatic fever in children. Med. Clin. N. Amer. **42**, 129—134 (1958). — EPSTEIN, W. V., E. P. ENGLEMAN and M. ROSS: Evaluation of qualitative precipitation reaktion for the detection of the rheumatoid factor. Ann. rheum. Dis. **16**, 448—453 (1957). — EWERBECK, H.: Rheumatische Erkrankungen im Kindesalter. In: Der Rheumatismus, S. 29—39. Stuttgart: Georg Thieme 1956.

FAHR, TH.: Die rheumatische Granulomatose (rheumatisches Fieber, Rheumatismus infectiosus specificus, Rheumatismus verus) vom Standpunkt des Morphologen. Ergebn. inn. Med. Kinderheilk. **54**, 357—396 (1938). — FANCONI, G.: Die Kollagenkrankheiten (Kollagenosen). Helv. paediat. Acta **12**, 1—19 (1957). — Die Kollagenosen und verwandte Reaktionskrankheiten. Münch. med. Wschr. **101**, 581—586 (1959). — FANCONI, G., u. G. WISSLER: Der Rheumatismus im Kindesalter. Teil I: Der Rheumatismus verus und seine Differentialdiagnose. Dresden u. Leipzig: Theodor Steinkopff 1943. — FASSBENDER, H. G.: Die Bedeutung des Endotoxins für den rheumatischen Gewebsschaden. Ärztl. Forsch. **15**, I, 221—234 (1961). — FELLINGER, K.: Einige Hinweise zur Diagnostik und Therapie rheumatischer Erkrankungen. Wien. klin. Wschr. **73**, 165—169 (1961). — FELLINGER, K., u. J. SCHMID: Klinik und Therapie des chronischen Gelenkrheumatismus. Wien: Wilhelm Maudrich 1954. — FRANCQ, J. C., A. EYQUEM, L. PODLIACHOUK et F. JACQUELINE: Immuno-elektrophoretische Untersuchungen bei chronisch entzündlichem Rheumatismus. Ann. Inst. Pasteur **96**, 413—420 (1959). — FRANKLIN, E. C., H. G. KUNKEL and J. R. WARD: Clinical studies of seven patients with rheumatoid arthritis and uniquely large amounts of rheumatoid factor. Arthr. and

Rheum. **1**, 400—409 (1958). — FRONTALI, G.: Endotheliale Konstitution und Rheumatismus. Münch. med. Wschr. **98**, 1018—1022 (1956). — FRÜHWALD, R.: Dermatologie und Rheumatismus. Dresden u. Leipzig: Theodor Steinkopff 1938.

GAMP, A.: Untersuchungen über das Verhalten eiweißgebundener Kohlenhydrate bei rheumatischen Erkrankungen. I. Der Glukosamingehalt des Serums. Z. Rheumaforsch. **14**, 167—179 (1955). — GEILER, G.: Morphologie und Pathogenese des rheumatischen Gewebsschadens. Dtsch. med. Wschr. **84**, 2259—2262 (1959). — GERHARDT, C.: Über Rheumatoid-Krankheiten. Verh. Kongr. inn. Med. **14**, 169—182 (1896). — GERLACH, W.: Studien über hyperergische Entzündung. Virchows Arch. path. Anat. **247**, 294—361 (1923). — GLANZMANN, E.: Die rheumatische Infektion. In: Handbuch der Kindesheilkunde, Ergänzungswerk hrsg. von v. PFAUNDLER, Bd. I, S. 399—410. Berlin: Springer 1942. GOEBEL, A.: — Die Pathologie des Rheumatismus. In: Der Rheumatismus, S. 8—22. Stuttgart: Georg Thieme 1956. — GOEHRS, H. R., A. H. BAGGENSTOSS and C. H. SLOCUMB: Cardiac lesions in rheumatoid arthritis. Arthr. and Rheum. **3**, 298—308 (1960). — GOLDBERGER, E.: The etiology and pathogenesis of rheumatic fever. Acta med. scand. **161**, 347—359 (1958). — GOOD, R. A., and J. ROTSTEIN: Rheumatoid arthritis and agammaglobulinaemie. Bull. rheum. Dis. **10**, 203—206 (1960). — GOTTRON, H. A.: Zur Pathogenese rheumatischer Hautreaktionen. Derm. Wschr. **132**, 1007—1015 (1955). — Haut und Rheuma. Mkurse ärztl. Fortbild. **1954**, Nr 2.— GRÄFF, S.: Rheumatismus und rheumatische Erkrankungen. Berlin u. Wien: Urban & Schwarzenberg 1936. — Rheumasymptom und rheumatische Erkrankungen. Z. Rheumaforsch. **3**, 461—479 (1940). — Rheumatismussymptom oder Rheumatismuserreger. Med. Welt **1951**, 1299—1303. — GRAHAM, G., and A. G. STANSFIELD: A case of a hitherto undescribed lipoidosis simulating rheumatoid arthritis. J. Path. Bact. **58**, 545—558 (1946). — GRAM, H. G., u. R. BÖHMIG: Experimentelle Untersuchungen mit Fraktionen der Leibessubstanzen der A-Streptokokken. Z. Immun.-Forsch. **119**, 1—94 (1960). — GRAMPA, G., e C. B. BALLABIO: Anatomia patologica dell'artrite reumatoide. Acta rheumat. (Documenta Geigy), p. 11—16. Basel 1961. — GRASER, F.: Die rheumatische Erkrankung bei Kindern. In: LINNEWEH, Die Prognose chronischer Erkrankungen. Long-term observations of chronic diseases, 375—378. Berlin-Göttingen-Heidelberg: Springer 1960. — GRENET, H.: La maladie de Bouillaud. Paris: Vigot 1949. — GUTHOF, O.: Bakteriologie und Serologie des Rheumatismus. In: Der Rheumatismus, S. 23—39. Stuttgart: Georg Thieme 1956.

HAGERMAN, G.: Infection, allergy and the pathogenesis of rheumatic disease. Acta rheum. scand. **1**, 209—234 (1956). — HALL, P.: Acute rheumatic fever. In: LINNEWEH, Die Prognose rheumatischer Erkrankungen. Long-term observations of chronic diseases, pp. 366—369. Berlin-Göttingen-Heidelberg: Springer 1960. — HALLIDIE-SMITH, K. A., and E. G. L. BYWATERS: The differential diagnosis of rheumatic fever. Arch. Dis. Childh. **33**, 350—357 (1958). — HANGARTNER, W.: Das Erbbild der rheumatischen und chronischen Gelenkerkrankungen. Dresden u. Leipzig: Theodor Steinkopff 1939. — HARTMANN, F.: Die Bedeutung humoraler Faktoren für den Verlauf des Rheumatismus. Z. Rheumaforsch. **11**, 65—79 (1952). — Serologische Reaktionen beim Rheumatismus. Z. Rheumaforsch. **16**, 150—182 (1957). — Die biochemischen und makromolekularen Grundlagen einer Pathologie der Bindegewebe. Internist **2**, 403—412 (1961). — HARTMANN, F., u. D. BERG: Versuche über die Wirkung intravenös gegebener Hyaluronidase auf die Eiweißdurchlässigkeit der Gefäße. Z. Rheumaforsch. **11**, 195—199 (1952). — HAUSS, W. H.: Ätiologische Vorstellungen über die akuten und chronischen Formen rheumatischer Erkrankungen. Med. Klin. **54**, 628—631 (1959). — HEATON, J. M.: Sjögren's syndrome and systemic lupus erythematodes. Brit. med. J. **1959 I**, 466—469. — HEILMEYER, L.: Lehrbuch der inneren Medizin, S. 214. Berlin-Göttingen-Heidelberg: Springer 1955. — HELLER, G., A. S. JAKOBSON and M. H. KOLODNY: A modification of the hemagglutination test for rheumatoid arthritis. Proc. Soc. exp. Biol. (N.Y.) **72**, 316—323 (1949). — HILLER, E.: Störungen des Wasser- und Zuckerstoffwechsels als Ausdruck einer diencephalen Störung bei chronischer Polyarthritis. Z. klin. Med. **146**, 569—577 (1950). — HOCHREIN, M.: Rheumatische Erkrankungen, Entstehung und Behandlung, 2. Aufl. Stuttgart: Georg Thieme 1952. — HORNSTEIN, O.: Zur nosologischen Stellung der Psoriasis arthropathica. Arch. klin. exp. Derm. **214**, 622—651 (1962). — HORNSTEIN, O., u. H. SCHUERMANN: Rheumatismus der Haut. In: GOTTRON-SCHÖNFELD, Dermatologie und Venerologie, Bd. II/1, S. 623—642. Stuttgart: Georg Thieme 1958. — HURMUZACHE, F., M. BURDEA, A. TUDURANU, S. BRĂTIANU, A. BRĂTIANU u. C. DOBRESCU: Die Haut- und Muskelbiopsie für die Diagnose der latenten Form des Rheumatismus bei Kindern. Probl. Reum. (Buc.) **5**, 83—84 (1958) [Rumänisch]. Ref. Zbl. inn. Med. **200**, 321 (1959).

JACQUELINE, F., E. EYQUEM et L. PODLIACHOUK: Hémagglutinations au cours des rhumatismes inflammatoires chroniques. Rév. rhum. (Paris) **24**, 385—398 (1957). — JESSAR, R. A.: Neue Fortschritte über Grundlagen und klinischen Verlauf der rheumatischen Polyarthritis. Klin. Wschr. **1958**, 998—1005. — JOHNSON, H. M., and I. L. TILDEN: Reticulo-histiocytic granulomas of the skin associated with arthritis mutilans: Report of a case followed 14 years. Arch. Derm. (Chic.) **75**, 405—417 (1957). — JUNG, A., u. A. BÖNI: Ist die primär-chronische

Polyarthritis eine Anpassungskrankheit im Sinne von SELYE? Schweiz. med. Wschr. 82, 852—857 (1952).

KAHLMETER, G.: De l'existence de lésions myocardiques et valvulaires dans les diverses formes de polyarthrites chroniques et des conclusions qu'on peut tirer touchant l'étiologie et le groupement clinique des polyarthrites chroniques. Acta med. scand. 59, 611—625 (1934). — KLEMPERER, P.: Der Begriff der Collagenkrankheiten. Wien. klin. Wschr. 67, 337—341 (1955). — KLINGE, F.: Der Rheumatismus. (Als Monographie.) Erg. allg. Path., Bd. 27. München: J. F. Bergmann 1933. — KLINGE, F., u. H. G. FASSBENDER: Pathologische Anatomie der experimentellen Grundlagen. In: K. HANSEN, Allergie, 3. Aufl., S. 86—118. Stuttgart: Georg Thieme 1957. — KÖHLER, W.: Die Serologie des Rheumatismus und der Streptokokkeninfektionen, 2. Aufl. Leipzig: Johann Ambrosius Barth 1959. — KÖTTGEN, U., u. W. CALLENSEE: Statistische Untersuchungen zum kindlichen Rheumatismus. Darmstadt: Theodor Steinkopff 1959. — KREBS, A.: Über Psoriasis arthropathica. Schweiz. med. Wschr. 92, 29—72 (1962). — KRESS, H. v.: Über das rheumatische Fieber und die chronischen Polyarthritiden. Münch. med. Wschr. 100, 1522—1525 (1958). — KÜSTER, F.: Nachweis eines Permeabilitäts- und eines Nekrosefaktors im Serum beim akuten Rheumatismus im Kindesalter. Klin. Wschr. 1952, 999—1000. — Akuter Rheumatismus und Scharlachrheumatismus. Arch. Kinderheilk. 148, 38—50 (1954). — Das rheumatische Fieber. Arch. Kinderheilk. 151, 113—132 (1955). — KÜSTER, F., u. E. LANGER: Beiträge zur Pathogenese des akuten Rheumatismus. II. Mitt. Die gewebsschädigenden Eigenschaften des Rheumatikerserums. Z. Kinderheilk. 74, 365—381 (1954). — KÜSTER, F., u. H. RODECK: Über die Eigenschaften des toxischen Serumfaktors beim rheumatischen Fieber. Klin. Wschr. 32, 739—740 (1954). — Beiträge zur Genese des akuten Rheumatismus. III. Mitt. Der Einfluß des Rheumatikerserums auf das isolierte Froschherz. Z. Kinderheilk. 74, 382—387 (1954). — KÜSTER, F., u. F. J. SCHULTE: Die Bildung biologisch aktiver Substanzen im Blut bei experimenteller Sensibilisierung (Modellversuch zur Entstehung der Gewebsschäden beim rheumatischen Fieber). Klin. Wschr. 35, 886—888 (1957). — KUSKE, H.: Rheumatismus und Haut. Praxis 10, 197—199 (1961).

LAYANI, F.: Le rhumatisme chronique déformant xanthomateux. Bull. Soc. méd. Hôp. Paris 55, 343—355 (1939). — LAYANI, F., V. MAY, L. DURUPT et Y. CHAOUAT: Du rhumatisme articulaires aigu à la polyarthrite chronique évolutive. (Sur les rapports de deux maladies.) Rev. rhum. 25 (Paris), 441—459 (1958). — LEIBER, B.: Altersbiologie des akuten Rheumatismus. Pathophysiologie einer Altersdisposition. In: Der Rheumatismus, hrsg. R. SCHOEN, Bd. 29. Dresden u. Leipzig: Theodor Steinkopff 1952. — LEICHTENTRITT, B.: Die rheumatische Infektion im Kindesalter. Ergebn. inn. Med. Kinderheilk. 37, 1—100 (1930). — LETTERER, E.: Die allergisch-hyperergische Entzündung. In: Handbuch der allgemeinen Pathologie, Bd. VII/1, S. 496—600. Berlin-Göttingen-Heidelberg: Springer 1956. — Allgemeine Pathologie. Stuttgart: Georg Thieme 1959. — LEWENFISZ-WOJNAROWSKA, T., S. JABLONSKA et B. ZAORSKA: Lésions de la peau apparamment saine au cours de la maladie rhumatismale chez les enfants. Arch. franç. Pédiat. 17, 655—663 (1960). — LOEBER, F., W. EICHLSEDER u. D. STUMPF: 5 Jahre Rezidivprophylaxe des rheumatischen Fiebers im Kinderkrankenhaus München-Schwabing. Münch. med. Wschr. 102, 1915—1920 (1960). — LUCHERINI, T., e C. CERVINI: Gli aspetti clinici della malattia reumatoide. Acta rheumat. (Documenta Geigy), pp. 42—62. Basel 1961. — LYELL, A., and A. J. CARR: Lipoid dermatoarthritis (Reticulohistiocytosis). Brit. J. Derm. 71, 12—21 (1959).

MASSELL, B. F.: The diagnosis and treatment of rheumatic fever and rheumatic carditis. Med. Clin. N. Amer. 42, 1343—1360 (1958). — MASSHOFF, W., u. H. F. REIMERS: Der rheumatische Gewebsschaden und die rheumatischen Erkrankungen aus der Sicht des Pathologen. Internist 2, 393—402 (1961). — MATHIES, H.: Der Rheumafaktor in der Rheumadiagnostik. Med. Klin. 55, 2028—2033 (1960). — MCCARTHY, M.: Nature of rheumatic fever. Circulation 14, 1138—1143 (1956). — MCEWEN, C.: Currier „Recent advances in diagnosis and treatment of rheumatic fever". Med. Clin. N. Amer. 39, 353—364 (1955). — MELLORS, R. C., R. HEIMER, J. CORCOS and L. KORNGOLD: Cellular origin of rheumatoid factor. J. exp. Med. 110, 875—886 (1959). — MENKIN, V.: Dynamics of inflammation. New York: MacMillan Comp. 1940. — MIEHLKE, K.: Fortschritte in der serologischen Rheumadiagnostik. Z. Rheumaforsch. 17, 362—365 (1958). — Die Rheumafibel. Berlin-Göttingen-Heidelberg: Springer 1961. — MIESCHER, P., u. K. O. VORLAENDER: Immunpathologie in Klinik und Forschung und das Problem der Autoantikörper, 2. Aufl. Stuttgart: Georg Thieme 1961. — MOESCHLIN, S.: Die Auto-Immunerkrankungen. Acta haemat. (Basel) 18, 13—32 (1957). — MOLL, W.: Klinische Rheumatologie. Pathogenese, Symptomatologie, Diagnostik und Therapie der Rheumaerkrankungen. Basel u. New York: Karger 1958. — MONTGOMERY, H., H. F. POLLEY and D. G. PUGH: Reticulohistiocytoma (Reticulohistiocytic Granuloma). Arch. Derm. (Chic.) 77, 61—72 (1958). — MÜLLER, W.: Die Serologie der chronischen Polyarthritis. Pathologie und Klinik in Einzeldarstellungen, Bd. XIII. Berlin-Göttingen-Heidelberg: Springer 1962. — MÜLLER-EBERHARD, H. J.: Der Rheumafaktor. Dtsch. med. Wschr. 84, 719—723 (1959). —

MURPHY, G. E., and H. F. SWIFT: Induction of cardiac lesions, closely resembling those of rheumatic fever in rabbits, following repeated skin infections with group A streptococci. J. exp. Med. **89**, 687—698 (1949).

NAEGELI, O.: Über Polyarthritis acuta (Rheumatismus verus). Schweiz. med. Wschr. **63**, 1197—1200 (1933). — NEERGAARD, K. v.: Die Katarrh-Infektion. Dresden u. Leipzig: Theodor Steinkopff 1939.

PALITZSCH, D.: Über den Wandel der Anschauungen von Pathogenese und Therapie akuter und chronischer Rheumatismusformen im Kindesalter. Münch. med. Wschr. **102**, 2585—2590 (1960). — POAL, J. M., and J. A. SARRÓ: New concepts about the pathology of psoriatic rheumatoid arthritis. Atti X. Congr. Lega Internaz. contro il Reumatismo, vol. II, pp. 339—340, Roma 1961.

QUINN, R. W.: The etiology and epidemiology of rheumatic fever. Trans. Amer. Coll. Cardiol. **6**, 15—27 (1956).

RAGAN, C.: The relationship in rheumatoid arthritis to periarteritis nodosa and systemic lupus erythematosus. J. chron. Dis. **5**, 688—696 (1957). — The history of the rheumatoid factor. Arthr. and Rheum. **4**, 571—573 (1961). — RAMMELKAMP, CH. H.: Epidemiology of streptococcal infections. Harvey Lect. **51**, 113—142 (1957). — Microbiologic aspects of glomerulonephritis. J. chron. Dis. **5**, 28—33 (1957). — RANTZ, L. A.: The streptococcal etiology of rheumatic fever. Med. Clin. N. Amer. **39**, 339—351 (1955). — RANTZ, L. A., E. RANDALL and D. KETTNER: Elektrophoretische Untersuchungen des für die serologische Reaktion verantwortlichen Serumfaktors beim Gelenkrheumatismus mit Nachweis von 2 Inhibitoren. Arthr. and Rheum. **2**, 104—113 (1959). — RAVAULT, P. P., et G. VIGNON: Klinische Rheumatologie. Paris: Masson & Cie. 1956. — REITER, H.: Die Reitersche Krankheit. Dtsch. med. Wschr. **82**, 1336—1337 (1957). — REJHOLEC, V., and V. WAGNER: Antimyocardial antibodies in rheumatic fever. Experientia (Basel) **11**, 278 (1955). — RICKER, G.: Das Zentralnervensystem und die rheumatisch genannte akute Polyarthritis mit ihrem Zubehör. Dresden u. Leipzig: Theodor Steinkopff 1938. — RIVA, G.: Allgemeine Diagnostik und Nomenklatur der rheumatischen Erkrankungen. Praxis **50**, 138—143 (1961). — ROBECCHI, A., e S. DI VITTORIO: Aspetti reumatologici delle artropatie psoriasiche. Atti X. Congr. Lega Internaz. contro il Reumatismo, vol. II, pp. 345—347, Roma 1961. — ROCH, M.: La maladie de Bouillaud de 1836 à aujourd'hui. Dialogue clinique. Praxis **37**, 943—945 (1961). — RÖSSLE, R.: Über den Formenkreis der rheumatischen Gewebsveränderungen mit besonderer Berücksichtigung der rheumatischen Gefäßentzündung. Virchows Arch. path. Anat. **288**, 780—832 (1933). — ROSE, H. M., C. RAGAN, E. PEARCE and M. O. LIPMAN: Differential agglutination of normal and sensitized sheep erythrocytes by sera of patients with rheumatoid arthritis. Proc. Soc. exp. Biol. (N.Y.) **68**, 1—6 (1948). — ROST, G. A.: Hautkrankheiten. Berlin: Springer 1926 (1. Aufl.), 1948 (2. Aufl.). — Pararheumatische Krankheiten (sog. Kollagenkrankheiten). Eine pathogenetische Studie. Arch. klin. exp. Derm. **210**, 581—624 (1960). — ROTSTEIN, J., and R. A. GOOD: The significance of the simultaneous occurrence of connective tissue disease and the agammaglobulinemic state. Atti X. Congr. Lega Internaz. contro il Reumatismo, vol. I, p. 277, Roma 1961. — RUBENS-DUVAL, A., et J. VILLIAUMEY: Esquisse de l'histogénèse des lésions de l'inflammation rhumatismale. Sem. Hôp. Paris **1953**, 2003—2008.

SACHSE, H. H., u. H. POSER: Zur Altersverteilung des sog. Rheumafaktors. Z. Alternsforsch. **15**, 191—200 (1961). — SASLOW, M. S., F. A. HERNANDEZ and S. C. WERBLOW: Conditions clinically confused with the rheumatic state. J. Pediat. **44**, 414—420 (1954). — SCHAUB, F.: Aktuelle Probleme des Rheumatismus acutus. Schweiz. med. Wschr. **91**, 129—134 (1961). — SCHEIFFARTH, F.: Experimentelle und klinische Studien zur Antistreptolysinreaktion und zur Waaler-Rose-Reaktion. Z. Rheumaforsch. **18**, 122—130 (1959). — SCHEIFFAHRT, F., W. FRENGER u. H. GRIMM: Untersuchungen zur klinischen Bedeutung der Haemagglutinationsreaktionen nach Waaler-Rose. Ärztl. Wschr. 575—577 (1958). — SCHEIFFARTH, F., u. F. LEGLER: Serologie und klinische Erfahrungen mit der Antistreptolysinreaktion bei akutem und chronischem Gelenkrheumatismus. Ärztl. Wschr. 660—666 (1951). — SCHLEGEL, B.: Die Therapie des chronischen Rheumatismus. Med. Welt **47**, 1—15 (1961). — SCHLEGEL, B., u. T. BEHREND: Die klinische Bedeutung der serologischen Reaktionen bei rheumatischen Erkrankungen. Z. Rheumaforsch. **16**, 182—196 (1957). — SCHMIDT, H.: Immunbiologische Bedeutung der Streptokokken. Z. Rheumaforsch. **11**, 1—16 (1952). — Allergie und Immunität. Dtsch. med. Wschr. **79**, 657—659 (1954). — Fortschritte der Serologie. Darmstadt: Theodor Steinkopff 1955. — SCHOEN, R.: Gemeinsame Grundlagen von Pathogenese und Therapie des entzündlichen Rheumatismus. Wien. klin. Wschr. **1953**, 889. — Zur Klinik und Pathogenese der Kollagenkrankheiten. Münch. med. Wschr. **100**, 1409—1415 (1958). — Einteilung und Begriffsbestimmung des Rheumatismus. Therapiewoche 8, 191—194 (1958). — SCHOEN, R., K. MIEHLKE u. G. BARGON: Die atypische subakute Polyarthritis. Internist **2**, 425—431 (1961). — SCHOEN, R., u. W. TISCHENDORF: Rheumatische und rheumatoide Krankheiten.

In: Handbuch der inneren Medizin, 4. Aufl., Bd. VI/1, S. 907—1042. Berlin-Göttingen-Heidelberg: Springer 1954. — SCHOTTMÜLLER, H.: Die Staphylokokken- und Streptokokkenerkrankungen in der inneren Medizin. Verh. Dtsch. Ges. Inn. Med., 37. Kongr. 1925, S. 150—179. — SCHUERMANN, H.: Hautkrankheiten mit Beziehungen zu Arthritis und Rheuma. Ärztl. Prax. **1953**, Nr V, 48. — SCHUERMANN, H., u. G. VELTMAN: Beziehungen zwischen Haut und Knochensystem. Verh. Dtsch. Orthop. Ges., 47. Kongr., Würzburg 1959, S. 209—228. — SEIDEL, K.: Über Erstmanifestationen verschiedener rheumatischer Erkrankungen des Bewegungsapparates. Ein Beitrag zur Altersdisposition des Rheumatismus. Z. Alternsforsch. **7**, 140—158 (1953). — Rheumatismus und Alter. Dtsch. Gesundh.-Wes. **15**, 664—670 (1961). — SEIFERT, H., u. H. TICHY: Die Anti-Staphylolysin-Reaktion bei chronischen Rheumatikern. Z. Rheumaforsch. **18**, 257—271 (1959). — SELYE, H.: The Physiology and Pathology of Exposure to Stress. Montreal 1950. — SHORT, C. L., W. BAUER and W. E. REYNOLDS: Rheumatoid arthritis. Cambridge (Mass.): Harvard Univ. Press 1957. — SIGLER, J. W., R. W. MONIO, D. C. ENSIGN, G. M. WILSON jr., J. W. REBUCK and J. D. LARETT: Vorkommen des L.E.-Zell-Phänomens bei Patienten mit rheumatischer Arthritis. (Eine 2jährige Beobachtung.) Arthr. and Rheum. **1**, 115—121 (1958). — SILVER, M., S. BERKOWITZ and O. STEINBROCKER: The „overlap syndrome": Observations on the coexistence of classical rheumatoid disease with systemic lupus erythematosus. Atti X. Congr. Lega Internaz. contro il Reumatismo, vol. II, pp. 582—583, Roma 1961. — SINGER, J. M., and C. M. PLOTZ: The latex fixation test for rheumatoid arthritis, using patients' own gamma-globulin. Arthr. and Rheum. **1**, 142—146 (1958). — SOKOLOFF, L.: The heart in rheumatoid arthritis. Amer. Heart J. **45**, 635—643 (1953). — SOTGIN, G., e G. CAVALLI: Rilievi biopsici epatici nell'artrite reumatoide. Acta rheumat. (Documenta Geigy), pp. 18—33. Basel 1961. — SPIETHOFF, B.: Rheuma und Hauterkrankungen. In: M. HOCHREIN, Rheumatische Erkrankungen, Entstehung und Behandlung. 1. Aufl., S. 215—219. Leipzig: Georg Thieme 1942. — STECHER, R. M., W. M. SOLOMON and R. WOLPAW: Heredity in rheumatoid arthritis and ankylosing spondylitis. In: C. H. SLOCUMB, Rheumatic Diseases, p. 66—67. (Proc. 7th Internat. Congr. Rheumat. Dis. 1952). — STEFFEN, C.: Bericht über den Nachweis sessiler Antikörper an Gewebs- und Blutzellen durch Antihumanglobulinablenkung. Klin. Wschr. **33**, 134—139 (1955). — Das Problem der Auto-Aggression. Wien. klin. Wschr. **68**, 865—872 (1956). — Untersuchung und Betrachtung der rheumatischen Erkrankungen als Auto-Aggressionskrankheiten. Acta neuroveg. (Wien) **15**, 154—168 (1956). — STEFFEN, C., and E. A. CHEESEMAN: Heredity and rheumatic fever. Study of 462 families ascertained by an affected child and 51 families ascertained by an affected mother. Ann. Eugen. (Lond.) **17**, 177—210 (1953). — STOLLERMANN, G. H.: The use of antibiotics for the prevention of rheumatic fever. Amer. J. Med. **17**, 757—767 (1954). — STUDER, A.: Rheumatismus als Problem der experimentellen Pathologie. Z. Rheumaforsch. **10**, 65—112 (1951). — STUDER, A., u. K. REBER: Rheumatismus als Problem der experimentellen Medizin. In: Der Rheumatismus, hrsg. R. SCHOEN, Bd. 33. Darmstadt: Theodor Steinkopff 1959. — SUTTON, V. R. L., and R. L. SUTTON jr.: Handbook of diseases of the skin. St. Louis: C. V. Mosby Comp. 1949. — SVARTZ, N.: Isolating the rheumatoid factor. Acta rheum. scand. **5**, 5—11 (1959). — Experimental studies on the rheumatoid factor. Atti X. Congr. Lega Internaz. contro il Reumatismo, vol. I, pp. 57—65, Roma 1961. — SVARTZ, N., u. A. EHRENBERG: Der Sedimentationskoeffizient des bei rheumatoider Arthritis vorkommenden Makroglobulins. Schweiz. med. Wschr. **37**, 1076—1084 (1961). — SVARTZ, N., and K. SCHLOSSMANN: A serum cold precipitable hemagglutination factor in rheumatoid arthritis. Acta med. scand. **149**, 83—89 (1954). — Agglutination of sensitized sheep erythrocyrtes in disseminated lupus erythematodes. Ann. rheum. Dis. **16**, 73—75 (1957). — SWIFT, H. F.: Bacterial and mycotic infections in man. Philadelphia: J. B. Lippincott Company 1948. — SWIFT, H. F., and B. E. HODGE: Type-specific anti-M-precipitins in rheumatic and non-rheumatic patients with hemolytic streptococcal infections. Proc. Soc. exp. Biol. (N.Y.) **34**, 849—854 (1936).

TACHAU, P.: Erythema exsudativum multiforme und nodosum. In: Handbuch der Haut- und Geschlechtskrankheiten, Bd. VI/2, S. 584—677. Berlin: Springer 1928. — TARANTA, A., M. SPAGNUOLO and A. R. FEINSTEIN: „Chronic" rheumatic fever. Atti X. Congr. Lega Internaz. contro il Reumatismo, vol. II, pp. 99—101, Roma 1961. — TARANTA, A., S. TOROSDAG, J. METRAKOS, W. JEGIER and I. UCHIDA: Rheumatic fever in monozygotic and dizygotic twins. Atti X. Congr. Lega Internaz. contro il Reumatismo, vol. II, pp. 96—98, Roma 1961. — TEDESCHI, C. G., B. M. WAGNER and K. C. PANI: Studies in rheumatic fever. In: The clinical significance of the Aschoff body based of morphologic observation. Arch. Path. **60**, 408—422 (1955). — TEODORI, U., e G. G. N. SERNERI: Il problema dell'eredità nelle malattie reumatiche. Reumatismo **9**, Suppl. 1, 3—63. Ref. Zbl. inn. Med. **190**, 111 (1957). — TICHY, H.: Streptokokken-Status, Antistreptolysin- und Waaler-Rose-Reaktion als Grundlagen einer systematischen Ordnung rheumatischer Krankheiten. Z. Rheumaforsch. **17**, 51—53 (1958). — TICHY, H., K. SEIDEL u. G. HEIDELMANN: Lehrbuch der Rheumatologie. Berlin: Volk u. Gesundheit 1959. Ref. Zbl. inn. Med. **213**, 208 (1960). — TÖNDER, O., and T. Quamme: Waaler-Rose-Test and activity of rheumatoid arthritis. Acta rheum. scand. **7**, 113—118 (1961).

Vargazon, B., u. S. Banic: Vergleichende Untersuchungen zwischen dem Latex-Rheumafaktor-Test und der Hämagglutinationsreaktion nach Waaler-Rose. Atti X. Congr. Lega Internaz. Contro il Reumatismo, vol. II, pp. 752—753, Roma 1961. — Vaughan, J. H.: Behaviour of the agglutination activating factor of rheumatoid arthritis with immune-praecipitates. Ann. rheum. Dis. **14**, 431—432 (1955). — Vaughan, J. H., and B. A. Good: Relation of a-gammaglobulinaemia-sera to rheumatoid agglutination reactions. Arthr. and Rheum. **1**, 99—111 (1958). — Veil, W. H.: Der Rheumatismus und die streptomykotische Symbiose. Stuttgart: Ferdinand Enke 1939. — Vilanova, X., J. Piñol et R. de Dalmases-Gosé: Sindromes cutaneo-articulares. Rev. esp. Reum. **6**, 169—179 (1955). Ref. Z. Rheumaforsch. **17**, 249 (1958). — Veil, W. H., u. A. Sturm: Pathologie des Stammhirns, 2. Aufl. Jena: Gustav Fischer 1946. — Voit, K.: Zur Differentialdiagnose der chronischen Polyarthritis. Münch. med. Wschr. **100**, 447—450 (1958). — Voit, K., u. H. Gamp: Der Rheumatismus, S. 66. Stuttgart: Ferdinand Enke 1958. — Zur Klinik des Rheumatismus. Med. Klin. **11**, 421—425 (1961). — Vorlaender, K. O.: Klinische Immunologie der entzündlich-rheumatischen Erkrankungen. In: Miescher-Vorlaender, Immunpathologie in Klinik und Forschung, 2. Aufl., S. 436—500. Stuttgart: Georg Thieme 1961. — Vorlaender, K. O., W. Fitting u. H. Blankenheim: Auto-Allergie und Rheumatismus. Z. Rheumaforsch. **13**, 276—296 (1954).

Waaler, E.: On the occurrence of a factor in human serum activating specific agglutination of sheep blood corpuscles. Acta path. microbiol. scand. **17**, 172—188 (1940). — Waller, M. V., B. Decker, E. C. Toone jr. and R. Irby: Evaluation of rheumatoid factor tests. Arthr. and Rheum. **4**, 579—591 (1961). — Walther, D.: Ein Beitrag zu dem Krankheitsbild der multiplen Reticulohistiocytome der Haut bei destruierenden Gelenkveränderungen. Hautarzt **9**, 77—81 (1958). — Wannamaker, L. W., F. W. Denny, W. D. Perry, C. R. Rammelkamp, G. E. Eckhardt, H. B. Houser and E. O. Hahn: The effect of Penicillin prophylaxis on streptococcal diseases. New Engl. J. Med. **249**, 1—7 (1953). — Wieland, R., J. Katz and H. K. Hellerstein: Prophylaxis against streptococcic infections in an adult rheumatic population. J. Amer. med. Ass. **173**, 350—353 (1960).— Wilson, M. G.: Present status of hormone therapy in rheumatic fever, with special reference to short-term treatment in active carditis. Advanc. Pediat. **11**, 243—262 (1960). — Wilson, M. G., and M. Schweizer: Pattern of hereditary susceptibility in rheumatic fever. Circulation **10**, 699—704 (1954). — Winblad, St.: Studies in hemolytic streptococcus. Kobenhavn: Munksgaard 1941. — Studies on agglutination of sensitized sheep cells in rheumatic diseases; agglutination titer after primary absorption of serum by sheep cells. Acta med. scand. **142**, 450 (1952). — Windom, R. E., J. P. Sanford and M. Ziff: Acne conglobata and arthritis. Arthr. and Rheum. **4**, 632—636 (1961). — Wöhler, F., W. Müller u. A. Hofmann: Über die Natur des Rheumafaktors. Z. Rheumaforsch. **19**, 85—92 (1960).

Zalesskij, G. D. u. R. S. Dreisen: Über einen spezifischen Rheumatismuserreger. Therapeut. Arch. (Moskau) **30**, 3—15 (1958). — Zalesskij, G. D., and R. S. Dreisen: On the special virus isolated from rheumatic patients. Atti X. Congr. Lega Internaz. contro il Reumatismo, vol. II, pp. 47—48, Roma 1961. — Ziff, M., P. Brown, D. Lospallutos, J. Badin and C. McEven: Agglutination and inhibition by serum globulin in the sensitized sheep cell agglutination reaction in rheumatoid arthritis. Amer. J. Med. **20**, 500—509 (1956).— Ziff, M., F. R. Schmid, A. J. Lewis and M. Tanner: Familial occurrence of the rheumatic factor. Arthr. and Rheum. **1**, 392—399 (1958).

II. Rheumatisches Fieber

1. (Vorwiegend) unspezifische Hauterscheinungen

Azua Dochao, L. de: Etiopatogenia de las afecciones cutaneas reumatoides (A.C.R.). Act. dermo-sifiliogr. (Madr.) **45**, 683—718 (1954).

Barlow, T.: Notes on rheumatism and its allies in childhood. Brit. med. J. **1883 II**, 509. — Bass, M. H.: The cutaneous manifestations of acute rheumatic fever in childhood. Med. Clin. N. Amer. **2**, 201—214 (1918). — Bock, H. E.: Zur Allergielage beim Erythema nodosum im Rahmen des Löfgren-Syndroms. Allergie u. Asthma **6**, 121—130 (1960).

Campbell, A. D., G. C. Griffith and W. H. Leake: Skin lesions of rheumatic fever. U.S. nav. med. Bull. **46**, 360—366 (1946). — Canizares, O.: Cutaneous lesions of rheumatic fever. Arch. Derm. **76**, 702—707 (1957). — Chester, W., and S. P. Schwartz: Skin lesions in rheumatic fever. Amer. Heart J. **9**, 105 (1933). — Cutaneous lesions in rheumatic fever. Amer. J. Dis. Child. **48**, 69—80 (1934).

Dahl, M., u. R. Nordman: Über den Morbus rheumaticus bei Kindern. Kinderärztl. Prax. **28**, 51—58 (1960). — Davis, E., and J. Landau: Capillary microscopy in rheumatic fever. The capillary patterns in conjunctiva and nailbed as clinical signs in rheumatic fever and rheumatic heart disease. Arch. intern. Med. **97**, 51—56 (1956).

EDSTRÖM, G.: Die Klinik des rheumatischen Fiebers. Ergebn. inn. Med. Kinderheilk. **52**, 439—503 (1937).

FANCONI, G., u. H. WISSLER: Der Rheumatismus im Kindesalter. I. Teil. In: Der Rheumatismus, hrsg. R. SCHOEN. Dresden u. Leipzig: Theodor Steinkopff 1943. — FEER, E.: Lehrbuch der Kinderheilkunde, 13. Aufl. Jena: Gustav Fischer 1941.

GARROD, A. E.: A treatise on rheumatism. Philadelphia: Blakiston's Son & Co. 1890. — On the nature of the connexion between erythemata and lesions of the joints. Lancet **1911 I**, 1411. — GREITHER, A.: Erythema nodosum und Erythema exsudativum multiforme. In: GOTTRON-SCHÖNFELD, Dermatologie und Venerologie, Bd. II/1, S. 445—460. Stuttgart: Georg Thieme 1958. — GRENET, H.: La maladie rhumatismale chez l'enfant. Arch. Méd. Enf. **40**, 329—356 (1937). — GRIFFITH, J. P. C., and A. G. MITCHELL: The diseases in infants and children, p. 474. Philadelphia: W. B. Saunders & Co. 1933. — GRINSPAN, D., y A. ZURITA: Livedo possreumático. (Enf. de Bouillaud.) Arch. argent. Derm. **5**, 277—278 (1955).

HOHLFELD, M.: Erythema exsudativum multiforme, Chorea, Rheumatismus nodosus, Endo-pericarditis. Berl. klin. Wschr. **10**, 701 (1903). — HOLBROOK, W. P.: The army air force rheumatic fever control program. J. Amer. med. Ass. **126**, 84—85 (1944). — HORNSTEIN, O., u. H. SCHUERMANN: Rheumatismus der Haut. In: GOTTRON-SCHÖNFELD, Dermatologie und Venerologie, Bd. II/1, S. 623—642. Stuttgart: Georg Thieme 1958.

INGERMAN, E., and M. G. WILSON: Rheumatism. Its manifestations on childhood today. J. Amer. med. Ass. **82**, 759—764 (1924).

JAMES, J. A., and F. G. BOLTON: Amyloidosis in Still's disease. Ann. rheum. Dis. **10**, 250—254 (1951). — JONES, T. D.: Diagnosis of rheumatic fever. J. Amer. med. Ass. **126**, 481—484 (1944).

KEIL, H.: The rheumatic erythemas. A critical survey. Ann. intern. Med. **11**, 2223—2272 (1938). — Relation of erythema nodosum and rheumatic fever: A critical survey. Ann. intern. Med. **10**, 1686—1707 (1937). — KÜSTER, F.: Das rheumatische Fieber. Arch. Kinderheilk. **151**, 113—132 (1955).

LANDAU, A.: Erythema nodosum und rheumatische Affektionen. Acta paediat. (Uppsala) **6**, 402—413 (1927). — LEWIN, G.: Erythema exsudativum multiforme. Charité-Ann. **111**, 622 (1876).

MEYER, A.: Akuter Gelenkrheumatismus mit Erythema pustulosum. Z. klin. Med. **117**, 413—424 (1931).

NAEGELI, O.: Über Polyarthritis acuta (Rheumatismus verus). Schweiz. med. Wschr. **63**, 1197—1200 (1933). — NATTENHEIMER, R.: Erythema annulare und Noduli rheumatici. Diss. Zürich 1939.

ORBANEJA, J. G.: Afecciones cutaneas reumatoides (Clinica). Act. dermo-sifiliogr. (Madr.) **45**, 719—773 (1954). Ref. Zbl. Haut- u. Geschl.-Kr. **92**, 71 (1954).

PAUNESCU-PODEANU, A., u. O. BALTACEANU: Rheuma-purpurische Zustände. Probl. Reum. (Buc.) **4**, 73—81 (1956) [Rumänisch]. Ref. Zbl. inn. Med. **177**, 539 (1957).

RIBOLD, G.: Zur Kenntnis der Komplikationen der Polyarthritis rheumatica von seiten der Haut. Dtsch. Arch. klin. Med. **82**, 272—293 (1905). — RIDLEY, C. M.: Still's disease with recrurrent uleration of the legs. Proc. roy. Soc. Med. **50**, 19 (1957). — RUTSTEIN, D. D., W. BAUER, A. DORFMAN, E. R. GROSS, J. A. LICHTY, H. B. TAUSSIG and R. WHITTEMORE: Jones criteria (modified) for guidance in the diagnosis of rheumatic fever. Report of the committee on standards and criteria for programs of care. Circulation **13**, 617—620 (1956).

SCHOEN, R., u. W. TISCHENDORF: Der akute Gelenkrheumatismus. In: Handbuch der inneren Medizin, Bd. VI/1, S. 907—949. Berlin-Göttingen-Heidelberg: Springer 1954. — SLATER, J. D. H., and S. ROSENBAUM: Acute rheumatic fever in young men. A clinical and epidemiologiacl study. Ann. rheum. Dis. **18**, 285—292 (1959). — STILL, G. F.: Common disorders and diseases of childhood, 5th ed.: Oxford University Press 1927. — STUCKI, P.: Über das Erythema nodosum und das Löfgren-Syndrom (Bilateral Hilar Lymphoma Syndrome). Praxis **50**, 271—275 1961). — SWIFT, H. F.: „Rheumatic Fever", in CECIL's Textbook of Medicine, p. 87. Philadelphia: W. B. Saunders & Co. 1930.

TOBIASCH, V.: Über die schwere Verlaufsform des Erythema exsudativum multiforme. Med. Wschr. **7**, 82—86 (1953). — TRAUB, E.: Über die Bedeutung der Hauterscheinungen beim akuten Gelenkrheumatismus. Z. Kinderheilk. **57**, 769—789 (1937).

VILANOVA, X., J. PIÑOL y J. ROTÉS QUEROL: Afecciones cutaneas reumatoides. Comentarios a nuestra casustica. Act. dermo-sifiliogr. (Madr.) **46**, 106—126 (1954). Ref. Zbl. Haut- u. Geschl.-Kr. **92**, 70 (1954).

WALLGREN, A.: Studies on erythema anulare rheumaticum. Acta paediat. (Uppsala) **17**, 447—468 1935). — Rheumatic eryhema nodosum. Amer. J. Dis. Child. **55**, 897—912 (1938). — WEST, S.: Rheumatic fever and rashes — clinical jottings No. 19. St. Bart.

Hosp. J. **19**, 218 (1911/12). — WIENER, K.: Skin manifestations of internal disorders, p. 37. St. Lois: C. V. Mosby & Comp. 1947. — WOLLHEIM, E. u. J. ZISSLER: Purpura rheumatica (Schönlein). In: Handbuch der inneren Medizin, 4. Aufl., Bd. IX/6, S. 564—566. Berlin-Göttingen-Heidelberg: Springer 1960. — WRIGHT, J. S. Experiences with rheumatic fever in the army. Bull. N.Y. Acad. Med. **21**, 419—432 (1,945).

II. 2. Erythema anulare Lehndorff-Leiner

ABLARD, G., et A. LARCAN: Érythèmes et purpuras au cours de la maladie rhumatismale de l'adulte. Presse méd. **1956**, 1970—1972. — ABT, A. F.: Erythema annulare rheumaticum. Amer. J. med. Sci. **190**, 824—833 (1935). — ALLEN, A. C.: The skin. A clinicopathologic treatise, pp. 142—190. St. Louis: C. V. Mosby Comp. 1954.

BARCAGLIA, A.: Eritema annulare di Lehndorff prodromico di grave cardiopatia reumatica. Osped. maggiore **26**, 255—259 (1938). — BARLOW, T.: Notes on rheumatism and its allies in childhood. Brit. med. J. **1883II**, 509. — BESNIER, E.: Étude sur les dermopathies rhumatismales ou arthritides rhumatismales. Ann. Derm. Syph. (Paris) **8**, 254—268, 320—337 (1876/77). — BINDSCHEDLER, J. J.: Érythème annulaire rhumatismal de Lehndorff et Leiner chez un garçonnet. Bull. Soc. franç. Derm. Syph. **43**, 856—859 (1936). — BIRKHAUG, K. E.: Rheumatic fever; skin hypersensitiveness of patients with rheumatic fever and chronic arthrides to filtrates actolysates and bacterial suspension of streptococci. J. infect. Dis. **44**, 363—377 (1929). — BOUISSOU, H.: Les lésions de la peau apparement saine au cours du rhumatisme articulaire aigu. Arch. franç. Pédiat. **14**, 322—326 (1957). — BRIGHT, R.: Reports of medical cases, vol. 2, pp. 468—509. London: Longman, Rees, Orme, Brown & Green 1831. — BURKE, J. B.: Erythema marginatum. Arch. Dis. Childh. **30**, 359—365 (1955).

CAMPBELL, A. D., G. C. GRIFFITH and W. H. LEAKE: Skin lesions of rheumatic fever. U.S. nav. med. Bull. **46**, 360—366 (1946). — CANIZARES, O.: Cutaneous lesions of rheumatic fever. A clinical study in young adults. Arch. Derm. **76**, 702—707 (1957). — CAROL, W. L. L., u. J. A. VAN KRIEKEN: Zur Histopathologie des Erythema anulare von Lehndorff-Leiner. Acta paediat. (Uppsala) **17**, 372—376 (1935). — CHEADLE, W. B.: The various manifestations of the rheumatic state as exemplified in childhood and early life. London: Smith, Elder & Co. 1889. — COCKAYNE, E. A.: Rheumatic rashes and their significance. Arch. Middx Hosp. Clin. **11**, 28 (1912).

DAHL, M., u. R. NORDMAN: Über den Morbus rheumaticus bei Kindern. Kinderärztl. Prax. **28**, 51—58 (1960). — DARRÉ, H.: Les symptomes cutanés de la Trypanosomiase humaine. Ann. Derm. Syph. (Paris) **9**, 673 (1908). — DEBRÉ, R., M. LAMY et M.-L. JAMMET: Érythème annulaire et streptococcémie à „Streptococcus viridans" au cours de la maladie de Bouillaud. Arch. Méd. Enf. **40**, 357—367 (1937). — DEBRÉ, R., et M. LELONG: Pédiatrie, Chap. VIII: Rhumatisme articulaire aigu. Paris: Éd. méd. Flammarion 1952. — DUKEN, J.: Reiz- und Giftempfindlichkeit im Ablauf der rheumatischen Infektion. Z. Kinderheilk. **59**, 583—599 (1938). — DYER, R. F.: The rheumatic erythemas. Med. Ann. D. C. **25**, 547—522 (1956).

ELGHAMMER, H. W.: Rheumatic fever in children. Med. Clin. N. Amer. **42**, 129—134 (1958).

FANCONI, G., u. H. WISSLER: Der Rheumatismus im Kindesalter. I. Der Rheumatismus verus und seine Differentialdiagnose. Dresden u. Leipzig: Theodor Steinkopff 1943. — FERRAND, E. A. A.: Les exanthèmes du rhumatisme. Thèse Paris 1862. — FINDLAY, L.: The rheumatic infection in childhood. London: E. Arnold & Co. 1931.

GANS, O.: Die Histopathologie polymorpher exsudativer Dermatosen in ihrer Beziehung zur speziellen Ätiologie. Arch. Derm. Syph. (Berl.) **130**, 15—135 (1921). — Histologie der Hautkrankheiten, Bd. I, S. 377. Berlin: Springer 1925. — GANS, O., u. G. KL. STEIGLEDER: Histologie der Hautkrankheiten, 2. Aufl., Bd. I, S. 411. Berlin-Göttingen-Heidelberg: Springer 1955. — GARROD, A. E.: A treatise on rheumatism and rheumatoid arthritis. London: Griffin & Co. 1890. — GLANZMANN, E.: Die rheumatische Infektion. In: Handbuch Kinderheilkunde, Ergänzungswerk, hrsg. von v. PFAUNDLER, Bd. I, S. 399—410. Berlin: Springer 1942. — GOTTRON, H. A.: Zur Pathogenese rheumatischer Hautreaktionen. Derm. Wschr. **132**, 1007—1015 (1955). — GREITHER, A.: Über das Erythema anulare rheumaticum. Arch. klin. exp. Derm. **204**, 205—212 (1957). — Das Erythema anulare rheumaticum. In: GOTTRON-SCHÖNFELD, Dermatologie und Venerologie, Bd. II/1, S. 469—471. Stuttgart: Georg Thieme 1958. — GRENET, H.: La maladie rhumatismale chez l'enfant. Arch. Méd. Enf. **40**, 329—356 (1937). — GRIMMER, H.: Erythema anulare (Lehndorff-Leiner 1922) (Histologischer Bildbericht). Z. Haut- u. Geschl.-Kr. **31**, H. 5, XVII—XX (1961).

HADLEY, H. G.: Rheumatic fever eruptions. Acta derm.-venereol. (Stockh.) **26**, 157—158 (1946). — HÄSSLER, E., u. L. MÖLLER: Klinik und Prognose des kindlichen Gelenkrheumatismus, der Chorea minor und der Endokarditis. (Bericht über 256 Erkrankungsfälle der Leipziger Kinderklinik aus den Jahren 1923—1930.) Jb. Kinderheilk. **136**, 257—301 (1932). — HAGERMAN, G.: Infection, allergy and the pathogenesis of rheumatic disease. Acta rheum.

scand. **1**, 209—234 (1956). — HORNSTEIN, O.: Zur Kenntnis des Erythema anulare rheumaticum. Hautarzt **9**, 120—125 (1958). — Über das Gewebsbild und die Pathogenese des Erythema anulare rheumaticum. Atti X. Congr. Lega Internaz. contro il Reumatismo vol. II, pp. 1067—1070, Roma 1961. — HORNSTEIN, O., u. H. SCHUERMANN: Rheumatismus der Haut. In: GOTTRON-SCHÖNFELD, Dermatologie und Venerologie, Bd. II/1, S. 623—642. Stuttgart: Georg Thieme 1958.

IACCHIA, P.: Eritema annulare precorrente una endocardite settica. Pediatria (Roma) **32**, 422—424 (1924). — ILLINGWORTH, R. S.: Rheumatic fever of the children. Lancet **1957 II** 653. Ref. Z. Rheumaforsch. **17**, 326 (1958).

JULKUNEN, H., and W. J. KAIPAINEN: Rheumatic fever and antistreptolysin-O titre. Ann. Med. intern. Fenn. **48**, 81—85 (1959). — JUSTIN-BESANÇON, L., A. RUBENS-DUVAL et J. VILLIAUMEY: Esquisse de l'histogénèse des lésions de l'inflammation rhumatismale. Sem. Hôp. Paris **1953**, 2003—2008.

KEIL, H.: The rheumatic erythemas: A critical survey. Ann. intern. Med. **11**, 2223—2272 (1938). — Dr. William Charles Wells and his contribution to the study of rheumatic fever. Bull. Inst. Hist. Med. Johns Hopk. Univ. (1936). — KLINKE, K.: Das rheumatische Fieber in heutiger Sicht. Ein kritischer Überblick. Medizinische **1958**, 12—15. — KLINGE u. FASSBENDER: s. S. 231. — KÖTTGEN, U.: Probleme der Nomenklatur bei den rheumatischen Erkrankungen des Kindesalters. Med. Welt **1960**, 959—962. — KRAMÁR, E.: Zur Klinik des akuten Rheumatismus. Jb. Kinderheilk. **149**, 108—120 (1937). — KÜSTER, F.: Das rheumatische Fieber. Arch. Kinderheilk. **151**, 113—132 (1955). — In: OPITZ-DE RUDDER, Pädiatrie. Ein Lehrbuch für Studierende und Ärzte, S. 377—391. Berlin-Göttingen-Heidelberg: Springer 1957.

LEHNDORFF, H.: Das Erythema annulare rheumaticum. Wien. med. Wschr. **1930 II**, 1449—1450. — Die Erythemkrankheiten im Kindesalter. Erythema annulare rheumaticum (Lehndorff-Leiner). In: Handbuch der Kinderheilkunde, hrsg. von v. PFAUNDLER-SCHLOSSMANN, Bd. 10, S. 584—588. Berlin: F. C. W. Vogel 1935. — LEHNDORFF, H., u. C. LEINER: Erythema annulare. Ein typisches Exanthem bei Endokarditis. Z. Kinderheilk. **32**, 46—53 (1922). — LEICHTENTRITT, B.: Zum Problem der rheumatischen Erkrankungen im Kindesalter. Mschr. Kinderheilk. **43**, 462—468 (1929). — Die rheumatische Infektion im Kindesalter. Ergebn. inn. Med. Kinderheilk. **37**, 1—100 (1930). — Der acute Gelenkrheumatismus als Teilerscheinung der rheumatischen Infektion, zugleich eine Darstellung des Rheumatismus nodosus und der Stillschen Krankheit. In: Handbuch der Kinderheilkunde, hrsg. von v. PFAUNDLER u. SCHLOSSMANN, Bd. II, S. 419—450. Leipzig: F. C. W. Vogel 1931.

MACKENZIE, S.: 3rd Intern. Congr. Dermat., p. 602, London 1896. — MENOZZI, R.: Eritema anulare di Lehndorff-Leiner. Clin. pediat. (Bologna) **23**, 280—288 (1941).

NATTENHEIMER, R.: Erythema annulare und Noduli rheumatici. Inaug.-Diss. Zürich 1939. — NESTEROV, A. I.: Fragen der Ätiologie, Therapie und Prophylaxe des Rheumatismus. Klin. Med. (Mosk.) **36**, H. 5, 3—18 (1958). — NITSCH, K.: Rheumatische Erkrankungen im Kindesalter. Ther. d. Gegenw. **97**, 409—413 (1958).

OSTAPJUK, F. E.: Über Hauterscheinungen bei Rheumatismus. Therap. Arch. (Mosk.) **30**, H. 5, 21—28 (1958).

PERROUD: De l'érysipèle rhumatismal. Ann. Derm. Syph. (Paris) **5**, 161—180 (1873). — PERRY, C. B.: Erythema marginatum (rheumaticum). Arch. Dis. Childh. **12**, 233—238 (1937). — PREUX, R. DE: Erythema annulare rheumaticum Lehndorff-Leiner. Derm. Wschr. **119**, 156—157 (1947).

RAYER, P. F.: Traité théorique et pratique des maladies de la peau. Éd. 2d. Paris: J. B. Baillière 1835. — RIEBOLD, G.: Zur Kenntnis der Komplikationen der Polyarthritis rheumatica acuta von seiten der Haut. Dtsch. Arch. klin. Med. **82**, 273—293 (1905). — RIETSCHEL, H.: Über acute Exantheme im Kindesalter. Kinderärztl. Prax. **5**, 246—251 (1934).

SCHLOSS, O. M.: Zit. nach BASS (s. II. *1.*). — SCHMIDEK, B.: Ein Fall von Erythema annulare. Med. Klin. **32**, 1048—1049 (1936). — SCHOEN, R., u. W. TISCHENDORF: Krankheiten der Knochen, Gelenke und Muskeln. In: Handbuch der inneren Medizin, 4. Aufl., Bd. VI/1, S. 918. Berlin-Göttingen-Heidelberg: Springer 1954. — SCHUERMANN, H.: Hautkrankheiten mit Beziehungen zu Arthritis und Rheuma. Ärztl. Prax. **5** (48) (28. 11. 1953). — SEVESTRE, A.: Erythème marginé et rhumatisme. Progr. méd. (Paris) **1**, 318 (1873). — SHELDON, W.: „Rheumatism". In: THURSFIELD and PATERSON's Diseases of Children, p. 1029. (1st ed., ed. by GARROD, BATTEN and THURSFIELD.) Baltimore: Wood & Co. 1934. — SINGER, G.: Die Hautveränderungen beim akuten Gelenkrheumatismus neben Bemerkungen über die Natur des Erythema multiforme. Wien. klin. Wschr. **1897**, 841. — STAMM, C.: Mitteilungen aus der Kinderpoliklinik in Hamburg. I. Rheumatismus nodosus. Arch. Kinderheilk. **60/61**, 706—709 (1913).

TARANTA, A.: Relationship of isolated recurrences of Sydenham's chorea to preceding streptococcal infections. New Engl. J. Med. **260**, 1204—1210 (1959). — TOBIASCH, V.: Die Klinik der rheumatischen Herzerkrankungen. Medizinische **1959**, 2026—2035. — TRAUB,

E.: Über die Bedeutung der Hauterscheinungen beim akuten Gelenkrheumatismus. Z. Kinderheilk. **58**, 769—789 (1937).

Urbach, E., u. A. Bleier: Erythema annulare rheumaticum (Lehndorff-Leiner). Arch. Derm. Syph. (Chic.) **41**, 515—520 (1940).

Vilanova, X., H. Piñol y J. Rotés Querol: Affecciones cutáneas reumatoides. Comentarios a nuestra casuistica. Acta dermo-sifiliogr. (Barcelona) **46**, 106—126 (1954).

Wallgren, A.: Studies on erythema annulare rheumaticum. Acta paediat. (Uppsala) **17**, 447—468 (1935). — The diagnosis of rheumatic fever. Ann. Paediat. Fenn. **3**, 548—554 (1957). — Wells, W. C.: Zit. nach Keil. – Wiener, K.: Skin manifestations of internal disorders, p. 37. St. Louis: C. V. Mosby Comp. 1947. — Winkler, W.: Erythema annulare Lehndorff-Leiner ohne andere rheumatische Manifestationen. Ann. paediat. (Basel) **168**, 303—310 (1947). — Woringer, F., et C. Lutz: Erythème rhumatismal de Lehndorff-Leiner chez une malade de vingt ans. Bull. Soc. franç. Derm. Syph. **58**, 67—68 (1951).

II. 3. Nodi (sive Noduli) rheumatici

Allen, A. C.: The skin. A clinicopathologic treatise, pp. 142—190. St. Louis: C. V. Mosby Comp. 1954. — Anderson, H. J. G.: Rheumatic nodules. J. Pediat. **12**, 91—94 (1938). — Audeoud, H.: Nodosités rhumatismales aigues. Schweiz. med. Wschr. **61**, 428—429 (1931).

Baldwin, J. S., J. M. Kerr, A. G. Kuttner and E. F. Doyle: Observations on rheumatic nodules over 30-year period. J. Pediat. **56**, 465—470 (1960). — Bang, B.: Zit. bei Fahr 1918. — Barlow, T., and F. Warner: On subcutaneous nodules connected with fibrous structures, occurring in children the subjects of rheumatism and chorea. Transact. 7th Intern. Med. Congr. **4**, 116 (London 1881). — Notes on rheumatism and its allieds in childhood. Brit. med. J. **1883 II**, 509—514. — Beatty jr., E. C.: Rheumatic-like nodules occurring in nonrheumatic children. Arch. Path. **68**, 154—159 (1959). — Bennett, G. A., J. W. Zeller and W. Bauer: Subcutaneous nodules of rheumatoid arthritis and rheumatic fever: pathologic study. Arch. Path. **30**, 70—89 (1940). — Berkowitz, R.: Rheumatismus nodosus im Kindesalter. Arch. Kinderheilk. **59**, 1—43 (1913). — Bollag, S.: Über die Beziehung des Rheumatismus nodosus zu den juxtaarticulären Knoten. Schweiz. med. Wschr. **65**, 702—704 (1935). — Bourcy, P.: Observation de nodosités rhumatismales. Bull. Soc. Clin. Paris **5**, 287 (1881). — Brennemann, J.: The incidence and significance of the rheumatic nodules in children. Amer. J. Dis. Child. **18**, 179—186 (1919). — Brocq, L.: Non-erythematous nodes in rheumatic subjects. J. cutan. vener. Dis. **2**, 281—283 (1884). — Bronson, E., and E. M. Carr: On subcutaneous fibroid nodules in rheumatism. Amer. J. med. Sci. **165**, 781—799 (1923).

Campbell, A. D., G. C. Griffith and W. H. Leake: Skin lesions of rheumatic fever. U.S. nav. med. Bull. **46**, 360—366 (1946). — Canizares, O.: Cutaneous lesions of rheumatic fever. Arch. Derm. **76**, 702—707 (1957). — Cerkovnaja, L. N., u. J. F. Škrudneva: Die prognostische Bedeutung der rheumatischen Knötchen bei Kindern. Pediatr. **1952**, H. 4, 28—31 [Russisch]. Ref. Zbl. Kinderheilk. **44**, 51 (1953). — Cheadle, W. B.: The acute rheumatism in childhood. In: Th. Cliff. Cellbutts, Systeme of medicine, vol. III, p. 46. London 1887. — Coates, V., and C. F. Coombs: Observations on the rheumatic nodule. Arch. Dis. Childh. **1**, 183—193 (1926). — Collins, D. H.: The subcutaneous nodule of rheumatoid arthritis. J. Path. Bact. **45**, 97—115 (1937).

Davaine, C.: Zit. nach Berkowitz. — Dawson, M. H., and R. H. Boots: Subcutaneous nodules in rheumatoid arthritis. J. Amer. med. Ass. **95**, 1894—1896 (1930). — A comparative study of subcutaneous nodules in rheumatic fever and rheumatoid arthritis. J. exp. Med. **57**, 845—858 (1933). — Draheim, J. H., L. C. Johnson and E. B. Helwig: Clinicopathologic analysis of „rheumatoid" nodules occurring in 54 children. (Abstr.) Amer. J. Path. **35**, 678 (1959).

Elias, H., A. Juster-Segal u. H. Fitzig: Atypische Formen des Rheumatismus Bouillaud-Sokolski (akuten Rheumatismus). Probl. Reum. (Buc.) **5**, 107—110 (1958). — Ewerbeck, H.: Rheumatische Erkrankungen im Kindesalter. In: Der Rheumatismus (hrsg. R. Hopmann), S. 29—39. Stuttgart: Georg Thieme 1956.

Fahr, T.: Zur Frage des Rheumatismus nodosus. Zbl. allg. Path. path. Anat. **24**, 625—630 (1918). — Die rheumatische Granulomatose (rheumatisches Fieber, Rheumatismus infectiosus specificus, Rheumatismus verus) vom Standpunkt des Morphologen. Ergebn. inn. Med. Kinderheilk. **54**, 375—396 (1938). — Fanconi, G., u. H. Wissler: Der Rheumatismus im Kindesalter, Teil I: Der Rheumatismus verus und seine Differentialdiagnose. In: Der Rheumatismus (hrsg. R. Schoen), Bd. 25. Dresden u. Leipzig: Theodor Steinkopff 1943. — Féréol, M.: Des nodosités cutanées éphémères chez les arthritiques. Zit. nach Wallace. Paris 1879. — French, H.: A case of multiple subcutaneous rheumatic nodules. Proc. roy. Soc. Med. **1**, 75 (1907/08).

GIBSON, ST.: Rheumatic fever and chorea. In: BRENNEMANNS Pract. of Pediatr., ed. by J. MCQUARRIE, vol. II, chapt. 19. Hagerstown, Maryland: W. F. Prior 1957. — Rheumatic heart disease. In: BRENNEMANNS Pract. of Pediatr., vol. III, chapt. 13, pp. 53—76. Hagerstown, Maryland: W. F. Prior 1957. — GOTTRON, H. A.: Zur Pathogenese rheumatischer Hautreaktionen. Derm. Wschr. **132**, 1007—1015 (1955). — GRASER, F.: Die rheumatische Erkrankung bei Kindern. In: F. LINNEWEH, Die Prognose chronischer Erkrankungen. Longterm observations of chronic diseases, S. 375—378. Berlin-Göttingen-Heidelberg: Springer 1960.

HÄSSLER, E., u. L. MÖLLER: Klinik und Prognose des kindlichen Gelenkrheumatismus, der Chorea minor und der Endokarditis. Jb. Kinderheilk. **136**, 257—301 (1932). — HALL, P.: Acute rheumatic fever. In: F. LINNEWEH, Die Prognose chronischer Erkrankungen. Longterm observations of chronic diseases, S. 366—369. Berlin-Göttingen-Heidelberg: Springer 1960. — HANSEN, A. E.: Rheumatic fever: Acute rheumatic fever and acute rheumatic heart disease. In: J. A. MEYERS and C. A. MCKINLAY, The chest and the heart, pp. 1543—1578. Springfield (Illinois): Ch. C. Thomas 1948. — Importance of early diagnosis in acute rheumatic fever. J. Amer. med. Ass. **148**, 1481—1485 (1952). — HAYES, R. M., and S. GIBSON: An evaluation of rheumatic nodules in children: Clinical study of 167 cases. J. Amer. med. Ass. **119**, 554—555 (1942). — HILLIER, T.: Diseases of children. Philadelphia: Lindsay & Blakiston 1868. — HIRSCHSPRUNG, H.: Eine eigentümliche Localisation des Rheumatismus nodosus im Kindesalter. Jb. Kinderheilk. **16**, 324—336 (1881). — HOPKINS, H. H.: Subcutaneous nodules of juxta-articular type. Bull. Johns Hopk. Hosp. **49**, 5—16 (1931). — HORNSTEIN, O., u. H. SCHUERMANN: Rheumatismus der Haut. In: GOTTRON-SCHÖNFELD, Dermatologie und Venerologie, Bd. II/1, S. 623—642. Stuttgart: Georg Thieme 1958.

INGERMAN, E., and M. G. WILSON: Rheumatism: Its manifestation in childhood today. J. Amer. med. Ass. **82**, 759—764 (1924).

JACKI, E.: Über rheumatische Knötchen in der Galea aponeurotica und ihre histologische Übereinstimmung mit den Aschoffschen Myokardknötchen. Frankfurt. Z. Path. **22**, 82—101 (1919).

KEIL, H.: The rheumatic subcutaneous nodules and stimulating lesions. Medicine (Baltimore) **17**, 261—380 (1938). — KÖTTGEN, U., u. W. CALLENSEE: Statistische Untersuchungen zum kindlichen Rheumatismus. Darmstadt: Theodor Steinkopff 1959. — KÜSTER, F.: Das rheumatische Fieber. Arch. Kinderheilk. **151**, 113—132 (1955).

LEICHTENTRITT, B.: Die rheumatische Infektion im Kindesalter. Ergebn. inn. Med. Kinderheilk. **37**, 1—99 (1930).

MASSELL, B. F., W. B. COEN and T. D. JONES: Observations regarding artificilly induced subcutaneous nodules in rheumatic fever patients. In: Rheumatic diseases,a pp. 27—42 (Proc. 7th Internat. Congr. Rheum. Dis.). Philadelphia and London: W. B. Saunders Company 1952. — MAYER, G.: 2 Fälle von Rheumatismus acutus im Kindesalter mit einer eigentümlichen Complication. Berl. klin. Wschr. **1882**, Nr 31. — MAZZONI, G.: Su un caso di reumatismo acuto nodoso con attegiamento delle mani a Dupuytren, trattato con cortisone. Reumatismo **6**, 392—397 (1954). — MERRITT, K.: Rheumatic nodules. Their incidence in rheumatic infections. Amer. J. Dis. Child. **35**, 823—836 (1928). — MEYER, A.: Die Stellung der Nodosis rheumatica im Ablauf der rheumatischen Infektion. Z. klin. Med. **123**, 142—153 (1933). — MEYNET, P.: Rhumatisme articulaire subaigu avec production de tumeurs multiples dans les tissus fibreux périarticulaires et sur le périoste d'un grand nombre d'os. Lyon. méd. **19**, 495—499 (1875). — MOLL, W.: Klinische Rheumatologie. Basel u. New York: Karger 1958.

NATTENHEIMER, R.: Erythema annulare und Noduli rheumatici. Diss. Zürich 1939. — NAVARRO, J. C.: Nodosità reumatiche. Scritti med. in onore Jensma **2**, 949—953 (1934). Ref. Zbl. Kinderheilk. **30**, 21 (1935).

POYNTON, F. J., and A. PAINE: Researches on rheumatism, p. 420. London: Macmillan Co. 1914.

ROY, P.: Les nodosités du rhumatisme articulaire. Thêse Paris 1910.

SCHLESINGER, B.: Public health aspect of heart disease in childhood (Milroy lecture). Lancet **1938 I**, 593. — SCHOEN, R., u. W. TISCHENDORF: Der akute Gelenkrheumatismus. In: Handbuch der inneren Medizin, 4. Aufl., Bd. VI/1, S. 918—949. Berlin-Göttingen-Heidelberg: Springer 1954. — STAMM, C.: Mitteilungen aus der Kinderpoliklinik in Hamburg. I. Rheumatismus nodosus. Arch. Kinderheilk. **60/61**, 706—709 (1913). — STILL, G.: Common disorders and diseases of childhood, 5th ed. London: Oxford Univ. Press 1927. — STRAUSS, H.: Über Nodosis rheumatica. Klin. Wschr. **9**, 1111—1113 (1930). — SUTTON, R. L., and R. L. SUTTON: Diseases of the skin, p. 155, 10th ed. St. Louis: C. V. Mosby Comp. 1939. — SYMMERS, D.: Zit. nach MERRITT sowie nach WALLACE.

TARANTA, A.: Occurrence of rheumatic-like subcutaneous nodules without evidence of joint or heart disease. Report of a case. New Engl. J. Med. **266**, 13—16 (1962). — THALHAMMER, O.: Rheumatismus nodosus im 7. Lebensmonat. Öst. Z. Kinderheilk. **4**, 201—209

(1950). — TIZARD, J. P. M.: Subcutaneous nodules: For diagnosis? Granuloma annulare. Proc. roy. Soc. Med. **41**, 301—303 (1948). — TROISIER, E., et L. BROCQ: Les nodosités sous-cutanés éphémères et le rhumatisme. Rev. Méd. (Paris) **1**, 297—308 (1881). — Les nodosités rhumatismales sous-cutanés. Progr. méd. **1883**, No 47, 48, 52; **1884**, No 1.

WALLACE, J. H.: A study of rheumatic nodules. Arch. Pediat. **41**, 731—742 (1924). — WEHSARG, F. K.: Der Rheumatismus nodosus (als Beitrag zur Rheumaforschung). Ergebn. inn. Med. Kinderheilk. **55**, 270—294 (1938). — WISHAHY, A. G., and M. RIDA: Rheumatic nodules in Egyptian children. J. Egypt. med. Ass. **41**, 18—21 (1958).

ZIEGLER, E.: Rheumatismus nodosus als einzige Manifestation der rheumatischen Krankheit. Arch. Kinderheilk. **122**, 1—6 (1941). — ZWEIG, H.: Über den Rheumatismus nodosus. Mschr. Kinderheilk. **29**, 131—133 (1924).

III. 2. u. 3. Primär-chronische Polyarthritis des Kindesalters einschließlich Stillsche Krankheit

ANSELL, B. M., and E. G. L. BYWATERS: Growth in Still's disease. Ann. rheum. Dis. **15**, 295—319 (1956). — Prognosis in Still's disease. Bull. rheum. Dis. **9**, 189—192 (1959). — Radiological abnormalities in the cervical spine in juvenile rheumatoid arthritis. Atti X. Congr. Lega Internaz. contro il Reumatismo, vol. II, pp. 241—243. Roma 1961. — ANSELL, B. M., E. G. L. BYWATERS and J. S. LAWRENCE: A family study in Still's disease. Atti X. Congr. Lega Internaz. contro il Reumatismo, vol. II, pp. 263—264. Roma 1961.

BAILEY, R. H., for Dr. PATERSON: Still's disease with erythema multiforme. Proc. roy. Soc. Med. (Sect. for Study of Dis. in Children) **28**, 157 (1934). — BOLDERS, H. E. A.: A case of Still's disease. Med. Soc. Trans. **16**, 55 (1933). — BONNET, P., et J. BONNET: Les manifestations oculaires dans les rhumatismes chroniques de l'enfance. Maladie de Still. Rhumatisme ankylosant et déformant. Arch. Ophtal. (Paris), N. S. **13**, 127—145 (1953). — BYWATERS, E. G. L., M. E. CARTER and T. E. T. SCOTT: Differential agglutination titre (D.A.T.) in juvenile rheumatoid arthritis. Ann. rheum. Dis. **18**, 225—232 (1959). — Comparism of differential agglutination (D.A.T.) in juvenile and adult rheumatoid arthritis. Ann. rheum. Dis. **18**, 233—238 (1959). — BYWATERS, E. G. L., L. E. GLYNN and A. ZELDIS: Subcutaneous nodules of Still's disease. Ann. rheum. Dis. **17**, 278—285 (1958).

CARTER, M. E.: Sacro-iliac joints in juvenile rheumatoid arthritis (Still's disease). Atti X. Congr. Lega Internaz. contro il Reumatismo, vol. II, pp. 212—214. Roma 1961. — COHEN, H.: The rarer arthritic syndromes. In: Textbook of the Rheumatic diseases, 2nd ed., p. 276. Edinburgh: Livingstone 1955. — COLLINS, D. H.: The subcutaneous nodule of rheumatoid arthritis. J. Path. Bact. **45**, 97—115 (1937). — COLVER, T.: The prognosis in rheumatoid arthritis in childhood. Arch. Dis. Childh. **12**, 253—260 (1937). — COSS jr., J. A., and H. R. BOOTS: Juvenile rheumatoid arthritis. J. Pediat. **29**, 143—156 (1946).

DAHL, M., u. R. NORDMANN: Über die Waaler-Rose-, Bentonit- und Latex-Reaktionen bei der Polyarthritis chronica im Kindesalter. Kinderärztl. Prax. **28**, 289—294 (1960). — DAWSON, M. H.: A comparative study of subcutaneous nodules in rheumatic fever and rheumatoid arthritis. J. exp. Med. **57**, 845—858 (1933). — DAWSON, M. H., and R. H. BOOTS: Subcutaneous nodules in rheumatoid (chronic infectious) arthritis. J. Amer. med. Ass. **95**, 1894—1896 (1930). — DEBRÉ, R., et M. LELONG: Pediatrie. Chap. X.: Rhumatismes chroniques de l'enfance. Paris: Éd. méd. Flammarion 1952.

Editorial: Prognosis in rheumatoid arthritis. Brit. med. J. **1956 I**, 1028—1029. — EDSTRÖM, G.: Rheumatoid arthritis and Still's disease in children. A survey of 161 cases. Arthr. and Rheum. **1**, 497—504 (1958). — EDSTRÖM, G., and P. O. GEDDA: Clinic and prognosis of rheumatoid arthritis in children. Acta rheum. scand. **3**, 129—153 (1957). — ELLMAN, P., and R. E. BALL: „Rheumatoid disease" with joint and pulmonary manifestations. Brit. med. J. **1948 II**, 816—820.

FAHR, T., u. H. KLEINSCHMIDT: Multiple chronische Gelenkerkrankung und rheumatische Infektion im Kindesalter. Klin. Wschr. **11**, 708 (1932). — FANCONI, G.: Reaktionskrankheiten und Allergie. In: FANCONI-WALLGREN, Lehrbuch der Paediatrie, 7. Aufl. Basel: Benno Schwabe & Co. 1961. — FORSYTH, C. C.: Calcification of the digital vessels in a child with rheumatoid arthritis. Arch. Dis. Childh. **35**, 296—301 (1960). — FRANCESCHETTI, A., J. D. BLUM and F. BAMATTER: Diagnostic value of ocular symptoms in juvenile chronic polyarthritis (Still's disease). Trans. ophthal. Soc. U. K. **71**, 17—27 (1952). — FRANÇOIS, J., et L. HAUSTRATE: Les manifestations oculaires de la maladie de Still. Ann. Oculist. (Paris) **187**, 1060—1080 (1954).

GAUCHAT, R. D., and C. D. MAY: Early recognition of rheumatoid disease with comments on treatment. Pediatrics **19**, 672—679 (1957).

HILTEMANN, H.: Periostitis ossificans bei Polyarthritis rheumatica im Kindesalter. Fortschr. Röntgenstr. **86**, 98—101 (1957).

ISDALE, J. C., and E. G. L. BYWATERS: The rash of rheumatoid arthritis or Still's disease. Quart. J. Med., N. S. **25**, 377—378 (1956).

JAMES, J. A., and F. G. BOLTON: Amyloidosis in Still's disease. Ann. rheum. Dis. **10**, 250—254 (1951).

KANTOR, T. G.: Is there a relationship between rubella arthritis and rheumatoid arthritis? Atti X. Congr. Lega Internaz. contro il Reumatismo, vol. II, pp. 251—252, Roma 1961. — KELLEY, V. C.: Rheumatoid disease in childhood. Pediat. Clin. N. Amer. **7**, 435—456 (1960).— KELSEY, W. M.: Rheumatoid disease in juvenile patients. J. Pediat. **59**, 227—233 (1961). — KLINKE, K.: Zur chronischen Polyarthritis im Kindesalter. Internist **2**, 431—435 (1960). — KÖLLE, G.: Anaemia in rheumatoid arthritis in childhood. Atti X. Congr. Lega Internaz. contro il Reumatismo, vol. II, pp. 247—249, Roma 1961. — KÖTTGEN, U., u. W. CALLENSEE: Statistische Untersuchungen zum kindlichen Rheumatismus. Darmstadt: Theodor Steinkopff 1959.

LANGMEAD: Diskussion zu BOLDERS. — LAYANI, F., V. MAY, L. DURUPT et Y. CHAOUAT: Du rhumatisme articulaire aigu à la polyarthrite chronique évolutive. (Sur les rapports de deux maladies.) Rev. Rhum. **25**, 441—459 (1958). — LEICHTENTRITT, B.: Gedanken zum Stillschen Symptomenkomplex. Kinderärztl. Prax. **25**, 464—474 (1957). — LOCKIE, L. M., and B. M. NORCROSS: Juvenile rheumatoid arthritis. Pediatrics **2**, 694—698 (1948).

MAYERHOFER, E.: Zur Ätiologie der infantilen Stillschen Erkrankung im Sinne einer „Adaption"-Stressorenwirkung im reticulo-endothelialen System. Ann. paediatr. (Basel) **183**, 203—218 (1954). — MCEWEN, C., M. ZIFF, PH. CARMEL, D. DITATA and M. TANNER: The relationship to rheumatic arthritis of its so-called variants. Arthr. and Rheum. **1**, 481—496 (1958). — MCMINN, F. J., and E. G. L. BYWATERS: Differences between the fever of Still's and that of rheumatic fever. Ann. rheum. Dis. **18**, 293—297 (1959).

PICKARD, N. S.: Rheumatoid arthritis in children. Arch. intern. Med. **80**, 771—790 (1947). — POTTER, T. A., R. BARKIN and S. J. STILLMAN: Occurrence of spondylitis in juvenile rheumatoid arthritis. Ann. rheum. Dis. **13**, 364—365 (1954).

RIDLEY, C. M.: Still's disease with recurrent ulceration of the legs. Proc. roy. Soc. Med. **50**, 19 (1957). — RÜMMELE, N.: Über die Beeinflussung allergischen Geschehens durch Cutivaccination, betrachtet an einem Fall Stillscher Erkrankung. Neue Öst. Z. Kinderheilk. **1**, 327—332 (1956).

SACREZ, R., et J. G. JUIF: Étude critique de quelques observations de rhumatisme chronique de l'enfant. Arch. franç. Pédiat. **14**, 623—645 (1957). — SCANO, V.: Contributo alla conoscenza dell'artrite reumatoide nell'infanzia. Ann. ital. Pediat. **11**, 557—602 (1958). — SCHLESINGER, B. E.: Rheumatoid arthritis in the young. Brit. med. J. **1949I**, 197—201. — SCHLESINGER, B., and J. A. B. CATHIE: Effect of Still's disease on the haemopoetic system. Ann. rheum. Dis. **10**, 412—417 (1951). — SCHLESINGER, B., C. C. FORSYTH, R. H. R. WHITE, J. M. SMELLIE and C. E. STROUD: Observations on the clinical course and treatment on one hundred cases of Still's disease. Arch. Dis. Child. **36**, 65—76 (1961). — SEITZ, L., u. K. BALLOWITZ: Die Infektionskrankheiten, p. 116. Berlin-München-Wien: Urban & Schwarzenberg 1947. — SPODICK, P. H.: Still's syndrome. Atypical juvenile rheumatoid arthritis. Arch. Pediat. **70**, 1—19 (1953). — STADLER. H. E.: Still's disease. A perplexing problem marked by pyrexia of six years duration. Arch. Pediat. **73**, 216—219 (1956). — STECHER, R. M., A. H. HERSH, W. M. SOLOMON and R. WOLPAW: The genetics of rheumatoid arthritis. Analyses of 224 families. Amer. J. hum. Genet. **5**, 118—138 (1953). — STEINER, G., H. A. FREUND, B. LEICHTENTRITT and M. E. MAUN: Lesions of skeletal muscles in rheumatoid arthritis: nodular polymyositis. Amer. J. Path. **22**, 103—130 (1946). — STILL, G. F.: On a form of chronic joint disease in children. Med.-chir. Trans. **80**, 47—59 (1897). — STOEBER, E.: Zur klinischen Sonderstellung des kindlichen Rheumatismus. Med. Klin. **1956**, 2153—2156. — Kombinierte Dauerbehandlung von Morbus Still und aktiver rheumatoider Arthritis des Kindes mit Prednisolon und Butazolidin. Z. Rheumaforsch. **16**, 283—285 (1957). — STOEBER, E., u. G. KÖLLE: Klinik und Therapie der primär-chronischen Polyarthritis im Kindesalter. Med. Klin. **1956**, 2197—2202. — SURY, B.: Rheumatoid arthritis in children: a clinical study (Thesis). Copenhagen: Munksgaard 1951. — The prognosis in rheumatic arthritis in children (Still's disease). Rev. esp. Reum., Sonderbd., 484—486 (1952). — Late prognosis in juvenile rheumatoid arthritis (Still's disease). Atti X. Congr. Lega Internaz. contro il Reumatismo, vol. II, pp. 238—240, Roma 1961. — SVĚRÁK, J., and J. ISERLE: Oculo-articular syndroms in children. Čs. Oftal. **13**, 420—425 (1957).

TOUMBIS, A., C. MCEWEN, E. C. FRANKLIN and A. G. KUTTNER: Clinical and serological observations in Still's disease. Atti X. Congr. Lega Internaz. contro il Reumatismo, vol. I, pp. 314—317, Roma 1961. — TRASOFF, A., N. SCHNEEBERG and M. SCARF: Arch. intern. Med. **74**, 4—10 (1944). Zit. nach JAMES und BOLTON.

VERDURA, G., e N. SVILOKOS: Considerazioni clinico-terapeutiche su due casi di morbo di Still. G. Mal. infett. **8**, 65—68 (1956). — VERDURA, G., N. SVILOKOS e L. SERAFINI: La malattia di Still e i suoi limiti nosologici. Minerva pediat. **10**, 1251—1267 (1958).

WEINER, E.: Zur Behandlung der primär-chronischen Polyarthritis rheumatica im Kindesalter. Medizinische **1953**, 1430—1431. — WOLFFERSDORFF, H. v.: Morbus Still und Iridocyklitis als Beitrag zur Genese der Iridocyklitis im Kindesalter. Klin. Mbl. Augenheilk. **123**, 530—536 (1933).

ZIFF, M., V. CONTRERAS and C. MCEWEN: Spondylitis in postpuberal patients with rheumatoid arthritis of juvenile onset. Ann. rheum. Dis. **15**, 40—45 (1956).

III. 1. Wissler-Fanconi-Syndrom

BALLOWITZ, L., G. FLEISCHHAUER u. A. LOESCHKE: Erfolgreiche Desensibilisierung einer Subsepsis allergica tuberculosa mit intravenösen Tuberkulineinspritzungen. Z. Kinderheilk. **76**, 586—592 (1955). — BERNHEIM, M., L. GAILLARD et G. EYSSERICH: Le syndrome de Wissler-Fanconi. Pédiatrie **7**, 229—234 (1952). — BIEDRZYCKA, R., et M. JANKOWSKA: Deux observations de syndrome de Wissler-Fanconi. Ann. Pédiat. **36**, 297—299 (1960). — BOUREL, M., G. GOUFFAULT, P. LENOIR, F. PIROT et J. GUINEBRETIÈRE: Fièvre, exanthème et polyarthrite rebelle. La maladie de Wissler-Fanconi. Sem. Hôp. (Ann. Pédiat.) **37**, 1295—1296 (1961).

CAMPANA, A., e G. RONCONI: Sulla sindrome di Wissler-Fanconi (Contributo clinico). Clin. pediat. (Bologna) **38**, 325—337 (1956). — CAUSSADE, L., N. NEIMANN, M. PIERSON et G. LASCOMBES: Le syndrome de Wissler-Fanconi et ses déterminations cutanées. Sem. Hôp. (Paris) (Ann. de Péd.) **32**, 3861—3866 (1956). — CORCOS, A., et J. HEURTEMATTE: Un cas de syndrome de Wissler-Fanconi. Arch. franç. Pédiat. **13**, 218—221 (1956).

DECASTELLO, A., u. O. WELTMANN: Febris maculosa intermittens. Wien. Arch. inn. Med. **1930 II**, 429. — DENYS, P., et P. PROVIS: Pseudosepsis allergica. Arch. franç. Pédiat. **15**, 1025—1029 (1958).

FANCONI, G.: Über einen Fall von Subsepsis allergica Wissler. Helv. paediat. Acta **1**, 532—537 (1945). — FANTUZZI, B., e G. GRANATA: Contributo alla conoscenza della sindrome di Wissler-Fanconi. Minerva pediat. **9**, 807—811 (1957). — FERRIER, P., et A. MÉGEVAND: Syndrome de Wissler-Fanconi. A propos de deux observations. Schweiz. med. Wschr. **91**, 881—895 (1961). — FISCHER, G.: Zur Subsepsis allergica. Dtsch. Gesundh.-Wes. **9**, 759—763 (1954). — FONTAN, R., et R. VERGER: Les formes atypiques de la maladie de Still: subsepsis allergica. Arch. franç. Pédiat. **4**, 359—362 (1948). — FRIEDEMANN, U., u. H. DEICHER: Über die Lenta-Form der Meningokokkensepsis. Dtsch. med. Wschr. **52 I**, 733—735 (1926).

GARBY, L.: Subsepsis allergica Wissler. A report on three cases. Acta paediat. (Uppsala) **42**, 351—356 (1953). — GILLOT, P., J. CLAUSSE et P. LALANNE: A propos d'un cas de syndrome de Wissler-Fanconi (pseudosepsis allergica). Pédiatrie **14**, 543—548 (1959). — GRISLAIN, J.-R., P. LEMOINE et J. GUILLON: Le syndrome de Wissler-Fanconi existe-t-il? Arch. franç. Pédiat. **12**, 843—855 (1955).

JANBON, M., L. BERTRAND et J. SALVAING: Un cas de maladie de Still avec érythèmes récidivant (ses rapports avec le syndrome décrit par Wissler). Arch. franç. Pédiat. **1**, 99—101 (1950).

KEMP, G.: Zur Subsepsis hyperergica. Z. Kinderheilk. **65**, 417—430 (1948). — KEYZER, J. L.: Primair chronische infectieuse polyarthritis en subsepsis hyperergica. Maandschr. Kindergeneesk. **14**, 145 (1946). — Een gevaal van Subsepsis allergica behandelt mit Pyramidon. Maandschr. Kindergeneesk. **20**, 112 (1952). — KIENITZ, M.: Zur Differentialdiagnose der chronischen Polyarthritis im Kindesalter mit besonderer Berücksichtigung der Subsepsis hyperergica (Wissler). Mschr. Kinderheilk. **104**, 371—374 (1956). — KLINKE, K.: Zur chronischen Polyarthritis im Kindesalter. Internist **2**, 431—435 (1961). — KÖLBL, H.: Subsepsis allergica mit akuter Erythroblastopenie und abnormer Riesenproerythroblastenbildung. Z. Kinderheilk. **75**, 525—531 (1954). — KÜSTER, F., u. F.-J. POTHMANN: Zur Pathogenese der sog. „Subsepsis hyperergica" (Wissler). Mschr. Kinderheilk. **102**, 13—17 (1954). — KUNDRATITZ, K., W. SWOBODA u. E. ZWEYMÜLLER: Zur Subsepsis allergica; Pathogenese, Klinik und Behandlungsmöglichkeit. Neue Öst. Z. Kinderheilk. **1**, 29—46 (1955).

LOTTI, F.: Contributo alla conoscenza della sindrome di Wissler-Fanconi. Clin. pediat. (Bologna) **40**, 513—521 (1958).

MONNET, P., P. DISSARD, S. PACAUD, J. BERTRAND et J.-J. VIALA: La maladie de Wissler-Fanconi. A propos de 2 observations. Pédiatrie **9**, 372—377 (1954). — MUSSO, E.: A propos d'un cas de subsepsis allergica (Syndrome de Wissler-Fanconi). Clin. lat. (Torino) **3**, 28—35 (1953).

NOWAK, T.: Die Überempfindlichkeit gegen Nahrungsmittel, Hausstaub und Pollen als Ursache des Wissler-Fanconi-Syndroms (Subsepsis allergica). Münch. med. Wschr. **103**, 366—368 (1961).

D'OELSNITZ, A., L. FABRE et TH. GIOANNI: Une forme particulière des polyarthrites infantiles. Le syndrome de Wissler-Fanconi. Arch. franç. Pédiat. **7**, 426—429 (1950). — ONYSKIEWICZ-BIELEWICZOWA, ST.: Wissler-Fanconi-syndrome caused probably by a virus infection. Pediat. pol. **33**, 1223—1227 (1958). Ref. Zbl. Kinderheilk. **69**, 158 (1959).

ROTTINI, G.: La sindrome de Wissler-Fanconi (pseudosepsi allergica eritemato-artralgica recidivante). Minerva pediat. **10** 432—448 (1958).

Spartà, D.: Studio istologico su di un caso di sindrome di Wissler-Fanconi ad evoluzione stilliana. Acta paediat. lat. (Reggio Emilia) **12**, 197—217 (1959). — Spartà, D., e A. Disertori: Contributo alla conoscenza del problema nosologico della sindrome di Still. Acta paediat. lat. (Reggio Emilia) **12**, 321—343 (1959).

Toscano, F., e N. Spinelli: Sindrome di Wissler-Fanconi. Aggiorn. pediat. 8, 371—384 (1957).

Vestermark, S.: Wissler's syndrome. Report of a case. Acta paediat. (Uppsala) **49**, 90—95 (1960).

Wedemeyer, F.-W.: Kälteagglutinine bei der sog. „Subsepsis hyperergica" (Wissler). Mschr. Kinderheilk. **104**, 193—195 (1952). — Wissler, H.: Über eine besondere Form sepsisähnlicher Krankheiten (Subsepsis hyperergica). Mschr. Kinderheilk. **94**, 1—16 (1944). — Subsepsis allergica. Helv. paediat. Acta **13**, 405—425 (1958). — Subsepsis allergica. Pediat. int. (Roma) **9**, 489—501 (1959).

Zardini, V.: Un caso di probabile sindrome di Wissler-Fanconi in lattante. Aggiorn. pediat. **11**, 39—45 (1960).

IV. 1 u. 3. Primär-chronische Polyarthritis des Erwachsenenalters (einschließlich monosymptomatischer „Rheumatismus nodosus")

Albertini, A. v., u. A. Vogel: Über wirkliche Kollagenosen. Dtsch. med. Wschr. **86**, 1421—1426 (1961). — Allen, A. C.: The skin. A clinicopathologic treatise, pp. 146—148. St. Louis: C. V. Mosby Comp. 1954. — Ayres jr., S., and S. Ayres: Gouty tophi (of ear, fingers, elbow etc. Arch. Derm. **73**, 614—615 (1956).

Ball, J.: Rheumatoid arthritis and polyarteritis nodosa. Ann. rheum. Dis. **13**, 277—290 (1954). — Ballabio, C. B., e G. Grampa: Il cuore nell'artrite reumatoide. In: III. Convivio internaz. su: Recenti aggiornamenti in tema di cardiovasculopatie, p. 291. Gonassini: Milano 1960. — Bannatyne, G. A.: Rheumatoid arthritis, its pathology, morbid anatomy and treatment, 2nd ed., 182 pp. Wright: Bristol 1898. — Barceló, P., C. Alegre-Marcet et J. Valls Serra: Exploration de vascularisation périphérique dans la polyarthrite chronique. Atti X. Congr. Lega Internaz. contro il Reumatismo, vol. II, p. 293, Roma 1961. — Bartfeld, H.: Chromosome studies of rheumatoid arthritis patients. Atti X. Congr. Lega Internaz. contro il Reumatismo, vol. II, p. 285, Roma 1961. — Bauer, W., and W. S. Clark: The systemic manifestations of rheumatoid arthritis. Trans. Ass. Amer. Phycns **61**, 339—342 (1948). — Bayles, T. B., R. J. Palmer, M. F. Massod and E. H. Judd: Vitamin B excretion studies in patients with rheumatoid arthritis. New Engl. J. Med. **242**, 249—252 (1950). — Bazex, A., A. Dupré et M. Parant: Granulome annulaire des mains et des oreilles, association à des nodules douloureux des oreilles. Bull. Soc. franç. Derm. Syph. **65**, 313 (1958). — Beninson, J., and D. C. Ensign: Leg ulcers in rheumatoid arthritis. Use of pressure-gradient theıapy, high-protein diet and other measures producing successful results. J. Amer. med. Ass. **175**, 437—440 (1961). — Bennett, G. A.: Medical criteria which govern relations of trauma to joint disease. Clinics **1**, 1448—1475 (1943). — Bennett, G. A., J. W. Zeller and W. Bauer: Subcutaneous nodules of rheumatoid arthritis and rheumatic fever: pathologic study. Arch. Path. **30**, 70—89 (1940). — Betz, E., u. R. Mauler: Periphere Kreislaufveränderungen beim chronischen Rheumatismus. Arch. phys. Ther. (Lpz.) 8, 257—262 (1956). — Bevans, M., J. Nadell, F. Demartini and C. Ragan: The systemic lesions of malignant rheumatoid arthritis. Amer. J. Med. **16**, 197—211 (1954). — Bianchi, V.: La patogenesi dell'artrite reumatoide. Acta rheum. (Documenta Geigy), No spec. 35—40 (1961). — Böni, A.: Klinik und Therapie der peripheren Durchblutungsstörungen bei rheumatischen Erkrankungen. Z. Rheumaforsch. **14**, 13—22 (1955). — Bolgert, M.: A propos de la pathogénie du granuloma annulaire. Ses analogies histologiques avec les nodosités rhumatismales sous-cutanées. Ann. Derm. Syph. (Paris) **1944**, 136—147. — Bolgert, M., et R. Poisson: Nodosités prérotuliennes bilatérales chez une enfant de 5 ans atteinte de granulome annulaire. Bull. Soc. franç. Derm. Syph. **63**, 322—323 (1956). — Bollag, S.: Über die Beziehung des Rheumatismus nodosus zu den juxtaarticulären Knoten. Schweiz. med. Wschr. **65**, 702—704 (1935). — Bowers, R. E.: The histology of granuloma annulare compared with that of the necrobiotic nodules of rheumatoid arthritis. Brit. J. Derm. **61**, 247—250 (1949). — Bürger, M.: Die Hand des Kranken. München: J. F. Lehmann 1956. — Bunim, J. J., L. Sokoloff, R. R. Williams and R. L. Black: Rheumatoid arthritis. A review of recent advances in our knowledge concerning pathology, diagnosis, and treatment. J. chron. Dis. **1**, 168—210 (1955). — Burnier, R.: Les nodosités juxta-articulaires et leurs rapports avec la syphilis. Presse méd. **49**, 995—997 (1933). — Burt, J. B., R. G. Gordon and A. R. Brown: The autonomic nervous system in rheumatoid arthritis. In: A survey of chron. rheum. Dis., pp. 137—147. London: Oxf. Univ. Press 1938. — Bywaters, E. G. L.: A variant of rheumatoid arthritis characterized by recurrent digital pad nodules and palmar fasciitis closely resembling palindromic rheumatism. Ann. rheum. Dis. 8, 1—30 (1949). — Peripheral vascular obstruction in rheumatoid arthritis and its relationship to other vascular lesions. Ann. rheum. Dis. **16**, 84—103 (1957).

CANEGHEM, P. VAN, et C. FIEVEZ: Granulomes annulaires superficiels et profonds. Arch. belges Derm. **13**, 230—232 (1957). — CATCHPOLE, B. N., R. P. JEPSON and J. H. KELLGREN: Peripheral vascular effect of cortisone in rheumatoid arthritis, scleroderma, and other related conditions. Ann. rheum. Dis. **13**, 302—306 (1954). — CERVINI, C.: Gli aspetti clinica della malattia reumatoide. Acta rheum. (Documenta Geigy), No. spec. 42—59 (1961). — CERVINI, C., e C. LONGO: Riposta cutanea all'acido nicotinico nell'artrite reumatoide. Gazz. int. Med. Chir. **58**, 493 (1953). — CHARCOT, J. M.: Études pour servir à l'histoire de l'affection décrite sous les noms de goutte asthénique primitive, nodosités des jointures, rhumatisme articulaire chronique (forme primitive) etc. Thèse Paris **44**, 58 pp. (1853). — CHEADLE, W. B.: The various manifestations of the rheumatic state as exemplified in childhood and early life. London: Lectures, Smithelder 1889. — CIVATTE, A.: Le granulome annulaire. Bull. Soc. franç. Derm. Syph. **45**, 1514—1517 (1938). — Les formes tuberculo-ulcéreuses et tuberculogommeuses du granulome annulaire. Ann. Derm. Syph. (Paris) **79**, 387—397 (1952). — CLEVE, H.: Neuere immunoelektrophoretische Untersuchungen im Serum Rheumakranker. Z. Rheumaforsch. **17**, 350—361 (1958). — COATES, V., and C. F. COOMBS: Observations on the rheumatic nodule. Arch. Dis. Childh. **1**, 183—193 (1926). — COATES, V., and J. L. DELICATI: Rheumatoid arthritis and its treatment. London: Lewis 1931. — COBB, S., F. ANDERSON and W. BAUER: Length of life and cause of death in rheumatoid arthritis. New Engl. J. Med. **249**, 553—556 (1953). — COBURN, A. F.: The factor of infection in the rheumatic states. Baltimore: Williams & Wilkins Company 1931. — COCHRANE, T.: Granuloma annulare: treatment with vitamin E. Brit. J. Derm. **62**, 316—318 (1950). — COLLINS, D. H.: The subcutaneous nodula of rheumatoid arthritis. J. Path. Bact. **45**, 97—115 (1937). — COMROE, B. I.: Arthritis and allied conditions, 3rd ed., 1359 pp. Philadelphia: Lea & Febiger 1944. — COSTE, F., et P. DESHAYES: Cœur et polyarthrite chronique évolutive. Rev. Rhum. **25**, 697—704 (1958). — CROCKER: Zit. nach GRAY. — CRUICKSHANK, B.: The arteritis of rheumatoid arthritis. Ann. rheum. Dis. **13**, 136—146 (1954). — Heart lesions in rheumatoid disease. J. Path. Bact. **76**, 223—240 (1958). — CURTIS, A. C., and H. M. POLLARD: Felty's syndrome; its several features, including tissue changes, compared with other forms of rheumatoid arthritis. Ann. intern. Med. **13**, 2265—2284 (1940).

DAM, G. VAN, A. LEZWIJN and J. G. BOS: Death-rate of patients with rheumatoid arthritis. Atti X. Congr. Lega Internaz. contro il Reumatismo, vol. I, pp. 161—164, Roma 1961. — DANNENBERG, A. M., J. YOUNG and M. T. TUNCALI: Granuloma annulare. Report of a case with lesions in the galea aponeurotica of a child. J. Dis. Child. **96**, 720—723 (1958). — DAVIS, E.: Purpura of the skin: a review of 500 cases. Lancet **1943** 245, 160—161. — DAWSON, M. H.: Chronic arthritis, chap. 29 in Nelson's New Loose Leaf Medicine, pp. 605—644. New York: Nelson & Sons 1935. — A note on the occurrence of psoriasis in rheumatoid arthritis. Med. clin. N. Amer. **21**, 1807—1808 (1937). — DAWSON, M. H., et R. H. BOOTS: Subcutaneous nodules in rheumatoid (chronic infections) arthritis. J. Amer. med. Ass. **95**, 1894—1896 (1930). — A comparative study of subcutaneous nodules in rheumatic fever and rheumatoid arthritis. J. exp. Med. **57**, 845—858 (1933). — DIETZ, V. H.: Intracutaneous tests using filtrates prepared from pathologic pulps of human teeth, with special reference to rheumatoid arthritis. Oral. Surg. **5**, 59, 199, 315, 418, 536, 646, 752 (1952). — DOUTHWAITE, A. H.: The treatment of rheumatoid arthritis and Sciatica. 2rd ed., 131 pp. London: Levis 1933. — DUPERRAT, B., et G. E. GOETSCHEL: Nodules juxta-articulaires du granulome annulaire chez un garçon de 4 ans. Bull. Soc. franç. Derm. Syph. **64**, 158—159 (1957). — DUTHIE, J. J. R., P. E. BROWN, L. H. TRUELOVE, F. D. BARAGAR and A. J. LAWRIE: Course and prognosis in rheumatoid arthritis (A further report). Atti X. Congr. Lega Internaz. contro il Reumatismo, vol. I, pp. 213—219, Roma 1961.

ELLIS, F. A., and H. KIRBY-SMITH: Necrobiosis lipoidica and granuloma annulare; comparative study. Arch. Derm. Syph. (Chic.) **45**, 40—60 (1942). — ELLMANN, P., et R. E. BALL: „Rheumatoid disease" with joint and pulmonary manifestations. Brit. med. J. **1948 II**, 816.

FAGGE, C. H., and P. H. PAYE-SMITH: General diseases affecting the joints. Text Book of Principl. and Pract. of Med., 3rd ed., vol. 2, pp. 669—732. London: J. & A. Churchill 1891. — FAHR, T.: Zur Frage des Rheumatismus nodosus. Zbl. allg. Path. path. Anat. **24**, 625—630 (1918). — Die rheumatische Granulomatose (rheumatisches Fieber, Rheumatismus infectiosus specificus, Rheumatismus verus) vom Standpunkt des Morphologen. Ergebn. inn. Med. Kinderheilk. **54**, 357—396 (1938). — FAWNS, H. T., and J. W. LANDELLS: Histochemical studies of rheumatic conditions. II. The nodule of rheumatoid arthritis. Ann. rheum. Dis. **13**, 28—34 (1954). — FELDAKER, M., H. O. PERRY and D. G. HANLON: Dermatologic manifestations associated with cryoglobulinemia. Arch. Derm. **73**, 325—335 (1956). — FEYRTER, F.: Über Probleme der peripheren Durchblutungsstörungen bei rheumatischen Erkrankungen. Z. Rheumaforsch. **14**, 1—13 (1955). — FIENBERG, R., and F. L. COLPOYS jr.: The involution of rheumatoid nodules treated with cortison and of non-treated rheumatoid nodules. Amer. J. Path. 27, 925—949 (1951). — FINDLAY, L.: The rheumatic infection in childhood. London: E. Arnold & Co. 1931. — FOX, R. F.: Arthritis in women. London: Lewis 1936. — The evolution of chronic rheumatism. London: Lewis 1938. — FRANÇON, F., R. BELOT et J. EXERTIER: Nodosités rhumatismales sous-cutanées par des traumatismes professionnels au cours du rhumatisme chronique progressif inflammatoire. Presse méd. 1957, 1935—1937. — FRANK, P.: Über den Rheumatismus nodosus mit besonderer Berücksichtigung des pathologisch-anatomischen Befundes. Berl. klin. Wschr. 1912, Nr 29. — FRANKLIN, E. C., H. G. KUNKEL and J. R. WARD: Clinical studies of seven patients with rheumatoid arthritis and uniquely large amounts of rheumatoid factor. Arthr. and Rheum. 1, 400—409 (1958). — FREUND, E.: Über rheumatische Knötchen bei chronischer Polyarthritis. Wien. Arch. inn. Med. 16, 73—96 (1928). — FRIEND, D. G., and E. A. EDWARDS: Use of "dibenzyline" as vasodilatator in patients with severe digital ischemia. Arch. intern. Med. 93, 928—937 (1954). — FRORIEP, R.: Beobachtungen über die Heilwirkung der Electricität bei der Anwendung des magnetoelectrischen Apparates. H. 1: Die rheumatische Schwiele. Ein Beitrag zur Pathologie und Therapie des Rheumatismus. Weimar 1843. — FURTADO, T. A.: Étiopathogénie des nodosités juxtaarticulaires. Ann. Derm. Syph. (Paris) 86, 638—654 (1959).

GADRAT, J., et SALVADOR: Nodosités juxta-articulaires et tuberculose. Bull. Soc. franç. Derm. Syph. 41, 669—673 (1934). — GARROD, A. E.: Treatise on rheumatism and rheumatoid arthritis, 342 pp. London: Charles Griffin 1890. — GEDDA, P. O.: Causes de mort dans la polyarthrite rhumatismale chronique. Méd. et Hyg. (Genève) 15, 195 (1957). — GINSBURG, P., u. W. STOJANOF: Über Knotenbildung an den Gelenken. Sovetsk. Vrac. Gaz. No 14, 1122—1125 (1935). Ref. Zbl. Haut- u. Geschl.-Kr. 52, 432 (1936). — GLEITZ, T., u. H.-J. HEITE: Das Krankheitsbild des Granuloma annulare in häufigkeitsanalytischer Betrachtungsweise. Arch. Derm. Syph. (Berl.) 199, 92—108 (1954). — GOEHRS, H. R., A. H. BAGGENSTOSS and C. H. SLOCUMB: Cardiac lesions in rheumatoid arthritis. Arthr. and Rheum. 3, 298—308 (1960). — GOLDSCHMIDT, N. W.: Case of granuloma annulare with subcutaneous nodules. Proc. roy. Soc. Med. 19, 11 (1925/26). — GOLDSTEIN, W.: Stillsches Krankheitsbild beim Erwachsenen. Med. Klin. 22, 1527—1529 (1926). — GOTTRON, H. A., u. G. W. KORTING: Chronische Hautgicht. Arch. klin. exp. Derm. 204, 483—499 (1957). — GRACIANSKY, P. DE, u. S. BOULLE: Granuloma anulare. In: Atlas der Dermatologie, Bd. III (dtsch. Übers. E. SCHEICHER-GOTTRON). Stuttgart: Gustav Fischer; Paris: Maloine 1962. — GRACIANSKY, P. DE, S. BOULLE et M. BOULLE: Atrophie en tâches après granulome annulaire. Bull. Soc. franç. Derm. Syph. 65, 585—586 (1958). — GRAMPA, G., e C. B. BALLABIO: Anatomia patologica dell'artrite reumatoide. Acta rheumat. (Documenta Geigy), No. spec. 11—16 (1961). — GRAUER, F. H.: Granuloma annulare: report of unusual case. Arch. Derm. Syph. (Chic.) 30, 785—789 (1934). — GRAY, A. M. H.: Generalized sclerodermia with subcutaneous nodules. Proc. roy. Soc. Med. 16, 107—108 (1922/23). — Granuloma annulare with subcutaneous nodules. Brit. J. Derm. 26, 157 (1914). — GRUENWALD, P.: Visceral lesions in a case rheumatoid arthritis. Arch. Path. 46, 59—67 (1948). — GRUPPER, C., et G. PLAS: Granulome annulaire et maladies du collagène. Bull. Soc. franç. Derm. Syph. 57, 178—179 (1950). — GSELL, O., u. P. MIESCHER: Die Beziehungen zwischen der primärchronischen Polyarthritis und dem visceralen Erythematodes auf Grund serologischer Reaktionen. Helv. med. Acta 25, 437—443 (1958). — GURLING, K. J.: Association of Sjögren's and Felty's syndromes. Ann. rheum. Dis. 12, 212—216 (1953).

HALL, F.: Granuloma annulare with dissemination following Calciferol therapy. Arch. Derm. Syph. (Chic.) 61, 145 (1950). — HARAGUS, ST., V. COSMA et D. ROSIN: Les artérites périphériques chez les cardiaques rhumatisants. Probl. reum. (Buc.) 2, 249—257 (1954). — HAWTHORNE, C. O.: Rheumatism, rheumatoid arthritis, and subcutaneous nodules, 53 pp. London: J. & A. Churchill 1900. — HAYGARTH, J.: A clinical history of diseases. Part first: being 1. A clinical history of acute rheumatism. 2. A clinical history of the nodosity of the joints, 168 pp. London: Cadell & Davies 1805. — HOFFMANN, H.: Juxtaartikuläre Knoten. In: JADASSOHNS Handbuch der Haut- und Geschlechtskrankheiten, Bd. 12, Teil I, S. 419—498. Berlin: Springer 1932. — HOLTZ, K. H.: Juxtaartikuläre Knoten bei primär chronischem Gelenkrheumatismus (Rheumatismus nodosus), Tendovaginitis rheumatica. Zbl. Haut- u. Geschl.-Kr. 92, 388 (1955). — HOPKINS, H. H.: Subcutaneous nodules of the juxtaarticular type. Arch. Derm. Syph. (Chic.) 49, 5—16 (1931). — HORNSTEIN, O., u. H. SCHUERMANN: Rheumatismus der Haut. In: GOTTRON-SCHÖNFELD, Dermatologie und Venerologie, Bd. II/1, S. 623—642. Stuttgart: Georg Thieme 1958. — HUDSON, E. H.: Juxta-articular nodes in Euphrates Arabs. Trans. roy. Soc. trop. Med. Hyg. 28, 511 (1935).

ISDALE, J. C., and E. G. L. BYWATERS: The rash of rheumatoid arthritis and Still's disease. Quart. J. Med., N. S. 25, 377—387 (1956).

JABLONSKA, S., B. BUBNOW u. B. LUKASIAK: Auswertung von Chronaxiemessungen bei Sklerodermie. Derm. Wschr. 136, 821—837 (1957). — Sklerodermähnliche Zustände. Die Differenzialdiagnose gegenüber Sklerodermie auf Grund von Sensibilitätschronaxiemessungen.

Derm. Wschr. **136**, 1201—1209 (1957). — Lésions pseudo-sclérodermiques dans le rhumatisme. Ann. Derm. Syph. (Paris) **87**, 241—257 (1960). — JACOBI, F.: Granuloma annulare. In: JADASSOHNs Handbuch der Haut- und Geschlechtskrankheiten, Bd. X/1, S. 796—822. Berlin: Springer 1931. — JONES, R. L.: Vasomotor and ocular phenomena in relation to rheumatoid arthritis. Bristol med.-chir. J. **20**, 328—332 (1902). — Arthritis deformans: comprising rheumatoid arthritis, osteo-arthritis, and spondylitis deformans, 365 pp. New York: Will. Wood 1909.

KAHLMETER, G.: De l'existence de lésions myocardiques et valvulaires dans les diverses formes de polyarthrites chroniques et des conclusions qu'on en peut tirer touchant l'étiologie et le groupement clinique des polyarthritis chroniques. Acta med. scand., Suppl. **59**, 611—625 (1934). — KATZ, G.: Subcutane Knoten bei chronischer Gelenkentzündung. Z. klin. Med. **129**, 363—376 (1936). — KELLGREN, J. H., and R. MOORE: Generalized osteoarthritis and Heberden's nodes. Brit. med. J. **1952I**, 181—187. — KERSLEY, G. D., and H. J. GIBSON: The histopathology of rheumatoid arthritis, especially in the extra-articular manifestations. In: C. H. SLOCUMB, Rheumatic diseases, pp. 280—287. (Proceed. 7th Intern. Congr. Rheum. Dis.) Philadelphia and London: W. B. Saunders Company 1952. — KLEMPERER, P., A. POLLACK and G. BAEHR: Diffuse collagen disease: acute disseminated lupus erythematosus and diffuse scleroderma. J. Amer. med. Ass. **119**, 331—332 (1942). — KLINGE, F., u. N. GRZIMEK: Das Gewebsbild des fieberhaften Rheumatismus. VI. Der chronische Gelenkrheumatismus (Infektarthritis, Polyarthritis lenta) und über „rheumatische Stigmata". Virchows Arch. path. Anat. **284**, 646-712 (1932). — KULKA, J. P., D. BOCKING, M. W. ROPES and W. BAUER: Early joint lesions of rheumatoid arthritis. Arch. Path. **59**, 129—150 (1955). — KUMER, L., u. F. LANG: Juxtaarticuläre Knoten und Rheumatismus nodosus. Arch. Derm. Syph. (Berl.) **174**, 533—540 (1936). — KWASNIEWSKI, S., and K. JASINSKI: Lesions in the peripheral vessels in rheumatic diseases. Pol. Tyg. lek. **10**, 918—925. Ref. Zbl. inn. Med. **164**, 119 (1956).

LEINBROCK, A.: Granuloma annulare giganteum (bei Spondylose etc.). Hautarzt **6**, 447—455 (1955). — LEWIS-FANING, E., and E. FLETCHER: Report on an enquiry into the aetiological factors associated with rheumatoid arthritis. Ann. rheum. Dis. **9** Suppl., 94 pp. (1950). — LIÈVRE, J. A.: Les débuts de la polyarthrite chronique évolutive. Vie méd. **37**, 1525—1528 (1956). — LÖVGREN, O.: Rheumatoid arthritis and the liver. Ann. Med. intern. Fenn. **42**, 42—51 (1953). — LÖVGREN, O., H. CASTENFORS, E. HULTMAN, A. FINDOR and S. OHLSSON: Liver studies in rheumatoid arthritis. Atti X. Congr. Lega Internaz. contro il Reumatismo, vol. II, pp. 275—277, Roma 1961. — LUCCHESI, M., and O. LUCCHESI: The significance of subcutaneous nodules in rheumatoid arthritis. Ann. rheum. Dis. **6**, 219—223 (1947). — LUCHERINI, T., e C. CERVINI: Reumatismo e gravidanza. Atti del Congr. Soc. Ital. Reumat. Napoli 1951, E.M.E.S., p. 138 (Roma 1951). — LUTZ, A.: Brief aus Honolulu. Mh. prakt. Derm. **13**, 488—490 (1891).

MAES, E.: Tophi goutteux avec exulcération d'aspect tuberculoide. Arch. belges Derm. **11**, 165 (1955). — MAHER, J. A.: Dural nodules in rheumatoid arthritis. Report of a case. Arch. Path. **58**, 354—359 (1954). — MARTIN, G. M., G. M. ROTH, E. C. ELKINS and F. H. KRUSEN: Cutaneous temperature of extremities of normal subjects and of patients with rheumatoid arthritis. Arch. phys. Med. **27**, 665—682 (1946). — MASSELL, B. F., W. B. COEN and T. D. JONES: Observations regarding artificially induced subcutaneous nodules in rheumatic fever patients. In: Rheumatic diseases, pp. 27—42. Proc. 7th Internat. Congr. Rheum. Dis. Philadelphia and London: W. B. Saunders Company 1952. — MATHER, H. G.: Unusual rheumatoid arthritis (arthritis mutilans). Proc. roy. Soc. Med. **47**, 457—460 (1954). — MATTA, A. DA: Primeiros casos de nodosidades de Lutz-Jeanselme. Brasil-méd. **35**, 26—28 (1921). — MCCRAE, T.: Arthritis deformans, chap. 25, in: W. OSLER and T. MCCRAE, Modern medicine, its theory and practice, 2nd ed., vol. 5, pp. 895—946. Philadelphia: Lea & Febiger 1915. — MELLORS, R. C., R. HEIMER, J. CORCOS and L. KORNGOLD: Cellular origin of rheumatoid factor. J. exp. Med. **110**, 875—886 (1959). — MEYER, A.: Die Stellung der Nodosis rheumatica im Ablauf der rheumatischen Infektion. Z. klin. Med. **123**, 142—153 (1933). — MICHELSON, H. E.: Nodular sub-epidermal fibrosis. Arch. Derm. Syph. (Chic.) **27**, 812—820 (1933). — MIEHLKE, K., u. G. SCHULZE: Klinische, histologische und serologische Befunde beim Fibrositis-Syndrom. Atti X. Congr. Lega Internaz. contro il Reumatismo, vol. II, pp. 535—537, Roma 1961. — MILIAN, G.: Rhumatisme chronique déformant développé au cours d'une ostéite tuberculeuse. Nodosités juxta-articulaires à structure tuberculoide. Bull. Soc. méd. Hôp. Paris **1**, 580 (1910). — MOLL, W.: Klinische Rheumatologie. Basel u. New York: Karger 1958. — MORITZ, U.: Muscular changes in rheumatoid arthritis (A preliminary report). Atti X. Congr. Lega Internaz. contro il Reumatismo, vol. II, pp. 224—225, Roma 1961. — MORRISON, L. R., P. M. CATTOGIO and W. BAUER: Observations on the histopathology of the neuromuscular system in rheumatoid arthritis. In: C. H. SLOCUMB, Rheumatic diseases, pp. 304—307. (Proceed. 7th Intern. Congr. Rheum. Dis.) Philadelphia and London: W. B. Saunders Company 1952. — MORRISON, L. R., C. L. SHORT, A. O. LUDWIG and R. S. SCHWAB: The neuromuscular system in rheumatoid arthritis: electromyographic and histologic observations. Amer. J. med. Sci. **214**, 33—49 (1947). — MOTULSKY, A. G., S. WEINBERG, O. SAPHIR and E. F. ROSENBERG: Lymph nodes in rheumatoid arthritis. Arch. intern. Med. **90**, 660—676 (1952). — MOVAT, H. Z.: Über das Fibrinoid im Subcutanknoten bei chronischem Rheumatismus nodosus. Virchows Arch. path. Anat. **330**, 425—435 (1957). — MOVITT, E. R., and A. E. DAVIS: Liver biopsy in rheumatoid arthritis. Amer. J. med. Sci. **226**, 516—520 (1953). — MUELLER, E. E., and S. MEAD: Electromyogram in rheumatoid arthritis. Amer. J. phys. Med. **31**, 67—73 (1952).

NASSIM, J. R., and H. BANNER: Skin response to local application of a nicotinic acid ester in rheumatoid arthritis; preliminary communication. Lancet **1952I**, 699. — NYSTRÖM, G.: Ann. Med. intern. Fenn. **42**, 52 (1953). Zit. nach SCOTT u. Mitarb. 1961.

OGRYZLO, M. A.: Diffuse systemic rheumatoid disease. Ann. rheum. Dis. **12**, 323—324 (1953). — OSHRAIN, H. I., and A. SACKLER: Involvement of the temporo mandibular joint in a case of rheumatoid arthritis. Oral Surg. 8, 1039—1043 (1955). — OTTEN, H. A., and F. WESTENDORP-BOERMA: Significance of the Waaler-Rose test, streptococcal agglutination, and antistreptolysin titre in the prognosis of rheumatoid arthritis. Ann. rheum. Dis. **18**, 24—28 (1959).

POTTER, J. L., and J. J. R. DUTHIE: Effects of environmental temperature upon capillary resistance in patients with rheumatoid arthritis and other individuals. Ann. rheum. Dis. **20**, 144—148 (1961).

RADNAI, B.: The significance of polyangitis in the pathogenesis of extra-articular manifestations of rheumatoid arthritis. Atti X. Congr. Lega Internaz. contro il Reumatismo, vol. II, p. 154, Roma 1961. — RAGAN, C.: The relationship of rheumatoid arthritis to periarteritis nodosa and systemic lupus erythematosus. J. chron. Dis. **5**, 688—696 (1957). — RATSCHOW, M.: Die Rolle der peripheren Durchblutungsstörungen bei rheumatischen Erkrankungen. Z. Rheumaforsch. **14**, 76—87 (1955). — REHN, H.: In C. GERHARDT, Handbuch der Kinderkrankheiten, Bd. 3, 1. 1878. — ROBINSON, W. D., A. J. FRENCH and I. F. DUFF: Polyarteritis in rheumatoid arthritis. Ann. rheum. Dis. **12**, 323 (1953). — ROEDERER, J., et F. WORINGER: Un cas de tophus goutteux de l'oreille. Bull. Soc. franç. Derm. Syph. **59**, 105—106 (1952). — ROLLIERS, M., R. ROLLIER et A. ZUITER: Purpura rhumatoide et Granuloma annulaire. Maroc. méd. **35**, 500—502 (1956). — ROSENBERG, E. F.: The visceral lesions of rheumatoid arthritis, Chap. 12 in COMROE's arthritis and allied conditions, 5th ed., pp. 171—185. Philadelphia: Hollander, Lea & Febiger 1953. — ROWNTREE, L. G., and A. W. ADSON: Bilateral lumbar sympathetic ganglionectomy and ramusectomy for polyarthritis of the lower extremities. J. Amer. med. Ass. **88**, 694—696 (1927). — RUITER, M.: Histologische Untersuchungen von Noduli rheumatici bei einem Fall von sog. atypischem (malignem) primär-chronischem Rheuma. Hautarzt **10**, 298—303 (1959).

SCHMID, J., u. F. WARUM: Pigmentveränderungen bei chronischer Polyarthritis und streuenden Herden. Wien. Z. inn. Med. **37**, 101—107 (1956). — SCHOEN, R., u. W. TISCHENDORF: Der akute Gelenkrheumatismus. In: Handbuch der inneren Medizin, 4. Aufl., Bd. VI/1, S. 918. Berlin-Göttingen-Heidelberg: Springer 1954. — SCHULHOF, Ö.: On the various types of course in rheumatoid arthritis. Atti X. Congr. Lega Internaz. contro il Reumatismo, vol. I, pp. 115—119, Roma 1961. — SCHULZE, G., u. K. MIEHLKE: Biochemische Befunde beim Fibrositissyndrom. Atti X. Congr. Lega Internaz. contro il Reumatismo, vol. II, p. 534, Roma 1961. — SCLATER, J. G.: An analysis of 388 cases of rheumatoid arthritis. Ann. rheum. Dis. **3**, 195—206 (1943). — SCOTT, J. T., D. O. HOURIHANE, F. H. DOYLE, R. E. STEINER, J. W. LAWS, A. ST. J. DIXON and E. G. L. BYWATERS: Digital arteritis in rheumatoid disease. Brit. med. Ass. **20**, 224—234 (1961). — SEIFERT, G., u. G. GEILER: Der Rheumatismus der Schleimbeutel und Sehnenscheiden. Z. Rheumaforsch. **17**, 337—350 (1958). — SEIFERT, H., u. H. TICHY: Die Anti-Staphylolysin-Reaktion bei chronischen Rheumatikern. Z. Rheumaforsch. **18**, 257—271 (1959). — SELYE, H.: Textbook of endocrinology, p. 135 and 260. Montreal: Acta Endocrin. 1947. — SHORT, C. L., W. BAUER and W. E. REYNOLDS: Rheumatoid arthritis. A definition of the disease and a clinical description on a numerical study of 293 patients and controls. Cambridge (Mass.): Harv. Univ. Press 1957. — SILVA, F.: Nodosidades juxta-articulares de Lutz-Jeanselme. Brasil.-méd. **34**, 687 (1920). — SMITH, M.: A study of 102 cases of atrophic arthritis. I. Instruction statistical data. New Engl. J .Med. **206**, 103—110 (1932). — SMYTH, C. J.: Bone absorption in rheumatoid arthritis: the opera-glass hand (la main en lorgnette). In: C. H. SLOCUMB, Rheumatic diseases (Proc. 7th Internat. Congr. Rheum, Dis.), pp. 196—208. Philadelphia and London: W. B. Saunders Company 1952. — SOILA, P., and K. BERGLUND: Angiographic findings in rheumatoid arthritis. Acta rheum. scand. **7**, 103—106 (1961). — SOKOLOFF, L.: The heart in rheumatoid arthritis. Amer. Heart J. **45**, 635—643 (1953). — SOKOLOFF, L., R. T. MCCLUSKEY and J. J. BUNIM: Vascularity of the early cutaneous nodule of rheumatoid arthritis. Arch. Path. (Chic.) **55**, 475—495 (1953). — SOKOLOFF, L., S. L. WILENS, J. J. BUNIM and C. MCEWEN: Diagnostic value of histologic lesions of striated muscle in rheumatoid arthritis. Amer. J. med. Sci. **219**, 174—182 (1950). — SOKOLOFF, L., S. L. WILENS and J. J. BUNIM: Arteritis of striated muscle in rheumatoid arthritis. Amer. J. Path. 27, 157—173 (1951). — Stecher, R. M., A. H. Hersh, W. M. Solomon and R. Wolpaw: The genetics of rheumatoid arthritis: analysis of 224 families. Amer. J. hum. Genet. 5, 118—138 (1953). — Steiner, G., H. Freund, B. Leichtentritt, and M. Mann: Amer- J. Path. 22, 103 (1946). Zit. nach Moritz. — Strauss, H.: Über Nodosis rheumatica. Klin. Wschr. 9, 1111—1113 (1930). — Sweitzer, S. E., and L. H. Winer: Fibrotic nodules of the skin. Arch. Derm. Syph. (Chic.) 45, 315—327 (1942). — Szabó, S. B.: Über die Thermoregulation der primär chronischen Polyarthritiker. Atti X. Congr. Lega Internaz. controil Reumatismo, vol. II, pp. 265—266, Roma 1961.

Tanasescu, R., V. Onojescu, G. Aldea u. J. Damian: Beitrag zum Studium der rheumatischen Phlebitiden. Probl. reum. (Buc.) 4, 139—146 (1956). Ref. Zbl. inn. Med. 179, 124 (1957). — Tappeiner, S.: Granuloma anulare der Ohrmuschelränder (nach Remission ?). Hautarzt 7, 374 (1956). — Tichy u- Mitarb. siehe S. 233. — Tizard, J. P. M.: Subcutaneous nodules: For diagnosis ? Granuloma annulare. Proc. roy. Soc. Med. 41, 301—303 (1948).

Uhlmann, W.: Zur Pathogenese und Differentialdiagnose des chronischen Rheumatismus nodosus. Dtsch. Z. Verdau.- u. Stoffwechselkr. 14, 24—31 (1954).

Vaughan, J. H., and R. A. Good: Relation of „agammaglobulinemia" sera to rheumatoid agglutination reactions. Arthr. and Rheum. 1, 99—111 (1958). — Verhoeff, F. H., and M. J. King: Scleromalacia perforans: report of a case in which eye was examined microscopically. Arch. Ophthal. 20, 1013—1035 (1938).

Wehsarg, F. K.: Der Rheumatismus nodosus (als Beitrag zur Rheumaforschung). Ergebn. inn. Med. Kinderheilk. 55, 270—294 (1938). — Weinberger, H. J.: Discussion. Ann. rheum. Dis. 12, 324—326 (1953). — Weintraub, A., u. S. Wyss: Über einen Fall von Lipoidgicht. Z. Rheumaforsch. 18, 137—143 (1959). — Willcox, R. R.: Njovera an endemic syphilis of Southern Rhodesia. Comparison with Bejel. Lancet 1951I, 558—560. — Wise, F.: Lepra with juxta-articular nodules. Arch. Derm. Syph. (Chic.) 41, 789 (1940). — Wood, M. G., and H. Beerman: Necrobiosis lipoidica, granuloma anulare and rheumatoid nodule. J. invest. Derm. 34, 139—147 (1960). — Wood, S. R.: Granuloma anulare of the scalp. Brit. J. Derm. 70, 179—180 (1958). — Woodmansey, A., and J. W. Beattie: Effect of cortisone and certain other steroids on the peripheral vasculature in arthritis. Ann. rheum. Dis. 14, 293—297 (1955). — Woodmansey, A., D. H. Collins and M. M. Ernst: Vascular reactions to the contrast bath in health and in rheumatoid arthritis. Lancet 1938II, 1350—1353.

Ziegler, E.: Rheumatismus nodosus als einzige Manifestation der rheumatischen Krankheit. Arch. Kinderheilk. 122, 1—6 (1941).

IV. 2. Felty-Syndrom

Aronson, A. R., and M. M. Montgomery: Chronic liver disease with a "lupus erythematosus-like syndrome". Arch. intern. Med. 104, 544—552 (1959). — Aslan, A., C. David, N. Gingold u. L. Hartia: Das Felty-Syndrom. Ätiopathogenetische und therapeutische Betrachtungen an Hand eines Beobachtungsfalles. Z. ges. inn. Med. 15, 79—84 (1960).

Beninson, J., and J. C. Ensign: Leg ulcers in rheumatoid arthritis. Use of pressure-gradient therapy, high protein diet and other measures producing successful results. J. Amer. med. Ass. 175, 437—440 (1961). — Bettley, F. R.: Leg ulcer and rheumatoid arthritis. Three cases. Proc. roy. Soc. Med. 50, 17—18 (1957). — Breu, W., u. H. Fleischhacker: Über das Feltysche Syndrom. Wien. klin. Wschr. 51, 1081—1087 (1938). — Bruegger, Y., et G. Majno: Étude clinique et anatomo-pathologique d'un cas de syndrome de Felty avec splénectomie. Helv. med. Acta 19, 501—519 (1952). — Buser, M.: Vergleichende Untersuchung über das Still- und das Felty-Syndrom. Dtsch. med. Wschr. 75, 818—823 (1950).

Chauffard, A., et F. Ramond: Des adenopathies dans le rhumatisme chronique infectueux. Rev. Méd. (Paris) 16, 345 (1896). — Conroe's Arthritis and Allied Conditions, 5th ed., completely revised and rewritten by J. L. Hollander and collaborators. Philadelphia: Lea & Febiger 1953. — Craven, E. B.: Splenectomy in chronic arthritis associated with splenomegaly and leukopenia (Felty's syndrome). J. Amer. med. Ass. 102, 823—826 (1934). — Curtis, A. C., and H. M. Pollard: Felty's syndrome: Comparison of Felty's syndrome with other forms of rheumatoid arthritis. Ann. intern. Med. 13, 2265—2284 (1940).

Denko, C. W., and C. W. Zumpft: Chronic arthritis in the adult, associated with splenomegalia and leukopenia. Atti X. Congr. Lega Internaz. contro il Reumatismo, vol. II, pp. 244—246, Roma 1961. — Donner, M.: Über das Felty-Syndrom (zugleich ein Beitrag zur Differentialdiagnose primär-chronischer Gelenkveränderungen). Dtsch. med. Wschr. 75, 1253—1254 (1950).

Ellmann, Ph., L. Cudkowicz and J. S. Elwood: Therapy of „Felty's syndrome". Ann. rheum. Dis. 14, 84—89 (1955).

Felty, A. R.: Chronic arthritis in the adult associated with splenomegaly and leukopenia. Bull. Johns Hopk. Hosp. 35, 16—20 (1924).

GEILER, G.: Über die gemeinsame Zuordnung von Felty- und Sjögren-Syndrom zum Rheumatismus. Dtsch. Gesundh.-Wes. **13**, 538—543 (1958). — GIGANTE, G., e A. GUARINO: La poliartrite cronica primaria adenosplenomegalia. Omnia med. (Pisa) **28**, 1—23 (1950). — GIGANTE, G., L. TROPEANO e A. GUARINO: Studio clinico ed ematologico di un caso di poli artrite cronica primaria adenosplenomegalica. G. Clin. med. **31**, 187—210 (1950). — GRANIRER, L. W.: Leg ulcer in rheumatoid arthritis. J. Amer. med. Ass. **169**, 1469—1470 (1959)-

HANRAHAN, E. M., and S. R. MILLER: Effect of splenectomy in Felty's syndrome. J. Amer. med. Ass. **99**, 1247—1249 (1932). — HASERICK, J. R.: Plasma L. E. test in systemic lupus. erythematosus: A study of 23 patients with a positive L.E. test. J. Amer. med. Ass. **146**, 16—20 (1951). — HIRSCHBOECK, J. S.: Haematologic effects of splenectomy in Still-Chauffard-Felty's syndrome: A report of 2 cases. Blood **1**, 247—255 (1946). — HJORTH, N.: Felty's syndrome with varicose ulcer. (Transactions Danish Dermat. Soc.) Acta derm.-venereol. (Stockh.) **35**, 236—238 (1955). — Felty's syndrome (Rheumatoid arthritis, neutropenia, splenomegaly) combined with ulcer of the leg. (Transactions Danish Dermat. Soc.) Acta derm.-venereol. (Stockh.) **36**, 213 (1956).

KEIL, H.: The rheumatic erythemas: A critical survey. Ann. intern. Med. **11**, 2223—2272 (1938). — KIRPILÄ, J.: Ovatko Nivelreumaa Sairastavien Ihohaavautumatkin Reumaattisia. Duodecim (Helsinki) **74**, 393—400 (1958). Zit. nach BENINSON u. ENSIGN. — KORTING, G. W., u. H. HOLZMANN: Dermatologische Veränderungen beim Felty-Syndrom. Arch. klin. exp. Derm. **210**, 472—484 (1960). — KÜHL, J.: Zur Pathologie des Felty-Syndroms und seiner Beziehungen zu rheumatischen Affektionen. Frankfurt. Z. Path. **65**, 271—283 (1954).

LARIZZA, P., u. F. ROVELLO: Das Felty-Syndrom. (Chronische Polyarthritis, Adenosplenomegalie, Leucopenie.) La sindrome di Felty. Zbl. inn. Med. **131**, 155 (1951). — LINDEBOOM, G. A.: Dysphagie beim Felty-Syndrom. Gastroenterologia (Basel) **75**, 129—137 (1949/50). — LODIN, A., and H. GENTELE: Demonstr. Case 92 and 93, 11th Internat. Congr. Dermat. Stockholm 1957. Acta derm.-venereol. (Stockh.), Suppl. 190—193 (1958). — LOUYOT, P., M. VINCENT et J. MATHIEU: Une observation de syndrome de Felty suivie pendant six ans. Rev. Rhumat. **26**, 696—706 (1959). — LUTZ, W.: Lehrbuch der Haut- und Geschlechtskrankheiten, 2. Aufl., S. 507. Basel: Benno Schwabe & Co. 1957.

MACCORMAC, H.: Chauffard-Still-Felty-Syndrom. Proc. roy. Soc. Med. **31**, 473 (1938). Zit. nach KORTING u. HOLZMANN. — MOTULSKY, A. G., S. WEINBERG, O. SAPHIR and E. ROSENBERG: Lymph nodes in rheumatoid arthritis. Arch. intern. Med. **90**, 660—676 (1952). — MÜLLER, H.: Das Felty-Syndrom. Z. ges. inn. Med. **15**, 8—17 (1960). — MÜLLER, R.: Zur Morphologie der Eiweißstoffwechselstörungen beim Felty-Syndrom. Z. Rheumaforsch. **16**, 129—145 (1957).

NYSTRÖM, G.: Associated rheumatoid arthritis, periarteritis nodosa and Felty's syndrome. Ann. med. intern. Fenn. **42**, 52—57 (1953).

PEDEN, J. C.: Hypersplenism: 2 cases with leg ulcers treated by splenectomy. Ann. intern. Med. **30**, 1248—1262 (1949). — PETRY, H.: Betrachtungen zum Felty-Syndrom. Z. Rheumaforsch. **9**, 73—85 (1950). — POLLITZER, H.: Über chronischen Gelenkrheumatismus mit Drüsenschwellungen und Milztumor (Typus Still-Chauffard). Med. Klin. **10**, 1511—1515 (1914).

ROGERS, H. M., and F. H. LANGLEY: Neutropenia associated with splenomegaly and atrophic arthritis (Felty's syndrome); report of a case in which splenectomy was performed. Ann. intern. Med. **32**, 745—754 (1950).

SCHOCH, E. P.: Ulcers of the leg in Felty's syndrome. Arch. Derm. Syph. (Chic.) **66**, 384—390 (1952). — SCHOEN, R., u. W. TISCHENDORF: Felty-Syndrom. Handbuch der inneren Medizin, 4. Aufl., Bd. VI/2, S. 980—983. Berlin-Göttingen-Heidelberg: Springer 1954. — SINGER, H. A.: Etiology of Felty's and ıelated syndromes. J. Amer. med. Ass. **101**, 2078 (1933). — STÖRMER, A.: Das Felty-Syndrom im Rahmen der chronischen Polyarthritis. Dtsch. med. Wschr. **77**, 161—165 (1952). — STOLTE, J. B.: Felty-Syndrom und Ulcera cruris bei Arthritis rheumatoidea als Äußerung des Erythematodes disseminatus. Folia med. neerl. **3**, 9—20 (1960). — STRAUSS, H.: Stillsche oder Mikuliczsche Krankheit? Med. Klin. **11**, 590—593 (1915). — SUTTON, R. L., and R. L. SUTTON jr.: Diseases of the skin, 10th ed., p. 547. St. Louis: C. V. Mosby Comp. 1939.

Die hämorrhagischen Diathesen

Von

H. Storck und E. G. Jung*-Zürich

Mit 40 Abbildungen

Einleitung

Hämorrhagische Diathesen bezeichnen Krankheitszustände mit abnormer Blutungsneigung aus Körperöffnungen oder in Haut, Schleimhaut, innere Organe: spontan (Mikrotraumen ?) oder nach geringgradiger Traumatisation. Der Begriff wurde 1854 von Virchow in die Medizin eingeführt.

Der Blutungsbereitschaft liegt eine Störung des normalen Blutstillungsmechanismus zugrunde, faßbar in Änderungen der Gerinnung, der Thrombocyten, der Gefäße sowie in kombinierter Störung deren Funktionen. Wenn auch nur ein kleiner Teil der Krankheiten, besonders der Dermatosen, mit hämorrhagischen Diathesen einhergehen, so ist doch die Blutungsbereitschaft ätiologisch und pathogenetisch besonders bedeutsam, weshalb sich Internisten, Pädiater, Chirurgen, Humangenetiker und nicht zuletzt Dermatologen speziell für diese Krankheitsgruppen interessieren.

Die gesamthafte Darstellung der hämorrhagischen Diathesen bereitete noch bis Ende der 40er Jahre große Schwierigkeiten, da an Stelle der heute relativ gut verstandenen pathogenetischen Prinzipien unübersichtliche kasuistische, nosologische und ätiologische Einteilungen verwendet wurden (s. F. Hammer in diesem Handbuch 1928, H. Gottron in Arzt/Zieler 1935, Jürgens 1938, 1955, M. A. Schoch 1940 u.a.m.). In neuerer Zeit hat sich die klarere und zweckmäßigere pathogenetische Einteilung in Koagulopathien, Thrombopathien und vasculäre Formen der hämorrhagischen Diathesen durchgesetzt (Jürgens 1949, 1955, Koller 1952, Croizat u.a. 1954, Storck 1955, Lehmann 1955, Quattrin 1957, W. Blaich 1958, Hegglin 1960).

Die vasculären, die thrombocytogenen hämorrhagischen Diathesen und die Koagulopathien sollen vorerst in ihren Beziehungen zu den betreffenden physiologischen Teilfaktoren der Blutstillung kurz dargestellt werden. Für ausführliche Angaben über Morphologie und Funktion der Blutgefäße sei auf andere Abschnitte des Ergänzungswerkes hingewiesen (z.B. E. Macher: Die gestörte Durchblutung); doch sollen die wesentlichen, für die hämorrhagische Diathese bedeutungsvollen Punkte im folgenden kurz erörtert werden.

Das *Elektronenmikroskop* hat neue Einblicke in die feinste Struktur und Morphologie von Capillaren, Thrombocyten, Fibrinogen und Fibrin ermöglicht, und die *Biochemie* ist heute imstande, mit ihren verfeinerten Methoden die chemischen Vorgänge an den Ultrastrukturen zu lokalisieren. Mit dem Vordringen in die Biochemie der kleinsten morphologischen Strukturen wurde das enge Ineinandergreifen der drei Faktoren der Blutstillung evident, und der Fortschritt in Pharma-

* Von E. G. Jung stammen Abschnitt B.II.1.: Hereditäre Thrombocytenstörung und Abschnitt B.III.: Die Koagulopathien.

kologie, Mikrobiologie, Immunpathologie, nicht zuletzt in der Erkennung der Autoaggression, gestattet, die Gefäßschädigung in ihren quantitativen Abstufungen bis zur Blutung zu erfassen.

Ein Teil der klinisch-histologischen Darstellung von Krankheitsbildern mit hämorrhagischen Diathesen soll im Nachfolgenden nur kurz geschehen, da sie bereits in der ersten Ausgabe dieses Handbuches ausgezeichnet bearbeitet wurde, z.B. F. HAMMER: „Hämorrhagische Krankheiten" Bd. VI/2, 512 (1928), I. HELLER: „Hämorrhagische Diathesen bei Tieren" Bd. XIV/1, 734 (1930), R. VOLK: „Hämorrhagie bei Tuberkulose" Bd. X/1, 425 (1931), E. MEIROWSKI: „Schamberg und verwandte Dermatosen" Bd. IV/2, 971 (1933), und R. L. MEYER: „Purpura bei Gold" Bd. IV/2, 87 (1933).

Neuere Krankheitsbilder wie thrombotisch-thrombopenische, thrombocytämische Purpura, Makro- und hyperglobulinämische Purpura Waldenström sowie einige andere, seltenere, z.T. auch hereditäre Formen sollen jedoch hier eingehender geschildert werden. Im übrigen mögen besonders die neueren pathogenetischen, wenn möglich auch ätiologischen Erkenntnisse, schließlich die neueren therapeutischen Konsequenzen speziell berücksichtigt werden.

Gesamthaft beurteilt erscheint bei den verschiedenen hämorrhagischen Diathesen charakteristisch, daß bei den hereditären Formen einzelne, spezifisch umschriebene Störungen auftreten, wie beispielsweise Fehlen eines bestimmten Koagulationsfaktors, einer besonderen Funktion der Thrombocyten oder umschriebene Gefäßveränderungen, daß demgegenüber bei erworbenen Formen meist Schädigungen mehrerer Faktoren auf breiterer Basis vorkommen (z.B. KOLLER 1952).

Die Dermatologen sehen hauptsächlich die vasculären hämorrhagischen Diathesen, seltener die Thrombopenien. Die Patienten mit hereditären Thrombopathien, ferner mit Koagulopathien suchen in der Regel den Pädiater und Internisten auf oder werden wegen pathologischen Blutungen nach Traumen von Chirurgen betreut. Deshalb sollen im folgenden zuerst und ausführlicher die Belange der vasculären, dann der thrombocytären und schließlich der plasmatischen hämorrhagischen Diathesen behandelt werden, im steten Bewußtsein, daß besonders bei den erworbenen Formen auch nur vorübergehende Abweichungen mehrerer Faktoren bereits zu pathologischen Blutungen führen können.

Nach FIEHRER (1958) z.B. verteilen sich die genannten drei Gruppen der hämorrhagischen Diathesen ungefähr folgendermaßen: 43% vasculäre, 37% thrombocytäre und 20% plasmatische Purpuraformen. Im dermatologischen Krankengut wird sich noch eine besondere Selektion der vasculären Formen finden.

A. Allgemeiner Teil

Die normale und pathologische Blutstillung wird nur verständlich, wenn die anatomischen und physiologischen Verhältnisse der drei Faktoren: Gefäße, Thrombocyten und Plasma (Gerinnungsfaktoren) bekannt sind. Es zeigt sich dann auch, wie eng diese verschiedenen Faktoren bei der Blutstillung und deren Störungen miteinander verflochten sind (siehe z.B. SPAET 1952, WITTE 1957, 1960).

So finden wir beispielsweise bei *thrombocytogenen hämorrhagischen Diathesen* verlängerte Blutungszeit, die nicht nur durch mangelnden Thrombusverschluß der angestochenen muskulären Arteriolen zu erklären ist, sondern auch noch durch Mangel eines plasmatischen Schutzfaktors. Dieser ist in der Plasmafraktion I nach COHN vorhanden und fehlt auch bei der Thrombopathie von WILLEBRAND-JÜRGENS (CAZAL u.a. 1956, S. WITTE u.a. 1957). Bei den *Koagulopathien* spielen andererseits bei der Krankheitsmanifestation ebenfalls Gefäßfaktoren im Sinne von schlechtem Verschluß der mikrotraumatisch bedingten Gefäßläsionen eine Rolle, wie beispielsweise die altersbedingte Degeneration bzw. Rigidität des perivasalen Bindegewebes.

Über die Frage von Anatomie und Physiopathologie der Capillaren, kleineren Arteriolen und Venolen stehen eine Reihe älterer und neuerer, wertvoller Übersichtsarbeiten zur Verfügung, die einen ausgezeichneten Einblick in das normale und pathologische Verhalten der Gefäße bis zur Blutung geben, in neuester Zeit unter Zuhilfenahme von elektronenmikroskopischen Untersuchungen (z. B. E. R. u. E. L. Clark 1932, I. F. Danielli u. Stock 1944/51, Th. H. Spaet 1952, 1955, R. Jürgens u. E. Deutsch 1958, W. Bargmann 1958, M. Ratschow u. a. 1959, S. Witte 1960, L. Illig 1961, W. Montagna u. R. A. Ellis 1962).

I. Anatomie und Physiopathologie

1. Zur Anatomie der Gefäße

Nachdem sich unsere anatomischen Kenntnisse in früheren Jahren aus makroskopischen und lichtmikroskopischen Untersuchungen entwickelten, haben neuerdings elektronenoptische Untersuchungen wichtige Kenntnislücken geschlossen und auch Irrtümer beseitigt (z. B. Nichtexistenz des Intercellularzementes von Zweifach). Neue Hautgefäßinjektionsmethoden mit indischer Tinte, histochemische Anfärbung der alkalischen Phosphatase für den Nachweis von Endothelien der Capillaren im Papillarkörper (Winkelmann 1960), Röntgenstrahlenprojektionsmikroskopie (nach Saunders) sowie spezielle Färbungen der feinsten Nervenfasern (Weddell u. a. 1960) lassen heute feine und feinste Strukturen der Hautgefäße erkennen. Ihre Variabilität mit großer Anpassungsfähigkeit an die Bedürfnisse der versorgten Organe ließ erkennen, daß die Blutstrombahn den Prototyp eines funktionellen Systems darstellt (Staubesand 1959). Der Arteriolenbaum der Haut als Widerstandsregler ist in Subcutis und Cutis als Netzarteriensystem gebaut und mündet erst in den Papillen in Endarterien mit nichtanastomosierten Capillaren. Entsprechend den Regionen der Körperstellen finden sich besondere Arteriolen- und Capillarenmuster (R. A. Ellis 1961), z. B. mit stärkerer Ausbildung von Arteriolen und Capillarschlingen in Bezirken mit breiter Epidermis und Hornschicht sowie abnehmender Vascularisation im Alter.

Der feinstrukturelle Bau von Arterien, Arteriolen, Capillaren, Venolen und Venen ist durch elektronenmikroskopische Untersuchungen bekannt. Bei den *kleinen Arterien* und *Arteriolen* beispielsweise findet sich ein zartes Relief der endothelialen Oberfläche (Moore u. Ruska 1957, Buck 1958, Staubesand 1959). Die Endothelien sind eng ineinander verzahnt, regelmäßig in der Jugend, zunehmend unregelmäßig im Alter. An den Membranen gegen das Gefäßlumen finden sich kleinste Invaginationen in Form kleinbläschenförmiger Gebilde. Fortsätze der Endothelzellen durchbrechen gegen außen die anschließende Elastica interna und stehen mit den Muskelzellen in inniger Verbindung. Auch hier finden sich wieder Taschen und Bläschen bis zur äußeren Grundmembran, so daß offensichtlich der Stofftransport von innen nach außen durch Pinocytose („self drinking“ nach Moore u. Ruska 1957) oder durch transendothelialen Stofftransport geschehen kann. In den Intercellulärspalten von 80—100 Å läßt sich kein Zement nachweisen (s. auch Witte 1960, Odland in Montagna u. Ellis 1961).

Der Feinbau der *Blutcapillaren* ist komplizierter als ursprünglich angenommen wurde und zeigt je nach Organ verschiedene Typen (Bargmann 1958). Trotz der neuesten elektronenmikroskopischen Fortschritte hält Zweifach (1962) die Verhältnisse für äußerst kompliziert und unübersichtlich, da Endothelialzellen und Membrane wahrscheinlich konstant Form und Dicke ändern.

Sämtliche Capillaren enthalten mindestens folgende Bauelemente:

1. Endothel mit Zellgrenzen, deren Cytoplasmen sich überlagern oder ineinander verzahnen.

2. Eine Polysaccharide, Proteine, wahrscheinlich auch Lipoide enthaltende Basalmembran. Diese ist z.T. faserig, besitzt keine Poren und zeigt im Polarisationsmikroskop intralamelläre Lipoideinlagerungen. Wahrscheinlich nehmen die lebenden Zellen der Capillarwand aktiv an den Permeabilitätsvorgängen teil (s. auch STAUBESAND, ROLLHÄUSER 1959).

Auch die Untersuchungen von ODLAND, neuerdings MACHER u. VOGELL, bestätigen die Existenz einer ununterbrochenen Basalmembran an den Hautcapillaren mit Fehlen der von PAPPENHEIMER (1953) angenommenen Poren. Diese Autoren fanden in den relativ dicken Endothelzellen Fasern, die den Tonofibrillen der Epidermis glichen und wahrscheinlich der Keratin-Myosin-Klasse fibröser Proteine angehören. Solche Fasern lassen aber nicht auf Kontraktilität schließen, sondern sind eher Resultat der großen Verschiebungskräfte der Haut. Um die Endothelien liegen pericapilläre Zellen mit einzelnen kollagenen Fibrillen. Auch hier finden sich in den Endothelzellen Plasmafortsätze mit taschen- und bläschenförmigen Gebilden als Ausdruck des Stofftransportes. Es finden sich keine Anhaltspunkte dafür, daß die Pericyten contractil sind. Das Fehlen von Lücken und Poren in der Basalmembran läßt den Mechanismus der Leukocytenauswanderung oder auch der Diapedesisblutung rätselhaft erscheinen. NIESSING u.a. (1954) studierten die Struktur des Grundhäutchens an Hirncapillaren polarisationsoptisch und fanden eine bimolekulare Lamelle mit einem faserigen Proteingerüst, in welchem Lipoidmoleküle radiär eingelagert sind.

2. Zur Physiopathologie der Gefäße

Bei Verletzung von muskulären Arterien und Arteriolen ziehen sich dieselben unmittelbar zusammen, bei Durchschneidung verschließt sich das Gefäß durch Invagination infolge des unterschiedlichen Elastizitätsmoduls von Muskel- und Elasticafasern (STAUBESAND 1959).

Die physiopathologischen Erkenntnisse über Arteriolen, Capillaren und Venolen (terminale Strombahn) wurden in den letzten drei Dezennien hauptsächlich durch Lebendbeobachtung am Tier gewonnen (z.B. Säugetier-Mesenterium, Hamsterbackentasche, Fledermausflügel, an der Chorion-Allantois-Membran des Embryos, Klarsichtkammermethode am Kaninchen- und Hundeohr [s. ILLIG 1961] sowie Nickhaut des Kaninchens [COPLEY u.a. 1953]). Am Menschen trugen besonders capillarmikroskopische Untersuchungen am Nagelfalz zur Kenntnis bei (MUELLER 1939, GILJE u.a. 1953), in neuerer Zeit auch an irgendeiner Körperstelle nach Entfernung der Hornschicht mit Abrißmethode (MICHAEL u.a. 1951, DAVIS und LAWLER 1958). Weniger aufschlußreich waren bis anhin physikalische Untersuchungsmethoden wie Temperaturmessungen, quantitativ schwierig beurteilbare Photo-Plethysmogramme usw., die allerdings für besondere physiologische Fragestellungen von Bedeutung sind (s. SCHOOP in RATSCHOW 1959).

Besonders untersucht wurden die Erregbarkeit von *Arterien und Arteriolen* mit rhythmischen Spasmen, mit nachfolgender Dilatation auf Witterungseinflüsse (BETTMAN 1930), Dilatation auf Milchsäure, CO_2, Adenosin-Mono- und -Triphosphat, Histamin, Acetylcholin, Kontraktion auf Noradrenalin und Adrenalin (hier allerdings Dilatation der Arterien in Muskulatur, die peripher zunimmt), ebenso die Reaktionen auf Stoffwechselprodukte, als Regler entsprechend dem Gewebsbedarf (s. SCHOOP 1959, ILLIG 1961).

Die *Capillaren* selbst reagieren als passives Rohr mit Erweiterung bei Arteriolendilatation und erhöhtem Blutzufluß (aktive Hyperämie) oder Stase der Venolen (passive Hyperämie) oder mit Verengerung bei Kontraktion der zuführenden Arteriolen (s. auch TAYLOR 1953).

Die Sphinctercapillaren am Zentralkanal, die ZWEIFACH ganz besonders untersucht hatte, können sich als Ausnahme aktiv verschließen, sind aber eine Spezialeinrichtung des Mesenteriums und kommen in der menschlichen Haut nur ausnahmsweise bei Abzweigungen von Arteriolen vor. Meist findet sich in der Haut das netzförmige Capillarbett nach SAUNDERS (ILLIG 1959). Die Blutdurchströmung der Hautcapillaren ist deshalb abhängig von Druck und Vasomotorik der benachbarten Arteriolen und Venolen.

Die örtlichen Kreislaufstörungen infolge motorischer Gefäßreaktionen, z.B. bedingt durch neurovegetative, myogene oder humorale Faktoren, haben lediglich Einfluß auf Diffusion und Ernährung des Gewebes, nicht aber auf Leukocytenauswanderung oder Erythrocytendiapedese, welche Vorgänge allerdings bei langsamer Strömung erleichtert, bei rascher Strömung erschwert werden.

Der *Stoffaustausch* in den Capillaren ist ein komplexes Geschehen, welches durch vitale Leistung der Endothelzellen äußerst rasch abläuft. Nach den Berechnungen von Renklin u. Pappenheimer (1957) findet der Blutumlauf im Körper in einer Minute statt, wobei sich das Blut weniger als 2 sec im Capillargebiet befindet, in welch kürzester Zeit der Stoffaustausch Blut—Gewebe und umgekehrt erfolgt. Gase, wasserlösliche Stoffe und Lipide verlassen das Blut entsprechend den Konzentrationsgradienten durch Diffusion via Endothelmembran, lipidunlösliche Stoffe und Elektrolyte jedoch durch die intercellulären Spalten, wofür maximal 0,1% der Capillaroberfläche zur Verfügung steht. Auf welche Weise aber die Pinocytose zustande kommt und wie das Grundhäutchen traversiert wird, ist noch nicht geklärt.

Örtliche Kreislaufstörungen mit Veränderung der Gefäßwand jedoch können zu Leukocytenauswanderung, Diapedesisblutung, prästatischer Strömungsverlangsamung, Stase und Thrombose führen (Illig 1959 u. 1961). Die *Leukocytenauswanderung* wird mit „Klebrigkeit" der Leukocyten und langsamem Rollen entlang der Capillarwand eingeleitet (evtl. eher vermehrter Adhäsivität der Endothelien?), dem sehr langsame Durchwanderung zwischen den Endothelien folgt, ohne daß aber Poren oder Lücken in der Basalmembran sichtbar würden. Die *Erythrocyten-Diapedese* hingegen geht rasch stoßweise vor sich und erfolgt offensichtlich zwischen den Endothelien, aber auch hier ohne sichtbare Lücken der Basalmembran. Nur bei Skorbut wurden dreieckige Membrandurchbrüche oder Lücken festgestellt. Die Blutaustritte erfolgen im allgemeinen am venösen Ende der Capillaren und nicht am arteriellen.

Die genannten örtlichen Störungen im Capillarbett, von welchen nur die Erythrocytendiapedese für die Kenntnis der hämorrhagischen Diathese direkt von Bedeutung ist, sind in Tabelle 1 nach Illig zusammengestellt.

Tabelle 1. *Die örtlichen Kreislaufstörungen des Capillarbettes*
(Aus L. Illig: Physiologie und Pathologie des Capillarbettes. In: M. Ratschow, Angiologie, S. 124—139. Stuttgart: Georg Thieme 1959)[1]
(Nach Illig und Weber, Klin. Wschr. **1958**)

A. Ausschließlich oder vorwiegend vasogene Störungen
(Ausgangspunkt der Störung in der Gefäßwand)

I. Motorische Form (durch Erregung oder Lähmung contractiler Elemente der Gefäßwand):

1. a) *arteriospastisch bedingte Strömungsverlangsamung (= Ischämie)*
Zuflußhemmung[2], Gefäßinhalt qualitativ unverändert;

b) *arteriospastisch bedingter Blutstillstand*
(bei Ausschwemmung der Erythrocyten = „Anämie")
Zuflußunterbrechung; Gefäßinhalt qualitativ unverändert;

c) *arterio-paretische Hyperämie*
Zuflußerhöhung; vermehrte Blutfülle der Capillaren und Venen mit druck-passiver Erweiterung;

2. *Funktionsstörungen der Capillarsphincter:*
Spasmen? Lähmung? Noch ungeklärt.

3. a) *venospastisch bedingte Strömungsverlangsamung:*
Abflußhemmung; Gefäßinhalt qualitativ nicht verändert; selten isoliert, meist in Verbindung mit arteriellen Spasmen;

b) *venospastisch bedingter Blutstillstand*
Abflußunterbrechung; Gefäßinhalt qualitativ unverändert[3]; selten isoliert, meist in Verbindung mit spastischen Arterienverschluß.

---

[1] Ausführliche Darstellung bei Illig 1959.

[2] Die hämodynamischen Angaben beziehen sich auf das Ziel der Blutversorgung, die Capillaren.

[3] Beobachtungen am Kaninchen-Pankreas sprechen dafür, daß es an stark durchbluteten Organen ohne Anastomosen zu *Stase* kommen kann.

Tabelle 1. (Fortsetzung)

c) veno-capilläre Hyperämie (Moon, Weber)
Vermehrte Blutfülle mit Strömungsverlangsamung auf der venösen Seite des Capillarbettes durch Erweiterung der kleinen Venen (selten).

II. Nicht-motorische Form

(Durch Schädigung oder funktionelle Störung der Gefäßwand ohne nachweisbare Änderung der Weite und Struktur[4]).

1. Leukocyten-Diapedese:
Beschränkt auf den venösen Abschnitt des Capillarbettes; häufig gekoppelt mit Strömungsverlangsamung, aber von dieser ursächlich unabhängig. Höhepunkt = Eiterung.

2. Erythrocyten-Diapedese: Vorwiegend an Capillaren und kleinen Venen; manchmal gekoppelt mit Strömungsverlangsamung, aber von dieser ursächlich unabhängig. Höhepunkt = Blutung.

3. Hämokonzentration (Landis)
(Viscositätserhöhung des Blutes durch Plasmaverarmung):
Durchflußhemmung; ob bis zur völligen Verstopfung der Gefäßlichtung möglich, ungeklärt und unwahrscheinlich. Keine Gerinnungsphänomene.

4. a) Prästase („peristatische Hyperämie")
(Viscositätserhöhung durch Plasma-Verarmung *und* Änderung der Suspensionsstabilität des Blutes):
im Bereich der Capillaren und kleinen Venen. Durchflußhemmung.

b) Stase (*Konglomeration*; Weber):
Plasmaverarmung und Änderung der Suspensionsstabilität des Blutes im Bereich der Capillaren und kleinen Venen. Verstopfung der Gefäßlichtung mit homogen erscheinenden Blutkörperchensäulen („Stasesäulen" bzw. „Stasezylinder"); keine Gerinnung.
Durchfluß-Unterbrechung. Bei längerer Dauer unter Umständen Untergang des zugehörigen Versorgungsgebietes.

5. Abscheidungs-Thrombose:
Abflußbehinderung auf der venösen Seite des Capillarbettes durch wandständige Thrombenbildung.

B. Vorwiegend sanguinogene Störungen

(Ausgangspunkt der Störung im strömenden Blut, *unabhängig* von eventuellen Veränderungen der Gefäßwand):
Durchflußhemmung oder Verstopfung durch Blutkörperchen-Aggregate („blood sludge"; Knisely, Harders).

[4] Beteiligung von Gewebsfaktoren (pathologische gefäß- oder blut-wirksame Stoffwechselprodukte aus dem mitgeschädigten Gewebe) und Blutfaktoren wahrscheinlich, aber mit den derzeitigen Methoden nicht in jedem Fall faßbar.

Im folgenden sollen noch einige Gesichtspunkte über den Blutaustritt aus der terminalen Strombahn erörtert werden. Daß es zum Blutaustritt kommt, stellt zweifelsohne etwas Besonderes dar und setzt eine spezielle Störung der terminalen Strombahn voraus. Erythrocytendiapedese wird beobachtet bei vermehrter Capillarfragilität (Spaet 1958). Sie erfolgt an den venennahen Capillarenden, an Venolen und kleinsten Venen im Gegensatz zu nur vereinzelten Blutaustritten aus den arteriolennahen Capillarenden (Humble 1949, Lit. s. Illig 1961).

Bei Lebendbeobachtung konnten Lee u.a. 1955 immer nur Blutaustritte aus den Venolen bzw. venösen Enden der Capillaren, nie aus Arteriolen oder arteriellem Capillaranteil feststellen. Dies galt sowohl bei Blutungen beim Meerschweinchen nach Vitamin C-freier Nahrung, beim Hamster nach Überschuß von Natrium, bei der Ratte nach Cholinmangel sowie beim Menschen bei Eklampsie.

Der „Gefäßfaktor" bei hämorrhagischer Diathese ist nach Witte (1957, 1958, 1960) nicht einheitlicher Natur. Bei Koagulopathien scheint mangelhafte Abdichtung der Gefäßwand nach Mikrotraumen von Bedeutung zu sein. Bei den vasculären hämorrhagischen Diathesen sind oft entzündliche Schädigungen, evtl. hereditäre Fehlentwicklung (z.B. Osler) oder auch biochemische Defekte an den Gefäßen vorhanden (z.B. Skorbut, Purpura senilis). Ein Gefäßschaden, besonders bei der vasculären hämorrhagischen Diathese, kann durch Antigen-Antikörper-Reaktionen zustande kommen (z.B. Sedormid-Purpura), evtl. durch das zweiphasische unspezifische Shwartzman-Sanarelli-Phänomen (z.B. bei Purpura fulminans) oder durch pathologische Einlagerungen (z.B. bei Paraproteinämien).

In Tierversuchen an der Hamster-Backentasche wurden von LUTZ u. FULTON (1954) petechiale Diapedesisblutungen durch Gefäßschaden nach örtlicher Anwendung von Streptokokkenfiltraten, Staphylokokkenkulturen, Formaldehyd, Terpentin, Crotonöl, verschiedenen Antikoagulantien, Röntgenstrahlen gesehen. Die Blutungen ließen sich durch Colchicin-Injektionen und Entfernung der Nebennieren steigern, durch Cortison herabsetzen. Gefäßerweiterungen, Prästase, Stase und andere vasomotorische Störungen allein führten nicht zur Blutung, doch kann die Erythrocytendiapedese durch verlangsamten Blutstrom und erhöhten Druck gesteigert werden.

CHAMBERS u.a. (1947) untersuchten eingehend in Lebendbeobachtung die Gefäßpermeabilität, meist mittels Adhäsion von intravasaler Tusche an den Endothelgrenzen. Sie fanden vermehrte Durchlässigkeit bei Ansäuerung, Calciummangel, Bakterientoxinen, Quetschung, Histamin, Acetylcholin, östrogenen Hormonen, Gewebsextrakten, Leukotoxin (MENKIN), „spreading factor" (Hyaluronidase). Eine Gefäßabdichtung war sichtbar bei Erhöhung der Calciumsalze, nach Einwirkung von Mineralo- und Glucocorticoiden, Vitamin D u.a.m. Der Zusammenhalt der Zellen vom Vitamin C war nur in Epithelgewebskulturen abhängig.

Stufenweise progressive Gefäßschädigungen beobachteten E. R. u. E. L. CLARK (1935) am Kaninchenohr, mit Anhaften von Leukocyten bei geringen Läsionen, mit Erythrocytenaustritten bei schwerer Schädigung durch Crotonöl oder Toxine.

Nach LUTZ u.a. (1954) werden *Petechien* beobachtet nach a) lokaler Entzündung durch Toxine von hämolytischen Streptokokken und Staphylococcus aureus, b) Formaldehyd, Terpentin, Crotonöl, Nitrogen mustard, c) Antikoagulantien in vivo, d) lokaler Röntgenbestrahlung mit 15000—25000 r, totaler Körperbestrahlung mit 100—1500 r, e) Implantation von DOCA-Tabletten, f) von Tumorzellen, g) Druck, h) Trauma.

Besondere, zu Blutung führende Gefäßschädigungen scheinen Endotoxine von gramnegativen Bakterien (z.B. Lipopolysaccharide von B. coli) zu erzeugen. So fanden L. THOMAS u.a. (1957) in Hautgefäßen von Kaninchen oder Mesenterialgefäßen der Ratte nach kleinsten intravenösen Endotoxingaben, eine Empfindlichkeitssteigerung auf aufgetropftes Adrenalin mit und ohne Serotonin, die zu schwerer hämorrhagischer Nekrose führte (s. auch Shwartzman-Sanarelli-Syndrom).

Die entscheidende Gefäßwandalteration bei der Diapedesisblutung scheint in der Basalmembran zu liegen, wenn auch licht- oder elektronenmikroskopisch entsprechende Poren oder Lücken nicht gefunden werden konnten. Nach CHAMBERS und ZWEIFACH tritt eine Blutung nach Auftragung von Hyaluronidase von außen mittels Mikropipette auf, was allerdings von anderen nicht bestätigt werden konnte (z.B. NIESSING u. ROLLHAEUSER 1954, BARGMANN 1958 u.a.). 1956 stellte WILHELM in Serum und Plasma von Meerschweinchen einen hitzelabilen, nur in der Serumverdünnung $^1/_{200}$—$^1/_{400}$ wirksamen „*Permeabilitätsfaktor*" fest, der ähnlich wie Histamin und Leukotaxin die Gefäßpermeabilität innerhalb von 3 min vorübergehend erhöhte. Die Bedeutung eines solchen Faktors für Hautblutungen bei Tier und Mensch wurde jedoch nicht weiter untersucht.

CH. J. SMYTH u. O. B. GUM machten 1961 auf das relativ massive Vorkommen von Mastzellen um Capillaren und größere Gefäße aufmerksam, die durch Ausschüttung von gefäß- und gerinnungsaktiven Substanzen (Heparin, Histamin, Hyaluronsäure, Serotonin) die Gefäßpermeabilität beeinflussen könnten. Wieweit Mastzellen bei der hämorrhagische Diathesen von Bedeutung sind, wäre noch abzuklären.

Der endocapillare Schutzfilm, welcher in seiner Bedeutung zur Gefäßabdichtung erstmals von CHAMBERS u. ZWEIFACH diskutiert wurde, scheint auch nach neueren Untersuchungen eine gewisse Rolle zu spielen. Er kann aber elektronenoptisch nicht nachgewiesen werden (E. MACHER u. W. VOGELL 1962). Nach COPLEY u.a. (1951, 1953, 1954, 1956, 1957) und WINTERSTEIN (1955) laufen am Endothel in einem solchen Schutzfilm ständig gerinnungsfördernde und hemmende Vorgänge ab, die zueinander in einem labilen Gleichgewicht stehen. Eine Störung dieser Vorgänge könnte ebenfalls die Erythrocytendiapedesis fördern.

Daß verschiedene Mechanismen zu Blutaustritt führen, geht aus den vier Bezeichnungen von COPLEY (1957) hervor, nämlich

1. Diarrhexis (Blutung durch traumatische Quetschung oder Verletzung des Endothels).

2. Diapedesis (Blutung zwischen den Endothelspalten).
3. Rhexis (Ruptur infolge Erkrankungen und Veränderung der Gefäßwand).
4. Diaprosis (Eröffnung der Gefäßwand durch Korrosionsprozesse in der Nähe der Gefäßwand, beispielsweise bei Ulcerationen).

Der verschiedene Mechanismus für den Durchtritt von Flüssigkeit, Leukocyten oder Erythrocyten aus dem Gefäß ist in Tabelle 2 nach Illig (1961) dargestellt.

Tabelle 2. *Der pathologische Austritt von Blutbestandteilen aus der Strombahn* (Aus L. Illig: Die terminale Strombahn, S. 147. Springer 1961)

Art	Ursache	Vermutlicher Sitz der Wandveränderung	Prädilektions-Ort	Eigenarten	Auswirkung
1. Flüssigkeits-Austritt	a) erhöhter Filtrationsdruck b) Gefäßwandschädigung	intercelluläre Spalträume, endocapillärer Eiweißfilm	Arteriolen, Capillaren und Venolen	von der Gefäßweite ziemlich unabhängig, u. U. sehr rasch	Ödem
2. Leukocyten-Auswanderung	Gefäßwandschädigung, chemotaktische Reize	Endothel (Gefäßwand im Ganzen ?)	Venolen und kleine Venen	langsam, Zelle für Zelle, unter typischer Deformierung	Eiterung
3. Erythrocyten-Diapedese	Gefäßwandschädigung	Grundhäutchen	Capillaren und Venolen, besonders Verzweigungsstellen	meist im Schwall, plötzlich und kurzdauernd. Keine Deformierung der Zellen beim Durchtritt	Blutung

R. Klima (1955) betont wahrscheinlich zu Recht, daß neben einer verminderten Capillarresistenz noch andere Faktoren für das Zustandekommen der Blutung mitverantwortlich sind; denn häufig werden klinisch Fälle mit verminderter Capillarresistenz, jedoch ohne vermehrte Blutungsneigung beobachtet.

Neben der Bedeutung von akuten oder chronischen Infektionen, Hepatopathien, Hyperglobulinämien, Dysproteinämien muß nach diesem Autor auch die Beziehung der Gefäße zu hormonalen Reaktionen unter Stresswirkung berücksichtigt werden, die unter anderem von Kramar (1953) tierexperimentell untersucht wurde. Durch Verminderung der adrenocorticalen Aktivität z. B. entstehen Capillarkrisen, die durch ACTH, Cortison vermindert und durch DOCA vermehrt werden können (Robson u. Duthie 1950/II, 1952/I). Wie die Blutung bei *Teleangiektasien* (Oslersche Krankheit, Purpura teleangiectodes Majocchi, Lebercirrhosen) zustande kommt, erscheint nicht gesichert, doch disponieren offenbar solche teleangiektatische Gefäße zu Blutungen, wie dies beispielsweise auch bei den maximal erweiterten Capillaren beim Shwartzman-Sanarelli-Phänomen festgestellt werden kann.

Klinisch unterscheidet Klima die echte Purpura bzw. die Purpura simplex mit Blutaustritten ohne weitere Veränderungen im umgebenden Gewebe, wie sie z.B. auch bei den Thrombopenien vorkommt, von der Purpura mit Veränderungen des perivasculären Gewebes in Form von Ödem, Entzündung usw. Wenn der Blutungsmechanismus bei der ersteren Form offensichtlich komplizierter ist und von mehreren Faktoren abhängt, erscheint die zweite Form durch entzündliche Gefäßschädigung verschiedenster Ätiologie zweifellos einfacher.

Wieweit das Nervensystem, insbesondere das vegetative, von Bedeutung ist, läßt sich noch nicht beurteilen, da offensichtlich rein neurovegetative vasomotorische Störungen experimentell lediglich zu Hyperämien mit Ödemen, nicht aber zu Blutungen führen. Nach Weddell finden sich vegetative Fasern nur in unmittelbarer Nähe der Capillaren, ohne aber direkt in denselben zu endigen. Immerhin wäre denkbar, daß nervale Einflüsse an Arteriolen und Venolen von Bedeutung für die Pathogenese von Hämorrhagien sein könnten, dies auch, trotzdem das Rickersche Stufengesetz nach neueren experimentellen Untersuchungen nicht mehr anerkannt wird (Lit. s. Illig 1959, 1961).

Nach Lecomte u. a. (1955, 1961) ist die Gefäßresistenz gegen toxische Stoffe, z. B. Crotonöl, welches bei Kaninchen und Mäusen zu petechialen Blutungen führt, von verschiedenen Faktoren abhängig, wie hämodynamischer Druck, Adrenalin und Serotonin, Stoffe wie Phenole und Polyphenole, Anaesthetica, synthetische Antihistaminica, Hydrocortison, Desoxycorticosteron, Testosteron, Oestradiol(mono)benzoat, Phenylbutazon, welche die Gefäßresistenz gegen Crotonöl erhöhen. Diese wird aber herabgesetzt durch Histamin, Natriumsuccinat, Tyramin und Calciumsalze. Wahrscheinlich liefert Adrenalin den Hauptschutz, verstärkt durch Nebennierenrindenhormone.

Wieweit außer den genannten Faktoren allergische Antigen-Antikörper-Reaktionen, unspezifische Shwartzman-Sanarclli-Phänomene, immunpathologische Autoaggressionen, toxische Schädigungen zu blutenden Gefäßläsionen führen können, soll in Abschnitt III besonders diskutiert werden.

3. Zur Struktur der Thrombocyten

Den Thrombocyten kommt zweifellos in der Blutstillung, damit beim Gerinnungsvorgang und in der Genese der Thrombosen, eine Schlüsselstellung zu,

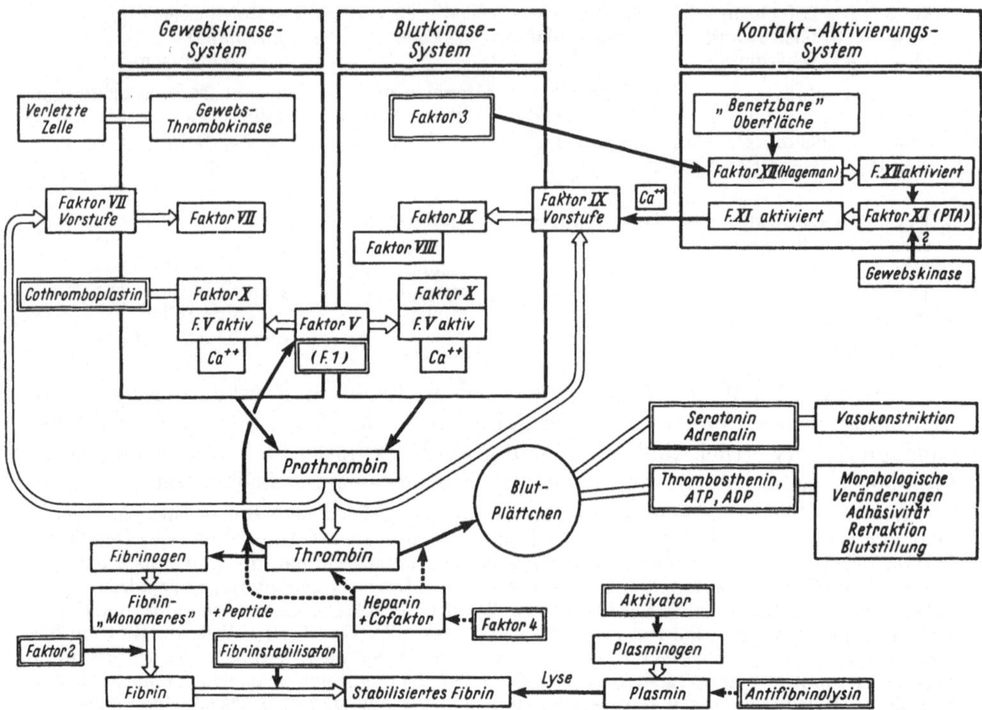

Abb. 1. Blutgerinnung und Gerinnungsfaktoren der Blutplättchen. Es bedeuten: schwarze Pfeile: Umwandlung in Thrombocytenfaktoren, durchbrochene Pfeile: Einwirkung auf Thrombocytenfaktoren, weiße Pfeile: Hemmung. — Die Plättchenfaktoren sind durch schattierte Felder hervorgehoben. [Aus E. F. Lüscher: in F. Linneweh: Erbliche Stoffwechselkrankheiten. München-Berlin: Urban & Schwarzenberg 1962

was bereits 1904 Morawitz mit seinem klassisch gewordenen Gerinnungsschema erkannt hatte.

Die Thrombocyten enthalten eine Reihe von fermentativ hochaktiven Stoffen, die am Gerinnungsvorgang und an der Gefäßabdichtung maßgeblich beteiligt sind (Faktor 1, 2, 3, 4, Thromboplastin, Fibrinstabilisator, Antifibrinolysin sowie Serotonin; Abb. 1 aus Lüscher 1962). Das Gerinnungssystem scheint auch beim Menschen vorwiegend auf die Thrombocyten und nicht auf das Fibrinogen-Fibrin ausgerichtet zu sein (Lüscher 1956).

Entwicklungsphysiologisch gesehen ist der Thrombocytenzerfall als hämostatischer Mechanismus älter als das Fibrinogen-Fibrin-System. Bei der Krabbe „limulus polyphenus" stellt die viscöse Metamorphose der Thrombocyten den einzigen Blutstillungsmechanismus dar. Es erscheint deshalb auch aus diesem Grunde berechtigt, die Thrombocyten vor den Gerinnungsfaktoren zu besprechen, wenn auch die genauere Kenntnis des komplizierten

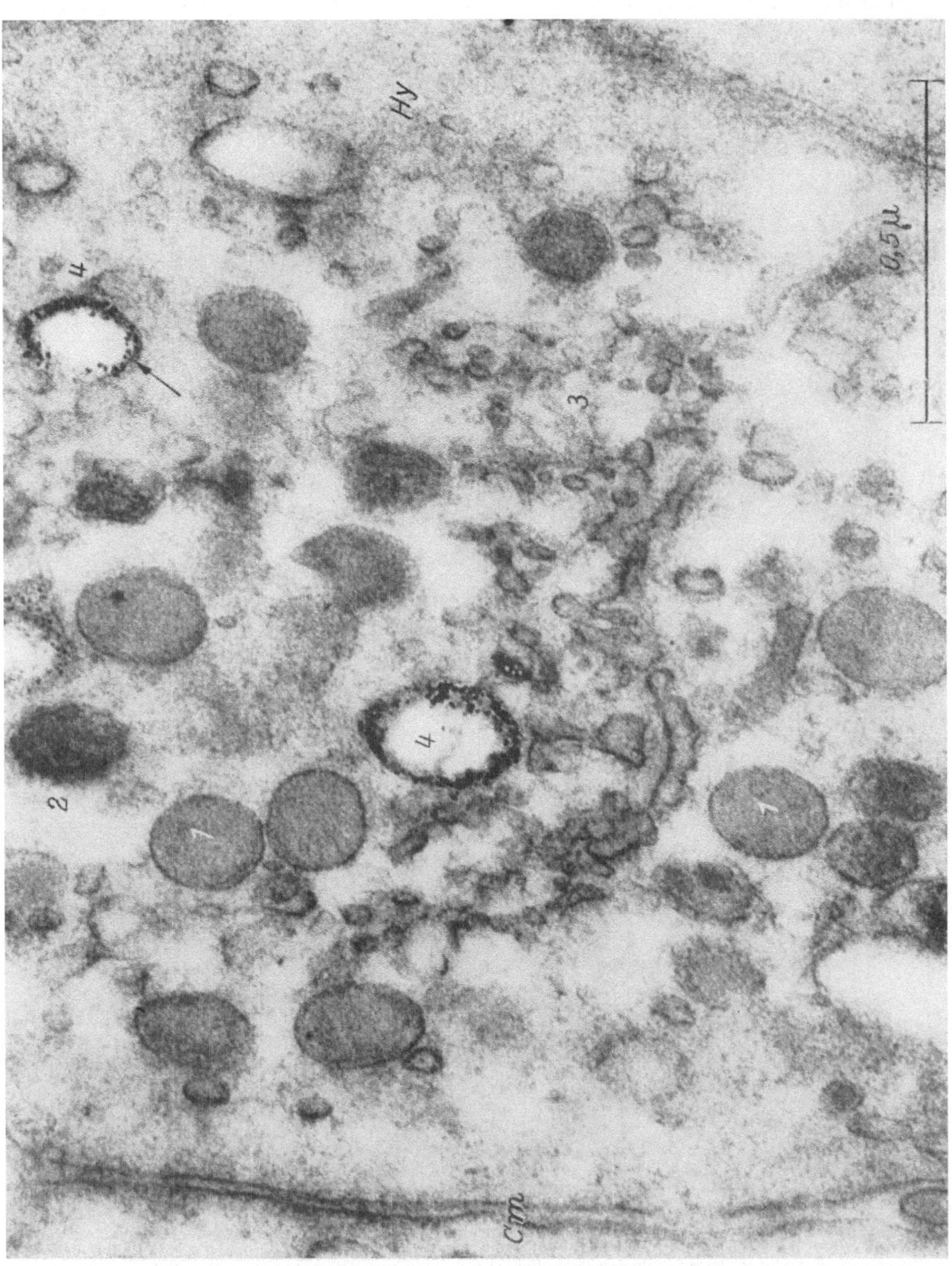

Abb. 2. Feinstruktur der Thrombocyten. Ausschnitt eines Thrombocyten. Normales menschliches Blut. *Cm* einfachkonturierte Zellmembran von zwei sich berührenden Thrombocyten. *Hy* homogene bis feingranuläre Grundsubstanz des Hyalomers. *1* Granulomer α, ovale Granula mit homogener Grundsubstanz. Die Granulamembran mißt 50 Å. *2* Granulomer β, Mitochondrium; *3* Granulomer γ, Zone aus Mikrobläschen und Tubuli (Golgi-Zone); *4* Gramulomer δ, Cytosomen mit zahlreichen kontrastreichen Körnchen, die sehr wahrscheinlich Ferritin darstellen. Die einzelnen liegenden Körnchen bei den Pfeilen messen 55 Å. [Aus H. Schulz u. H. Hiepler:. Lokalisierung von gerinnungsphysiologischen Aktivitäten in submikroskopischen Strukturen der Thrombocyten Klin. Wschr. **37**, H. 6 (1959)]

Gerinnungsvorganges hauptsächlich auf Ergebnissen der modernen Gerinnungsphysiopathologie im Plasma beruht.

Die Thrombocyten sind kleinste, plasmatische, kernlose, runde bis ovale, scheibchenförmige Blutbestandteile, welche nach Blutentnahme und Zugabe von

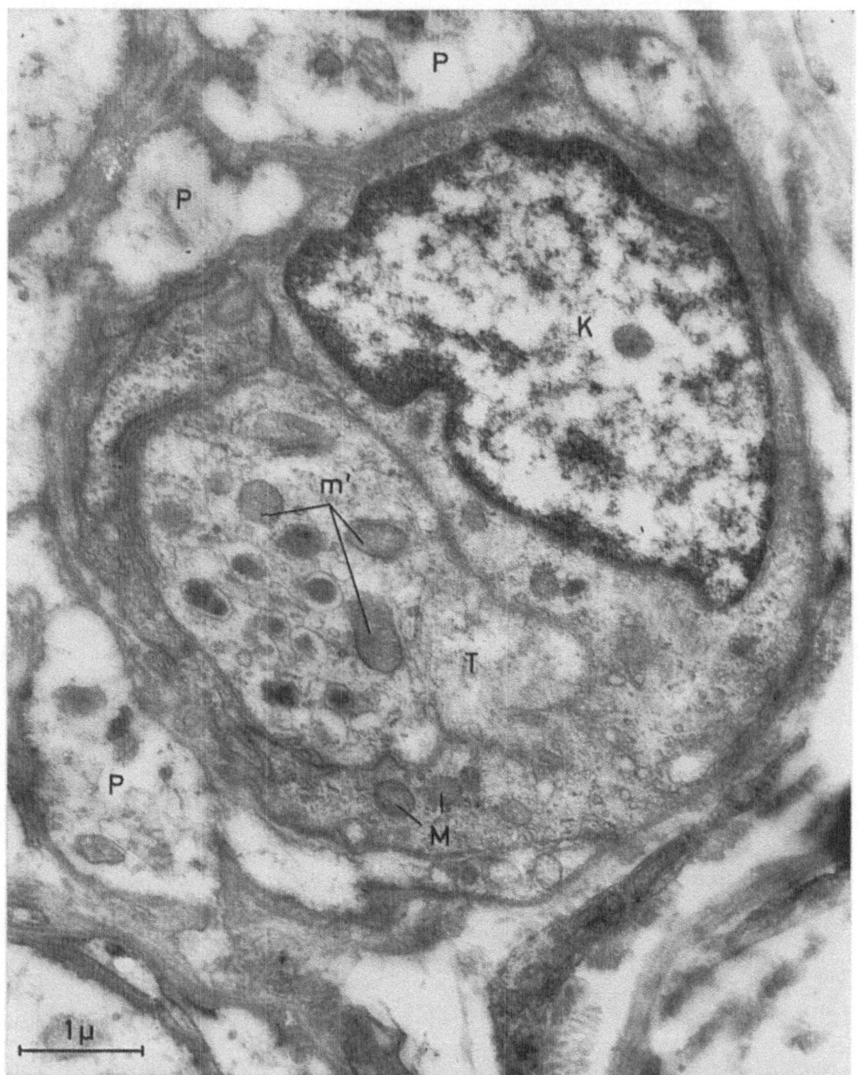

Abb. 3. Feinstruktur von Thrombocyten und Capillaren. Capillarquerschnitt mit Thrombocytenausschnitt (*T*), der das Lumen der Capillare ausfüllt. *K* Endothelkern, *M* Mitochondrien mit Cytoplasma des Endothels. Im Thrombocytenanschnitt Bestandteile des Granulomers, darunter auch Mitochondrien (*m'*). *P* Pericytenplasma. Vergrößerung 1:18000 *γ*. [Aus E. MACHER u. W. VOGELL: Elektronenmikroskopische Untersuchungen an Hautcapillaren. Dermatologica (Basel) **124**, 101 (1962)]

gerinnungshemmenden Mitteln zipflige Ausstülpungen am Zellrand oder sternförmige Gestalt zeigen. Die Thrombocyten ändern die Form je nach gerinnungshemmendem Zusatz; sie sind z.B. kugelig in Komplexon-Lösung und bei Magnesiumüberschuß, scheibchenförmig nach Oxalat- und Citratzugabe bei 37°C. Im Zentrum läßt sich ein körniges Granulomer, umgeben von einem strukturlosen

Tabelle 3. *Die wichtigsten Gerinnungsfaktoren der Thrombocyten*
(Aus R. JÜRGENS: Pathophysiologie und Klinik der Thrombopathien, S. 4—22. Internat. Symposium. Wien: Springer 1955)

Name	Synonyma	Allgemeine Eigenschaften und Funktionen	Wasserlöslichkeit	Fällung mit	Sedimentierung in Ultrazentrifuge	Hitzebeständigkeit	Adsorption
Plättchen-Faktor 1. (SEEGERS)	Plateletaccelerator (SEEGERS) Platelet-Ac-Globulin (JOHNSON et al.)	Wirkt auf die Umwandlung von Prothrombin auf Thrombin ähnlich z. B. Faktor V	löslich	$(NH_4)_2SO_4$ 50%	sedimentiert bei 32000 g in 30 min	weitgehend zerstört bei 53°	*nicht an* $BaSO_4$ oder $Ca_3(PO_4)_2$
Plättchen-Faktor 2. (SEEGERS)	Thrombinaccelerator (SEEGERS)	Wirkt auf die Umwandlung von Fibrinogen zu Fibrin (Unterstützung von Thrombin)	löslich	$(NH_4)_2SO_4$ 50%	sedimentiert *nicht* bei 32000 g in 45 min resp. 43000 g in 20 min	bei 53° in 30 min kein Verlust	adsorbiert an $BaSO_4$ und $Ca_3(PO_4)_2$
Plättchen-Faktor der Thrombokinase (JÜRGENS und DIALER)	Plättchen-Faktor 3 (SEEGERS) Platelet-Thromboplastic-Factor (STEFANINI) Thromboplastinogenase (QUICK) TCC = Thromboplastic Cell Component (SHINOWARA) Platelet-Factor 4 (BASERGA)	Bildet mit einem oder mehreren Plasmafaktoren zusammen die aktive Plasma-Thrombokinase	unlöslich	/	sedimentiert bei 32000 g in 30 min resp. 43000 g in 20 min	relativ beständig bei 56° zerstört bei 53° in 30 min	?
Heparin-Inhibitor (JÜRGENS und DIALER)	Plättchen-Faktor 4 (SEEGERS) Platelet-Factor 3 (VAN CREVELD)	Phosphatid, das die Antithrombinwirkung von Heparin hemmt	unlöslich	/	sedimentiert *nicht* bei 43000 g in 20 min	beständig bei 53° in 30 min	*nicht* an $Ca_3(PO_4)_2$ oder $BaSO_4$

Hyalomer, nachweisen (S. WITTE u.a. 1958, ZUCKER 1961). Die Strukturänderungen bei verschiedenen Blutzusätzen oder beim Gerinnungsvorgang lassen sich besonders gut im Phasenkontrast, Dunkelfeld- oder Fluorescenz-Mikroskop beobachten (FONIO 1957, D. DANON u.a. 1961, ACHENBACH u. RYSSEL 1962).

In neuerer Zeit wurden die Thrombocyten mehrfach mit dem Elektronenmikroskop untersucht (C. H. BRAUNSTEINER 1951, W. BERNHARD u.a. 1955, D. DANON u.a. 1961, H. SCHULZ u.a. 1962), wobei im Granulomer verschiedene Einschußkörperchen (α, β, γ s. Abb. 2 u. 3) festgestellt wurden (MARX 1955, FEISSLY u.a. 1957), deren Gehalt an gerinnungsaktiven Substanzen nach Ultrazentrifugation biologisch bestimmt werden konnten (SCHULZ u. HIEPLER 1959).

Es wurde festgestellt, daß die Thrombocyten außerdem die verschiedensten Metalle (Na, K, Ch. Mg, Cu, Fe, Me), kleinmolekulare Verbindungen, freie Aminosäuren, Thaurin, Hypoxanthin, Adenin, Nucleotide, Adenosintriphosphorsäure, Histamin, Adrenalin, Carotinoide, die verschiedensten Fermente und schließlich, außer den genannten thrombocytenspezifischen Faktoren, noch hochmolekulare Stoffe enthalten wie Polysaccharide, Mucopolysaccharide, Mucoproteine, Blutgruppensubstanzen, Ribonucleinsäure, Serumproteine. Desoxyribonucleinsäure fehlt. Man kann also sagen, daß die Thrombocyten außerordentlich reich ausgestattete Plasmateilchen darstellen, mit einer Anzahl von Gerinnungsfaktoren (Lüscher 1959, Gerok u.a. 1959), die sich gegenseitig beeinflussen (Abb. 1) und welche chemisch verschiedene Eigenschaften besitzen (Tabelle 3) (Jürgens 1955).

Die Thrombocyten stammen aus den Megakaryocyten im Knochenmark und sind Cytoplasmateilchen derselben.

Die Entstehung der Thrombocyten aus den Megakaryocyten, z.T. durch Abschnürung, wurde 1957 von M. Albrecht in menschlichen Knochenmarkkulturen studiert. Die Ausreifungszeit der Blutplättchen beträgt nach D. Hess (1958) durchschnittlich 6—8 Tage; ihre Lebensdauer nach Messungen mit P^{32} wahrscheinlich 6—14 Tage (E. Adelson u.a. 1957, M. B. Zucker u.a. 1961).

Die Thrombocytenzahl ist nicht konstant, sondern ändert sich unter verschiedenen Einflüssen, so im Tag- und Nachtrhythmus mit höchsten Werten um 15 Uhr und tiefsten zwischen 21—23 Uhr (Goldeck u.a. 1950), durch den Verdauungsprozeß (Benhamou u. Nouchy, Matis u.a. 1951), durch Arbeit, Saisonwechsel, operative Eingriffe (Goldeck), je nach der Reaktionslage des vegetativen Nervensystems, abhängig vom vierten Ventrikel und der tubero-infundibulären Region, nach Glucose-Injektionen (Dyke 1924) und Menstruation Dameshek, z.T. zit. nach Beis 1960).

Die Thrombocyten machen etwa 2% des Blutvolumens aus; ihre Zahl beträgt durchschnittlich 250000/cm³. Auf benetzbarer Oberfläche, z.B. Glas, breiten sich die Thrombocyten unmittelbar unter Pseudopodienbildung auf das Mehrfache ihres Originaldurchmessers aus (Zucker 1961). Sie haben wahrscheinlich einen nur geringen Metabolismus. Die osmotische Resistenz der Thrombocyten entspricht derjenigen der Erythrocyten und nimmt bei verschiedenen Tierarten progressiv zu, von Schaf, Maus, Kaninchen, Ratte, Meerschweinchen bis zum Menschen (Gilboa u.a. 1960, Nelken u.a. 1961).

4. Zur Physiopathologie der Thrombocyten

Den Thrombocyten kommen zwei wichtige Funktionen zu, nämlich

1. Blutstillung,
2. Erhaltung der Funktionstüchtigkeit der Gefäße.

Grundlage der physiologischen Funktion der Blutstillung ist die *viscöse Metamorphose*, in deren Verlauf die Plättchen unter Einfluß von Thrombin und einem niedermolekularen Plasmafaktor unbekannter Herkunft charakteristisch zerfallen und anschließend retrahieren (Lüscher 1956, Mason u.a. 1962). Statt Retraktion schlägt neuerdings Lüscher den Ausdruck Agglutination und Verfestigung der Aggregate vor (persönliche Mitteilung). Bei der viscösen Metamorphose nach Kontakt mit benetzbaren Oberflächen lagern sich die Thrombocyten zusammen, breiten sich aus und die Zellgrenzen verschwinden (im Gegensatz zu einem reinen Agglutinationsvorgang) (Abb. 4). Das für diesen Vorgang notwendige Thrombin bildet sich in unmittelbarer Nähe der Thrombocyten als Endprodukt eines komplizierten Gerinnungsablaufes aus dem Prothrombin unter Einwirkung von Thrombokinase und Calcium. Die rasch wirksame und in großer Menge bei Gewebsverletzung frei werdende Gewebskinase benötigt zur Wirksamkeit die Gerinnungsfaktoren V und VII; die in unmittelbarer Nähe der Thrombocyten entstehende Blutkinase benötigt zu ihrer Entstehung außerdem Thrombocyten-Faktor 3 die Gerinnungsfaktoren V, VIII, IX und Calcium (s. auch Abschnitt III).

Die erwähnten Thrombocytenumwandlungen lassen sich bei bestimmten Laboratoriumsuntersuchungen außer durch Citrat, Heparin, Oxalat, EDTA durch Silikonisierung der Glaswaren verhindern (E. LEPPS 1949).

Die mit dem Phasenmikroskop ausgezeichnet verfolgbare viscöse Metamorphose und Verklumpung ist bei der Thrombasthenie Glanzmann-Nägeli stark gestört, nicht aber bei der Angiohämophilie von WILLEBRAND-JÜRGENS. Starke Plättchenanisocytose, Riesenformen mit retraktionslosen Plättchen zeigt sich bei myeloproliferativen Erkrankungen und bei symptomatischen Thrombocytosen. Die verschiedensten Störungen der Thrombusstruktur können auf einem Mißverhältnis zwischen Plättchenzahl und Fibrinmenge, mangelnder Haft- und Kontaktfähigkeit der Thrombocyten und ihrer verminderten oder erhöhten Zerfallsbereitschaft beruhen (ACHENBACH u. RYSSEL 1962).

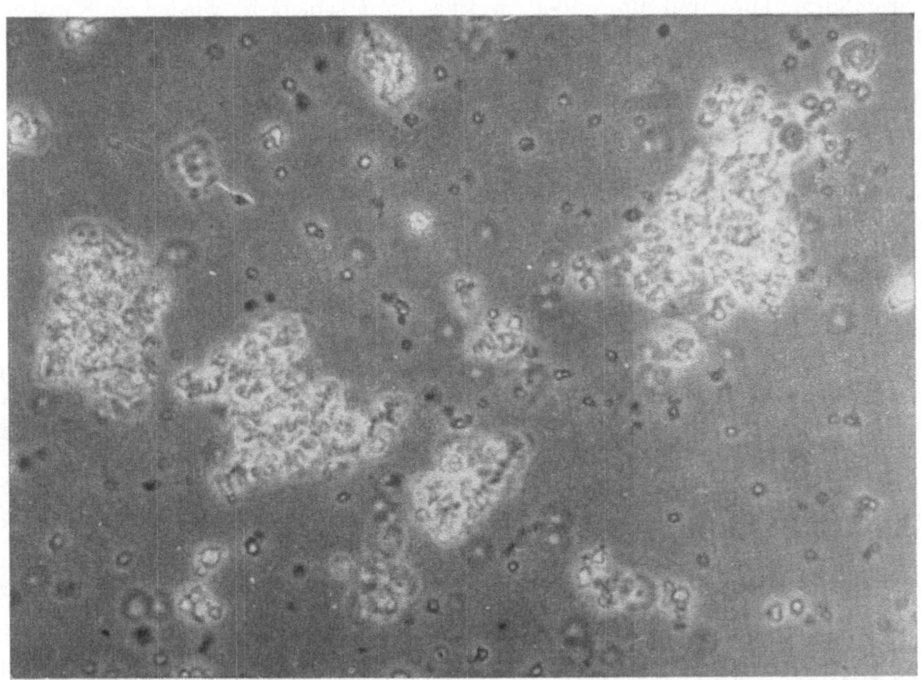

Abb. 4. Viscöse Metamorphose der Thrombocyten: die individuelle Struktur der Plättchen geht völlig verloren. (Aus F. KOLLER: Über die Wirkung der Antikoagulantien auf die Blutplättchen. In: Nebenwirkungen von Arzneimitteln auf Blut und Knochenmark. Symposium Malmö 1957, herausgeg. von R. JÜRGENS u. J. WALDENSTRÖM. Schattauer-Verlag Stuttgart

Die neueren Mikroanalysen mittels Ultrazentrifugation und elektronenoptischer Identifizierung der isolierten Bestandteile zeigten, daß die α-Granula den Plättchenfaktor 1 und 3 enthalten, das β-Granulomer die Mitochondrien und das bläschenförmige γ-Granulomer der Plättchen Faktor 1. Im Hyalomer sind weiterhin die Plättchenfaktoren 2 und 4 enthalten (Abb. 2), (Allgemeine Eigenschaften und Funktionen dieser Faktoren s. Tabelle 3.)

Außer Faktor 2 und 4 enthält das Hyalomer fünf elektrophoretisch abtrennbare Eiweißfraktionen, worunter das für die Erzeugung der Klebrigkeit wichtige Protein S (LÜSCHER 1956), ferner das die Gefäßkontraktion vermittelnde 5-Hydroxytryptamin (ZUCKER u. BORELLI) und eine noch nicht definierte gefäßabdichtende Substanz (LÜSCHER), welche bei Thrombopenie und Thrombocytose verringert ist (BIGELOW 1954), ferner noch reichlich Adenosintriphosphorsäure (ZUCKER u.a. 1961). Die Oberfläche der Thrombocyten scheint absorptiv außerordentlich aktiv zu sein und enthält wahrscheinlich Calcium, Prothrombin, vermutlich auch Faktor V (BOUNAMEAUX 1957). Es zeigte sich, daß zudem noch ein Fibrinstabilisator sowie ein Antifibrinolysin anwesend ist (Abb. 1) (LÜSCHER 1962).

Nach neuesten Untersuchungen (W. O. REID u.a. 1962) kommt aber den Blutplättchen in der Fibrinolyse eine bivalente Rolle zu, nämlich einerseits die erwähnte Fibrinstabilisation, andererseits erhöhte fermentative Fibrinolyse. Eine solche erhöhte Fibrinolyse wurde mit einer neuen standardisierten Thrombinzeitbestimmungsmethode post mortem bei 20 Thrombopenie-Patienten mit hämorrhagischer Diathese gefunden, nicht aber bei 20 Thrombopenien ohne Blutungen. Nach GROSS u.a. (1962) ist ein solcher Proaktivator der Fibrinolyse nicht mit dem Plättchenaktivator und Plasminogen identisch.

Diese komplizierten und reichlich ausgestatteten kernlosen Plasmateile sind unter Einwirkung von Calcium und den Gerinnungsfaktoren V, VIII und IX entscheidend an der Entstehung der Blutthrombokinase beteiligt, welche das Prothrombin in Thrombin umwandelt, welches dann seinerseits wieder als Substrat für Thrombocyten und Fibrinogen dient (Abb. 1).

Die vasokonstriktive Aktivität der Thrombocyten ist an den Arterien deutlicher als an den Venen sichtbar und beruht auf dem Gehalt an 5-Hydroxytryptamin (Serotonin). Das direkt in das Gewebe diffundierende Serotonin hat eine unmittelbare Wirkung, wobei dann der Gefäßkontraktionsimpuls wahrscheinlich neurogen weitergeleitet wird. Bei der Blutstillung der peripheren Arterien kommt zum Plättchenagglutinat (Weißthrombus) zusätzlich Vasoconstriction, an den größeren peripheren Venen jedoch lediglich Plättchenagglutinate, ebenso an den Capillaren, hier zudem Gefäßkollaps mit Zusammenkleben. (Diese Vorgänge konnten im Lebendpräparat eingehend studiert werden; s. ILLIG 1961.) Dem Fibrin kommt nach LÜSCHER u.a. lediglich eine Verstärkung des primären Wundverschlusses zu. Daß die Thrombocyten neben der Kontraktionsförderung noch capillarabdichtend wirksam sind, zeigt sich in der 1000mal höheren ödemverhindernden Aktivität von Plättchenpräparaten verglichen mit Seren (LÜSCHER 1956).

Bei der Thrombose sind die Plättchen sekundär von Bedeutung. Durch Überschießen des an sich durchaus physiologischen Prozesses der Plättchenanlagerung an das irgendwie geschädigte Endothel entsteht die Thrombose. Begünstigend wirken erhöhte allgemeine Gerinnungsbereitschaft des strömenden Blutes bei Stauung und Verlangsamung der Blutströmungsgeschwindigkeit, bei erhöhter Agglutinationsbereitschaft der Plättchen oder Anhaften der Plättchen an veränderten Endothelien, evtl. auch Erhöhung einzelner Gerinnungsfaktoren.

Bei Lebendbeobachtung am Rattenmesenterium kreisen die Thrombocyten scheibchenbis spindelförmig im strömenden Blut ohne engere Beziehung zur Gefäßwand. Bei der viscösen Metamorphose sind Volumzunahme, Pseudopodienbildung, Klebrigwerden und Festhaften gegenseitig an Leukocyten sowie am Gefäßendothel zu beobachten (WITTE u.a. 1958). Dieser Vorgang kann ausgelöst werden durch intravenöse Injektion von Thrombin, Trypsin oder auch durch lokale Thrombinapplikation sowie Endothelschädigung. Eine Gerinnung des Fibrinogens im Blutplasma ist nicht sichtbar, sondern alle intravasalen Gerinnungsvorgänge scheinen sich an den wichtigen Thrombocyten abzuspielen.

Die Retraktion des Fibringerinnsels ist physiologisch von größter Bedeutung, weil dadurch die entstandene Blutthrombokinase und das Serotonin aus dem Faserwerk des Gerinnsels ausgedrückt wird und zur Wirkung kommt. Das retraktile Material wird durch die Thrombocyten selbst geliefert und das Fibrin spielt beim Retraktionsprozeß nur eine passive Rolle (LÜSCHER 1956). Der Thrombocytenfaktor, welcher für die Kontraktion des Gerinnsels verantwortlich ist, konnte von BETTEX-GALLAND u. LÜSCHER (1959) als Protein mit den Eigenschaften von Muskelactomyosin isoliert werden.

Das contractile Protein „Thrombosthenin" beträgt nach BETTEX u.a. (1962) 15% des Plättchenproteins, ist nicht mit dem Muskelactomyosin identisch und kann mit einer besonderen Methode sauber extrahiert werden. (Weitere Arbeiten über Fibrinkontraktion und Thrombocyten s. FONIO 1947, 1950, LÜSCHER 1956, FIEHRER 1957, BETTEX-GALLAND u.a. 1959, 1960, 1961, WALLER u.a. 1959.) Die Energie für die Fibrinretraktionsprozesse wird glykolytisch aus Adenosintriphosphat (ATP) gewonnen, und zwar mittels der Phosphoglyceraldehyddehydrogenase. Diese ist bei der Thrombasthenie Glanzmann-Nägeli verändert (GROSS u.a. 1960), nicht aber im Alter (DETWYLER u.a. 1962).

Die für die Blutstillung wichtige Fibrinretraktion ist nicht nur bei thrombopenischen Zuständen, sondern auch bei pathologischen Veränderungen des Eiweiß-Stoffwechsels (γ-Plasmocytom, M. WALDENSTRÖM) und reaktiven Änderungen der Serumeiweiße (Lebercirrhosen, GARBE u.a. 1961) gestört.

Mit der Immunofluorescenz nach COONS läßt sich nachweisen, daß im Zentrum der Plättchen Fibrinogen enthalten ist, welches bei der Thrombocytenagglutination die Fibrinknoten bildet (SOKAL 1962).

Gerinnungsprozesse unter Beteiligung der Thrombocyten spielen nicht nur bei der Blutstillung nach Verletzung eine Rolle, sondern scheinen in kleinem Maßstabe fortwährend an den Gefäßendothelien abzulaufen, wie dies besonders WINTERSTEIN (1955), COPLEY (1957), LAKI (1962) u.a. betonen. Pseudopodienbildung, Agglutination und viscöse Metamorphose der Thrombocyten wurden elektronenmikroskopisch von FEISSLY u.a. (1957) verfolgt.

Die Thrombocyten spielen bei den idiopathischen (essentiellen) und symptomatischen (sekundären) thrombopenischen hämorrhagischen Diathesen eine besondere Rolle. Obwohl kein strenger Parallelismus zwischen Thrombocytenzahl und Ausmaß der Hautblutung besteht, scheint die kritische Zahl zur Bildung von Suffusionen und Petechien zwischen 30000—40000/mm^3 zu liegen. Der Gefäßfaktor läßt sich mit der Verlängerung der Blutungszeit, mit dem Rumpel-Leedeschen Phänomen und mit den positiven Kneif-Saug-Stichproben nachweisen. Der Gerinnungsvorgang verläuft meist ungestört, die direkte Retraktion des Blutkuchens ist aber oft verspätet oder fehlt. Im Knochenmark finden sich häufig vermehrte und unreife Megakaryocyten ohne sichtbare Plättchenbildung. Die Milz kann mäßig vergrößert sein.

Als Zeichen einer gestörten Plättchenfunktion kann oft mangelhafte Spontanagglutination festgestellt werden. Der Prothrombinverbrauch ist dann im Konsumptions-Test herabgesetzt (P. DE NICOLA).

Die Mechanismen der Funktionen der Blutplättchen bei der Blutstillung und der Thrombose können also folgendermaßen zusammengefaßt werden:

1. Unmittelbar nach Durchtrennung oder Läsion eines kleineren Gefäßes beginnen die Plättchen an die Schnittstelle anzuhaften; dieses Anhaften ist wahrscheinlich ein passiver Vorgang und die Frage, ob der „Intercellulärzement" klebriger wird, wie dies CHAMBERS u. ZWEIFACH 1947 u.a. annehmen, ist nicht mit Sicherheit zu beantworten.

2. Durch fortlaufendes Anhaften weiterer Plättchen an den bereits angelagerten kommt es zur Bildung eines lockeren, oft recht voluminösen Plättchenpfropfes. Dieser ist für das ausströmende Blut noch durchlässig; seine mechanische Festigkeit ist gering, und häufig werden Fragmente vom Blutstrom weggerissen (LÜSCHER 1959). Während dieser Phase durchlaufen die Plättchen die „viscöse Metamorphose" mit den entsprechenden Formveränderungen. Die für die Einleitung der „viscösen Metamorphose" wirksame Thrombinmenge ist außerordentlich gering und liegt unter einer Einheit pro Kubikmillimeter. Der Thrombinangriff bewirkt eine tiefgreifende Permeabilitätsstörung der Plättchenmembran; wahrscheinlich tritt in dieser zweiten Phase aus dem verletzten Gefäßendothel etwas Gewebskinase, wodurch weiteres Thrombin gebildet wird, welches die viscöse Metamorphose der passiv angelagerten Plättchen unterstützt.

3. Die Konsolidierung dieses primären Gefäßverschlusses setzt ein. Der Plättchenpfropf wird fest und undurchlässig. Die Blutung kommt endgültig zum Stillstand. Bei der Verfestigung des Plättchenpfropfes spielt die Kontraktion des Blutgerinnsels mit Hilfe des neuerdings isolierten Muskelactonomyosin-artigen Proteins, welches unter Wirkung von ATP kontrahiert, die entscheidende Rolle.

4. Serotonin der Plättchen sowie noch andere Faktoren unterstützen die Blutstillung durch Gefäßkontraktion und Gefäßabdichtung.

Die gegenseitigen engen Beziehungen zwischen Gerinnungsmechanismen und Plättchenfunktionen sowie deren Einfluß auf die verschiedenen Krankheitszustände können nun recht übersichtlich dargestellt werden, und auch die Folgen des Ausfalles einzelner Komponenten dieser Systeme werden gut verstanden (s. Abb. 5, LÜSCHER 1959).

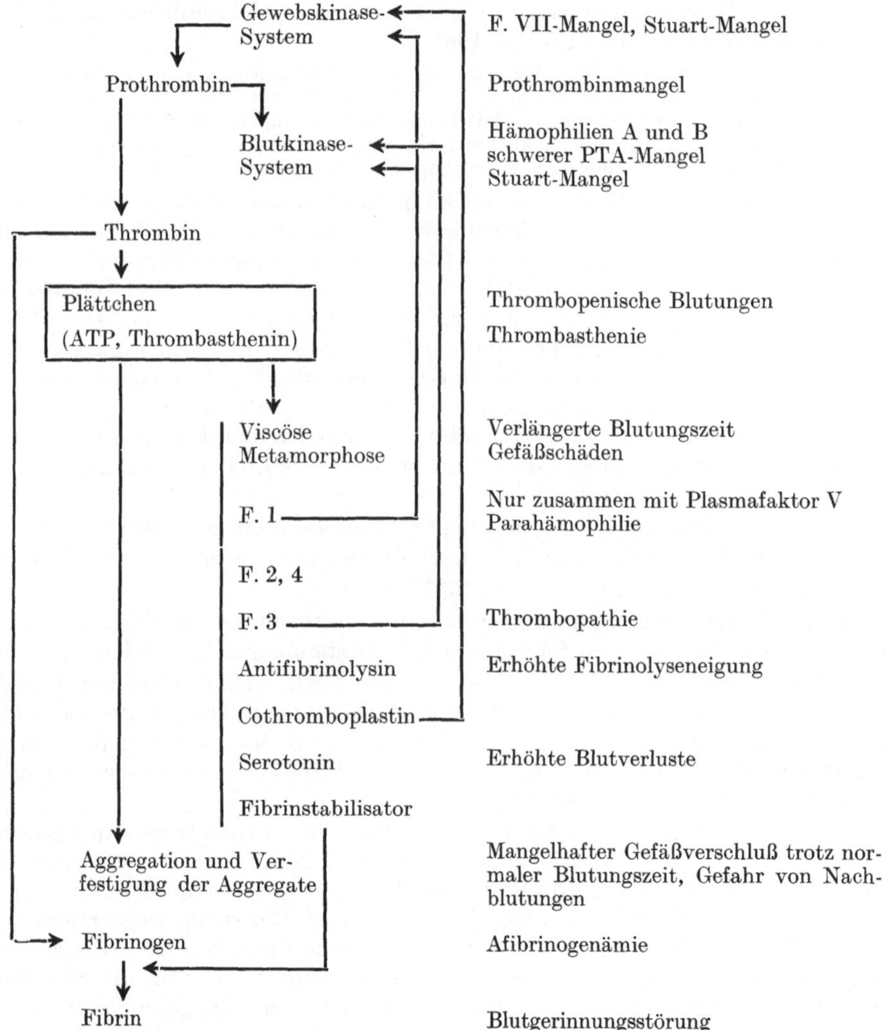

Abb. 5. Gegenseitige Beziehungen zwischen Gerinnungsmechanismus und Plättchenfunktionen und die Folgen des Ausfalls einzelner Komponenten dieses Systems. [Aus E. F. LÜSCHER: Biochemische Eigenschaften und physiologische Bedeutung der Blutplättchen (1959)]

Es besteht also eine funktionelle Einheit zwischen Capillarwand, Thrombocyten und plasmatischen Gerinnungsfaktoren (FLEISCHHACKER u. STACHER 1962). Bei normalen Verhältnissen läuft ständig an der Gefäßwand ein Gerinnungsvorgang ab und bildet einen ultravisiblen Film. Durch gerinnungshemmende plasmatische Wirkstoffe und vor allem durch die gleichfalls stetig ablaufende Fibrinolyse wird verhindert, daß sich die Gerinnung pathologisch verstärkt.

Diese komplexen und wichtigen Funktionen können die Thrombocyten nur in frischem Zustand erfüllen, wie Tierversuche an röntgenbestrahlten Ratten mit strahlenbedingter Markthrombocytopenie (RACCUGLIA 1962) zeigten. Bei -20^{0}C und $+6^{0}$C während 24 Std in

Gelatine-Elektrolyt-Medium oder NaCl konservierte Rattenthrombocyten konnten die verlängerte Blutungszeit nicht normalisieren.

Selbstverständlich ist es im Rahmen dieses Handbuchbeitrages nicht möglich, die außerordentlich komplizierten Verhältnisse der Thrombocyten vollständig darzustellen. Die besprochenen wichtigen Erkenntnisse können an Hand von weiteren Übersichtsarbeiten ergänzt werden, so von HITTMAIR 1938, DEBRAY 1959, OSTEN 1959, LÜSCHER 1959).

5. Zur Physiopathologie der Gerinnung

Der lebenswichtige Gerinnungsvorgang ist ein komplizierter fermentativer Prozeß, bei welchem das lösliche Faserprotein Fibrinogen in monomeres Fibrin

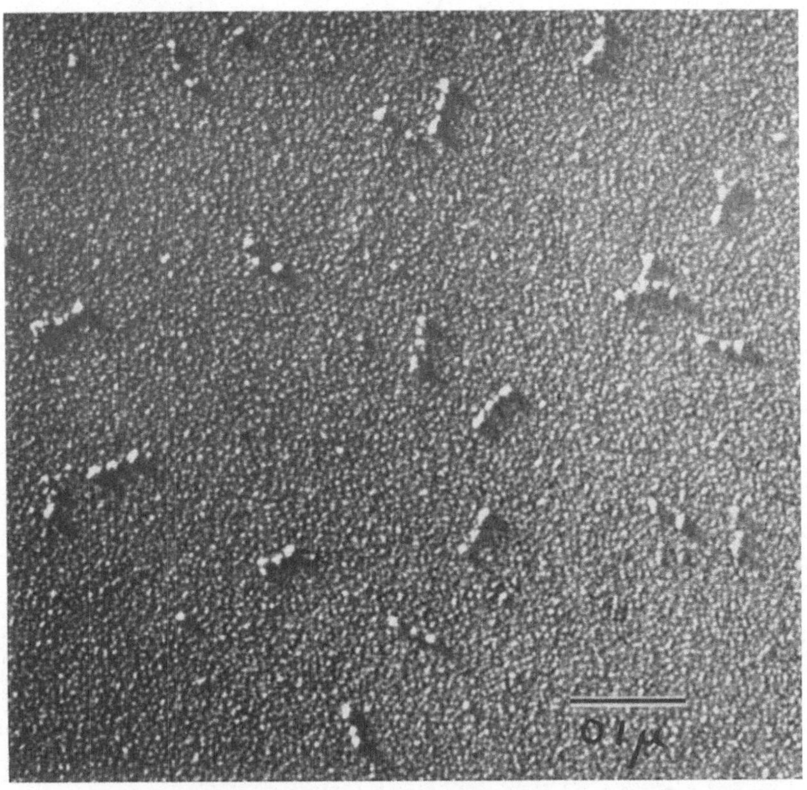

Abb. 6. Feinstruktur der Fibrinogenmoleküle. Fibrinogenmoleküle (hier ungefähr 150000mal vergrößert) erscheinen als Kügelchentriaden ohne Spirale dazwischen. (Elektronenphotographie von C. E. HALL und H. S. SLAYTER, Massachusetts Institute of Technicology.) [Aus K. LAKI: The Clotting of fibrinogen (1962). Nachdruck der Abb. 6—8 mit Genehmigung des Verlages Scientific American Inc.]

unter dem Einfluß des proteolytischen Enzyms Thrombin umgewandelt wird, das sich dann unter dem Einfluß des „Fibrin stabilizing factors" (FSF) zu den langen Fibrinfasern polymerisiert (LAKI 1962).

Die Fibrinogenmoleküle enthalten 18 Aminosäuren, haben ein Molekulargewicht von 330000—400000 und messen ungefähr 600 Å. Elektronenmikroskopisch sind die Moleküle in der Mitte und endständig kugelförmig verdickt (Abb. 6). Unter dem Einfluß des proteolytischen Ferment-Riesenmoleküls Thrombin werden von der mittleren, elektronenoptisch kugeligen Stelle zwei Aminosäuren, nämlich Threonin (Peptid B) und von einer endständigen kugeligen Struktur zwei Glutaminsäuremoleküle (Peptid A) unter Verlust von 14 negativen Ladungen abgetrennt, wodurch sich eine vierte kleinere kugelige Struktur am Molekül bildet unter leichter Verlängerung derselben (Abb. 7). Diese neugebildeten monomeren Fibrinmoleküle verbinden sich dann endständig mittels Wasserstoffbrücken unter Einfluß des Laki-Lorand-(Fibrinstabilisierung-)Faktors (FSF) zu langen Fasern, verfestigen sich auch quer mittels Wasserstoffbrücken, so daß ein solides Fibringerüst entsteht (Abb. 8). Durch Färbung mit Phosphorwolframsäure läßt sich eine regelmäßige Querstreifung mit dickeren Färbungen im Abstand von 240 Å und von 120 Å nachweisen. Im Gegensatz zum monomeren Fibrin ist das polymere nicht mehr harnstofflöslich und relativ elastisch.

Verhältnismäßig kompliziert beim ganzen Gerinnungsvorgang ist der fermentative Prozeß der Thrombinbildung aus Prothrombin *(erste Gerinnungsphase)*, in welchem sich dieses lösliche Glucoprotein (enthaltend 18 Aminosäuren, Acetyl-

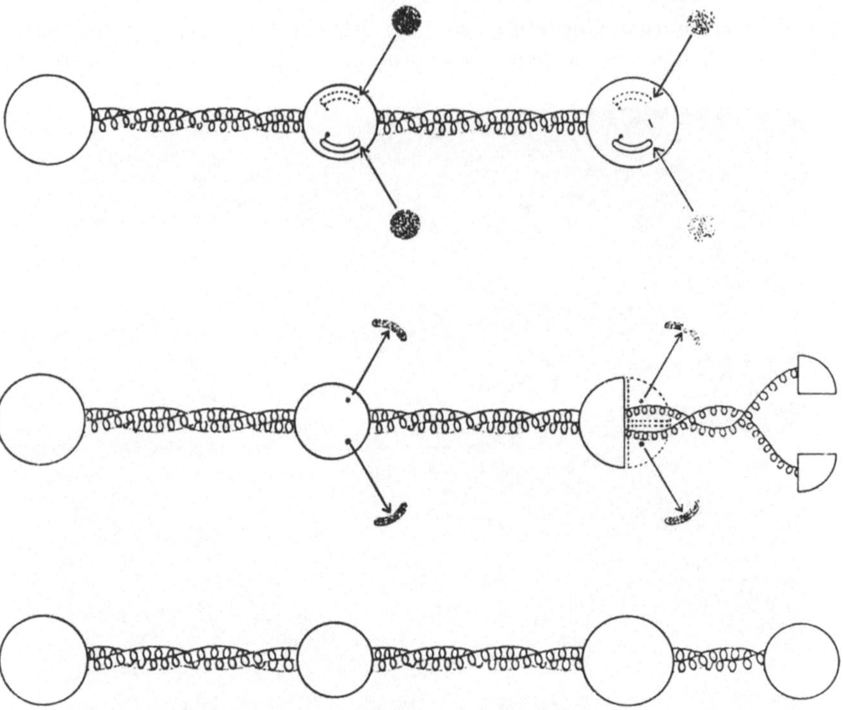

Abb. 7. Umwandlung von Fibrinogen in Fibrin. *Fibrinogen* verwandelt sich in *Fibrin* durch die Einwirkung des Enzyms Thrombin. Thrombinmoleküle (graue Kreise obere Reihe) greifen (s. Pfeile) die 4 Peptide an, indem sie die 2. und 3. Kügelchen des Fibrinogenmoleküls zusammenbringen. Die schwachen Wasserstoffbindungen, welche das andere Ende der Peptide zusammenhalten, brechen dann leicht auf und 2 Peptide (*A*) werden dem 2. Kügelchen, ferner 2 Peptide (*B*) dem 3. Kügelchen weggenommen. Ein 4. Kügelchen beginnt sich zu bilden (mittlere Reihe). Das fertige Fibrinmolekül (unten) besteht aus 4 Kügelchen und ist ein wenig länger als das ursprüngliche Fibrinogen. [Aus K. Laki: The clotting of fibrinogen (1962)]

hexosamin und Pentose) in das lösliche proteolytische Ferment Thrombin (mit 16 Aminosäuren) umwandelt. Dieses Ferment läßt sich mit anderen proteolytischen Enzymen wie Pepsin oder Trypsin vergleichen, ist aber viel spezifischer und begnügt sich mit der erwähnten Abspaltung der vier Aminosäuren aus einem Fibrinogenmolekül.

Die Umwandlung von Prothrombin in Thrombin geschieht fermentativ entweder im Blut selbst, unter dem Einfluß der unter besonderen Umständen gebildeten Blutthrombokinase, oder vasculär unter Einwirkung der Gewebsthrombokinase (Thromboplastin, Faktor III).

Beide Arten von Thrombokinase entstehen *(Vorphase)* unter Einwirkung von spezifischen Lipoproteiden (bei Gewebsthrombokinase Gewebsextrakt, bei der Blutthrombokinase Plättchenfaktor 3), den Plasmafaktoren V und X (Stuart-Prower-Faktor) sowie Calcium, ferner aus unterschiedlichen Plasmafaktoren, bei der Gewebsthrombokinase F. VII, bei der Blutthrombokinase F. VII und F. IX. Außer den genannten Lipoproteinen und Calcium bestehen diese Faktoren

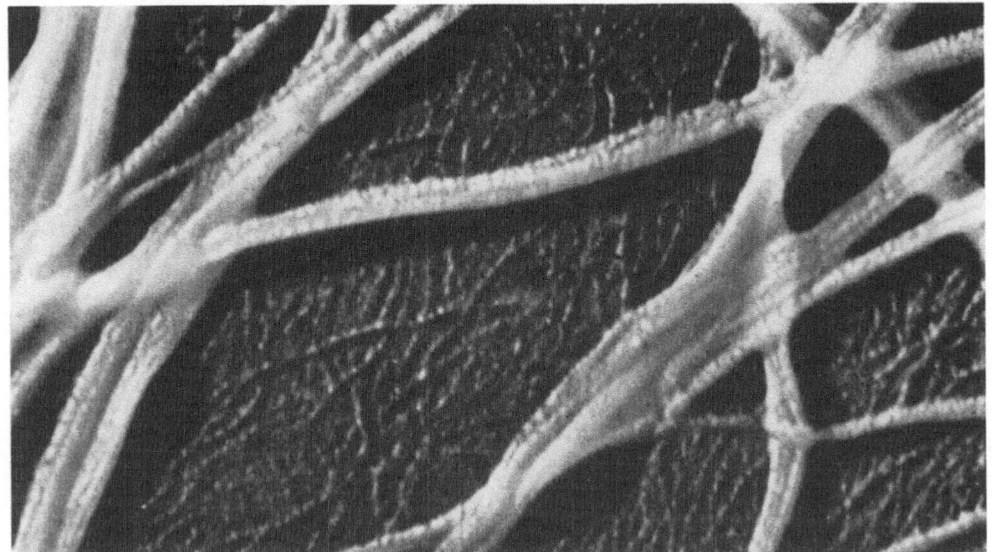

Abb. 8. Feinstruktur der Fibringerinnsel. Fibringerinnsel (Vergrößerung ungefähr 80000mal) zeigt sowohl dicke, verzweigte Stränge wie auch End-zu-End-Bildungen (feine Filamente im Hintergrund) des Fibrinmoleküls Elektronenphotographie von HAWN und PORTER, Rockefeller-Institute, New York). [Aus K. LAKI: The clotting of fibrinogen (1962)]

im allgemeinen aus Sphäroproteinen und wirken teils katalytisch ohne Verminderung während des Gerinnungsvorganges oder werden teils verbraucht oder entstehen erst während des Gerinnungsvorgangs (Abb. 9).

So bleiben bei der Gewebsgerinnung Calcium und F. VII konstant, F. I, II, V und X verschwinden. Bei der Blutgerinnung bleiben Calcium, F. X und plasma thromboplastin-antecedent (PTA) konstant, F. I, II, V und VIII werden verbraucht, wogegen F. IX und Hageman-Faktor entstehen.

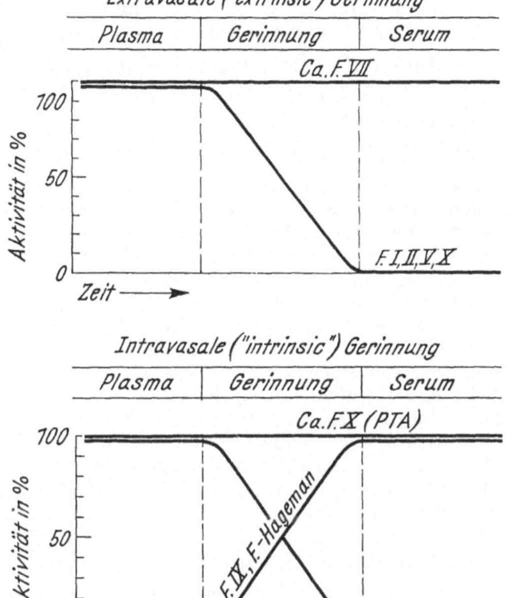

Abb. 9. Quantitatives Verhalten der Gerinnungsfaktoren während der Gerinnung. [Aus F. KOLLER: La conception actuelle de la coagulation du sang (1961)]

In Abb. 10 sind die drei Phasen der intra- und extravasalen Blutgerinnung (Vorphase, erste und zweite Phase) nach KOLLER (1958) dargestellt.

Nach internationalem Übereinkommen wurde der Großteil der bis heute bekannten gerinnungsphysiologischen Faktoren ohne Präjudiz über ihre Funktion von I—XII fortlaufend numeriert. Nomenklatur, chemische Natur und physiologische Wirkung all dieser Faktoren sind in Tabelle 4 aufgestellt (z.T. nach KOLLER 1958, ROOS 1959).

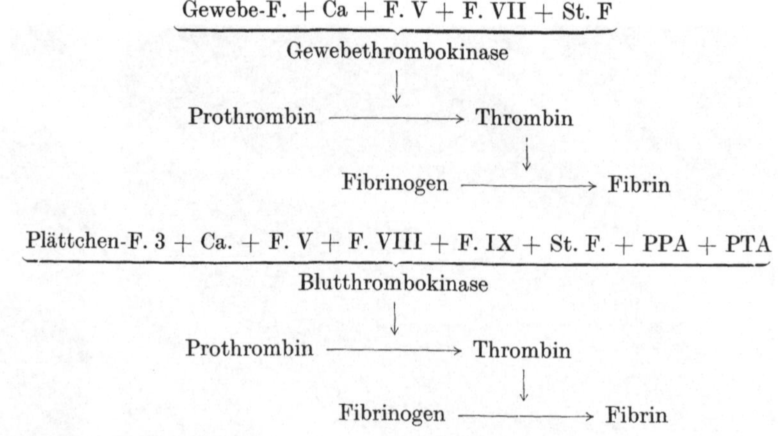

Abb. 10. Phasen der Blutgerinnung. [Aus F. KOLLER: Der heutige Stand der Gerinnungsforschung (1958)]

Die „Kinetik" der Blutgerinnung, d.h. die Reihenfolge des Eingreifens der verschiedenen Faktoren bis zur Generation der Thrombokinasen, ist noch nicht sicher geklärt. Nach KOLLER (1958) entsteht die Gewebsthrombokinase zweistufig, die Blutthrombokinase dreistufig (Tabelle 5), wobei nur bei der Gewebsthrombokinase der Lipoproteingewebsfaktor zu Beginn eingreift, bei der Blutthrombokinase erst in der zweiten Phase, in Form des Plättchenfaktors 3.

In vitro, d.h. in Blutkonserven, sind die Faktoren verschieden lang haltbar (Halbwertzeit: F. V etwa 5 Tage, F. VIII etwa 10 Tage, F. I, II, VII, IX, X mehr als 18 Tage). Auch die Blutplättchen nehmen relativ rasch ab (KOLLER 1958). Aus diesem Grund sind bei Hämophilie, Thrombopenien und Thrombopathien frische Blutkonserven (nicht über 8 Tage alt) zu verwenden. In vivo sind die Faktoren viel labiler (Halbwertzeit von F. VII 4 Std, F. II 24—30 Std, F. VIII 2 Std, F. IX über 30 Std, F. X 24—30 Std (KOLLER 1958).

Im Gegensatz zu den vorgängig erwähnten mehr auf die Thrombocyten ausgerichteten Theorien könnten die Auslösung des Gerinnungsprozesses wahrscheinlich auch folgendermaßen verstanden werden: Bei der „extravasalen" Gerinnung (mit Gewebsthrombokinase) tritt sie innerhalb von wenigen Sekunden ein. Die „intravasale" Gerinnung erfolgt etwas langsamer; sie benötigt einige Minuten. Die erste Stufe mit Bildung des intermediären Produktes I findet ohne Beteiligung der Plättchen statt (Tabelle 5); erst in der zweiten Stufe mit Bildung des intermediären Produktes II greifen die Plättchen ein, indem sie hier hämostatisch agglutinieren („verfallen"), mit vollständiger Verschmelzung der einzelnen Thrombocyten im Sinne der „viscösen Metamorphose" (nach EBERTH u. SCHIMMELBUSCH, zit. KOLLER 1958). Dieser Vorgang läuft nicht nur bei Endothelverletzungen, Kontakt mit benetzbaren Oberflächen bis zur völligen Gerinnung ab, sondern es finden wahrscheinlich fortlaufend geringgradige Gerinnungsvorgänge in kleiner Menge auch an den normalen Endothelien statt (s. WITTE), was ROSE (zit. KOLLER 1958) elektronenmikroskopisch durch Feststellung eines feinen Endothelüberzuges der Gefäßwand mit einem Fibrinnetz bestätigen konnte. Die Übergänge von normaler intravasaler geringgradiger Gerinnung bis zur blutstillenden Koagulation bei Verletzungen und anderen Vorgängen und schließlich bis zur übermäßigen Gerinnung mit dem Thrombose-Embolie-Syndrom sind also fließend.

Bei der *Thrombosebereitschaft* mag die Vermehrung bestimmter Faktoren von Bedeutung sein, wie F. II und VII am Ende von Gravidität und Wochenbett, F. I bei Infektionskrankheiten und schließlich postoperative Vermehrung der Blutplättchen, besonders nach Splenektomie (KOLLER 1957), doch können diese Faktorenschwankungen mit der Thrombelastographie und dem Heparintoleranztest nicht sicher erfaßt werden.

Herabsetzung oder Fehlen einzelner oder mehrerer Faktoren ist für die Entstehung von hämorrhagischen Diathesen wichtig. Einzelne Gerinnungsfaktoren

Tabelle 4. *Nomenklatur, Chemie und Wirkung der Gerinnungsfaktoren*

Nomenklatur	Chemische Natur	Physiologische Wirkung
Faktor I Fibrinogen	lösliches zirkulierendes fibrilläres Protein, 18 Aminosäuren Mol.-Gew. 330000 bis 400000, 600 Å lang	Vorläufer für Fibrin. Gibt unter Thrombin Fibrinopeptid ab, polymerisiert zu Fibrin-polymer und wird unter Fibrin stabilizing factor zu Fibrin
Faktor II Prothrombin	lösliches Glucoprotein: 18 Aminosäuren + Acetylhexosamin + Pentose	Proenzym: durch Verlust von zwei Aminosäuren und KH-Fraktion → Thrombin (= proteolytisches Enzym)
Faktor III (Gewebs-)Thrombokinase, Thromboplastin	Phospholipoidkomplex aus Gewebe (Lipoproteid)	beteiligt sich mit Calcium und drei Plasmafaktoren an der Bildung der Gewebsthrombokinase
Faktor IV Calcium	Mineral Ion	beschleunigt Bildung von Blut- und Gewebs-Thrombokinase
Faktor V Proaccelerin Acc. Globulin Plasma Accelerator Globulin	Sphäroprotein	labiler Accelerator für Konversion von Prothrombin in Thrombin (Blut- und Gewebsthrombokinase). Bildet unter Thrombin Faktor VI
Faktor VI Accelerin Serum accelerator	Sphäroprotein	durch Thrombin aktiviertes Proaccelerin. Beschleunigt Bildung der Gewebsthrombokinase
Faktor VII SPCA, stable factor (Serum prothrombin conversion factor)	Sphäroprotein	Faktor notwendig bei der Bildung der Gewebsthrombokinase
Faktor VIII Antihämophil. factor (AHF) Anti-Hämophil.-A-Faktor, Plättchenfaktor	Sphäroprotein	notwendiger Faktor bei der Bildung der Blutthrombokinase. Fehlt bei klassischer Hämophilie (A)
Faktor IX PTC (plasma thromboplastin component) Antihämophil. B-Faktor	Sphäroprotein	notwendiger Faktor für Bildung der Blutthrombokinase. Fehlt bei „Christmas disease" (Hämophilie B)
Faktor X Stuart-Prower Factor	Sphäroprotein	notwendiger Faktor für Bildung von Blut- und Gewebsthrombokinase
Faktor XI PTA (Plasma-Thromboplastin Antecedent)	Sphäroprotein	Plasma Factor in einer der hämophiloiden Krankheiten fehlend
Faktor XII Hageman-Faktor	Sphäroprotein	notwendig für normale Gesamtblut-Koagulation? Kontakt-Faktor?

Tabelle 5. *Kinetik der „Blutgerinnung"*
(Nach F. Koller: Der heutige Stand der Gerinnungsforschung, 1958)

1. *Bildung der Gewebsthrombokinase*

Gewebe-F. + F. VII + St. F. + Ca	→ Intermediär-Produkt (Convertin)
Intermed.-Prod. (Convertin) + F. V	→ Gewebethrombokinase (Prothrombinase)

2. *Bildung der Blutthrombokinase*

F. VIII + F. IX + St. F. + PPA + Ca	→ Intermediär-Prod. I
Intermediär-Prod. I + Plättchen-F. 3	→ Intermediär-Prod. II
Intermediär-Prod. II + F. V	→ Blutthrombokinase

fehlen bei den hereditären Koagulopathien, mehrere Faktoren können bei den erworbenen Koagulopathien herabgesetzt sein (s. späterer Abschnitt). Auch Überwiegen von physiologischen oder therapeutischen Antikoagulantien spielen bei den Blutungsübeln eine wichtige Rolle (Blutplättchen-Faktor 4, Heparin [Antithrombin], Dicoumarin) (Tabelle 4, s. auch Koagulopathien C.III.).

II. Klinisches Bild und Untersuchungsmethoden der hämorrhagischen Diathesen

Entsprechend Verlauf und klinischem Bild (Abb. 11) kann mit einiger Wahrscheinlichkeit eine Diagnose der mutmaßlich vorliegenden pathogenetischen Störungen gestellt werden.

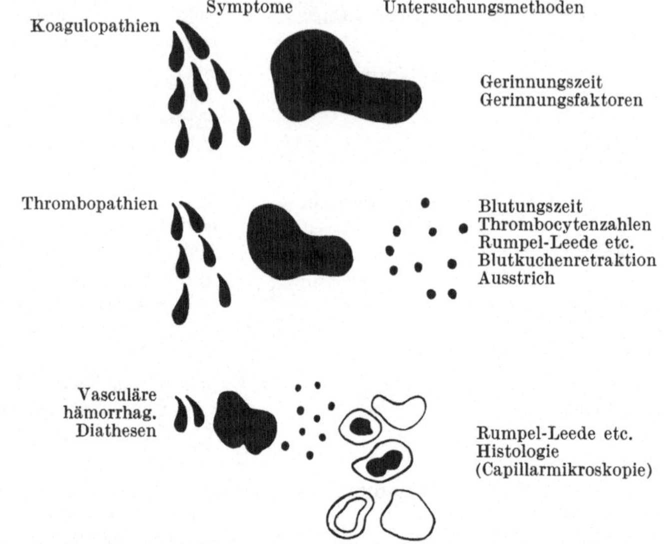

Abb. 11. Symptome und Untersuchungsmethoden bei hämorrhagischen Diathesen

1. Vasculäre hämorrhagische Diathesen

Bei den vasculären *hämorrhagischen Diathesen* (Vasopathien) finden sich meist nur unbedeutende Blutungen nach Verletzungen. Suffusionen treten weniger hervor, dagegen finden sich neben Petechien in der Regel polymorphe, primär- oder sekundär-hämorrhagische Hautefflorescenzen verschiedensten Aspektes, meist papulös-exsudativ, oft an Erythema exsudativum multiforme erinnernd. Oft sind die Efflorescenzen nur fakultativ-hämorrhagisch und vergesellschaften sich mit nicht-hämorrhagischen exsudativen Hautveränderungen (Abb. 11, 12). Bei *M. Schamberg* und *Purpura annularis Majocchi* beschränken sich die Veränderungen auf umschriebene, teils annuläre hämorrhagische ekzematoide Flecken. Als wichtigstes typisches Beispiel dieser vorwiegend vasculären hämorrhagischen Phänomene sei auf die anaphylaktoide Purpura (Abb. 12) verwiesen mit ihren hämorrhagischen, exsudativen, oft an Erythema exsudativa multiforme erinnernden Efflorescenzen besonders an Streckseiten der Extremitäten, lateralen Partien von Stamm und Glutäen, bei Fehlen von Blutungen in die Mundschleimhaut und spontanen Blutflüssen. Rheumatoide Gelenkbeschwerden können auf die anaphylaktoide Genese deuten (Storck 1955).

Bei den teleangiektatischen Vasopathien finden sich Blutungen an bestimmten lokalisierten Stellen der Gefäßveränderungen (Locus Kieselbachii, Augenhintergrund) bei Skorbut am Zahnfleisch, bei Morbus Möller-Barlow am Periost (JÜRGENS 1955). Aus dem klinischen Bild und den relativ einfachen Routine-Untersuchungen ist es dem Arzt meist möglich, eine Diagnose der hämorrhagischen Diathesen mit dem vorwiegend pathogenetischen Mechanismus zu stellen, um

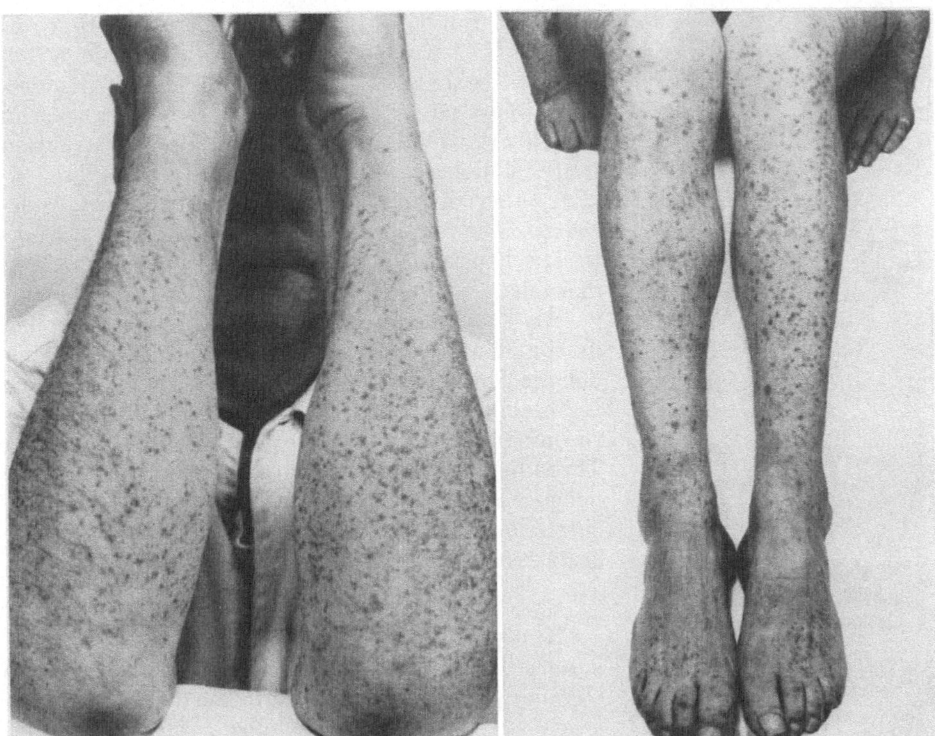

Abb. 12. Anaphylaktoide Purpura

sich weiterhin Rechenschaft darüber abzulegen, ob es sich um ein hereditäres oder erworbenes Leiden handelt, mit toxischer, allergischer, stoffwechsel- oder hormonbedingter, evtl. idiopathischer Ätiopathogenese (s. später).

2. Thrombocytogene Purpura (Thrombopenien, Thrombopathien)

Bei der *thrombocytogenen Purpura* finden sich unterhalb des meist kritischen Thrombocytenabfalles auf 30000/cm³ oder bei funktionsuntüchtigen Thrombocyten in normaler Zahl neben schwer stillbaren Blutungen aus kleinsten Verletzungen von Haut und Schleimhaut Suffusionen und Sugillationen, ferner typische Petechien als Ausdruck mangelnder sofortiger Abdichtung der verletzten Capillaren (Abb. 11, 13, 36). Das charakteristische klinische Bild für diese Form der hämorrhagischen Diathesen ist der nach WERLHOF, dem Mitbegründer der Göttinger Fakultät des Jahres 1737, benannte M. maculosus, mit Petechien, planen Ecchymosen und handtellergroßen cutanen Blutungen sowie Blutaustritten aus den Schleimhäuten, meist nach stumpfen Traumen (Abb. 13). Durch Abbau des Blutfarbstoffes älterer cutaner Hämorrhagien kann die Haut ein buntscheckiges Bild zeigen.

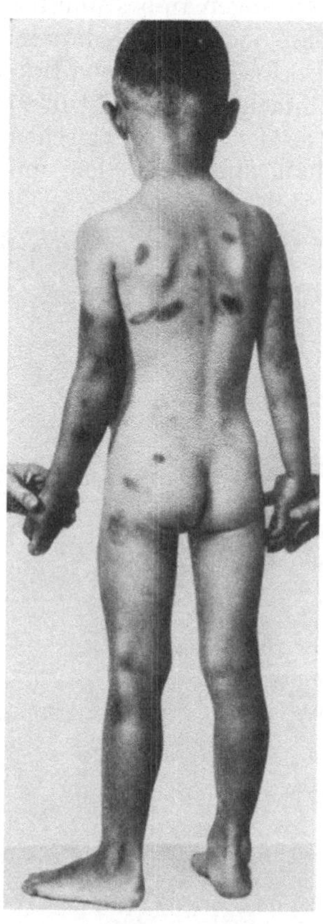

Abb. 13. Sugillationen bei essentieller Thrombopenie

Die verlängerte Blutungszeit über 2 min erweist den ungenügenden Gefäßabschluß infolge mangelnder Thrombocyten. Die Retraktion des Blutkuchens ist vermindert, die Gerinnungszeit normal. Positiver Rumpel-Leede- oder Kneif-Phänomen nach JÜRGENS weisen auf die sekundäre Gefäßschädigung hin.

Die *Thrombopathien* neigen mehr zum hämophilen als zum thrombopenischen Blutungstypus (JÜRGENS 1955). Hier werden ausgesprochene Blutungen in Schüben beobachtet, entweder im frühesten Kindesalter, meist mit letalem Ausgang, vermehrt auch in der Pubertät (Verbluten bei der ersten Menstruation junger Mädchen), dann im beginnenden Erwachsenenalter, aber oft mit Persistieren in späteren Lebensjahren. Die für thrombopenische Blutungen charakteristischen Haut- und Schleimhautblutungen fehlen meistens.

Als Untersuchungsmethoden kommen neben den in Abb. 11 angegebenen neuere Methoden hinzu, nämlich die Thrombelastographie nach HARTERT (s. auch G. MARCHAL u. a. 1959, P. DE NICOLA 1959), der Prothrombinkonsumptionsteste (nach QUICK) und der Thromboplastingenerationsteste (nach BIGGS), die neben verfeinerten Untersuchungen der Thrombocyten im Ausstrichpräparat eine exaktere Analyse gestatten.

3. Koagulopathien

Klinisch äußern sich *Koagulopathien* in schweren, kaum stillbaren Blutflüssen nach außen und in innere Organe. Bei der Hämophilie erfolgen die Blutungen in Schüben, meist während besonderer Altersperioden, z.B. im frühen Knabenalter, in der Pubertät, im frühen Mannesalter, mit Abflauen der Symptome im späteren Leben. Es handelt sich hier um schwer stillbare Blutungen aus Verletzungen (z.B. anläßlich von Zahnextraktionen), Blutungen in innere Organe (Nieren, Muskeln, Gelenke), bei stumpfen Traumen oft ringförmige Suffusionen unter die Haut, ebenso nach Sternalpunktion oder Schnepperstich (Abb. 14) (STORCK 1955, JÜRGENS 1955). An der Haut können sich mehr oder minder ausgedehnte, nichtentzündliche Suffusionen und Sugillationen finden, bei vollständigem Fehlen der für Thrombopathien und vasculäre hämorrhagische Diathesen

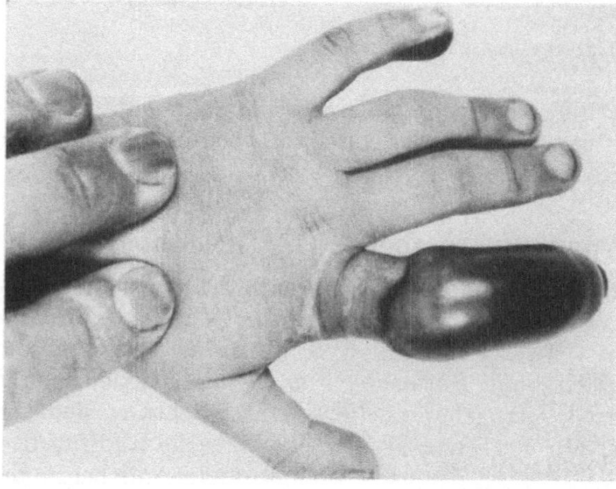

Abb. 14. Hautblutung nach Schnepperstich bei Hämophilie

typischen Petechien (Abb. 11). Die normalen Gefäßreaktionen mit funktionstüchtigen Endothelien und Thrombocyten genügen, um trotz schwerster Gerinnungsstörung nach Mikrotraumen die Gefäße abzudichten, weshalb Petechien und Ecchymosen ausbleiben. Die labormäßigen Untersuchungsmethoden ergeben Verminderung einzelner oder mehrerer Gerinnungsfaktoren, die Gerinnungszeit ist über 8 min verlängert, wogegen die Blutungszeit normal bleibt.

4. Spezielle Untersuchungsmethoden

Für die Gruppendiagnose sind neben dem klinischen Aspekt und der Anamnese relativ einfache Untersuchungsmethoden von Bedeutung (s. Abb. 11).

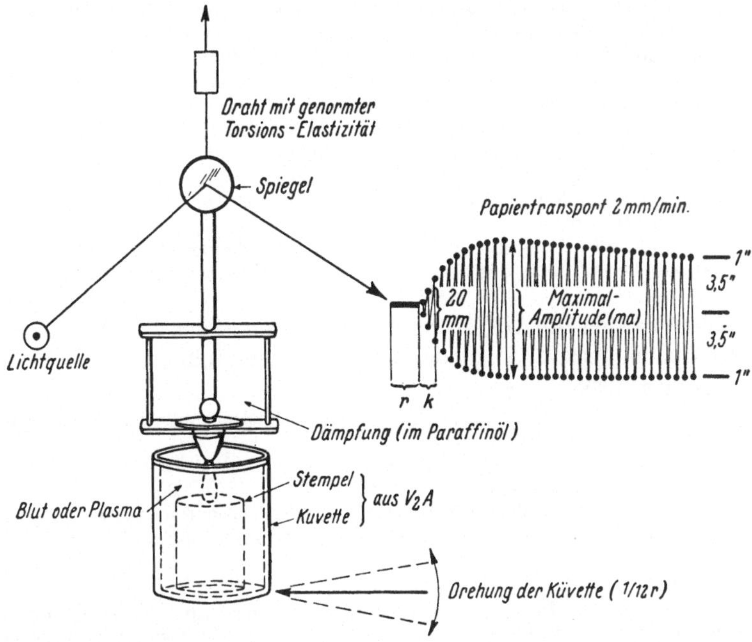

Abb. 15. Schematische Darstellung der Registrierungsvorgänge und der Kurvenentstehung im Hartertschen Thrombelastographen. (Aus R. GROSS: Hämorrhagische Diathesen. In: Klinik der Gegenwart, Bd. 9. München u. Berlin: Urban & Schwarzenberg u. Klin. Wschr. **1958**, 112)

Die *Gefäßbrüchigkeit* (vasculäre und thrombocytogene Purpura, Capillarfragilität) kann am Arm mit dem Stauversuch nach RUMPEL-LEEDE, durch den Kneif-Versuch nach JÜRGENS, durch Abheben und Drehen einer Hautfalte, evtl. durch dosierten Unterdruck (Saugglocke) geprüft werden.

Für die *Thrombocytenzählung* wurden mehrere Methoden entwickelt, so eine indirekte mit Beziehung zur Erythrocytenzahl (FONIO, LENGGENHAGER 1936) oder direkte Zählungen (O. THOMSEN 1919) nach Formaldehyd oder Citratzusatz (REES u. ECKER 1923), nach Cocainzusatz (FEISSLY u. LÜDIN 1949, MARMONT u. CIACCA 1957, BEIS 1960), mit Verwendung von Sequestrennatrium und hypotoner Cocainlösung (W. OSTEN 1959). Neuerdings gelang M. C. MORGAN u.a. (1961) nach Zusatz von Silicon und Zentrifugation die Isolierung und Zählung funktionstüchtiger Thrombocyten.

Eine grobe Prüfung der *Blutkuchenretraktion* ist möglich nach Aufenthalt des Vollblutes während 2 Std im Brutschrank oder 6 Std bei Zimmertemperatur, die *Blutungszeit*, z.B. mit Technik nach DUKE, läßt sich gut beurteilen und erleichtert die Diagnosestellung in Richtung der thrombocytogenen Purpura. Neuerdings hat sich die Prüfung der *Scheer-Elastizität* des gebildeten Gerinnsels mittels der *Thrombelastographie* nach HARTERT (1952) bewährt, welche auch eine krankhaft gesteigerte Fibrinolyse messen läßt (Abb. 15). Es zeigen sich z.B. typische Thrombelastogramme bei Hämophilie A, Thrombocytopenie, Hyperfibrinogenämie, gesteigerter Fibrinolyse (GROSS 1959).

Als zusätzliche Untersuchungsmethoden wird heute mit Gewinn der Prothrombinkonsumtion-Test nach QUICK und der Thromboplastingenerationstest von BIGGS durchgeführt (s. JÜRGENS und R. SCHOEN, Hämorrhagische Diathesen 1955).

Ein Einblick in die *Gerinnungsstörung* kann durch die Bestimmung der Gerinnungszeit, z.B. nach BÜRKER, ferner der verschiedensten Gerinnungsfaktoren gewonnen werden, hier besonders der Prothrombinzeit (Thromboplastinzeit) nach QUICK, die aber nicht nur vom Mangel an Prothrombin, sondern weiterhin an Faktor VII, V, Fibrinogen sowie Vermehrung gerinnungshemmender Substanzen abhängt (KOLLER 1952, GROSS 1959).

Die weitere Differenzierung der verschiedensten Gerinnungsfaktoren nach sorgfältiger Blutentnahme und Zusatz von Antikoagulantien geschieht am besten durch ein geschultes Gerinnungslaboratorium. Eine relativ einfache übersichtsmäßige Bestimmung geschieht mit dem Prinzip der Einstufung, wobei sämtliche Faktoren mit Ausnahme des zu bestimmenden Faktors im Gerinnungssystem konstant gehalten werden. Dazu kommen Bestimmung des Antithrombins (KOLLER 1952), evtl. der Prothrombinverbrauchstest (Konsumtionstest nach QUICK), Thromboplastingenerationstest nach DOUGLAS und BIGGS, Heparintoleranztest usw.

Die orientierenden Laboratoriumsteste zur Untersuchung einer hämorrhagischen Diathese werden ungefähr nach folgenden Richtlinien vorgenommen (GROSS 1959):

1. Die Teste sollen möglichst einfach sein, so daß sie bei vielen Kranken ohne allzu großen technischen Aufwand durchgeführt werden können.
2. Die Teste sollen möglichst empfindlich sein, damit fälschlich positive oder zweifelhafte Befunde eher zu weiteren Untersuchungen mit schließlich negativem Ergebnis führen und damit auch leichte Störungen nicht übersehen werden.
3. Die Teste sollen möglichst unspezifisch sein, d.h. einen möglichst breiten Bereich von Streuungen erfassen *(Globalteste)*.
4. Für die definitive Feststellung, welcher Mangelzustand einer etwaigen hämorrhagischen Diathese zugrunde liegt, sollen dann hochspezifische Laboratoriumsmethoden angewendet werden.

Demzufolge werden zur Abklärung der hämorrhagischen Diathesen von einigen Autoren routinemäßig z.B. folgende Reaktionen empfohlen:

Von A. FIEHRER (1958):

1. Blutgerinnungszeit, Retraktion des Blutkuchens, Bestimmung der Fibrinolyse.
2. Prothrombinzeit nach QUICK.
3. *Rumpel-Leede*, evtl. Saugglockenversuch.
4. Blutungszeit am Ohrläppchen.
5. Auszählung der geformten Blutelemente, d.h. Erythrocyten, Leukocyten und Blutplättchen, mit Beurteilung derselben bezüglich Größe, Gruppierung und Form im Ausstrichpräparat.

Von GROSS (1959):

Kneif-Versuch (RUMPEL-LEEDE), Blutungszeit, Heparingerinnungszeit, Quick im Plasma und im Serum, Gerinnung mit Thrombin, mit Normalplasma (ein Teil normales zu vier Teilen pathologisches Plasma).

Von HEGGLIN (1960):

Gerinnungszeit, Retraktion des Koagulums. Prothrombin-„Konzentration".

Wir selbst untersuchen z.B. die in Abb. 11 dargestellten Werte sowie die besonderen Gerinnungsfaktoren in Zusammenarbeit mit dem Gerinnungslaboratorium der Medizinischen Universitätsklinik Zürich.

Selbstverständlich können klinisch-dermatologische und histologische Untersuchungsmethoden besonders bei den vasculären Formen der hämorrhagischen Diathese wichtige differentialdiagnostische Hinweise geben, wie im speziellen Teil besprochen werden soll.

III. Besondere pathogenetische Prinzipien

Abgesehen von hereditären, toxischen, hormonellen und stoffwechselbedingten Störungen, welche an Gefäßen, Thrombocyten und Gerinnungsfaktoren, hereditär oder erworben, angreifen, kommen einzelne übergeordnete pathogenetische Prinzipien zur Wirkung. Es sind dies vor allen Dingen

1. immunpathologische Reaktionen mit Sensibilisierungen gegenüber körperfremden oder körpereigenen Stoffen und

2. unspezifische Reaktionen, wie das besonders gefäßaktive Shwartzman-Sanarelli-Phänomen.

Diese beiden Reaktionsformen sollen hier als pathogenetische Prinzipien kurz erörtert werden.

1. Immunpathologische Reaktionen

a) Anaphylaxie und Arthus-Phänomen

Nach spezifischer Sensibilisierung gegenüber körperfremden oder körpereigenen Antigenen (Allergenen) können nach Wiederkontakt mit den betreffenden Stoffen Schädigung der Gefäße, der Thrombocyten und der Gerinnungsfaktoren auftreten, mit hämorrhagischem Phänomen bei stärkster Ausprägung. Im Tierexperiment lassen sich solche Vorgänge am anaphylaktischen Grundversuch und am Arthus-Phänomen studieren.

α) Reaktionen an den Gefäßen

Beim anaphylaktischen Versuch und beim Arthus-Phänomen werden die Tiere spezifisch gegen ein Antigen (z.B. artfremdes Serum) mittels wiederholter parenteraler Injektionen in Intervallen von mehreren Tagen sensibilisiert. Je nach Antigen kann der anaphylaktische Schock durch intravenöse Reinjektion schon nach wenigen sensibilisierenden Applikationen oder erst später ausgelöst werden.

Die besondere Gefäßbeteiligung beim *anaphylaktischen Geschehen* erweisen unter anderem die Versuche von KNEPPER (1936), gemäß welchen mit zirkulationswirksamen Mitteln, wie Wärme, Kälte, Verabreichung von kreislaufaktiven Pharmaka und Hormonen, die anaphylaktische Reaktion nach der Auslösungsinjektion willkürlich an die Gefäße verschiedenster Körperregionen geleitet werden kann. Durch Verlangsamung des Blutstromes kommt dann an diesen Stellen das zirkulierende Antigen ausgiebiger mit den „zellständigen" Antikörpern, wahrscheinlich besonders an den Endothelien in Kontakt und löst die Reaktion lokalisiert aus.

Das *Arthus-Phänomen* kann durch subcutane oder intracutane Injektionen des Antigens nach vorangegangener spezifischer Sensibilisierung ausgelöst werden, tritt aber erst dann in Erscheinung, wenn durch wiederholte Antigen-Injektionen bereits ein hoher Titer an zirkulierenden Antikörpern erreicht wurde.

Auch *Antigen-Antikörperkomplexe* spielen wahrscheinlich eine Rolle (WEIGLE, DIXON u.a.).

Klinisch zeigen sich beim Arthus-Phänomen an der Reinjektionsstelle entzündliche Infiltrate, bei starken Reaktionen hämorrhagische Nekrosen. Bei den genannten Versuchsbedingungen tritt gegenüber dem Antigen eine spezifische Sensibilisierung durch Antikörperbildung ein. Gefäßschädigungen und Blutungen treten jedoch nur bei starken Reaktionen, gleichsam fakultativ in Erscheinung (STORCK 1951).

Daß die kleinsten Gefäße nicht nur bei der Antigen-Antikörper-Reaktion mitbeteiligt sind, sondern möglicherweise auch bei der Antikörperbildung selbst, lassen elektronenoptische Untersuchungen von v. ALBERTINI (1959) an Serum sensibilisierten Pferden vermuten. Er fand zwischen Endothelzellen der Netzcapillaren in nicht eitrigem, chronisch-entzündlichem Gewebe Plasmazellen, die dort sehr wahrscheinlich aus lymphoiden Vorstufen entstanden sind.

Die Kontraktion der glatten Muskulatur beim *anaphylaktischen Schock* ist das augenfälligste Symptom, nicht nur der Gefäße, sondern auch anderer Organe (Lebendbeobachtungen im Tierexperiment, MCMASTER 1959, ILLIG 1961). Bei intensivem Schock führen die Spasmen zum Stop der Blutströmung mit Asphyxie, bei starker Schädigung und Blutung. Die schädigende Antigen-Antikörper-Reaktion kann vom Blutstrom aus an den Endothelien zur Wirkung kommen. Als reaktionsauslösende Übermittlungssubstanzen bei solchen Antigen-Antikörper-Reaktionen wurden Histamin und histaminähnliche Substanzen, „slow reacting substances", Pepton, Proteinabbauprodukte, proteolytische Enzyme, weniger Acetylcholin diskutiert. Nach neueren Untersuchungen sind besonders lösliche

Antigen-Antikörperkomplexe im anaphylaktischen Versuch ausgesprochen gefäßaktiv (WEIGLE, DIXON u.a. 1958, 1960, 1961, MCCLUSKEY und BENACERRAF 1959).

Bei der *lokalen Anaphylaxie* von geringem Ausmaße ist die Quaddelbildung, die wahrscheinlich durch maximale Arteriolenkontraktion — dadurch Rückstauung aus dem Venolenanteil der Capillaren mit Transsudation — zustande kommt, von Bedeutung, führt aber nur in seltenen und intensiven Reaktionen zu Hämorrhagien.

Wichtiger als der generalisierte Schock ist für die Blutung das *Arthus-Phänomen*, welches nach OVARY und BIER (1953) durch lokale spezifische Reaktion der zirkulierenden Antikörper mit dem lokal injizierten Antigen oder umgekehrt zustande kommt. Ausmaß der Reaktion ist vom Sensibilisierungszustand, also besonders von der Quantität der Antikörper abhängig, was sich mit der passiven anaphylaktischen Übertragung beweisen läßt (FISHEL u. KABAT 1947 und BENACERRAF u. KABAT 1950, P. G. H. GELL u. T. HINDE 1954). Auch lösliche Antigen-Antikörperkomplexe scheinen hier von Bedeutung zu sein (SIQUEIRA u. BIER 1961). Beim Arthus-Phänomen entsteht in den ersten 20 Std Ödem, dann Blutung. Spasmen der Arteriolen, Verlangsamung des Blutstromes in Capillaren und erweiterten Venolen führen zu Stase und Thrombose, im Bindegewebe zu Ödem mit Leukocyteninfiltration, in den äußeren ischämischen und nekrotischen Bezirken zu Blutaustritten. Die Blutung ist je nach Intensität der Reaktion mehr oder weniger ausgeprägt (C. GERLACH 1923). Wahrscheinlich ist auch hier das Endothel der Capillaren primärer Reaktionsort (LETTERER 1956, MOON 1938).

Hier führt also die Arteriolenkonstriktion zur ischämischen Schädigung mit Änderung von Endothelpermeabilität, die Stase zu Thrombose. Folge ist Erythrocyten-Diapedese, evtl. ausgedehnte Hämorrhagie, Nekrose, dies möglicherweise infolge sekundärer infektiöser Gangrän.

Wenn also durch Antigen-Antikörper-Reaktion Endothelien und Gefäße einfach mittelbar bis zur Blutung geschädigt werden können, dann scheint dies um so mehr unmittelbar dann zu geschehen, wenn Tiere gegen die Endothelien selbst sensibilisiert sind, wenn sich also die Reaktionen direkt gegen die Endothelien als Antigene richten (KATSURA zit. nach CLARK und JACOBS 1950).

Für die spezifische Sensibilisierung mit möglicher Gefäßbeteiligung bei der auslösenden Reaktion kommt neben der anaphylaktischen Überempfindlichkeit auch die *infektionsallergische Sensibilisierung* (vom Tuberkulin-Typ) in Frage, die sich allerdings in wichtigen Punkten von der ersteren unterscheidet. Während sich im Tierexperiment die anaphylaktische Überempfindlichkeit und das lokalisierte Arthus-Phänomen durch Injektion von gelösten Antigenproteinen herbeiführen lassen, verlangt die infektionsallergische Sensibilisierung den parenteralen Kontakt mit vollständigen Mikroben oder mit besonderen mikrobeneigenen Substanzen, z.B. Lipopolysacchariden (RAFFEL). Im Cutantest zeigt sich die typische Spätreaktion. Antikörper lassen sich nicht mobil im Serum durch passive Übertragung, sondern lediglich sessil durch Übertragung von Lymphocyten nachweisen. Mikrobielle Sensibilisierungen von diesem Typus scheinen bei einem Teil der anaphylaktoiden Purpura (s. später) von Bedeutung zu sein, wobei Staphylo- und Streptokokken, Tuberkelbacillen u.a.m. das Antigen liefern.

Daß Sensibilisierung vom Spätreaktionstypus, ähnlich wie vom anaphylaktischen Sofort-Reaktionstypus, die Gefäßpermeabilität erhöht, jedoch in anderen Zeitintervallen, erwiesen Versuche von G. A. VOISIN (1960) unter anderem am Meerschweinchen. Ob allerdings solche Schädigungen bis zur Hämorrhagie führen, wurde von diesen Autoren nicht weiteruntersucht. Teils scheinen solche immunologische Gefäßschädigungen vom Tuberkulintyp durch Vermittlung von Histamin, Serotonin, Thrombocyten, Leukocyten zu entstehen, teils durch Antigen-Antikörper-Reaktionen direkt (J. H. HUMPHREY 1959).

Bei sensibilisierten Kaninchen ist nach S. IJIMA allgemein eine erhöhte Gefäßreagibilität auf unspezifische Reize (mechanisch, Kälte, Histamin) im Sinne von stärkeren und längeren Kontraktionen mit länger dauernder Nachdilatation zu beobachten, möglicherweise abhängig vom vegetativen Nervensystem (IJIMA 1958).

Auch MANWARING u.a. (1923), PETERSEN u. LEVINSON (1923), STORCK (1951) betonen, daß bei starken anaphylaktischen Reaktionen Blutextravasate entstehen. Häufig kommen aber Mischformen von Früh- und Spättypus in Frage (GELL u. HINDE 1954).

Mit mehr oder weniger Erfolg wurde versucht, auch histologisch eine Parallele zwischen den Veränderungen des anaphylaktischen Experimentes oder der infektionsallergischen Sensibilisierung bei den menschlichen Vasopathien zu ziehen (STORCK 1951).

β) Reaktionen an den Thrombocyten

Sowohl tierexperimentell als auch in der menschlichen Pathologie können Immunothrombopenien erzeugt oder beobachtet werden. Wie solche gewebsschädigende spezifische Reaktionen klassifiziert werden können, zeigt ein Schema

Tabelle 6. *In vivo-Auswirkungen von Antigen-Antikörper-Reaktionen*[1]
(Aus P. MIESCHER u. K. O. VORLAENDER: Immunopathologie in Klinik und Forschung, 2. Aufl. Stuttgart: Georg Thieme 1961)

	Phylakogene Wirkungen		Pathogene Wirkungen oder Folgen				
	Antitoxische	Antibakterielle	Unmittelbare	Einfache mittelbare	Indirekte		
					Frühreaktionstypus	Intermediärreaktionstypus	Spätreaktionstypus
Mechanismen oder Beispiele	Neutralisation von toxischen Substanzen usw.	Zerstörung von Mikroorganismen durch Opsonisierung, Bakteriolyse, Bakteriostase usw.	Cytotrope oder cytotoxische Wirkungen von gegen genetisch determinierte Gewebsantigene gerichteten Hetero-, Iso- oder Auto-Antikörpern; Transfusionszwischenfälle	Passive Hämagglutination mit Hämolyse (Anämie!); medikamentöse Leukopenien und Thrombopenien	Anaphylaktischer Schock; urticarielle Reaktion; Heufieber; Asthma; passive cutane Anaphylaxie	Arthus-Phänomen; Periarteritis nodosa	Tuberkulin-Reaktion; allergisches Ekzem
Latenzzeit bis zum Manifestwerden der Reaktion	Minuten	Minuten bis Stunden	Minuten	Minuten bis Stunden	Minuten	Stunden	Tage
Mitwirkung von: Komplement	0	+	0 (oder +)	+	+	0	0[2]
Mitwirkung von: Histamin usw.	0	?	0	vielleicht (?)	+	0	0[2]
Passive Übertragung durch	Serum	Serum	Serum	Serum	Serum	Serum	Zellen
Antikörper-Eigenschaften: Präcipitierend	+	+	+	+	+	+	Wahrscheinlich spezielle Antikörper
Antikörper-Eigenschaften: Nichtpräcipitierend	+	+ (?)	+	+	+	0	

[1] Vereinfacht und abgeändert nach B. H. WAKSMAN (unveröffentlicht) und P. MIESCHER (unveröffentlicht).
[2] Wahrscheinlich andere, noch unbekannte Substanzen.

von B. H. WAKSMAN und P. MIESCHER (1961), in welchem zwischen unmittelbaren cytotropen oder cytotoxischen und einfach mittelbaren (z.B. medikamentöser Thrombopenie) Immunoreaktionen unterschieden wird (Tabelle 6).

Vom anaphylaktischen Tierexperiment ist bekannt, daß Thrombocyten bei der Auslösungsreaktion abfallen (E. W. SCHULTZ 1924, STORCK 1951). Möglicherweise agglutinieren die Thrombocyten unspezifisch bei der Antigen-Antikörper-Reaktion und werden im Capillarbett von Lunge, Leber, Milz, evtl. auch anderer Organe, abgefangen. Sie würden beim vorerwähnten Schema bei der einfach mittelbaren oder bei der indirekten Immunreaktion (Anaphylaxie = Frühreaktionstyp, Arthus-Phänomen = Intermediärtyp) indirekt in Mitleidenschaft gezogen. Möglicherweise ist beim anaphylaktischen Thrombocytenabfall auch der Anstieg des Heparins im Blut von Bedeutung (MARMONT u.a. 1954). Solche Reaktionen können in der Humanpathologie bei bestimmten Formen von thrombopenischer Purpura auf Arzneimittel entstehen, so bei Chinidin, Chinin usw., evtl. in seltenen Fällen auch bei mittelbaren thrombopenischen Reaktionen auf Nahrungsmittel und Infektionsallergene.

Im Tierversuch an Meerschweinchen und Kaninchen führen nach SIQUEIRA u. NELSON (1961) Antigen-Antikörper-Komplementkomplexe zu Thrombocytenagglutination, indem sich diese möglicherweise an besonderen Receptoren der Plättchenoberfläche fixieren. Diese Agglutination geht nach Erhitzung (während 15 min auf 56°C) oder nach Behandlung mit Trypsin oder Chymotrypsin verloren, ebenso nach EDTA. Die Agglutination kann mit S. typhosa, aber auch mit gewissen Dextranen, die als „präparierend“ oder „auslösend“ beim Shwartzman-Phänomen wirken, studiert werden. Neuerdings wurden besondere Techniken zum Nachweis von Thrombocytenagglutininen (z.B. Schüttelmethode mit Hilfe formalinisierter Thrombocyten) ausgearbeitet (MAJSKY u.a. 1960, sowie weitere Techniken von DAUSSET u.a. 1958). Nach PAGE (1954) wird durch Antigen-Antikörper-Reaktionen aus den Thrombocyten das gefäßwirksame Histamin und Serotonin liberiert (s. auch HUMPHREY 1959).

Durch Verminderung der Thrombocyten mit Abnahme des Thromboplastins sowie des Antithrombins kommt es im Tierversuch zur bekannten Abnahme der Blutkoagulabilität im anaphylaktischen Schock (SCHULTZ 1924).

Von größerer Bedeutung scheinen in zunehmendem Maße die unmittelbaren cytotropen Immunreaktionen mit Beteiligung von Iso- und Autoantikörpern zu werden. Die von ACKROYD beschriebene Thrombocytolyse unter Komplementeinwirkung bei Sedormid, in welchem nach seiner Hypothese ein Antikörper gegen den Thrombocyten-Sedormid-Komplex entstehe, stellt wohl einen Intermediärfall dar.

Immunisierungsversuche an Kaninchen gegenüber gewaschenen Thrombocyten von Meerschweinchen wurden schon früh durchgeführt, so von MARINO (1905), COLE (1908), LEDINGHAM (1914 u.a., 1915), GOTTLIEB (1919) (zit. nach P. MIESCHER 1961). Mittels solcher Tierversuche konnten sowohl Hetero- als auch Isoantikörper nachgewiesen werden, die zu Thrombocytolyse führten, mit und ohne Purpura. Man hat erkannt, daß die Thrombocyten besondere antigene Strukturen haben und mindestens in vier bis sechs blutgruppenähnliche Klassen differenziert werden können.

Besonders schöne Versuche führten TOCANTINS u. STEWART (1939, 1940) mit Antiplättchenseren am Hunde durch. Sie fanden am 1.—5. Tag nach Seruminjektion ein erstes akutes Stadium mit Thrombopenie, verlängerter Blutungszeit, Hämorrhagie in die Gewebe, Ödem und Pigmentablagerung, vom 5.—10. Tag ein intermediäres Stadium mit Anstieg der Plättchen, verkürzter Blutungszeit, mit vielen vasculären Thromben in diversen Organen, besonders in der Milz, und schließlich nach dem 10. Tag ein Reaktionsstadium mit hoher Plättchenzahl, hyperplastischer Reaktion in Knochenmark, Milz, Lymphknoten und Thymus.

Nach WITTE (1956) kommt es nach Antithrombocytenreaktionen bei der Ratte nicht nur zu intravasaler Agglutination der Plättchen, sondern auch zur Schädigung der Megakaryocyten im Knochenmark mit thrombopenischer Purpura.

Von 1938—1953 wurden durch verschiedene Forscher wichtige experimentelle Untersuchungen durchgeführt, welche die Natur der cytotoxischen Thrombopenien erwiesen (Tabelle 7). Es folgten mehrere Arbeiten, die den Nachweis erbrachten, daß Immunothrombopenien vorkommen, welche durch einen Serumfaktor von der Art eines Thrombocytenantikörpers bedingt sind. Wie aber solche Autoantikörper entstehen und durch welchen Mechanismus die Thrombocyten bis zur Antigenität denaturiert werden, ist noch unbekannt. P. MIESCHER denkt an

Tabelle 7. *Entwicklung der Forschung über die Natur des thrombocytopenogenen Faktors bei der essentiellen Thrombopenie*

(Aus P. MIESCHER: Immunothrombopenien. In: JÜRGENS u. DEUTSCH, Hämorrhagische Diathesen, S. 44. Internat. Symposium. Wien: Springer 1955)

		Cytotoxische Thrombopenien
1938	TROLAND u. LEE	„*Thrombocytopen*" (Aceton-Milzextrakt)
1949	EVANS u. DUANE	Vermuten erstmals das Vorhandensein von *Thrombocyten-Autoantikörpern* in Analogie zu den Erythrocyten-Autoantikörpern
1950	EPSTEIN u. Mitarb.	*Thrombopenie von Neugeborenen*, deren Mütter an einer chronischen idiopathischen Thrombopenie erkrankt sind (Immunkörper)
1951	EVANS u. Mitarb.	Nachweis eines *Thrombocytenagglutinins*
1951	HARRINGTON u. Mitarb.	Transfusionsversuche: *thrombocytopenogener Faktor*
1951	STEFANINI u. CHATTERJEA	*Verkürzte Lebensdauer* transfundierter Thrombocyten bei Fällen von idiopathischer Thrombopenie
1952	MIESCHER, CRUCHAUD, HEMMELER	*Spezifität des Plättchenagglutinins* bei idiopathischer Thrombopenie durch *Absorptionsversuch* bewiesen. Wirkung auf *Kaninchen-Thrombocyten* analog der Aktion eines experimentellen Antithrombocytenserums
1953	STEFANINI u. Mitarb.	Anwendung des *Coombs-Testes* für Thrombocyten-*Absorptionsversuche.* Wirkung auf Kaninchen-Thrombocyten. *Antikörper in β_2-Fraktion*

die Möglichkeit, daß es sich dabei um eine Fehlleistung der Eiweißproduktion wie bei den Paraproteinen handeln könnte.

Zweifellos kommen nicht nur immunologisch bedingte Schwankungen der peripheren Thrombocytenzahl vor.

So erhöhen nach H. P. WRIGHT (1944) Pyridin-Injektionen und Adrenalin die Thrombocytenzahl, und nach BUTLER u.a. (1950) führt Histamin durch Plättchenzerfall zur Verminderung. Auch die in ihrer Pathogenese noch umstrittene thrombocytenverändernde Wirkung der Milz läßt sich nach COONEY u.a. (1961) bei Mäusen, Kaninchen und Hunden durch Injektionen von gereinigtem Extrakt aus normaler Rindermilz nachahmen.

γ) Mitbeteiligung von Gerinnungsfaktoren

Auch diese können im anaphylaktischen Tierexperiment verändert werden, wie dies schon früher an der Ungerinnbarkeit des Blutes beobachtet wurde. Beim anaphylaktischen Schock zeigt sich ein steiler Anstieg des Heparins, etwa 1—2 Std dauernd, der alsdann wieder abfällt bis zur Norm. Beim Arthus-Phänomen hingegen ist ein solcher Anstieg des Heparins flach und deutlich protrahiert (HOIGNÉ 1951, STORCK 1951). Solche Steigerungen des Antithrombintiters vorübergehender Natur finden sich auch in der Humanpathologie, z.B. bei der anaphylaktoiden Purpura (STORCK 1955, Tabelle 10).

b) Das Shwartzman-Sanarelli-Phänomen

Beim Sanarelli-Shwartzman-Phänomen werden die Tiere durch Injektion von endotoxinhaltigen Bakterienfiltraten unspezifisch umgestimmt. Ähnlich wie für das Arthus-Phänomen eignen sich zum Versuch am besten Kaninchen, weniger Meerschweinchen, und schlecht Ratten sowie Mäuse.

Die *Präparierung* gelingt besonders gut mit Filtraten von gramnegativen Bakterien, aber auch alte Kulturen von grampositiven Bakterien, Viren sowie spezifische Antigen-Antikörper-Reaktionen (z.B. infektionsallergische Vorgänge) können die Umstimmung herbeiführen. Beim lokalisierten Shwartzman-Phänomen geschieht die Präparation durch intracutane Injektion oder durch Injektion in Organe oder Gelenke (G. SHWARTZMAN 1928, 1935). Beim generalisierten Sanarelli-Phänomen (1924) wird die Vorbereitung durch eine oder mehrere, kurz aufeinanderfolgende intravenöse oder intraperitoneale Injektionen der präparierenden Substanz durchgeführt.

Wenn zur *Auslösung* beim lokalen Shwartzman-Phänomen dasselbe Filtrat oder auch ein mit der Präparierung nicht verwandtes Bakterienfiltrat, Stärke, Agar, Kaolin oder bei spezifisch sensibilisiertem Organismus das Antigen 20—48 Std nach Präparierung intravenös injiziert wird, treten nach wenigen Stunden akute Blutungen auf. Beim Shwartzman-Phänomen beschränkt sich die Blutung auf die präparierte Hautstelle oder auf das präparierte Organ, beim generalisierten Sanarelli-Phänomen betreffen diese Blutungen innere Organe, wie Nieren, Lungen, Darm, Lymphdrüsen und Leber (zit. s. STORCK 1951).

Tabelle 8. *Anaphylaxie (Arthus-Phänomen) und Sanarelli-(Shwartzmann-)Phänomen* [Aus H. STORCK, Dermatologica (Basel) 102, 197 (1951)]

	Anaphylaxie (Arthus)	Sanarelli (Shwartzman)
1. Vorbereitende Injektion	einmal bis mehrmals	einmal
2. Intervall Vorbereitung — Auslösung	Minimum 8—14 Tage	2—72 Std
3. Spezifität	spezifisch	unspezifisch
4. Auslösung	antigene Substanzen	auch nichtantigene Substanzen
5. Passive Übertragung	möglich	nicht möglich
6. Desensibilisierung	möglich	nicht möglich

Die zweite Injektion kann auch mit synthetischen sauren großmolekularen Polymeren, wie Na-Polyantylsulfat, Na-Polyvinylalkohol-Sulfonat, Dextran-Sulfonat usw. geschehen, und zwar hier bereits 4 Std nach der ersten Injektion (THOMAS 1958).

Diese hämorrhagischen Umstimmungen sind unspezifisch, zeitlich begrenzt und passiv nicht übertragbar. Die Blutung ist nicht, wie beim Arthus-Phänomen, von der Stärke der Reaktion abhängig, sondern tritt als Hauptsymptom auch bei schwachen Reaktionen obligat in Erscheinung. Der Unterschied zwischen Anaphylaxie (Arthus-Phänomen) und Sanarelli-Shwartzman-Phänomen ist auf Tabelle 8 dargestellt (STORCK 1951).

Das Shwartzman-Sanarelli-Phänomen ist für das Verständnis der hämorrhagischen Diathesen besonders interessant, da sich hier maximale Schädigungen der kleinen Gefäße mit obligaten Blutungen einstellen, wie erwähnt beim Shwartzman-Phänomen lokalisiert an vorbehandelter Haut, beim Sanarelli-Phänomen generalisiert in den verschiedensten parenchymatösen Organen. Der Mechanismus, der zu solchen maximalen Gefäßstörungen führt, scheint beim Shwartzman-Phänomen auf leukocytär-thrombocytären Gefäßverschlüssen und fibrinoiden Thromben zu beruhen, bei welchen allerdings leukocytäre Prozesse Vorbedingung sind (s. auch H. T. KARSNER u.a. 1934).

Beide Phänomene lassen sich durch leukocytenvermindernde Maßnahmen wie Behandlung mit Nitrogen mustard, Röntgenbestrahlungen, antileukocytären Seren verhindern, ebenso durch thromboseverhindernde Mittel wie Heparin, Dicumarol u. a. m. Die conditio sine qua non für beide Phänomene ist mindestens einmalige Einwirkung von Toxin aus gramnegativen Bakterien (Endotoxin, Lipoide oder Lipopolysaccharide), die nicht allergisierend, sondern rein toxisch bzw. umstimmend auf die verschiedensten Körperzellen oder biologischen

Systeme wirken (THOMAS 1958). Daß die erste oder zweite Phase, besonders beim lokalisierten, weniger beim generalisierten Phänomen, durch spezifische Antigen-Antikörper-Reaktionen, insbesondere vom Tuberkulintypus, ersetzt werden kann, besagt jedoch nicht, daß das Phänomen allergischer Natur ist.

Wenn auch noch vieles in der Pathogenese des Shwartzman-Sanarelli-Phänomens nicht geklärt ist, sei dasselbe doch wegen seiner möglichen Bedeutung besonders für die vasculären hämorrhagischen Diathesen kurz in den wesentlichen Erforschungsphasen dargestellt (s. auch THOMAS 1958, MCMASTER 1959).

METTLER u. Mitarb. fanden 1958, daß das Shwartzman-Phänomen durch Dämpfung der blutbildenden Organe, d.h. durch Leukopenie (z.B. mittels Benzol), Röntgenganzbestrahlung (800 r 3—4 Tage vor Präparierung), Nitrogen mustard (0,5—2 mg/kg Körpergewicht i.v. 3—5 Tage vor Präparierung) unterdrückt werden kann.

Das Shwartzman-Phänomen entsteht durch *einmalige Injektion*, wenn beim spezifisch sensibilisierten Tier gleichzeitig mit dem Endotoxin das Antigen injiziert wird (BLACK-SCHAFFER u.a. 1950), wenn die Kaninchen unter Cortison stehen (THOMAS u. GOOD 1952), wenn Thorotrast oder Trypanblau unmittelbar vor der Toxininjektion eingespritzt werden (GOOD u. THOMAS 1952), wenn die Kaninchen von einer lokalen oder generalisierten Streptokokkeninfektion befallen sind (THOMAS, DENNY, FLOYD 1953), oder wenn das Toxin mit Tuberkulin beim tuberkulinisierten Tier injiziert wird (STETSON 1955).

Die Steigerung der Reagibilität beim Shwartzman-Sanarelli-Phänomen durch Thorotrast und Trypanblau beruht wahrscheinlich auf Blockierung des Reticuloendothelialsystems (WIZNITZER u.a. 1960), welches dadurch die bakteriellen Endotoxine ungenügend inaktiviert.

Daß die *periphere Leukopenie* und *Thrombopenie* für Vorbereitung oder Auslösung des Shwartzman-Phänomens von Bedeutung ist, geht aus den Versuchen von STETSON u.a. 1951 hervor, die zeigten, daß die verschiedensten Agentien wie Glucogen, Agar, Antigen-Antikörperkomplexe sowohl periphere Leuko- und Thrombopenie erzeugen, als auch das Shwartzman-Phänomen vorbereiten oder auslösen. Bei peripheren Leuko- und Thrombopenien finden sich Agglutinate dieser Zellen in den kleinen Gefäßen von Haut oder parenchymatösen Organen und verstopfen die Capillaren (STETSON 1951). Kurz nach der auslösenden Injektion lassen sich dann an diesen Stellen Leukocytentrümmer mit Capillarschädigung bis zur Hämorrhagie nachweisen. Durch die Präparierung wird unter notwendiger Mitwirkung der Leukocyten das intracelluläre Katepsin aktiviert mit Veränderung des lokalen Redoxpotentials, Vermehrung der aeroben Glykolyse, Anreicherung von Milchsäure, Absinken des p_H (STETSON u. GOOD 1951). Mittels Injektion von Tusche läßt sich nachweisen, daß Gefäßdilatation und Stase in den Nierenglomeruli eine wesentliche Voraussetzung für die Auslösung des Sanarelli-Phänomens darstellen (MCKAY, ROWE 1960).

Neben peripherer Leukopenie und Thrombopenie finden sich nach Auslösung des Shwartzman-Phänomens Anstieg des Antithrombins, Steigerung der Prothrombinaktivität, beim Sanarelli-Phänomen Mangel an Faktor V (HOIGNÉ 1951). Neue Untersuchungen von RODRIGUEZ-ERDMANN u.a. (1961) beim Sanarelli-Shwartzman-Phänomen ergaben einen Aktivitätsverlust der Faktoren V, IX, Prothrombin, Fibrinogen und PTA im Sinne einer Verbrauchskoagulopathie. Daneben fand sich die bekannte Verminderung der Thrombocyten im strömenden Blut mit Verminderung der Thrombocytenfaktoren 1 und 3.

Entsprechend der Wirkung von ACTH auf Blutplättchen, Antithrombin, Prothrombin und Capillarresistenz läßt sich das Shwartzman-Phänomen durch dieses Hormon tierexperimentell abschwächen oder vollständig unterdrücken (HOIGNÉ/KOLLER/STORCK 1951). Daß die Mikrothrombose in den Capillaren für die Blutung bei Reinjektion von Bedeutung ist, erweisen die Versuche von GOOD u. THOMAS (1953), nämlich Verhinderung des Phänomens durch Heparin in einer Dosis, die das Blut für 4 Std ungerinnbar macht. Auch durch Dicumarol läßt sich das Shwartzman-Sanarelli-Phänomen unterdrücken (SPANONDIS u.a. 1955).

Eine eigenartige Beziehung zwischen Änderung des Fibrinogen-Fibrin-Komplexes und Entstehung von Blutungen erforschten beim Sanarelli-Phänomen THOMAS u.a. (1955, 1958). Das besonders in den Capillaren der Nieren zur Blutung führende Fibrinoid entsteht nach diesen Autoren wahrscheinlich durch qualitative Änderung des Fibrinogenmoleküls mit anschließender Präcipitation durch ein saures Polymer. Durch die erste Toxininjektion komme das veränderte präcipitable Fibrinogen zustande und erscheine vorübergehend im Blut, wodurch Leukocytenänderung und ein saures Polymer, möglicherweise ein Polysaccharid auftreten. Bei der zweiten Endotoxininjektion werde erneut das präcipitable Fibrinogen gebildet, mit anschließender intravasculärer Präcipitation.

Die zweite Toxininjektion kann durch Dextransulfonat, Natriumpolyanetholsulfonat, Natriumpolyvinylalkoholsulfonat ersetzt werden. Dies kann so interpretiert werden, daß diese sauren Polymere die Funktion der Leukocyten beim Sanarelli-Phänomen übernehmen, denn durch Nitrogen mustard läßt sich diese blutungsauslösende Endotoxin-Polymer-Kombination nicht unterdrücken. Daß tatsächlich die Präcipitation des pathologischen Fibrinogens für die Blutung eine Rolle spielt, zeigt bei der Auslösung der abrupte Fibrinogenabfall im Blut, welcher mit dem das Sanarelli-Phänomen verhindernden Heparin aufgehoben werden kann. Bei der Ausscheidung des Fibrins oder Fibrinoids spielt wahrscheinlich das RES eine bedeutende Rolle, denn das Shwartzman-Sanarelli-Phänomen läßt sich durch Thrombininfusion nur nach Blockierung desselben erzeugen (Lee 1962). Auch mit thrombelastographischen Untersuchungen konnte gezeigt werden, daß beim Sanarelli-Shwartzman-Phänomen nicht Fibrinogenabbauprodukte auftreten (also keine Fibrinolyse), sondern daß eine intravasale Gerinnung (Verbrauchskoagulopathie) von entscheidender Bedeutung ist (Müller-Berghaus u.a. 1963).

Das beim Sanarelli-Shwartzman-Phänomen wirksame Fibrinoid kann jedoch gegenüber der Norm nicht sehr verändert sein, denn elektronenmikroskopisch zeigt sich, daß das in den Capillaren beim Sanarelli-Phänomen auftretende Fibrinoid in der Periodik dem gewöhnlichen Fibrin gleicht (Bohle u.a. in „Immunopathologie“ 1959).

Beim Shwartzman-Sanarelli-Phänomen wird durch das präparierende oder auslösende bakterielle Endotoxin auch die Reaktionsfähigkeit von Arteriolen und Venolen gegenüber Adrenalin oder Norepinephrin beeinflußt (Thomas 1959), denn durch einseitige sympathische Denervation der Niere beim Kaninchen, 5—21 Std vor der auslösenden Injektion, kann das Sanarelli-Phänomen an der operierten Niere in der Regel unterdrückt werden. Das intakte, sympathische Nervensystem scheint also für die Reaktion notwendig zu sein (Palmerio u.a. 1962). Die Bedeutung des zentralen autonomen Nervensystems ist noch umstritten (Alechinsky 1958). Durch Trypsin läßt sich das Shwartzman-Phänomen potenzieren (Antopol u.a. 1960). Die Schwierigkeit der passiven Übertragung des Shwartzman-Sanarelli-Phänomens wurde neuerdings nochmals von Nagler u. Zweifach (1961) betont und weiter untersucht.

Das generalisierte Shwartzman-Sanarelli-Phänomen scheint nach neuesten Untersuchungen bei der trächtigen Ratte auch diätetisch auslösbar zu sein. Werden nämlich trächtige Ratten zuerst mit einer tocopherolfreien Diät, dann mit einer Diät reich an oxydierten Lipiden gefüttert, entstehen Fibrinthrombi mit Sanarelli-ähnlichen Blutungen in Glomeruli, Lungen, Leber, Milz, Nebennieren und Uterus. Die Todesrate kann hier aber durch Antibiotica um das Vierfache vermindert werden (Kaunitz u.a. 1962). Ob diese Beobachtungen mit der Permeabilitätssteigerung der Capillaren beim Kücken bei Vitamin E-Mangel in Beziehung stehen (Dam u. Glavind 1940), muß weiter untersucht werden. Auch Vitamin K scheint für das Shwartzman-Phänomen von Bedeutung zu sein (Oswald 1956).

So wie dies heute beurteilt werden kann, stellt das Shwartzman-Sanarelli-Phänomen also ein zweiphasisches hämorrhagisches Phänomen dar, an welchem Thrombocyten, Leukocyten, Gerinnungsfaktoren, Fibrinogen, Polysaccharide und weitere Substanzen, möglicherweise auch die vegetative Innervation beteiligt sind, und das umschrieben zur massiven Gefäßschädigung führt. Nach Bernard (1963) ist das Primum movens dieser anfänglich thrombopenischen, dann hämorrhagischen, schließlich nekrotischen Reaktion noch unbekannt (s. auch Alechinsky 1957).

Es finden sich aber auch gewisse Ähnlichkeiten zwischen *Arthus-Reaktion* und *Shwartzman-Phänomen*, indem beispielsweise bei beiden Vorgängen eine Verminderung der polymorphkernigen Leukocyten, z.B. durch Nitrogen mustard oder Antileukocytenseren den Gewebs- oder Gefäßschaden verhindert (Stetson 1951, Humphrey 1955, 1959). Trotz dieser unbedeutenden Gemeinsamkeiten erscheint es aber nicht gerechtfertigt, diese fundamental verschiedenen Phänomene zu vermengen.

Wieweit das „*Phänomen von Reilly*“ evtl. dem Shwartzman-Sanarelli-Phänomen gleicht, ist noch nicht genügend untersucht. Reilly u.a. hatten 1934 bei Meerschweinchen, Mäusen, Ratten, Hunden, Ziegen und Katzen durch Injektion von verschiedensten Noxen (Toxin von Typhus, Paratyphus, Diphtherie, ferner Bleiacetat, Nickel, Chrom) nach operativer Freilegung unmittelbar in den linken Splanchnicus hämorrhagische Reaktionen im Verdauungstractus erzeugt. Innerhalb von wenigen Stunden nach der Injektion in kleinen Dosen entstanden progressive Hämorrhagien in Magen, Dünn- und Dickdarm sowie Mesenterialdrüsen. Histologisch waren Endothelveränderungen mit Nekrosen und Thrombosen, in Capillaren und Arteriolen nachweisbar. Anscheinend war die Reaktion von der Schädigung des Sympathicus abhängig, denn intraarterielle Injektionen zeitigten keine Ergebnisse.

2. Weitere Mechanismen

Zweifellos sind noch weitere allgemein-pathogenetische Prinzipien bei der Entstehung hämorrhagischer Diathesen von Interesse, so *Leberstörungen*, und zwar bei den erworbenen Koagulopathien im Sinne von Störungen der Prothrombinsynthese, ferner *Avitaminosen* (Vitamin C- und P-Mangel) bei der Entstehung gewisser vasculärer hämorrhagischer Diathesen (s. spezieller Teil).

Aber auch Stoffwechselstörungen verschiedenster Genese können zu Blutungsübeln mit verschiedenartigen Angriffspunkten führen. So wurde schon bei chronischen und akuten Urämien auf das gehäufte Vorkommen von hämorrhagischen Diathesen hingewiesen (Kendall u.a. 1961). Auch hier werden verschiedene Angriffspunkte diskutiert, nämlich

1. Capillarschaden (Rumpel-Leede oft positiv), erkennbar in maximaler Capillardilatation im Magen-Darmtrakt mit Blutungen, verlängerter Blutungszeit bei normalen Thrombocyten, erniedrigtem Serotoningehalt in den Thrombocyten.
2. Thrombocytenschädigung (Schädigung von Faktor 3, abnormer Phosphatidgehalt der urämischen Plättchen, allerdings bei elektronenoptisch normalen Thrombocyten, Unterdrückung der Knochenmarkmegakaryocyten).
3. Verlängerung der Prothrombin-Gerinnungszeit.

Auch die interessanten Beziehungen zwischen Nieren-Hormone-Stoffwechsel und hämorrhagischen Diathesen wurden neuerdings tierexperimentell untersucht. Masson u.a. (1962) erzeugten bei Ratten, die mit Aldosteron und NaCl vorbehandelt worden waren, durch Injektion von Renin Okklusionen der Glomeruli mit Niereninsuffizienz, Wasserretention, Gefäßläsion und Hämorrhagien.

B. Spezieller Teil

I. Die vasculären hämorrhagischen Reaktionen

Die vasculären hämorrhagischen Diathesen stellen ein komplexes, pathogenetisch z.T. noch wenig geklärtes Geschehen dar. Neben den eingangs erwähnten neueren Erkenntnissen über Struktur, Ultrastruktur, physiopathologischen Reaktionen der terminalen Strombahn haben besonders die von Mueller (1939) in zwei Bänden dargestellten capillarmikroskopischen Untersuchungen wichtige Einblicke in physiologische und pathologische Reaktionen des Capillarbettes geliefert, und weitere Resultate sind möglicherweise durch Capillarmikroskopie an anderer Hautstelle nach Abrißtechnik oder mit anderen neueren Untersuchungsmethoden zu erwarten.

Die vasculären hämorrhagischen Reaktionen können in kongenitale (hereditäre) und erworbene gruppiert werden (Tabelle 9).

Allgemein handelt es sich bei den seltenen kongenitalen, in der Regel umschriebenen Gefäßläsionen um lokalisierte, rezidivierende Blutungen, meist infolge angeborener, circumscripter Gefäßbrüchigkeit bei Teleangiektasien, wogegen bei den erworbenen vasculären hämorrhagischen Krankheiten die verschiedensten disseminierten Schädigungen der feinen Gefäße durch Strukturänderung (Avitaminosen), durch Entzündung (z.B. anaphylaktoide Purpura), evtl. vorübergehend kombiniert mit leichten Störungen von Thrombocyten und Gerinnungsfaktoren, entstehen. Als besondere Mechanismen kommen in Frage: allergische Reaktionen, unspezifische Umstimmung im Sinne des Shwartzman-Sanarelli-Phänomens, Anoxämie, Sklerose, Störungen der Elastica, unspezifische Entzündungen, unbekannte neuropathische Einflüsse, hormonelle Einwirkungen,

Tabelle 9. *Vasculäre hämorrhagische Diathesen*

I. Kongenital
1. *Hereditäre Teleangiektasien* (Morbus Osler)
2. *Angiomatosis retinae* (VON HIPPEL-LINDAU)
3. *Hereditäre familiäre Purpura simplex* (DAVIS)

II. Erworben
1. *Avitaminosen* (Vitamin C und P)
2. *Möglicherweise allergische vasculäre hämorrhagische Diathese*
   a) Purpura rheumatica (SCHÖNLEIN)
   Purpura abdominalis (HENOCH)
   anaphylaktoide Purpura (GLANZMANN)
   b) Periarteriitis nodosa cutanea (Hypersensitivity angiitis)
   c) Purpura bei Erythrocyten-Sensibilisierung (GARDNER-DIAMOND)
3. *Möglicherweise unspezifische vasculäre hämorrhagische Diathese* (Shwartzman-Sanarelli-Phänomen)
   a) Purpura fulminans
   b) Waterhouse-Friderichsen-Phänomen
4. *Anoxämie, Sklerose*
   a) Purpura senilis
   b) Purpura orthostatica
   c) Ehlers-Danlos-Syndrom
5. *Unbestimmte vasculäre hämorrhagische Diathesen*
   a) Purpura pigmentosa progressiva (KALKOFF)
   Morbus Schamberg, Morbus Gougerot
   Purpura annularis teleangiectodes (MAJOCCHI) und
   Purpura téléangiectasique arciforme (TOURAINE)
   b) ekzematoide Purpura
   epidemische purpurisch-lichenoide Dermatitis (DOUCAS und KAPETANAKIS)
   itching Purpura (LOEWENTHAL)
   Dermatitis caused by shirts (HODGSON und HELLIER)
   sekundär hämorrhagische Ekzeme (Aldrich-Syndrom)
   Purpura bei „Margarine-Krankheit"
6. *Verschiedene weitere vasculär-hämorrhagische Diathesen*
   a) Purpura hyperglobulinaemica Waldenström
   b) Purpura macroglobulinaemica Waldenström und
   Purpura kryoglobulinaemica
   c) epidemische, hauptsächlich vasculäre, fieberhafte hämorrhagische Erkrankungen
   d) hormonell bedingte vasculäre Purpura
   bei Morbus Cushing und Hypercortisonismus
   bei Schilddrüsenstörungen
   e) Neuropathenflecken (Stigmatisation)
   f) Purpura nach Fettembolie

Virusinfektionen, Strukturänderungen durch Globuline, insbesondere Makroglobulineinlagerungen.

Die vasculären hämorrhagischen Diathesen lassen sich selbstverständlich auch noch anders gruppieren, so wie dies z.B. OSGOOD u.a. 1954, FIEHRER 1959, HEGGLIN 1960 getan haben.

OSGOOD u. Mitarb. (1954) z.B. teilen die capillären Purpura-Fälle ätiologisch ein, nämlich in *1. mechanische* (z.B. Keuchhusten), *2. infektiöse* (z.B. Meningokokken-Sepsis), *3. embolische* (z.B. subakute bakterielle Endokarditis), *4. allergische* (z.B. nutritive und medikamentöse Allergie), *5. vitamindefizitäre* (z.B. Skorbut), *6. auf Verlust des elastischen Gewebes* beruhende (z.B. Senilität, Ehlers-Danlos-Syndrom), *7. Nicht-Kontraktibilität* der Capillaren (z.B. vererbte Capillarbrüchigkeit), *8. metabolische* (Urämie, Hypothyreoidismus, Anoxie), *9. teleangiektatische* (z.B. hereditäre capilläre Teleangiektasien).

FIEHRER (1959) ordnet die vasculären Purpurafälle in solche

1. ohne vermehrte Capillarbrüchigkeit (Purpura senilis von BATEMAN, Purpura bei EHLERS-DANLOS, pigmentierte und purpurische Angiodermitis von FAVRE u. CHAIX, Purpura annularis teleangiectodes von MAJOCCHI, benigne inflammatorische Purpura mit polynucleärer Leukocytose von P. CHEVALLIER, Purpura rheumatica, Purpura fulminans).

2. *Mit vermehrter Capillarfragilität* (konstitutionelle hämorrhagische Diathesen, Arteriosklerose mit und ohne Hypertonie, Skorbut, Endocarditis maligna Osler) und schließlich

3. *mit Verlängerung der Blutungszeit* (M. v. WILLEBRAND-JÜRGENS, atonische Angiopathie, ferner konstitutionelle Capillaratonien bei postoperativen, neurovegetativen Blutungen).

R. HEGGLIN (1963) gruppiert die hämorrhagischen Diathesen infolge von Gefäßstörungen in

1. *allgemeine Gefäßschädigungen* bei vorwiegend primär extravasculären Erkrankungen (Hypertonie, infektiös-toxisch, rheumatisch, allergischer Formenkreis mit Purpura Schönlein-Henoch, Purpura Majocchi, hormonelle Störungen, Skorbut, neurovasculäre Störungen, Ehlers-Danlos-Syndrom, Purpura hyperglobulinaemica, bei abnormen Proteinen [Makroglobulin und Kryoglobulin], Pseudohämophilie [Angiohämophilie]).

2. *Umschriebene Gefäßwandläsionen* (hereditäre hämorrhagische Teleangiektasie, M. Osler, Angiomatosis retinae [Morbus von HIPPEL-LINDAU], Leptomeningosis interna [CATEL], hereditäre familiäre Purpura simplex [DAVIS]).

Im folgenden seien die kongenitalen und erworbenen Krankheitsgruppen entsprechend unserem Schema vom klinischen und ätio-pathogenetischen Standpunkt aus dargestellt.

1. Kongenitale vasculäre hämorrhagische Diathesen

a) Hereditäre Teleangiektasien (OSLER-RENDU)

Das Leiden wurde 1864 von SUTTON, 1876 von LEGG beschrieben, später aber nach RENDU (1896), OSLER (1901), teils WEBER (1907) benannt.

Wie OSLER 1907 berichtete, bestehen die Haut- und Schleimhautveränderungen aus kleinen, teleangiektatischen Maculae, Spiders und Knötchen. Nach den Beobachtungen von BIRD u.a. (1957) an einem ausgedehnten Stammbaum sind die meist nach dem 20. Altersjahr gehäuft auftretenden Efflorescenzen zuerst maculös und wandeln sich später in Spiders und Knötchen um. Am häufigsten werden die Veränderungen im 3. bis 5. Dezennium manifest; sie sind in abnehmender Häufigkeit lokalisiert am Gesicht (Lippen, Nase, Zunge, Ohren), an Brust, Händen und Füßen (Abb. 16) sowie inneren Organen. Die Läsionen können zu Blutungen führen, hauptsächlich aus Nase, wesentlich seltener aus Mund, gastrointestinalem und genitourinealem Tractus sowie Lungen. Selbst epileptische Anfälle und pathologisches EEG infolge abnormer intrakranieller Gefäße können beobachtet werden (BLOOM u.a. 1960). Ungefähr ein Drittel aller Patienten zeigte nach diesen Autoren ausgedehnte Teleangiektasien und litt zeitweise an schweren, lebensbedrohlichen Blutungen. In selteneren familiären Fällen scheinen sich Teleangiektasien auf den Verdauungstrakt zu konzentrieren. Gelegentlich entstehen im kleinen Kreislauf zahlreiche kleine arteriovenöse Aneurysmen, die in ihrer Vielzahl wie ein einzelner großer Shunt wirken, mit Hämoptysis, Blässe, Cyanose, Polyglobulie und Trommelschlegelfingern. In einer Familie von 93 Mitgliedern, 5 Generationen angehörend, stellten BERGQVIST u.a. 1962 bei 17 von 22 Patienten solche arteriovenöse Aneurysmen fest.

Die plasmatischen Gerinnungsfaktoren sowie die Thrombocytenzahlen sind normal, doch zeigen die Plättchen pathologische Formen bei Fehlen der Agglutinationsfähigkeit (QUATTRIN 1955). GARLAND u.a. (1950) halten die Krankheit bei Semiten für häufiger. SMITH u.a. (1954) beobachteten die Krankheit auch bei einer Negerfamilie.

Genetisch handelt es sich um ein autosomal-dominant vererbtes Leiden, wahrscheinlich mit starker Penetranz (GARLAND u.a. 1950). Es findet sich keine regelmäßige Koppelung mit den Blutgruppen des A—B—0-, Rh-, MNS-, Lewis- oder Kelly/Duffy-Systems. (Weiterer Stammbaum bei PROPPE 1938.)

Histologisch finden sich Teleangiektasien mit ausgesprochener Dünnwandigkeit der erweiterten und geschlängelten Capillaren und Venolen, bei Verminderung der elastischen und muskulären Elemente (s. GROSS 1959).

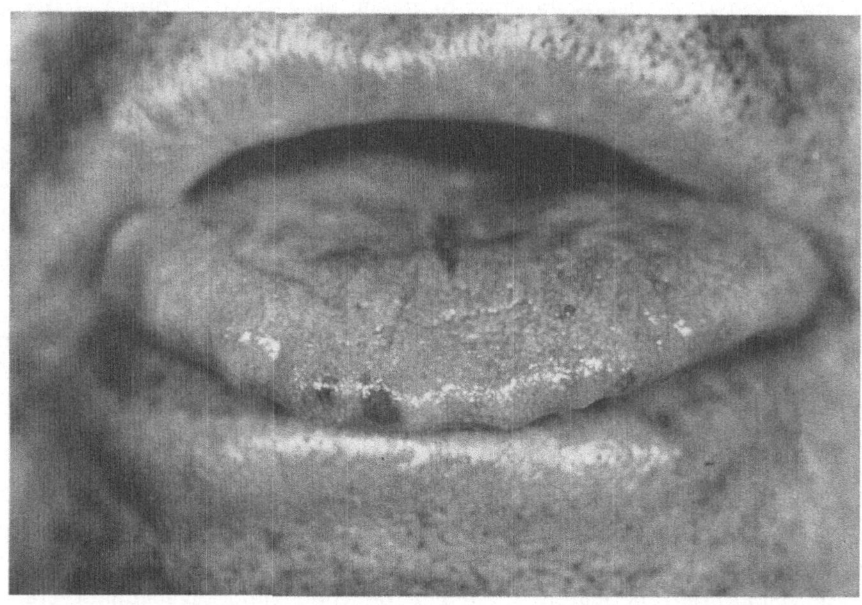

a

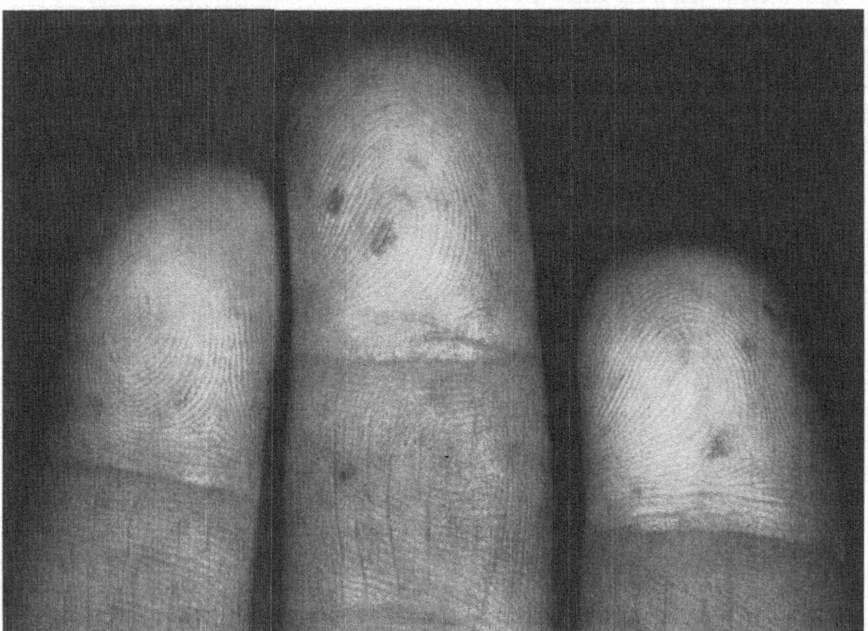

b

Abb. 16a u. b. Morbus Osler. [Aus R. M. BIRD et al.: A family reunion. A study of hereditary hemorrhagic teleangiectasia. New Engl. med. J. 257, 105 (1957)]

Differentialdiagnostisch kommen die Venulae stellatae (Eppinger-Faltitschek-sche Sternchen, Spinnennaevi, Spiders) bei chronischen Leberleiden, Avitaminosen, Schwangerschaft, Morbus Cushing, Hyperthyreose, chronischem Gelenkrheumatismus und Xeroderma pigmentosum in Frage, die aber meist im Zentrum pulsieren, sozusagen nie an Schleimhäuten vorkommen und klinisch nicht zu Blutungen neigen. Ferner sind differentialdiagnostisch „senile Angiome“ abzugrenzen.

Pathogenetisch stellten GOTTRON u. KORTING (1958) den Einfluß der arteriovenösen Anastomosen und Sperrgefäße auf die Durchblutung (Blutströmungsgeschwindigkeit und Capillarenweite) für die Blutungen in den Vordergrund, mit Permeabilitätsstörungen infolge der verschiedensten Noxen. Hormonale Einflüsse wie Pubertät, Gravidität, Klimakterium, Morbus Basedow können die Blutungsneigung einleiten.

KLUG (1949) unterschied zwei Typen von sternförmigen Teleangiektasien, nämlich 1. rasch auftretende und wieder verschwindende, 2. solche, die langsam in Erscheinung treten und persistieren, so bei chronischer Nephritis, Magencarcinom, Schwangerschaft usw., Veränderungen, die auch an Handrücken, Gesicht und Schleimhaut vorkommen, histologisch ein gewuchertes Endothel und verdickte Media mit aufgesplitterter Elastica zeigen und möglicherweise infolge pathologischer Bluteiweiße bei Leberstörungen entstehen. Die Autoren unterscheiden drei Entstehungsarten der Teleangiektasien, nämlich

1. infolge anderer Krankheit (Lebercirrhose, Nephritis) entstandene Paraproteinämie,
2. erbliche „Paraproteinämie“ (M. Osler),
3. als Folge einer diencephalen Störung, wofür auch die Schübe von Oslerschen Blutungen nach psychischen Traumen (W. RICHTER 1933) oder nach Aufregungen (CICOVACKI u.a. 1939) sprechen.

Therapeutisch sind nach OSGOOD u.a. (1954) besonders die Blutungen aus Urogenital- und Gastrointestinaltrakt schwer zu beeinflussen (Versagen von Rutin, Oestrogenen, Adrenochrom, Monosemicarbazon, Natriumsalicylatkomplex [Adrenosan]).

Weitere klinische und genetische Hinweise auf M. Osler finden sich im Ergänzungsband III/1 im Kapitel „Hämangiome“ von U. W. SCHNYDER (S. 540) 1963.

b) Angiomatosis retinae (v. HIPPEL-LINDAU) (retinocerebrale Angiomatose)

Diese umschriebene, teils auf Teleangiektasien, teils auf Angiombildung beruhende Krankheit wurde von v. HIPPEL u. LINDAU 1927 beschrieben. Prädilektionsstelle sind Augenhintergrund, Cerebellum, aber auch andere Stellen können befallen sein. Der Vererbungsmodus ist unregelmäßig-dominant, 20% der Fälle sind familiär. Die intrafamiliären klinischen Erscheinungen können variieren.

Die retinale Angiomatose stellt sich bei der ophthalmoskopischen Untersuchung in zwei- bis dreifach erweiterten Arterien und Venen dar, zentral mit ausgesprochenen Windungen, die peripher in mehrere gelbliche oder rötlichgraue Tumörchen münden. Meist werden Exsudate, seltener Hämorrhagien angetroffen. Gelegentlich gesellen sich Retinitis, Glaskörperhämorrhagie und sekundäres Glaukom hinzu, vereinzelt auch Angiome der Iris.

Die cerebrale Angiomatose betrifft Cerebellum und vierten Ventrikel mit intrakranieller Hypertension. Seltener liegt die Angiomatose in Hirnstamm oder Rückenmark. Klinisch findet sich meist psychische Alteration, Epilepsie und Demenz.

Gelegentlich werden auch *teleangiektatische Cysten* an *inneren Organen*, so hauptsächlich an Nieren, seltener Nebennieren, Ovarien, Leber, Milz angetroffen (LINDAU 1927, APPLEMANS 1947, FRANÇOIS u. COFFYN 1951).

c) Hereditäre, familiäre Purpura simplex

1939 berichtete DAVIS über elf Familien mit spontanen Ekchymosen, z.T. orthostatisch bedingt, am Stamm gelegentlich mit Petechien. Die Krankheit trat meist während des Klimakteriums auf, in späteren Generationen früher. Capillarresistenz z.T. erniedrigt, Koagulationsfaktoren, Thrombocyten, Blutungszeit normal. Zum Teil fand sich gehäuft rheumatische Arthritis. Im Gegensatz zur

Thrombasthenie Glanzmann konnten keine ausgedehnten Blutungen nach minimen Traumen oder Blutungen in den Magen-Darmtrakt festgestellt werden. In drei Familien wurde leichtes Nasenbluten und Menorrhagien beobachtet.

Frauen erkranken häufiger als Männer; das Leiden wird autosomal dominant vererbt. In einer Familie war nach FISHER u. a. (1954) das Leiden über vier Generationen noch mit einer dominanten kongenitalen Augenlidptose gekoppelt.

2. Erworbene vasculäre hämorrhagische Diathesen

Übersichtsweise sind die verschiedenen Formen in Tabelle 9 aufgeführt.

a) Vasculäre hämorrhagische Diathesen bei Avitaminosen

Nach neueren Erkenntnissen sind es hauptsächlich die Vitamine C und P, welche für die Abdichtung der Gefäßendothelien von Bedeutung sind. Die Blutungen bei Vitamin C-Mangel sind besonders unter dem Krankheitsbild des Skorbuts im Erwachsenenalter, der Möller-Barlowschen Krankheit bei Kindern bekannt und wurden von F. HAMMER 1928 (Bd. VI/2, S. 523—527) der ersten Ausgabe dieses Handbuches behandelt.

α) Vitamin C-Mangelkrankheiten

Zur Zeit der Herausgabe des oben erwähnten Handbuchbeitrages (1928) war der Skorbut noch nicht als C-Avitaminose erkannt. Wohl wurden richtigerweise für die schweren hämorrhagischen Störungen besonders bei Expeditionsteilnehmern Mangelzustände infolge einseitiger Ernährung vermutet und zusätzliche Komplikationen durch Infektion angenommen, doch nach der experimentellen Erzeugung der Krankheit beim Meerschweinchen durch einseitige Ernährung mit Cerealien (HOLST u. FRÖLICH 1907, 1910) brachte erst die Reindarstellung des skorbutverhütenden Faktors durch A. v. SZENT-GYÖRGY (1927—1932) und schließlich die Aufklärung der Konstitution des Vitamins C durch HAWORTH, HIRST, KARRER, MICHEL, sowie die Synthese durch REICHSTEIN (1933 u. 1934) vollständige Klarheit. Es zeigte sich dann auch, daß lediglich die petechialen Blutungen und Ekchymosen an den abhängigen Körperpartien, die Zahnfleischblutungen, die Knochenschmerzen durch subperiostale Blutungen, die allgemeine Müdigkeit und die Infektionsabwehrschwäche auf Vitamin C-Mangel beruhen, nicht aber die häufig gleichzeitig vorkommende Nachtblindheit, die follikuläre Hyperkeratose, die Magendarmstörungen, welche durch Mangel anderer Vitamine entstehen, z. T. infolge Resorptionsstörungen. Dies auch bei der oft beobachteten Anämie, die vermutlich durch Eisenresorptionsstörung bei Vitamin C-Mangel auftritt.

Das voll ausgebildete Krankheitsbild des Skorbuts wird heute kaum mehr gesehen, hingegen Skorbut-Vorstadien, z. B. bei Vitamin C-konsumierenden chronischen Infekten (Typhus, Rheumatismus), bei unterernährten Landstreichern, schlecht gepflegten Geisteskranken, auch bei älteren Menschen mit Resorptionsstörungen des Magen-Darmkanals, ferner möglicherweise bei erhöhtem Vitamin C-Verbrauch während Schwangerschaft und Wochenbett. Solche Zustände werden besonders während der gemüsearmen Frühjahrsmonate (Frühjahrsmüdigkeit) im Sinne von Appetitabnahme, ziehende Wadenschmerzen, Neigung zu Zahnfleischblutungen, Nervosität usw. beobachtet. Rumpel-Leede kann positiv sein, Thrombocyten und Gerinnungsfaktoren sind normal.

Pathogenetisch wird heute angenommen, daß die „Kittsubstanz" zwischen den Endothelien der Gefäße bei Vitamin C-Mangel ungenügend ausgebildet ist, wie dies Versuche mit Gewebskulturen von JENAY u. TÖRÖ (1938) nahelegten.

Neben dem Gefäßfaktor scheinen aber auch Gerinnungsstörungen, ähnlich dem angeborenen Mangel an plasmatischem „prothromboplastin antecedent“ und „Hageman-Faktor“ beim experimentell erzeugten Meerschweinchenskorbut vorzukommen (FLUTE u. HOWARD 1959).

Therapeutisch kommen synthetische Vitamin C-Präparate per os in Frage, ferner früchte- und gemüsereiche Diät.

β) Vasculäre hämorrhagische Diathesen bei Vitamin P-Mangel

Die erhöhte Blutungsbereitschaft bei Skorbut ist wahrscheinlich zusätzlich auf das gleichzeitige Fehlen von *Vitamin P* zurückzuführen. S. SZENT-GYÖRGY konnte nachweisen, daß Citronensaft und Paprika bei Skorbut eine bessere Heilwirkung zeigen als Ascorbinsäure allein. Wahrscheinlich ist es das Rutin, welches einen ausgesprochen capillarabdichtenden Effekt aufweist. Es ist aber nicht gesichert, ob das Rutin tatsächlich das Permeabilitätsvitamin der Gefäße darstellt.

Das Rutin ist eines der unzähligen pflanzlichen Substanzen, der sog. „Flavone“, ein Derivat des γ-Benzopyrons. Es kommt in Blüten, Blättern und Früchten verschiedenster Pflanzen vor, so Buchweizen, Paprika, Citrone, Holunderbeeren, Leguminosen, Korbblütlern. Seine Bruttoformel ist $C_{27}H_{30}O_{16}$.

Die Wirkungen des Rutins (Vitamin P) bestehen in 1. Erhöhung der Capillarresistenz und 2. Herabsetzung der Permeabilität der Zellmembranen; 3. vermindert es die Aktivität der Hyaluronidase und fördert bei Anwesenheit von Calcium das Wachstum.

Im Tierexperiment kann Vitamin P die Blutungszeit verkürzen, die Wirkung des Dicumarols z.T. aufheben und z.T. die Gerinnungszeit verkürzen (zit. nach JOBÉ 1954).

Bei Ratten, die mit antithrombocytären Immunseren von Kaninchen behandelt wurden, konnte durch Rutin eine Verminderung der Capillarläsionen, nicht aber Verhütung des Thrombocyten- und Erythrocytenabfalles erzielt werden (WITTE u.a. 1952).

Wegen der günstigen Wirkung des Rutins auf Capillarresistenz und Permeabilität der Zellmembranen ist verständlich, daß es als Therapeuticum bei hämorrhagischen Diathesen mit beteiligter Gefäßkomponente empfohlen wird, in der Regel zusammen mit Vitamin C.

b) Möglicherweise allergische vasculäre hämorrhagische Diathesen

α) Purpura (Peliosis) rheumatica (SCHÖNLEIN), Purpura abdominalis (HENOCH), anaphylaktoide Purpura (GLANZMANN)

Bei der anaphylaktoiden Purpura handelt es sich um eine erworbene, vasculäre hämorrhagische Diathese, die in ihren hauptsächlichsten klinischen Verlaufsformen von SCHÖNLEIN, HENOCH und GLANZMANN beschrieben wurde. Es ist eine entzündliche, fakultativ hämorrhagische, schubweise auftretende Krankheit, bei welcher die Gefäße durch den entzündlichen Prozeß bis zur Blutung geschädigt werden.

Allergische Reaktionen scheinen bei diesen Affektionen das pathogenetische Prinzip zu sein, möglicherweise sekundär verstärkt durch das zweiphasische Shwartzman-Sanarelli-Phänomen. Allerdings muß zugegeben werden, daß in etwa einem Drittel der Fälle der sichere Nachweis eines schädigenden Allergens nicht gelingt. Da in der Regel bei diesen Krankheiten entzündliche Prozesse an den cutanen kleinen Gefäßen zur Blutung führen, bei intensiven Reaktionen auf die größeren und tieferliegenden Gefäße übergreifend, ist eine Abgrenzung von anderen, z.T. verwandten Krankheitsbildern, wie Periarteriitis nodosa cutanea gelegentlich nicht leicht.

So werden z.B. von WINKELMANN (1959) die anaphylaktoide Purpura mit allergischer Angiitis, nekrotisierender Angiitis, hypersensitiver Periarteriitis nodosa, nodulärer Allergie von GOUGEROT und allergischem Mikrobid in nahe Beziehung gebracht und mit der Gruppe der systematisierten Angiitiden, letalem Mittelliniegranulom des Nasopharynx (Granulome centrofacial, Wegener-Granulome) sowie der temporalen Arteriitis verglichen. Tatsächlich können bei der anaphylaktischen Purpura neben kleineren auch größere Gefäße in den Entzündungsprozeß einbezogen sein, mit histologisch nachweisbaren Gefäßveränderungen, ähnlich einer Panarteriitis, wie wir dies selbst mehrmals beobachten konnten (Storck 1951).

Nachdem *klinisches Bild* und Verlauf durch F. Hammer (1928) bereits unter den „idiopathischen essentiellen Purpuraformen" eingehend beschrieben wurde, sollen diese hier nur kurz gestreift und hauptsächlich neuere, ätiopathogenetische Erkenntnisse berücksichtigt werden.

Die schubweise, in gewissen Fällen rezidivierend auftretenden Hautefflorescenzen finden sich hauptsächlich an Streckseiten der Extremitäten, an den lateralen Stamm- und Glutäalgebieten, selten in Gesicht, Hals, Rücken und an Mundschleimhaut. Sie stellen entzündliche, maculopapulöse, z.T. urticarielle, seltener blasig nekrotisierende oder rein maculöse petechiale Läsionen dar, die sich zu Beginn oder erst später, gelegentlich nur vereinzelt purpurisch umwandeln (Abb. 12 u. 17). Da sich auch Gefäße anderer Organe an der krankhaften Reaktion beteiligen können, entstehen gelegentlich arthritische Störungen, besonders der größeren Gelenke, abdominelle Beschwerden mit Krämpfen und Blutungen (dies besonders bei Kindern; Conca u.a. 1962, Feldt u.a. 1962), ferner angedeutete oder intensive Nierenblutungen (dies besonders bei Abdominalbeschwerden) mit Zeichen von Nephritis, in seltenen Fällen mit letalem Ausgang. Durch rezidivierende Beteiligung der Lungencapillaren kann es zur Lungenfibrose mit Hämochromatose (z.B. Siegenthaler, Dvorak 1959) bei Befall der Gehirngefäße zu Cerebralblutungen kommen.

Besonders bei Kindern scheint die Nierenbeteiligung nicht harmlos zu sein. So fanden Derham u.a. 1956 unter 94 Kindern mit Schönlein-Henoch in mehr als 50% Nierenschädigungen und zwei Todesfälle mit Urämie, viermal Übergang in chronische Nephritis.

Histologisch findet sich in den purpurischen Hautelementen entsprechend dem klinischen Bild Entzündung mit Infiltration und Exsudation, hauptsächlich perivasculär um Capillaren, Venolen und Arteriolen der oberen Cutispartien gelegen. Die Infiltrate bestehen hauptsächlich aus polynucleären Leukocyten, welche, wie G. Miescher betonte, meist außerordentlich leukoclasisch sind (leukoclasisches Mikrobid, G. Miescher 1946) (Abb. 17). In weniger ausgeprägten oder älteren Herden bestehen die Infiltrate mehr aus Lymphocyten und monocytoiden Zellen (P. Miescher 1961). Die Infiltrate können bei dichter Lagerung die Blutung verdecken. Meist zeigen Capillaren, Arteriolen und Venolen leichte Schädigung mit Endothelschwellung. Bei besonders akuten Reaktionen weist das umgebende Bindegewebe mandelförmig fibrinoide Deneration oder Infiltrate mit fibrinoider Substanz auf, bei größeren Arteriolen Medianekrosen, gelegentlich auch granulomatöse Umwandlung von Intima und Adventitia, die oft das Bild einer Periarteriitis nodosa imitieren. In einzelnen Efflorescenzen kann die Blutung klinisch und histologisch trotz dichten leukocytären oder leukoclasischen Infiltraten fehlen, was die fakultative Natur der hämorrhagischen Komponente erweist.

Pathogenetisch wurden schon früh allergische Mechanismen zur Diskussion gestellt, so von Glanzmann Infektionen des Respirationstraktes, später von den verschiedensten Autoren Reaktionen auf Infektions-, Nahrungsmittel- und Arzneimittel-Allergene. Meist wurden solche ursächlichen Zusammenhänge mit vorgängigen akuten, subakuten oder chronischen Infektionen des Respirationstraktes oder anderer Foci, gelegentlich mit Tuberkulose, angenommen.

Nicht-thrombopenische Purpurafälle nach Medikamenten wurden ebenfalls beobachtet, so z.B. nach Jodiden, Copaiba, Belladonna, Atropin, Chinin, Bismut, Quecksilber, Acetophenetidin (Phenacetin), Aspirin, Salicylsäure, Chloralhydrat, Phenylbutazon, Penicillin (Wintrobe 1951, Jensen 1955, Arrighi 1955, Huriez u.a. 1955, Fleischhacker 1955). (Purpura auf Grund medikamentöser Allergie s. auch Burckhardt, in diesem Handbuch, Ergänzungsband II/1, S. 564, 1963.)

Selten wurden zur ätiologischen Aufklärung besondere Testungen, Expositions- und Eliminationsversuche oder besondere immunpathologische (allergologische) Untersuchungsreihen angestellt.

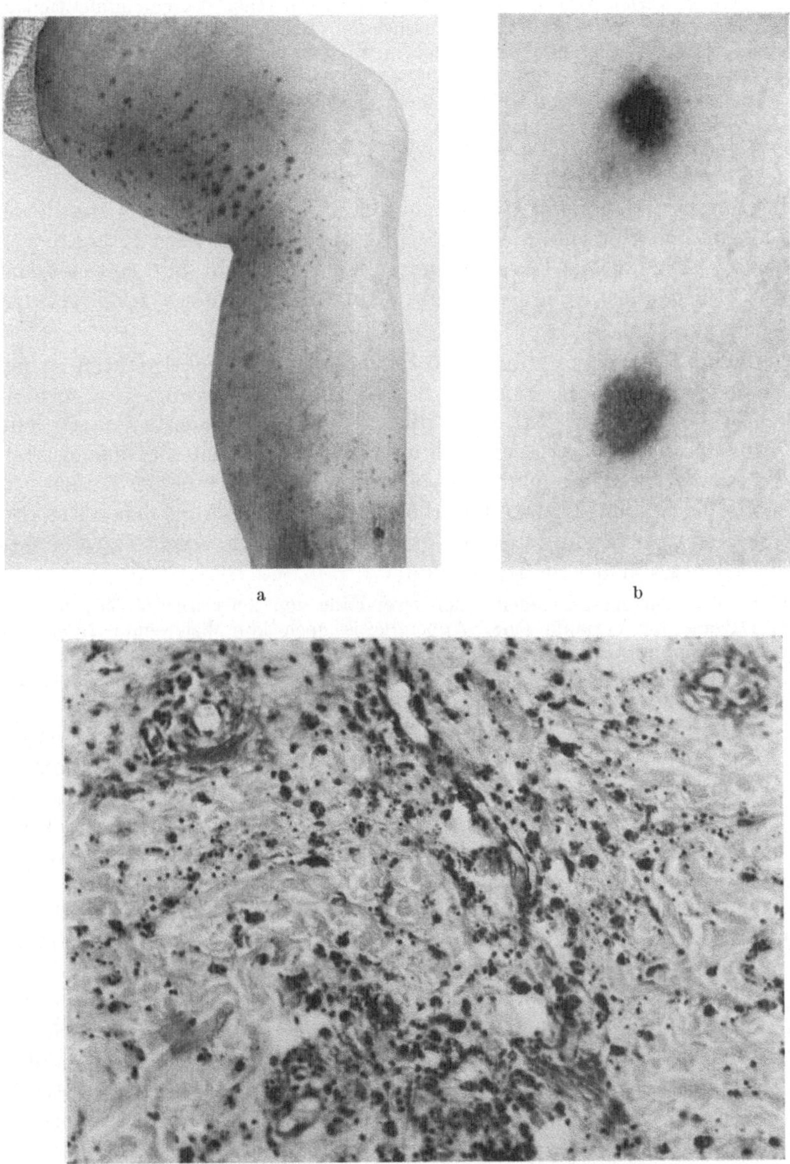

Abb. 17 a—c. Hämorrhagisches Mikrobid (als Focus chronische Tonsillitis) (a), hämorrhagische Filtratproben auf Staphylococcus aureus und Streptococcus haemolyticus (b), histologisch leukoklasisches Mikrobid (c)

Folgende infektionsallergischen Ursachen wurden in Erwägung gezogen: *Tuberkulose:* von Bochsler 1933, Fox u. Enzer 1938, Dalgleish u.a. 1950, Racine u.a. 1952, Mathé 1954, Bauch 1916. *Scharlach:* Osgood u.a. 1954. *Pertussis:* Burnet 1923, Smith-Bertram 1926, Coke 1931, Bartley u.a. 1936, Kugelmans 1936. *Fokalinfekte:* Fiaschi 1949, 1950, Storck u.a. 1951, P. Miescher u. Reymond 1954 (besonders chronische Bronchitis), Ball 1954, Stüttgen 1955, Ruiter 1956, G. Miescher, Reymond u. Ritter 1956, Ablard u. Larcan 1956, Pratesi u. Rizzuto 1956 (49% Rachen- und Mandelinfekte, 51% Fokalherde in anderen Organen), LISSIA 1956 (Tonsillen), BYWATERS u.a. 1957 (Antistreptolysintiter in 33% erhöht), P. MIESCHER u. VORLAENDER 1957, P. MIESCHER 1957, NICOLAU u.a. 1958, FIEHRER 1958, WINKELMANN 1958, STÜTTGEN 1959, NORKIN u. WIENER 1960, CONCA u. KEHYAYAN 1961.

Unspezifische Infektionen, besonders der oberen Luftwege, Allgemeininfektionen wie Scharlach, Masern, Diphtherie, Malaria, Mononucleose, Brucellose, Varicellen, Bakteriämien nach Pneumo-, Strepto-, Meningokokkeninfektionen wurden ebenfalls mehrfach diskutiert (GAIRDNER 1947/48, s. auch MIESCHER u. VORLAENDER 1960).

Vasculäre hämorrhagische Hautschübe nach Vaccine-Injektionen wurden erstmals von COKE 1931 beschrieben, dann mehrmals von anderen Autoren beobachtet, so von STORCK 1951, 1952, G. MIESCHER 1961. Einen Fall nach Immunisierung mit asiatischer Influenza-Vaccine beschrieben STEFANINI u.a. 1958).

Da die Purpura Schönlein-Henoch häufig mit arthritischen Veränderungen einhergeht, untersuchten einige Autoren die Häufigkeit dieser Krankheit beim *Rheumatismus*. Eine solche Koinzidenz scheint aber ein nur seltenes, unterhalb von 2% liegendes Ereignis zu sein (ABLARD u. LARCAN 1956, CANIZARES 1957).

Die *Pathogenese* der Entstehung von Hautblutungen nach Infekten ist jedoch noch nicht sicher geklärt. Es ist möglich, daß toxische Wirkungen zu vermehrter Capillarbrüchigkeit führen. Daß zusätzlich allergische Momente von Bedeutung sind, ist wahrscheinlich, steht aber noch nicht fest. Nach den Versuchen über das Shwartzman-Sanarelli-Phänomen, bei welchem wenigstens eine der beiden Phasen durch spezifische, besonders infektionsallergische Antigen-Antikörper-Reaktionen übernommen werden kann, sind möglicherweise auch solche zweiphasische, unspezifische Reaktionen von Bedeutung.

In diesem Sinne sprechen vielleicht auch zwei Fälle von STÜTTGEN (1959), bei welchen mikrobielle Ekzeme im Verlaufe einer Appendicitis nach komplizierender Lymphangitis sekundär hämorrhagische Umwandlungen zeigten, gleichzeitig mit Entwicklung einer intestinalen Purpura Schönlein-Henoch. Zu einem mikrobiell-allergischen Geschehen kam also ein zweiter bakterieller Prozeß, welcher die Hämorrhagie auslöste.

ACKROYD (1953) äußert sich besonders wegen des meist normalen Antistreptolysintiters zurückhaltend und skeptisch gegenüber der infektionsallergischen Hypothese und stellt allergische Reaktionen auf *Nahrungs-* und *Arzneimittel* in den Vordergrund, die nach ihm vor allem den vasculären Purpuratypus Schönlein-Henoch bevorzugen. Nahrungsmittelallergische Reaktionen waren schon früh in Erwägung gezogen worden, so von SACHS (1916, Sardellenbutter), ALEXANDER u.a. (1929, Eier, Milch, Weizen, Bohnen), BARTHELME (1929, Weizen, Eiweiß), KAHN (1929, spanische Nüsse), wurden aber in letzter Zeit weniger in Betracht gezogen, wohl wegen der Schwierigkeit eines exakten Allergennachweises.

Einzelne Autoren versuchten, die Purpura vom Schönlein-Henoch-Typus auf *Autosensibilisierungen* gegenüber Gefäßendothelien zurückzuführen. Die Autoantikörperhypothese bei solchen vasculären Purpuraformen scheint jedoch vorläufig experimentell nicht genügend gestützt, weil die Resultate der bisherigen Forschung widersprechend ausfielen, und praktisch meist nur in vitro fragliche Reaktionen gefunden wurden.

Japanische Autoren wie KATSURA (1924), OKANA u.a. (1938), HIRAMATSU (1941—1948) versuchten als erste, z.T. erfolgreich, durch Injektion von „antivascular endothelium serum" tierexperimentell Diapedesis von Erythrocyten mit erhöhter Capillarpermeabilität zu erzeugen. CLARK u. JACOBS stellten 1950 Kaninchen-Immunserum gegen Blutplättchen, Milz, Knochenmark, ferner Gefäßendothelien von Meerschweinchen und Mäusen her. Mit den meisten Antiseren ließen sich nach Zugabe des homologen Antigens in vitro Agglutinationen oder Komplementfixationen, in vivo Thrombopenien, jedoch keine vasculären Hämorrhagien erzeugen. Eine vasculäre Purpura fand sich lediglich in einem Versuch bei zwei Hunden, denen Antigefäßendothelien-Immunserum injiziert worden war. An der Injektionsstelle sowie an Rücken und Flanken dieser Tiere entstanden Ekchymosen, ferner Blutungen des Gastrointestinaltraktes mit Vergrößerung der Milz.

STEFANINI u.a. (1950) sowie DAMASHEK (1950) versuchten mittels der Ring-Präcipitationsmethode antiendotheliale Antikörper nachzuweisen. 1956 glaubten ISRAEL/MATHÉ/BERNARD, durch intracutane Injektion von 0,2—0,3 cm³ Serum von Patienten mit Purpura Schönlein-Henoch beim Meerschweinchen hämorrhagische Reaktionen hervorgerufen zu haben, was aber P. MIESCHER 1961 nicht bestätigen konnte. STEFFEN (1956) zeigte bei Patienten mit der Antiglobulinkonsumtion-Testmethode gegen Gefäßendothelien gerichtete Antikörper, und auch SNEDDON (1957) fand eine spezifische Antikörperbildung. BERNARD/MATHÉ/ISRAEL (1957) konnten jedoch mittels Coombs-Test bei 65 Patienten keine Antikörper gegen Erythrocyten, Leukocyten, Plättchen oder Endothelien nachweisen. Auch CRUICKSHANK fand 1959 in einer sorgfältig durchgeführten experimentellen Arbeit weder präcipitierende noch agglutinierende oder komplementbindende Antikörper in Seren von Patienten mit anaphylaktoider Purpura. Als Antigen dienten hier Extrakte aus normalen menschlichen Arterien, Nierenglomeruli oder auch von zellfreiem arteriellem Reticulin. Selbst mit der Immunfluorescenz nach COONS fielen die Resultate negativ aus.

Um ein gefäßaktives Prinzip im Serum von Patienten mit vasculärer Purpura nachzuweisen, machten NICOLAU und BADANOIU 1960 folgende Versuche: Sie entnahmen 103 Patienten, wovon 63 mit vasculären Allergiden, Blut und injizierten Meerschweinchen intradermal das Serum. Mit 68 Patientenseren erzeugten sie starke erythemato-ödematöse Infiltrate mit zentraler Nekrose, nicht aber mit Seren von Patienten ohne Purpura, z.B. mit Ekzem, Urticaria, Prurigo, Neurodermitis. Histologisch waren an der Reaktionsstelle des Meerschweinchens Veränderungen an Capillaren und Arteriolen mit polynucleären Infiltrationen bis tief in der Cutis festzustellen. Auf Grund dieser Übertragungsversuche (von Patientenseren auf Tiere) glaubten die Forscher, passiv übertragbare, gefäßaktive Substanzen, wahrscheinlich Heparinoide oder proteolytische Fermente, nachgewiesen zu haben.

STEFANINI u.a. erörterten 1959 eingehend die Autosensibilisierungstheorie, ohne jedoch weitere Beweise beibringen zu können und lehnten 1962 mit PIOMELLI deshalb die Autoimmunhypothese der anaphylaktoiden Purpura gänzlich ab. Denn sie konnten mit Antiseren gegen Endothelien von Kaninchen, Meerschweinchen und Hunden bei den ersteren Tieren lediglich anaphylaktischen Schock, beim Hund zudem Reaktionen vom Masugi-Nephritis-Typus erzeugen, nie aber Purpura, obwohl mit der Immunfluorescenz nach COONS die Antikörper an den Gefäßen verankert waren.

Bis jetzt scheint die *infektionsallergische Hypothese* experimentell am besten untersucht und soll hier kurz besprochen werden.

Nachdem G. MIESCHER an Hand eines Falles von rezidivierender anaphylaktoider Purpura mit der von ihm als charakteristisch erkannten leukoclasischen perivasculären Infiltration auf die Bedeutung chronischer Fokalinfekte hingewiesen hatte, versuchten STORCK/HOIGNÉ u. KOLLER in tierexperimentellen Modellversuchen (Arthus-Phänomen, anaphylaktischer Schock, Shwartzman-Sanarelli-Phänomen) die hämatologischen, gerinnungsphysiologischen und histologischen Veränderungen zu erforschen, um möglicherweise Parallelen zu den klinischen vasculären hämorrhagischen Diathesen zu ziehen.

Sie fanden im Tierversuch bei sämtlichen experimentellen Versuchsanordnungen eine akute oder protrahierte Senkung der Thrombo- und Leukocytenzahl mit anschließendem kompensatorischem Anstieg über die Norm, dazu spiegelbildlich Anstieg, dann Abfall des Antithrombins im Blut. Zudem fand sich beim Sanarelli-Phänomen ein deutlicher Faktor V-Mangel. Es schien also, daß die allergische vasculäre Blutung durch vorübergehende Thrombocytopenie mit Heparinanstieg, beim Sanarelli-Phänomen zusätzlich durch Faktor V-Mangel gefördert werde.

Ein Parallelismus von klinischen Fällen mit anaphylaktoider Purpura zu den genannten Tierversuchen (vorübergehender Abfall der Thrombocyten und Anstieg des Antithrombins) zeigte sich dann auch in einzelnen Fällen (Tabelle 10).

Daß bei Purpura Schönlein-Henoch nicht nur Gefäßschädigungen, sondern auch Störungen von Thrombocyten und Gerinnungsfaktoren vorkommen, lassen weiterhin Beobachtungen von KORTING u.a. (1957) vermuten. Diese Autoren fanden bei einem Fall von „Schönlein-artigem Mikrobid" eine kompensierte Gerinnungsstörung im Sinne eines Faktor IX-Mangels und zudem elektronenoptisch eine vermehrte Adhäsion und Konzentration der Thrombocyten zu Riesenagglutinaten, die möglicherweise die Ausbildung eines geordneten Fibringerüstes störten.

Die bei Purpura Schönlein-Henoch häufig hämorrhagisch ausfallenden Intracutanspätreaktionen auf Bakterienfiltrate (Strepto. haem., Staph. aur.) deuten

Tabelle 10. *Zusammenstellung der Fälle mit hämorrhagischem Mikrobid*
[Aus H. Storck, Dermatologica (Basel) 102, 211 (1951)]

Pat. Nr.	Senkungs-reaktion	Leuko-cyten	Thrombo-cyten	Heparin (Anti-thrombin)	Faktor V	Pro-throm-bin (Quick)	Blu-tungs-zeit	Gerin-nungs-zeit	Capillar-resistenz	i.cut Test Bakt. Filtr.
1	5/12	6100	202000			100%	1′30″	4′15″	normal	*hämorrhag.*
2	*55/65*	*15700*	*350000*	*erhöht*		60%	2′	7′15″	normal	*hämorrhag.*
3	4/10	4920	*143000*	normal		95%	1′	7′30″	normal	*hämorrhag.*
4	5/12	*15500*	206000	*erhöht*	normal	95%	45″	2—5′	normal	*hämorrhag.*
5	*13/28*	4500	48000	*erhöht*	normal	60%	1′30″	*18′*	*vermindert*	*hämorrhag.*
6	*34/50*	*11700*	*385000*				2′30″	3′15″	*vermindert*	*hämorrhag.*
7	*26/46*	6520	300000			100%	2′	3′	*vermindert*	positiv nicht häm.
8	*24/38*	5200	*66000* (225000)	normal	normal	90%	2′15″	7′	*vermindert*	positiv nicht häm.
9		*14400*	*960000*	*erhöht*	normal	90%	normal	normal	normal	positiv nicht häm.
10	*58/62*	*14200*	*372480*			70%	2′	3′	*vermindert*	
11	*46/54*	5700	*24000* (340000)				2′30″	5′30″	*vermindert*	
12	10/18	6700	*93000*			90%	1′	3′	*vermindert*	
13	*14/22*	6000	190000			60%	2′30″	3′30″	normal	negativ
14	10/15	6680	*103000*			90%	2′30″	5′45″	*vermindert*	positiv nicht häm.

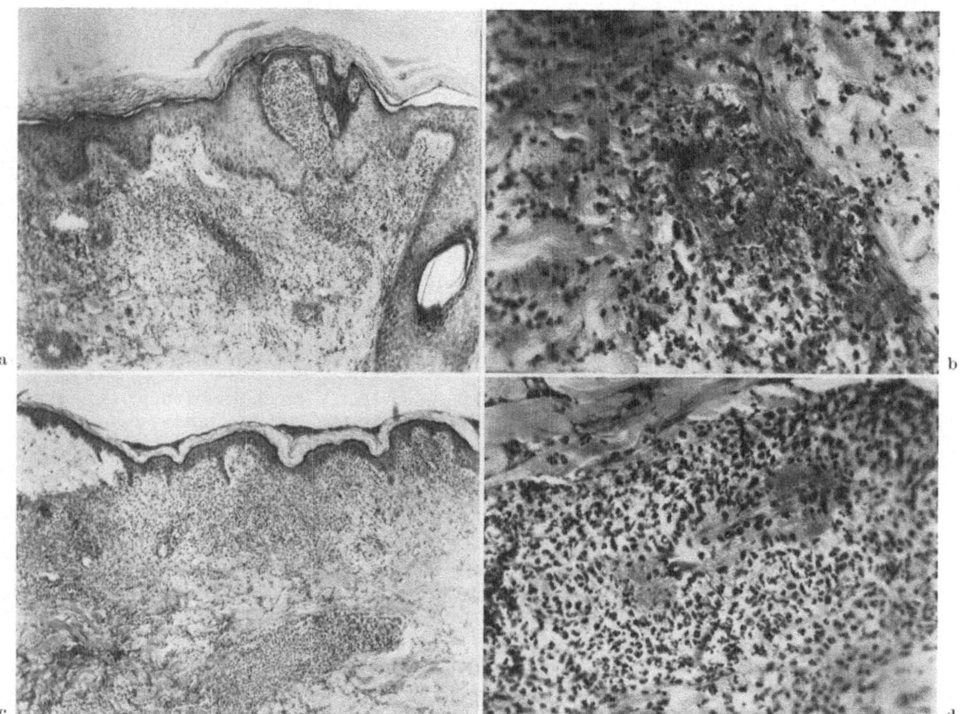

Abb. 18a—d. Leukoklasisches Mikrobid bei anaphylaktoider Purpura. a und b: Hämorrhagische Primärefflorescenz. c und d: Hämorrhagische Spätreaktion auf Filtrat von Staphylococcus aureus

ferner auf eine spezifische infektionsallergische Umstimmung gegenüber Erregern aus Fokalherden, welche bei diesen Erkrankungen anamnestisch und klinisch häufig vorhanden sind (Abb. 17). Gelegentlich waren Intracutanteste nur auf die fokalen Eigenstämme hämorrhagisch, nicht aber auf Mischfiltrate. Histologisch zeigten solche hämorrhagischen Spätreaktionen auf Bakterienfiltrate ebenfalls perivasculäre Infiltrate aus polynucleären Leukocyten, z.T. mit Leukoclasie, die den Primäreffloreszenzen der Purpura Schönlein-Henoch glichen (STORCK 1951) (Abb. 18). Durch diese Versuche war aber nicht geklärt, ob es sich um toxische oder allergische Reaktionen handle. P. MIESCHER gelang aber 1957 bei acht Fällen von Purpura Schönlein-Henoch mit hämorrhagischen Spätreaktionen auf Bakterienfiltrate, die passive Übertragung der Empfindlichkeit mittels Leukocyten auf gesunde Personen, was eher für ein infektionsallergisches Geschehen spricht.

P. MIESCHER verwendete zur passiven Übertragung dreimal gewaschene Leukocyten der Patienten, welche gesunden Versuchspersonen als Empfängern intracutan injiziert wurden. Nach Auslösung der vorbehandelten Hautstelle mit den Filtraten zeigte sich in jedem Fall eine verzögerte Spätreaktion vom Tuberkulin-Typus, die in zwei histologisch untersuchten Fällen eine starke perivasculäre, vorwiegend mononucleäre Entzündung ergab. Eine passive Übertragung mit dem Serum nach PRAUSNITZ-KÜSTNER im Sinne einer urticariellen Frühreaktion gelang nur zweimal. P. MIESCHER schloß aus diesen Beobachtungen, daß es sich bei der Purpura Schönlein-Henoch tatsächlich um eine infektionsallergische, mit Leukocyten übertragbare Spätreaktion handle, nicht aber um eine Sofortreaktion im Sinne eines Arthus-Phänomens. Intensive Reaktionen führen nach seiner Ansicht zur Leukoclasie, milde Reaktionen zu lymphomonocytären Infiltraten.

Therapeutisch kommen neben spezifischer Eliminationstherapie (Fokalsanierung, Arzneimittelentzug, Diät) Cortison, ACTH, Vitamin C und P, adrenalinartige Stoffe (Adrenochrom, Adrenoxyl) und Röntgenweichstrahlen in Frage (s. auch KLIMA 1955, HARRINGTON 1957, MENZI 1958, GROSS 1959, SCHREINER 1959).

β) Periarteriitis nodosa cutanea (Arteriitis allergica cutis)

Wenn auch diese Affektionen nur in vereinzelten Fällen zu Blutungen führen und, im Gegensatz zur anaphylaktoiden Purpura, klinisch hauptsächlich knotige, blaurote, dem Erythema nodosum ähnliche (Abb. 19), z.T. nekrotisierend-ulcerative Hautveränderungen aufweisen, nur selten vergesellschaftet mit Erythema exsudative multiforme-artigen, blasigen Efflorescenzen, gelegentlich mit Hautzeichnungen ähnlich der Livedo racemosa, sollen sie doch hier kurz erörtert werden. Denn es handelt sich sehr wahrscheinlich ebenfalls um allergische Störungen an den Gefäßen, diesmal aber vor allem an den größeren Arteriolen und Venolen, und nicht an der terminalen Strombahn. Solche Übergänge von reinen anaphylaktoiden Purpuraformen bis zu nodulär-nodösen, gefäßbedingten, hauptsächlich an den unteren Extremitäten auftretenden Knoten wurden schon häufig beobachtet, so von MACAIGNE-NICAUD (1932), LINDBERG (1932 u. 1933), CAROL u. PRAKKEN (1937, z.T. zit. nach G. MIESCHER 1946); sie können als cutane Formen der Periarteriitis nodosa aufgefaßt werden.

Da bei den verschiedensten Krankheiten an den cutanen, hauptsächlich tiefer liegenden größeren Gefäße nekrotisierende entzündliche granulomatöse Vorgänge mit fibrinoider Degeneration (Abb. 19) vorkommen können, wurden diese Krankheitsbilder unter dem Leitsymptom der nekrotisierenden Angiitis von STRAUSS u.a. (1951) sowie ZEEK (1953) neu gruppiert. Diese Autoren beschrieben als besondere Formen das Krankheitsbild der allergischen Granulomatosis, ein Syndrom mit Fieber, Eosinophilie und systematisierten Gefäßstörungen an Herz, Lungen, Magendarmtrakt, Niere, dazu noduläre, hämorrhagische oder Erythema multiforme-ähnliche Hautläsionen. Anatomisches Substrat stellen Gefäßstörungen mit granulomatöser Entzündung, starker Eosinophilie, nekrotisierendem Exsudat im umgebenden Bindegewebe mit Histiocyten und Riesenzellen dar.

ZEEK unternahm 1953 folgende weitere, allerdings nicht durchwegs anerkannte Unterteilung, nämlich:

1. Periarteriitis nodosa cutanea mit den bekannten typischen Veränderungen an den großen Arterien, gelegentlich Venen, besonders an deren Verzweigungen in den verschiedensten Organen, mit ausgedehnter fibrinoider Nekrose, Wandveränderungen bis zu Aneurysmabildung. Das Geschehen verläuft nach ADKIN in folgender Reihenfolge: Medianekrose, Degeneration, Leukocyteninfiltration, Granulombildung.

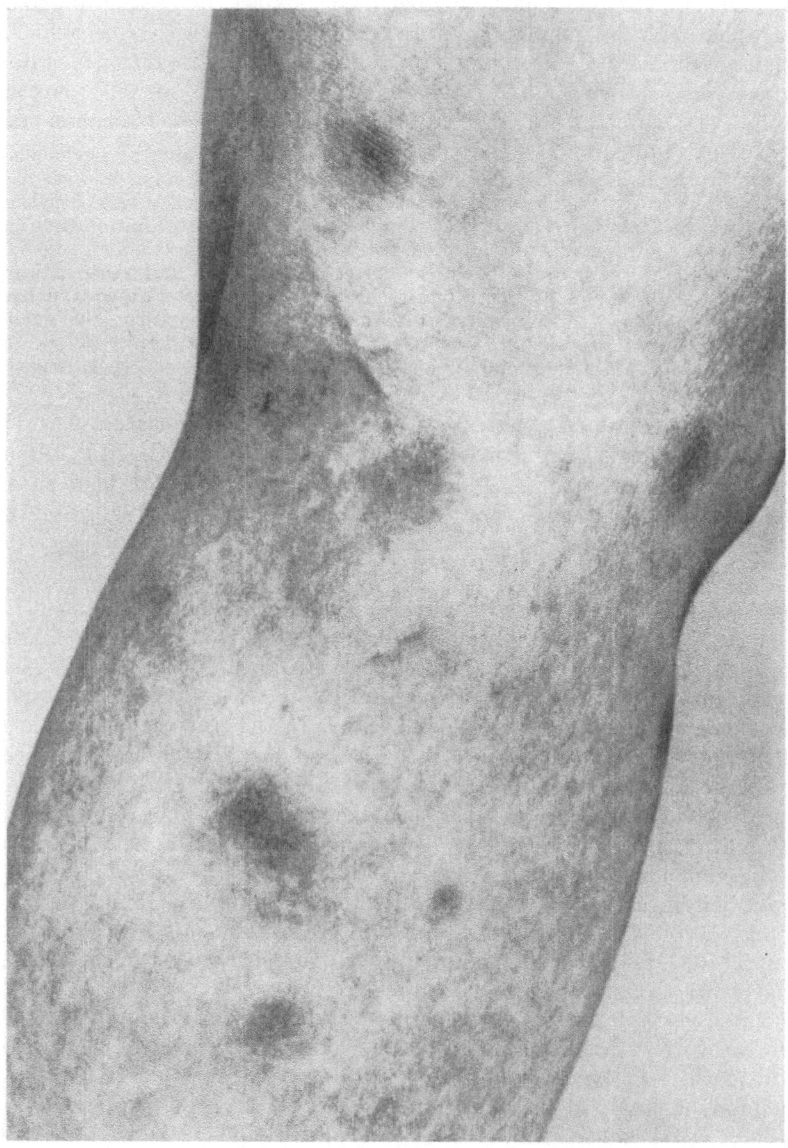

a

Abb. 19a u. b. Periarteriitis nodosa cutanea

2. „Hypersensitivity angitis" mit akuter nekrotisierender Entzündung in und um die kleinen Äste der Arteriolen und Venolen in Viscera und Dermis, möglicherweise mit Übergreifen auf die größeren Gefäße. Nach KABAT (zit. nach HARKAVY 1952) kann bei zunehmender Allergisierung stets die Tendenz zum Befall nicht nur von Capillaren, sondern auch von größeren Gefäßen festgestellt werden, was den Übergang von anaphylaktoider Purpura zu solchen Krankheitszuständen erklären könnte. Nach ZEEK beginnt die fibrinoide Nekrose zunächst subendothelial in der Intima, dehnt sich dann bis auf die ganze Arterienwand aus, gefolgt von polymorpher Entzündung, meist mit starker Eosinophilie. Hier sind Gefäße mehrerer Organe wie Haut, Nieren, Lungen betroffen. Die Krankheit verläuft häufig akut und letal infolge Niereninsuffizienz. Ursächlich sind meist Fokalinfekte im Spiel.

3. *Rheumatische Arteriitis* mit charakteristischen fibrinoiden Nekrosen an den kleinen Gefäßen von Herz und Lungen, dazu typische Aschoffsche Knötchen kardial.

4. *Allergische granulomatöse Angiitis,* mit Befall der kleinen Gefäße mit eosinophilen, epitheloiden Granulomen und Riesenzellen, meist am Herzen.

5. *Temporale Arteriitis,* mit besonderem granulomatösem Befall der Arteria temporalis.

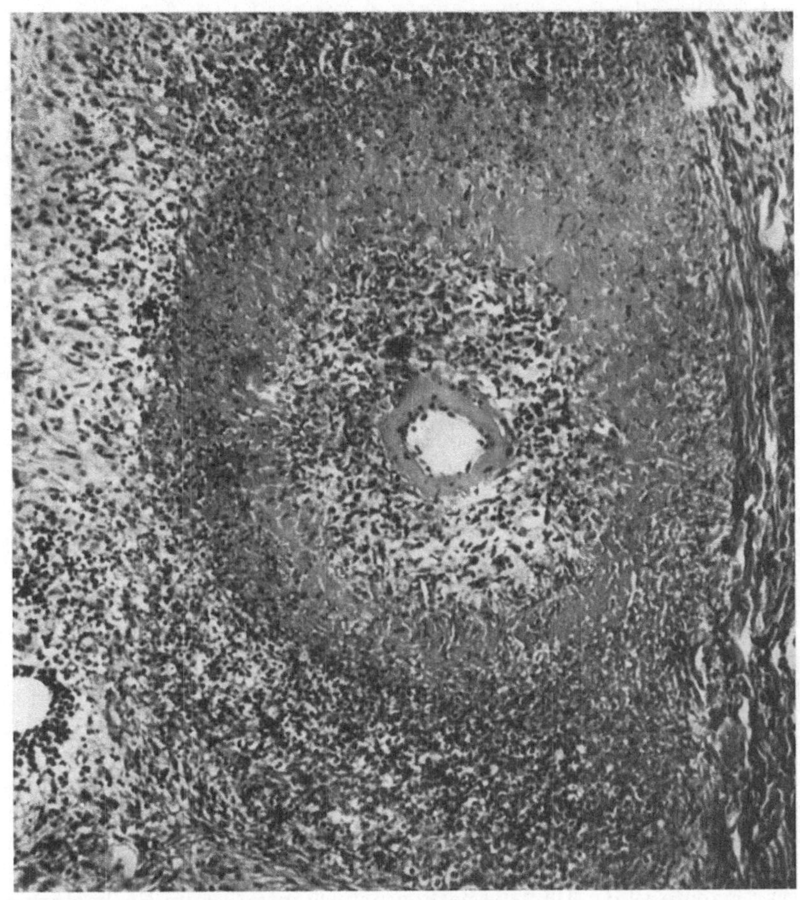

Abb. 19 b

Seither haben viele Forscher diese gefäßgebundenen, vermutlich allergischen Krankheiten mit unterschiedlichem Verlauf und Prognose studiert (z.B. Ruiter 1948, 1953—1954, 1957, 1958, 1960, 1962, Randerath 1954, Blankenhorn u. Knowles 1954, Kaemmerer u. Michel 1956, McCombs 1958, Duperrat u. Montfort 1958, McCarthy u. Kesten 1959, Knoth u. Meyhoefer 1959, Portwich 1959, Winkelmann u. Montgomery 1960, Cruchaud u.a. 1960, Orbaneja u. Puchol 1960, Bittersoll 1961, Heinlein u.a. 1961, Puchol 1962 u.a.m.).

Wie schon G. Miescher festgestellt hatte, können neben rein cutanen, benignen, schubweise auftretenden Hautveränderungen Übergänge mit Beteiligung innerer Organe bis zur letalen Periarteriitis nodosa cutanea vorkommen, so daß eine exakte Unterteilung der Krankheiten in die verschiedenen Gruppen oft auf größte Schwierigkeiten stößt.

WINKELMANN u. MONTGOMERY (1960) charakterisieren die cutane Periarteriitis nodosa cutanea folgendermaßen:

1. Die Krankheit kann auch ohne Therapie gutartig verlaufen.
2. Häufigste Cutanveränderung: Livedo mit anderen Hauterscheinungen.
3. Die allgemeinen Untersuchungs- und Laboratoriumsbefunde geben keine Anhaltspunkte für innere Veränderungen.
4. Die Histologie der Arterien von muskulärem Typ entsprechen dem klassischen Bild der Periarteriitis nodosa cutanea der anderen Organe.
5. Der Prozeß kann durch Corticoid-Therapie unterdrückt und in Grenzen gehalten werden.

DUPERRAT u. MONTFORT (1958) fügen zu den allergisch bedingten Angiitiden (nach RUITER „Arteriolitis allergica cutis") noch die „allergides nodulaires de Gougerot" (1914 bis 1918) hinzu und setzen die „vascularite nodulaire" (MONTGOMERY u.a. 1945) den Erythema induratum Bazin-ähnlichen Veränderungen gleich. Schließlich wird auch das Granuloma gangraenescens (WEGENERS Granulomatose) mit dieser Gruppe in Beziehung gebracht (s. auch NEUSS 1960, KINNEY u.a. 1961).

Das Granuloma gangraenescens (Wegenersche Granulomatose, evtl. auch „granulome malin centro-facial Woods, Degos") scheint nach verschiedenen Autoren zu den Periarteriitis nodosa-artigen Affektionen der Sinus-Nase-Augen-Region zu gehören (WEGENER 1939, GEIST u.a. 1953, ROGERS 1956, FELSON u.a. 1958) oder zu den Reticuloendotheliosen sowie zum rheumatischen Formenkreis (NEUSS 1960). Die progredienten Granulomatosen der Sinus-Nase-Augen-Region, oft mit Pneumopathie und Glomerulonephritis, führen jedoch nicht zu Blutungen, sondern zu Gangrän. Auf der Haut können sich allerdings zusätzlich polymorphe Veränderungen wie bei der Periarteriitis nodosa zeigen.

Therapeutisch scheinen bei diesem Krankheitsbild Corticoide, ACTH sowie lokal kleindosierte Röntgenbestrahlungen am ehesten Erfolg zu versprechen (NEUSS 1960). Oft verbirgt sich aber unter dem Krankheitsbild des Wegenerschen Granuloms ein progredientes Epipharynx-Malignom, wie wir es selbst in einem Fall beobachteten, bei dem dann nur frühzeitige, hochdosierte Röntgenbestrahlung Heilung bringen kann.

ORBANEJA u. PUCHOL (1960) versuchten durch eigene Klassifizierung eine bessere Übersicht über die komplexe Gruppe der nekrotisierenden Angiitiden mit fibrinoider Nekrose der Gefäßwände zu schaffen.

Ätiopathogenetisch wurden bei den möglicherweise auf allergische Mechanismen zurückzuführenden nodulären, teils hämorrhagischen Veränderungen, ähnlich wie bei der bereits erwähnten anaphylaktischen Purpura, folgende Substanzen in Erwägung gezogen: Streptokokken (METZ 1932, v. ALBERTINI u. GRUMBACH 1938), Staphylo- und Streptokokken-Fokalinfekte (MIESCHER 1946, STORCK 1951, 1960, RUITER 1956, GERBAUT u.a. 1957, BELISARIO 1960), Streptokokkensepsis (RUITER 1957), Meningokokkensepsis (GERBAUT u.a. 1957), Parahaemophilus influenzae (RUITER 1957), Grippevirus (KRESBACH 1959), Varicellen (GERBAUT 1957), Tuberkulose (HERZBERG u. SCHULZ 1957, RUITER 1958). Serum (RICH 1942), Sulfonamide (RICH 1942, RUITER 1958), Butazolidin (HORLER/TRUELOVE 1955, KINDERMANN 1961), Eumed (GERTLER 1960), Penicillin (PETERS u.a. 1960), Tabak (HARKAVY 1941, 1943). Auch genetische Faktoren werden diskutiert (ANDERSON u. HECKAMAN 1962).

RUITER machte 1961—1962 die pathogenetisch interessante Beobachtung, daß die fibrinoide Nekrose wahrscheinlich bei erhöhter Gefäßpermeabilität durch Infiltration der Gefäßwand und der umgebenden Fibrillen mit Fibrinogen oder Fibrinogenderivat zustande kommt mit Ausfällung als Fibrin. Diese präcipitierende Substanz stammt aus einer Blutplasmafraktion (HPF), die in hepariniertem Plasma bei 4^0C präcipitiert (Abb. 20). Semiquantitative Methoden zeigen, daß solche Plasmafraktionen anscheinend zu Beginn der Purpuraschübe erhöht sind und parallel zum Krankheitsverlauf, der Blutsenkung und der C-reaktiven Proteine quantitativ wechseln (RUITER 1963). Das HPF ist aber nicht für eine allergische Vasculitis spezifisch, sondern kommt auch bei anderen Krankheitszuständen vor.

Tierexperimentell wurden zur Abklärung dieser Krankheitsgruppen neben den unter rheumatoider Purpura erwähnten Versuchen noch folgende durchgeführt:

METZ (1932) sensibilisierte Ratten auf Streptokokken und erzeugte bei diesen Tieren durch Reinjektion von Keimen, Toxinen oder unspezifischen Eiweißkörpern Periarteriitis nodosa-ähnliche Läsionen. Analoge Veränderungen ließen sich auch durch Sensibilisierung gegenüber Serum produzieren, doch reagierten hier nur konstitutionell besonders veranlagte Tiere. GRUMBACH u. v. ALBERTINI (1938) infizierten Kaninchen mit Streptokokken, die aus menschlichen Foci gezüchtet worden waren. Sie fanden bei einem Teil der Tiere in verschiedenen Organen Gefäßänderungen, die Züge von Periarteriitis nodosa aufwiesen. RICH rief beim Kaninchen Periarteriitis nodosa-ähnliche Gefäßveränderungen hervor durch Sensibilisierung auf Fremdserum. C. C. SMITH u.a. erzeugten 1944 bei Ratten und Hunden Periarteriitis nodosa, indem sie durch Drosselung der Nierengefäße mit Seide eine Hypertonie verursachten. COHEN u.a. (1957) beobachteten beim Kaninchen Peri- und Panarteriitiden in den Lungengefäßen, wenn sie hochtitriges, Staphylokokken-agglutinierendes Antiserum sorgfältig fraktioniert während 60 min intravenös injizierten. Bei rascher Injektion trat erwartungsgemäß ein tödlicher anaphylaktischer Schock auf. NICOLAU u. BADANOIU (1960) erzeugten an Ohrvenen von Kaninchen polymorphe, allergidähnliche Veränderungen, wenn sie Staphylokokken-, Eiweiß- oder Tuberkulin-Antiseren in 2tägigen Intervallen mehrmals in dieselbe Ohrvene langsam injizierten. Klinisch zeigten die Veränderungen an den Injektionsstellen meist Erythem, Ödem, Infiltration mit Nekrose, histologisch Ödem und Leukocytendiapedese, später Endothelproliferation bis zu Gefäßverschluß mit mono- und histiocytären, perivasculären Granulationen.

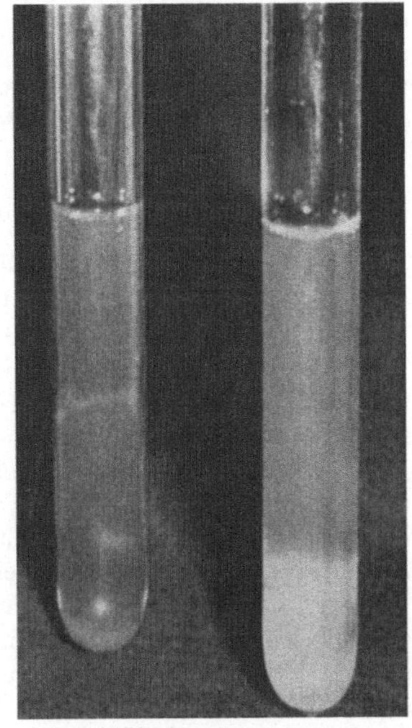

Abb. 20. Kältepräcipitate im Plasma bei „Arteriolitis allergica" Ruiter. [Aus M. RUITER: Possible connection between an abnormal plasma fraction (HPF) and vascular fibrinoid in arteriolitis (vasculitis „allergica" cutis]

Mit der Technik der umgekehrten passiven anaphylaktischen Sensibilisierung im Kaninchenversuch erzeugten COHEN und SAPP (1961) mittels gereinigten Rinderplasmaproteins Arteriitiden, Glomerulitiden und Myokarditiden und versuchten, diese pathologischen Veränderungen durch hämostatisch und fibrinolytisch wirksame Arzneimittel wie Heparin, Coumarin, EDTA, Natriumcitrat, Protamin, Fibrinolysin, Streptokinase, Trypsin, Hydroxychloroquin zu verhindern; aber nur die Streptokinase hemmte signifikant die Bildung von Arteriitis und Myokarditis.

Neben den erwähnten spezifischen Sensibilisierungen gegenüber *mikrobiellen Antigenen, Seren* und *Arzneimitteln* scheinen bei Patienten mit Periarteriitis nodosa allgemeine Änderungen im Immunmechanismus vorzuliegen, mit gelegentlichem Auftreten von unspezifischer Wa.R., selten mit antinucleären Antikörpern (L.E. Zell-Test). Eine solche Änderung des Immunmechanismus, die besonders bei den Kollagenosen beobachtet wird, ist nach ZIFF (1961) wahrscheinlich genetisch bedingt.

Neuerdings wurden die von STEFANINI und MEDNICOFF (1955) festgestellten Antikörper gegen *Autoantigene der Gefäßwand* nach zunächst negativen Befunden von FABIUS mittels einer modifizierten Agargeldiffusionsmethode von VORLAENDER bestätigt.

Als Antigen wirken hier unter Komplementbindung Extrakte aus Organen, die reich an kleineren und größeren Arterien sind. Im Gegensatz zum L.E. Zell-Phänomen wird dieser präcipitierende Serumfaktor durch Nucleoproteine und DNS nicht absorbiert bzw. neutralisiert. Ob dieser Serumfaktor gegen eines der von SCOTT (1959) postulierten Antigene (Basalmembran, Reticulin, fibrinöses Bindegewebe) gegen einzelne von FUCHS festgestellten Bindegewebsproteine oder gegen das von WATSON u.a. (1954), ROTHBARD und WATSON (1962) als Antigen erkannte Kollagen gerichtet ist, kann noch nicht gesagt werden. Ebensowenig weiß man, durch welche äußere Faktoren (Infekt, Medikament, Antigen-Antikörper-Reaktion) solche Autoantigene entstehen könnten bzw. aktiviert werden, um dann die starke immunologische Reizbeantwortung gegen gewebsfixierte Antigene in Gang zu setzen, und ob solche Vorgänge tatsächlich pathogen sind oder lediglich einen serologischen Begleitprozeß darstellen.

Ausführliche Darstellung von Klinik, Histologie, Ätiologie, Pathogenese, Diagnose und Therapie s. R. SCHUPPLI: Periarteriitis nodosa in diesem Ergänzungsband.

γ) Purpura bei Erythrocytensensibilisierung (Gardner-Diamond)

1955 publizierten Gardner u. Diamond Beobachtungen an fünf Patienten, die meist nach Traumen rezidivierende Ekchymosen aufwiesen. Später traten die Blutungen auch nach physiologischen Mikrotraumen auf. Einmal schien Splenektomie die Krankheit für 3 Jahre zum Stillstand zu bringen.

Offenbar handelte es sich um eine Störung der Gefäße mit pathologischer Reaktion auf Blutextravasate. Intracutanteste mit Erythrocytenstroma, Hämoglobin, Plasma und verschiedenen Plasmafraktionen ergab nur mit Erythrocytenstroma eine hämorrhagische Reaktion. Nach Gottlieb u.a. (1957) handelt es sich hierbei um eine verzögerte Reaktion, die nicht nur durch Erythrocytenstroma von Eigen-, sondern auch von Fremdblut ausgelöst werden kann und bei nichtsensibilisierten Kontrollpersonen negativ verläuft. Es liegt also hier eine gefäßschädigende, erworbene Sensibilisierung auf Erythrocyten vor, meist nach schweren Traumen.

c) Möglicherweise unspezifische vasculäre hämorrhagische Diathesen (Shwartzman-Sanarelli-Phänomen)

α) Purpura fulminans

Die Purpura fulminans ist ein relativ seltenes, schweres Leiden, das besonders Kinder nach Scharlachinfektion befällt mit akut, innerhalb von wenigen Stunden auftretenden und sich symmetrisch an Streckseiten der Extremitäten ausbreitenden Hämorrhagien mit Blasenbildung und Nekrosen (Abb. 21). Gelegentlich kann die Purpura fulminans mit einem erythemato-maculösen Rash beginnen (Turin u.a. 1959). Kürzlich wurde sogar ein Fall von Purpura fulminans bei einem Neugeborenen mit Tod nach 8 Tagen veröffentlicht (van der Horst 1962). Selten kommt die Affektion bei Erwachsenen vor.

Das Leiden wurde erstmals von Quelliot-Henoch (1884), dann von Henoch (1886) beschrieben und erhielt Bezeichnungen wie „Purpura fulminans", „Purpura haemorrhagica", „Purpura gangraenosa", „Purpura necrotica", von französischen Autoren den Namen „purpura infectieux foudroyant". Schließlich empfahl Little (1959) die pathogenetisch vielleicht bessere Benennung einer „postinfektiösen intravasalen Thrombose mit Gangrän".

Der Krankheit scheint in der Regel eine Infektion vorauszugehen, meist Scharlach, aber auch Varicellen (Radl u. Hekele 1957), Masern, Pneumonie (zit. Gutheil 1958), banale Anginen (Stüttgen 1955), Pneumokokkensepsis (Storck 1951). Obwohl Glanzmann 1916, König 1922, Jastremski u. Hoyt 1952, Heinild 1947 Purpura fulminans bei Meningo- und Streptokokkensepsis beschrieben haben, möchten einige Autoren (Schultz 1918, Frank 1925, Baar u. Stransky 1928) diese septischen schweren hämorrhagischen Erscheinungen von der eigentlichen Purpura fulminans absondern (zit. nach Gutheil 1958).

Die *Pathogenese* schien zunächst zweifelhaft, obwohl Glanzmann schon 1916 die Purpura fulminans als Folge einer hochgradigen Sensibilisierung der Haut auf konstitutioneller Basis, wahrscheinlich als schwerste Form der anaphylaktoiden Purpura, auffaßte und selbst eine Analogie zum Shwartzman-Sanarelli-Phänomen erwog. Moravitz (1930) rechnete sie in seiner ätiologischen Einteilung der hämorrhagischen Diathesen zum toxischen Hämorrhagie-Typus durch unbekannte Gifte (zit. nach Jürgens 1955), und Jürgens zählte sie zu den neurovasculären Blutungskrankheiten auf Grund unbekannter Noxen.

Obwohl bei der Purpura fulminans schon mehrfach Thrombopenien, Fibrinogen- und Prothrombin-Mangel beobachtet worden waren, zeigten zwei Fälle von Purpura fulminans nach Scharlach (Koller u.a. 1950) einen Mangel bzw.

völliges Fehlen von Faktor V und einen Antithrombin-Überschuß, die den Störungen von Thrombocyten und Koagulationsfaktoren beim bereits erwähnten tierexperimentellen Shwartzman-Sanarelli-Phänomen glichen (Storck 1951, Hoigné 1952). Nach Radl/Hekele (1957) u.a.m. kann zusätzlich ein Faktor VIII-Mangel vorkommen, capillarmikroskopisch sind oft Erweiterungen der Haargefäße am Übergang vom arteriellen zum venösen Schenkel beobachtet worden.

Wenn auch gewiß mit Recht wegen der Symmetrie der Läsionen und Fehlen von Schleimhautblutungen besonders an neurovasculäre Störungen gedacht wurde (Gasser, de Muralt 1950), dies auch in Anbetracht von histologischen Veränderungen an sympathischen Ganglien (Castex, zit. nach Gasser/de Muralt) oder aber wegen der topographischen Verteilung an zentralnervöse Mechanismen (L. Suender 1943), so erscheinen doch die Parallelen mit dem Shwartzman-Sanarelli-Phänomen sehr auffällig (akutes Auftreten, Sekundärerkrankung, vorübergehende Thrombopenie, Veränderungen der Gerinnungsfaktoren, histologische Veränderungen). Allerdings läßt sich eine Mitbeteiligung des neurovegetativen Systems nicht ausschließen, wie z.B. Denervationsversuche an den Nieren mit Unterdrückung des Shwartzman-Sanarelli-Phänomens zeigten (Palmiero u.a. 1962). Little betrachtet die Herabsetzung von Fibrinogen und Faktor V als sekundäres Phänomen nach ausgedehnten intravasalen Koagulationen mit peripherer Fibrinverarmung und setzt die histologisch nachweisbaren Fibrinthromben zu den experimentellen Befunden von Thomas u. Stetson beim Shwartzman-Sanarelli-Phänomen in Beziehung.

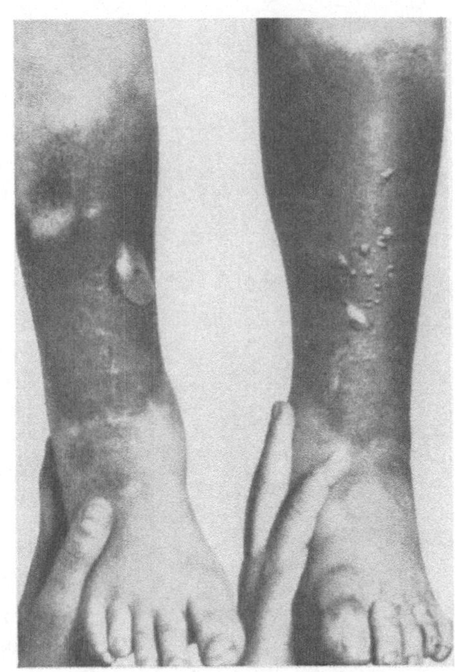

Abb. 21. Manschettenförmige Blutungen bei Purpura fulminans nach Scharlach

Therapeutisch erwies sich gemäß der letztgenannten Auffassung eine 12tägige Heparininfusion in einem Fall als lebensrettend (Little 1959), wogegen nach Gasser u. de Muralt (1950) totaler Blutaustausch, nach anderen Beobachtungen Gaben von ACTH, Cortison (Schreiner 1959), Antibiotica, Bluttransfusionen entscheidend für die Heilung sein können. Teils wurden auch Vitamin C, K und P empfohlen (Gutheil 1958), ebenso antiallergische Behandlung (Radl u. Hekele (1957).

β) Waterhouse-Friderichsen-Syndrom

Ein besonders heftiges, meist tödliches Geschehen stellen die schweren Blutungen mit leichenfleckartigen Hautveränderungen und schwerstem Kreislaufkollaps beim Waterhouse-Friderichsen-Syndrom dar, meist bei Meningo- oder Pneumokokkensepsis (Friderichsen 1955, v. Rechenberg 1953, Grumbach 1958, Berkson u. a. 1959, Kutschera-Eichberger 1959, Bohn/Winter 1960).

Entscheidend für Verlauf und Therapie ist hier die sog. „Nebennierenapoplexie“ durch Blutung, wobei therapeutisch besonders die Glucocorticoide, weniger die Mineralocorticoide, wirksam sind (Wolter/Loeb 1956, Schreiner 1959). Ausnahmsweise kann das Syndrom auch bei Staphylokokkensepticämie vorkommen (Rambert u. a. 1959). Wahrscheinlich handelt es sich auch hier um den zweiphasigen Mechanismus des Shwartzman-Sanarelli-Phänomens (Storck 1953). Staude berichtete 1960 allerdings über eine interessante Gruppenerkrankung bei fünf Kindern, von denen drei mit autoptisch gesichertem Befund an diesem Syndrom starben. Erstaunlicherweise konnten jedoch trotz größter Sorgfalt bei keinem dieser Fälle Meningokokken oder andere Keime gezüchtet werden, so daß diese Ätiologie hier in Frage gestellt ist.

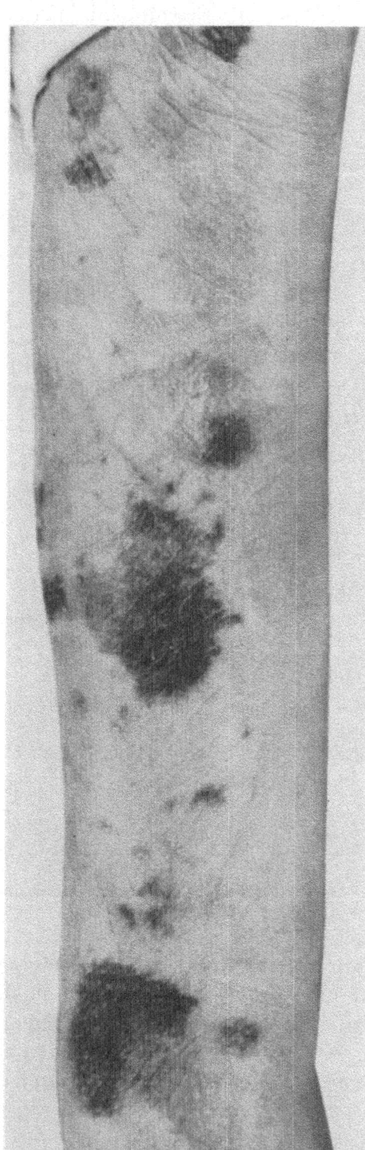

Abb. 22. Purpura senilis

d) Vasculäre hämorrhagische Diathese infolge Anoxämie oder Altersdegeneration

α) Purpura senilis

Wir hatten 1955 die Purpura senilis mit der Purpura orthostatica bei den vasculären hämorrhagischen Reaktionen durch Anoxämie und Sklerose eingereiht. In der ätiologischen Einteilung der hämorrhagischen Diathesen von Morawitz (1930) erscheint die Purpura senilis zusammen mit der Purpura cachecticorum bei den allgemeinen Ernährungsstörungen. Bei der nosologischen Einteilung nach Jürgens (1955) ist sie unter den Blutungskrankheiten bei Mangelzuständen, bei der pathogenetischen Klassifikation durch denselben Autor unter den Gefäßdegenerationen zu finden.

Das von Bateman 1836, dann von Unna 1895 und später von vielen anderen beschriebene purpurische Altersleiden entsteht in Schüben, gleicherweise bei Frauen und Männern, meist nicht vor dem 60. Altersjahr. Die Ekchymosen sind vorzugsweise an der radialen Streckseite der Vorderarme und an Handrücken, seltener an Gesicht und Beinen lokalisiert, meist in Form von 1—4 cm messenden, unregelmäßig begrenzten, dunkelroten Flecken, in der Regel in altersdegenerierten, pigmentierten, weichen, dünnen, unelastischen Hautbezirken. Die Blutungen können wenige Tage bis einige Wochen bestehen bleiben und machen den üblichen, allerdings stark verzögerten Farbwechsel des Hämoglobinabbaues durch (Abb. 22).

Die *histologischen* Untersuchungen zeigen die für das Alter charakteristische Verdünnung der Epidermis mit verstrichenen Papillen, feiner subpapillärer elastischer Faserschicht, gedehnten oder geschlängelten Blutgefäßen, Rarifizierung der Kollagenfasern, jedoch mit ausgeprägter seniler elastoider Degeneration. Die elastoid-degenerierten Bindegewebsbalken sind vermehrt geschlängelt und fraktioniert, in höherem Maße als dies normalerweise im Alter der Fall ist.

Pathogenetisch scheint nicht allgemeine Capillarbrüchigkeit oder Arteriosklerose das Leiden auszulösen (TATTERSALL u.a. 1950), denn es können typische purpurische Läsionen willkürlich innerhalb von 1—10 min durch stumpfen Druck auf der Haut der befallenen Extremitäten erzeugt werden, nicht aber am Stamm ohne degenerative Veränderung des Bindegewebes. OSGOOD u.a. (1954) schreiben der Verwitterung des elastischen Gewebes bei älteren Patienten die Hauptverantwortung in der Genese der flachen Ekchymosen zu. Möglicherweise spielt zusätzlich bei der Purpura senilis neben der altersbedingten Degeneration eine Lebererkrankung eine Rolle, wie dies DEBRAY/KERNOSKI (1959) an Hand von Leberbiopsien bei zehn Fällen vermuteten. Diese Autoren empfahlen deshalb Leberfunktionsprüfungen, wenn auch die Koagulationsfaktoren bei diesen Patienten nicht verändert sind. Neben der senilen Degeneration von Gefäß- und Bindegewebe, möglicherweise zusammen mit dem elektronenmikroskopisch im Alter nachweisbaren unregelmäßigen Aufbau der Endothelien (s. früher), scheinen also noch zusätzliche Faktoren (Vitamin E-Mangel, Leberstörungen?) eine Rolle zu spielen.

SHUSTER/SCARBOROUGH (1961) haben bei über 80 älteren Patienten interessante experimentelle Versuche durchgeführt. Danach werden die Gefäße in der lockeren Altershand (elastoide Degeneration) an den Prädilektionsstellen vermehrt traumatisiert und lädiert. Das ausgetretene Blut breitet sich im schlaffen Gewebe aus und wird im senilen histiocytenarmen Gewebe nur verzögert resorbiert. Durch Armut der Histiocyten geschieht auch der Hämoglobinabbau nur verzögert, was das fehlende intracelluläre Hämosiderin erweist. Diese Annahmen konnten an Hand von artifiziellen Läsionen nach intracutaner Blutquaddel mit und ohne vorgängiger Hämolyse experimentell bestätigt werden.

Therapeutisch scheinen Rutin, Ascorbinsäure und Nicotinsäure das Leiden nicht zu beeinflussen (TATTERSALL u. SEVILLE 1950). Hingegen soll Vitamin E in hohen Dosen, während 1—2 Monaten täglich 200—400 mg parenteral, dann einen Monat per os (MARS u.a. 1957) gegeben, die Purpuraschübe unterdrücken, allerdings nur während der Behandlungsperiode.

β) Purpura orthostatica

Im Gegensatz zur senilen Purpura findet sich die *Purpura orthostatica* hauptsächlich an den orthostatisch belasteten unteren Extremitäten. Sie entwickelt sich ebenfalls vorzugsweise im Bereich von altersveränderter Haut und scheint durch entzündliche Prozesse verschiedenster Ursache, Stauungen im Abdomen, sowie durch venöse Insuffizienz zur Manifestation zu kommen (KALKOFF 1962).

γ) Purpura bei Ehlers-Danlos-Syndrom

Ein Symptom des Ehlers-Danlos-Syndroms ist vermehrte Verletzlichkeit von Haut- und Blutgefäßen, neben der bekannten Hyperelastizität der Cutis und Hyperextensibilität der Gelenke, Pseudotumoren über den knöchernen Prominenzen, calcifizierten subcutanen Knoten und Skeletanomalien. Die leicht eintretenden Quetschungen mit Bildung von Hämatomen und Ekchymosen führten schon mehrfach dazu, daß eine hämorrhagische Diathese angenommen wurde mit genauen hämatologischen Untersuchungen. Thrombocyten und Koagulationsfaktoren sind jedoch im allgemeinen normal, doch kann vermehrte Gefäßfragilität mit positivem Rumpel-Leede-Phänomen gefunden werden (Klinik, Blutungsbereitschaft, Histologie und ausführliche Literatur s. Kapitel „Cutis laxa“

[Ehlers-Danlos-Syndrom] von G. W. KORTING in Ergänzungsband III/1, S. 413 bis 423 dieses Handbuches).

Auch mit neuesten gerinnungsphysiologischen Untersuchungsmethoden fanden P. G. FRICK u.a. (1956) bei drei Patienten mit Ehlers-Danlos-Syndrom keine pathologischen Veränderungen, indem Blutungs-, Gerinnungs-, Prothrombin-, Recalcifizierungszeit, Plättchenzahl, Blutkuchenretraktion, Fibrinogen, Thrombinzeit und Prothrombinkonsumptionszeit im Bereiche der Norm lagen. Lediglich der Rumpel-Leede-Test war positiv, als einziges Zeichen einer vererbten Blutungsdisposition in zwei Generationen. Es handelt sich also um eine vasculäre Purpura, ähnlich wie bei der Purpura senilis, bedingt durch das mangelhafte Bindegewebe (mangelhafte Verflechtung oder Entflechtung der straffen Netzstruktur des kollagenen Gewebes), mangelhaften kollagenen Halt der Blutlymphgefäße mit auffallender Windung und Schlängelung (KORTING), Verfilzung, Zusammenballung der elastischen Fasern, wodurch Blutungen per rhexim entstehen.

e) Unbestimmte vasculäre hämorrhagische Diathesen. Verschiedenes

α) Purpura pigmentosa progressiva (KALKOFF)

Eine Reihe hämorrhagischer pigmentierter Dermatosen kann unter diesem 1962 von KALKOFF vorgeschlagenen Begriff zusammengefaßt werden, nämlich M. Schamberg, M. Gougerot-Blum, Purpura annularis teleangiectodes Majocchi, Purpura téléangiectasique arciforme Touraine, ferner Abarten, die unter anderen Bezeichnungen publiziert wurden, wie Angioma serpiginosum (HUTCHINSON u. CROCKER) usw.

Wenn auch die einzelnen Krankheitsbilder klinisch gewisse Besonderheiten aufweisen mögen, finden sich doch häufig Übergänge, so daß es fraglich erscheint, ob die verschiedenen Typen überhaupt nosologisch voneinander abgetrennt werden sollen (ARNDT, HAGERMAN, RANDALL u.a. 1951, KALKOFF 1959, 1962).

Diese Krankheitsgruppen zeigen alle ein chronisch-progressives Auftreten von umschriebenen petechialen Blutungen mit knötchenförmiger, ekzematoider Entzündung und Übergang des ausgetretenen Blutfarbstoffes von Purpurrot, Braunrot in Braun als fleckige Pigmentierung infolge intracellulär gespeichertem Hämosiderin (Abb. 23). Meist beginnt das Leiden an der Fußknöchelregion mit Ausbreitung auf Bein, Stamm, evtl. auch auf obere Extremitäten. Bei einer Krankheitsgruppe (Purpura Majocchi, Purpura téléangiectasique arciforme Touraine) findet sich Tendenz zu annulärer Ausbreitung der Herde mit Abheilung, evtl. angedeuteter Atrophie im Zentrum (Abb. 24). Der Juckreiz tritt meist zurück. Eine Beteiligung innerer Organe fehlt. Die Geschlechtsverteilung ist uncharakteristisch, Erkrankungsalter meist zwischen 30—60 Jahren.

Schwere Störungen von Koagulationsfaktoren und Thrombocyten fehlen. Die Purpura beruht auf erhöhter Capillarverletzlichkeit, nachweisbar mittels Capillarmikroskopie, Rumpel-Leede-Test und Saugglocken-Versuch, der aber nur bei generalisierter Capillarstörung positiv ist.

Histologisch finden sich nichtreaktionslose Erythrocytenaustritte (wie z.B. bei thrombopenischer Purpura, 1. Grundform) oder serös-exsudative, polymorphkernige Leukocyteninfiltrate und Erythrocytenextravasate bei dilatierten und degenerierten Gefäßen (wie bei der anaphylaktoiden Purpura, 2. Grundform), sondern nur diskrete Gefäßveränderungen, Degeneration und Proliferation der Capillarendothelien mit Erythrocytenaustritten meist um die Schaltstücke (wie dies capillarmikroskopisch bestätigt werden kann), mit lymphohistiocytären Infiltraten und auffallender intracellulärer Hämosiderin-Ablagerung bei Fehlen von Fibrin (3. Grundform, KALKOFF 1959) (Abb. 24).

Ätiopathogenetisch ist diese Gruppe der vasculären hämorrhagischen Diathesen noch wenig geklärt, obwohl bereits einzelne versprechende Hypothesen aufgestellt wurden. Wie KALKOFF mit Recht betont, ist die außerordentlich auffällige

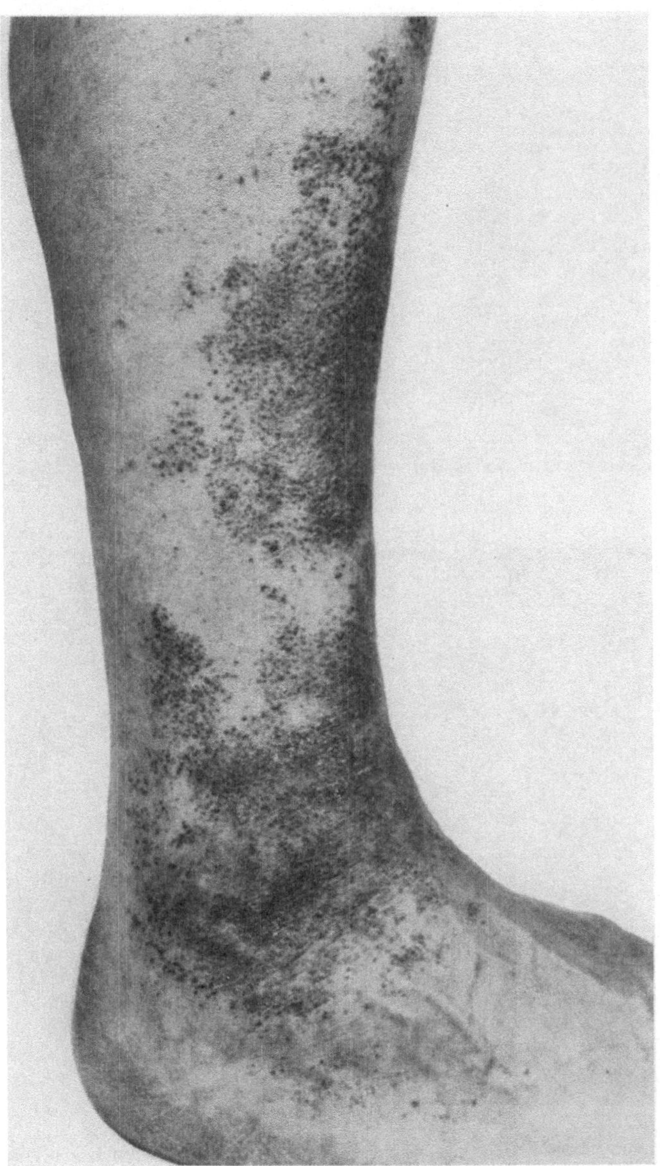

Abb. 23. Morbus Schamberg

Hämosiderinspeicherung bei diesen Krankheitsformen von besonderem Interesse, wobei hier der Blutabbau den Weg des mit höherem Eisengehalt an eiweißgebundenen Hämosiderins und nicht des Ferritins wählt (HEILMEYER u. WEISSENBACH). Die verschiedensten Realisationsfaktoren werden diskutiert, so konstitutionell bedingte Störungen des peripheren Kreislaufs mit Blutdrucklabilität und Akrocyanose (VILMAR 1948), allgemeine Disposition zu Gefäßschädigung und lang anhaltender Speicherung eisenhaltigen Pigmentes (STEIGLEDER 1953), angioneurotisch-vegetative Dysregulationen, z.B. mit Fingertremor und Lidflattern (SCHUPPENER 1954), Polyglobulie, labiler Hochdruck (GOTTRON 1935), Vorliegen

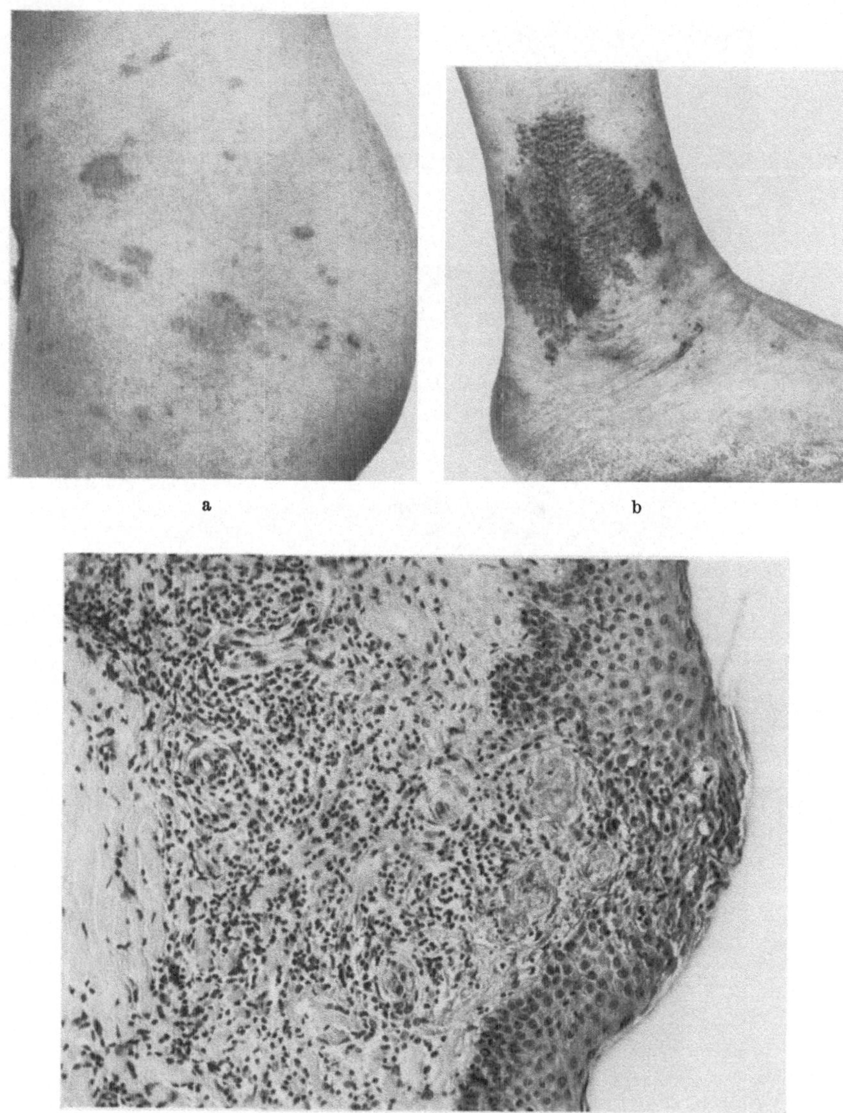

Abb. 24a—c. a Purpura Majocchi. b Morbus Schamberg. c Auch bei letzterem neben lymphocytären Infiltraten gelegentlich teleangiektatisch erweiterte, von Erythrocyten vollgepfropfte Capillaren

einer diffusen Capillaropathie, z.T. mit vorübergehender Hypofibrinogenämie, sogar flüchtigem Fehlen von Faktor VIII und IX (LEOVEY u.a., VEZEKENYI 1960).

BECHELLI u.a. (1952) suchten auf Grund klinischer und histologischer Veränderungen die genannten Krankheiten in *drei Gruppen zu unterteilen*, nämlich 1. in progressiv pigmentierende Dermatosen mit capillären Blutungen und diskreter Entzündung der Capillarregion der oberen Cutis, 2. in pigmentierende purpurische lichenoide Dermatitis mit gleichen Veränderungen, aber zusätzlich mit ausgesprochener Infiltration bis zur Ausbildung typischer lichenoider Papeln, und 3. in annuläre teleangiektatische purpurische Herde mit tieferer und intensiverer Entzündung bis zur dermo-hypodermatischen Grenze, wobei die annulären Läsionen oft eine cutane Atrophie bedingen.

Besonders schöne und interessante *capillarmikroskopische Untersuchungen* haben 1941 SCHOCH und 1958 DAVIS u.a. angestellt.

SCHOCH fand capillarmikroskopisch bei drei Fällen von Purpura Majocchi in den Krankheitsherden Eröffnung der Capillaren mit geringer Strömungsgeschwindigkeit in den erweiterten Gefäßen. Der venöse Schenkel war außerordentlich weit, der arterielle eng, so daß venöse Stase, im arteriellen Schenkel deutlich körnige Strömung zu sehen war. Diese Besonderheiten traten jeweils in rhythmischem Wechsel auf. In der Umgebung der feinsten Capillaren konnte oft ausgetretenes Blut in großen Mengen, an mehreren Stellen auch Hämosiderin festgestellt werden. Der Blutungsvorgang wurde meist durch eine starke Verengerung des arteriellen Schenkels bei weitem venösen Schenkel eingeleitet, dann schien auch dieser etwas enger zu werden. SCHOCH beobachtete gelegentlich, „daß plötzlich, etwa am Übergang des venösen in den arteriellen Schenkel, eine geringe Menge Blut aus den Gefäßen austrat und in Form einer kleinen Wolke liegen blieb. Die ausgetretene Menge vermehrte sich nicht, es schien also kein Blut mehr nachzufließen. Die Stase im venösen Schenkel war nach dem Blutaustritt behoben, und die Blutströmung in den Capillaren nahm an Geschwindigkeit wieder zu. Auch der arterielle Schenkel wurde deutlicher sichtbar und stärker erweitert. Im Zentrum der ringförmig angeordneten Blutung waren sämtliche Capillaren außerordentlich eng. Die Unterscheidung der arteriellen und venösen Schenkel bereitete oft Schwierigkeiten. In der Umgebung solcher atrophisch erscheinender Haargefäße, wie auch in ihnen selbst, lag Hämosiderin in Schollen, anscheinend von früheren Blutungen.“ SCHOCH machte auf Grund dieser Beobachtungen auf die pathogenetische Bedeutung der Vasomotoren aufmerksam. Da die Blutungen jeweils durch Vasoconstriction des arteriellen Anteils eingeleitet wurden, wäre auch an allergische Mechanismen im Sinne des Arthus-Phänomens oder der umschriebenen Anaphylaxie zu denken.

DAVIS u. LAWLER (1958) fanden in zwölf Fällen von pigmentierter purpurischer Dermatose capillarmikroskopisch Erweiterung des Capillarlumens dort, wo die petechialen Hämorrhagien stattfanden mit Bildung von Hämosiderin. An den Stellen wiederholter Petechien blieb jedoch Capillarregeneration aus, mit Rarifizierung der Haargefäße und Atrophie der Dermalpapillen sowie anschließender teleangiektatischer Erweiterung des darunter liegenden Venengeflechtes.

Obwohl ein Großteil der progressiven purpurischen und pigmentierten Dermatosen bereits von MEIROWSKI (E. VBJ IV/2) in diesem Handbuch 1933 geschildert wurde, sollen hier zusätzlich einzelne neuere Beobachtungen und Auffassungen kurz dargestellt werden.

αα) Morbus Schamberg und Purpura angiosclćreux et prurigineux avec éléments lichénoïdes Gougerot-Blum. SCHAMBERG hatte 1901 unter der Bezeichnung „peculiar progressive pigmentary disease of the skin“ die nach ihm benannte Krankheit, und GOUGEROT mit BLUM 1925 eine Abart unter „purpura angiosclćreux prurigineux avec éléments lichénoïdes“ beschrieben.

Zum *Syndrom Gougerot und Blum* wurden verschiedene weitere Einzelfälle publiziert, so von PECK 1938, GROSS 1939, PROSSER, THOMAS u. ROOK 1949, KORTING u. EISSNER 1958 u.a.m. 1950 fügten GOUGEROT u. BLUM eine weitere Variante unter dem Namen „*Trisymptome*“, dann „*Pentasymptome*“ hinzu, wobei die Haut beim Trisymptom kleine Nodositäten, kokardenähnliches Erythema multiforme und Purpura aufwies, beim selteneren Pentasymptom zusätzlich Urticaria, selbst Blasenbildung an den Extremitäten.

Ätiopathogenetisch wurden neben den vorgängig erwähnten Mechanismen lokalisierte Kreislaufstörungen der terminalen Strombahn im Sinne des Stufengesetzes von RICKER angenommen (PFLEGER 1954), vereinzelt verlängerte Nativblutgerinnungszeit (SPIER u. MARX 1953), neurogene Faktoren wie Paraesthesien, Fehlen von Patellarsehnenreflex, tiefe Sensibilitätsstörungen (SPENCER 1951). Zusammenhänge mit toxischen bzw. allergischen Reaktionen nahmen bei dieser Krankheitsgruppe KRUIZINGA (1951) an, anläßlich der Beobachtung einer 65jährigen

Patientin mit Adalin-Unverträglichkeit, einem brom- und harnstoffhaltigen Schlafmittel, welches relativ häufig durch Capillarschädigungen hämorrhagische Exantheme hervorrief. Wegen gehäuften Vorkommens im 2. Weltkrieg, meist 10 Tage nach Infektion der oberen Luftwege bei marschungewohnten Rekruten, erwog Slepyan (1951) toxisch-infektiöse Capillarschädigungen und Manifestation an den orthostatisch belasteten unteren Extremitäten. Krueger (1961) vermutete ebenfalls Herdinfekte und Hy u. Lamotte (1959) hepatische Virusinfektion mit positivem Nachweis verschiedener Agglutinine bei Vermehrung der α_2-Globuline.

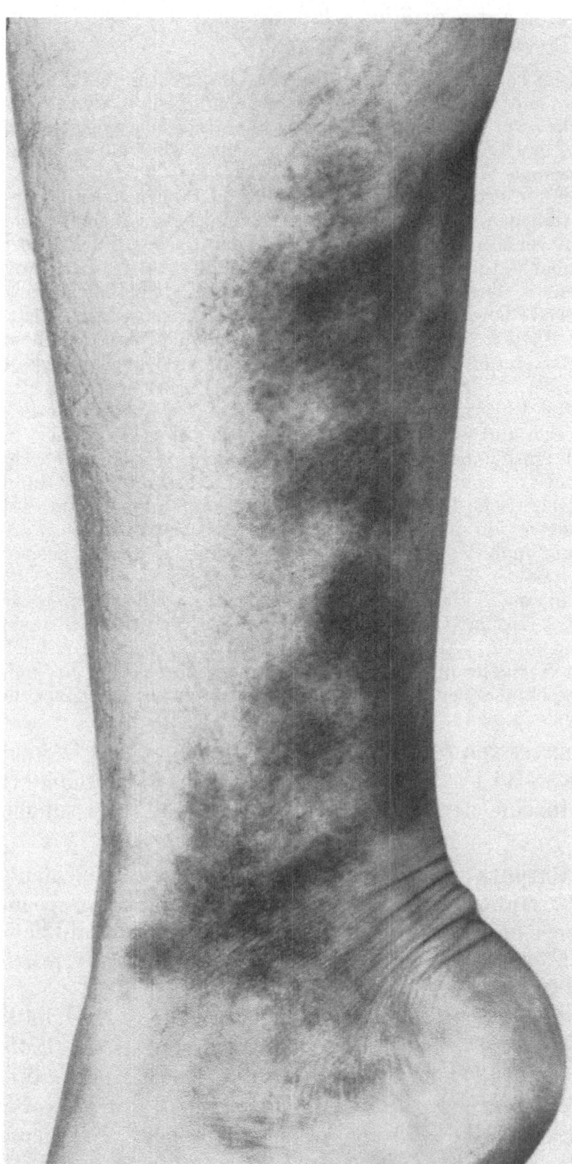

Abb. 25. Purpura téléangiectasique arciforme Touraine

Beim Morbus Schamberg konnte der zunächst angenommene Zusammenhang des Leidens mit Hypercholesterinämie oder Tuberkulose nicht bestätigt werden (Guilaine 1956). Das „Angioma serpiginosum" scheint mit dem Morbus Schamberg nicht identisch zu sein (Miedzinski u.a. 1956).

ββ) Purpura annularis teleangiectodes (Majocchi) und Purpura téléangiectasique arciforme (Touraine). Zu dem von Majocchi 1896 beschriebenen Krankheitsbild fügte Touraine eine Variante hinzu (Abb. 25). Das klinische Bild der Purpura annularis teleangiectodes Majocchi (Abb. 24) wurde eingehend in der ersten Ausgabe dieses Handbuches beschrieben (Band IV/2, S. 986, VI/2, S. 555).

Pathogenetisch wurden auch hier einige besondere Mechanismen erwogen, so von Gottron (1930) hauptsächlich eine *Kreislaufstörung*, die besonders auf konstitutioneller Minderwertigkeit des Capillarsystems, Erythrocytose und Einwirkung von Mikrotraumen beruhe. Im Vordergrund stehe die funktionelle Kreislaufstörung, wobei nicht an jeder Ektasie Blutaustritt stattfinde, die Hämorrhagie also kein notwendiges Stadium der Dermatose, sondern nur einen möglichen

Ausgang derselben darstelle. Ähnliche Gedanken über eine Angioneurose hatte bereits MAJOCCHI geäußert. GOTTRON gibt allerdings zu, daß sich die zugrunde liegenden, funktionellen Kreislaufstörungen nur schwer objektivieren lassen. Auch SCHOCH (1941) denkt, wie erwähnt, hauptsächlich an nervöse, vasomotorisch bedingte Zirkulationsstörungen, vor allem auf Grund seiner capillarmikroskopischen Untersuchungen. Zusätzlich kommen aber auch gastrointestinale Störungen mit toxisch-allergischer Capillarschädigung in Frage. Die Adalingenese wurde von MULZER u. HABERMANN (1930) an einigen Fällen von Purpura Majocchi demonstriert, wobei sich allerdings diese Fälle durch ungewöhnlichen Pruritus auszeichneten. Wahrscheinlich *nutritive Allergie* (auf Milch- und Milchprodukte) demonstrierte STORCK 1959, an einem Fall von hartnäckiger Purpura Majocchi, wobei der Milchgenuß jeweils eine klar registrierbare, vorübergehende Tachykardie erzeugte; auch klang das Leiden nach Eliminationsdiät allmählich ab.

BORN beschrieb 1956 gehäuftes Vorkommen von hämorrhagischen pigmentierten Dermatosen im Sinne von Purpura Majocchi, Morbus Schamberg und Gougerot-Blum bei Soldaten, bei welchen anscheinend *Kontakt mit Textilien* (Khaki-Uniform, neue Zivilkleidung) und Mikrotraumen für das Leiden verantwortlich gemacht werden, obwohl Teste mit solchen Stoffen negativ ausfielen. Die Abheilung erfolgte jeweils nach Weglassen der betreffenden Kleidungsstücke (s. auch später: „Dermatitis caused by shirts").

Beim Purpura annularis-Typ Touraine diskutierte 1954 BREHM die verschiedensten pathogenetischen Aspekte, wie vorübergehende Störungen des Gerinnungsmechanismus, gesteigerte Capillarpermeabilität, Stauung im venösen Kreislauf, infektiös-toxische Prozesse, Systemerkrankungen des Reticuloendothelialsystems und vermutete die ursächliche Bedeutung des Neurovegetativums.

Infolge mannigfacher Variationen und Atypien lassen sich einzelne Fälle nicht sicher in eine der genannten Gruppen einreihen, wie beispielsweise Fälle von TÉMINE (1954), von GRUPPER u.a. (1955), von PEGUM (1957), von LE COULANT u.a. (1960) usw., bei welchen dann auch die Differentialdiagnose der „dermites pigmentées purpuriques et téléangiectasiques en plaques" von DEGOS in Frage kommt.

Therapeutisch werden bei sämtlichen der genannten progressiven pigmentierten hämorrhagischen Dermatosen einerseits Vitamine wie Vitamin C und P, Calcium-Injektionen, diätetische Maßnahmen, gelegentlich in schweren Fällen Bluttransfusionen, in neuester Zeit Prednison und Röntgenbestrahlungen empfohlen (z.B. mit weichen Strahlen 4—6mal 60 r, 30 kV, 0,5 Al.-Filter, einmal wöchentlich gegeben). Da die Krankheit häufig schubweise verläuft, ist aber eine sichere Beurteilung des Therapieerfolges schwierig. Oft erweist sich der progressive Verlauf als sehr hartnäckig, so daß intensivere Behandlungsmethoden wie Corticoide und Röntgenstrahlen durchaus am Platze sind; dies um so mehr, als nur in einer relativ kleinen Anzahl der Fälle eine Kausaltherapie (Fokalsanierung, Eliminationsdiät, Ausschaltung gewisser Medikamente) durchgeführt werden kann.

β) Ekzematoide Purpuraformen

Unter den ekzematoiden, in der Regel vasculären Purpuraformen sollen kurz die Ekzematid-ähnliche Purpura von DOUCAS u. KAPETANAKIS (1952, 1953), die „Itching Purpura" von LOEWENTHAL (1954), die „Dermatitis caused by shirts" (HODGSON u. HELLIER 1946), die „sekundär-hämorrhagischen Ekzeme" und schließlich das Aldrich-Syndrom Erwähnung finden.

αα) Epidemische purpurisch-lichenoide Dermatitis (eczematid-like Purpura Doucas and Kapetanakis). DOUCAS u. KAPETANAKIS beschrieben 1952 pigmentierte, purpurisch-lichenoide Dermatitiden, ähnlich dem Morbus Schamberg oder Morbus Gougerot-Blum, beginnend an den Beinen mit Ausbreitung in die Inguinal- und Glutäalbezirke innerhalb von 15—20 Tagen, epidemisch auftretend (Abb. 26). Die Affektion wurde in den Jahren 1940—1951, in den Monaten März bis August besonders bei erwachsenen Frauen im Alter von 40—50 Jahren beobachtet. Die Krankheit verlief in Schüben rezidivierend über mehrere Monate bis

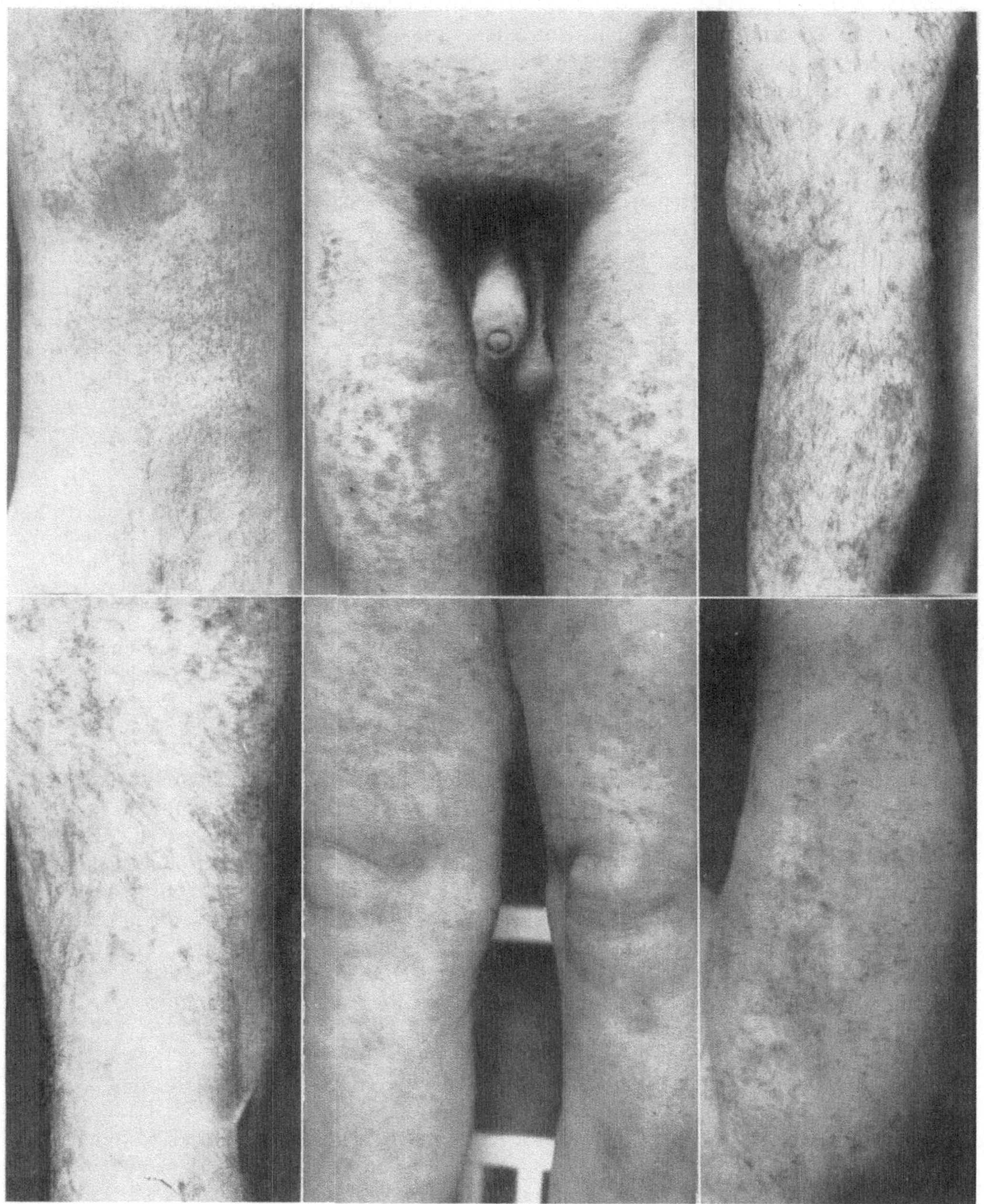

Abb. 26. „Eczematid-like purpura“ Doucas und Kapetanakis. [Aus C. DOUCAS and J. KAPETANAKIS: Eczematidlike Purpura. Dermatologica (Basel) **106**, 86 (1953)]

2 Jahre und heilte unter Hinterlassung von Pigmentierung (Hämosiderin) der Unterschenkel ab. Die Blutbefunde waren normal, jedoch war die Capillarfragilität erhöht.

Pathogenetisch konnte die Affektion nicht mit Sicherheit abgeklärt werden, doch fand sich in 85% der Fälle im Stuhl Entamoeba histolytica.

Ähnliche Beobachtungen folgten von CASALA/SANTIAGO u.a. (1955), CSERMELY (1955, 1957), VILANOVA u. a. (1956), BINAZZI u.a. (1958). Wenn auch DOUCAS u.a.

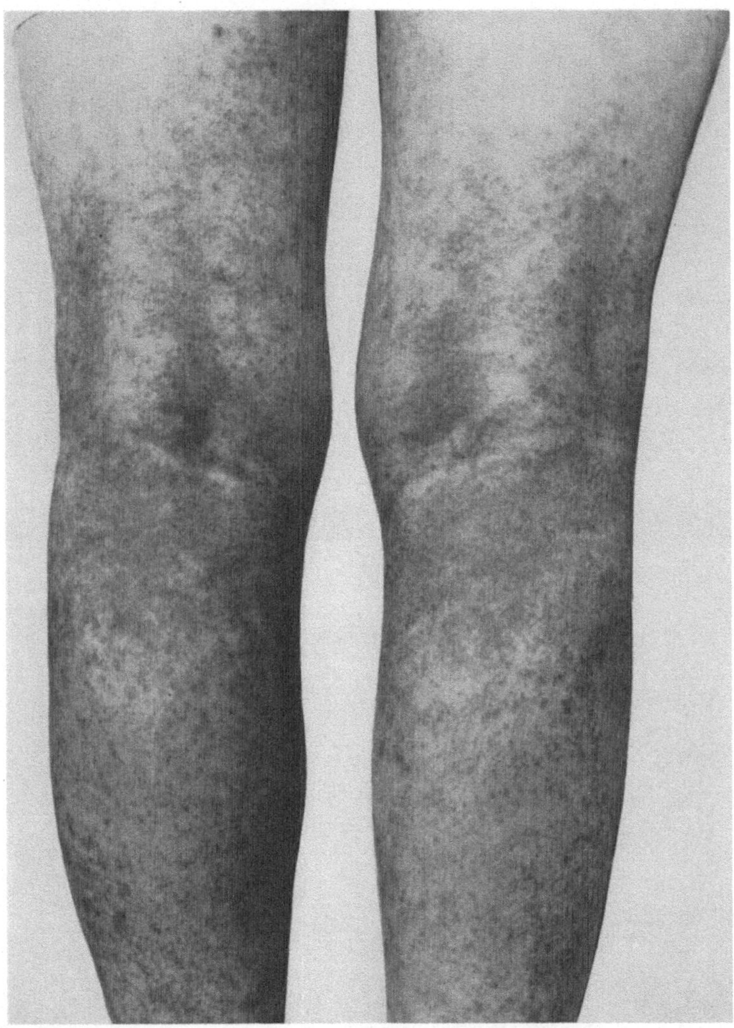

Abb. 27. „Itching-Purpura" Loewenthal. [Aus L. J. A. LOEWENTHAL: Itching purpura. Brit. J. Derm. **66**, 95 (1954)]

zunächst den Juckreiz nicht besonders erwähnten, wurde dieser von CASALA u.a. hervorgehoben. VILANOVA fand in seinem Fall ebenfalls Parasiten, nämlich Trichocephalen. CZERMELY stellte besonders noch die Differentialdiagnose mit serpiginösem Angioma Hutchinson in den Vordergrund. BINAZZI u. FINZI dachten in erster Linie an Dental- oder Tonsillarfoci, da die Haut sehr stark gegen Streptokokken- und Staphylokokken-Antigene reagierte. Allerdings hatten Breitspektrum-Antibiotica keinen Erfolg, wohl aber Prednisolon.

Die *histologischen* Veränderungen entsprachen ungefähr denen der anderen progressiven hämorrhagischen pigmentierten Dermatosen.

Therapeutisch bewährten sich meistens Ascorbinsäure und Rutin.

ββ) Itching Purpura (Loewenthal). Der einzige Unterschied der von Loewenthal beschriebenen Fälle von „Itching Purpura" gegenüber den vorher erwähnten Gruppen besteht im Vorhandensein eines nagenden Juckreizes, welcher nur

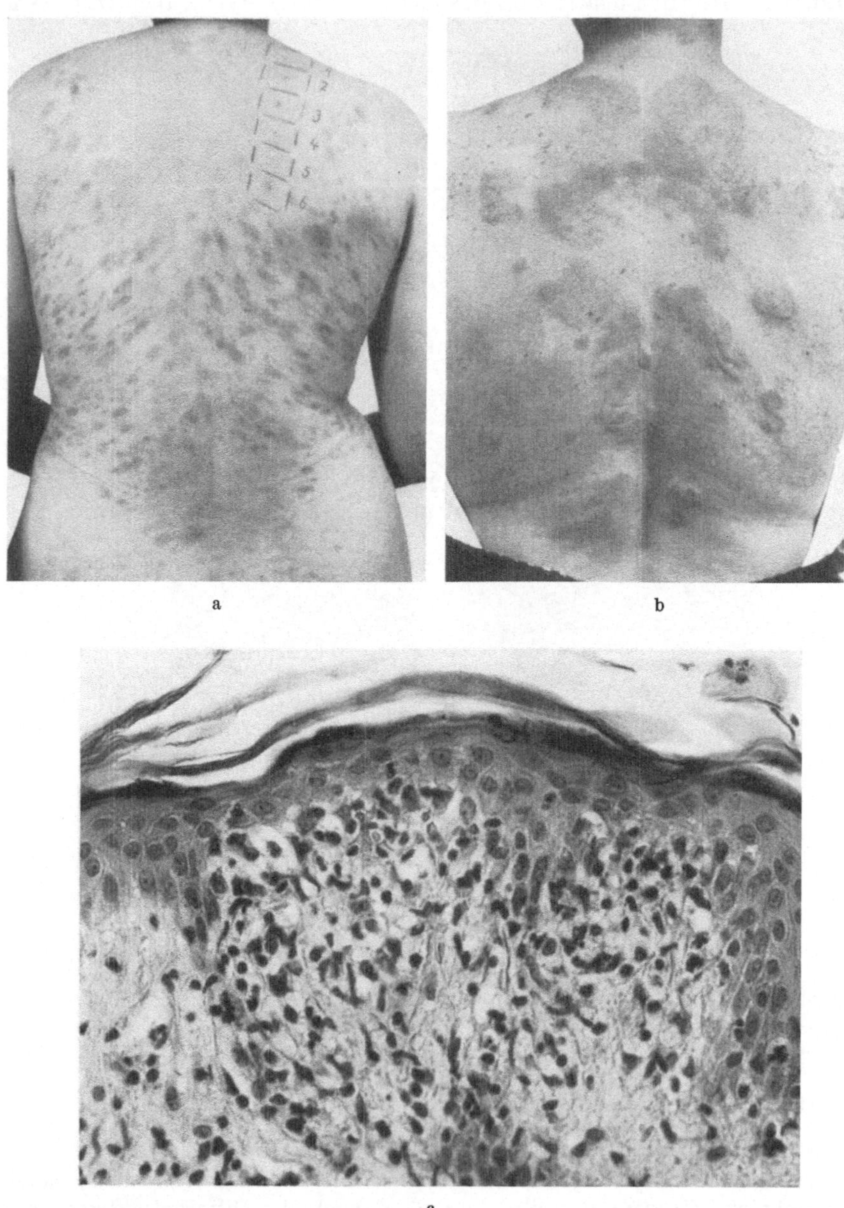

Abb. 28a—c. a Sekundär-hämorrhagisches Ekzem nach Urticaria. b Sekundäre hämorrhagische Urticaria bei Allergie auf Hydantal. c Histologisch Spongiose und Mikroblutung in den Papillarkörper

gelegentlich auch bei den anderen Gruppen erwähnt wurde (Abb. 27). Auch hier kommen sämtliche differentialdiagnostische Erwägungen gegenüber den erwähnten pigmentierten purpurischen Krankheiten in Frage.

Therapeutisch bewährte sich nach Loewenthal Liquor Fowleri, wogegen Vitamin C und Antihistaminica unwirksam blieben.

γγ) Dermatitis „caused by shirts“. Die von Hodgson u. Hellier beschriebene *Dermatitis „caused by shirts“* wurde unter den britischen Truppen während des Krieges 1944/45 in der Normandie gehäuft beobachtet. Ekzemproben mit Seifen, Farbstoffen und DDT erwiesen sich negativ. Trotzdem wurde die neue Wolle der amerikanischen Hemden als ätiologischer Faktor angesehen. Ähnliche Beobachtungen machte 1953 Sneddon bei sechs Patienten, wovon allerdings nur einer Khaki-Kleidung getragen hatte. Die papulösen purpurischen Herde befanden sich bei allen Patienten hauptsächlich an den Stellen des Kleidungskontaktes, breiteten sich aber später auf andere Körperpartien aus.

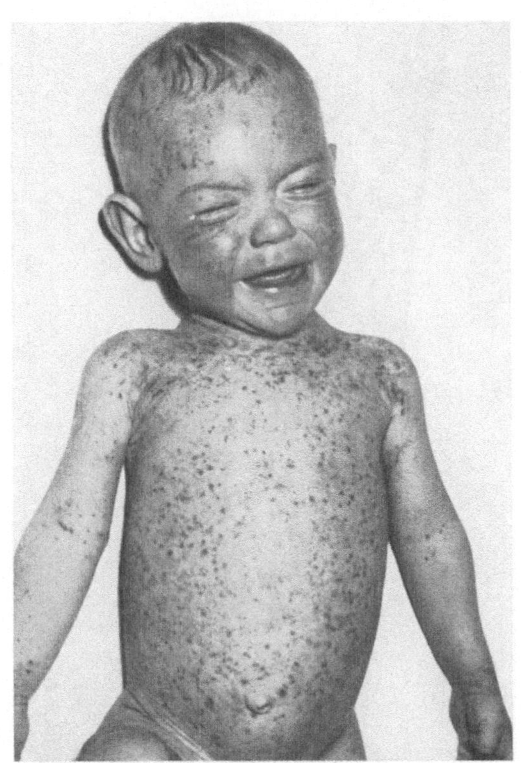

Abb. 29. Aldrich-Syndrom mit Eczema varicelliforme Kaposi. [Aus J. Gelzer u. C. Gasser: Wiskott-Aldrich-Syndrom. Helv. paediat. Acta **16**, 17 (1961)]

Neuerdings scheinen die Untersuchungen von Greenwood (1960) auf die Ursache dieses Krankheitsbildes neues Licht zu werfen, indem Fälle mit Schamberg-ähnlichen Läsionen eine Hautempfindlichkeit zeigten gegenüber Ölen, die in der Wollappretur verwendet werden (positive Reaktionen bei sechs von sieben Fällen). Sollten sich diese Untersuchungsbefunde bestätigen, bestünde die Möglichkeit, daß ein Großteil der genannten Affektionen auf einer Kontaktnoxe beruht.

δδ) Sekundär-hämorrhagische Ekzeme. Kontaktekzeme und endogen-mikrobielle Ekzeme können bei den verschiedensten, das Capillarbett schädigenden Faktoren fakultativ hämorrhagisch werden, wie wir dies z. B. bei einem Fall mit rezidivierenden Anginen und Überempfindlichkeit gegenüber den eingenommenen Kopfschmerztabletten schon sahen (Abb. 28) (Storck 1955). Allergische Sensibilisierungen gegenüber Arzneimittel (z. B. Hydantal, erwiesen durch einen positiven thrombopenischen Index) können selbst urticarielle Schübe sekundär hämorrhagisch umwandeln. Auch die bereits erwähnten Fälle von Stüttgen mit hämorrhagischem Ekzem bei Appendicitis dürften zu dieser Gruppe gehören. Die sekundär-hämorrhagischen Exantheme bei Infektionskrankheiten wurden bereits erwähnt.

εε) Das Aldrich-Syndrom. Das von Aldrich u. a. (1954) beschriebene Syndrom umfaßt die Trias: Thrombocytopenie, oft purpurisches Ekzem und rezidivierende Infektionen bei männlichen Säuglingen und Kleinkindern. Es ist ein geschlechtsgebundenes Leiden mit recessivem Erbgang, in der Regel mit letalem Ausgang. (Dieses Syndrom sollte vielleicht trotz der ekzematoiden Hautveränderungen eher zu den hereditären thrombocytopenischen Affektionen gerechnet werden, und wird auch dort nochmals erwähnt.)

Als rezidivierende Infektionen werden oft Otitis media, Mastoiditis, Sinusitis, Pneumonie, Pyodermie und multiple Hautabscesse gefunden. Dazu kommen rebellische Säuglingsekzeme mit purpurischen Schüben (Abb. 29), mit Petechien an Haut und Mucosa (MILLS u. WINKELMANN 1959), bei welchen der Gefäßfaktor unsicher, die Thrombocytopenie aber wahrscheinlich von Bedeutung ist. Ein γ-Globulinmangelsyndrom konnte bisher nicht gefunden werden, doch vermutete M. SCHWARZ (1961) eine verspätete Reifung der β-Globuline.

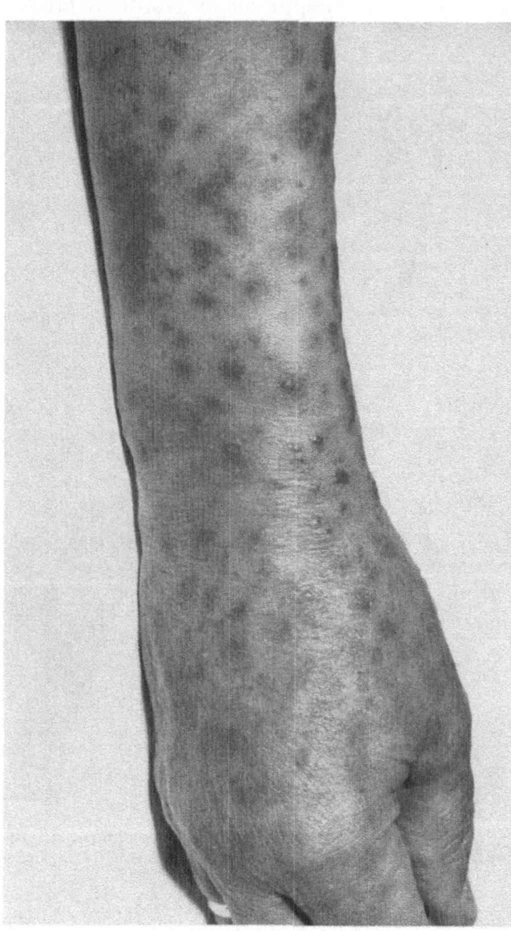

a

Abb. 30a u. b. Margarine-Krankheit. [Aus J. W. K. MALI, K. E. MALTEN u. C. J. VAN NEER: Die holländische Margarine-Krankheit. Hautarzt **13**, 152 (1962)]

NOSSEL u.a. (1962) fanden neben den genannten, typischen klinischen Zeichen Fehlen des lymphoiden Gewebes im Nasopharynx selbst bei Kindern, bei denen sonst dieses Gewebe stark entwickelt ist. Aber die lymphoide Antwort auf Infektion wird durch Lymphgewebe anderer Lokalisation ersetzt, bei normalen γ-Globulinen.

Wenn auch HUNTLEY u.a. (1957) allergische Mechanismen (Milch, Infekte) diskutierten, so konnten nach anderen Autoren für ein allergisches Geschehen keine Anhaltspunkte gefunden werden. Wiederholt wurde eine Hypoaminacidurie festgestellt, was einen ,,inborn error of metabolism" nahelegt (GELZER u. GASSER 1961).

Therapieversuche mit Cortison, ACTH, Oestrogenen, Progesteron, Antiallergica, Antibiotica waren nach bisherigen Erfahrungen erfolglos [s. auch späterer Abschnitt: ,,Komplexe hereditäre Syndrome mit Begleitthrombopenie" sowie H. J. BANDMANN, ,,Wiskott-Aldrich-Syndrom" in Ergänzungsband II/1 dieses Handbuches (1962).

ζζ) Purpura bei ,,Margarine-Krankheit". 1961—1962 wurde in Holland eine ,,epidemische" Hautkrankheit mit multiforme-ähnlichem Exanthem und Purpura beobachtet (Abb. 30). Die Abklärung ergab, daß es sich um eine Schädigung der oberflächlichen Cutispartien mit Schwellung und Schwund von Endothelzellen, perivasculären, lymphocytären Infiltraten, z.T. Erythrocyten-Extravasaten handelt, sehr wahrscheinlich hervorgerufen durch einen Emulgator (M.E. 18), der der Margarine beigemischt war.

Im Tierversuch zeigte dieser Emulgator eine starke Affinität zum Serumalbumin und eine außerordentliche Potenz zur Erzeugung granulomatöser Entzündung nach subepidermaler Injektion. Nach Inkorporierung per os schien sich bei diesen Patienten eine Überempfindlichkeit von cellulärem „delayed"-Typ einzustellen, doch waren bei einem Teil der Kranken auf dem Höhepunkt der Affektion mobile Antikörper nachweisbar, die sich mit Serum passiv auf Kontrollen übertragen ließen. Nach Abklingen der akuten Erkrankung waren solche Antikörper verschwunden und die Intracutanteste negativ. Nach ALEXANDER u. GRELL (1963) konnte bei einzelnen, nach Jahren nachkontrollierten Patienten mit erhitztem Emulgator im Scratchtest Spätreaktionen vom Tuberkulintypus ausgelöst werden.

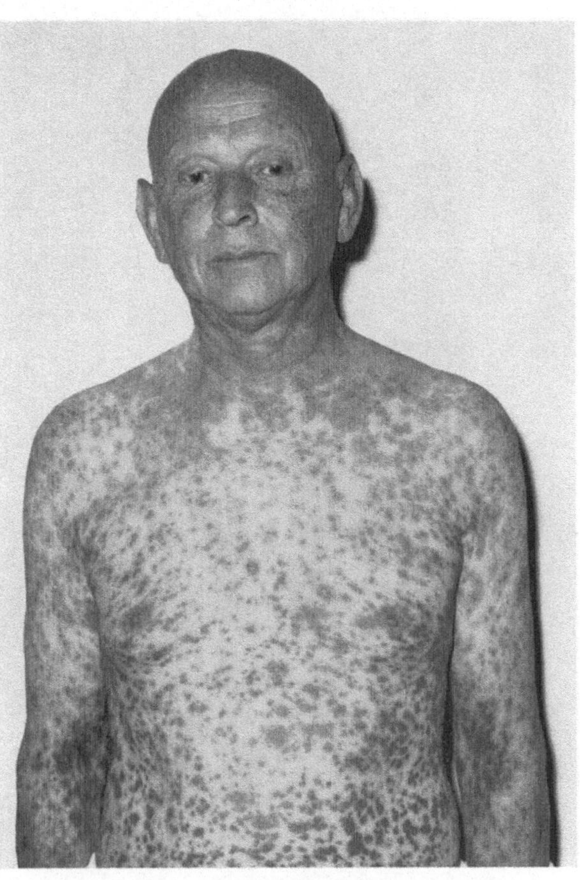

Abb. 30 b

Bei Ferkeln konnten durch Verfütterung des Emulgators ähnliche Krankheitserscheinungen wie beim Menschen erzeugt werden, mit klinisch und histologisch ähnliche Hautläsionen. Auch Fütterung von Meerschweinchen mit erhitztem Emulgator führte zu Hauterscheinungen und positiven Hauttesten vom Tuberkulin-Typus (ALEXANDER u. GRELL 1963).

Es liegt also bei dieser „Margarine-Krankheit" mutmaßlich ein vasculäres, purpurisches Exanthem vor, ausgelöst durch Sensibilisierung auf einen Emulgator mit starker Avidität zu Serumalbumin (MALI u.a. 1962), Anhaltspunkte für eine Virusinfektion konnten nicht gefunden werden, obwohl SIMONS die Margarine-Genese für unwahrscheinlich hält.

γ) Purpura hyperglobulinaemica

1943/44 beschrieb I. WALDENSTRÖM nach einer groß angelegten Untersuchungsserie über Hyper- und Dysproteinämien Arbeiten zwei interessante Krankheitsbilder, die nach ihm benannt wurden, nämlich 1. Purpura hyperglobulinaemica, 2. Purpura makroglobulinaemica.

Beide Affektionen gehen mit Proteinerhöhung, sehr hoher Blutsenkungsgeschwindigkeit und hämorrhagischen Diathesen einher, wobei aber bei der Purpura hyperglobulinaemica nur die γ-Globuline vermehrt sind, mit chronischrezidivierender, vasculärer, hauptsächlich an den Beinen auftretender Purpura, wogegen bei der Purpura makroglobulinaemica besondere Makroglobuline der

β_2-M-Fraktion erhöht sind und die Blutungen eher dem koagulopathischen Typus entsprechen, mit Epistaxis, Sickerblutungen aus Mundschleimhaut sowie Retinalblutungen. Die Gefäßstörungen sind hier noch fraglich und die Störungen der Gerinnungsfaktoren nicht einheitlicher Natur. Diese Krankheit sollte deshalb von

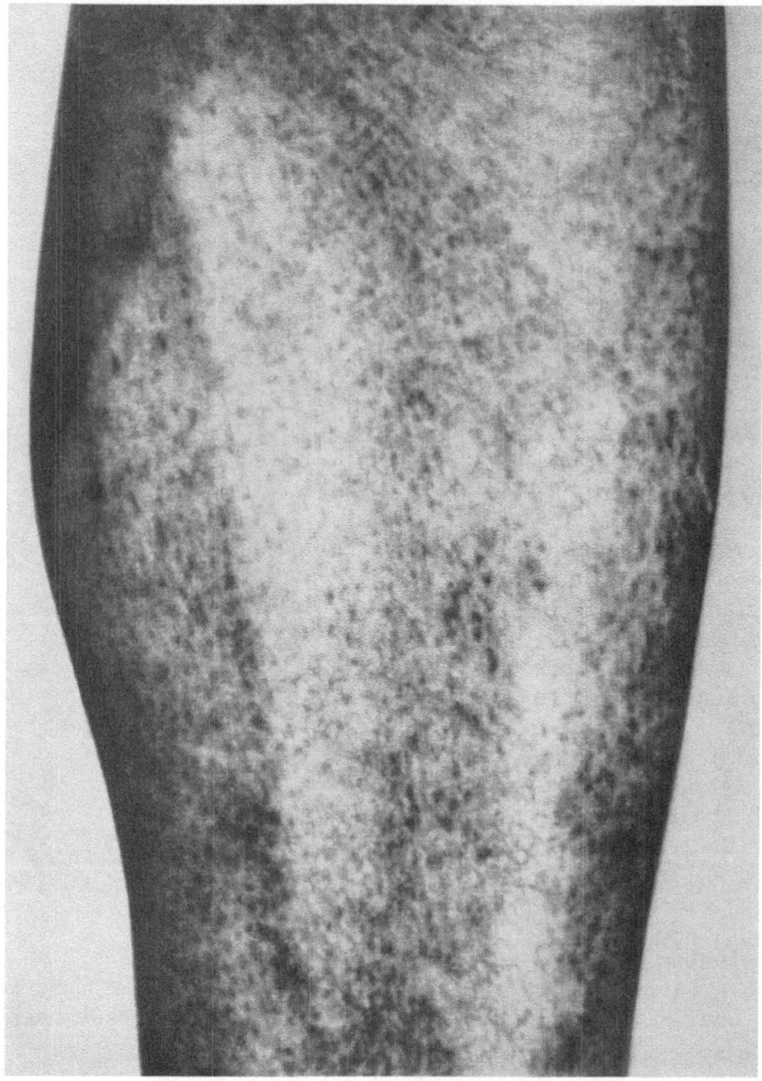

Abb. 31. Purpura hyperglobulinaemica. [Aus J. Waldenström: Three new cases of purpura hyperglobulinaemica. Acta med. scand., Suppl. (1952)]

der hyperglobulinämischen Form strikte abgetrennt werden und wäre vielleicht richtiger im Abschnitt der Koagulopathien zu erörtern. (Gute, relativ ausführliche Arbeiten über die Differentialdiagnose dieser beiden Krankheitsbilder wurden unter anderem von Weinreich 1955, Quattrin u.a. 1956, Hambrick 1958, Allegra 1959 u.a. veröffentlicht.)

Quattrin trennt von der Purpura hyperglobulinaemica Waldenström noch eine schwere Purpura mit Hypergammaglobulinämie ab, die aber klinisch mehr der Purpura makroglobulinaemica Waldenström gleicht. Eine exakte Differentialdiagnose kann nur mittels Ultrazentrifugation des Serums und anschließenden immunologischen Testen gestellt werden. QUATTRINS differentialdiagnostische Merkmale sind in Tabelle 11 zusammengestellt.

Klinisch tritt die *Purpura hyperglobulinaemica* in Schüben, meist in Form von Blutpunkten an den Beinen, gelegentlich an den oberen Extremitäten, auf, wobei infolge der häufigen Rezidive eine pigmentierte (hämosiderinhaltige) gefleckte Haut entsteht (Abb. 31). Als Realisationsfaktoren wirken offensichtlich statische und mechanische Momente und wahrscheinlich spielt auch die Muskeltätigkeit eine Rolle. Blutungen der Schleimhäute und inneren Organe treten in der Regel nicht auf. Meist kann eine generalisierte Lymphdrüsenschwellung, gelegentlich Milz- und Lebervergrößerung beobachtet werden.

Die Purpura tritt am häufigsten zwischen dem 20.—60. Altersjahr auf. Frauen sind fünf- bis sechsmal häufiger als Männer befallen.

Als Folge einer hochgradigen Zunahme der elektrophoretisch identifizierbaren γ-Globuline findet sich eine sehr hohe Blutsenkungsreaktion. Die Ultrazentrifugation ergibt zusätzlich eine Erhöhung der Lipoproteine mit Sedimentationskonstante S_f 7 (FLEISCHMAJER u.a. 1957). Die γ-Globulinwerte schwanken zwischen 22—78%, das Gesamteiweiß ist in 50% der Fälle auf über 8,7 g-% erhöht, in 20% der Fälle an der oberen Grenze der Norm.

Der chronische Verlauf ist für das Krankheitsbild charakteristisch. Es konnten Fälle von über 10jähriger Dauer beobachtet werden, wie einer der ersten beschriebenen Fälle von WALDENSTRÖM. Die Capillarresistenz ist meist herabgesetzt (positiver Rumpel-Leede), die Koagulationsfaktoren sind normal. Häufig findet sich gleichzeitig eine normocytär-normochrome Anämie mäßigen Grades, eine leichte Autoagglutination der Erythrocyten sowie Verminderung der Serumalbumine (SYMON 1957).

Häufig liegt eine Trockenheit der Schleimhäute vor, ähnlich wie beim Sjögren- oder Mikulicz-Syndrom, wie dies z.B. DOERKEN (1954), SIEMS u. RAUSCH-STROOMANN (1955), SYMON u.a. (1957), MUELLER (1958), GOLTZ u. GOOD (1961), BOUSSER u.a. (1961) betonten.

Da die Hautveränderungen bei der hyperglobulinämischen Purpura sowohl klinisch wie histologisch in hohem Maße den Hautläsionen der anaphylaktoiden Purpura gleichen, ist die Frage umstritten, ob es sich tatsächlich um ein nosologisch-selbständiges Krankheitsbild handle und nicht um eine spezielle Verlaufsform der Purpura Schönlein-Henoch. Für die letztere Auffassung traten PRIBILLA (1951), KORTING u. BREHM (1956), BENDER u. GERLACH (1955), JADASSOHN u. PAILLARD (1955), MUELLER (1958) ein. Dementsprechend wird auch die Hyperglobulinämie bei diesem Krankheitsbild lediglich als sekundäre Folge eines langdauernden Reizzustandes durch immunisatorische Einwirkung auf das reticuloendotheliale System angesehen (SYMON u.a. 1957, MUELLER 1958, EHLERS u. HEINZE 1962). Ein positiver Coombs-Test mit Erythrocyten wurde von KORTING u. BREHM (1956) sowie von KUHN (1956) gefunden, weshalb auch autoimmunisatorische Prozesse pathogenetisch diskutiert werden.

DOERKEN schlug 1954 vor, bei der Purpura hyperglobulinaemica *primäre* und *sekundäre* Formen zu unterscheiden, welcher Anregung sich mehrere Autoren anschlossen (BERTHOUD u.a. 1956, BOLLIGER 1958, HAMBRICK 1958). Der sekundären hyperglobulinämischen Purpura können z.B. Myelome, Lebercirrhosen, Morbus Boeck, Kryoglobulinämie (DOERKEN 1954), Diabetes, Granulomatose, Lungentuberkulose, Lebercarcinome, Emphysembronchitis (BERTHOUD 1956) als ursächliche Faktoren zugrunde liegen, wobei nun allerdings spätere biochemische Analysen gezeigt haben, daß die Eiweißvermehrung bei Myelomen und

Tabelle 11. *Differentialdiagnose der hämorrhagischen Makroglobulinämie und der Purpuras mit Hypergammaglobulinämie.* (Nach persönlicher Mitteilung von N. QUATTRIN 1963)

Syndrome	Hämorrhagische Makroglobulinämie (WALDENSTRÖM)	Schwere Purpura mit Hypergammaglobulinämie	Purpura hyperglobulinaemica (WALDENSTRÖM)	Purpura cryoglobulinaemica
Geschlecht	unmaßgeblich	unmaßgeblich	weibliches bevorzugt	unmaßgeblich
Alter	Früh- oder Spätadoleszenz	unmaßgeblich	unmaßgeblich	Erwachsene
Verlauf	letal	schwer oder letal	mild	gut- oder bösartig
Begleitkrankheiten	idiopathische oder lymphoreticuläre Blastome	Myelome Kryoglobulinämie hyperproteinämische Lebercirrhose	Sarkoidose chron. Rheumatismus Sjögren-Syndrom usw.	idiopathisch, Myelomatose lymphatische Leukämie lymphoreticuläre Blastome
Klinisches Bild	schwere hämorrhagische Diathese (besonders der Retina). Störungen des zentralen und peripheren Nervensystems. „Febris paraproteinaemica"	schwere hämorrhagische Diathese, besonders der Haut (Mikro- und Makropetechien)	Purpura der Beine (auch bei Kryoglobulinämie)	polymorphe hämorrhagische Diathese mit Bevorzugung der Beine. Rezidivierende Mikro- und Makropetechien Kälteempfindlichkeit unbeständig
Blutbefunde	normochrome Anämie, Leukopenie mit Lymphocytose. Gelegentlich Thrombopenie und Thrombopathie. Lymphoreticuläre Mastzellenproliferation im Knochenmark	wie bei der hämorrhagischen Makroglobulinämie	leichte Veränderungen	wie bei der hämorrhagischen Makroglobulinämie
Blutchemismus	auffallende Steigerung der Viscosität; schwere Veränderungen der Serumkolloide und besonders des Brahhama-Sachari-Sia-Tests. Mäßige Häufigkeit der Kryoglobuline	wie bei der hyperglobulinämischen Purpura oder der Makroglobulinämie	erhöhte Viscosität Veränderung des Serumkolloids	wechselnde, aber meist milde Veränderungen
Proteinämie und Papierelektrophorese	Hyperproteinämie mit sehr auffallender homogener β-, γ- oder „Fi"-Globulinämie	wie bei der Purpura Waldenström	milde Hyperproteinämie und nur Hypergammaglobulinämie	in der Regel Hypergamma- oder -betaglobulinämie
Ring-Test	positiv	negativ	negativ	negativ
Immunoelektrophorese	schwere Abnormitäten der β_2-M-Linie	nicht spezifisch	nicht spezifisch	spezifische Änderungen nur in der Kryomakroglobulinämie

Tabelle 11. (Fortsetzung)

Syndrome	Hämorrhagische Makroglobulinämie (Waldenström)	Schwere Purpura mit Hypergammaglobulinämie	Purpura hyperglobulinaemica (Waldenström)	Purpura cryoglobulinämica
Ultrazentrifugation	Makroglobuline (16—20 S = 20 bis 30%)	wie bei der Purpura Waldenström	normal	nicht spezifisch
Bence-Jones-Proteinurie	sehr selten	möglich	fehlt	möglich
Pathogenese der hämorrhagischen Diathese	verschieden (Hypoprothrombinämie, Serotoninopenie, gestörte Plättchenagglutination, Thrombocytopenie	wie bei hämorrhagischer Makroglobulinämie	nur vasculär?	vasculär? Thrombocytopenie häufiger

Kryoglobulinämien anderer Natur ist. Gegen eine Unterteilung in primäre und sekundäre Form wandte sich unter anderem MUELLER (1958).

Die *Pathogenese* ist noch nicht sicher geklärt. Die zumindest nahe Verwandtschaft dieser Affektionen mit Purpura Schönlein-Henoch läßt alle dort erwähnten pathogenetischen Prinzipien auch hier diskutierbar erscheinen. Neben infektiös-allergischen Mechanismen, Abwehrschwäche gegenüber banalen Infektionserregern werden allgemein-allergische Prozesse erörtert (z.B. ESSER u. SCHMENGLER 1952), ferner endoallergische Immunreaktionen (mit reaktiver Retikulose; SCHMENGLER u. ESSER 1952, HAENSCH 1954), autoimmune Vorgänge (G. W. KORTING u. G. BREHM 1953, positiver Coombs-Test, BOUSSER u.a. 1961). KORTING u. ADAM (1955) empfahlen eine Abgrenzung der sekundären hyperglobulinämischen Purpura bei Lebercirrhose.

FLEISCHMAJER u.a. (1957) diskutieren ferner als pathogenetische Faktoren: *1.* vorübergehende Thrombopenie durch Invasion des Knochenmarks mit pathologischen Zellen, *2.* Infiltration der Gefäßwand mit pathologischen Proteinen, und *3.* vorübergehende Abnormität der Blutkoagulationsfaktoren. HENSTELL u. KLIGERMAN (1959) untersuchten über 1000 Fälle mit Makroglobulinämie, Kryoglobulinämie, viscerale Leishmaniosis, verschiedenen Hyperglobulinämien, wobei sie in 63—94% Fällen der verschiedenen Krankheitsgruppen als allgemeines Symptom Purpura bei erhöhten Plasmaglobulinwerten fanden, dazu Thrombosen in 3—21%. Die beiden Autoren schlagen deshalb den Namen einer *hyperglobulinämischen thrombohämorrhagischen Diathese* vor.

Laboratoriumsuntersuchungen zeigten, daß sich einige Globuline auch mit einzelnen Koagulationsfaktoren verbinden können, so daß deren Inaktivierung zu Blutungen führen kann. Nach Dissoziation solcher Komplexe würden dann aber große Mengen Koagulationsfaktoren frei, mit entsprechender, gelegentlich beobachteter Thrombosebildung. Weitere Fälle von Purpura hyperglobulinaemica wurden von LINDEBOOM (1948), WALDENSTRÖM (1948—1952), GAUTHIER u.a. (1953), LAPIÈRE u.a. (1962), publiziert.

Therapeutisch wurde neuerdings von WEISS u.a. (1963) die Anwendung von Thioguanin empfohlen, welches aber die Blutungsbereitschaft nur vorübergehend hemmte, ohne die erhöhten γ-Globulinwerte zu normalisieren.

δ_1) Makroglobulinämie Waldenström

Die zweite von WALDENSTRÖM entdeckte Gruppe von hämorrhagischen Veränderungen betrifft Paraproteinämien (Vermehrung von Makroglobulinen), die sich klinisch manifestieren durch Schleimhautblutungen aus Mund und Nase, gelegentlich auch Blutungen in das Zentralnervensystem (ESSER u. SCHMENGLER 1948), Veränderungen des Augenhintergrundes mit Netzhautablösung (Einlagerung von Makroglobulinen, Thrombosen), ferner durch Müdigkeit, Kurzatmigkeit, Ödeme, häufig generalisierten Lymphknotenschwellungen, selten auch Milz- und Leberschwellung. Regelmäßig findet sich normochrome Anämie, stark beschleunigte Blutsenkung, hochpathologisches Serum, Labilitätsreaktionen, insbesondere Formogel-Reaktionen, positive SIA-Reaktionen (WALDENSTRÖM), selten leichte Thrombocytopenie (R. KAPPELER u.a. 1958). In neuerer Zeit wurde vermehrt auf periphere Neuritiden hingewiesen (DARNLEY 1962, GARCIN u.a. 1962, 1963).

Elektrophoretisch findet sich im Serum eine meist hohe und schmale pathologische Zacke mit Wanderungsgeschwindigkeit der β_2-M-γ-Globuline (P. BURTIN u.a. 1957). Von den normalen Globulinen unterscheidet sich dieses Globulin durch das hohe Molekulargewicht von etwa 1 Million. Bei Ultrazentrifugierung zeigt sich eine Sedimentationskonstante von 25 (HAESSIG 1961), selten sogar 35 (NORDÖY 1962) Swedberg-Einheiten (H. ISLIKER 1958).

Mit *immunbiologischen* Versuchsanordnungen läßt sich nachweisen, daß es sich um ein immunologisch spezifisches Makroglobulin handelt (KANZOW 1956, KANZOW u.a. 1961, HAESSIG 1961), welches sich von den beim Plasmocytom oder sonst vorkommenden Makroglobulinen unterscheidet, aber identisch ist mit den normalerweise in kleiner Menge vorkommenden β_2-M-Globulinen (KANZOW u.a. 1961). Die Makroglobuline Waldenström lassen sich also von den Myeloproteinen und Bence-Jonesschen Uroproteinen differenzieren. Sämtliche genannten Paraproteine stellen funktionell inerte Eiweißkörper dar. Die Myeloproteine sind in den γ- und β_2-A-Globulinfraktionen enthalten, die Waldenströmschen Makroglobuline jedoch in der β_2-M-Globulinfraktion, die Bence-Jonesschen Uroproteine in den seltenen intermediären Fraktionen (BURTIN u.a. 1957, J. J. SCHEIDEGGER u.a. 1958, HERRMANN 1960, GRABAR 1960, HAESSIG u.a. 1961). In einem Teil der Fälle fanden sich auch Kryoglobuline (LERNER, BARNUM, WATSON u.a. 1947).

Auf die Differentialdiagnose gegenüber hyperglobulinämischer Purpura wurde bereits hingewiesen (Tabelle 11).

Die exzessiv vermehrte Globulinfraktion in β- und γ-Stellung, die schmalbasisch und steil ist, kann auch papierelektrophoretisch nachgewiesen werden (WALDENSTRÖM 1959, WEISE 1961). Die Paraproteine lassen sich auch im Harn feststellen. Paraproteinämien kommen in höherem Lebensalter, und zwar bei Männern gehäuft vor (HEILMEYER 1950, WALDENSTRÖM 1958, IMHOF u.a. 1959, MICHON u.a. 1960, QUATTRIN u.a. 1961, BENKÖ u. TIBOLDI 1961). 1961 zeigten BUTLER u.a., daß sich Makroglobuline auch mit der Stärke-Gel-Elektrophorese nachweisen lassen, sofern zum Buffer 2-mercaptoäthanol zugesetzt wird.

Die bei der Makroglobulinämie vorkommenden Gerinnungsstörungen sind nicht einheitlicher Natur. Es wurden Störungen sowohl in der zweiten Phase (Fibrinogen-Fibrin) gefunden (UEHLINGER 1949, LÜSCHER/LABHART 1949) als auch in der Vor- und ersten Gerinnungsphase (Verlängerung der Gerinnungs- und Recalcifizierungszeit, Verminderung der Heparintoleranz, Verminderung der Thrombusretraktion, der Thrombenfestigkeit, Verkürzung der Prothrombinzeit, der Accelerationsfaktoren, Herabsetzung der Thrombokinasebildung [ACHENBACH u. KANZOW 1956]). Es wurde aber auch eine Hemmkörperwirkung durch die Paraproteine diskutiert (HAENSCH 1954, 1959) sowie Adsorption der verschiedensten Koagulationsfaktoren an die Makroglobuline (MENACHÉ 1960). Durch das Vorhandensein der Makroglobuline wird die normale Immunisierung, gemessen an der Bildung von Präcipitinen gegen Antigene, oder an der Abstoßung von Hauttransplantaten, gestört (R. HONG u.a. 1962).

Auch die Thrombocyten sind bei den Makroglobulinämien an den Hämorrhagien beteiligt, obwohl sie allgemein in normaler Zahl vorhanden sind; sie sind jedoch minderwertig, indem sie kein Blutthrombopastin bilden und eine herabgesetzte Adhäsivität besitzen (Jürgens 1956, Haensch 1959).

Neben den unregelmäßig gestörten plasmatischen Koagulationsfaktoren und Thrombocyten hebt Achenbach (1960) auch die Bedeutung von Gefäßfaktoren hervor, die wahrscheinlich auf Grund von Blutviscosität, Hämodynamik und immunbiologischen Prozessen pathologisch zur Auswirkung kommen, ähnlich wie bei der Paramyloidose oder Amyloidose, bei welchen gelegentlich ähnliche Purpuraformen gefunden werden (Zahnd u.a. 1959).

Die *Pathogenese* der vasculären Blutungen ist jedoch noch nicht gesichert. Im Gegensatz zur Gefäßinfiltration bei Amyloidose findet sich beim Gefäßschaden der Makroglobulinämie kein anatomisches Substrat (Haensch 1959).

Auch bei *Polycythämie* können in seltenen Fällen Hämorrhagien aus Schleimhäuten und in innere Organe, besonders subdural oder urethral, erfolgen, die ähnlich wie bei Amyloidose, vielleicht auch bei Makroglobulinämien durch hyaline Umwandlungen der Gefäßwände mit starker plasmatischer Durchtränkung und Dissezierung zustande kommen, wie dies Lienhard (1962) feststellte.

Zum Gefäßfaktor kommen die funktionellen Störungen der Thrombocyten und die Gerinnungsstörungen mit oben genannter Wirkung, aber ohne tatsächliches Defizit an Gerinnungsfaktoren (Haensch 1959).

Mutterzellen der genannten pathologischen Makroglobuline sind wahrscheinlich lymphocytoide Reticulumzellen im Knochenmark (Tischendorf u. Hartmann 1950, Braunsteiner u.a. 1956, Kanzow 1956, Ascenzi u.a. 1957, Wuhrmann u. Wunderly 1957, Waldenström 1958, Zollinger 1958, Haensch 1959, Nordöy 1962). Diese lymphocytoiden Reticulumzellen wurden genauer untersucht (Dutcher u. Fahey 1959, Samarcq 1960).

Daß die erwähnten Lymphoreticulumzellen nicht nur im Knochenmark, sondern Mycosis fungoides-ähnlich auch in der Haut bei Makroglobulinämie Waldenström als Reizhyperplasie auftreten können, zeigte eine Beobachtung von Röckl u.a. (1962).

Wohl die interessantesten Versuche zur Aufklärung des Blutungsmechanismus bei Makroglobulinämien führten Berneaud u. Nover (1957, 1958) durch. Sie sensibilisierten Kaninchen mit einem heterologen Antigen und injizierten später ein hochviscöses Fremdkolloid (Kollidon 60) in die Nickhaut der Augen. Mit der Spaltlampe wurden nun ausgeprägte Fraktionierung der Blutsäule beobachtet, Verlangsamung des Blutstromes, dann Blutaustritt. Zur hämorrhagischen Diathese bei bestimmten Paraproteinämien braucht es deshalb eine Störung der Hämodynamik (z.B. Viscositätserhöhung) und einen die Gefäßwand schädigenden Faktor (z.B. Sensibilisierung auf Fremdkolloid).

Auf welche Weise es zur Bildung von lymphocytoiden Reticulumzellen, und damit von Makroglobulinen, kommt, ist noch nicht geklärt. Waldenström hat einmal einen Vergleich mit Störungen der pflanzlichen Proteinsynthese nach „Virusinfektionen“ gezogen und denkt bei den Makroglobulinämien besonders an eine erworbene Erkrankung der Matrize für die Synthese der Proteinmoleküle, welche dann zur Bildung von abnormen Serumproteinen führe. Es komme aber auch eine „genetisch“ bedingte „molekulare“ Störung der Globulinsynthese durch Mutation in Frage (Waldenström 1958).

Kint (1961) weist besonders auf purpurische Hautläsionen beim Plasmocytom *(Morbus de Kahler)* hin, die aber als Petechien, Ekchymosen und gingivale Blutungen in Erscheinung treten. Dazu gesellen sich häufig lichenoide oder urticarielle Papeln sowie follikuläre Hyperkeratosen.

Therapeutisch kommen Bluttransfusionen und Infusionen von Plasma, besonders von Fraktion I, in Betracht (Achenbach 1960). Steroide haben relativ wenig Erfolg; immerhin erwiesen sich diese in den Tierversuchen von Berneaud u.a. (1959) wirksamer als Kastanienextrakte. Bayrd (1961) berichtet über vier Patienten, die gut auf protrahierte Behandlung mit Chlorambucil (Leukeran) ansprachen, nachdem Steroide, Stilbamidin, Röntgenbestrahlungen usw. ohne

Wirkung angewendet worden waren, ebenso Plasmapheresis (Schwab u. Fahey 1960, Conway u.a. 1962). Nur vereinzelt wurde über vorübergehende Erfolge mit Plasmapheresis-Therapie berichtet (Solomon u. Fahey 1963).

δ_2) Purpura bei Kryoglobulinämien

Da ein Teil der Makroglobuline auch bei Kälteeinwirkung als Kryoglobuline ausfallen kann, sollen hier einzelne Fälle von Purpura bei Kryoglobulinämie Erwähnung finden.

Es existieren anscheinend verschiedene kälteaktive Bluteiweiße, so Kryoglobuline, Kryofibrinogene und Makroglobuline (Harders 1958), so daß diese Gruppe nicht einheitlicher Natur ist. An der Haut können hauptsächlich bei Kälteeinwirkung Nekrosen, Purpura und Raynaud-ähnliche Läsionen entstehen (Abb. 32). Aber auch Magen-Darmstörungen mit schwersten Blutungen, apoplektiforme Anfälle und Exitus letalis kommen vor (Braumann u.a. 1956). Rezidivierende Blasenblutungen, Blutungen nach Zahnextraktion, Anämie sowie die eigenartige Serumpräcipitation bei Kälte können auf das Leiden hinweisen, wie dies McFarlane u.a. (1952) mitteilte. Möglicherweise spielt nach F. Allegra (1963) auch der Rheumafaktor in der Genese der Kryoglobulinämien eine Rolle.

Neben rezidivierender Purpura können auch schmerzhafte Geschwüre nach Thrombosen, Pruritus, Pigmentationen und lichenoide Knötchen auftreten (Duperrat 1957/58). Schwere Magen-Darmstörungen unter dem Bilde einer Dysphagia arteriosclerotica abdominalis intermittens (Sladky u.a. 1959) werden gelegentlich beobachtet, bei welchen als Auslösungsfaktoren der Koliken Abkühlung der Haut gelten kann.

Gelegentlich scheinen sich die Patienten auf die präcipitable Fraktion des Serums in Form von Kälteurticaria zu sensibilisieren, wobei alsdann mit dem Kältepräcipitat positive Intracutanteste erhalten werden (Steinhardt u. Fisher 1954). Hier entstehen bei Kälte ausgesprochen urticarielle Reaktionen.

Pathogenetisch beruht die vorübergehende Capillarbrüchigkeit mit Purpura wahrscheinlich auf einer Hyperviscosität des Blutes, ähnlich der Auffassung von Berneaud u. Nover bei der Makroglobulinämie. Braumann u.a. (1956) stellten die Hypothese auf, daß durch die intravasale Präcipitation der Kryoglobuline der Blutfluß verlangsamt werde, wobei Geldrollenbildung der Erythrocyten an den kälteexponierten Stellen das Endothel durch Anoxämie schädige. Rorwick u. Lepoff (1949) konnten histochemisch in der Gefäßwand Proteinpräcipitate nachweisen. Kryoglobuline fallen bereits bei 37°C in großer Menge, bei 4°C in kleiner Menge aus. Die Kristalle sind bei 10—30°C in physiologischem NaCl wieder löslich.

Im Knochenmark werden in der Regel Plasmazellen gefunden. Bei der Kryogelifikation können 0,25—25‰ der Proteine ausfallen (Duperrat 1957, 1958).

Möglicherweise stellen noch Arzneimittelreaktionen eine zusätzliche auslösende Ursache dar, wie Phenacetin (Nödl 1960), Irgapyrin und Phenacetin (Blume u.a. 1960). Fleury u.a. glauben, daß sogar beim Thomson-Syndrom Kryoglobuline beteiligt sind. Weitere Einzelfälle wurden von McKenzie u.a. (1960), Roder (1961), Allegra (1963) publiziert.

Was die Herkunft der Makroglobuline, Kryoglobuline und Amyloide anbetrifft, so nimmt Cairns (1962) bei den ersten zwei Hyperreaktivität der Lymphocyten, bei den letzteren hauptsächlich der Plasmazellen an.

Histologisch gelang Nödl in den Gefäßen der Nachweis von „sludged"-Erythrocyten sowie von Eiweißpräcipitaten in Venen und Capillaren, darstellbar als fadenförmige Niederschläge innerhalb von Erythrocytenhaufen oder als Ablagerung in der Capillarwand (Abb. 33).

Es ist zu erwarten, daß nächstens auch die molekulare und fermentchemische Ausfällung der Kryoglobuline so exakt erforscht wird, wie dies heute schon am Kryoprofibrin durch SHAINOFF u. PAGE (1962) durchgeführt worden ist.

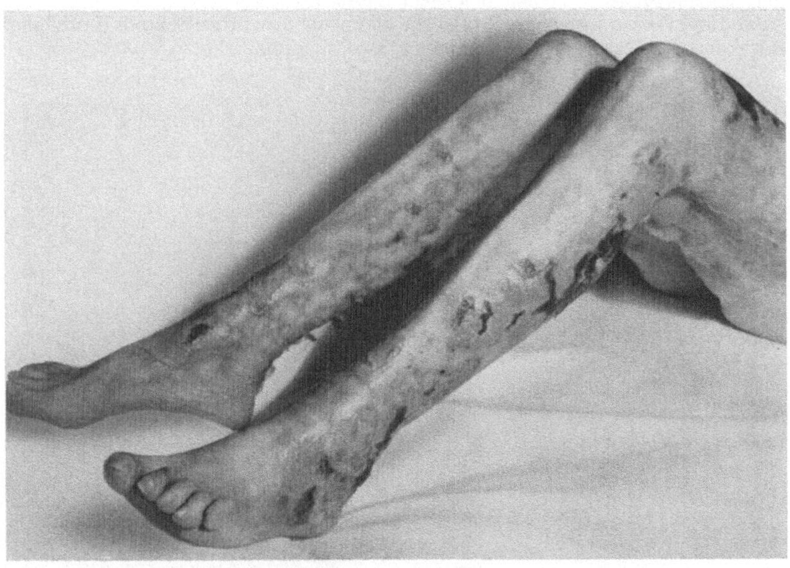

a

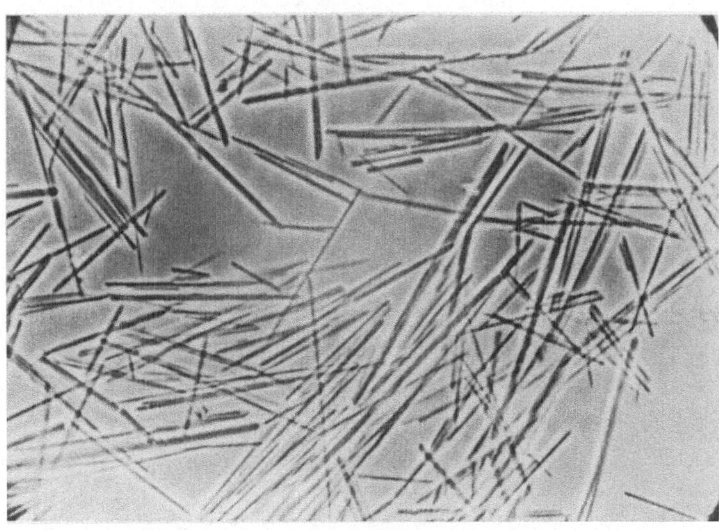

b

Abb. 32a u. b. Purpura cryoglobulinaemica. a Aussehen der unteren Extremitäten vor Prednisonbehandlung. b Kryoglobulinkristalleyim Serum einige Stunden nach Blutentnahme. [Aus J. BRAUMAN et al.: Myélome à croglobuline spontanément cristallisable. Acta clin. belg. 518 (1956)]

Die *Therapie* scheint schwierig zu sein. ACTH, Corticoide sind wenig wirksam. STEINHARDT u.a. berichten über Erfolge mit intravenöser Injektion von 50 mg Benadryl. Sollte es sich bei einzelnen Fällen um eine symptomatische bzw. durch Arzneimittelwirkung geförderte Kryoglobulinämie handeln, könnte sich gezielte Elimination günstig auswirken.

Nicht nur Kälte, sondern auch andere physikalische Einwirkungen können zu wahrscheinlich vasculär bedingten Purpuraformen führen. So beschrieb Lindemayr (1961) vier Fälle von *Lichtdermatosen*, die mit Purpura einhergingen. Vermutlich ist hier der langwellige Anteil des Sonnenspektrums auslösender Faktor, ähnlich wie bei Eczema solare, allerdings mit zusätzlichen Hautblutungen. Vielleicht spielen unterschwellige Sensibilisierungen auf Arzneimittel- und Infektionserreger eine Rolle, die dann an den unbedeckten Hautstellen durch Lichteinwirkung zur Manifestation kommen.

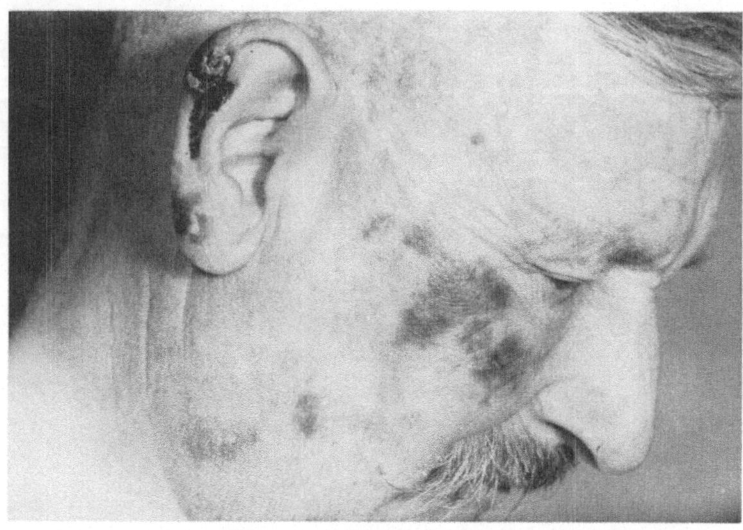

a

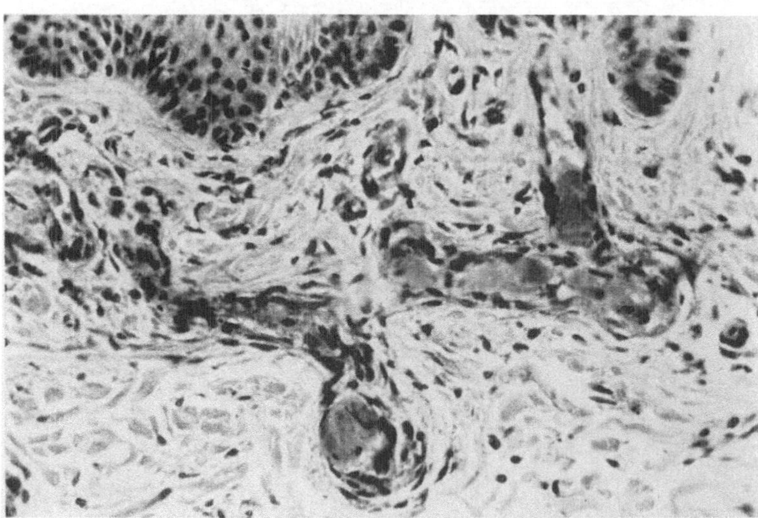

b

Abb. 33a u. b. Purpura bei essentieller Kryoglobulinämie (HE-Gefrierschnitt, 225fach). Intravasale Präcipitate, die sich stellenweise kontinuierlich in den venösen Capillarschenkel der Papille fortsetzen. [Aus F. Nödl: Purpura bei essentieller Kryoglobulinämie. Arch. klin. exp. Derm. **210**, 76 (1960)]

ε) Epidemische, hauptsächlich vasculär-hämorrhagische fieberhafte Erkrankungen

Schon wiederholt wurde beobachtet, daß verschiedene Infektionskrankheiten z.T. durch Capillarläsionen, z.T. durch kleinste Cutanembolien, zu Blutungen führen können, so subakute bakterielle Endokarditis, Meningokokkensepsis,

Rochy Mountain Fever und Typhus. Neuerdings sind zudem vermehrt epidemisch auftretende hämorrhagische febrile Krankheiten beschrieben worden.

1951/52 wurde zunächst in Korea, später in anderen fernöstlichen Gebieten wie Thailand und Rußland über solche Affektionen, z.T. mit Nierenbeteiligung, berichtet.

Der Beginn der Erkrankungen in *Korea* war meist unspezifisch fieberhaft mit kardiovasculären, gastrointestinalen und renalen Symptomen. Am 2. Krankheitstag traten Hautläsionen auf, zuerst mit Petechien in Axillen und am weichen Gaumen, später mit ausgedehnten hämorrhagischen Exanthemen unter vermehrter Capillarfragilität, z.T. mit Thrombocytenabfall (100000—20000, evtl. weniger) und Verlängerung der Blutungszeit. Nach GUDGEL u.a. (1955) bestehen die Hautmanifestationen aus einer Trias, nämlich 1. in hellroten, scarlatiniformen, fleckigen Exanthemen an Gesicht, Nacken, Brust, meist ab 3.—20. Tag der Krankheit, gefolgt von feiner Schuppung, 2. konjunktivaler und pharyngealer Injektion oder Hämorrhagie, und 3. Ödem des Gesichtes, besonders der Periorbitalgegend. Dazu gesellte sich häufig vom 2. bis 4. Tag an Mikrohämaturie und Albuminurie mit Einschränkung der Diurese, Nephrose und Rest-N-Erhöhung, in gewissen Fällen bis zu schwerer Urämie. Gegen Ende der 2. Woche bildeten sich Krankheitsgefühl, Fieber, hämorrhagische Läsionen zurück (BARBERO u.a. 1953, ANDREW 1953, POWELL 1953). In allen Organen wurden Petechien gefunden, des ferneren subkapsuläre Blutungen an Leber, Endokard, außerdem lymphocytäre Entzündungen in Milz, Lymphknoten, Lungen und im interstitiellen Bindegewebe anderer Organe.

Auch das epidemische hämorrhagische Fieber in *Thailand* (PIYARATN 1961) schien ähnlich zu verlaufen und wird wahrscheinlich durch ein von Arthropoden übertragenes Virus (möglicherweise vom Dengue 2-Typ) erzeugt. Unter den Fällen von *Singapore* fanden CHEW u.a. (1961) neben der mutmaßlich „hämorrhagischen Variante" des Dengue-Virus gelegentlich unspezifisch positive Widal- und Weil-Felix-Agglutinationen.

Die *Pathogenese* des Gefäßschadens ist noch nicht gesichert. Entsprechend der histologisch nachgewiesenen Gefäßerweiterung mit vermehrter Permeabilität wird ein direkter Endothelschaden durch das Virus oder Schädigung des nervösen Terminalreticulums diskutiert. Dafür spricht auch die intensive reticuloendotheliale Zellproliferation. Möglicherweise stellt die Thrombocytopenie nur eine Begleiterscheinung dar.

Die neuerdings im Fernen Osten beschriebenen hämorrhagischen Fieber (hämorrhagisches Fieber mit Renalsyndrom aus *Nordrußland*, südsowjetisches hämorrhagisches Fieber, russisches Frühling/Sommer-hämorrhagisches Fieber mit Encephalitis, die hämorrhagischen fieberhaften Erkrankungen von Thailand (Singapore, Philippinen) scheinen durch Moskitos übertragen zu werden und besonders Kinder zu befallen.

In der Regel verlaufen diese Krankheiten fünfphasig, nämlich *1.* febrile Phase mit feinen Petechien an druckexponierten Körperstellen, positivem Rumpel-Leede-Phänomen, beginnendem Plättchenabfall, *2.* hypotensive Phase mit starkem Plasmaverlust durch die geschädigten Capillaren, erhöhtem Hämatokritwert, Ekchymosen, Hämatomen und anderen Cutanblutungen, auch an Stellen von kleinen Traumen, Hämaturie, Hämatemesis, Melaena, *3.* oligurische Phase, evtl. mit schwerer Nieren- und Lungenblutung, gelegentlich auch Hirnblutung, *4.* diuretische Phase und *5.* Phase der Rekonvaleszenz.

Obwohl die schweren Schädigungen der kleinen Gefäße klinisch offensichtlich sind, finden sich *histologisch* keine charakteristischen Veränderungen derselben. In der 1. Phase scheint es sich hauptsächlich um eine neuro-vasculäre Instabilität zu handeln (nach russischen Autoren Capillartoxikose). In der febrilen Phase scheint bei erhöhter Capillarfragilität die Blutung durch Thrombocytopenie und maximale Capillardilatation begünstigt zu werden (Gajdusek 1962).

Es ist wahrscheinlich, daß das hämorrhagische Syndrom bei diesen fiebrigen hämorrhagischen Virusinfektionen ähnlich entsteht wie bei hämorrhagischen Masern, Rubeolen, Varicellen, infektiösen Hepatitiden und Mononucleosis bei Kindern, die ebenfalls häufig mit Thrombocytopenien einhergehen. Vermutlich ist das „hämorrhagische Fieber" nicht eine nosologische Einheit.

Hämorrhagische, z.T. febrile, virusbedingte Krankheiten werden auch im Tierreich, so beim Pferd (Equine arteritis virus) und beim Hirsch (Epizootic hemorrhagic disease; R. E. Hope u. a. 1960) beobachtet. Der Erreger, der N. Jersey-Stamm oder S. Dakota-Stamm des EDH-Virus, läßt sich intracerebral auf weißen Mäusen oder auf He-La-Zellen züchten (Mettler u. a. 1962). Ähnliche Affektionen lassen sich auch an Kleintieren, so z.B. beim Hamster, mit dem Polyoma-Virus erzeugen (Barski u. a. 1962).

ζ) Hormonell bedingte, vasculäre Purpura

Purpura wird bei endokrinen Störungen relativ selten gesehen, am ehesten bei M. Cushing und Hypercortisonismus, gelegentlich bei Myxödem. Die Pathogenese solcher Blutungen ist jedoch noch nicht geklärt.

1. Blutungen bei M. Cushing und Hypercortisonismus

Neben den bekannten Hautveränderungen bei *M. Cushing* (Marmorierung, Pigmentierung, Striae rubrae, Acne) kann Blutungsbereitschaft beobachtet werden mit Petechien und flächenhaften Suffusionen, besonders an Streckseiten der Vorderarme, gelegentlich auch an anderen, dem Druck ausgesetzten Körperstellen. Selten kommen auch Blutungen ins Darmlumen vor. Die Gerinnungsfaktoren, Blutungs- und Gerinnungszeiten sind stets normal, doch kann das Rumpel-Leede-Phänomen positiv ausfallen, was auf das Vorliegen vasculärer Störungen hinweist. Nur selten ist Fibrinogen verändert.

Pathogenetisch wird die antianabole Eigenschaft des Cortisons diskutiert.

Auch beim medikamentösen Hypercortisonismus können Ekchymosen und Purpura beobachtet werden. Der Hinweis auf die Wirkung der Corticoide scheint jedoch für die Erklärung dieser Nebenerscheinungen ungenügend, da diese bei Verwendung der Δ_1-Verbindungen erheblich an Häufigkeit zugenommen haben. Die Blutungen sind meist kleinfleckig und zahlreich; sie betreffen hauptsächlich Ober- und Unterschenkel (Abb. 34a), können aber auch an Stamm und oberen Extremitäten auftreten, z.T. als Ekchymosen (Abb. 34b). Leichte Traumen begünstigen die Hämorrhagien. An den Schleimhäuten wurden bis anhin keine Blutungen beobachtet. Besonders anfällig sind ältere Frauen. Bei sehr hoher Dosierung der Corticoide werden aber auch Männer befallen, wie wir dies selbst z.B. bei Prednison-behandelten Pemphigusfällen sahen. Die Häufigkeit dieser Komplikation scheint bei den einzelnen Corticosteroiden verschieden zu sein: mit Cortison und Hydrocortison wurden Blutungen in 2—5% der Fälle beobachtet (Slocumb u. a. 1957); bei Prednison und Prednisolon in 18—34% der Fälle (Boland 1956, Denko und Schroeder 1957). Die Blutungen können sich schon nach 20 Behandlungstagen oder aber erst später einstellen (Adam 1960).

Pathogenetisch halten Winer u. a. (1962) an Hand ihrer Beobachtung an 81 rheumatischen Patienten mit vasculärer Purpura bei langdauernder Cortisontherapie die histologisch nachweisbare medikamentbedingte Fragmentierung der elastischen Fasern, die elastoide Degeneration der Kollagenfasern oder ihr Fehlen in den pericapillären Spalten für entscheidend. Das cortisonbedingte Fehlen der entzündlichen Infiltratzellen läßt die Blutungen länger bestehen, ähnlich wie bei Purpura senilis (SHUSTER u. SCARBOROUGH 1961, zit. nach WINER 1962).

2. Blutungen bei Schilddrüsenstörungen

Bei Hypothyreose wurde gelegentlich eine vermehrte Capillarfragilität gefunden (BLACKBURN 1959), z.T. mit cutanen und ausgedehnten intestinalen Blutungen (ORR 1962). Neben der erhöhten Gefäßbrüchigkeit liegt in seltenen Fällen eine Thrombocytenstörung vor. Wie weit myxödematöse Einlagerungen zur Schädigung der Capillaren führen, ist noch ungeklärt.

Auch bei Hyperthyreose kann eine vermehrte Capillarfragilität vorkommen, möglicherweise verstärkt durch Vitamin C-Defizit, welches oft bei Patienten mit Morbus Basedow entsteht (BICKEL u.a. 1942). Gelegentlich kommen aber auch schwerste hämorrhagische Diathesen mit ausgedehnten Suffusionen, Schleimhautblutungen und rezidivierenden visceralen Blutungen vor. Hier handelt es sich sehr wahrscheinlich um eine hepatogene Störung der Prothrombinbildung, wobei das Vitamin K durch die thyreogen schwer insuffiziente Leber nicht mehr verwertet werden kann (BICKEL u.a. 1942).

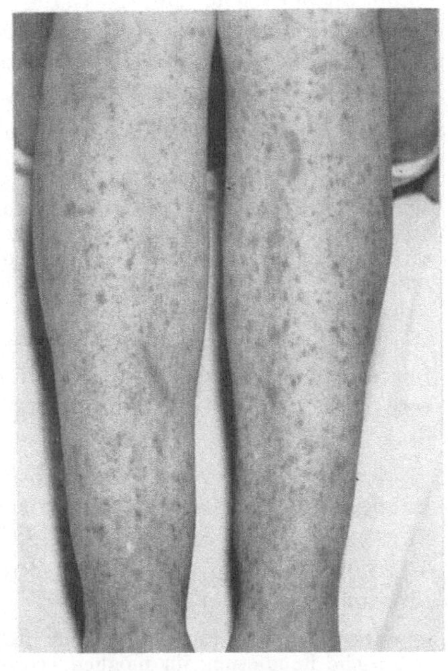

a

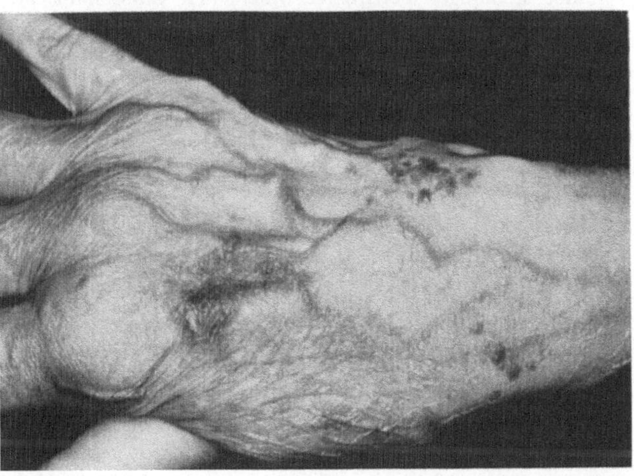

b

Abb. 34a u. b. a Purpura Schönlein während Prednison-Langzeitbehandlung. (Aus W. ADAM: In: Klinik und Therapie der Nebenwirkungen, S. 787. Stuttgart: Georg Thieme 1960.) b Ecchymosis bei Patient mit Arthritis nach Langzeitbehandlung mit Corticosteroiden. [Aus L. H. WINER, D. H. KLING and G. H. LEVIN: Ecchymosis in arthritis patient on prolonged corticosteroids. Arch. Derm. **86**, 654 (1962)]

η) Stigmatisierung (Neuropathenflecken)

Die wahrscheinlich vasculären Blutungen der Stigmatisierten, von welchen die katholische Kirche seit dem heiligen Franziskus von Assisi im 12. Jahrhundert bis heute über mehr als 300 Fälle berichtet, sind medizinisch nicht geklärt. Solche Stigmatisationen wurden erneut anläßlich der Ereignisse um Therese Neumann in Konnersreuth 1926 und später durch mehrere Ärzte eingehender untersucht und diskutiert. Wesentlich neue Erkenntnisse sind aber seit der Abfassung des Handbuch-Beitrages von W. TH. SACK, „Psyche und Haut" (Band IV/2, Springer 1933, über Stigmatisierung S. 1361/62) nicht gewonnen worden.

Die üblichen Auffassungen gehen von den Virchowschen Antipoden: „Wunder oder Betrug" über die moderneren Begriffe „Suggestion und Autosuggestion" bis zu den etwas vagen Ausdrücken „Vasoneurose, reizbare Konstitution" mit und ohne unspezifische Herabsetzung der Reizschwelle gegenüber Traumen. Der Psychiater und Philosoph C. JASPERS (1953) hat die möglichen Beziehungen Seele und Leib unter dem Begriff: „vegetative Stigmatisation" wohl richtig formuliert, wenn er schrieb:

„Die Beziehung der Seele zu den groben Anfällen, zu den Organstörungen, zu den komplexen Handlungsfunktionen ist ungemein verwickelt, so einfach sie im Einzelfall manchmal zu sein scheint. Überall ist hier der Zusammenhang zwischen Seele und Leib bei aller Plausibilität im Einzelnen, im Ganzen doch undurchsichtig und sehr verschiedener Art. Die außerbewußten Mechanismen sind offenbar mehrere. Die Organe und leiblichen Voraussetzungen müssen der Seele gleichsam entgegenkommen. Es ist, als ob die Seele die Organe wähle, in denen sie durch Störungen sich kundgibt, oder die Funktion, in deren Vollzug sie sich verwirrend einschaltet."

Es sei daher verziehen, wenn ein psychologisch relativ Ungeschulter, wie der Schreibende, bei der angedeuteten Komplexität der Leib-Seele-Verhältnisse den roten Faden zum ebenso komplexen Gebiet der hämorrhagischen Diathesen nicht findet.

Sehr gründlich verarbeiteten BORELLI u. FÜRST (1960) die älteren und neueren Publikationen über die Stigmatisierung (z.B. POLLACK 1938, v. TSCHERMAK-SEYSENEGG 1940, SCHLEYER 1948, SIMON 1953, OBERMAYER 1955, KLEINSORGE u. KLUMBIES 1955 und 1959). BORELLI u. FÜRST haben wohl recht, wenn sie zusammenfassend schreiben:

„Die zitierten Autoren halten eine Stigmatisation sui generis und die Hautblutungen ohne organische Fundierung für möglich. Gegen einen im Rahmen des organisch Möglichen verlaufenden Mechanismus sprechen nur PETERS, URBAN, LHERMITTE und BON. Die Verschiedenheit der Meinungen betrifft vor allem den Entstehungsmechanismus, während die Frage: ‚Wunder oder Betrug' fast ausschließlich abgelehnt wird. Die allgemein neurovegetative Disposition (Hysterie, Neurose) wird von jedem Autor als eine Vorbedingung angesehen. Wichtig ist jedoch, daß auf Grund von Experimenten und klinischen Beobachtungen objektiviert worden ist, daß sich im Organismus Vorgänge abspielen können, die unter Dazwischengreifen eines oder mehrerer Schaltneuronen die ‚Seele' des Individuums als maßgebliches Agens erkennen lassen. Die ätiopathologischen Hypothesen über die Stigmatisierung, d.h. Suggestion, Autosuggestion, Schrankendurchlässigkeit, Engramme, Projektion, Erregungswellen, Schmerzsuggestion, bleiben vorerst noch Forschungsinhalt."

Biologisch fällt es nach den im allgemeinen Teil erwähnten Experimenten und Erkenntnissen schwer, an rein neurohormonale, lokalisierte Blutungen zu glauben (s. auch AGLE u. RATNOFF 1962).

ϑ) Purpura nach Fettembolie

Auftreten von Petechien oder anderen Zeichen einer allgemeinen hämorrhagischen Diathese nach systematisierter Fettembolie sind klinisch seit langer Zeit bekannt (F. BUSCH 1866, CAMMERMEYER 1953, I. C. EBERTH 1951, zit. nach SESSNER u.a. 1962 und STEPHENS u.a. 1962). Meist wird ein Schub kleinster Petechien an den vorderen Schulter- und Brustpartien, an Halsansatz, in Axillen und auf Konjunktiven beobachtet, mit Farbwechsel von Rot zu Bräunlich, in der Regel 24—36 Std nach der Fettembolie (z.B. traumatische Fraktur von Röhrenknochen), wobei sich die Veränderungen in den ersten 24 Std zuerst ausbreiten, um dann nach 3—4 Tagen spontan zu verschwinden. Aber auch andere Körperregionen wie Abdomen und untere Extremitäten können befallen sein. Oft sind diese charakteristischen Petechien nach Trauma das einzige Zeichen einer Fettembolie, können aber nach schwereren Unfällen mit cerebralen und neurologischen Symptomen, Respirationsstörungen, Fieber und Tachykardien einhergehen, so daß meist irrtümlicherweise an Infekt (Blutkulturen aber steril) oder allergische Reaktionen gedacht wird.

Histologisch werden Blutaustritte um die kleinen Gefäße gefunden, selten Fibrinniederschläge, z.T. subendothelial, z.T. perivasal und nur außerordentlich selten sudanophile Einschlüsse.

Pathogenetisch wird von SESSNER u.a. (1962) auf Grund ihrer tierexperimentellen Untersuchungen an Kaninchen mit Fettembolie nach intravenöser Injektion von Olivenöl eine *Verbrauchskoagulopathie* angenommen, mit Hypokoagulabilität auf Grund eines gesteigerten Verbrauchs von Gerinnungsfaktoren und Thrombocyten im strömenden Blut. Pathologisch-anatomisch fanden die Autoren neben den Fetttröpfchen Blutungen und Fibrinniederschläge in den Gefäßwänden. Sie vergleichen diese Verbrauchskoagulopathie auch mit den Verhältnissen beim Shwartzman-Sanarelli-Phänomen mit ähnlichen gerinnungsanalytischen Befunden. Das Nebeneinander von Fettembolus, Blutungen und vasculären Fibrinniederschlägen infolge Einschwemmung nicht-emulgierten Fettes in die Blutbahn ist charakteristisch.

II. Thrombocytogene, hämorrhagische Diathesen

Die heute bekannten thrombocytenbedingten hämorrhagischen Diathesen sind als hereditär oder erworben übersichtsweise in Tabelle 12 dargestellt.

Tabelle 12. *Thrombocytogene hämorrhagische Diathesen*

I. Hereditäre Thrombocytenstörungen
1. *Thrombopathia Glanzmann-Naegeli* (Thrombasthenie)
2. *Polyphile Reifestörung* (MAY-HEGGLIN)
3. *Thrombopathia v. Willebrand-Jürgens*
4. *Thrombopathia haemophilica* (Morbus van Creveld)
5. *Familiäre Thrombopathie* (HEMMELER)
6. *Komplexe hereditäre Syndrome mit Begleitthrombopenie*
Aldrich-Syndrom
Dyskeratosis congenitalis mit Myelopathie (Typus Zinsser-Cole-Engman)
Fanconi-Syndrom
Chediak-Steinbrinck-Anomalie

II. Erworbene Thrombopathien
1. *Essentielle Thrombopenie* (Morbus maculosus Werlhof)
2. *Thrombocytogene Purpura bei Neugeborenen und Kindern*
3. *Symptomatische allergische thrombopenische Purpura*
4. *Unbestimmte immunopathologische Thrombocytopenien*
a) Thrombotisch-thrombocytopenische Purpura
b) Idiopathische thrombotische Purpura mit erworbener hämolytischer Anämie (Evans-Syndrom)
c) Onyalai
5. *Symptomatische Thrombocytopenie bei Panmyelophthise*
a) toxisch und allergisch
b) bei Tumoren
c) durch Strahlen und Verschiedenes
6. *Symptomatische Thrombopenie bei Hypersplenismus*
7. *Verschiedenes*
a) thrombocytopenische hämorrhagische Diathese bei Myeloblastenanämie
b) kongenitales Hämangiom mit Thrombopenie
c) thrombocytämische Purpura (Dispiastrinemia di Guglielmo, hyperthrombocytäre Myelose (REVOL)
d) thrombopenische Purpura bei endokrinen Störungen
e) unbestimmte Fälle

1. Hereditäre Thrombocytenstörungen

Hier gelangen die erblichen, angeborenen Störungen der Blutgerinnung zur Darstellung, insofern sie auf einer pathologischen Veränderung der Blutplättchen beruhen oder durch einen Mangel derselben hervorgerufen sind: also die qualitativen und quantitativen Thrombopathien mit hereditärem Charakter.

a) Thrombopathie Glanzmann-Naegeli (Thrombasthenie)

Glanzmann beschrieb 1918 eine hereditäre hämorrhagische Diathese als Thrombasthenie, da er in Einzelfällen funktionell minderwertige und morphologisch veränderte Thrombocyten in annähernd normaler Zahl fand. Während hier die Blutungszeit als normal angegeben wurde, beobachtete Naegeli 1931 bei entsprechenden Fällen eine verlängerte Blutungszeit. Symptomatisch handelt es sich um frühkindlich beginnende, typisch thrombocytäre Hämorrhagien aller Art; Petechien, Suffusionen, Schleimhautblutungen und auch sog. Nach- oder Spätblutungen. Bei annähernd normaler Zahl wird mikroskopisch eine Anisocytose der Plättchen beschrieben, Mikro- und Makroformen imponieren auch durch pathologische Vacuolen und stark verwaschene Mitochondrien. Während die plasmatische Blutgerinnung (inklusive Plättchenfaktor 3) normal abläuft, kann immer wieder eine gestörte Agglutination der Thrombocyten und eine vollständig fehlende Retraktion beobachtet werden (Bucher u. Baumgartner 1958, dort reichlich Lit.). Diese Tatsache führte mehrere Autoren zur bis jetzt immer noch unbewiesenen Annahme eines für die Retraktion verantwortlichen Eiweißes (Retraktozym), das bei der Thrombopathie angeblich fehlen soll. Bis jetzt konnte aber ein Retraktozym nie nachgewiesen werden, vielmehr gehen die biologischen Untersuchungen in den letzten Jahren mehr in Richtung der Fermentchemie der Plättchen.

Bettex-Galand u. Luescher (1959/60/61) zeigten zunächst, daß die Retraktion eines Gerinnsels vom Adenosintriphosphat-(ATP)-Gehalt der Plättchen abhängt. Sie fanden auch ein retraktiles Plättcheneiweiß (Thrombosthenin), das zusammen mit ATP entsprechend dem Muskel-Actomyosin wirksam ist. Weitere Beobachtungen, auch an pathologischen Thrombocyten, zeigen, daß die Zugabe von ATP und Magnesiumionen deren Retraktion zu normalisieren vermag (Larrieu u.a. 1961). Gross u.a. (1960) vermochten bei fünf von acht untersuchten Patienten eine Erniedrigung der glykolytischen Fermente (Glycerinaldehyd-3-Phosphat-Dehydrogenase und Pyruvatkinase) nachzuweisen. Damit kann eine ungenügende Regeneration des ATP erklärt werden. Marx u. Jean 1958 fanden bei zwei schweren Fällen und weiteren zwei Abortivformen in einer süddeutschen Familie wohl eine Verwertungsstörung des ATP, jedoch keine meßbare Verminderung der glykolytischen Fermentreihen. Im Elektronenmikroskop fanden diese Autoren eine Verarmung an Mitochondrien und besonders dichte Granula im Plättchengranulomer. Eine wahrscheinlich nahe verwandte Störung beschrieb Bernard 1957 mit abnormen Thrombocyten, gestörter Thromboplastinbildung und Serotoninverminderung. Kreuzversuche erlaubten eine Abgrenzung gegenüber der Thrombopathie Glanzmann-Naegeli.

Während Glanzmann seinerzeit einen dominanten Erbgang postulierte, sind in letzter Zeit daran einige Zweifel wach geworden. Bucher berichtete nur über Solitärfälle, Gross untersuchte zwei Schwestern und mehrere Solitärfälle, Larrieu zwei Brüder und drei solitäre Fälle. Aus diesen Tatsachen glauben letztere Autoren auf einen recessiv-autosomalen Erbgang schließen zu können.

b) Polyphile Reifestörung May-Hegglin (May-Hegglinsche Protoplasmaanomalie)

Diese anscheinend dominant vererbte Reifestörung betrifft die Neutrophilen, Basophilen, Eosinophilen und Monocyten, die alle einen bis zwei basophile Schlieren im Cytoplasma (Doehlesche Körper) aufweisen. Daneben sind die Thrombocyten vermindert auf Werte zwischen 4000—30000/mm^3, und es besteht morphologisch eine Anisocytose mit vorwiegend Makroformen. Klinisch imponiert eine leichte hämorrhagische Diathese thrombopenischer Art, ohne andere Erscheinungen. Die morphologische Beschreibung stammt von May (1909), die genetische Beobachtung von Hegglin (1945). Letzterer erwähnt auch, daß möglicherweise doch eine psychische Komponente vorliegen könnte. Seither sind von Scholer u.a. (1960) ein Solitärfall, von Oski (1962), von Wassmuth u.a. (1963) und von Hegglin weitere Familien bekannt geworden.

c) Thrombopathie von Willebrand-Jürgens (Vasculäre Hämophilie, Angiohämophilie, Hämophiloid, Pseudohämophilie)

Da nach den neueren Untersuchungen bei diesem autosomal-dominant vererbten Blutungsübel die plasmatische Störung pathogenetisch gegenüber der Plättchenstörung in den Vordergrund gerückt wird, verweisen wir auf die Besprechung der vasculären Hämophilie unter den kombinierten Defekten der plasmatisch bedingten hämorrhagischen Diathesen. Dort wird auch auf die noch nicht gesicherte Plättchenstörung eingegangen (vgl. S. 365).

d) Thrombopathia haemophilica (Morbus van Creveld)

Van Creveld beschreibt 1953 vier solitäre Fälle, wovon drei Kinder, die an einer mittelschweren hämorrhagischen Diathese mit allen Erscheinungsformen der Blutung leiden. Besonders sind die unteren Extremitäten befallen. Es sind Knaben und Mädchen betroffen, jedoch bis anhin keine familiären Fälle bekannt.

Gerinnungsphysiologisch konnte eine verzögerte plasmatische Gerinnung neben normalen Plättchenzahlen gefunden werden, wobei die einzelnen Gerinnungsfaktoren genügend vorhanden sind. Es kann ein isolierter Defekt des Plättchenfaktors 3 beschrieben werden (verzögerte Heparinneutralisation).

e) Familiäre Thrombopathie Hemmeler

1958 beschreibt Hemmeler eine anscheinend dominant vererbte Störung der Megakariocyten und Plättchen. Diese sind, obschon in normaler Zahl vorhanden, funktionell minderwertig und als Ursache der hämorrhagischen Diathese anzusehen. Mikroskopisch fehlen im Megakariocytenplasma die Granula, die Plättchen sind klein und ohne Granulomer. Nach Undritz sind bis 1960 keine analogen Fälle bekannt.

f) Komplexe hereditäre Syndrome mit Begleitthrombopenie

Die essentielle Form der Thrombopenie, der eigentliche Morbus maculosus Werlhof, ist nach Frank (1958) keine vererbbare, kongenitale Störung. Allerdings beschreiben Bernard u.a. einen Fall von kongenitaler Thrombopenie mit Blutungen bei angeborener Megakariocytopenie. Die übermäßige Vermehrung der Thrombocyten, ein ebenfalls zu Blutungen führendes Krankheitsbild, Thrombocytosis haemorrhagica, ist als erworbene Störung anzusehen. Einzig Beretta (1961) stellt einen möglicherweise kongenitalen Fall zur Diskussion.

Hingegen tritt bei mehreren komplexen hereditären Syndromen eine hämorrhagische Diathese als Begleitsymptom auf, deren Ursache zumeist in einer Thrombopenie zu suchen ist:

α) Aldrich-Syndrom (Wiskott-Aldrich-Syndrom)

Es handelt sich um ein recessives, X-chromosomal vererbtes Leiden mit Thrombopenie (30000—80000/mm³), wechselnder hämorrhagischer Diathese, Infektanfälligkeit und einem in den ersten Lebensmonaten auftretenden, teils fleckigen, teils flächigen Ekzem vom seborrhoischen Typus, das mit der Zeit lichenifiziert. Das Syndrom wurde 1954 von ALDRICH an Hand eines ausführlichen Stammbaumes neu beschrieben, nachdem WISKOTT (1937) schon früher ähnliche Fälle publizierte. GELZER u. GASSER (1961) faßten die neueren Untersuchungen an Hand fünf eigener Fälle zusammen. Bis jetzt sind nur etwa 60 Fälle beschrieben worden (vgl. RIVERA u.a. 1960, BAKER u.a. 1962, KILDEBERG 1961). Die ausführliche Besprechung erfolgte durch H. J. BANDMANN im Ergänzungsband II/1 dieses Werkes, S. 355—357 (1962).

β) Dyskeratosis congenitalis mit Myelopathie (Typus Zinsser-Cole-Engman)

BAZEX und DUPRÉ beschrieben 1957 einen Fall von Dyskeratosis congenitalis mit reticulärer Pigmentierung, Nageldystrophien und oralen Leukoplakien. Daneben besteht eine schwere hämorrhagische Diathese, die auf einer Thrombopenie von 6000—45000/mm³ beruht. Gleichzeitig fanden die Autoren als weiteren Ausdruck der Myelopathie eine leichte normochrome Anämie und eine Leukopenie. Von solchen Dyskeratosen sind bis anhin elf Fälle bekannt, alles Knaben. Diese verteilen sich auf drei Brüderpaare und fünf Solitärfälle. KOSZEWSKI u.a. (1956), GARB u.a. (1958) und auch McKUSICK (1962) postulieren einen recessiven, X-chromosomalen Erbgang. Außer dem zitierten Fall fanden auch GARB (1947) und JANSEN (1950) bei Solitärfällen die Blutungstendenz im Vordergrund des klinischen Geschehens.

γ) Fanconi-Syndrom

Diese Fälle sind recht nahe verwandt mit der von FANCONI (1927) beschriebenen konstitutionellen, infantilen Panmyelopathie, die mit Anämie, Leukopenie und Thrombopenie klinisch als hämorrhagische Diathese mit Infektanfälligkeit imponiert. Bei diesen Fällen ist ein besonderer Habitus mit Kleinwuchs, Mikrocephalie, Hypogenitalismus und Melanodermie auffällig. Das Leiden soll auch familiär auftreten (GASSER 1961).

δ) Chediak-Steinbrinck-Anomalie

Bei der Chediak-Steinbrinck-Anomalie mit konstitutionellen Riesengranula der Leukocyten, Infektanfälligkeit, Hepatosplenomegalie und Drüsenschwellungen wird zuweilen eine terminale Thrombopenie zusammen mit einer Anämie gesehen. Dieses Leiden ist vielfach mit Albinismus vergesellschaftet und erscheint autosomal-recessiv vererbt. Es sind bis jetzt nach UNDRITZ (1958, 1960) etwa 20 Fälle eingehend beschrieben worden. Seither sind noch einige Beiträge hinzugekommen von BERNARD u.a. (1960), PIERINI u.a. (1958), HANSSON u.a. (1959) und auch von PAGE u.a. (1962).

2. Erworbene Thrombocytopathien

a) Essentielle Thrombopenie (Morbus maculosus Werlhof)

α) Klinik

Dieses sog. idiopathische, essentielle thrombocytogene Blutungsleiden wurde vom Göttinger Internisten WERLHOF als Morbus maculosus eingehend beschrieben. In der ersten Ausgabe dieses Handbuches wurden die klinischen Belange von S. HAMMER ausführlich gewürdigt (Bd. VI/2, S. 512—583, 1928).

Die idiopathische thrombopenische Purpura bevorzugt das jugendliche Alter (nach LOZNER 1954 bis zum 15. Altersjahr 45%, über 16 Jahre 55% der Fälle); sie kann akut, meist aber chronisch verlaufen. Klinisch finden sich in der Regel wie bei den meisten thrombocytopenischen Purpuraformen petechiale Blutungen an Haut und Schleimhaut, besonders an den abhängigen Körperpartien, daneben flächenhafte, oberflächliche Ekchymosen, seltener tiefliegende Sugillationen (Abb. 13). Entzündliche Reaktionen oder Ödeme fehlen im allgemeinen. Dazu kommen schwer stillbare Blutungen aus Zahnfleisch und Nase, Magendarmtrakt, Harnwegen, Genitalien. Hämarthrosen und intrakranielle Blutungen sind ungewöhnlich. Wir sahen aber solche cerebrale Hämorrhagien z.B. bei einem Mädchen mit idiopathischer thrombopenischer Purpura und Blutungen im Herde eines Lupus erythematodes chronicus discoides (STORCK 1950).

Die Blutungen entstehen bei Traumatisierungen (Verletzungen, Quetschungen, Zahnextraktionen), aber auch bei sekundär das Knochenmark und RES-belastenden Erkrankungen wie banale Infekte, Menstruation usw. Sie können besonders im Kindesalter akut auftreten, mit meist guter, spontaner Rückbildung, aber auch chronisch-rezidivierend verlaufen, dies sowohl im Kindes- wie auch Erwachsenenalter (SCHOEN 1955, LOZNER 1954, SCHÄFER u.a. 1958, 1960). Es besteht kein strenger Parallelismus zwischen Grad der Thrombopenie und Schwere der Hämorrhagien (DEBRAY 1958), was vielleicht auf den im „Allgemeinen Teil" erwähnten, für die Blutungsentstehung zusätzlich notwendigen Faktor des Fibrolysins zurückzuführen ist.

Allgemein ist die Gruppe der thrombopenischen Purpuraformen unter den thrombocytogenen hämorrhagischen Diathesen wohl die wichtigste (BERNARD 1959, WURZEL 1961), doch ist die idiopathische thrombopenische Purpura relativ selten. Von 867 Thrombopenie-Patienten waren z.B. im Beobachtungsgut von WURZEL nur 65 Fälle (1,9%) idiopathische Thrombopenien (s. auch STOEGER 1942, NEALE 1955, HAYHOE 1957, GUAY 1957, GENTILI u.a. 1959, BALLERINI 1961).

Die *Diagnose* läßt sich neben Klinik und Anamnese auf Grund der verlängerten Blutungszeit, der verminderten Thrombocytenzahl, der verminderten Faktor III-Aktivität, des direkten Coombs-Testes, der verlängerten Recalcifizierungszeit, der pathologischen Blutkuchenretraktion und des positiven Rumpel-Leede- bzw. Saugglockenversuchs stellen. Die Milz ist nicht immer, gelegentlich nur unwesentlich vergrößert.

Pathogenetisch von Interesse sind besonders die Befunde von Knochenmark und Milz sowie die immunbiologischen Verhältnisse an den Thrombocyten.

Bei jeder thrombopenischen Purpura sollte das *Knochenmark* untersucht werden. Bei der idiopathischen thrombopenischen Purpura werden meist pathologische Abweichungen mit Vermehrung der Riesenzellen, mäßiger Vermehrung unreifer Zellvorstufen, Anisocytose der Megakaryocyten, unterschiedlich starker Kernsegmentierung gefunden. Das Cytoplasma der Megakaryocyten ist häufig stark basophil, zeigt manchmal diffuse, außerordentlich feine Azurgranulationen. Diese Befunde sprechen nach CLEVE u.a. (1958) für Proliferation mit Linksverschiebung der Megakaryopoese des Knochenmarks und Beeinträchtigung des Ausreifungsprozesses der Megakaryocyten. Diese Reifungshemmung betrifft hauptsächlich die Funktion der normalen Plättchenbildung.

Eine solche Reifungshemmung der Megakaryocyten wurde auch von anderen Autoren festgestellt, so von LOZNER (1953), hier gelegentlich auch Eosinophile, deren Anwesenheit besonders für die Erfolgsprognose einer Splenektomie günstig sei (STEFANINI u. DAMESHEK 1953, SCHAEFER u.a. 1958, 1960).

Da sich diese leichten Störungen des Knochenmarks auch noch wenige bis viele Stunden nach erfolgreicher Splenektomie finden, zieht SCHOEN folgende Schlußfolgerungen:

1. Das System der Knochenmark-Riesenzellen leidet bei der idiopathischen thrombopenischen Purpura an einer konstitutionellen Minderwertigkeit, welche mit der Bildung besonders fragiler Plättchen einhergeht und so lange manifest bleibt, als die Milz die Abbauprodukte der Thrombocyten entfernt.

2. Die Megakaryocyten werden durch vermehrten peripheren Verschleiß der Plättchen zu einer kompensatorischen Hyperplasie veranlaßt, die bei längerem Bestehen zu einer irreversiblen Verminderung der thrombopoetischen Aktivität führt.

3. Die peripher angreifenden Noxen der gesteigerten Thrombocytenzerstörung wirken gleichzeitig auch auf die Megakaryocyten und werden auch durch die Splenektomie grundsätzlich nicht beseitigt.

Da erfahrungsgemäß die Milz in der Genese der Thrombocytopenien eine wichtige Rolle zu spielen scheint (Hypersplenismus), interessierten auch die feingeweblichen Befunde dieses bei der idiopathischen thrombopenischen Purpura oft mäßig vergrößerten Organs, dessen Exstirpation häufig einen guten therapeutischen Erfolg zeitigt. Die Befunde sind aber nicht einheitlich.

Histologisch konnten CLEVE u.a. (1958) in der Milz keine Vermehrung der Follikel und überhaupt kein für idiopathische thrombopenische Purpura charakteristisches Substrat feststellen. Hingegen fanden sie oft umfangreiche Thrombocytenhaufen bei Untersuchung von Tupfpräparaten, worauf sie auf die hervorragende Bedeutung dieses Organs beim Abbau der durch Antikörper geschädigten (und agglutinierten ?) Thrombocyten schlossen. Splenektomie beseitige diesen Ort der Thrombocytenzerstörung und entferne damit auch ein wichtiges antikörperbildendes Organ. Im Gegensatz zu LOZNER, welcher Sekretion einer megakaryocytenhemmenden Substanz durch die Milz für möglich hält, glauben CLEVE u.a. bei der idiopathischen thrombopenischen Purpura nicht an eine spezifisch lienale Hemmungsfunktion auf die Thrombopoese. BOWMAN u.a. fanden demgegenüber 1955 bei 45 exstirpierten, leicht bis mäßig vergrößerten Milzen von Patienten mit idiopathischer thrombopenischer Purpura erweiterte Sinusoide, deutliche Vermehrung der Keimzentren, unspezifische Vermehrung der Megakaryocyten, hingegen keine besondere Änderung des Gehaltes an Eosinophilen oder neutrophilen Leukocyten. SALTZSTEIN beschrieb 1961 vermehrtes Vorkommen von Lipiden (wahrscheinlich Phospholipiden) in den Histiocyten der Milzpulpa bei idiopathischen thrombopenischen Purpura-Patienten.

Pathogenetisch sprechen das Fehlen von spezifischen und unspezifischen Ursachen bei idiopathischer Thrombopenie, die erwähnten Knochenmarks- und Milzbefunde sowie die im nachfolgenden Abschnitt zu erörternden immunpathologischen Erkenntnisse am ehesten für die Bedeutung von *Autoantikörpern* gegenüber Blutplättchen (s. Tabelle 13 unter III. 1. a), was nach WAKSMAN u. MIESCHER (s. Tabelle 6 allgemeiner Teil) als unmittelbare pathogene Wirkungen durch cytotrope oder cytotoxische Auto-Antikörper gedeutet werden kann.

β) Immunpathologie

Zunächst wurde während längerer Zeit die medulläre Hemmung der Thrombopoese durch die Milz diskutiert (FRANK 1915, DAMESHEK 1932 u.a.), doch erklärte TIDY bereits 1926 die Thrombopenie durch ein Übermaß des Thrombocytenverbrauches in den Capillaren. Seither wurde der alten Theorie von KAZNELSON (1916) einer vermehrten peripheren Destruktion der Thrombocyten durch Lyse oder Phagocytose, und zwar im Sinne einer Autoimmunreaktion (Autoaggression), wieder mehr Aufmerksamkeit geschenkt.

EPSTEIN u.a. (1950) zeigten als erste Thrombocytenagglutinine in Seren von sieben idiopathischen thrombopenischen Purpura-Patienten. 1950—1951 wurde beobachtet, daß Blut von Patienten mit idiopathischer thrombopenischer Purpura bei den Empfängern einen Thrombocytenabfall hervorrief, wahrscheinlich durch einen plasmatischen Antiplättchenfaktor (DAUSSET u.a. 1952, 1953). MIESCHER u.a. (1952) sowie STEFANINI u.a. (1953) zeigten in einzelnen Fällen von idiopathischer thrombopenischer Purpura hochtitrige Thrombocytenagglutinine. In der Folge konnten im Serum von Patienten mit idiopathischer thrombopenischer Purpura Antiplättchenfaktoren mit folgenden antithrombocytären Wirkungen gefunden werden: Lyse, Agglutination, positiver Plättchen-Coombs-Test, Opsonisation, Verhinderung der Blutkuchenretraktion, passive Hämagglutination, in vivo-Hemmung im Tierversuch und beim Menschen (zit. nach DAUSSET 1956, R. JUERGENS u. DEUTSCH 1955,

Tabelle 13. *Unterteilung der Thrombocytopathien*
[Aus K. H. SCHÄFER, G. LANDBECK u. K. FISCHER: Neue Erkenntnisse auf dem Gebiet der thrombocytär bedingten hämorrhagischen Diathesen. Dtsch. med. Wschr. **85**, 781 (1960)]

I. Thrombocytopathien durch Verminderung der Thrombocytenzahl (Thrombocytopenien mit Ausnahme der Antikörperformen):

1. Thrombocytopenien durch physikalische Einwirkung: ionisierende Strahlen (Röntgen, Radium, Radioisotope).
2. Thrombocytopenien durch chemisch-toxische Einwirkung:
   a) infolge Schädigung der Thrombocytopoese: endogene Giftstoffe (s. auch Gruppe II, 2), Cytostatica, Chloramphenicol, Hydantoin, Benzol, Arsen, DDT u.a.;
   b) infolge erhöhten Thrombocytenabbaus: Benzol, Pilzgifte, allergische Antigen-Antikörperreaktionen (s. III).
3. Thrombocytopenien durch mikrobiell-toxische Einflüsse:
   a) bakteriell: z.B. Sepsis, toxische Diphtherie;
   b) viral: z.B. Cytomegalie, Grippe, Rickettsiosen (Fleckfieber).
4. Thrombocytopenien durch Wirkstoffmangel oder endokrine Störungen: z.B. Vitamin B_{12}-Mangel, Skorbut, Thyreotoxikose(?).
5. Thrombocytopenien durch Verdrängung der Thrombocytopoese (z.T. wohl auch thrombocytolytisch): Leukämie, Erythroleukämie (DI GUGLIELMO), in das Knochenmark metastasierende maligne Tumoren, Lymphogranulomatose, Plasmocytom, Retikulosen, partielle Markhyperplasien (z.B. bei schweren hämolytischen Anämien, gehören z.T. wohl auch in die nachfolgende Untergruppe 6).
6. Thrombocytopenien durch „Hypersplenie": bei chronischen Infektionen (Malaria, Lues, Kala-Azar, Brucellosen, Histoplasmose, Milztuberkulose; Milz-Boeck), bei portalen Zirkulationsstörungen, bei Speicherkrankheiten (Morbus Gaucher).
7. Passagere Thrombocytopenien durch mechanische Zerstörung bei extrakorporalem Kreislauf: z.B. bei Einsatz der Herz-Lungenmaschine oder künstlicher Niere.
8. Kongenitale nichterbliche Thrombocytopenien, z.T. in Kombination mit multiplen Abartungen.
9. Genetisch bedingte Thrombocytopenien:
   familiärer Morbus Werlhof(?), Fanconi'sche Panmyelopathie,
   Chediak-Steinbrinck-Anomalie, Dyskeratosis congenita,
   Aldrich-Syndrom, Hegglin-Syndrom.
10. Thrombocytopenien unbekannter Ursache und Entstehung.

II. Thrombocytopathien durch Störung der Thrombocytenfunktion:

1. Konstitutionelle Thrombopathie v. Willebrand-Jürgens (konstitutioneller Thrombocytenfaktor 3-Mangel ohne, bzw. mit Verminderung der Plasma-Gerinnungsfaktoren VIII und bzw. oder V).
2. Erworbene Störung der Thrombocytenfaktor 3-Aktivität, z.B. bei Urämie oder Makroglobulinämie Waldenström.
3. Thrombasthenie Glanzmann (konstitutioneller Mangel an Retraktionsfunktion der Thrombocyten).

III. Thrombocytopathien durch Verminderung der Thrombocytenzahl und gleichzeitige Störung der Thrombocytenfunktion:

1. Antikörper-Thrombocytopenien (Immun-Thrombocytopenien):
   a) durch Autoantikörper[1]: ein mehr oder weniger hoher Prozentsatz des Morbus Werlhof (idiopathische, chronische Thrombocytopenie, auch im Rahmen der akuten Erythroblastopenie [GASSER]);
   b) durch allergische Antikörper: ausgelöst durch verschiedenste Medikamente, vor allem — früher — Sedormid, viele Fälle von akuter Thrombocytopenie, gewisse Fälle der akuten Erythroblastopenie (GASSER);
   c) durch Isoantikörper: fetale Thrombocytopenie, bisweilen nach Bluttransfusionen.
2. Thrombocytopenien fraglicher Antikörperentstehung:
   gewisse Fälle von Panmyelophthise, thrombotische thrombocytopenische Purpura (MOSCHCOWITZ), Evans-Syndrom, hämolytisch-urämisches Syndrom (GASSER), Hämangiom-Thrombocytopenie-Syndrom (KASABACH-MERRITT).

[1] Unter Autoantikörper verstehen wir „autoaggressive Substanzen" (DAUSSET), die sich physikochemisch wie echte Antikörper verhalten.

J. Bernard u.a. 1956, P. Miescher 1957, Dausset 1957, G. Miescher 1960, Damerow 1961, Deutsch 1961, P. Miescher u. R. Vorlaender 1961).

Die immunologische Autoaggressionshypothese beruht auf direkten und indirekten Befunden (Tabelle 7 und 14).

Zu den *direkten Befunden* gehört der Nachweis von cytotoxischen, gegen Plättchen gerichteten Antikörpern, und zwar nachweisbar *in vitro* im Sinne von *Agglutininen*, welche in rund 50% der Fälle von idiopathischer thrombopenischer Purpura vorhanden sind und z.T. wichtige Funktionen der Thrombocyten behindern (Evans u.a. 1951, Stefanini u.a. 1952, Dausset u.a. 1952, Harrington u.a. 1953, Tullis 1953, Stefanini u.a. 1953, Miescher u.a. 1954, Pfeiffer u.a. 1956, Hennemann 1958); ferner im Sinne von *Lysinen* (Tullis 1953), *komplementbindenden Antikörpern* (Hennemann 1958, van de Wiel 1961), *Phagocytosen* (P. Miescher 1953), *direkter Coombs-Test* (Flückiger 1953, Pfeiffer u.a. 1956, Schaefer u.a. 1958, Hennemann u.a. 1958) und *Antiglobulinkonsumptionstest* nach Moulinier u. Steffen (Steffen 1958, Dausset 1959, 1961, Nelken u.a. 1961, van de Wiel 1961).

Schließlich sind zu erwähnen *in vivo-Teste*, nämlich

1. an *Kaninchen, Thrombocytensturz,* evtl. anaphylaktischer Schock nach intravenöser Injektion des Serums von Patienten mit idiopathischer thrombopenischer Purpura (P. Miescher u.a. 1953, Steffen 1958, Hennemann 1958). Nach dem letztgenannten Autor scheint dieser Test empfindlicher als die in vitro-Thrombocytenagglutination- oder Komplementbindungsreaktionen zu sein.

2. beim *Menschen,* indem idiopathische thrombopenische Purpura-Patienten als Empfänger von transfundiertem, thrombocytenreichem Blut die Plättchen bei akuter idiopathischer thrombopenischer Purpura rasch, d.h. innerhalb von Minuten bis zu 3 Std zerstören (Stefanini u.a. 1951, 1962), bei chronischer idiopathischer thrombopenischer Purpura langsamer, innerhalb von 12—36 Std (Tabelle 14). Das von idiopathischen thrombopenischen Purpura-Patienten gespendete Blut oder Plasma erzeugt andererseits bei normalen Individuen eine *vorübergehende Thrombopenie,* evtl. unter vorübergehendem Auftreten von Agglutininen und Vacuolisierung der Megakaryocyten im Empfänger-Knochenmark (Harrington u.a. 1951, Stefanini u.a. 1952). Durch solche Autoantikörper können die Thrombocyten eine Einschränkung ihrer Funktion erleiden, wie verminderte Adhäsivität und Faktor 3-Mangel (Bounameaux 1957, Schaefer 1958). Die Autoagglutinine bleiben auch nach Splenektomie bestehen (Lozner 1953, Steffen u.a. 1953).

Der thrombocytenschädigende Faktor ist in der β_2-Globulinfraktion enthalten (Harrington u.a. 1951, Stefanini u.a. 1952, 1953, Dausset 1959) oder in der Cohnschen dritten Fraktion (P. Miescher 1954), ist bei 5°C 9 Tage haltbar (Harrington u.a. 1951, Stefanini u.a. 1952), relativ thermostabil, d.h. übersteht Erhitzung auf 56°C, nicht aber auf 65°C (Miescher u.a. 1954). Die verschiedenen Spezifitäten der Thrombocytenantigene wurden erfolgreich 1956 von Dausset untersucht.

Als *indirekter Hinweis* auf das Vorliegen von Thrombocytenantikörpern können angesehen werden: die vorgängig besprochenen Reizzustände der Megakaryocyten im Knochenmark, die Veränderungen in der Milz mit Thrombocytenagglutination im Tupfpräparat sowie die raschere Thrombocytenzerstörung bei idiopathischer thrombopenischer Purpura, verglichen mit normalen, nachweisbar mit radioaktiv markierten Plättchen.

So gingen beispielsweise nach Najean (1961) bei 24 idiopathischen thrombopenischen Purpura-Patienten markierte und übertragene, gruppengleiche Fremdthrombocyten in einem Tag zugrunde, bei 11 weiteren idiopathischen thrombopenischen Purpura-Patienten in 2—4 Tagen, bei 16 gesunden Kontrollpersonen erst in 7 Tagen.

Antithrombocytäre Autoantikörper wurden schon mehrmals bei *Lupus erythematodes disseminatus,* meist mit klinisch manifester Thrombopenie, festgestellt, so Cytolysine von

Tabelle 14. *Differenzierung zwischen akuter und chronischer idiopathischer thrombocytopenischer Purpura*
(Nach M. STEFANINI u. W. DAMESHEK: Idiopathic, thrombocytopenic Purpura. Lancet **1955 II**, 209)

	Akute idiopathische thrombopenische Purpura	Chronische idiopathische thrombopenische Purpura
Familienanamnese	gelegentlich Hämatome nach leichten Prellungen	gelegentlich Thrombocytopenie. Tendenz zur Hämatombildung
Vorgeschichte	keine	seit Jahren Neigung zu abnormen Blutungen
Ätiologische Faktoren	Infektionen, Medikamente, Antibiotica, Antihistaminica usw.	Plättchenagglutinine? Unbekannt
Klinische Befunde	schwere Purpura	weniger schwere Purpura. Splenomegalie in 20—30% der Fälle
Blutbefunde außer Thrombopenie	Lymphocytose, besonders bei Kindern, oft Eosinophilie; seltene Plättchen, normale Morphologie	Plättchen groß, seltsam geformt, ohne Granula. Sonst keine diagnostisch verwertbare Befunde
Knochenmarksbefunde	Lymphocytose und gelegentlich Eosinophilie. Megakaryocytenzahl normal oder leicht erhöht. Keine Zeichen von Plättchenbildung und ungenügende Granulierung des Megakaryocytencytoplasma, mit Tendenz zu Vorstufen (Megakaryoblasten, Promegakaryocyten)	Megakaryocytenzahl erhöht, zeitweilig in starkem Maße. Keine Zeichen von Plättchenbildung und Granulierung in der Zellperipherie, sonst normal in perinucleären Zonen; Megakaryocyten reifer (intermediäre und reife Formen)
Überlebenszeit der injizierten Plättchen	1—2 Std	12—36 Std, selten länger
Elektrophoretische Muster (BERNFELD u. STEFANINI 1951)	Vorhandensein von α_x-Globulin	keine charakteristischen Befunde
Thrombopenischer Effekt von Patientenplasma auf gesunde Personen	in den meisten Fällen keiner (nicht größer als der übliche thrombopenische Effekt von Normalplasma in den meisten Fällen)	wechselnd; oft vorhanden (in rund 60% der Fälle)
Zirkulierende Plättchenagglutinine	keine (mit seltenen Ausnahmen)	in etwa 50% der Fälle
Verlauf	akut, zeitlich beschränkt. Tod durch unstillbare Blutung oder Spontanheilung innerhalb von 4 Monaten	chronisch, Plättchenzahl erreicht kaum Normalwerte; häufige Exacerbationen, besonders bei Menstruation
Therapie	stützend, Cortitrophin und Plättchenübertragung. Wert der Splenektomie schwer einschätzbar	Splenektomie erfolgreich in $^2/_3$ der Fälle. Corticosteroide und Plättchenübertragung nützlich zur Überbrückung von Krisen oder Vorbereitung zur Splenektomie

TAMPONI (1958), Agglutinine von DAUSSET (1959) und komplementbindende Antikörper von DAMESHEK u.a. (1956), SIGUIER u.a. (1961). Es ist deshalb wohl mit Recht von verschiedenen Autoren darauf hingewiesen worden, daß ein Teil der sog. idiopathischen thrombopenischen Purpura Vorläufer eines Lupus erythematodes sein könne, besonders dann, wenn es sich um eine nicht purpurische, aber ungeklärte Thrombopenie handle. Der Lupus erythematodes kann in solchen Fällen erst Monate bis Jahre später manifest werden (MICHAEL u.a. 1951, EVERSOLE 1955, DAMESHEK u.a. 1956, KRUG u. WELLER 1960, SIGUIER u.a. 1961, ZIFF 1961).

γ) Therapie

Die Behandlung der idiopathischen thrombopenischen Purpura stellt wegen der Plättchenautoaggressinen, die auch nach Milzexstirpation nicht unbedingt verschwinden, ein schwieriges Problem dar. Glücklicherweise zeigen vor allem die akuten Purpuraformen, besonders bei Jugendlichen, Neigung zur Spontanheilung. Grosso modo kann hier in rund 38% der Fälle mit einer Spontanheilung gerechnet werden (ROSENTHAL 1939, HANLON 1952, DAMESHEK 1952, WATSON-WILLIAMS u.a. 1958, BERNARD 1959).

Die beste Therapie stellt wohl die *Splenektomie* dar, die aber als symptomatische Maßnahme angesehen werden muß, nicht immer erfolgreich ist und bei verkapptem visceralem Lupus erythematodes sogar zu schweren, ja letalen Krisen führen kann. Auch ist der Eingriff nicht harmlos, da sich schwere Blutungen in das Milzbett einstellen können (HARRINGTON 1957, MIALARET u.a. 1962). Es wird deshalb vielerorts als Vorbehandlung ACTH- oder Corticoid-Verabreichung empfohlen (BERNARD u.a. 1956, 1958, MEYERS 1961). Bei größeren Beobachtungsserien werden Heilungen oder Remissionen nach Milzexstirpation in 50—80% der Fälle mitgeteilt (CARPENTER u.a. 1959 81%, WATSON-WILLIAMS u.a. 50%, MEYERS 1961 83%, BUNTING u.a. 1961 in akuten Fällen 67%, in chronischen Fällen 52%). Gute Erfolge meldeten ebenfalls HANLON (1952), GUAY (1957), GROSS (1961).

Die Behandlung mit ACTH und Cortison allein wird eher zurückhaltend beurteilt:

ACTH und Cortison bei HANLON (1952), BRUSH u.a. (1954), HARRINGTON (1957), HOERDER (1957), der aber ACTH-Gaben vor Splenektomie befürwortete (GROSS 1958). Mit Prednison, allerdings in relativ hohen Dosen, z.B. 20—150 mg pro Tag, dann Erhaltungsdosen von 2,5—15 mg, scheinen verhältnismäßig gute Erfolge erzielt worden zu sein (z.B. in 22 von 30 Fällen von DAMESHEK u.a. 1958, COOPERBERG 1959). Besonders günstig reagieren frische, weniger gut ältere Fälle (BERNARD u.a. 1959, WATSON-WILLIAMS u.a. 1959). Auch hier sind bei akuten Schüben die Heilungen häufiger (z.B. in 25%) als bei chronischen Fällen (in 8%, BUNTING u.a. 1961). CARPENTER (1958) sah in 38% Heilung. HARDER (1957) ist hingegen eher skeptisch. COHEN u.a. (1961) fanden besonders mit kleinen Prednisongaben einen befriedigenden Anstieg der Thrombocytenzahl, ihrer Ansicht nach infolge der anabolen Wirkung der Steroide auf die verschiedensten Körperzellen (s. auch SCHREINER 1959).

Des weiteren kommen in Frage Transfusionen von thrombocytenreichem Polycythämikerblut (DAMESHEK 1952, HANLON 1952, HIRSCH 1952, HARRINGTON 1957), thrombocytenreichem Plasma oder Thrombocytenextrakten unter Berücksichtigung der Isogruppen (BENHAMOU 1959), Cohnsche Fraktion 1 (GROSS 1958, HAESSIG u.a. 1958), Fibrinogen (BELLER 1959 nach BAUMGARTNER 1960 weniger erfolgreich). Bei der idiopathischen thrombopenischen Purpura haben aber diese Maßnahmen wegen der Persistenz der Autoantikörper, wie gesagt, nur vorübergehenden Effekt.

Als weitere Mittel kommen in Frage: Adrenalinderivate, Vitamin C und P, Frischvollblut, Gewebsthrombokinase (GROSS 1958), bei Frauen nach Splenektomie physiologische Ovarialhormone (KAYE u.a. 1961), evtl. auch BAL (2,3-Dimercaptopropanol) und N-Acetyl-Cysteamin (BIGLIARDI u.a. 1952, WEICKER u.a. 1953).

b) Thrombocytogene Purpura bei Neugeborenen und Kindern

Differentialdiagnostisch und immunpathologisch sind die thrombocytogenen Purpuraformen bei Neugeborenen besonders interessant, da einerseits iso-autoallergische Antikörper gegen die kindlichen Thrombocyten von der Mutter via Placenta auf den Fetus übergehen können, andererseits die verschiedensten Purpuraformen bereits früh bei Säuglingen zur Manifestation kommen.

α) Beim Neugeborenen

Die verschiedenen Möglichkeiten der kongenitalen und neonatalen thrombocytopenischen Purpura sind in Tabelle 15 nach KAPLAN (1959) zusammengestellt.

Danach können *Autoantikörper bei mütterlicher idiopathischer Thrombopenie* mit und ohne manifester Purpura der Mutter auf das Kind übertragen werden, aber auch allergische Antikörper bei medikamentöser Allergie der Mutter. Diese passiv, via Placenta übertragenen, gegen die Thrombocyten gerichteten Aggressine beim Säugling sind meist nur vorübergehend aktiv (CLEMENT u. DIAMOND 1953,

Tabelle 15. *Kongenitale und neonatale thrombocytopenische Purpura*
[Nach E. KAPLAN: Congenital and neonatal thrombocytopenic Purpuras. J. Pediat, 54, 644 (1959)]

A. Akute Formen

1. ausgelöst durch mütterliche Antikörper
   bei mütterlicher Purpura
   mütterliche idiopathische thrombopenische Purpura
   mütterliche Arzneimittel-Allergie
   ohne mütterliche Purpura
   mütterliche Isoimmunisation auf Plättchen
   mütterliche Isoimmunisation auf Erythrocyten
2. Transfusionelle Thrombocytopenie
3. Neonatale Infektion
   durch Bakterien, Viren, Spirochäten
4. Akute neonatale Thrombocytopenie unklarer ätiologischer Genese

B. Chronische Formen

1. Megakaryocytenhypoplasie
   Kongenitale hypoplastische Thrombocytopenie
   Kongenitale hypoplastische Anämie (FANCONI)
   Kongenitale Leukämie
   Kongenitale Reticuloendotheliose (LETTERER-SIWE)
2. Periphere Plättchenerschöpfung
   Familiäre Purpura mit chronischem Ekzem und Otitis media (Wiscott-Aldrich-Syndrom)
   Riesenhämangioendotheliom (Kasabach-Merritt-Syndrom)
   Chronische idiopathische thrombocytopenische Purpura

STENING 1953, KAPLAN 1959, GERMAIN 1959). Dauern die purpurischen Erscheinungen beim Kinde länger an, dann stellen sie meistens keine passiven Sensibilisierungen dar, sondern es liegt eine primäre thrombopenische Purpura mit Frühmanifestation vor (KAPLAN 1959).

Klinisch zeigen sich im allgemeinen Petechien, Melaena, intracerebrale Blutungen (MORRIS 1954). Bei idiopathischer thrombopenischer Purpura der Mutter kommen in 15% der Fälle Aborte vor, in 50—75% vorübergehende thrombopenische Purpura beim Kind (PETERSON u. LARSSON 1954). Es sind auch Fälle bekannt, bei welchen Mütter mit idiopathischer thrombopenischer Purpura mehrmals Kinder mit thrombopenischer Purpura gebaren, wobei im Blut der Mutter nach jeder Gravidität ein ansteigender Titer von Autoantikörpern mittels Thrombocytenagglutinations- und Antiglobulinkonsumptionstest festgestellt werden konnte.

Fehlt bei der Mutter eine klinisch manifeste Purpura, dann handelt es sich häufig um *mütterliche Isoimmunisation gegenüber den Plättchen des Fetus*, wie dies bei der mütterlichen Sensibilisierung gegenüber den Erythrocyten (Erythroblastosis fetalis) seit längerer Zeit bekannt ist. Wiederholte Schwangerschaften sowie Bluttransfusionen fördern eine solche Immunisierung.

Solche Fälle wurden bis jetzt z. B. von HARRINGTON u.a. 1953, SCHULMAN u.a. 1954, MORRIS 1954, STEFANINI u. DAMESHEK 1955, TULLIS 1956 publiziert, wobei der Isoantikörpernachweis mittels des technisch schwierigen Plättchenagglutinationstests mit mütterlichem Serum versucht wurde. Mahon u.a. (1957), Moulinier u.a. (1958) führten erfolgreich den Antiglobulinkonsumtionstest durch. Besonders interessant ist die Mitteilung von Shulman u.a. (1962), laut welchen bei sechs Kindern von vier Müttern mittels Komplementbindung Anti-TLA_1 und TLB_1-Antikörper nachgewiesen werden konnten, ferner die Fälle von Garrett u.a. (1960) mit Isoantikörpern, festgestellt mit einer neuen „mixt antiglobulin reaction" nach Chalmers u.a. (1962). Bei diesem Test werden Plättchen mit dem zu prüfenden Serum inkubiert, gewaschen, dann mit Antiglobulinserum-sensibilisierten Erythrocyten zusammengebracht. Bei positivem Ausfall entstehen gemischte Agglutinate von Plättchen und Erythrocyten.

Therapeutisch werden in solchen Fällen ACTH, Corticoide, gelegentlich auch Blutaustauschtransfusion (Stening 1955) empfohlen, hier allerdings mit dem Risiko, daß wegen Vorhandenseins von Isoantikörpern Schockreaktionen auftreten können (Shulman u.a. 1962).

Purpura bei Neugeborenen infolge *allergischer Antikörperbildung der Mutter*, z.B. bei Arzneimittelallergie, kommt seltener vor und setzt eine Nachwirkung des resorbierten Antigens beim Säugling oder Neuresorption via Muttermilch voraus. Ein solcher Fall wurde beispielsweise von Mauer u.a. (1957) bei Chinin-Purpura der Mutter, beim Kind am 2. Lebenstag beschrieben. Auch diese Purpuraformen sind nur vorübergehender Art und nicht bedrohlich.

Hält die Purpura beim Säugling länger an oder entsteht sie erst eine Woche nach der Geburt, so handelt es sich größtenteils um eine *„aktive" thrombopenische Purpura*, meist nach *neonataler Infektion*, in der Regel des Respirationstraktes (Clement u.a. 1953, z.B. Streptokokken-Tonsillitis, Pharyngitis, Otitis). Die Prognose ist auch hier meist günstig.

Aber auch eine *primäre idiopathische thrombopenische Purpura* mit schlechterer Prognose kann beim Neugeborenen früh zur Manifestation kommen (Tabelle 15, B.2., Kaplan 1959, Garrett u.a. 1960). Therapeutisch sind hier Cortison, Splenektomie, evtl. Plättchentransfusion angezeigt (Stening 1955, Mills 1956). Die idiopathische thrombopenische Purpura kann besonders bei Neugeborenen

Tabelle 16. *Übersicht der Thrombocytopathien im Kindesalter*
Erworbene Thrombocytopenien. (Nach C. Gasser 1956)

A. Ohne Megakaryocytenschwund im Mark:
1. Essentielle chronische Thrombocytopenie (Immuno-Thrombocytopenie, Morbus Werlhof)
2. Symptomatische Thrombocytopenien:
   a) akute allergische Thrombocytopenie (postinfektiös, medikamentös)
   b) splenomegale Thrombocytopenie (Hypersplenie)
   c) Thrombocytopenie bei Mangel an Reifungsfaktoren (Perniciosa)
3. Thrombocytopenie des Neugeborenen

B. Mit Megakaryocytenschwund im Mark:
1. Essentielle chronische aplastische Thrombocytopenie
2. Akute, toxisch-aplastische Thrombocytopenie
3. Symptomatische Thrombocytopenie bei Knochenmarkserkrankungen (Leukämie usw.)

C. „Thrombotisch-thrombocytopenische Purpura" (Moschkowicz-Singer-Symmers)

Hereditäre Thrombocytopathien

Hereditäre hämorrhagische Thrombasthenie Glanzmann
Konstitutionelle Thrombocytopathie Willebrand-Jürgens
Thrombocytopathie Typus Naegeli
Thrombocytopathie Typus Jürgens
Thrombocytopathia haemophilica van Creveld
Dystrophie thrombocytaire hémorragipare congénitale (Bernard-Soulier)
Hemorrhagic diathesis due to a qualitative platelet defect (Sussman-Wald-Rosenthal)
Thrombocytopathie bei polyphiler Reifungsstörung (Hegglin)
Aldrich-Syndrom

mit cyanotischer kongenitaler Herzkrankheit gehäuft vorkommen (D. VEREL u.a. 1962) und gebietet Vorsicht bei chirurgischen Eingriffen.

Man kann z. B. auch mit DEUTSCH (1961) bei Thrombopenien der Neugeborenen vier Formen mit unterschiedlicher Prognose differenzieren: *1.* Die hereditäre Thrombopenie. *2.* Die diaplacentare Übertragung von Autoantikörpern von der Mutter auf das Kind. Die Mutter selbst leidet an einer durch Autoantikörper bedingten Thrombopenie (idiopathische thrombopenische Purpura). Das Kind ist nach Ablauf von 3 Monaten gesund. *3.* Die diaplacentare Übertragung von Isoantikörpern. Die Mutter wurde durch Bluttransfusionen oder frühere Schwangerschaften gegenüber Thrombocyten sensibilisiert und leidet selbst nicht an einer Thrombopenie. Die maximale Krankheitsdauer beträgt beim Kinde 3 Monate. *4.* Purpura infolge Markaplasie (Fanconi-Anämie).

Neuerdings wurde thrombopenische Blutungen infolge mütterlicher Isoimmunisation auch beim Schwein beobachtet (STORMORKEN u.a. 1963).

β) Beim Kleinkind

Hier kommen die meisten, auch beim Erwachsenen auftretenden thrombocytogenen Purpuraformen vor. Sie wurden von GASSER (1956) klassifiziert (Tabelle 16), nach persönlicher Besprechung mit dem Autor (1963) abgeändert. Wie daraus ersichtlich, ist unter A.3. wohl mit Recht die Thrombocytopenie des Neugeborenen auf Grund der speziellen immunpathologischen Verhältnisse besonders aufgeführt.

c) Symptomatische allergische thrombopenische Purpura

(Allergische Immunoreaktion von intermediärem Typus, MIESCHER 1958; allergische Antikörper, Typus akute Thrombopenie, SCHAEFER 1960; einfache mittelbare pathogene Antikörperwirkung, WAKSMAN u. MIESCHER 1961),

Klinik. Es handelt sich in der Regel um ein akutes, innerhalb von wenigen Stunden nach Einnahme des betreffenden Allergens (meist *Arzneimittel*) auftretendes schweres Krankheitsbild mit fast völligem Verschwinden der Thrombocyten im peripheren Blut, massenhaft Hautpetechien und Suffusionen an den abhängigen Körperpartien (Abb. 35), Blutungen aus Mund, Nase, Genitalien, gelegentlich Exitus infolge cerebraler Blutung. Bei günstigem Verlauf kann nach Tagen oder Wochen vollständige Remission eintreten. Bei starken Blutungen kommt es zu schwerer sekundärer Anämie mit Hämoglobinabfall unter 50%. Im allgemeinen fehlt ein Milztumor. Bei *Infekten* als Allergenquelle verläuft die Krankheit milder und protrahierter, wobei die Differentialdiagnose mit einer idiopathischen thrombopenischen Purpura oft schwierig zu stellen ist.

Histologisch finden sich Erythrocytenextravasate ohne entzündliche Gefäßreaktionen mit nur gelegentlicher geringgradiger Vermehrung von monohistiocytären Elementen um die Gefäße (GROSS 1958, DEUTSCH 1961, MIESCHER 1961).

Diagnostisch sind entscheidend: Verlängerung der Blutungszeit, Verminderung der Thrombocytenzahl im peripheren Blut, gelegentliche Verminderung von Faktor III, meist negativer Coombs-Test, normale Recalcifizierungszeit, in Einzelfällen pathologische Blutkuchenretraktion, positiver Rumpel-Leede-Versuch. Oft werden passagere Riesenthrombocyten beobachtet, im Gegensatz zum Befund bei Patienten mit Thrombopenie bei Lupus erythematodes, wo diese abnormen Formen konstant vorhanden zu sein scheinen (STÜTTGEN u.a. 1962).

Für den *Nachweis spezifischer Antikörper* ist mit mehr oder weniger Erfolg viel Zeit und Mühe verwendet worden. Am gründlichsten ist wohl die thrombopenische Sedormid-Purpura durch ACKROYD (1949–1962) bearbeitet und abgeklärt worden, mit dem erfolgreichen Nachweis von Thrombocytenagglutininen und Lysinen, hervorgerufen durch einen relativ thermolabilen, in der γ-Fraktion enthaltenen Antikörper. Ohne Komplement tritt in vitro Thrombocytenagglutination, mit Komplement Lyse der Thrombocyten auf. Die Thrombocytolyse erfolgt rasch, innerhalb von wenigen Sekunden (SPIELMANN u.a. 1957).

Für den spezifischen *Nachweis von solchen thrombocytenschädigenden Antikörpern* vom allergischen Typus kommen mehrere Untersuchungsmethoden in Frage, von welchen aber keine mit Sicherheit in allen Fällen befriedigende Resultate ergibt (Miescher 1961).

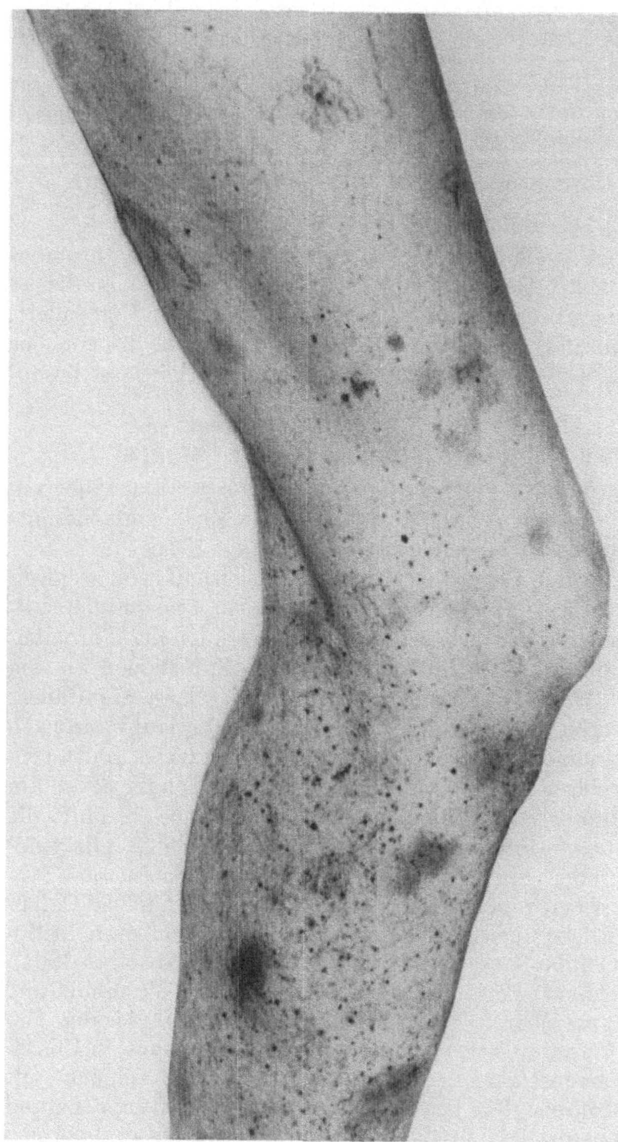

Abb. 35. Arzneimittelallergische, akute thrombopenische Purpura

Es sind dies: *1. Reexposition* mit dem verdächtigen Medikament, wobei allerdings wegen möglichen schweren thrombopenischen Zwischenfällen Vorsicht in der Dosierung geboten ist (Spielmann u.a. 1957). Im allgemeinen fallen die Thrombocytenzahlen innerhalb von $1^1/_2$ Std ab, bei der thrombopenischen Purpura bis auf tiefe, zu Blutungen führende Werte, d.h. unter $50000/cm^3$. Dies stellt zweifellos ein anaphylaktisches Geschehen dar, welches bekanntlich auch im Tierversuch als mittelbare Reaktion beobachtet wird. Solche vorübergehende, durch Antigen-Antikörper-Reaktionen bedingte Thrombopenien wurden von Storck u. a. 1951, 1955, 1956, Hoigné u. a. 1953, 1954, 1957, Nilzén 1959, Heijer u.a. 1960 für den diagnostischen Nachweis von Allergenen benutzt, selbst wenn diese klinisch nicht zu Thrombopenien führten.

2. Hautproben. Diese sind nur gelegentlich adäquat (im Patch-Test und Intracutan- oder Scratch-Test). Sie geben bei der Arzneimittelallergie in der Regel unzuverlässige Resultate. Ackroyd (1949) sah bei der Sedormid-Purpura mit dem Patch-Test von den Thrombocyten unabhängige Gefäßschädigungen (Ackroyd 1949).

3. Thrombocytenagglutination nach Serum- und Antigenzugabe, meist in der Verdünnung, welche natürlicherweise im Blutspiegel vorkommt. Diese Reaktionen sind aber technisch nicht einfach durchführbar und geben häufig unspezifische Resultate. Sie wurden unter anderem mit Erfolg von Ackroyd (1958), Schen u.a. (1958) angewendet. Thromboagglutinationen fielen nach Tullis (1953) meist negativ aus, waren aber nach van de Wiel (1961) unter 353 Patienten mit sekundärer thrombopenischer Purpura in 6% der Fälle positiv (worunter auch Fälle mit erworbener hämolytischer Anämie, Lupus erythematodes, idiopathischer Pancytopenie, Leukämie, Lebercirrhose usw.).

4. Reduktion der Blutkuchenretraktion nach Antigenzusatz. Es wird meist $2 cm^3$ Blut in silikonisierte Röhrchen gegeben, in welchen sich $0{,}05 cm^3$ geeigneter Antigenverdünnung befindet. Der Test kann auch indirekt durchgeführt werden (s. SCHEN u.a. 1958). WEINTRAUB führte diese Methode 1952 erfolgreich mit Chinin, Chinidin und Dilantin durch.

5. Komplementbindungsreaktion, welche aber relativ unempfindlich ist und selten positive Reaktionen gibt, wohl deshalb, weil für die Thrombocytenagglutination zu wenig Komplement gebunden wird (SHULMAN 1958).

6. Es wurden noch folgende Testversuche gemacht: Der *indirekte Antihumanglobulinconsumptionstest* war nur in 8,8% der Fälle positiv, hingegen der *direkte AHGL* in 27% der Fälle (gegenüber 56% bei idiopathischer thrombopenischer Purpura) (s. auch GUREVITCH u. NELKEN 1956, BAUMGARTNER u.a. 1956). Der *direkte Coombs-Test* war nur in vereinzelten Fällen positiv (z.B. D'ESHOUGUES 1959).

Neuerdings untersuchte SHULMAN (1958) am Chinidin, welches Versuchspersonen zweimal innerhalb von mehreren Wochen infundiert worden war, das Verhalten der Thrombocyten in vitro (Agglutination, Komplementbindung) und in vivo. Bei der zweiten Infusion sank die Zahl der Blutplättchen, erreichte aber die Normalwerte wieder innerhalb von 4 Tagen. Die Megakaryocyten im Knochenmark zeigten keine Besonderheiten, der Rumpel-Leede blieb negativ. Nach SPIELMANN u.a. (1957) führte aber eine rasche Antigen-Antikörper-Reaktion zu peripherer Plättchenlyse, die ihrerseits das Knochenmark reizte.

ACKROYD (1962) schließt aus seinen gründlichen Untersuchungen bei medikamentöser Purpura mit Sedormid (= Allylisopropyl-acetyl-carbamid) und Antazolin (2-N-phenyl-benzyl-aminoäthyl-imidazolin) folgendes: *1.* Die Purpura ist eine gelegentliche Komplikation bei der Behandlung mit einer großen Zahl von Arzneimitteln. *2.* Fast immer bilden solche Arzneimittel sehr labile Komplexe mit den Blutplättchen. *3.* Diese Arzneimittel-Plättchen-Komplexe sind möglicherweise antigen, wobei das Arzneimittel das Hapten darstellt. Da die Kombination sehr labil ist, bleibt sie selten lange genug mit den antikörperbildenden Geweben in Kontakt, um Antikörper zu bilden. *4.* Wenn einmal die Antikörper gebildet sind, stellt sich beim Patienten eine Thrombopenie ein, jedoch nur, wenn er das Medikament einnimmt, weil sich die Arznei mit den Plättchen verbindet und dadurch erst antigen wird. Die Lyse dieser Arzneimittel-Plättchen-Komplexe durch die Antikörper führt zu Thrombopenien. *5.* Selten führt ein solches Arzneimittel zur Bildung von Immunpräcipitaten, deren Bedeutung unbekannt ist. *6.* Über die Natur der Gefäßschädigung bei arzneimittelbedingter Purpura ist wenig bekannt. Auch bei thrombopenischen Fällen scheint die Capillarläsion unabhängig von Plättchendefekten einzutreten. Es wäre denkbar, daß auch hier Antikörper gegen Komplexe von Gefäßendothel und Arzneimittel entstehen.

Art der Allergene

Bei den symptomatischen, thrombopenisch-allergischen Purpuraformen können Nahrungsmittel, Medikamente und Infektionserreger allergen sein.

α) Nahrungsmittelallergene

Wenn auch diese Allergenart zuerst untersucht wurde (z.B. Kuhmilch: LANZBERGER 1925, zit. nach MIESCHER 1961), so ist diese doch relativ selten. Die verschiedensten Nahrungsmittel wurden als Allergene angeschuldigt, z.B. auch Obst, und zwar hier spezifisch die Apfelsäure, wobei allerdings ein Fokalinfekt in Form von Appendicitis als Realisationsfaktor auftrat (SONNECK 1957). Weitere nahrungsmittelbedingte, thrombopenische Purpura s. SQUIER u.a. (1937), HAMPTON (1941), POHLE u.a. (1947), ACKROYD (1953), PETRIDES (1963), HOIGNÉ (1960) u.a.m.

β) Arzneimittel als Allergene

Seit den 50er Jahren wurden die verschiedensten Medikamente als Allergene bei akuten thrombopenischen Purpurafällen erkannt. Die große Zahl der allergenen Arzneimittel wird in Zukunft zweifellos noch zunehmen.

Ganz besonders untersucht wurden die Reaktionen mit *Chinin* (BAERMANN 1909, BEIGLBÖCK 1937, STEINKAMP u.a. 1955, KISSMEYER 1956, SCHEN u.a. 1958,

Danilovic u.a. 1960), *Sedormid* (Ackroyd 1952, 1959, Hening, Blessing u. Heni [Erythrocytenballungen 1953], Calo u.a. 1954, Dausset u.a. 1954, Gottron 1956), *Arsphenamin* (Rumpel 1910, Haynes u.a. 1950, Stüttgen 1951) und *Chinidin* (Spielmann u.a. 1957, Bolton u.a. 1957, Hunt u.a. 1958; z.T. zit. nach P. Miescher 1961).

Des weiteren wurden noch andere Arzneimittel als Allergene eruiert, wie Heparin, Gold, Bismut, Nirvanol, Phenobarbital, Hydantoin, Atebrin, Sulfonamide, Chloromycetin, Streptomycin, Diamox, Antazolin, Digitoxin, ferner Insulin, Phenacetin, Dicumarol, Tetraäthylaminchlorid, Natriumsalicylate, Thioharnstoff, Sulfonoxal (zit. nach Miescher 1961). Außerdem kommen als Allergene in Frage: Sulfanylharnstoff, Tolbutamin (Schaefer 1960), Trinitrin (Shmushkovich u.a. 1955), Phenylbutazon (Miescher 1961, Lüllmann 1962, d'Eshougues u.a. 1956), Phenyldimethylisopropylpyrazolon (Dausset u.a. 1954, Miescher 1961), Salicylamid (Greig 1955), Gantrisin (Nash 1956, Green 1956), Merfen (Portwich 1959), Aspirin (d'Eshougues u.a. 1956), Doriden (Kirchmaier 1958), Chlorothiacid (Horowitz u.a. 1959, Nordqvist u.a. 1959), Corticosteroid (Winer u.a. 1962), Thalidomid (Schulz u.a. 1963).

(Weitere Übersichten über medikamentös bedingte, thrombopenische Purpura s. Carr 1954, P. Miescher 1955, Dausset 1956, Petrides 1957, Dacie 1962, Ackroyd 1962, Burckhardt 1963 in diesem Handbuch, Ergänzungsband II/1.)

γ) Infektionsallergische thrombopenische Purpura

Im allgemeinen verlaufen die infektionsbedingten thrombopenischen Purpuraformen wie erwähnt milder und protrahierter als die durch Arzneimittel ausgelösten Reaktionen und stellen deshalb für die Differentialdiagnose mit der idiopathischen thrombopenischen Purpura gewisse Schwierigkeiten dar (Deutsch 1961, Miescher 1961). Der Antigen-Antikörper-Nachweis in vitro mit bakteriellen Allergenen gelingt im allgemeinen nicht, entweder weil Antikörper nur flüchtig vorhanden sind oder weil bei den thrombopenischen Krisen nur wenige Plättchen für die Untersuchung zur Verfügung stehen. Es ist auch keineswegs gesichert, ob die infektionsbedingten thrombopenischen Purpuraformen toxischer oder allergischer Natur sind (Ackroyd 1953, Schaefer 1960).

Thrombopenische Purpuraschübe wurden unter anderen bei folgenden Infektionskrankheiten beobachtet: Varicellen, Masern, Röteln, Keuchhusten, Erkältungskrankheiten (zit. nach Miescher 1961), Diphtherie, Ikterus, Tuberkulose, Malaria, Brucellose (Ackroyd 1953, Kalinowski u.a. 1956), Mononukleose (Pader u.a. 1956, Verheij u.a. 1959), Katzenkratzkrankheit (Billo u.a. 1960), Vaccinierung (Mandersma 1962), Coli-Infektionen (Cereczky u. Vajda 1962), ,,Bläschenkrankheit" (Schaefer 1960).

Therapeutisch kommt hauptsächlich spezifische Elimination in Frage, evtl. zusätzlich die bei idiopathischer thrombopenischer Purpura erwähnten Maßnahmen, inklusive Desensibilisierungen, Corticosteroide, ACTH, Reizkörpertherapie (z.B. Pyrifer), Transfusionen, Vitamin C und P, Splenektomie, BAL (s. auch Petrides 1953).

d) Unbestimmte immunopathologische Thrombocytopenien

α) Thrombotisch-thrombocytopenische Purpura

(thrombohämolytische thrombopenische Purpura, akute febrile Anämie mit thrombopenischer Purpura (Nussbaum u. Dameshek 1957).

1925 beschrieb Moschcowitz unter der Bezeichnung ,,akute pleiochrome Anämie mit hyaliner Thrombose der terminalen Arteriolen und Capillaren" den ersten Fall. Seither sind über 60 Fälle publiziert worden, hauptsächlich im Erwachsenenalter, seltener bei Kindern aufgetreten (WILE u.a. 1956, CLEMENT u.a. 1957, ROBINOW u.a. 1958, LORBER u.a. 1959, MACWHINNEY u.a. 1962). Wenn aber auch die Fälle mit Thrombopenie ohne manifeste Purpura dazu gerechnet werden, scheint dieses Syndrom relativ häufig zu sein (FOSSGREEN 1962).

Das Leiden kann entweder akut mit Exitus letalis innerhalb von Tagen oder Wochen, oder chronisch mit Exacerbationen und Remissionen während Jahren und Spätexitus verlaufen. Es besteht aus der *Trias: thrombopenische Purpura, hämolytische Anämie* und *transitorische neurale Störungen.* Häufig wird es nach Infektionen des Respirationstraktes, seltener nach anderen Infekten, z.B. Rubeolen (SWAIMAN u.a. 1961) oder auch nach Pockenschutzimpfung, Sulfonamidtherapie beobachtet. Meist befällt es Frauen.

Die Prodrome bestehen in Cephalgie, Anorexie, Darmbeschwerden, Erbrechen, Diarrhoe, Müdigkeit, Schwindel, Arthralgien. Es schließt sich ein febriles Stadium an mit Temperaturen von 39,8—41°C. Neben den klinischen Zeichen einer hämolytischen Anämie (Blässe, diskreter Ikterus) finden sich als Hinweise der thrombopenischen Purpura Petechien, Blutungen aus Nase, Zahnfleisch, Lunge, Magen-Darmtrakt, Niere, Genitalien. Dazu kommen verschiedene Organstörungen (Herzmuskel, Nebennierenrinde-Kapselzone, Pankreas, Gehirn, verifizierbar auf Grund der histologischen Gefäßveränderungen). Leber und Milz sind meist vergrößert, und es finden sich Zeichen von Glomerulonephritis und bakterieller Endokarditis (MOSCHCOWITZ 1925, BAEHR u.a. 1936, KORNFELD 1958, ANTES 1958, BERNSTOCK u.a. 1960, FOSSGREEN 1962, MCWHINNEY u.a. 1962).

Die *histologischen Veränderungen* an den Gefäßen verschiedener Organe zeigen charakteristischerweise Verschluß von Arteriolen und Capillaren, seltener von Venolen durch amorphes oder granuliertes, acidophiles Material, an dessen Rand stellenweise einzelne Blutplättchen feststellbar sind. An den Übergängen von Arteriolen und Capillaren finden sich aneurysmaartige Erweiterungen. Oft ist acidophile Substanz unter dem Endothel in Intima, Media sowie Adventitia sichtbar. Um die befallenen Gefäße sind keine entzündlichen Reaktionen feststellbar. Später kann in den thrombosierten Gefäßen fibröse Organisation, in gewissen Fällen Rekanalisation beobachtet werden (WILE 1956, SYMMERS 1956), MCCORMACK u.a. 1963).

Die *Pathogenese* ist unklar. Auf Grund des gelegentlichen Auftretens von visceralem Lupus erythematodes oder Periarteriitis nodosa zählt CRIEP (1959) das Krankheitsbild zu den Kollagenosen. Auch allergische Reaktionen wurden diskutiert (SIEGEL u.a. 1958), ferner leukämoide Zustände mit Reiz des Knochenmarks (SHARNOFF 1957) sowie Meningokokkensepsis (NUSSBAUM u. DAMESHEK 1957). Eine solche Ätiologie wurde hauptsächlich durch Tierversuche an Kaninchen mit Meningokokkeninfektionen von BRUNSON u.a. (1955) erforscht.

Es ist aber auch denkbar, daß es sich um ein Syndrom und nicht um eine nosologische Einheit handelt, da ähnliche Veränderungen bei Sepsis, bakterieller Endokarditis und Tuberkulose beobachtet wurden (SHARNOFF 1957). SWAIMAN u.a. denken an die pathogenetische Bedeutung des Phospholipidgehaltes von Erythrocyten und Blutplättchen.

Obwohl WILE u.a. (1956) Autoimmunisierungen gegen Erythrocyten, Thrombocyten und Endothelien diskutieren, finden sich nach BRITTINGHAM u.a. (1957) keine Leukocyten- oder Plättchenagglutinine. Auch der direkte und indirekte Coombs-Test ist negativ (SYMMERS 1959), Transfusionen von Patientenplasma auf Kontrollpersonen führen nicht zu Thrombocytenabfall (BRITTINGHAM u.a.).

Die *Diagnose* wird anamnestisch, klinisch und hämatologisch gestellt. Probeexcisionen, besonders aus den Randpartien von Lymphknoten, können die erwähnten charakteristischen Gefäßveränderungen zeigen.

Therapeutisch ist das Leiden außerordentlich schwer anzugehen; ACTH, Cortison und Splenektomie können die Blutbefunde verbessern, den Verlauf aber nicht entscheidend beeinflussen (SIEGEL 1958).

β) Idiopathische thrombotische Purpura mit erworbener hämolytischer Anämie (Evans-Syndrom)

Es scheint sich um eine relativ seltene Kombination von immunohämolytischer Anämie und Immunocytothrombopenie zu handeln, die EVANS u.a. (1951) beschrieben. Bisher wurden 25 Fälle publiziert, davon 19 als sekundäres Syndrom bei Leukämie, Lymphom, Tuberkulose, Lupus erythematodes, Cirrhosis hepatica, chronischer Glomerulonephritis, thrombopenisch-thrombolytischer Purpura (SILVERSTEIN u.a. 1962). BRUNNER u. FRICK (1962) beobachteten dieses Syndrom, d.h. hämolytische Anämie, bei Patienten mit idiopathischer thrombopenischer Purpura nach Splenektomie.

Mutmaßlich erzeugt ein autoimmunologischer Prozeß die hämolytische Anämie und Thrombopenie mit inkompletten Wärmeantikörpern. Diese Kombination der Autoantikörper ist aber selten, denn in der Mayo-Clinic wurden von 1950—1958 unter 399 hämolytischen Anämiefällen und 367 Fällen thrombopenischer Purpura nur in sechs Fällen die beiden Symptome kombiniert gefunden. Der Coombs-Test fällt meist negativ aus.

Die Affektion ist wohl nicht prinzipiell von der idiopathischen thrombopenischen Purpura abzugrenzen und stellt wahrscheinlich nur eine Variante mit zusätzlich erworbener autoimmuner hämolytischer Anämie dar. Die Krankheit verläuft meist chronisch-rezidivierend mit Remissionen und Exacerbationen; im Krankengut der Mayo-Clinic wurden vier Todesfälle beobachtet. Splenektomie hatte nur einmal eine günstige Wirkung.

γ) Onyalai

1904 wurde von WELLMAN diese unter den Bantu-Negern von Westzentralafrika vorkommende Krankheit erstmals erwähnt. Sie wurde seither in über 90 Publikationen beschrieben (Lit. s. SNYMAN u.a. 1956, FERNEX 1962).

Das Leiden verläuft ähnlich wie eine idiopathische thrombopenische Purpura, zeigt jedoch ausgesprochene hämorrhagische Blasenbildung an Schleimhaut und Haut. Die Patienten, wie erwähnt, größtenteils Bantuneger, standen meist in mittlerem Lebensalter.

Klinisch treten nach unbestimmten Prodromen (meist Leibschmerzen) Blutungen in Darm, Nieren und Uterus wie auch Gehirn auf. Charakteristisch sind die erbs- bis taubeneigroßen Blutblasen in Mund, Nase und Pharynx, welche aufbrechen und dann während Stunden bis Tagen Sickerblutungen hervorrufen. Auch auf der Haut, meist in der Pectoralisregion und an den Oberschenkeln, entstehen Blutblasen, allerdings kleineren Ausmaßes. Exitus tritt in der Regel infolge Cerebralblutungen, in gewissen Fällen durch Schock nach akutem Blutverlust ein.

Das *Blutbild* zeigt bei stärkeren Hämorrhagien normochrome Anämie, dazu deutliche Thrombopenie, verlängerte Blutungszeit, gestörte Blutkuchenretraktion, erhöhte Capillarfragilität bei normalen Gerinnungsfaktoren, Prothrombinzeit, Fibrinogen und Calcium (SNYMAN 1956).

Histologisch erscheinen die Capillaren in der Nähe von Blutungsherden gedehnt und gewunden, mit sinusartigen Ausbuchtungen, spontanen Rupturen mit Blutungen zwischen Bindegewebsbalken ohne entzündliche Reaktion (FERNEX 1962).

Im Knochenmark finden sich gelegentlich Vermehrung aller blutbildenden Zellen, Megakaryocyten inbegriffen, ferner Metaplasie der blutbildenden Zellen in Lymphdrüsen, Leber, Milz und Myokard, oft mit atypischen Megakaryocyten (FERNEX 1962).

Die *Ätiologie* ist unbekannt. Medikamentöse oder infektiöse Allergie ist unwahrscheinlich (SNYMAN u.a. 1956).

Die *Therapie* stößt meist auf Schwierigkeiten. Bluttransfusionen, Gaben von Vitaminen, Antibiotica, Cortison sind oft nur von fraglichem Wert (FERNEX 1962).

1953 beschrieben BERNARD u.a. unter der Bezeichnung „purpura thrombopénique aigu avec bulles sanglantes buccales et hématuries" bei vier Franzosen in Europa eine Onyalai-artige Krankheit, die ebenfalls mit blutigen, kirschstein- bis traubenkerngroßen, angiomähnlichen Blasen im Mund (Zunge, Wangenschleimhaut, Gingiva, Gaumen), Fieber und Abgeschlagenheit einherging. Gleich nach Beginn der Erkrankung traten rezidivierende Hämaturien mit dunklem Urin, diskreten Petechien und Ekchymosen, gelegentlich auch blutigen Blasen der Haut, Epistaxis, Melaena, cerebrale Hämorrhagien auf. Die Thrombocyten waren auf 32000—62000 vermindert, Blutungszeit bis 15 min verlängert, Blutkuchenretraktion gestört, Rumpel-Leede positiv, Prothrombinkonsumation pathologisch, ebenso Heparintoleranz; mäßige bis starke Anämie, in einzelnen Fällen Eosinophilie. Milz, Lymphknoten, Knochenmark o. B. (WATRIN 1955).

Die Krankheit verlief akut innerhalb von 10—12 Tagen, die Thrombocyten normalisierten sich nach 15—20 Tagen.

Die Autoren verglichen wohl mit Recht diese Affektion mit Onyalai und bezeichneten sie als „Onyalai nostra". Differentialdiagnostisch kommt aber auch eine idiopathische thrombopenische Purpura in Frage.

e) Symptomatische Thrombocytopenie bei Panmyelophthise

Eine Panmyelophthise mit Thrombopenie kann infolge verschiedener Ursachen beobachtet werden, nämlich als Folge toxischer und allergischer Einwirkungen sowie Strahlenschäden, wie auch bei Tumoren.

α) Toxische und allergische Einwirkungen

Es läßt sich oft nicht entscheiden, ob eine Schädigung toxischer oder allergischer Natur ist, dies um so weniger, als der Nachweis von Antikörpern, wie erwähnt, oft außerordentlich schwierig ist, selbst mittels modernster in vitro-Methoden.

Allgemein spricht ein langsam auftretender Schaden nach längerer Einwirkungsdauer eines Stoffes oder Medikamentes eher für eine toxische Schädigung, außer bei rascher wirkenden Cytostatica (STICH 1950, hier auch Lit.). Zweifellos kommen auch Mischformen von toxischen und allergischen Mechanismen in Frage. Sämtliche unter den allergischen symptomatischen Thrombocytopenien aufgeführten Arzneimittel kommen auch für eine allergische Knochenmarkschädigung in Frage, weshalb hier ergänzend auf die vor allem toxisch wirkenden Medikamente hingewiesen werden soll.

Klinisch finden sich meist Ekchymosen, seltener Petechien, bei intensivem Schaden massive Blutungen aus Nase, Mund, Darm, Nieren, Uterus, gelegentlich aus Hirngefäßen. Bei der Knochenmarkpunktion sind die Megakaryocyten vermindert oder fehlen und weisen in der Regel pathologische Formen auf. Häufig finden sich zusätzlich Störungen der Myelo- und Erythropoese. Wahrscheinlich schädigt ein Teil der Substanzen nicht nur die Thrombocytopoese, sondern auch peripher toxisch die Thrombocyten (Dysthrombocytose). Folgende Substanzen kommen hauptsächlich in Frage (z.T. nach MOESCHLIN 1962):

αα) Wahrscheinlich direkt chemisch-toxische Wirkung:

a) *Benzol* (SCHATZMANN 1959) und seine Abkömmlinge: Nitrobenzol, Toluol, Xylol, Trinitrotoluol, Chloramphenicol (MOESCHLIN 1962).

b) *Cytostatica*, besonders Stickstofflost und seine Derivate, aber auch Arsen, Urethan, Myleran, Colcemid, Leukoblastin, Podophyllin.

c) Die neueren, *antimetabolisch* wirkenden Substanzen Aminopterin, 6-Mercaptopurin, Methotrexat usw.

d) Durch *Strahlung* wirkende Gifte.

ββ) Indirekte, durch Sensibilisierung bedingte, d. h. allergisch-toxische Wirkung:

a) Aplastische Anämie und Panmyelophthise (Gold, Salvarsan usw.).

b) Immunocytopenien (Sedormid, Chinidin usw.). Dazu wahrscheinlich noch folgende Substanzen: Antiepileptica (Hydantoine); einzelne Antibiotica (Chloramphenicol u.a.m.), *Sulfonamide* (Storck 1955) (einschließlich Antidiabetica, Diuretica), Antihistaminica; Tuberkulostatica (PAS, Thiosemicarbazone); Antirheumatica (Pyrazolon, Phenylbutazon u.a.); Thyreostatica (Lit. s. Stich 1960, Moeschlin 1962).

Daß tatsächlich toxische Megakaryocytenschädigungen mit Thrombopenien auftreten können, wurde tierexperimentell beim Kaninchen mit Germanin nachgewiesen (Dietrich u.a. 1930).

Therapeutisch kommen in Frage: 1. Elimination der schädlichen Substanz oder des Arzneimittels. 2. Bluttransfusionen (Frischblut, Blutkonserven, Thrombocytentransfusionen). Bei Markaplasien überleben die transfundierten Plättchen 5—6 Tage, jedoch nur kürzere Zeit bei akuter Leukämie, Lymphosarkom, Myelom, metastasierenden Carcinomen. 3. ACTH, Cortison. 4. Allgemeine und okale hämostyptische Behandlung (s. auch Petrides 1953).

β) Tumoren

Bei den verschiedensten Geschwulstkrankheiten kann das Knochenmark durch Verdrängung bis zur Myelophthise geschädigt werden, so bei akuter und chronischer Leukämie, bei Lymphomatose und Myelomatose sowie bei Carcinomatose. Bei diesen tumorbedingten Knochenmarkverdrängungen können die schwersten thrombopenischen Blutungen auftreten. Mittels des Thrombelastogramms lassen sich bei myeloischer Leukämie Gerinnungsstörungen nachweisen, die an die Thrombocytenfunktion gebunden sind (Marchal u.a. 1958).

Interessant sind die Fälle von Ebbe u.a. (1962), in welchen trotz chronisch-lymphatischer Leukämie oder Lymphosarkomatose mit schwerster peripherer Thrombopenie im Knochenmark noch reichlich Megakaryocyten vorhanden waren. Die Autoren nehmen in diesen Fällen einen autoimmunen Aggressionsprozeß an, welcher zusätzlich bei diesen Lymphomatosen die peripheren Thrombocyten schädigen. Hoefer (1954) beschrieb einen eigenen, eigenartigen Fall, in welchem 3 Monate nach einer „Lymphadenosis benigna cutis" im Gesicht, die durch Bestrahlung erfolgreich behandelt worden war, ein Rezidiv mit schwerster Thrombopenie und Exitus, wahrscheinlich infolge medullärer Lymphomatose eintrat (s. auch Hirsch u.a. 1952, Bernard 1959).

Nach Hubler u.a. (1947) gehen 25% der monocytären Leukämien mit Purpura einher.

γ) Myelophthise nach verschiedenen Schädigungen

Außer den genannten knochenmarkverdrängenden Prozessen wurden Knochenmarkschädigungen beispielsweise bei perniziöser Anämie, Tuberkulose, Fanconi-Syndrom, idiopathischer akuter und chronisch-idiopathischer Pancytopenie, vor allen Dingen aber nach Röntgen- oder Radiumbestrahlungen beobachtet.

So beschrieben z.B. Böhme u.a. (1955) zwei Röntgenassistentinnen, welche eine knochenmarkbedingte thrombopenische Purpura aufwiesen, bei Arbeitsaussetzung remittierend, bei Wiederexposition rezidivierend. Es wurde eine Schädigung durch Summation zahlreicher kleinster Strahlendosen angenommen.

Therapeutisch sind strahlenbedingte Markthrombopenien kaum zu beeinflussen, wie dies Raccuglia u.a. (1962) bei röntgenbestrahlten Ratten feststellten. Hydrocortisonsuccinat, adrenochrom-Monosemicarbazone-Salicylate-Komplex, Oestrogene „citrus bioflavonoide" mit Ascorbinsäure waren unwirksam.

f) Symptomatische Thrombopenie bei Hypersplenismus

Splenomegalien verschiedensten Ursprungs können zu Hypersplenismus führen und damit zur Thrombopenie mit und ohne hämorrhagische Diathese. Die Pathogenese der Thrombocytenschädigung durch Hypersplenismus ist jedoch noch nicht gesichert.

Der Hypersplenismus kann sich folgendermaßen manifestieren (Moeschlin 1956): 1. Splenomegalie. 2. Cytopenie eines oder mehrerer Blutzellensysteme,

3. Knochenmarkhypertrophie mit Vorherrschen der unreifen Vorstufen, 4. eventuell positiver Erfolg der Splenektomie, 5. bei Jugendlichen evtl. verzögerte Pubertät mit Persistieren des Längenwachstums.

Der Begriff des Hypersplenismus stammt von FRANK u. EPPINGER (1915). Folgende Ursachen der Splenomegalie können zu Hypersplenismus führen (MOESCHLIN 1956): *a)* Stauung im Pfortadersystem: M. Banti (primär oder als Syndrom), Lebercirrhose (nach WURZEL 1961, BREDDIN u.a. 1962 wohl die häufigste Ursache); Milzvenenverschluß durch Thrombose oder Kompression. *b)* Speicherkrankheiten: M. Gaucher, M. Niemann-Pick. *c)* Chronische Infekte: Kala-Azar, Malaria, Brucellose, Tuberkulose und Morbus Boeck der Milz, chronische Mononukleose. *d)* Primärer Erythrocytendefekt; familiäre hämolytische

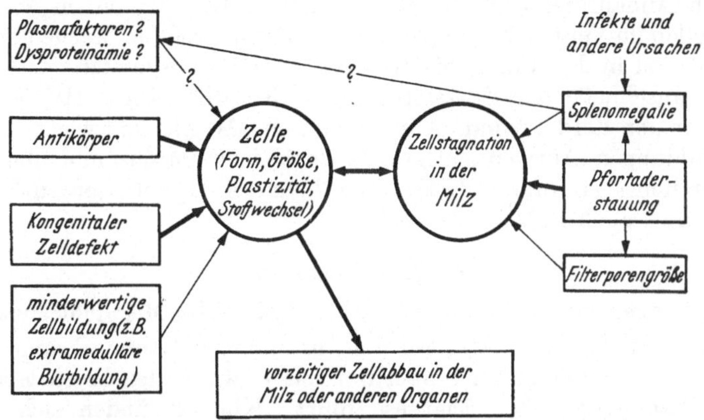

Abb. 36. Gesicherte und mögliche Einflüsse der Milz, des Pfortadersystems, der Blutzellen selbst und exogener Faktoren auf den vorzeitigen Abbau von Blutzellen als mögliche Ursache des sogenannten „Hypersplenismus". [Aus J. WEINREICH: Neuere Untersuchungsergebnisse zur Frage des Hypersplenismus. Med. Klin. **58**, 81 (1963)]

Anämie, M. Cooley, Sichelzellanämie. *e)* Unbekannte Mechanismen (idiopathische Formen), Hämangiome, chronische lymphocytäre Leukosen, Lymphoblastoma Brill-Symmers, Lymphosarkome, Morbus Hodgkin, maligne Reticuloendotheliosen, Sarkome.

Nach LOZNER (1954) führen noch das Felty-Syndrom und disseminierter Lupus erythematodes zu Splenomegalie, nach MARCHAL u.a. (1957) in seltenen Fällen auch myeloische Leukämie. WURZEL (1961) sah unter 150 Patienten mit Lebercirrhose in 15 Fällen Thrombocytenzahlen unter 100000. Häufig fand er Thrombopenien kombiniert mit Abfall von Prothrombin und Faktor V. BREDDIN (1962) fand bei 54 von 84 Patienten mit Lebercirrhose und in 16 von 23 Fällen mit chronischer Hepatitis eine Störung der Thrombocytenfunktion, hauptsächlich mit Verminderung der Blutkuchenretraktion und der Thrombusfestigkeit, gemessen mit dem Thrombelastographen, wodurch gelegentlich selbst bei normaler Blutplättchenzahl Hämorrhagien auftraten. Das Ausmaß der Thrombocytenfunktionsstörung geht aber der Schwere der Lebercirrhose nicht parallel. Diese Thrombocytenfunktionsstörungen gleichen nach BREDDIN der erblichen Thrombasthenie. Neben Thrombopenie und den erwähnten Thrombocytenfunktionsstörungen wurden auch Thrombokinasebildungsstörung, Verminderung des Prothrombins, der Acceleratoren, des Fibrinogens und Steigerung der Fibrinolyse beobachtet.

Bei einem Fall von TOMSI u.a. (1955) erzeugte ein infolge Morbus Hodgkin vergrößerter Lymphknoten am Hilus der Milz den Hypersplenismus.

Die *Differentialdiagnose* der hypersplenischen Thrombopenie ist eine internistische Aufgabe und kann durch Milz- und Knochenmarkfunktionsprüfung, Messung der Überlebenszeit von Erythro- und Thrombocyten, evtl. ex iuvantibus aus der Wirkung von ACTH und Cortison geschehen.

Der Hypersplenismus kann zur Erythropenie (Färbeindex normal oder leicht erhöht), Leukopenie, evtl. mit mehr oder minder ausgesprochener Lymphocytopenie, Thrombocytopenie, in gewissen Fällen Auftreten von atypischen großen und kleinen Thrombocyten führen. Gelegentlich kommen kombinierte Formen vor (Pancytopenien). Das Knochenmark ist meist hypertrophisch mit Vermehrung der unreifen Zellvorstufen.

Pathogenetisch wurden besonders folgende Hypothesen für die Entstehung des Hypersplenismus diskutiert: *1.* Bildung eines knochenmarkhemmenden Hormons in der Milz mit Reifungshemmung im Knochenmark und Ausschwemmungsblockierung. Diese Hypothese konnte im Tierexperiment nicht mit Sicherheit bestätigt werden. *2.* Zerstörung einer das Knochenmark stimulierenden Substanz durch die vergrößerte Milz. Diese Hypothese ist unwahrscheinlich, da nach Splenektomie oder bei Sprue keine Überproduktion des Knochenmarks beobachtet werden kann. *3.* Gesteigerte Zellsequestration, Phagocytose und Lysis in der Milz. Durch Anhäufung von Thrombocyten und Leukocyten im Milzsinusblut sind diese Zellen im Vergleich zum peripheren Blut in größerer Menge und während längerer Zeit den in der Milz gebildeten Antikörpern ausgesetzt. *4.* Antikörperbildung mit anschließender Zellzerstörung in der Milz. Diese Hypothese rückt immer mehr in den Vordergrund. Abb. 36 gibt eine Möglichkeit wieder, sich solche Antikörperbildungen, Antigen-Antikörper-Reaktionen im Zusammenhang mit der Milz vorzustellen (WEINREICH 1963). Die 3. und 4. Hypothesen sind am wahrscheinlichsten (s. auch P. MIESCHER 1960).

g) Verschiedenes

α) Thrombocytopenische hämorrhagische Diathese bei Megaloblastenanämie

1962 macht M. D. SMITH u.a. auf die Thrombopenie aufmerksam, die häufig bei Megaloblastenanämie auftritt, aber nur selten, wie in den beschriebenen neun Fällen, zur hämorrhagischen Diathese führt. Klinisch finden sich Epistaxis, gingivale, retinale, gastrointestinale Blutungen mit Hämatemesis, Hämaturie, Menorrhagie und schließlich Petechien mit gelegentlichen Hautsuffusionen. Die Thrombocytenzahl kann auf 5000—70000 absinken, mit entsprechender Verlängerung der Blutungszeit. Daß bei Perniciosa Retinablutungen und Petechien auftreten können, hat BIERMER bereits 1872 beobachtet (zit. nach DAVIS u. BROWN 1953).

Thrombopenische Zustände bei Megaloblastenanämie wurden verschiedentlich gesehen (MINOT 1918, DAVIS u.a. 1953, TORREY 1953, BISGEIER 1954, WHITBY u.a. 1957, WINTROBE 1956, GRUCHY 1958, COSNETT u. MACLEOD 1959). Megaloblastenanämie verschiedenster Genese, z.B. bei Perniciosa, Schwangerschaft, Steatorrhoe, können zu solchen Zuständen führen. Die Thrombocytopenie wird in diesen Fällen als dyshormopoetische Lage infolge Mangel an Vitamin B_{12} oder Folsäure aufgefaßt.

Therapeutisch kommen neben Bluttransfusionen Vitamin B_{12} und Leberextrakt in Frage.

β) Kongenitales Hämangiom mit Thrombopenie

1940 beschrieben KASABACH u. MERRITT den Fall eines Kleinkindes mit ausgedehntem capillärem planem Hämangiom der unteren Stammhälfte und des linken Beines, mit schwerer thrombocytopenischer Purpura vergesellschaftet. Bis 1961 wurden über 20 ähnliche Fälle publiziert (Lit. s. JAMES u.a. 1961); z.T. handelte es sich um planotuberöse oder kavernöse Hämangiome, doch kann aus den Publikationen die Art der Hämangiome nicht immer mit Sicherheit rekonstruiert werden. Voraussetzung für die Entstehung der thrombopenischen Purpura ist offensichtlich eine große Ausdehnung der Hämangiome (DARGEON u.a. 1959, DOOREN u.a. 1961) (Abb. 37).

Nachdem zunächst eine bloße Koincidenz des Hämangioms mit einer thrombopenischen Purpura angenommen wurde, wird seit kurzem die enge Beziehung zwischen Größe des Hämangioms und thrombopenischer Purpura als besonderes klinisches Syndrom anerkannt. Nach GOOD u.a. 1955, DARGEON u.a. 1959 werden die Blutplättchen im Hämangiom abgefangen, sequestriert, verbraucht und zerstört. Das Hämangiom scheint eine ähnliche Funktion auszuüben wie die Milz bei Hypersplenismus (STUBER 1956). Antigen-Antikörper-Reaktionen spielen keine Rolle. Gelegentlich findet sich auch eine Vermehrung und Linksverschiebung der

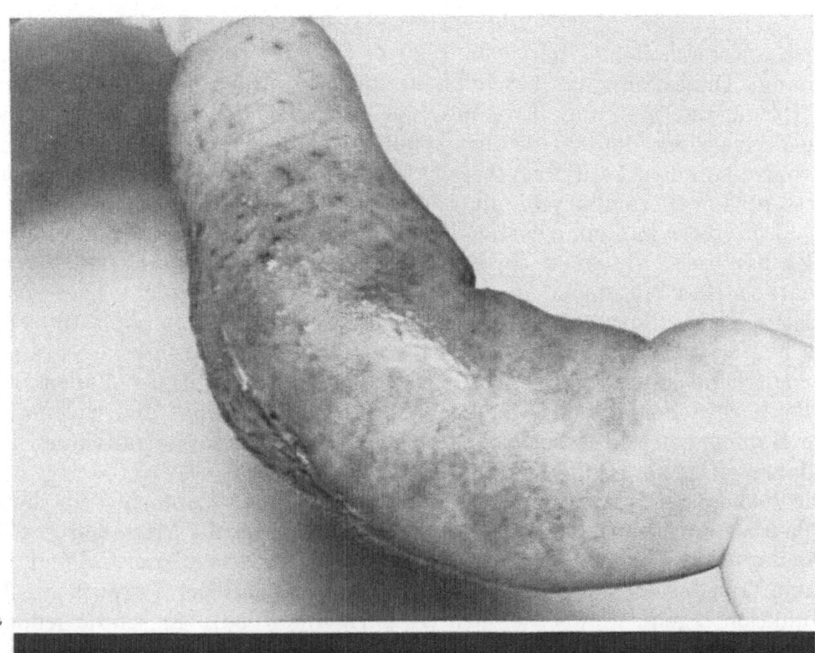

a

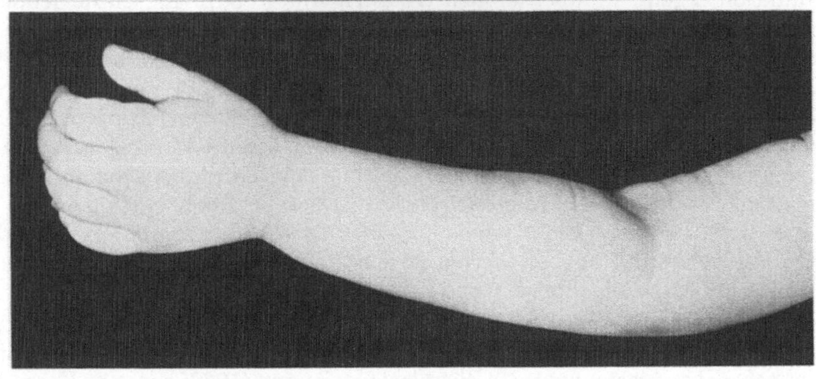

b

Abb. 37a u. b. Hypertrophisches Hämangiom mit thrombopenischer Purpura vor und nach Röntgentherapie. [Aus H. W. DARGEON, A. C. ADIAO and G. T. PACK: Hemangioma with Thrombocytopenia. J. Pediat. **54**, 285 (1959)]

Megakaryocyten im Knochenmark, ähnlich wie bei der idiopathischen thrombopenischen Purpura (GOOD u.a. 1955).

Histologisch lassen sich in den Gefäßen des Hämangioms wesentlich mehr Thrombocyten feststellen als in den peripheren Blutgefäßen oder im peripheren Blut.

Daß das Hämangiom für die Thrombopenie von entscheidender Bedeutung ist, zeigt die Rückbildung derselben nach erfolgreicher Röntgenbestrahlung des Primärtumors. Röntgenbestrahlung ist in diesen Fällen die Therapie der Wahl, denn vor Rückbildung des Hämangioms haben auch Transfusionen von frischen konzentrierten Plättchen keinen Effekt (James u.a. 1961). Splenektomie hatte nur in einem von sechs Fällen Erfolg (Dargeon u.a. 1959). Die thrombopenischen Blutungen können bis zum Bestrahlungseffekt durch Corticoide symptomatisch unterdrückt werden.

γ) Thrombocythämische Purpura (Dispiastrinemia di Guglielmo), hyperthrombocytäre Myelose (Revol)

Dieses Krankheitsbild hat wohl 1920 di Guglielmo erstmals unter der Bezeichnung „Dipiastrinemia" beschrieben. Seither wurden gegen 100 Fälle publiziert (Revol 1962). Mäßige Erhöhung der Thrombocyten führt zu Thrombosen, starke Vermehrung (500000 bis über 1000000) zu Hämorrhagien. Solche Thrombocytämien kommen bei Polycythämia vera, chronischer Granulocytenleukämie und essentieller Thrombocythämie vor (Spaeth u.a. 1956, Stecher u.a. 1961).

Klinisch treten hämophilieartige Blutungen in Erscheinung, weniger Petechien und Ekchymosen, wie sonst bei thrombopenischer Purpura. Es entstehen nur gelegentlich Hautblutungen, in der Regel nach Traumen, nicht aber spontan. Capillarfragilität, Blutungs- und Gerinnungszeit normal, Thromboplastintest nach Biggs häufig pathologisch (Bousser 1959). Auch das Thrombelastogramm ist pathologisch (Marchal u.a. 1958). Meist finden sich bei diesen Fällen Splenomegalie, leichte Polyglobulie, Leukocytose, im Myelogramm und Splenogramm dichte Haufen von Thrombocyten. Das Leiden befällt meist Individuen in den 50er Jahren (Ozer u.a. 1960, Revol 1962).

Die *Pathogenese* ist noch ungeklärt. Einzelne Momente sprechen für die Blutplättchen als Auslösungsfaktor bei den Blutungen, obwohl Plättchen von Polycythämikerno der Patienten mit Thrombocythämie funktionell normal sind, indem sie nach Transfusionen bei idiopathischer thrombopenischer Purpura die Plättchenfunktion regelrecht übernehmen (Spaeth u.a. 1956). Es wurde jedoch bei solchen Fällen schon Hypofibrinogenämie festgestellt, und zudem wird eine antikoagulative Aktivität von Thrombocyten in großer Zahl angenommen. Koller u. Bounameaux (1956) fanden eine ungenügende Thrombokinasebildung, wahrscheinlich infolge des Mißverhältnisses zwischen der hohen Konzentration des Plättchenfaktors 3 zu den übrigen, bei der Blutthrombokinasegeneration notwendigen Gerinnungsfaktoren: sie beobachteten eine Thrombocythaemia haemorrhagica auch reaktiv nach Milzexstirpation. Dieselbe Beobachtung wurde auch von Binswanger u.a. (1955) gemacht. Vuille (1960) nimmt auf Grund von in vitro-Versuchen mit angereicherten normalen Thrombocyten an, daß dieselben in großer Zahl sämtliche Phasen und auch die Fibrinretraktion hemmen.

Nach Gimeno-Alfos u.a. (1959) ist die Lebensdauer der Blutplättchen (bestimmt mit P^{132}) verlängert, möglicherweise durch Störung des Mechanismus zur Plättcheneliminierung aus der Zirkulation. Revol (1962) hält das Krankheitsbild für ein myelo-proliferatives Syndrom, ähnlich der leukämischen Myelose. Er empfiehlt deshalb die Bezeichnung „hyperthrombocytäre Myelose".

Therapeutisch scheint die Behandlung mit radioaktivem Phosphor am ehesten erfolgversprechend, ähnlich wie bei der Polyglobulinämie (Tubiana u.a. 1957, Bousser 1959, Shaw 1961, Shechter u.a. 1962), oder auch Busulfan = MyPeran (Webb u.a. 1963).

δ) Thrombopenische Purpura bei endokrinen Störungen

Roberts publizierte 1948 einen Fall von Morbus Basedow, bei welchem 6 Monate nach Krankheitsbeginn Nasenbluten, Menorrhagie sowie Petechien und Ekchymosen an den Beinen auftraten bei vollständigem Fehlen der Blutplättchen.

Es schien, daß die Schilddrüse einen hemmenden Effekt auf das Knochenmark ausübte mit totaler Knochenmarkaplasie des Thrombocytensystems. ITEN u.a. publizierten 1956 den Fall einer 60jährigen Frau mit Cushing-Syndrom, Guillain-Barré-Syndrom und thrombopenischer Purpura. Interessanterweise bewirkte eine doppelseitige Nebennierenhyperplasie vermehrte Sekretion von Nebennierenrindenhormonen. Dies ist um so bemerkenswerter, als sonst NNR-Hormone therapeutisch bei thrombocytopenischer Purpura angewandt werden.

Auch die Ovarialdysfunktion (Hypo-, evtl. Hyperfollikulinämie, Hyperluteinämie) kann einen Einfluß auf die Blutungsbereitschaft, besonders im Sinne von thrombopenischer Purpura haben. Neben cyclischen Blutungen bei *Morbus Werlhof* beobachteten PAVLOWSKY u.a. (1953) vier Fälle mit prämenstrueller oder menstrueller thrombopenischer Purpura, die auf Behandlung mit Testosteronpropionat ausgezeichnet ansprachen.

ε) Unbestimmte Fälle

Zweifellos können nicht sämtliche Fälle von thrombopenischer Purpura mit Sicherheit eingereiht werden, wie beispielsweise der von HOLZMANN u. KORTING (1959) publizierte Fall mit thrombopenischer Purpura, mangelnder Thrombocytenfunktion, gestörter Blutkuchenretraktion, aber vollkommen negativen immunbiologischen Reaktionen (Thrombocyten- und Coombs-Test sowie Thrombocytenagglutinationstest). Hier schien Adalin eine chronisch-toxische Schädigung der Thrombocytopoese verursacht zu haben bei labilem Hypertonus, wobei jeweils die niedrigen Blutdruckphasen synchron mit dem Thrombocytenabfall waren. Es wäre denkbar, daß die Milzdurchblutung bei den Blutdruckschwankungen von Bedeutung sein könnte.

Ebenfalls schwer einzureihen ist der Fall von BERNARD u.a. (1962) mit cyclischer Hemmung der Megakaryocytopoese, jedoch ohne nachweisbare Plättchenautoantikörper.

Tabelle 17. *Übersicht der plasmatisch bedingten hämorrhagischen Diathesen (Koagulopathien)*

Gerinnungsfaktoren	Fehlen bei folgenden Krankheiten	
	kongenital	erworben
Fibrinogen (Faktor I)	Afibrinogenämie	Fibrinolyse (Proteolyse) Intravasale Gerinnung (Defibrinierung) Schwerster Leberschaden Generalisierte Malignome
Prothrombin (Faktor II)	Prothrombinmangel	Leberschaden K-Avitaminose Dicoumaroltherapie Intravasale Gerinnung
Faktor V	Faktor V-Mangel	Fibrinolyse (Proteolyse) Intravasale Gerinnung Schwerster Leberschaden Purpura fulminans
Faktor VII	Faktor VII-Mangel	Leberschaden K-Avitaminose Dicoumaroltherapie
Faktor VIII	Hämophilie A	Fibrinolyse (Proteolyse) Intravasale Gerinnung Purpura fulmimans
Faktor IX	Hämophilie B	Leberschaden K-Avitaminose Dicoumaroltherapie
Faktor X	Faktor X-Mangel (Stuart-Prower-Mangel)	Leberschaden K-Avitaminosen Dicumaroltherapie
Faktor XI	PTA-Mangel	—
Faktor XII	Hageman Trait	—
Fibrin Stabilising Factor (FSF)	FSF-Mangel	(Schwere Dysproteinämien)

III. Die Koagulopathien

Klinisches Bild und Untersuchungsmethoden wurden übersichtsweise im allgemeinen Teil besprochen (II.3.). Hier sollen die speziellen Krankheitsbilder mit den speziellen diagnostischen Verhältnissen besprochen werden und wiederum wie bei den vorgängigen Abschnitten, in hereditäre und erworbene Koagulopathien gegliedert werden. Die Krankheitsbilder sind übersichtsweise in Tabelle 17 dargestellt.

1. Hereditäre Koagulopathien

a) Historischer Überblick

Bis vor wenigen Jahrzehnten wurden alle Patienten mit angeborener, erblicher Blutungsneigung einheitlich als „Bluter" bezeichnet. Die Kenntnis dieser Krankheit geht bis ins Mittelalter zurück und hat in Geschichte und Literatur Eingang gefunden. Am besten bekannt ist die Blutersippe, die, ausgehend von der Königin Viktoria von England, die meisten Fürstenhäuser Europas durchsetzte und auch literarisch mehrmals gewürdigt wurde (VERSCHUER). Eine andere Sippe ist Gegenstand des Romans „Die Frauen von Tanno" (Tenna, Graubünden/Schweiz) von ERNST ZAHN. In seinen Vorlesungen (1828—1832) prägte J. L. SCHÖNLEIN für diese Krankheit den Namen „Hämophilie".

1920 beschrieben RABE und SALOMON einen kongenitalen Fibrinogenmangel und grenzten erstmals ein streng umschriebenes Krankheitsbild vom Sammelbegriff der Hämophilie ab. Eine weitere Gruppe von Blutungsübeln kann seit 1935 dank der von QUICK eingeführten „Prothrombinbestimmung" gesondert erfaßt werden. Diese Gruppe umfaßt den 1944 von OWREN erstmals beschriebenen Faktor V-Mangel, den Mangel an Faktor VII (KOLLER et al. 1950) und den 1956 von HOUGIE und TELFER getrennt entdeckten Faktor X-Mangel (Stuart-Prower-Mangel). Aber auch die Hämophilie erwies sich nicht als einheitliches Krankheitsbild, seit KOLLER et al. 1950 durch Kreuzversuche zeigen konnten, daß bei der klassischen Hämophilie A (Faktor VIII-Mangel) eine andere Proteinfraktion fehlt, als bei der seither so bezeichneten Hämophilie B (Faktor IX-Mangel, PTC-deficiency, Christmas disease). 1953 beschrieben ROSENTHAL et al. noch eine dritte Hämophilieform, den PTA-Mangel (Faktor XI-Mangel).

Während die Unterscheidung aller dieser kongenitalen, erblichen Koagulopathien auf Grund der klinischen Erscheinungsbilder nicht oder nur andeutungsweise gelingt, kann durch gerinnungsphysiologische Analyse der jeweils vorliegende Defekt erfaßt und eine eindeutige Diagnose gestellt werden (KOLLER, QUICK).

b) Ätiologie und funktionelle Erörterung

Bei den Gerinnungsfaktoren handelt es sich durchwegs um Globuline, die sich in der elektrophoretischen Trennung zwischen den α_2-Globulinen und den γ-Globulinen bewegen. Mengenmäßig steht das Fibrinogen (Normalwert 200—400 mg/ml Plasma) weitaus an der Spitze. Die anderen Faktoren sind nur in Mengen von weniger als 3 mg/ml Plasma vorhanden (DUCKERT). Bei den kongenitalen Mangelzuständen ist meistens ein isolierter Gerinnungsfaktor bedeutend erniedrigt oder fehlt ganz. Dies beruht auf nur teilweiser oder fehlender Synthese desselben und ist genetisch kontrolliert. Man spricht deshalb folgerichtig von Defektdysproteinämien oder von Enzymopathien, je nachdem, ob das fehlende Protein als Substrat oder als Ferment in den Gerinnungsvorgang eingreifen sollte. Entsprechend der Bezeichnung von GARROD kann man diese Fälle auch bei den „inborn errors of metabolism" einreihen (HSIA). Zur besseren Übersicht seien hier kurz Ablauf und

Reaktionskinetik des Gerinnungsvorganges angeschnitten. Daraus ist verständlich, wo beim Fehlen eines Faktors der Stop im Gesamtablauf liegt (Schema, Abb. 38, Nomenklatur und Krankheitsbilder, Tabelle 17, Synonyma, Tabelle 18).

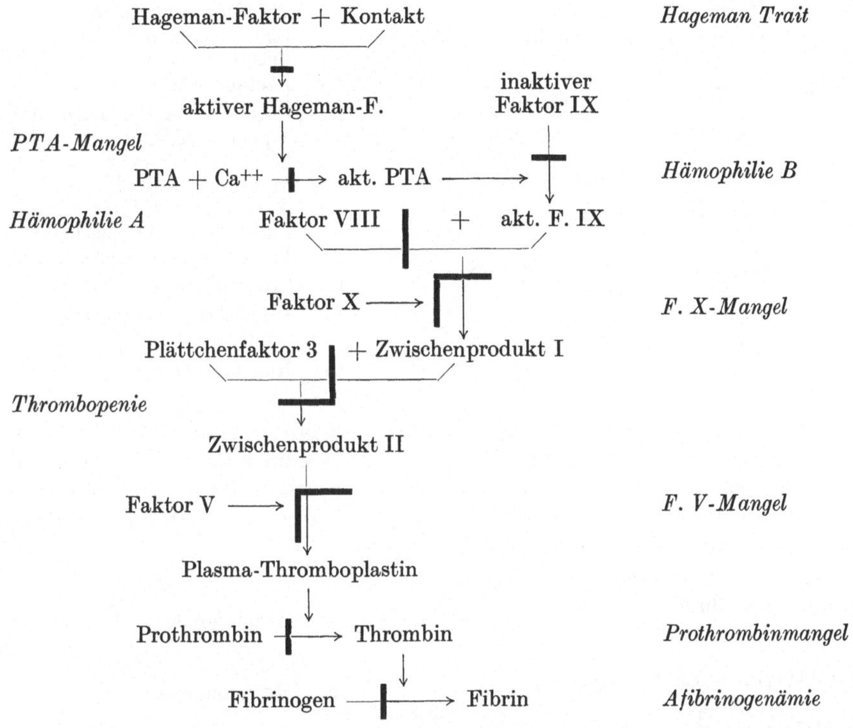

| Gibt den Stop im Gerinnungsablauf an, der eintritt, wenn kongenitale oder erworbene Mangelzustände (*Kursivdruck*) der entsprechenden Plasma- oder Plättchenfaktoren vorliegen.
→ Deuten Reaktionen oder Einwirkung von Acceleratoren an. (Abkürzungen vgl. Liste der Synonyma.)

Abb. 38. Ablauf der Gerinnung im „intrinsic system" (Plasma- und Plättchenfaktoren)

Das auch heute noch anerkannte Gerinnungsschema beruht auf den grundlegenden Arbeiten von A. SCHMIDT (1892), der damals folgende Gliederung machte:

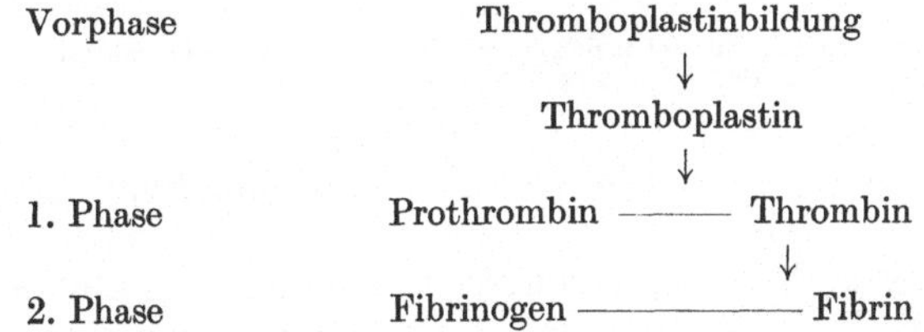

Durch kinetische Studien und Analysen an gesunden und pathologischen Individuen konnte seither vor allem die Bildung des Thromboplastins weitgehend aufgeklärt werden. Heute muß zwischen Blut-(Plasma-)Thromboplastin und Gewebe-Thromboplastin unterschieden werden. Bei der Blutthromboplastinbildung werden mehrere Zwischenprodukte erfaßt (BERGSAGEL u. HOUGIE, FISCH u. DUCKERT, BIGGS, TOCANTINS). So wirken blutstromfremder Kontakt, die Faktoren VIII, IX, X, XI, XII und Calciumionen in gegenseitiger Aktivierung zusammen zur Zwischenprodukt I-Bildung.

Tabelle 18. *Synonyma der Gerinnungsfaktoren*

Faktor	Synonyma
Faktor I	Fibrinogen
II	Prothrombin
III	Thromboplastin (Gewebethromboplastin)
IV	Calcium
V	Proaccelerin Labile factor Accelerator globulin (AcG)
(VI	Accelerin)
VII	Proconvertin Serum prothrombin conversion accelerator (SPCA) Stable factor Autothrombin I
Faktor VIII	Antihemophilic factor (AHF) Antihemophilic globulin (AHG) Thromboplastinogen Platelet cofactor I Plasma thromboplastic factor A Facteur antihémophilique A
IX	Plasma thromboplastin component (PTC) Christmas factor Platelet cofactor II Autoprothrombin II Plasma thromboplastic factor B Facteur antihémophilique B
X	Stuart-Prower factor
XI	Plasma thromboplastin antecedent (PTA)
XII	Hageman factor

Dieses wiederum bildet mit Plättchenfaktor 3 ein Zwischenprodukt II, und dieses erst wird unter dem Einfluß von Faktor V zum aktiven Blut-Thromboplastin (Schema, Abb. 38). Die Gewebe-Thromboplastinbildung durch Gewebefaktor, die Gerinnungsfaktoren V, VII, X und Calciumionen wurden von HJORT; STRAUB u. DUCKERT u. a. genauer erforscht (vgl. auch TOCANTINS) (Schema, Abb. 39a).

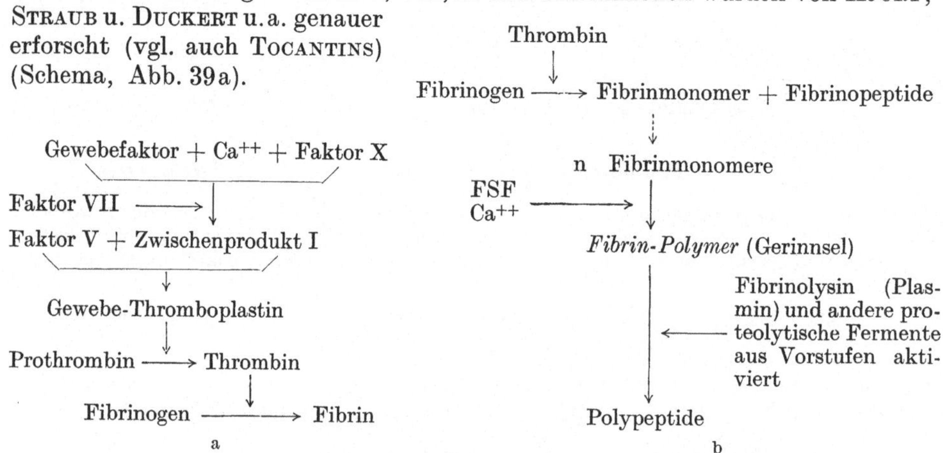

Abb. 39. a Ablauf der Gerinnung im „extrinsic system“ (Plasma- und Gewebefaktoren). b Ablauf der Fibrinbildung (gemeinsame Endphase)

Aber auch die gemeinsame Endphase, die Fibrinbildung, ist seit der Entdeckung des „fibrin stabilising factor“ durch LAKI u. LORAND und durch die Studien von LOEWY u. EDSALL, DUCKERT u. a. besser bekannt geworden (vgl. Schema, Abb. 39b). Durch Aktivierung der proteolytischen Systeme (Thrombolyse, Fibrinolyse) werden gebildete Gerinnsel oder Thrombosen wieder aufgelöst. Dieser Vorgang wird unter physiologischen Verhältnissen durch Antagonisten kontrolliert, kann aber unter pathologischen Umständen oder durch therapeutische Beeinflussung stark in den Vordergrund treten (KOLLER, SHERRY).

Erst auf Grund dieser physiologischen Vorgänge und deren Beeinflussung oder Beeinträchtigung durch pathologische Zustände oder fehlerhafte genetische Steuerung können die einzelnen Krankheitsbilder verstanden werden, die nachstehend beschrieben werden.

c) Spezielle Klinik und Genetik der einzelnen Krankheitsbilder

Die Darstellung der einzelnen hereditären Koagulopathien erfolgt nach pathogenetischen Gesichtspunkten: vgl. hierzu die Tabelle 17 und die Liste der Synonyma (Tabelle 18).

α) Afibrinogenämie (Fibrinogenmangel, Faktor I-Mangel)

Es handelt sich um eine schwere Blutungsneigung, da das Blut infolge Fehlens des Fibrinogens praktisch nicht gerinnbar ist. Nicht selten tritt schon eine fast unstillbare Nabelschnurblutung auf, und in der Folge löst eine Blutung die andere ab. Im Gegensatz zu den Hämophilien sind auch Hirnblutungen beschrieben, während MACFARLANE und auch PRENTICE ausdrücklich das Fehlen der Gelenkblutungen unterstreichen. Nur selten erreicht ein Patient das Erwachsenenalter. Aus diesen Gründen umfaßt die Literatur neben Einzelfällen (PINNINGER u. PRUNTY, GITLIN u. BORGES, FRICK u. MCQUARRIE, ALEXANDER et al., SOULIER et al., HARDISTY u. PINNINGER, MORITA u. KAGAMI, V. CREFELD u. LIEM) nur wenige familiäre Afibrinogenämien (CAUSSADE et al., HITZIG, MAUPIN et al.). Der Defekt muß auf einem Autosom lokalisiert sein. Über den Vererbungsmodus kann an Hand der wenigen Fälle noch nichts Zuverlässiges ausgesagt werden, immerhin postuliert HASSELBACK für die Hypofibrinogenämie auf Grund von fünf Fällen in zwei Generationen einen dominanten Erbgang mit variabler Penetranz.

Mehrere Autoren führten an solchen Patienten gerinnungsphysiologische Studien durch; so konnten ASTRUP und V. CREFELD normales fibrinolytisches System nachweisen und RAUSEN et al. bestimmten bei Normalpersonen wie bei Fibrinogen-Mangelpatienten die Halbwertzeit des Fibrinogens mittels J^{131}-markiertem Fibrinogen zwischen 2,8—3,6 Tagen. Dem gegenüber steht eine verkürzte Halbwertezeit bei Patienten, die zusätzlich einen transfusionsbedingten Hemmkörper gegen das wiederholt zugeführte Fibrinogen entwickelten. Bei einem 16jährigen Mädchen konnten DE VRIES et al. solche Fibrinogen-Antikörper im Präcipitintest nachweisen. Sowohl Patientenplasma bei Normalpersonen wie Normalfibrinogen bei der Patientin bewirkt intracutan gespritzt eine starke Reaktion vom Soforttypus. Klinisch standen immer stärker ausgeprägte Schocksymptome im Vordergrund, die schließlich ad exitum führten. Ähnliche Beobachtungen stammen von BRÖNNIMANN und von DE SILVA et al.

β) Prothrombinmangel (Hypoprothrombinämie, Faktor II-Mangel)

Bei den meisten der als Prothrombinmangel beschriebenen Fällen ergaben Nachkontrollen und Kreuzversuche, daß nicht eine Prothrombinverminderung, sondern ein Mangel an Faktor X (Stuart-Prower-Faktor) vorliegt. Die Fälle von V. CREFELD (1954) und QUICK (1955) sind somit als die ersten gesicherten Hypoprothrombinämien anzusehen. Nachuntersuchungen von DUCKERT zeigten eine sichere Verminderung von Faktor II auf 5—8% der Norm. Es handelt sich um ein extrem seltenes Krankheitsbild, das noch ungenügend untersucht ist. Einzelfälle werden von RADHAKISHUN, JOSSO, POOL und BORCHGREVINK beschrieben, wobei klinisch immer Hämatome, Nachblutungen, Epistaxis und auch Gelenkblutungen (POOL) als Zeichen der manifesten Blutungsneigung beschrieben werden. Obschon der Restgehalt von Prothrombin im Plasma (3—12% der Norm, je nach Fall) normal verbraucht wird, genügen die Mengen Thrombin nicht, um eine normale Hämostase zu gewährleisten. POST beschreibt eine Mutter mit drei Kindern, die alle einen tiefen Prothrombinspiegel aufweisen; Mutter und zwei Kinder neigen zu Blutungen.

γ) Faktor V-Mangel (Parahämophilie, Hypoproaccelerinämie)

Der erste Fall von kongenitalem Faktor V-Mangel wurde 1944 von OWREN in Norwegen gefunden und 1947 in einer ausführlichen Monographie beschrieben. Weitere Einzelfälle und Familienuntersuchungen ließen erkennen, daß es sich bei den manifest erkrankten Patienten um ein klinisch kaum von der Hämophilie zu unterscheidendes Bild handelt. Epistaxis, Zahnblutungen, Hämatome und Gelenkblutungen stehen im Vordergrund (SAILER, GOBBI). Gerinnungsphysiologische Untersuchungen und genetische Studien an ganzen Familien liegen ebenfalls vor: KINGSLEY, HOERDER, LEWIS und FERGUSON, FRIEDMAN et al. zeigen, daß homozygot kranke, heterozygote und normale Familienmitglieder mit Gerinnungsuntersuchungen genau erfaßt werden können. Die Heterozygoten und Normalen zeigen klinisch keine Blutungsneigung. Die zahlenmäßige Verteilung entspricht recht gut derjenigen eines autosomal-intermediären Erbganges mit Variation in Expressivität und Penetranz (BACHMANN, dort auch Literaturübersicht bis 1958). Auch bei diesem Leiden kann bei einzelnen Patienten, die häufig mit Bluttransfusionen behandelt wurden, ein Auftreten von spezifischen Hemmkörpern gegen Faktor V beobachtet werden. Solche Fälle wurden von HOERDER, von FERGUSON et al. und von MARGOLIUS et al. beschrieben.

δ) Faktor VII-Mangel (SPCA-Mangel, Hypoproconvertinämie)

1951 wurde der Faktor VII von KOLLER et al. entdeckt, charakterisiert und dessen klinische Bedeutung abgegrenzt. Im selben Jahre wurde von ALEXANDER et al. auch der erste Fall von kongenitalem Faktor VII-Mangel beschrieben. Seit 1956 wurden die bis jetzt beschriebenen Fälle neu gegen den Faktor X-Mangel abgegrenzt (RAK, MILLER). 1958 gibt BACHMANN eine vollständige Literaturübersicht und kritische Würdigung dieser Unterteilung. Ausgedehnte Familienuntersuchungen von ZOLLINGER in der Schweiz und von VOSS und WAALER in Norwegen zeigen eindeutig, daß neben den manifest erkrankten, den Patienten mit hämorrhagischer Diathese, die 0—1% des Normalgehaltes an Faktor VII aufweisen, die phänotypisch Gesunden nochmals aufgetrennt werden können. Mit Sicherheit kann man dank der exakten Bestimmungsmethode die homozygot Gesunden mit Normalgehalt von den Heterozygoten mit einem Gehalt von etwa 30—70% Faktor VII unterscheiden. Der Erbgang wird als autosomal mit intermediärer Expressivität und hoher Penetranz angegeben (DISCHE). Klinisch treten bei den manifest Kranken schon in den ersten Lebenstagen massive Haut- und Schleimhautblutungen auf, die meist in den ersten Lebensjahren ad exitum führen. Gelenkblutungen treten eher selten auf (CHOREMIS et al.). Diese Patienten haben eine sehr schlechte Prognose, da auch zugeführter Faktor VII innerhalb 1—2 Tagen wieder unter eine hämostatisch wirksame Konzentration im zirkulierenden Blut sinkt. Halbwertszeitbestimmungen ergeben ein T/2 von nur 2—4 Std (HITZIG und ZOLLINGER, CAEN et al., HOAG et al.). Weder bei den homozygot Erkrankten noch bei den Heterozygoten kann durch Vitamin K-Gabe eine Steigerung der Faktor VII-Produktion erreicht werden. Der genetisch fixierte Spiegel läßt sich nicht verändern. Dies kann vor allem in der sicheren Erkennung von Heterozygoten nützlich sein und eine Abgrenzung gegenüber den Synthesestörungen erlauben (DUCKERT). Weitere Fallberichte von CLETON und von KUPFER bestätigen diese Tatsachen.

ε) Hämophilie A (klassische Hämophilie, AHG-Mangel, Faktor VIII-Mangel)

Das Krankheitsbild der Hämophilie ist durch immer wiederkehrende Blutungen gekennzeichnet. Schon kurz nach der Geburt, spätestens bei den ersten Gehversuchen (KÜNZER), erleiden die Kinder nach geringfügigen, alltäglichen

Traumen übermäßig starke Blutungen, meistens in die Haut oder Muskulatur oder aber in die Gelenke. Bei Erwachsenen kann man feststellen, daß die Häufigkeit der Blutungsepisoden gegenüber denen der Kindheit zurückgeht. Dies beruht auf vermehrter Vorsicht durch Erfahrung und Kenntnis der Krankheit und ist nicht Folge von Besserung oder gar Ausheilung des Leidens. Trotz aller Vorsicht können sich Bluter aber selten längere Zeitspannen frei von Blutungen halten. Prognostisch sind die großen und kleinen Blutungen in Haut und Muskulatur recht gut zu bewerten, während Schleimhaut- oder Organblutungen durch den enormen Blutverlust und durch Organschäden wesentlich ernster erscheinen und einer intensiven Therapie bedürfen. Kleinchirurgische Eingriffe, ja auch geringste Verletzungen durch Schnepperstiche usw. zu diagnostischen Zwecken, sind oft Ausgangspunkte von starken Blutungen und Anlaß zu gefürchteten Nachblutungen (Abb. 14). Die Vermeidung unnötiger Verletzungen, die sorgfältige prophylaktische Behandlung von Blutentnahmestellen usw. ist gerade aus diesen Gründen von größter Bedeutung. Auch sind subcutane und intramuskuläre Injektionen soweit wie möglich zu umgehen. Ebenfalls von eminenter Bedeutung ist eine sorgfältige konservative und fortlaufende Zahnpflege zur Vermeidung der Notwendigkeit einer Zahnextraktion (Wishart et al.). Gelenkblutungen treten erstmals meist nach kleinen Traumen wie Quetschungen, Stauchungen, Prellungen oder Verstauchungen auf und rezidivieren dann „spontan" nach geringsten Gelenkbeanspruchungen. Wegen langsamem Abbau und recht hingezogener Heilung erfolgt die nächste Blutung oft schon vor der Abheilung der ersten, also noch während der Reparationsphase. So wird das einmal lädierte Gelenk immer wieder weiter geschädigt und kann nicht mehr zur Ruhe kommen. In unaufhaltbarer Entwicklung reihen sich die pathologischen Veränderungen aneinander und führen zu versteiften Gelenken in Fehlstellung und oft schmerzhafter Auftreibung. Vgl. Deutsch, Wilkinson et al., Jürgens, Nelson und Mitchell, Biggs. Durch die Blutungen können aber auch indirekte Schäden entstehen, vor allem durch Druck auf benachbarte Organe oder durch Beeinträchtigung von Hohlorganen durch die Blutmassen. Douglas beobachtet bei 10% seiner Hämophilie-Patienten druckbedingte Nervenschäden. Es handelt sich meist um periphere Lähmungen und nur in vereinzelten Fällen um cerebrale Störungen infolge Hirnblutung. Wenn die Hämophilen auch sinngemäß keine thrombotische Krankheiten erleiden, so sind sie doch gegen andere Erkrankungen keineswegs gefeit. Dies führt denn auch hin und wieder zur Notwendigkeit eines operativen Eingriffs mit der damit verbundenen großen Gefahr einer lebensbedrohlichen Blutung. Diese Probleme werden von chirurgischer und internistischer Seite ausführlich dargelegt von Macfarlane et al., Jkkala et al., Brown et al. Obschon mehrfach Notfalloperationen nach besonders geleiteter Vorbereitung gelungen sind (vgl. Handley, Fross, Bachmann et al.), so gibt Pieper 1959 in einer Übersicht die Mortalität bei operativen Eingriffen an Hämophilen mit 20% an.

Bei der klassischen Hämophilie wird gerinnungsphysiologisch ein isolierter Defekt von Faktor VIII gefunden. Entsprechend dem klinischen Schweregrad der Erkrankung können auch labormäßig ähnliche Abstufungen gefunden werden. Innerhalb einer Sippe wird bei den manifest Erkrankten sowohl klinischer Schweregrad wie auch Restgehalt an Faktor VIII in engen Grenzen konstant gefunden. Danach kann angenommen werden, daß einerseits der klinische Grad der Erkrankung direkt vom Restgehalt des Faktor VIII abhängt, und andererseits auch, daß dieser Restgehalt genetisch festgelegt ist. Brinkhaus et al. haben diese Tatsache als multiple Allelie gedeutet. Damit wurde die frühere Auffassung einer Variation der Expressivität widerlegt. Die verschiedenen Schweregrade können etwa folgendermaßen umschrieben werden (Deutsch, Jung):

Schwere Hämophilie. Faktor VIII-Gehalt unter 1% der Norm. Wiederholte schwere Blutungen führen meist zu Invalidität und oft zu Bewegungseinschränkung wegen Gelenkveränderungen. Die Schul- und Berufsausbildung ist durch die langen und häufigen Krankenlager empfindlich gestört, die Arbeitsfähigkeit meist aufgehoben (Allel h).

Intermediäre Form. Gehalt an Faktor VIII zwischen 2—6% der Norm. Durch vorsichtige Lebensweise können die Patienten Blutungsepisoden teilweise vermeiden und sind dadurch in der Regel zu einem eigenen Broterwerb befähigt (Allel hi).

Milde Form. Bei einem Gehalt an Faktor VIII zwischen 6—20% der Norm leben die Patienten ungestört. Die latente Blutungsneigung kommt aber bei kleinen Verletzungen, Zahnextraktionen oder operativen Eingriffen zum Vorschein und führt zu ungewöhnlich starken Blutungen oder oft erst zu schweren Nachblutungen (Allel h^m).

Seit langem ist bekannt, daß nur Männer an Hämophilie erkranken. Die Kinder eines Bluters sind klinisch alle gesund. Allerdings sind die Töchter als Konduktorinnen Träger des pathologischen Gens und geben dieses theoretisch an die Hälfte der männlichen Nachkommen (Bluter) und auch an die Hälfte der weiblichen Nachkommen (Konduktorinnen) weiter. Dieser Erbmodus entspricht einem recessiv geschlechtsgebundenen Erbgang (X-chromosomal). Das pathologische Gen liegt im Differentialsegment des X-Chromosoms (Koller). Infolge der Recessivität des Gens ist eine manifeste hämorrhagische Diathese nur bei homozygoten Frauen zu erwarten. Solche können nur aus einer Ehe zwischen einem Hämophilen und einer Konduktorin hervorgehen. Dieses ohne Zweifel äußerst seltene Zusammentreffen pathologischer Gene wurde jedoch schon mehrmals beobachtet und eingehend beschrieben, wobei jeweils die Vaterschaft überprüft wurde (Merskey, Merskey und MacFarlane, Pinninger und Franks, Israels et al., Choremis et al., Taylor und Biggs, Pola und Svojitka, Quick und Hussey, McGovern und Steinberg, Stefanovic). Nilsson et al. beschrieben dann 1959 bei einem 16monatigen Mädchen mit schwerer Hämophilie A, dessen Mutter Konduktorin, der Vater aber gesund war, trotz weiblichen äußeren Genitalien ein männliches chromosomales Geschlecht. Damit konnte die angebliche Ausnahme von der X-chromosomalen Vererbung erklärt werden. Seither sind aber auch chromosomal gesicherte, weibliche Hämophilie-Patienten beschrieben worden, ohne daß immer die theoretische Konstellation der Eltern gefunden wurde (Mellmann et al., Braun und Stollar, Chapelle et al.). Da trotz Blutgruppenstudien jeweils eine unbekannte Vaterschaft nicht ausgeschlossen werden konnte, erübrigen sich Diskussionen über Neumutationen.

Bei Konduktorinnen liegen ausgedehnte Untersuchungen, vor allem gerinnungsphysiologischer Art vor, die alle versuchen, den latenten Defekt nachzuweisen, also die Konduktorin eindeutig als solche zu entlarven. Mit der Verfeinerung der Bestimmungsmethoden häufen sich in den letzten Jahren die Mitteilungen, wonach bei den Konduktorinnen ein deutlich erniedrigter Faktor VIII-Spiegel festgestellt werden kann. Nilsson et al. besprechen die damals zur Verfügung stehende Literatur (1959) und fügen selber die Befunde von 27 genetisch sicheren Konduktorinnen an, von denen 24 einen Gehalt an Faktor VIII von etwa 50% der Norm aufweisen. Seither bestätigen Rapaport et al. (1960) diese Ergebnisse an Hand von 16, Bentley und Krivit an Hand von 21 untersuchten Konduktorinnen. Diese Autoren sprechen an Hand ihrer Ergebnisse von „incompletely recessive trait", Nilsson sogar von semidominantem Erbgang. Weitere Literatur bei Deutsch und Brüster.

An Hand eines Kollektivs von 267 Blutern fanden WILKINSON et al. eine Verteilung der Blutgruppen, die sehr genau derjenigen der Normalbevölkerung entspricht. Über Koppelung mit anderen geschlechtsgebundenen, recessiven oder dominanten Krankheiten oder Merkmalen ist noch wenig bekannt. Immerhin sind nach FRANÇOIS 20 Stammbäume bekannt, in welchen sich Rotgrünblindheit und Hämophilie A entweder koppeln oder repulsieren. Es werden etwa 10% crossing over geschätzt (WHITTAKER). SINISCALCO et al. berichten über die Beobachtungen in Inzuchtgebieten in Sardinien, wo die Rotgrün-Farbsehstörung eher gehäuft mit dem Favismus (Glucose-6-phosphat-dehydrogenase-Defekt) auftritt und gibt eine Repulsion von Favismus und Hämophilie an.

Eine eigentümliche Komplikation im Verlauf einer Hämophilie beschreibt 1950 DEUTSCH erstmals zusammenfassend als *Hemmkörper-Hämophilie*. Ohne erkennbare Auslösung tritt bei Hämophilie-Patienten ein zirkulierender Hemmkörper gegen den fehlenden Gerinnungsfaktor auf. Es handelt sich um Globuline, die in Mischversuchen eindeutig erfaßt und bestimmt werden können. Diese Hemmkörper neutralisieren den aus therapeutischen Gründen zugeführten, eben fehlenden Faktor oder senken den genetisch bedingten Restgehalt von Faktor VIII durch Neutralisation noch mehr. MARCHAL glaubt, daß wiederholte Transfusionen von demselben Spender einer solchen Hemmkörperbildung Vorschub leisten könnten. Oft verschwindet der Hemmkörper nach Monaten oder Jahren ebenfalls wieder spontan und ohne Beziehung zur Behandlung. Es macht jedoch den Anschein, daß wiederholte Transfusionen den Gehalt an Hemmkörper steigern oder seine Dauer verlängern könnte. Zumeist wird ein Fremdempfinden des zugeführten Faktors durch den Empfänger als pathogenetische Ursache angenommen. Eigentümlicherweise werden aber auch Hemmkörper gebildet bei Patienten, die noch einen relativ guten Restgehalt an Faktor VIII aufweisen, also bei relativ leichten Hämophilen. Hier zumindest wird diese Erklärung den Tatsachen nicht vollauf gerecht. MASURE gibt an, daß bei 26% (15 Fälle) von seinen 58 Hämophilie A-Patienten eine Hemmkörperbildung beobachtet werden konnte. Er berichtet auch über weitere 40 Fälle aus der Literatur. In neuerer Zeit beschreiben auch BIGGS und BIDWELL, HALL, EGEBERG weitere Fälle. BACHMANN et al. beschreiben einen Hämophilie A-Patienten, bei welchem infolge Magen-Darmblutungen mit anschließender erfolgreicher Operation große Mengen von Plasma und Faktor VIII-Konzentrat zugeführt werden mußten und konnten eine Hemmkörperbildung gegen menschliches, bovines und porcines antihämophiles Globulin nachweisen.

ζ) Hämophilie B (Christmas-Disease, PTC-Deficiency, Faktor IX-Mangel)

Die Hämophilie B kann nur gerinnungsphysiologisch von der Hämophilie A unterschieden werden. Demnach gelten die klinischen und genetischen Erörterungen, die letztere kennzeichnen, sinngemäß auch für die Hämophilie B. BARROW et al. konnten bei Konduktorinnen eine Verminderung des Faktos IX-Gehaltes feststellen, und COOK und DOUGLAS fanden eine Hämophilie B bei zwei Schwestern. SIMPSON und BIGGS beobachteten auch Sippen mit unterschiedlichen, aber auch familiär konstanten Restgehalt von Faktor IX und postulierten auch hier eine multiple Allelie. Die Monographie von MOOR-JANKOWSKI et al. gibt eine umfassende Beschreibung einer ausgedehnten Sippe, wobei keine Koppelung mit Farbsehstörungen oder Störungen der Geruchsempfindung gefunden werden konnte.

Auch bei der Hämophilie B wurden verschiedentlich Hemmkörper beobachtet und von O'BRIEN, LEWIS et al. (1956), GOLDSTEIN et al. ausführlich beschrieben.

BÜTLER et al. beschreiben ein familiäres Hämophilie-Syndrom, das sich gerinnungsphysiologisch wenig von der Hämophilie B unterscheidet. STOCKER et al. konnten durch Nachuntersuchungen eine Faktor IX-Aktivität feststellen. Gleichzeitig fanden sie eine pathologische Eiweißfraktion (M-Zacke) in der Elektrophorese und diskutieren die Möglichkeit einer Hemmwirkung derselben auf den Gerinnungsablauf.

η) Faktor X-Mangel (Stuart-Prower-Mangel)

1956 beschrieben Hougie und Graham einen Patienten mit neuartigem Gerinnungsdefekt, der klar vom Mangel an Faktor VII abgegrenzt werden konnte (Stuart-Fall). Gleichzeitig beschrieben Telfer et al. eine analoge Gerinnungsstörung bei einer Frau (Prower-Fall). Bachmann findet denselben Defekt auch in der Schweiz (1957) bei zwei Kindern und kann sowohl bei den beiden Eltern wie auch bei 11 der 60 untersuchten Verwandten, die alle klinisch gesund waren, gerinnungsphysiologisch eindeutig erniedrigte Faktor X-Werte nachweisen. Dies deckt sich mit den Untersuchungen von Hougie et al., die bei den fünf Kindern des Stuart-Patienten Faktor X-Werte zwischen 11% und 44% der Norm angeben. Alle diese Heterozygote sind klinisch gesund, jedoch ist der niedrige Gehalt an Faktor X genetisch so festgelegt, daß auch durch übermäßige Gaben von Vitamin K keine Mehrproduktion erreicht werden kann. Die homozygot Erkrankten leiden an einer schweren und klinisch kaum von einer Hämophilie zu unterscheidenden hämorrhagischen Diathese. Die oben genannte ausführliche Studie von Bachmann weist auf einen autosomal intermediären Erbgang hin. Seither sind von Roos et al., Hörder, Chevalier et al., Rabiner und Kretschmer noch weitere Fälle bekannt geworden, die auch durch Kreuzversuche mit den ersten Fällen gesichert werden konnten.

ϑ) Faktor XI-Mangel (Plasma Thromboplastin Antecedent Deficiency, PTA-Mangel, Hämophilie C)

1953 wurde von Rosenthal et al. an Hand von drei Patienten eine hämophilieartige hämorrhagische Diathese beschrieben und diese von den bekannten Gerinnungsstörungen abgegrenzt. Seither wurden verschiedene Fälle beschrieben (Caen, Cavins, Bistoffa), wovon wir die eingehenden Untersuchungen von Bachmann et al. an zwei schweren Fällen und die Studien von Ràk und Kovacs an zwei leicht Erkrankten besonders nennen. Es handelt sich zumeist um Patienten israelitischer Abstammung. Schon klinisch kann gegen die klassischen Hämophilien eine Abgrenzung erfolgen, da die PTA-Patienten kaum Spontanblutungen erleiden, jedoch nach Traumen oder Operationen schwere Blutungen und Nachblutungen durchmachen. Die Frauen verlieren vor allem in den jüngeren Jahren viel Blut durch Menorrhagien. Der Erbgang ist autosomal. Rapaport et al. beschrieben in acht Familien 15 manifest erkrankte Patienten und 30 sog. „minor"-Fälle mit vermindertem Gehalt an Faktor XI, klinisch jedoch normalem Bilde. Diese Autoren glauben, daß es sich bei diesen „minor"-Fällen um Heterozygote handelt und postulieren einen intermediär-recessiven Erbgang, dies im Gegensatz zu Rosenthal, der ursprünglich eine dominante Übertragung annahm. Eine vorübergehende Hemmkörperbildung beschreibt Josephson et al. bei einem PTA-Patienten.

Der Vollständigkeit halber sei hier auch noch der sog. *Hageman-Trait* (Faktor XII-Mangel) genannt, der zwar eine deutlich verlängerte Gerinnungs- und Recalcifizierungszeit bewirkt, klinisch jedoch nicht zu einer hämorrhagischen Diathese Anlaß gibt. Dieses Merkmal ist 1954 von Ratnoff entdeckt worden und dient seither vor allem zur Untersuchung der Initialphase der Blutgerinnung (weitere Literatur s. bei Loeliger und bei Soulier).

ι) FSF-Mangel (Mangel an Fibrin Stabilising Factor, Fibrinasemangel)

1960 konnten SHMERLING, JUNG und DUCKERT zwei Brüder und ein weiter verwandtes Mädchen untersuchen, welche an einer hämorrhagischen Diathese mit ausgesprochen schlechter und verzögerter Wundheilung leiden. Gerinnungsphysiologisch konnte ein solitärer Defekt der Fibrinstabilisierung gefunden werden und auf einen Mangel des von LAKI und LORAND als Fibrin stabilising factor bezeichneten Globulins zurückgeführt werden. Entsprechend der unstabilen Fibrinstruktur (Patientengerinnsel sind in 5 M Harnstoff löslich) leiden die Patienten an Nabelblutungen in der zweiten Lebenswoche, an andauernden Nachblutungen nach Verletzungen, an Zahnblutungen und verzögerter Hämatomrückbildung, jedoch nicht an sog. Spontanblutungen. BECK et al. zeigten an Hand von Zellkulturen, daß Fibroblasten im Patientenplasma angesetzt qualitativ und quantitativ schlechter wachsen. DUCKERT et al. untersuchten die Fibrinstruktur elektronenmikroskopisch und sahen bei den Patienten eine gröbere Textur des Gerinnsels und nach kurzer Harnstoffbehandlung auch einen Verlust der spezifischen Querstreifung der Fibrinfasern. Der Erbgang ist autosomal, wahrscheinlich recessiv. Einen Solitärfall beschrieb auch IKKALA.

κ) Hyperheparinämie

1956 berichten HEINI und KRAUS über eine kongenitale Vermehrung eines heparinartig wirkenden Hemmkörpers der Thrombokinasebildung und der Thrombinwirkung, dessen Wirkung durch Protaminsulfat aufgehoben werden kann. Vater und Tochter leiden seit der Kindheit an starker Blutungsneigung mit mehreren bedrohlichen Episoden. Über einen ähnlichen Fall berichten QUICK und HUSSEY 1957.

d) Kombinierte Defekte

Vasculäre Hämophilie (Angiohämophilie, Hämophiloid, Konstitutionelle Thrombopathie v. WILLEBRAND-JÜRGENS, Pseudohämophilie)

1926 beschrieb v. WILLEBRAND bei Leuten der Åland-Inseln eine dominant-autosomal vererbte hämorrhagische Diathese, die charakterisiert wird durch verlängerte Blutungszeit, schlechten Prothrombinverbrauch im Serum, positiven Rumpel-Leede-Versuch bei normaler Plättchenzahl. Zusammen mit JÜRGENS wurde 1931 eine gestörte Blutthromboplastinbildung gefunden und ein partieller Defekt an Plättchenfaktor 3 postuliert. Dies führte dann zum Namen der konstitutionellen Thrombopathie.

Klinisch und genetisch wurde von ALEXANDER und GOLDSTEIN 1953 ein sehr ähnliches Krankheitsbild, dem ein Faktor VIII-Mangel und eine gestörte Gefäßfunktion zugrunde liegt, als Angiohämophilie beschrieben. Auch die vasculäre Hämophilie, von SCHULMAN et al. angegeben, deckt sich damit weitgehend. Diese Autoren fanden als Substrat eine Veränderung der Nagelfalzcapillaren. Seither wurden von mehreren Autoren weitere Fälle beschrieben und abgeklärt. Durchwegs konnte eine Verminderung des Faktors VIII (bzw. IX) auf etwa 5—50% der Norm und eine deutlich verlängerte Blutungszeit als Charakteristikum des Gefäßdefektes gefunden werden. Die Thrombocyten waren meistens zahlenmäßig und funktionell genügend (BUCHANAN et al., BLACKBURN, LARRIEU und SOULIER, RACCUGLIA et al. 1960, PITNEY und ARNOLD, BACHMANN). Ausgedehnte Familienuntersuchungen bestätigen den autosomal-dominanten Erbgang und die Variationen in Expressivität und Penetranz (NEVANLINNA et al., MARX, CORNU et al.). Die Patienten leiden bei immer gleichbleibendem Gerinnungsdefekt an saisonabhängigen Blutungen, wobei Epistaxis, Haut-, Schleimhaut- und Muskelblutungen im Vordergrund stehen. Es handelt sich vor allem um Blutungen nach kleineren Verletzungen und subklinischen Traumen, seltener um sichere Spontanblutungen. 1957 gelang NILSSON et al. die Trennung einer Unterfraktion I—0 der üblichen Cohnschen Fraktionierung vom Fibrinogen, welche, diesen Patienten zugeführt, eine vorübergehende Besserung des Gefäßdefektes bewirkte. Auch bei Patienten der ursprünglichen Åland-Familien ist dies den Autoren gelungen (NILSSON et al.). Bei diesen Nachuntersuchungen konnte ein sicherer Plättchendefekt dieser Patienten nicht bestätigt werden.

JÜRGENS und auch ERIKSSON et al. berichten an Hand eigener Nachuntersuchungen jedoch über elektronenmikroskopische Thrombocytenstudien bei diesen Åland-Familien, die neben dem Faktor VIII-Mangel eine deutliche Veränderung der Plättchen ergaben, nämlich Anisocytose, Mikroformen, Veränderung der Granula usw. Diese Autoren und auch BRÜSTER stellen deshalb den Plättchendefekt wieder in den Vordergrund des pathogenetischen Geschehens und können teilweise auch pathophysiologisch eine gestörte Blutthromboplastinbildung nachweisen (LANDBECK).

Zusammenfassend kann gesagt werden, daß man sich über die Natur des sicher komplexen Vorganges, der zur Åland-Thrombopathie führt, noch nicht im klaren ist. Vor allem ist die Frage der Plättchenveränderung noch zu wenig untersucht und der Einfluß der Fraktion I—0 als „antibleeding factor" noch nicht vollständig gesichert. Um allen Möglichkeiten gerecht zu werden, hat QUATTRIN auch den Namen Angio-Plasma-Thrombopathie vorgeschlagen. Wahrscheinlich handelt es sich bei den Fällen der Literatur (mit Ausnahme der Åland-Fälle) um einen nahe verwandten Defekt, wenn nicht um denselben, sind doch Genetik und Klinik durchaus übereinstimmend (MARCHAL, DE VRIES).

Gefäßdefekte kombiniert mit Faktor IX-Mangel (GUGLER, LATALLO) und PTA-Mangel (FRICK) werden ebenfalls berichtet.

Sehr selten werden andere Kombinationen von kongenitalen Defekten gefunden:

Bei zwei Brüdern fanden OERI et al. einen Mangel der Faktoren V und VIII, was zu einer schweren hämorrhagischen Diathese führte. Gleiche Fälle wurden seither auch noch von IVERSEN, SEIBERT und auch von JONES mitgeteilt. Kombiniertes Fehlen der Faktoren VIII und IX (Hämophilie A und B) wurde ebenfalls beobachtet, doch sind einzelne Untersuchungen nicht mit allen nötigen Kreuzversuchen durchgeführt worden (SOULIER, HILL, VERSTRATE, SJØLIN). NOUR-ELDIN berichtet ferner über den kombinierten Mangel von Faktor VII und IX, GASTON über eine Kombination von Faktor VII- und Faktor VIII-Mangel.

e) Häufigkeit und Verteilung der hereditären Koagulopathien

Im Untersuchungsgut der gerinnungsphysiologischen Zentren stehen thrombocytäre Störungen und erworbene Blutungsneigungen an erster Stelle (DEUTSCH, WURZEL). Koagulopathien sind weit seltener, so daß WURZEL unter 3342 untersuchten Patienten nur etwa 3% mit kongenitalen Gerinnungsfaktoren findet. Unter diesen wiederum ist die Hämophilie weitaus am häufigsten, während die übrigen Koagulopathien sehr seltene Krankheiten sind. Von einzelnen Formen sind nur wenige Fälle oder Familien bekannt, von den anderen vielleicht bis 100 Fälle. Die Hämophilie ist keineswegs eine Krankheit nur der weißen Rassen, obschon weitaus die meisten Fälle in Europa und Amerika beschrieben wurden. Doch BOYLES und CURRIE, BULLOCK et al. und auch NESBITT et al. konnten typische Hämophilien bei Negern beobachten, und FELDMAN et al. beschreibt die Krankheit auch bei Bantus. Die Häufigkeit der Hämophilie wird etwas unterschiedlich mit zwei bis fünf Patienten pro 10000 Einwohner angegeben. JUNG konnte in einer Zusammenstellung bis 1959 über 1353 Fälle aus der Literatur berichten. Seither wurden uns noch weitere 798 Fälle bekannt (Thomas et al., Hoerder, Sjølin, Ikkala, Fonio, Wilkinson, Wurzel, Deutsch), so daß Ende 1961 insgesamt 2151 Hämophiliepatienten bekannt sind. Diese verteilen sich folgendermaßen:

Hämophilie-Patienten	Hämophilie A	Hämophilie B
2151 (100%)	1751 (81,4%)	400 (18,6%)

Gerinnungsstörungen werden aber nicht nur bei den Menschen, sondern auch bei Tieren gefunden. Graham et al. züchten seit 1949 einen Hundestamm mit Hämophilie A und verwenden diese Zucht zu gerinnungsphysiologischen und genetischen Studien. 1960 berichteten Mustard et al. über einen Hundestamm mit Hämophilie B und 1962 auch über einen solchen mit kongenitalem Faktor VII-Mangel. Nossel et al. berichten über eine equine Hämophilie A.

2. Erworbene Koagulopathien

Im Gegensatz zu den kongenitalen Koagulopathien, bei welchen fast immer ein Gerinnungsfaktor fehlt, beruhen die erworbenen Koagulopathien größtenteils auf Veränderungen an einer Gruppe solcher Gerinnungsfaktoren. Es handelt sich zumeist um indirekte Gerinnungsstörungen, die durch mangelhafte Bildung, beschleunigten Abbau oder Hemmung der Wirkung der gerinnungsaktiven Eiweiße oder einzelner Wirkgruppen bedingt sind.

In der *Leber* tritt eine Synthesestörung der Faktoren II, VII, IX und X mit daraus resultierenden entsprechenden Mangelzuständen auf, wenn entweder das dazu nötige Vitamin K fehlt, wenn die Synthese durch kompetitive Hemmung blockiert ist oder wenn die Leberzellen selber erkrankt und in der Leistung eingeschränkt sind.

Andererseits bewirkt *übersteigerte proteolytische Aktivität* im zirkulierenden Blut einen raschen Abbau von Fibrinogen und den Faktoren V und VIII, was ebenfalls zu deren Mangel führt. *Pathologische Hemmkörper*, die bei vorbestehenden Gerinnungsstörungen oder bei irgendeinem Grundleiden als Komplikation auftreten, greifen hemmend in den Gerinnungsvorgang ein, wodurch eine verzögerte Gerinnung und eine insuffiziente Hämostase hervorgerufen werden.

Vorerst sollen die *medikamentös bedingten erworbenen Koagulopathien* kurz besprochen werden. Allen voran an Wichtigkeit und an Häufigkeit sind hier die *Antikoagulantienblutungen* zu nennen, die auf Unregelmäßigkeiten der heute sehr verbreiteten und segensreichen Möglichkeit der Thromboseprophylaxe mit verschiedenen Antikoagulantien beruht. Zur Anwendung gelangen entweder eigentliche Hemmkörper (Heparin oder Heparinoide), die eine sofortige Wirkung haben, andererseits jedoch auch rasch wieder neutralisiert und ausgeschieden werden, oder die *Cumarin*-Präparate, die sich vor allem für die Dauerbehandlung eignen. Letztere wirken indirekt, nämlich durch kompetitive Hemmung der Synthese in den Leberzellen, wobei Vitamin K nicht mehr verwendet werden kann. Bei vorsichtiger Dosierung und laufenden Kontrollen kann damit eine Hypokoagubilität eingehalten werden, die einerseits noch nicht zu Blutungen führt, andererseits jedoch die Möglichkeit der intravasalen Gerinnung und Thrombosierung weitgehend ausschließt. Trotz guter Kontrollen und sachgerechter Dosierung werden in 3—6% der so behandelten Patienten Blutungen, meist harmloser Art, hervorgerufen (Venho, Koller). Es sind dies Hämaturien, Hautblutungen, Epistaxis, Hämatome an Injektionsstellen, Hämatemesis, Melaena usw., wobei diese Reihenfolge auch der Häufigkeit entspricht (Jakob). Durch sorgfältige Einstellung und Kontrolle können solche Blutungen weitgehend vermieden oder doch rasch wieder behoben werden. Über Detailfragen verweisen wir auf die Fachliteratur: KOLLER, BIGGS, THIES und OERI, ZUKSCHWERDT und THIES. Es werden aber auch immer wieder *Vergiftungen* durch massive Überdosierung (evtl. in suicidaler Absicht) solcher Antikoagulantien beschrieben (GERTENBACH, GROSS). Diese haben neben dem relativen Späteffekt der Blutungsneigung eine eigentlich *toxische Wirkung*, welche teils letal sein kann. Die entsprechende Literatur und experimentelle Studien sind bei VENHO angegeben. Diese primär-toxische Wirkung kann auch durch Vitamin K nicht beeinflußt werden. Eine weitere, evtl. durch *lokal-hyperergische Vorgänge* eingeleitete Komplikation besteht aus cutan-subcutanen, umschriebenen Nekrosen, die zumeist am 3.—5. Tag der Behandlung mit Cumarinen auftritt, obschon die Gerinnungsfähigkeit im Quick-Test noch im optimalen Bereich liegt (STÖCKLI, LEYPOLD et al., FRIES, STEFANELLI et al.). BEAMICH et al. beschrieben sieben Fälle von akutem Ileus infolge solcher, teils hämorrhagischer, teils auch nekrotischer Veränderungen der Darmwand. Außer diesen unerwünschten Nebenwirkungen und Komplikationen steht einer Antikoagulantienbehandlung wenig im Wege.

Als *Kontraindikationen* gelten Blutungsneigungen jeder Genese, maligner Hochdruck und schwere Leberaffektionen. Unter letztere muß auch die übermäßige Belastung der Leber durch Alkoholexzesse und durch Vergiftungen gerechnet werden.

Einige Medikamente können durch eine *unerwünschte Wechselwirkung* eine solche Antikoagulantientherapie stören. So beschrieb SIGG et al. eine Verzögerung der Cumarin-Ausscheidung durch Butazolidin, weshalb eine gleichzeitige Behandlung mit diesen beiden Prinzipien vermieden werden sollte. Aber auch Salicylate und Barbiturate haben, wenn auch in geringerem Ausmaße, eine ähnliche Wirkung. Ebenfalls bei den neuen Medikamenten, die den Cholesterinspiegel im Blut senken, konnte OWEN eine Beeinflussung der Antikoagulantieneinstellung bzw. einen Spareffekt beobachten. Eher bekannt sind die akuten hämorrhagischen Episoden nach Propylthiouracil-Behandlung der Hyperthyreosen, welche auch auf einem Prothrombinmangel basieren (GREENSTEIN et al., D'ANGELO et al.).

Neben diesen therapeutischen Prothrombinmangelzuständen kann es aus mehrfacher Ursache auch im *Verlauf einer Allgemeinerkrankung* zu entsprechender Symptomatik kommen. Die mangelnde Synthese durch die Leber wird dann nicht durch Synthesehemmung, sondern durch *Fehlen des nötigen Vitamin K* ausgelöst (SCHIMKE, KORSAN-BENGTSEN, GROSS, LASCH). Solche *Blutungen als Begleiterscheinungen von Allgemeinerkrankungen* sind durch *schlechte Fettresorption* im Darm bedingt, da dann auch eine ungenügende Vitamin K-Aufnahme vorliegt, wie bei *Sprue, Sprue-Syndrom* (MOORE), *Cöliakie* oder bei einer richtigen *K-Avitaminose* durch einseitige, fettarme Ernährung. Solche können allerdings auch bei stark gestörter oder *fehlender Darmflora* auftreten, da erst die präresorptive Aufspaltung des Vitamins eine Passage ermöglicht. Solches kann bei *langdauernder Antibioticatherapie* auftreten.

Eine Sonderstellung nimmt hier der *Morbus haemorrhagicus neonatorum* ein, der ebenfalls auf mangelhafter Lebersynthese der Gerinnungsfaktoren beruht. Bei der termingerechten Geburt besteht eine physiologische, mäßige Erniedrigung der in der Leber unter Verwertung von Vitamin K synthetisierten Gerinnungsfaktoren, ohne daß es aber zu einer Blutung kommen sollte (Schema, Abb. 40). Nach FANCONI und WALLGREN treten nur bei 0,5% der ausgewachsenen Neugeborenen während der ersten 3—5 Tage Melaena oder andere Blutungen auf. Wesentlich stärker gestört erweist sich die Synthese jedoch bei den Frühgeborenen, die denn auch in weit höherem Prozentsatz Blutungen aufweisen (v. CREVELD). Ausgedehnte Untersuchungen zeigten, daß Gaben von fettlöslichen Vitamin K-

Präparaten bei Mutter und Kind eine wirksame Prophylaxe dieser in seltenen Fällen tödlichen Komplikationen darstellt. Andererseits zeigte WILLI und auch VEST, daß die synthetischen, wasserlöslichen Präparate weniger wirksam sind und zudem zu toxischen Reaktionen führen (Innenkörperanämie, Ikterus usw.).

Gleichfalls als schwerwiegende Begleiterscheinung von allgemeinen Erkrankungen muß eine meist zeitlich begrenzte, pathologisch *gesteigerte Aktivität der proteolytischen Fermentsysteme* im Blute aufgefaßt werden. Diese werden durch Ausschwemmung von Fibrinolysinen und Aktivatoren derselben in Gang gesetzt und führen neben der *Fibrin-(Thrombus-)Auflösung* auch zur *proteolytischen Aufspaltung* und damit *Inaktivierung der Gerinnungsfaktoren Fibrinogen, Faktor V und VIII* sowie teilweise von *Prothrombin* und von *Serumkomplement* (JUNG). Solche Episoden führen zu einer akuten Blutungsgefahr infolge der Defibrinierung. Oft ist noch eine gewisse intravasale Gerinnung dabei oder vorangegangen, die durch gewebsaktive Stoffe ausgelöst wurde.

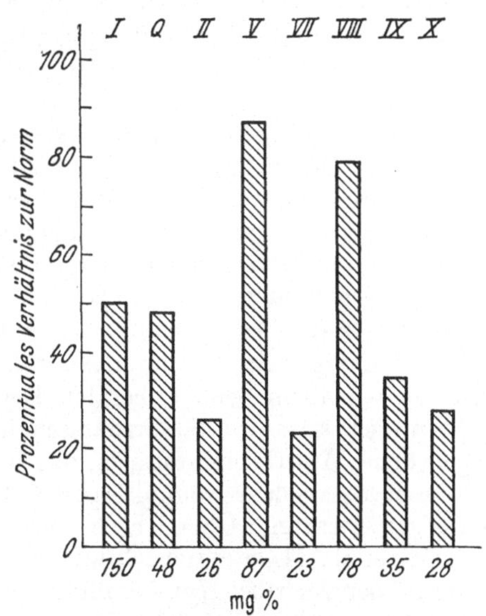

Abb. 40. Gerinnungsfaktoren im Nabelschnurblut von Neugeborenen. Mittlere Werte Quick (*Q*) und Gerinnungsfaktoren (*I—X*) bei 36 gesunden Neugeborenen (Blut aus der Nabelschnur). [Aus E. G. JUNG: A rapid quantitative assay of Factor VIII without the use of hemophilia A plasma. Thrombos. Diathes. haemorrh. (Stuttg.) 4, 323 (1960)]

Recht bekannt ist dieser Vorgang bei *metastasierenden Malignomen*, vor allem bei solchen der Prostata (COTTIER et al., STEFAN, BREDT), bei Melanomalignomen (LOELIGER), bei verschiedenen Leukosen (ZOLLINGER und HITZIG, SCHREIBER), bei Cystinspeicherkrankheit (BURGSTEDT und MARX), aber auch bei anderen Malignomen (WALTHER) und bei *Lebercirrhosen* (ausgedehnte Übersichten bei SHERRY et al.). Das Defibrinierungs-Syndrom durch intravasale Gerinnung und anschließende Steigerung der Proteolyse wird in der Frauenheilkunde nicht selten beobachtet, und zwar im Anschluß an die *Lösung der normal sitzenden Placenta*, wenn es zu Blutungen und Nekrosen kommt (Utero-placentare Apoplexie). Durch Ausschwemmung von Placentarteilen werden sowohl Gewebefaktor zur intravasalen Gerinnung wie auch Aktivatoren der Fibrinolyse in großen Mengen frei und leiten die pathologischen Phänomene ein. Solche Zwischenfälle können auch als Folge von Fruchtwasserembolien (amniotic fluid embolism) oder von intrauterinem Fruchttod (retention of dead fetus) auftreten und zu schweren, kaum stillbaren Blutungen führen. Für Einzelheiten sei auf die betreffende Fachliteratur verwiesen (HELD, STAMM, SHERRY et al., SCHNEIDER, WRIGHT et al., SCOTT, REGAN).

Ebenfalls zu solchen induzierten proteolytischen Zwischenfällen kommt es im Anschluß an *Streptokokkeninfekte*, wobei dem klinischen Bild der *Purpura fulminans* experimentell das Shwartzman-Sanarelli-Phänomen entspricht. Klinisch kann dabei in den wenigen Fällen, die überlebten, eine vorübergehende Senkung der Gerinnungsfaktoren I, V, VIII und ein Anstieg des aus dem Fibrinogenabbau entstehenden Antithrombin VI beobachtet werden (s. Abschnitt III.1b).

Eine weitere vorübergehende Komplikation bei verschiedenen Krankheitsbildern, die *Hemmkörperbildung*, führt zu akuten Blutungsepisoden. Bei den kongenitalen Blutungsübeln kann eine solche das Grundleiden noch verstärken (s. auch kongenitale Koagulopathien). Bei Allgemeinerkrankungen können solche Hemmkörper als Ausdruck einer weit gefaßten *Autoimmunisierung* in die Reihe der anderen gleichgesinnten Reaktionen eingereiht werden. Gerinnungsphysiologisch sind eigentliche Antithrombine von den Hemmkörpern gegen einzelne Gerinnungsfaktoren und von solchen gegen die gebildeten Zwischenprodukte zu unterscheiden.

Heparinartige Antikoagulantien (Antithrombine) beobachtete MASURE in 58% der schweren Leberzellschäden. Vereinzelte Beobachtungen wurden auch gemacht bei primär chronischer Polyarthritis (LOELIGER und HERS), bei Myelomen (EYGONNET), bei Schwangerschaftskomplikationen (BAKER et al., KLEINMANS) und nach ausgedehnten Bestrahlungen (ALLEN et al., STENDER, SISE).

In letzter Zeit wurden von BRAUN-FALCO et al. und von LANDBECK mehrere Fälle von diffusen Haut-Mastocytosen untersucht. Dabei konnten diese Autoren eine leichte Vermehrung von zirkulierendem, heparinähnlichem Antikoagulans feststellen. Durch Frottieren der Haut und auch durch eine Probeexcision (VILANOVA) wurde einerseits ein urticarieller Dermographismus mit Blasenbildung und andererseits eine starke Vermehrung des Antikoagulans induziert. Daneben kann auch eine verstärkte Ausscheidung von 5-oxy-Indolessigsäure im Urin (Serotonin-Metabolit) gefunden werden. Die Autoren diskutieren den Zusammenhang von Mastocytose und Vermehrung von Heparin und Serotonin.

Hemmkörper der Gerinnungsvorphase und der gebildeten Zwischenprodukte wurden vor allem beim visceralen Erythematodes immer wieder gefunden und führen nicht selten zu hämorrhagischen Komplikationen. Es handelt sich um ein eigentliches Antithromboplastin, das bei der Hemmung Komplement verbraucht (JUNG et al.). Solche Hemmkörper sind bei etwa 10% der akuten Erythematodes-Fälle zu erwarten (Übersichten über Literatur und Kasuistik finden sich bei CONLEY et al., MARGOLIUS, GOBBI, FRICK, LOELIGER et al. 1959, RAPAPORT et al. 1960). Aber auch bei Hyperglobulinämien konnten LÜSCHER und LABHART sowie LAURELL und NILSSON solche Hemmkörper finden, wobei letztere Autoren elektrophoretisch dieses Antikoagulans in derselben Fraktion wie die Wassermann-Reagine der unspezifisch positiven Wa.R. fanden. Weiter können entsprechende Antikoagulantien bei vereinzelten Fällen von Myelomen (FRICK), Makroglobulinämien, Pancytopenien, hämolytischen Anämien, Sepsis lenta (MASURE) und bei verschiedenen Dermatosen gefunden werden. So fanden QUICK et al., DIETER, BENTHAUS, KLINGMÜLLER, GASSER, BJÖRNBERG bei Pemphigus vulgaris und BJÖRNBERG auch beim Senear-Usher solche Hemmkörper, während TZANCK et al. und PAVLOWSKY entsprechende Beobachtungen bei Dermatitis herpetiformis Duhring machten.

Literatur

ABLARD, G., et A. LARCAN: Erythèmes et purpuras au cours de la maladie rhumatismale de l'adulte. Presse méd. **64**, 1970 (1956). — ACHENBACH, W.: Über die hämorrhagische Diathese bei Paraproteinämien. Schweiz. med. Wschr. **90**, 1491 (1960). — ACHENBACH, W., u. KANZOW: Zur hämorrhagischen Diathese bei der Makroglobulinämie Waldenström. 5. Kongr. Europ. Ges. Hämat. 1956, S. 631. — ACHENBACH, W., u. U. RYSSEL: Phasenoptische Thrombocytenstudien während der Gerinnung in vitro. Med. Welt **1962**, Nr 17, 947. — ACKROYD, J. F.: The pathogenesis of thrombocytopenic purpura due to hypersensitivity to sedormid. Clin. Sci. **7**, 249 (1948); **8**, 235, 269 (1949). — Sedormid purpura, an immunological study in form of drug sensitivity. In: P. KALLOS, Progress in allergy, vol. III, S. 531. Basel: S. Karger 1952. — Allergic purpura, including purpura due to food, drugs and infection. Amer. J. Med. **14**, 605 (1953). — Thrombocytopenic purpura due to hypersensitivity to the antihistaminic drug antazone. Sang **26**, 115 (1955). — Sensitivity reactions due to drugs. Oxford: Rosenheim & Moulton 1958. — The immunological basis of purpura due to drug hypersensitivity. Proc. roy. Soc. Med. **55** (1), 30 (1962). — ADAM, W.: Anticoagulantien. In: Klinik und Therapie der Nebenwirkungen von KÜMMERLE u.a. Stuttgart: Georg Thieme 1960. — ADELSON, E., J. J. RHEINGOLD and W. H. CROSBY: Studies of platelet survival by tagging in vivo with P^{32}. J. Lab. clin. Med. **50**, 570 (1957). — AGLE, D. P., and D. O. RATNOFF: Purpura as psychosomatic entity. Arch. intern. Med. **109**, 685 (1962). — ALBERTINI, A. v.: Zur Morphologie der terminalen Strombahn im Granulationsgewebe. Schweiz. Z. allg. Path. **22**, 285 (1959). — ALBERTINI, A. v., u. A. GRUMBACH: Ergebnisse experimenteller Forschung zur Frage der Herdinfektion. Schweiz. med. Wschr. **1938**, 1308. — ALBRECHT, M.: Studien zur Thrombocytenbildung an Megakaryocyten in menschlichen Knochenmarkkulturen. Acta haemat. (Basel) **17**, 160 (1957). — ALDRICH, R. A., A. G. STEINBERG and D. C. CAMPBELL: Pedigree demonstrating a sex-linked recessive condition characterized by draining ears, eczematoid dermatitis and bloody diarrhea. Pediatrics **13**, 133 (1954). — ALECHINSKY, A.: A propos de l'allergie vasculaire. Acta derm.-venereol. (Stockh.) Proc. 11th. Intern. Congr. Derm. 1957, vol. II, p. 191. — Allergie vasculaire et système nerveux. Arch. belges Derm. **14**, 170 (1958). — ALEXANDER, B., and R. GOLDSTEIN: Dual hemostatic defect in pseudohemophilia. J. clin. Invest. **32**, 551 (1953). — ALEXANDER, B., R. GOLDSTEIN, G. LANDWEHR and D. D. COOK: Congenital SPCA deficiency. J. clin. Invest. **30**, 596 (1951). — ALEXANDER, B., R. GOLDSTEIN, L. RICH, A. G. LE BOLLOCH, L. K. DIAMOND and W. BORGES: Congenital afibrinogenemia. A study of some basic aspects of coagulation. Blood **9**, 843 (1954). — ALEXANDER, H. L., and C. H. EYERMANN: Allergic purpura. J. Amer. med. Ass. **92**, 2092 (1929). — ALEXANDER, M., u. J. GRELL: Klinische Beobachtungen und tierexperimentelle Untersuchungen zur sog. Margarinekrankheit. Med. Klin. **58**, 1550 (1963). — ALLEGRA, F.: Porpore disproteinemiche. Minerva derm. **34**, 69 (1959). — Zwei Krankheitsfälle mit Kryoglobulinämie. Arch. klin. exp. Derm. **217**, 363 (1963). — ALLEN, J. G., P. E. MOULDER and D. M. ENERSON: Pathogenesis and treatment of postirradiation syndrome. J. Amer. med. Ass. **145**, 704 (1951). — ANDERSON, A. B.: Anaphylactoid purpura following i.m. penicillin therapy. Med. J. Aust. **34**, 305 (1947). — ANDERSON, P. C., and J. H. HECKAMAN: Erythema, hypersensitivity and vasculitis. Amer. Practit. **13**, 285 (1962). — ANDREW, R.: Epidemic haemorrhagic fever. Brit. med. J. **1953I**, 1053. — ANTES, E. H.: Purpura thrombocytopénique thrombosant. Ann. intern. Med. **48**, 512 (1958). — ANTOPOL, W., and C. CHRYSSANTHOU: Potentiation of the local Shwartzman phenomenon by trypsin. Proc. Soc. exp. Biol. (N.Y.) **103**, 25 (1960). — APPLEMANS, M.: L'angiomatose de la rétine chez l'enfant. Arch. ophtal. (Paris), N. s. **7** (5), 489 (1947). — ARKIN, A.: A clinical and pathological study of periarteritis nodosa. Amer. J. Path. **6**, 401 (1930). — ARNDT, G.: Purpura annularis. 7e. Intern. Congr. Derm. Rom 1912. — Purpura annularis teleangiectodes. Derm. Z. 14. Zit. MEIROWSKY in JADASSOHNs Handbuch der Haut- und Geschlechtskrankheiten, Bd. IV/2. Berlin: Springer 1935. — ARRIGHI, F.: Purpura bulleux et nécrotique provoqué par l'aspirine. Bull. Soc. franç. Derm. Syph. **62**, 447 (1955). — ASCENZI, A., F. FABIANI e L. LUCENTINI: Studio anatomopatologico di un caso di macroglobulinemia di Waldenström. Haematologica **42**, 153 (1957). — ASTRUP, T., and S. VAN CREVELD: Normal fibrinolytic system in blood in congenital afibrinogenemia and its significance. Thrombos Diathes. haemorrh. (Stuttg.) **6**, 188 (1961). — ASTRUP, T., and P. OLLENDORF: Estimation of thromboplastin activation in plasma. Scand. J. clin. Lab. Invest. **13**, 377 (1961).

BAAR, H., u. E. STRANSKY: Klinische Hämatologie des Kindesalters. Leipzig u. Wien: F. Deuticke 1928. — BACHMANN, F.: Familienuntersuchungen beim kongenitalen Stuart-Prower-Faktormangel. Arch. Klaus-Stift. Vererb.-Forsch. **33**, 1 (1958). — Vasculäre Hämophilie und Thrombopathie v. Willebrand-Jürgens. Schweiz. med. Wschr. **89**, 1036 (1959). — BACHMANN, F., E. BECK, A. AKOVBIANTZ u. F. DUCKERT: Richtlinien für die Operation bei schwerer Haemophilie A. Die Verwendung von tierischem AHG. (Faktor VIII.) Dtsch. med. Wschr. **87**, 1527 (1962). — BACHMANN, F., F. DUCKERT, U. FISCH, F. STREULI, D. GERBER u. F. KOLLER: Der Gerinnungsdefekt beim kongenitalen PTA-Mangel. Schweiz. med. Wschr. **88**, 1037 (1958). — BACHMANN, F., F. DUCKERT, P. FLÜCKIGER u. W. H. HITZIG: Hämorrhagische Diathesen, verursacht durch Mangel des Stuart-Prower-Faktors. Schweiz. med. Wschr. **87**, 1221 (1957). — BAEHR, G., P. KLEMPERER and A. SCHIFRIN: An acute febrile anemia and thrombocytopenic purpura with diffuse platelet thromboses of capillaries and arterioles. Trans. Ass. Amer. Phycns **51**, 43 (1936). — BAERMANN, G.: Über Chinin-Tod. Münch. med. Wschr. **56**, 2319 (1909). — BAGRATUNI, L.: The incidence of cryoglobulinaemia as determined by a turbidimetric method. J. clin. Path. **15**, 569 (1962). — BAKER, H. D., E. A. PARMER and J. A. WOLFF: Roentgen manifestation of the Aldrich syndrome. Amer. J. Roentgenol. **88**, 458 (1962). — BAKER, S. J., and E. JAKOB: A hemorrhagic disorder in pregnancy due to an anticoagulant preventing the conversion of fibrinogen to fibrin. J. clin. Path. **13**, 214 (1960). — BALF, CHS.: Anaphylactoid purpura. Med. Press Nr 6023, 338 (1954). — BALLERINI, G.: Il morbo di Werlhof. Minerva med. **52**, 3095 (1961). — BANDMANN, H. J.: Wiskott-Aldrich-Syndrom. In JADASSOHNs Handbuch der Haut- und Geschlechtskrankheiten, Erg.-Bd. II/1. Berlin-Göttingen-Heidelberg: Springer 1962. —

Barbero, G. J., S. Katz, H. Kraus and Sh. Leedham: Clinical and laboratory study of 31 patients with hemorrhagic fever. Arch. intern. Med. **91**, 177 (1953). — Bargmann, W.: Über die Struktur der Kapillaren. Dtsch. med. Wschr. **83**, 1704 (1958). — Barrow, E. M., W. R. Bullock and J. B. Graham: A study of the carrier state for PTC-deficiency, utilizing a new assay procedure. J. Lab. clin. Med. **6**, 936 (1960). — Barski, G., Z. Chlap, T. Gotlieb and M. Charlier: Neoplasms and haemorrhagic disease induced in adult hamster with polyoma virus. Nature (Lond.) **193**, No 4812, 298 (1962). — Barthelme, F. L.: Allergic purpura (Schönlein-Henoch). J. Allergy **1**, 170 (1929). — Bartley, C. A. D., and A. D. C. Bell: The allergic basis of primary purpura in children. Lancet **1936 II**, 231, 359. — Bateman, T.: Delineation of cutaneous diseases. London 1817, 1836. Zit. Shuster u.a. 1961. — Bauch, S.: Three cases of purpura hemorrhagica in chronic tuberculosis. Arch. intern. Med. **17**, 444 (1916). — Baumgartner, W.: Klinische Demonstrationen (thrombozythämische Purpura). Helv. med. Acta **23**, 311 (1956). — Zur Hämotherapie hämorrhagischer Krankheiten. Ther. Umsch. **17**, 90 (1960). — Bayrd, E. D.: Continuous chlorambucil therapy in primary macroglobulinaemia of Waldenström. Report of 4 cases. Proc. Mayo Clin. **36**, 135 (1961). — Bazex, A., et A. Dupré: Dyskératose congénitale (type Zinsser-Cole-Engman) associée à une myélopathie constitutionnelle (Purpura thrombopénique et neutropénie). Ann. franç. Derm. **1957**, 497. — Beamish, R. E., and N. D. McCreath: Intestinal obstruction complicating anticoagulant therapy. Lancet **1961 II**, 390. — Bechelli, L. M., L. Batista and F. L. Alayon: Observations on various cases of hemosiderosis (progressive pigmentary dermatosis, purpura annularis telangiectodes and pigmented purpuric lichenoid dermatitis. Arch. argent. Derm. **2**, 281 (1952). — Beck, E., F. Bachmann, J. Müller and F. Duckert: Formation of an inhibitor against Factor VIII as a postoperative complication in a severe case of hemophilia A. Thrombos. Diathes. haemorrh. (Stuttg.) **7**, 27 (1962). — Beck, E., F. Duckert and M. Ernst: The influence of fibrin stabilizing factor on the growth of fibroblasts in vitro and wound healing. Thrombos. Diathes. haemorrh. (Stuttg.) **6**, 485 (1961). —Beiglböck, W.: Ein Fall von thrombopenischer Purpura bei echter Chininüberempfindlichkeit. Z. klin. Med. **131**, 308 (1937). — Beis, L.: The novocain method of counting thrombocytes in premature babies, in new-borns and in young children. Diss. Basel 1960. — Belisario, J. C.: Cutaneous manifestations in polyarteritis (periarteritis) nodosa. Report of 1 case with livedo reticularis. Arch. Derm. **82**, 526 (1960). — Beller, F. K.: Fibrinogeninfusionen als allgemein hämostatisches Prinzip bei schweren Blutungen. Medizinische **25**, 1198 (1959). — Benacerraf, B., and E. A. Kabat: A quantitative study of the Arthus phenomenon induced passively in the guinea pig. J. Immunol. **64**, 1 (1950). — Bender, F., u. U. Gerlach: Zur Kenntnis der Purpura hyperglobulinaemica. Hautarzt **6**, 456 (1955). — Benhamou, E.: L'utilisation thérapeutique des plaquettes sanguines. Rev. Prat. (Paris) **9**, 2101 (1959). — Benhamou, E., et A. Nouchy: Les plaquettes sanguines chez le nouveau-né. C. R. Soc. Biol. (Paris) **107**, 171 (1931). — Benkö, S., and T. Tiboldi: The pathoproteinaemias. Acta med. Acad. Sci. hung. **17**, 224 (1961). — Benthaus, J.: Über die Retraktion des Blutgerinnsels. Thrombos. Diathes. haemorrh. (Stuttg.) **3**, 311 (1959). — Benthaus, J., u. W. C. Richter: Zum Krankheitsbilde der Hemmkörperhämophilie. Dtsch. Arch. klin. Med. **203**, 1 (1956). — Bentley, P., and W. Krivit: An assay of antihemophilic globulin activity in the carrier female. J. Lab. clin. Med. **4**, 613 (1960). — Beretta, Anguissola, A., e V. Prato: Trombocitosi ereditaria (prima osservazione). Minerva med. **52**, No 103, 4545 (1961). — Bergqvist, G., I. Hessén and M. Hey: Arteriovenous pulmonary aneurysms in Osler's disease. Telangiectasia hereditaria haem. Report of 4 cases in the same family. Acta med. scand. **171**, 301 (1962). — Bergqvist, G., and A. Nilzén: The thrombocyte index after injection of staphylococcous vaccine in man. Acta derm. venereol. (Stockh.) **40**, 58 (1960). — Bergsagel, D. E., and C. Hougie: Intermediate stages in the formation of blood thromboplastin. Brit. J. Haemat. **2**, 113 (1956). — Berkson, D. M., L. Perlman and I. J. Miller: Fulminating meningococcemia (Waterhouse-Friderichsen syndrome). J. Amer. med. Ass. **170**, 1387 (1959). — Bernard, J.: Le syndrôme de Schönlein-Henoch. Rev. Hémat. **12**, 3 (1957). — Thrombopénie. Caractères généraux. Rev. Prat. (Paris) **9**, 2061 (1959a). — Traitement des purpuras thrombopéniques idiopathiques. Sem. Hôp. Paris **34**, 28/6 (1959b). — Etat actuel du traitement des purpuras thrombopéniques idiopathiques. Algérie méd. **63**, 13 (1959c). — Le phénomène de Sanarelli-Shwartzman. Rev. franç. Allerg. **3**, 17 (1963). — Bernard, J., J. L. Beaumont et J. Caen: Le traitement des purpuras thrombopéniques idiopathiques par la cortisone et l'ACTH. J. thér. Paris **1956a**, 229. — Indications actuelles de l'hormonothérapie et de la splénectomie dans le traitement des purpuras thrombopéniques idiopathiques. Sang **27**, 882 (1956b). — Bernard, J., M. Bessis, M. Seligmann, J. Chassigneux et J. Chomé: Un cas de maladie de Chediak-Steinbrinck-Higashi. Presse méd. **1960 I**, 15, 68. — Bernard, J., P. Boivin et J. Caen: Les cytopénies hypoplastiques congénitales dissociées. Sem. Hôp. Paris **1956a**, 1597. — Les cytopénies hypoplastiques congénitales dissociées. Purpura thrombopénique congénital avec mégacaryocytopénie. Sem. Hôp. Paris **1956b**, 1597. — Bernard, J., et J. Caen: Purpura thrombopénique et mégacariocytopénie cycliques mensuels. Rev. franç. hémat. **2**, 378 (1962). — BERNARD, J., J. CAEN et P. MAROTEAUX: La dystrophie thrombocytaire hémorragipare congénitale. Rev. Hémat. **12**, 222 (1957). — BERNARD, J., M. J. LARRIEU, J. CAEN et P. MAROTEAUX: Maladies hémorrhagiques familiales associant un allongement du temps de saignement à un déficit en facteur prothromboplastique plasmatique. Haematologica **42**, 7 (1957). — BERNARD, J., G. MATHÉ et L. ISRAEL: Etudes cliniques et biologiques du syndrome Schönlein-Henoch. Presse méd. **65**, 759 (1957). — BERNARD, J., G. MATHÉ et J. TOULOUSE: Conditions étiologiques et évolution des thrombopénies idiopathiques. Sang **27**, 907 (1956). — BERNARD, J., et A. NENNA: Le purpura thrombopénique aigu avec bulles sanglantes buccales et hématuries. Sem. Hôp. Paris **1953**, 3422. — BERNARDT, W., et R. LEPLUS: La méthode des coupes ultrafines et son application à l'étude de l'ultrastructure des cellules sanguines. Schweiz. med. Wschr. **85**, 897 (1955). — BERNEAUD-KÖTZ, G., u. A. NOVER: Klinische und experimentelle Beobachtungen über Augenveränderungen bei der Makroglobulinämie Waldenström. Klin. Wschr. **35**, 472 (1957). — Zur Wirkung von Cortison und Roßkastanienextrakten auf eine experimentell ausgelöste Blutungsbereitschaft. Thrombos. Diathes. haemorrh. (Stuttg.) **3**, 428 (1959). — BERNSTOCK, L., and C. HIRSON: Thrombotic thrombocytopenic purpura. Remission on treatment with heparin. Lancet **1960I**, 28. — BERTHOUD, E., G. FALLET et J. J. SCHEIDEGGER: Le purpura hyperglobulinémique de Waldenström. Sem. Hôp. Paris **1956**, 2135. — BETTEX-GALLAND, M., and E. F. LÜSCHER: Extraction of an actomyosin-like protein from human thrombocytes. Nature (Lond.) **184**, 276 (1959). — Studies on the metabolism of human blood platelets in relation to clot retraction. Thrombos. Diathes. haemorrh. (Stuttg.) **4**, 178 (1960). — Thrombosthenin, a contractile protein from thrombocytes, its extraction from human blood platelets and some of its properties. Biochim. biophys. Acta (Amst.) **49**, 536 (1961). — BETTEX-GALLAND, M., H. PORTZEHL and E. F. LÜSCHER: Dissociation of thrombosthenin into 2 components comparable with actin and myosin. Nature (Lond.) **193**, 777 (1962). — BETTMANN, S.: Zur atmosphärischen Beeinflussung der Hautgefäße. Münch. med. Wschr. **1930**, 2003. — BICKEL, G., et S. DICKER: Considération sur le purpura hémorrhagique des basédowiens. Schweiz. med. Wschr. **1942**, 411. — BIGELOW, F. S.: Serotonin activity in blood, measurements in normal subjects and in patients with thrombocythemia haemorrhagica and other hemorrhagic states. J. Lab. clin. Med. **43**, 759 (1954). — BIGELOW, F. S., and J. F. DESFORGES: Platelet agglutination by an abnormal plasma factor in thrombocytopenic purpura associated with quinidine ingestion. Amer. J. med. Sci. **224**, 274 (1951). — BIGGS, R., and E. BIDWELL: A method for the study of antihaemophilic globulin inhibitors with reference to 6 cases. Brit. J. Haemat. **5**, 379 (1959). — BIGGS, R., E. BIDWELL, D. A. HANDLEY, R. G. MACFARLANE, J. TRUSTA, A. ELLIOT-SMITH, G. W. R. DIKE and B. J. ACH: The preparation and assay of a Christmas factor concentrate and its use in the treatment of 2 patients. Brit. J. Haemat. **7**, 349 (1961). — BIGGS, R., and R. G. MACFARLANE: Human blood coagulation and its disorders. Oxford: Blackwell Scientific Publ. 1957 und 1962. — Hemophilia and related conditions. A survey of 187 cases. Brit. J. Haemat. **4**, 1 (1958). — BIGLIARDI, P., G. QUADBECK u. H. WEICKER: Vergleichende Untersuchungen über den Thrombocytensteigernden Effekt von BAL (2,3-Dimercaptopropanol) und N-Acetyl-Cysteamin. Klin. Wschr. **1952**, H. 23/24, 567. — BILLO, O. E., and J. A. WOLFF: Thrombocytopenic purpura due to cat-scratch-disease. J. Amer. med. Ass. **174**, 1824 (1960). — BINAZZI, M., e A. F. FINZI: Eczematid-like purpura. G. ital. Derm. **99** (2) (1958). — BINSWANGER, D., F. SCHAUB u. W. SCHEITLIN: Zur hämorrhagischen Diathese bei extremer Vermehrung der Thrombozyten. Acta haemat. (Basel) **14**, 382 (1955). — BIRD, R. M., J. F. HAMMERSTEN, R. A. MARSHALL and R. R. ROBINSON: A family reunion. A study of hereditary hemorrhagic telangiectasia. New Engl. J. Med. **257**, 105 (1957). — BISGEIER, G. P.: Hemorrhage in pernicious anemia. J. med. Soc. N.J. **51**, 94 (1954). — BISTOFFA, R., e S. GARBIN: Un caso di malattia da deficit di PTA. Haematologica **46**, 741 (1961). — BITTERSOLL, R.: Zur Kenntnis nekrotischer Formen der Purpura Schönlein-Henoch-Glanzmann. Hautarzt **12**, 121 (1961). — BJÖRKMAN, S. E., and I. M. NILSSON: Demonstration of a fibrinolytic activator in red bone marrow. Acta haemat. (Basel) **26**, 273 (1961). — BJÖRNBERG, A.: Circulating anticoagulant and bullous dermatoses. Acta derm.-venereol. (Stockh.) **38**, 251 (1958). — BLACKBURN, E. K.: Haemorrhagic states. Postgrad. med. J. **35**, 519 (1959). — Primary capillary haemorrhage (incl. von Willebrand's disease). Brit. J. Haemat. **7**, 239 (1961). — Antihaemophilic factor deficiency, capillary defect of v. Willebrand type and idiopathic thrombocytopenia occurring in one family. J. clin. Path. **14**, 540 (1961). — BLACK-SCHAFFER, B., J. W. MILAM, D. D. BROCKMAN, E. V. COONRAD and S. B. SILVERMAN: Production of the Shwartzman phenomenon by a single injection. J. exp. Med. **91**, 539 (1950). — BLAICH, W.: Hämorrhagische Diathesen. In: Handbuch der Dermatologie und Venerologie v. GOTTRON u. SCHÖNFELD, Bd. II/2, S. 796—831. Stuttgart: Georg Thieme 1958. — BLANKENHORN, M. A., and H. C. KNOWLES jr.: Periarteritis nodosa: recognition and clinical symptoms. Ann. intern. Med. **41**, 867 (1954). — BLIX, S.: The fibrinolysis of plasma clots under various conditions. Acta med. scand. **169**, 495 (1961). — BLOOM, R. V., and E. J. MOYNAHAN: Hereditary haemorrhagic telangiectasia

(Study of a family with 6 children). Brit. J. Derm. **72**, 312 (1960). — BLUME, H. G., u. H. LIEBESKIND: Rezidivierende Purpura bei Kryoglobulinämie. Dtsch. med. Wschr. **85**, 377 (1960). — BÖHME, A., u. Dr. OBERSTE-BERGHAUS: Thrombopenische Purpura bei Röntgenassistentinnen. Strahlentherapie **97**, 292 (1955). — BOHLE, A., H. J. KRECKE, F. MILLER u. H. SITTE: Über die Natur des sog. Fibrinoids bei der generalisierten Shwartzman-Reaktion. In: Immunopathologie, S. 339. Basel: Benno Schwabe & Co. 1959. — BOHN, H., u. H. WINTER: Zum Problem des perakuten NNR-Versagens beim Waterhouse-Friderichsen-Syndrom (am Beispiel von 2 geretteten Kranken). Med. Welt **1960 I**, 13. — BOIVIN, A., I. MESROBEANU u. L. MESROBEANU: Technique pour la préparation des polysaccharides microbiens spécifiques. C. R. Soc. Biol. (Paris) **113**, 490 (1933). — BOLAND, S. W.: Prednisone and prednisolone therapy in rheumatoid arthritis. J. Amer. med. Ass. **160**, 611 (1956). — BOLLIGER, A.: Purpura hyperglobulinaemica bei Lebercirrhose. Schweiz. med. Wschr. **46**, 1158 (1958). — BOLTON, F. G., and J. E. CLARK: A method of assaying Christmas factor; its application to the study of Christmas disease (Factor IX-deficiency). Brit. J. Haemat. **5**, 396 (1962). — BOLTON, F. G., and W. DAMESHEK: Thrombocytopenic purpura due to quinidine. I. Clinical studies. Blood **11**, 527 (1956). — BON, H.: Précis de Médecine catholique. Paris 1935. — BOND, T. P., W. C. LEVIN, D. R. CELANDER and M. M. GUEST: „Mild hemophilia" affecting both males and females. New Engl. J. Med. **266**, 220 (1962). — BONNIN, J. A., and K. CHENEY: The PTF test: an improved method for estimation of platelet thromboplastic function. Brit. J. Haemat. **7**, 512 (1961). — BORCHGREVINK, C. F., O. EGEBERG, J. G. POOL, T. SKULASON, K. STORMOREN and B. WAALER: A study of a case of congenital hypoprothrombinemia. Brit. J. Haemat. **5**, 294 (1959). — BORCHGREVINK, C. F., and P. A. OWREN: The hemostatic effect of normal platelets in hemophilia and factor V deficiency. Acta med. scand. **179**, 375 (1961). — BORCHGREVINK, C. F., and B. A. WAALER: Secondary bleeding time: new method for differentiation of hemorrhagic diseases. Acta med. scand. **162**, 361 (1958). — BORELLI, S., u. R. FÜRST: Die Stigmatisation — das extreme Beispiel einer psychogenen Dermatose. Praxis **49**, 389 (1960). — BORN, W.: Purpura Majocchi im Bereich definierter Kontaktflächen. Hautarzt **7**, 516 (1956). — BOUNAMEAUX, Y.: Valeur fonctionnelle des thrombocytes dans le purpura idiopathique thrombopénique. Sang **28**, 127 (1957). — Recherches sur le mécanisme de la formation de la thromboplastine sanguine. Acta haemat. **17**, 65 (1957). — L'accolement des plaquettes aux fibres sous-endothéliales. C. R. Soc. Biol. (Paris) **153**, 865 (1959). — BOUSSER, J.: Thrombocytémies et thrombocytose. Rev. Prat. (Paris) **9**, 1071 (1959). — BOUSSER, J., D. CHRISTOL et R. ZITTOUN: Purpura hyperglobulinique de Waldenström et syndrome de Sjögren-Gougerot. 2 nouveaux cas. Sem. Hôp. Paris **37**, 2531 (1961). — BOWMAN, H. E., V. D. PETTIT, F. T. CALDWELL and E. B. SMITH: Morphology of the spleen in idiopathic thrombocytopenic purpura. Lab. Invest. **4**, 206 (1955). — BOYLES, P. W., and J. CURRIE: Classic hemophilia in a negro infant. Amer. J. med. Sci. **235**, 452 (1958). — BRADFORD, W. D., C. D. COOK and G. F. VAWTER: Livedo reticularis: a form of allergic vasculitis. J. Pediat. **60**, 266 (1962). — BRADLOW, B. A.: Liberation of material with platelet-like coagulant properties from intact red cells and particularly from reticulocytes. Brit. J. Haemat. **7**, 476 (1961). — BRAUMAN, J., R. DURET, G. GRAY, P. POTVLIEGE, P. BURTIN, J. VAN CUTSEM et P. P. LAMBERT: Myélome, à cryoglobuline spontanément cristallisable. Acta clin. belg. **11** (II), 517 (1956). — BRAUN, E. H., and D. B. STOLLAR: Spontaneous hemophilia in a female. Thrombos. Diathes. haemorrh. (Stuttg.) **4**, 369 (1960). — BRAUN-FALCO, O., u. J. JUNG: Über klinische und experimentelle Beobachtungen bei einem Fall von diffuser Haut-Mastocytose. Arch. klin. exp. Derm. **213**, 639 (1961). — BRAUNSTEINER, H.: Über Morphologie, Physiologie und Pathologie der Thrombocyten. Klin. Wschr. **29**, 335 (1951). — BRAUNSTEINER, H., E. OSWALD, F. PAKESCH u. E. REIMER: Lymphoretikulosen mit Makroglobulinämie. Wien. Z. inn. Med. **37**, **349** (1956). — BREDDIN, K.: Hämorrhagische Diathesen bei Lebererkrankungen unter besonderer Berücksichtigung der Thrombocytenfunktion. Acta haemat. (Basel) **27**, 1 (1962). — BREDT, J.: Hyperfibrinolyse bei Prostatakarzinom. Blut 8, 22 (1962). — BREHM, G.: Zur Purpura teleangiectatica arciformis (Touraine). Z. Haut- u. Geschl.-Kr. **17**, 331 (1954). — BRITTINGHAM, T. H., and H. CHAPLIN jr.: Attempted passive transfer of thrombotic thrombocytopenic purpura. Blood **12**, 480 (1957). — BRÖNNIMANN, R.: Kongenitale Afibrinogenämie. Acta haemat. (Basel) **11**, 40 (1954). — BROWN, I. W., W. W. SMITH and R. M. HOWSE: Surgical management in hemophilia and the hemophiloid diseases. Ann. Surg. **149**, 721 (1959). — BRÜSCHKE, G., W. THIELE u. F. H. SCHULZ: Die Abhängigkeit der Retraktion des Fibringerinnsels vom Alter. Z. Alternsforsch. **15**, 185 (1961). — BRÜSTER H.: Untersuchung zum v. Willebrand-Jürgens-Syndrom unter besonderer Berücksichtigung elektronenoptischer Studien. Mschr. Kinderheilk. **107**, 18 (1959). — Die Erkennung hämophiler Konduktorinnen mit Hilfe des osmotischen Resistenztests der Blutplättchen. Dtsch., med. Wschr. **87**, 2588 (1962). — BRUNNER, H. E., u. P. G. FRICK: Simultane thrombopenische Purpura und autoimmune hämolytische Anämie. Dtsch. med. Wschr. **87**, 1002 (1962). — BRUNSON, J. A., C. N. GAMBLE and L. THOMAS: Morphologic changes in rabbits following the intravenous administration of meningococcal toxin, I. and II. Amer. J. Path. **31**, 489—655 (1955). — BRUSH, B. E., R. W. MONTO, J. ABRAHAM, E. J. GORDON and J. R. CALDER: Use of cortisone in thrombocytopenic purpura. Preoperative and postoperative management of patients. Arch. Surg. **68**, 787 (1954). — BUCHANAN, J. C., and B. S. LEAVELL: Pseudohemophilia. Ann. intern. Med. **44**, 241 (1956). — BUCHER, U., u. W. BAUMGARTNER: Die Thrombozytopathie „Glanzmann-Naegeli". Schweiz. med. Wschr. **88**, 753 (1958). — BUCK, R. C.: The fine structure of endothelium of large arteries. J. biophys. biochem. Cytol. **4**, 187 (1958). — BÜTLER, R., S. RÖHRIG, P. SIEGENTHALER and S. MOESCHLIN: A special haemophilic syndrome. Acta haemat. (Basel) **22**, 292 (1959). — BULLOCK, W. H., J. B. JOHNSON and T. W. DAVIS: Hemophilia in negro subjects. Arch. intern. Med. **100**, 759 (1957). — BUNTING, W. L., J. M. KIELY and D. C. CAMPBELL: Idiopathic thrombocytopenic purpura. Arch. intern. Med. **108**, 733 (1961). — BURDON, K. L., J. P. McGOVERN, G. D. BARKIN and W. M. MEYERS: Fibrinolysis and anaphylaxis. J. Allergy **32**, 55, 63 (1961). — BURGSTEDT, H. J., u. R. MARX: Afibrinogenämie, Parahämophilie und Hypoproteinämie bei Zysteinspeicherkrankheit. Klin. Wschr. **34**, 31 (1955). — BURKE, E. O., S. D. MILLS and G. B. STICKLER: Nephritis associated with anaphylactoid purpura in childhood. Clinical observations and prognosis. Proc. Mayo Clin. **35**, 641 (1960). — BURNET, J.: Bacillus coli infection in children. Int. Clin. **3**, 198 (1923). — BURTIN, P., L. HARTMANN, J. HEREMANS, J. J. SCHEIDEGGER, F. WESTENDORP-BOERMA, R. WIEME, CH. WUNDERLY, R. FAUVERT et P. GRABAR: Etudes immunochimiques et immuno-électrophorétiques des macroglobulinémies. Rev. franç. Étud. clin. biol. **2**, 161 (1957). — BUTLER, E. A., F. V. FLYNN, H. HARRIS and E. B. ROBSON: The laboratory diagnosis of macroglobulinaemia with special reference to starch-gel electrophoresis. Lancet **1961 II**, 289. — BUTLER, S., R. HALL and H. SANFORD: Observations on the influence of i.v. histamine on qualitative platelet activity in coagulation. J. Lab. clin. Med. **36**, 710 (1950). — BYWATERS, E. G. L., I. ISDALE and J. J. KEMPTON: Schönlein-Henoch purpura. Evidence for a group Aβ-haemolytic streptococcal aetiology. Quart. J. Med., N. s. **26**, 161 (1957).

CAEN, J., et J. BERNARD: Syndrome hémorragique dû au défaut du facteur prothromboplastique de Rosenthal (PTA). Sang **27**, 249 (1956). — CAEN, J., S. YANOTTI, J. VARANKOT et J. BERNARD: Etude d'un cas d'hypoproconvertinémie vraie congénitale. Sang **30**, 535 (1959). — CAIRNS, R. J.: Amyloidosis — a tissue proteinosis. Trans. St. Johns Hosp. derm. Soc. (Lond.) **48**, 145 (1962). — CALNAN, C. D., and D. J. M. LISTER: Anaphylactoid purpura from tetracycline. Trans. St. John's Hosp. derm. Soc. (Lond.) **44**, 69 (1960). — CALO, A., et G. DIACONO: Purpura hémorragique thrombocytopénique par l'intolérance à l'allyl-isopropyl-acetyl-carbamide (Sedormid). Sang **25**, 85 (1954). — CANIZARES, O.: Cutaneous lesions of rheumatic fever. Clinical study in young adults. Arch. Derm. **76**, 702 (1957). — CAROL, W. L. L., u. J. R. PRAKKEN: Die kutane Form der Periarteriitis nodosa. Acta derm. venereol. (Stockh.) **18**, 102 (1937). — CARPENTER, A. F., M. M. WINTROBE, E. A. FULLER, A. HAUT and G. E. CARTWRIGHT: Treatment of idiopathic thrombocytopenic purpura. Amer. J. med. Ass. **171**, 1911 (1959). — CARR jr., E. A.: Drug allergy. Pharmacol. Rev. **6**, 365 (1954). — „Group III" reactions to drugs: apparently allergic reactions occurring almost exclusively with drugs. In: Current problems in allergy and immunology, pp. 485—504. 1959. — CASALÀ Y SANTIAGO, A. M., y J. MOSTO: Angiodermitis pruriginosa disseminada „eczematid-like purpura" (Doucas & Kapetanakis), „Itching purpura" (Loewenthal). Arch. argent. Derm. **5**, 209 (1955). — CASTEX, M. R.: La pathogénie du purpura hémorrhagique. Presse méd. **1924**, 277. — CAUSSADE, L., N. NEIMAN, M. PIERSON et M. MANCIAUX: L'afibrinogénémie congénitale familiale. Presse méd. **62**, 1040 (1954). — CAVINS, J. A., and R. L. WALL: Clinical and laboratory studies of plasma thromboplastin antecedent (PTA). Amer. J. Med. **29**, 444 (1960). — CAZAL, P., R. GRAAFLAND, P. IZARN, M. MATHIEU, G. PELEIRAC et J. FISCHER: Hémorragies thrombocytopéniques arrêtées par injections intraveineuses de fibrinogène humain. Sang **27**, 84 (1956). — CHALMERS, D. G., R. R. A. COOMBS and B. W. GURNER: Antiglobulin reaction in the detection of human iso-antibodies against leucocytes, platelets and He-La cells. Brit. J. Haemat. **5**, 225 (1962). — CHAMBERS, R., and G. CAMERON: The effect of 1-ascorbic acid on epithelial sheets in tissue cultures. Amer. J. Physiol. **139**, 21 (1943). — CHAMBERS, R., and B. W. ZWEIFACH: Intercellular cement and capillary permeability. Physiol. Rev. **27**, 436 (1947a). — CHEVALLIER, P., J. BERNARD, G. BILSKI-PASQUIER, J. DE GROUCHY et N. SAMAMA: Déficience congénitale et familiale en facteur Stuart. Sang **30**, 525 (1959). — CHEVALLIER, P., A. FIEHRER, G. BILSKI-PASQUIER et P. FUNEL: Hémogénie avec excès d'antithrombine physiologique. Sang **26**, 589 (1955). — CHEW, A., G. A. LENG, H. YUEN, K. O. TEIK, L. Y. KIAT, H. CHENG and R. WELLS: A haemorrhagic fever in Singapore. Lancet **1961 I**, 307. — CHOREMIS, C., C. PADIATELLIS, I. TSEVRENIS, E. HADJIDIMITRIOU, I. PRIOVOLOS et T. MANDALAKI: A propos d'un cas d'hypoproconvertinémie congénitale. Helv. paediat. Acta **11**, 301 (1956). — CHOREMIS, C., N. ZERVOS, H. TSEVRENIS, E. APOSTOLOPOULO et T. MANDALAKI: Hémophilie A chez une fille agée de deux ans. Helv. paediat. Acta **11**, 305 (1956). — CHURG, J., and L. STRAUSS: Allergic granulomatosis, allergic angitis and periarteritis nodosa. Amer. J. Path. **27**, 277 (1951). — ČIČOVAČKI, D., u. R. STOEGER: Über die Osler'sche Krankheit. Wien. klin. Wschr. **1939 II**, 708. — CLARK, E. R., and E. L. CLARK: Observations on living preformed blood vessels as seen in a transparent chamber inserted into the rabbits ear. Amer. J. Anat. 49, 441 (1932). — Observations on changes in blood vascular endothelium in the living animal. Amer. J. Anat. 57, 385 (1935). — Clark, W. G., and E. Jacobs: Experimental nonthrombopenic vascular purpura. Blood 5, 320 (1950). — Clauss, A.: Gerinnungsphysiologische Schnellmethode zur Bestimmung des Fibrinogens. Acta haemat. (Basel) 17, 237 (1957). — Clement, D. H., and L. K. Diamond: Purpura in infants and children. Amer. J. Dis. Child. 85, 259 (1953). — Clément, R., J. Bernard, M. G. Papaioannou, R. Habib et M. Designolle: Purpura thrombotique thrombocytopénique. (Maladie de Moschkovitz chez un enfant de 10 mois.) Arch. franç. Pédiat. 14, No 10 (1957). — Cleton, F. J., and E. A. Loeliger: Two typical hereditary charts of congenital factor VII deficiency. Thrombos. Diathes. haemorrh. (Stuttg.) 5, 87 (1960). — Cleve, H., F. Heckner u. R. Schoen: Das morphologische Substrat der idiopathischen thrombopenischen Purpura im Lichte neuer pathogenetischer Erkenntnisse. Schweiz. med. Wschr. 88, 323 (1958). — Cohen, Ph., and F. H. Gardner: The thrombocytopenic effect of sustained high-dosage prednisone therapy in thrombocytopenic purpura. N. Engl. J. Med. 265, 611 (1961). — Cohen, S. G., D. S. Dzury and F. J. Michelini: Staphylococcus aureus antigens in hypersensitivity reactions and experimental arterial sensitization. J. Allergy 28, 531 (1957). — Cohen, S. G., and T. M. Sapp: Hemostatic- and fibrinolytic-affecting agents in experimental vascular sensitization. Circulat. Res. 9, 851 (1961). — Coke, H.: Two interesting cases of purpura. Brit. med. J. 1931, 535. — Cole, R. I.: Note on the production of an agglutinating serum for blood platelets. Bull. Johns Hopk. Hosp. 18, 261 (1907). — Conca, G., e E. Kehyayan: Osservazioni su 18 casi di sindrome die Schönlein-Henoch. Minerva pediat. 13, 1562 (1961). — Conley, C. L., and R. C. Hartmann: A hemorrhagic disorder caused by circulating anticoagulant in patients with disseminated lupus erythematodes. J. clin. Invest. 31, 621 (1952). — Conway, N., and J. M. Walker: Treatment of macroglobulinaemia. Brit. med. J. 1962 (4), 1296. — Cook, I. A., and A. S. Douglas: Demonstrable deficiency of Christmas factor in two sisters. Brit. med. J. 1960 (1), No 5171, 479. — Cooney, D. P., W. F. Blatt and H. Jensen: Studies on thrombopoiesis. I. Effect of a dialysable spleen preparation on the thrombocyte level. Acta haemat. (Basel) 26, 317 (1961). — Cooperberg, A. H.: The management of idiopathic thrombocytopenic purpura. Canad. med. J. 80, 937 (1959). — Copley, A. L.: A new concept and studies of capillary hemorrhagic diseases. Proc. 3rd. Internat. Congr. Intern. Soc. Haemat. New York: Grune & Stratton 1951, p. 541. — Neue Auffassungen über Hämorrhagie, Hämostase und Thrombose. Ärztl. Forsch. 11, 114 (1957). — Copley, A. L., and R. Chambers: Experimentally induced petechial hemorrhage and white embolization in the rabbits nictitating membrane. Amer. Heart J. 45, 237 (1953). — Cornu, P., M. J. Larrieu, J. Caen et J. Bernard: Maladie de Willebrand. Etude clinique, génétique et biologique. Nouv. Rev. franç. Hémat. 1, 231 (1961). — Cottier, P., R. Leupold u. W. Scheitlin: Die hämorrhagische Diathese bei Prostatakarzinom und ihre Behandlung. Schweiz. med. Wschr. 85, 781 (1955). — Crawford, S. E., and J. G. Riddler: Purpura fulminans. Amer. J. Dis. Child. 97, 198 (1959). — Creveld, S. van: Congenital idiopathic hypoprothrombinemia. Acta paediat. (Uppsala), Suppl. 100, 245 (1954). — Creveld, S. van, et K. H. Liem: Congenital afibrinogenemia. Étud. néo-natales 7, 89 (1958). — Coagulation disorders in the newborn period. J. paediat. 54, 633 (1959). — Creveld, S. van, and I. A. Mochtar: Modern aspects of the treatment of haemophilia. Canad. med. Ass. J. 87, 993 (1962). — Creveld, S. van, and M. M. Paulssen: A form of haemorrhagic diathesis characterized by the lack of the third clotting-factor, normally present in blood platelets. Ann. paediat. (Basel) 181, 193 (1953). — Creyssel, R.: Les thrombopathies et la thrombasthénie. Rev. Prat. (Paris) 9, 2079 (1959). — Criep, L.: A consideration of the so-called collagen and systemic connective tissue diseases. In: Current problems in allergy and immunology, p. 587. 1959. — Crocker, H. R.: Angioma serpiginosum, Lymphoderma perniciosa. Brit. J. Derm. 6, 367 (1894). — Croizat, J., et J. Favre-Gilly: Classification des purpuras. Rev. Prat. (Paris) 1954, 3883. — Cruchaud, A., C. A. Bouvier et L. Humair: Les artérites nécrosantes par sensibilisation. Schweiz. med. Wschr. 90, 298 (1960). — Cruickshank, B.: The role of „auto-antibodies" in anaphylactoid purpura. Immunology 2, 123 (1959). — Csermely, E.: A proposito della cosidetta „eczematid-like purpura". Minerva Derm. 30 (4), Suppl. 2, 105 (1955). — Considerazioni su alcuni casi di „eczematid-like purpura". G. ital. Derm. 98, 265 (1957).

Dacie, J. V.: Haemolytic reaction to drugs. Proc. roy. Soc. Med. 55, 28 (1962). — Dalgleish, P. G., and B. M. Ansell: Anaphylactic purpura in pulmonary tuberculosis. Brit. med. J. 1950 I, 225. — Dam, H., u. J. Glavind: Vitamin E und Kapillarpermeabilität. Naturwissenschaften 28, 207 (1940). — Damerow, R.: Über die thrombocytären Autosensibilisierungen. Z. Kinderheilk. 85, 493 (1961). — Dameshek, W.: Method for simultaneous enumeration of blood platelets. Arch. intern. Med. 50, 579 (1932). — Dameshek, W., and E. B. Miller: Megakaryocytes in idiopathic thrombocytopenic purpura. Blood 1, 27 (1946). — Dameshek, W., and W. H. Reeves: Exacerbation of lupus erythematosus following splenectomy in „idiopathic" thrombocytopenic purpura and autoimmune hemolytic anemia. Amer. J. Med. 2, 560 (1956). — Dameshek,

W., F. Rubio jr., J. P. Mahoney, W. Reeves and L. A. Bürgin: Treatment of idiopathic thrombocytopenic purpura with prednisone. J. Amer. med. Ass. **166**, 1803 (1958). — Dameshek, W., and M. Stefanini: Idiopathic thrombocytopenic Purpura: Some ideas on its pathogenesis and treatment. Med. Clin. N. Amer. **37**, 1395 (1953). — d'Angelo, G., and L. Ph. de Gressley: Severe hypoprothrombinemia after propylthiouracil therapy. Canad. med. Ass. J. **81**, 479 (1959). — Danielli, J. F., and A. Stock: The structure and permeability of blood capillaries. Biol. Rev. **1944/45**, 19, 81. — Danilovic, V., et M. Ljaljevic: Nos expériences dans l'allergie médicamenteuse. Acta allerg. (Kbh.) **15**, Suppl. 7, 250 (1960). — Danon, D., N. Gilboa-Garber and D. Nelken: Reversible and irreversible changes in normal human thrombocyte membranes by slow and rapid swelling. J. cell. comp. Physiol. **57**, 21 (1961). — Dargeon, H. W., C. Amparo, A. C. Adiao and G. T. Pack: Hemangioma with thrombocytopenia. J. Pediat. **54**, 285 (1959). — Darnley, J. D.: Polyneuropathy in Waldenström's macroglobulinemia. Neurology (Minneap.) **12**, 617 (1962). — Dausset, J.: Immunohématologie biologique et clinique. Paris: Ed. méd. Flammarion 1956. — Les auto-anticorps dans les purpuras thrombopéniques et les leucopénies. Strasbourg méd., N. s. **8**, 545 (1957). — Les auto-anticorps antiplaquettaires et les tests immunologiques. Rev. Prat. (Paris) **9**, 2087 (1959a). — Le test de consommation directe de l'antiglobuline sur les plaquettes et les leucocytes desm alades atteints de purpura thrombopénique et de pancytopénie. Rev. franç. Étud. clin. biol. **4**, 495 (1959b). — Dausset, J., B. Bilski-Pasquier, G. Malinvaud, J. R. Davy et St. Tara: Syndromes hémorragiques par sensibilisation médicamenteuse. Etat actuel de la question à propos d'un cas de purpura thrombopénique à l'allyl-isopropyl-acétyl-carbamide. Sang **25**, 911 (1954). — Dausset, J., et M. Colin: Technique de recherche des thromboagglutinines immunologiques (Influence du chauffage préalable de la suspension plaquettaire). Rev. franç. Étud. clin. biol. **3**, 60 (1958). — Dausset, J., and M. Colombani: Study of leucopenias and thrombocytopenias by the direct antiglobulin consumption test on leucocytes and/or platelets. Blood **18**, 672 (1961). — Dausset, J., P. Delafontaine, G. Damiens et Y. Fleuriot: Purpura thrombopénique aigu d'auto-agression. Mise en évidence in vitro d'une agglutinine antiplaquettaire. Sem. Hôp. Paris **29**, 1334 (1953). — Dausset, J., P. Delafontaine et Y. Fleuriot: Agglutination et destruction in vitro de plaquettes normales par le sérum d'une malade atteinte de purpura thrombocytopénique aigu. Sang **23**, 373 (1952). — Dausset, J., G. Malinvaud et F. Layani: Purpura thrombopénique aigu au phényldiméthyl-isopropyl-pyrazolone. Sem. Hôp. Paris **1954**, 3055. — Davis, E.: Hereditary familial purpura simplex. Lancet **1939 II**, 1110. — Davis, L. J., and A. Brown: The megaloplastic anaemias. Oxford: Blackwell 1953. — Davis, M. J., and J. C. Lawler: The capillary circulation of the skin. Arch. Derm. **77**, 690 (1958). — Capillary alterations in pigmented purpuric diseases of the skin. Arch. Derm. **78**, 723 (1958). — Debray, J.: Les purpuras thrombopéniques. Presse méd. **66**, 29, 642 (1958). — Introduction à la physiopathie des plaquettes. Rev. Prat. (Paris) **9**, 2057 (1959). — Denko, C. W., and L. R. Schroeder: Ecchymotic skin lesions in patients receiving prednisone. J. Amer. med. Ass. **164**, 41 (1957). — Derbes, V. J., and M. E. Chernosky: Senile purpura and liver disease. Arch. Derm. **80**, 529 (1959). — Derham, R. J., and M. M. Rogerson: Schönlein-Henoch syndrome with particular reference to renal sequelae. Arch. Dis. Childh. **31**, 364 (1956). — Detwilder, T. C., T. T. Odell jr. and T. P. McDonald: Platelet size, ATP content and clot retraction in relation to platelet age. Amer. J. Physiol. **203**, 107 (1962). — Deutsch, E.: Die Hemmkörperhaemophilie. Wien: Springer 1950 u. Schweiz. med. Wschr. **81**, 74 (1951). — Hereditäre Koagulopathien. Ref. 5. Kongr. Europ. Ges. Hämatol. 1955. Stuttgart: Georg Thieme 1956, p. 369. — Coagulopathien. In: Prognose chronischer Erkrankungen von F. Linneweh. Berlin: Springer 1960. — Blutungsübel. Wien. med. Wschr. **111**, 69 (1961a). — Langzeitprognose hämorrhagischer Diathesen. Neue öst. Z. Kinderheilk. **6**, 23 (1961b). — Deutsch, E., u. M. Koch: Beitrag zur Objektivierung der Diagnose der hämophilen Konduktorin. Wien. klin. Wschr. **74**, 793 (1962). — Dieter, D. H., M. Spooner and F. I. Pohle: Studies on an indetermined circulating anticoagulant. Blood **4**, 120 (1949). — Dietrich, A., u. M. Nordmann: Versuche zur hämorrhagischen Diathese. Verh. dtsch. Ges. Path., 25. Tagg zu Berlin, S. 46 (1930). — Dische, F. E., and V. Benfield: Congenital factor VII deficiency. Acta haemat. (Basel) **21**, 257 (1959). — Doerken, H.: Die Purpura hyperglobulinaemica (Waldenström) und ihre Zuordnung. Verh. dtsch. Ges. inn. Med. **60**, 761 (1954). — Dooren, L. J., u. K. F. Kerrebijn: Hemangioom met thrombocytopenie. Maandschr. Kindergeneesk. **29**, 136 (1961). — Doucas, C., and J. Kapetanakis: Eczematid-like purpura. Dermatologica (Basel) **106**, 86 (1953). — Douglas, A. S., and S. G. McAlpin: Neurological complications of hemophilia and christmas disease. Scot. med. J. **1**, 270 (1956). — Duckert, F.: Le diagnostic des coagulopathies. Mécanisme de la coagulation. Röntgen- u. Lab.-Prax. **13**, 156, 203 (1960). — Persönliche Mitteilung 1962. — Duckert, F., E. Beck, R. Rondez and A. Vogel: Fibrin stabilising factor and fibrin properties. 8th. Congr. Europ. Soc. Haem. Wien 1961. — Duckert, F., P. Flückiger, M. Matter and F. Koller: Clotting factor X. Physiologic and physicochemical properties. Proc. Soc. exp. Biol. (N.Y.) **90**, 17 (1955). — Duckert, F., E. Jung and D. H. Shmerling: A hitherto undescribed congenital hemorrhagic diathesis probably due to fibrin stabilising factor deficiency. Thrombos. Diathes. haemorrh. 5, 179 (1960). — DUCKERT, F., T. E. YIN and W. STRAUB: Separation and purification of the blood clotting factors by means of chromatography and electrophoresis. VIII Coll. protides of biologic fluids. Brügge 1960. — DUNN, W. J., and W. M. MCCONAHEY: Cushing's syndrome complicated by Guillain-Barré-syndrome and thrombocytopenia with purpura. Report of a case. Proc. Mayo Clin. 31, 322 (1956). — DUPERRAT, B.: Manifestations cutanées de la cryoglobulinémie. Arch. belges Derm. 13/14, 310 (1957/58). — DUPERRAT, B., et J. MONFORT: Les allergides vasculaires hypodermiques. Ann. Derm. Syph. (Paris) 85, 385 (1958). — DUTCHER, T. M., and J. L. FAHEY: Histopathology of macroglobulinemia of Waldenström. J. Nat. Cancer Inst. 5, 887 (1959). — DUTTON, L. O.: Thrombocytopenic purpura due to food allergy. J. Amer. med. Ass. 111, 1920 (1938). — DVORAK, K.: Idiopathische Lungenhämosiderose mit Schönlein-Henoch'scher Purpura. Z. ges. inn. Med. 14, 113 (1959). — DYKE, S. C.: The blood platelets and their place in medicine. Lancet 1924II, 714.

EBBE, S., B. WITTELS and W. DAMESHEK: Autoimmune thrombocytopenic purpura („ITP"-type with chronic lymphocytic leukemia). Blood 19, 23 (1962). — EBERT, R. H., and R. W. WISSLER: In vivo observations of the effects of cortisone on the vascular reaction to large doses of horse serum using the rabbit ear chamber technique. J. Lab. clin. Med. 38, 497 (1951). — EGEBERG, O.: Acquired circulating anticoagulant in classical hemophilia. Scand. J. clin. Lab. Invest. 13, 535 (1961). — The effect of unspecific fever induction on the blood clotting system. Scand. J. clin. Lab. Invest. 14, 471 (1962a). — The effect of serum infusion on the blood clotting system. Scand. J. clin. Lab. Invest. 14, 475 (1962b). — EGLI, H., K. KESSELER u. R. KLESPER: Über die Inaktivierung von Blutthrombokinase (zugleich ein Beitrag zur Unterscheidung von Blut- und Gewebsthrombokinase). Acta haemat. (Basel) 17, 338 (1957). — EHLERS, G., u. H. HEINZE: Zur Symptomatologie und Pathogenese der Purpura hyperglobulinaemica Waldenström. Derm. Wschr. 145, 428 (1962). — ELLIS, R. A.: Vascular patterns of the skin. In: Blood vessels and circulation Montagna and Ellis. Oxford-London: Pergamon Press 1961. — ELLIS, R. A., and W. MONTAGNA: Histology and chemistry of human skin. J. Histochem. Cytochem. 6, 201 (1958). — EPSTEIN, R. D., E. L. LOZNER, T. S. COBBEY and C. S. DAVIDSON: Congenital thrombopenic purpura. Purpura haemorrhagica in pregnancy and in the new-born. Amer. J. Med. 9, 44 (1950). — ERIKSSON, A. W., E. HIEPLER, R. JÜRGENS, W. LEHMANN u. H. SCHULZ: Untersuchungen zur Thrombopathie (v. Willebrand-Jürgens). Klin. Wschr. 38, 32 (1961). — ESHOUGUES, J. R. D', et P. GRIGUER: Purpura thrombopénique aigu mortel avec thrombo-agglutinines hétérophiles, consécutif à l'absorption de pyramidon 5 mois après cure de phénylbutazone. Sang 27, 138 (1956). — ESHOUGUES, J. R. D', P. GRIGUER et A. TADÉI: Aspirine et purpura. Bull. Soc. méd. Hôp. Paris 75, 862 (1959). — ESHOUGUES, J. R. D', et A. TADEI: Les accidents hémorragiques des médications antirhumatismales. Algérie méd. 63, 32 (1959). — EVANS, R. S., K. TAKAHASHI, A. B. DUANE, R. PAYNE and C. K. LIU: Primary thrombocytopenic purpura and acquired hemolytie anemia. Arch. intern. Med. 87, 48 (1951). — EVERSOLE, ST. L.: Cases of disseminated lupus erythematodes diagnosed as thrombocytopenic purpura. Bull. Johns Hopk. Hosp. 96, 210 (1955). — EYGONNET, J. P.: Les anticoagulants circulants dans la maladie de Kahler. Diss. Lyon 1960.

FANCONI, G.: Familiäre, infantile, perniciosaartige Anämien. Jb. Kinderheilk. 117, 257 (1927). — FANCONI, G., u. A. WALLGREN: Lehrbuch der Paediatrie. Basel: Benno Schwabe 1954. — FAVRE-GILLY, J. E., A. BEAUDOING et J. P. THOUVEREZ: Les différents types génétiques de la maladie de Willebrand. 5. Kongr. Europ. Haemat. Ges. Freiburg 1955. Stuttgart: Georg Thieme 1956, p. 432. — FEISSLY, R., A. GAUTIER et I. MARCOVICI: Nouveau procédé d'examen des thrombocytes au microscope électronique (Note préliminaire). Rev. Hémat. 12, 397 (1957). — FEISSLY, R., et H. LÜDIN: Microscopie par contrastes de phases. Rev. Hémat. 4, 481 (1949). — FELDMAN, N., and S. N. LEWIS: Hemophilia in a South-African Bantu child. S. Afr. J. med. Sci. 17, 13 (1952). — FELDT, R. H., and G. B. STRICKLER: The gastrointestinal manifestations of anaphylactoid purpura in children. Staff Mayo Clin. 37, 465 (1962). — FELSON, B., and H. BRAUNSTEIN: Noninfectious necrotizing granulomatosis (Wegener's syndrome, lethal granuloma and allergic angiitis and granulomatosis). Radiology 70, 326 (1958). — FERGUSON, J. H., C. L. JOHNSTON and D. A. HOWELL: Anti-Accelerator globulin. Proc. Soc. exp. biol. (N.Y.) 95, 567 (1957). — FERNEX, M.: L'Onyalai: Une maladie hémorragipare d'Afrique. Une réticulose réactionelle gigantocellulaire. Acta trop. (Basel) 18, 289 (1961). — FIASCHI, E.: Le porpore emorragiche da infezione focale. Arch. E. Maragliano Pat. Clin. 14, 331 (1949). — L'etiopatogenesi focale de alcune porpore emorragiche. Settim. med. 38, 133 (1950). — FIEHRER, A.: Le facteur plasmatique normal antirétractant (F.A.R.). Trans. 6th. Congr. Europ. Soc. Haemat. Copenhagen 1957. — Clinique et laboratoire des purpuras. Conf. du 13. 11. 1958. Soc. Franç. d'Angéiologie, Paris. — Nouvelle classification des purpuras. Ann. Biol. clin. 17, 43 (1959). — FISCH, U., and F. DUCKERT: Some aspects of kinetics of the first stages of thromboplastin formation. Thrombos. Diathes. haemorrh. (Stuttg.) 3, 98 (1959). — FISCHBACHER, W.: Beitrag zur Fibrinolyse. Diss. Zürich 1960. — FISCHEL, E. E., and E. KABAT: Quantitative study of the Arthus phenomenon induced passively in the rabbit. J. Immunol. **55**, 337 (1947). — FISHER, B., G. H. ZUCKERMAN and R. C. DOUGLASS: Combined inheritance of purpura simplex and ptosis in 4 generations of one family. Blood **9**, 1199 (1954). — FISHER, EDW. R., and D. L. CREED: Thrombotic thrombocytepenic purpura. Report of one case with discussion of its tinctorial features. Amer. J. clin. Path. **25**, 620 (1955). — FLEISCHHACKER, H.: Medikamentös bedingte hämorrhagische Diathesen. Häm. Diath. Intern. Symposium. Wien: Springer 1955, S. 142. — FLEISCHHACKER, H., u. A. STACHER: Leitsymptom: Spontanblutungen. Münch. med. Wschr. **104**, 305 (1962). — FLEISCHMAJER, R., C. R. REIN, F. PASCHER and C. F. SIMS: Purpura of idiopathic hyperglobulinemia. Arch. Derm. **76**, 575 (1957). — FLÜCKIGER, P.: Ein Beitrag zur Genese der idiopathischen Thrombopenie. Diss. Zürich 1953. — FLUTE, P. T., and A. N. HOWARD: Blood coagulation in scorbutic guinea pigs. A defect in activation by glass contact. Brit. J. Haemat. **5**, 421 (1959). — FODOR, O., F. SURIANU, F. BARBARINO u. CH. ABEL: Autoimmun-hämatologische Erscheinungen bei Erkrankungen des reticulo-hystiozytären Systems und Kollagenkrankheiten. Dtsch. Gesundh.-Wes. **17**, 634 (1962). — FONIO, A.: Neuere Untersuchungen über die retraktionsauslösende Funktion der Thrombocyten. Praxis **36**, 725 (1947). — Über die Einwirkung quantitativer und qualitativer Schädigung auf die Funktion der Thrombocyten in bezug auf die Retraktion des Blutgerinnsels bzw. Thrombus. Bull. schweiz. Akad. med. Wiss. **6**, 115 (1950). — Zytologie und Physiologie der Thrombocyten. In: Handbuch der gesamten Hämatologie, 2. Aufl., Bd. 1. Wien: Urban & Schwarzenberg 1957. — Die Gerinnungsfaktoren bei der Haemophilie. Basel u. Stuttgart: Benno Schwabe & Co. 1961 (a). — Über vorzeitigen Fibrinausfall bei 2 Hämophilen. Acta haemat. (Basel) **25**, 372 (1961 b). — FOSSGREEN, J.: Trombotisk trombocytopenisk purpura. Nord. Med. **67**, 51 (1962). — FOX, M. J., and N. ENZER: A consideration of the phenomenon of purpura following scarlet fever. Amer. J. med. Sci. **196**, 321 (1938). — FRANÇOIS, J., et J. COFFYN: Angiomatose rétino-cérébello-viscérale de von Hippel-Lindau. Ann. Oculist. (Paris) **184**, 206 (1951). — L'hérédité en ophtalmologie. Paris: Masson & Cie. 1958. — FRANK, E.: Die essentielle Thrombopenie nach 40 Jahren. Münch. med. Wschr. **100**, 940 (1958). — FRICK, P. G.: Acquired circulating anticoagulant in systemic collagen disease. Blood **10**, 691 (1955 a). — Inhibition of conversion of fibrinogen to fibrin by abnormal proteins in multiple myeloma. Amer. J. clin. Path. **25**, 1263 (1955 b). — FRICK, P. G., F. BACHMANN and F. DUCKERT: Vascular anomaly associated with plasma thromboplastin antecedent deficiency. J. Lab. clin. Med. **54**, 680 (1959). — FRICK, P. G., and C. H. HITZIG: Simultaneous thrombotic thrombocytopenic purpura and agammaglobulinaemia. Schweiz. med. Wschr. **89**, 58 (1959). — FRICK, P. G., and J. D. KRAFCHUK: Studies of hemostasis in the Ehlers-Danlos syndrome. J. invest. Derm. **26**, 453 (1956). — FRICK, P. G., and I. MCQUARRIE: Congenital afibrinogenemia. Paediatrics **13**, 44 (1954). — FRIDERICHSEN, C.: Waterhouse-Friderichsen syndrome. Acta endocr. (Kbh.) **18**, 482 (1955). — FRIEDMAN, I. A., A. J. QUICK, F. HIGGINS, C. V. HUSSEY and M. E. HICKEY: Hereditary labile factor (F. V) deficiency. J. Amer. med. Ass. **175**, 370 (1961). — FROSS, J. D., R. C. HARTMANN, J. B. GRAHAM and C. B. TAYLOR: Splenectomy in hemophilia. Bull. Johns Hopk. Hosp. **100**, 223 (1957). — Hemophilia complicated by an acquired circulating anticoagulant. Brit. J. Haemat. **7**, 340 (1961). — FULTON, G. P., R. P. AKERS and B. R. LUTZ: White thrombo-embolism and vascular fragility in the hamster cheek pouch after anticoagulants. Blood **8**, 141 (1953).

GAIRDNER, D.: The Schönlein-Henoch syndrom (anaphylactoid purpura). Quart. J. Med. **17**, 95 (1948). — GAJDUSEK, D. C.: Virus hemorrhagic fevers. J. Pediat. **60** (6), 841 (1962). — GARB, J.: Dyskeratosis congenita with pigmentation, dystrophia unguium and leukoplakia oris. Arch. Derm. Syph. (Chic.) **55**, 242 (1947). — Dyskeratosis congenita with pigmentation, dystrophia unguium and leukoplakia oris. Arch. Derm. **77**, 704 (1958). — GARBE, CH., G. BRÜSCHKE u. F. H. SCHULZ: Das Retraktionsvermögen des Fibrins bei verschiedenen Krankheiten. Dtsch. Gesundh.-Wes. **16**, 661 (1961). — GARCIN, R., J. MALLARMÉ et P. RONDOT: Névrites dysglobulinémiques. Presse méd. **70**, 111 (1962). — GARCIN, R., et P. RONDOT: Les aspects névritiques initiaux de la macrobulinémie de Waldenström. Psychiat. Neurol. Neurochir. (Amst.) **66**, 318 (1963). — GARDNER, F. H., and L. K. DIAMOND: Autoerythrocyte sensitization. A form of purpura producing painful bruising following autosensibilisation in red cells blood in certain women. Blood **10**, 675 (1955). — GARLAND, H. G., and S. T. ANNING: Hereditary hemorrhagic telangiectasia. Genetic and bibliographic study. Brit. J. Derm. **62**, 289 (1950). — GARRETT, J. V., H. McC. GILES, R. R. A. COOMBS and B. W. GURNER: Neonatal purpura with platelet isoantibody in maternal serum. Lancet **1960 I**, 521. — GARROD, A. E.: Inborn errors of metabolism. Oxford: Frowde, Hodxer & Stoughton. — GASSER, C.: Klinik und Therapie der hämorrhagischen Diathesen im Kindesalter. Period. Mitt. Schweiz. Lebensversich. Nr 32, 579 (1956). — Panmyelopathien im Kindesalter. Helv. paediat. Acta **16**, 752 (1961). — GASSER, C., u. G. DE MURALT: Purpura fulminans mit Faktor-V-Mangel und Heilung durch Blutaustauschtransfusion. Helv. paediat. Acta **5**, 364 (1950). — GASSER, H.: Über Hemmkörperhämophilie bei Pemphigus vulgaris. Dtsch. Arch. klin. Med. **203**, 617 (1957). — GASTON,

L. W.: Hemophilia A and concurrent factor VII deficiency. New Engl. J. Med. **21**, 1078 (1961). — GAUTHIER, A., et P. A. MAURICE: Purpura hyperglobulinémique de Waldenstroem et maladie de Besnier-Boeck-Schaumann. Schweiz. med. Wschr. **1953**, 1110. — GEIST jr., R. M., and W. H. MULLEN jr.: Roentgenologic aspects of lethal granulomatous ulceration of the midline facial tissues. Amer. J. Roentgenol. **70**, 566 (1953). — GÉLIN, G.: Purpuras thrombocytopéniques aigus traités par la cortisone. Acta haemat. (Basel) **13**, 298 (1955). — GELL, P. G. H., and I. T. HINDE: Observations on the histology of the Arthus reaction and its relation to other known types of skin hypersensitivity. Int. Arch. Allergy **5**, 23 (1954). — GELZER, J., u. C. GASSER: Wiskott-Aldrich-Syndrom. Helv. paediat. Acta **16**, 17 (1961). — GENTILI, A., e G. GELLI: Sulle trombopatie pure essenziali. Minerva pediat. **11**, 171 (1959). — GERBAUT, P., M. PIERSON, J. LORRAIN et M. T. WAUTHIER: Purpura gangréneux au cours de maladies infectieuses. Bull. Soc. franç. Derm. Syph. **64**, 485 (1957). — GERLACH, W.: Studien über hyperergische Entzündung. Virchows Arch. path. Anat. **247**, 294 (1923). — GERMAIN, D.: Purpuras du nouveau-né. Méd. infant. **66**, 23 (1959). — GEROK, W., u. R. GROSS: Aminosäuren in normalen menschlichen Thrombocyten. Thrombos. Diathes. haemorrh. (Stuttg.) **3**, 654 (1959). — GERTENBACH, H. W., u. K. JAHNKE: Vortäuschung einer hämorrhagischen Diathese mit einem Anticoagulans. Ärztl. Wschr. **1955**, 463. — GILBOA-GARBER, N., D. NELKEN and J. GUREVITCH: The osmotic fragility of thrombocytes of laboratory animals. Experientia (Basel) **16**, 542 (1960). — GILJE, O., P. A. O'LEARY and ED. BALDES: Capillary microscopic examination in skin diseases. Arch. Derm. Syph. (Chic.) **68**, 136 (1953). — GILLY, R.: Purpura rhumatoïde. Méd. infant. **66**, 33 (1959). — GIMENO-ALFOS, L., E. O. FIELD and E. M. LEDLIE: Clinical studies with $DF^{32}P$ on the lifespan of platelets. Lancet **1959 II**, 941. — GITLIN, D., and W. H. BORGES: Studies on the metabolism of fibrinogen in two patients with congenital afibrinogenemia. Blood **8**, 679 (1953). — GLANZMANN, E.: Familiäre haemorrhagische Thrombasthenie. Jb. Kinderheilk. **88**, 1 (1918). — GLÜECK, H. J., L. WAYNE and R. GOLDSMITH: Abnormal calcium binding associated with hyperglobulinemia, clotting defects, and osteoporosis. A study of this relationship. J. Lab. clin. Med. **59** (1), 40 (1962). — GOBBI, F.: Deficit congenito di proaccelerina. Minerva med. **51**, 78 (1960). — GOBBI, F., and M. STEFANINI: Circulating anticoagulant in a patient with lupus erythematosus. Acta haemat. (Basel) **28**, 155 (1962). — GOLDECK, H., G. HERRNING u. U. RICHTER: Die 24 h-Periodik der Thrombocyten. Dtsch. med. Wschr. **75**, 702 (1950). — GOLDSTEIN, R., M. GELFAND, M. SANDERS and R. ROSEN: Anticoagulant appearing in plasma thromboplastin component deficiency. J. clin. Invest. **35**, 707 (1956). — GOLLUB, S., H. BOLTON, E. HESSERT and A. ULIN: Acquired hemophilia B. J. Amer. med. Ass. **171**, 1333 (1959). — GOLTZ, R. W., and R. A. GOOD: Benign hyperglobulinemic purpura. Relation to Mikulicz's disease, Sicca syndrome and epidermolysis bullosa dystrophica. Arch. Derm. **83**, 80 (1961). — GOOD, R. A., and L. THOMAS: Studies on the generalized Shwartzman-reaction. J. exp. Med. **96**, 625 (1952). — Studies on the generalized Shwartzmann-reaction. IV. Production of the local and generalized Sh.-reaction with heparin. J. exp. Med. **97**, 871 (1953). — GOOD, THS. A., S. F. CARNAZZO and R. A. GOOD: Thrombocytopenia and giant hemangioma in infants. Amer. J. Dis. Child. **90**, 260 (1955). — GORECZKY, L., and G. VADJA: Autoagressive thrombopenia and the megacaryocytic changes. Path. et Microbiol. (Basel) **25**, 184 (1962). — GORMSEN, J.: Thrombelastography and hypercoagulability. Acta med. scand. **170**, 313 (1961). — GOTTLIEB, M. S.: Experimental purpura. J. Immunol. **4**, 309 (1919). — GOTTLIEB, PH. M., S. STUPNIKER, H. SANDBERG and J. WOLDOW: Erythrocyte autosensitization. Amer. J. med. Sci. **233**, 196 (1957). — GOTTRON, H.: Purpura Majocchi. Arch. Derm. Syph. (Berl.) **159**, 355 (1930). — Kreislaufstörungen und Hämorrhagien der Haut. In: Haut- und Geschlechtskrankheiten von ARZT u. ZIELER, Bd. II. Wien: Urban & Schwarzenberg 1935. — Therapieschäden an der Haut. Regensburg. Jb. ärztl. Fortbild. **5**, 295 (1956). — GOTTRON, H. A., u. G. W. KORTING: Über Ablagerung körpereigener Stoffe (Amyloidosis, Calcinosis) bei Morbus Osler. Arch. klin. exp. Derm. **207**, 177 (1958). — GOUGEROT, H., et P. BLUM: Purpura angiosclèreux prurigineux avec éléments lichenoides. Bull. Soc. franç. Derm. Syph. **32**, 161 (1925). — Un nouveau cas de trisymptôme ou plutôt pentasymptôme. Bull. Soc. franç. Derm. Syph. **57**, 336 (1950). — GRABAR, P.: Die Immunoelektrophorese: Untersuchung normaler und pathologischer Komponenten des Blutes. Triangel (Basel, Sandoz) **4**, 185 (1960). — Grundbegriffe der Immunologie. In: Immunpathologie in Klinik und Forschung. Stuttgart: Georg Thieme 1961. — GRAHAM, J. B., J. A. BUCKWALTER, L. J. HARTLEY and K. M. BRINKHOUS: Canine hemophilia. J. exp. Med. **90**, 97 (1949). — GREEN, TH. W., and J. Q. EARLY: Thrombocytopenic purpura resulting from sulfisexazole (Gantrisin) therapy. J. Amer. med. Ass. **161**, 1563 (1956). — GREENSTEIN, R. H.: Hypoprothrombinemia due to propylthiouracil-therapy. J. Amer. med. Ass. **173**, 1014 (1960). — GREENWOOD, K.: Dermatitis with capillar fragility. Arch. Derm. **81**, 947 (1960). — GREIG, H. B. W.: Salicylamide purpura. S. Afr. med. J. **1955**, 269. — GRETLER, H.: Arzneimittelexanthem unter dem Bilde der Arteriolitis allergica cutis bei hochgradiger Arteriosklerose. Derm. Wschr. **15**, 369 (1960). — GROMOTKA, R., u. S. WITTE: Zur Behandlung der Thrombasthenie. Dtsch. med. Wschr. **85**, 1398 (1961). —

GROSS, P.: Lichenoid purpuric dermatitis of Gougerot and Blum. Arch. Derm. **39**, 770 (1939). — GROSS, R.: Hämorrhagische Diathesen (mit besond. Berücksichtigung der Störungen der Thrombocytopoese. Aus: Klinik der Gegenwart (Handbuch der praktischen Medizin), Bd. IX, S. 167. 1959a. — Blutgerinnungsfaktoren. Klin. Wschr. **37**, 405 (1959b). — Pathophysiologie und Klinik der Thrombocytopathien. Verh. Dtsch. Ges. inn. Med. 66. Kongr. 1960, S. 813. — Beurteilung und Behandlung von Blutungen. Internist (Berl.) **2**, 1 (1961). — Blutungen durch Mißbrauch von Cumarinen und ihre Differentialdiagnose. Med. Welt **1962**, 745. — GROSS, R., W. GEROK, G. W. LÖHR, W. VÖGELI, H. D. WALLER u. W. THEOPOLD: Über die Natur der Thrombasthenie (Thr. Glanzmann u. Naegeli). Klin. Wschr. **38**, 193 (1960). — GROSS, R., u. W. HARTL: Antistreptokinase und Streptokinaseresistenz. Klin. Wschr. **40**, 813 (1962). — GROSS, R., u. E. LECHLER: Weitere Untersuchungen über den Plättchen-Proaktivator der Fibrinolyse. Klin. Wschr. **40**, 818 (1962). — GROSS, R., G. W. LÖHR and H. D. WALLER: Zur Biochemie der Thrombocyten. 4th intern. Congr. of Biochem. London: Pergamon Press 1951, Bd. 10. — GROSS, R., H. NIETH u. E. MAMMEN: Blutungsbereitschaft und Gerinnungsstörungen bei Urämie. Klin. Wschr. **36**, 107 (1958). — GRUCHY, G. C. DE: Clinical haematology in medical practice. Oxford: Blackwell 1958. — GRUMBACH, A.: Die Infektionskrankheiten des Menschen und ihre Erreger. In: W. KIKUTH u. A. GRUMBACH, Bd. I. Stuttgart: Georg Thieme 1958. — GRUPPER, CH., MLLE. WETZLAR et J. DE BRUX: Dermite pigmentée purpurique et téléangiectasique en plaques (Cas pour diagnostic). Bull. Soc. franç. Derm. Syph. **62**, 43 (1955). — GUAY, M.: Purpura. Considérations sur l'étiologie, le diagnostic et le traitement. Laval méd. **22**, 186 (1957). — GUDGEL, ED. F., and F. H. GRAUER: Epidemic hemorrhagic fever with emphasis on dermatologic manifestations. Arch. Derm. **71**, 89 (1955). — GUGLER, E.: Angiohämophilie. Schweiz. med. Wschr. **90**, 563 (1960). — GUILAINE, J.: A propos d'un cas de maladie de Schamberg. Bull. Soc. franç. Derm. Syph. **63**, 21 (1956). — GUILLOT, M., et A. FIEHRER: Recherches sur quelques facteurs de la rétraction du caillot. I. L'action de certains facteurs physiques. Sang **28**, 196 (1957a). — Recherches sur quelques facteurs de la rétraction du caillot. II. Hypothèses sur la nature des différents facteurs de la rétraction. Sang **28**, 372 (1957b). — GUREVITCH, J., et D. NELKEN: Osmotic fragility of human blood platelets. Blood **11**, 924 (1956). — GUTHEIL, H.: Zur Purpura fulminans (Heilung bei 2 Kindern). Kinderärztl. Prax. **26**, 432 (1958).

HABERMANN: Schamberg'sche Krankheit. Zbl. Haut- u. Geschl.-Kr. **21**, 559 (1926). — HAENSCH, R.: Purpura hyperglobulinaemica (Waldenström) und andere Hyperglobulinämien mit hämorrhagischer Diathese. Hautarzt **5**, 241 (1953). — Dys- und Paraproteinämien und hämorrhagische Diathesen. Hautarzt **10**, 97 (1959). — HÄSSIG, A., S. BARANDUN u. U. STAMPFLI: Zur therapeutischen Verwendung von Plasmafraktionen. Bibl. haemat. (Basel), Fasc. 9, 42 (1958). — HÄSSIG, A., H. STIRNEMANN u. R. BÜTLER: Immunoplasmopathien. In: Immunopathologie in Klinik und Forschung (P. MIESCHER u. O. VORLAENDER), S. 270. Stuttgart: Georg Thieme 1961. — HALL, M.: Haemophilia complicated by an acquired circulating anticoagulant. Brit. J. Haemat. **7**, 340 (1961). — HAMBRICK, G. W.: Dysproteinemic purpura of the hypergammaglobulinemic type. Clinical features and differential diagnosis. Arch. Derm. **77**, 23 (1958). — HAMMER, FR.: Haemorrhagische Krankheiten. In: Handbuch der Haut- und Geschlechtskrankheiten, Bd. VI/2, S. 512. Berlin: Springer 1928. — HAMPTON, S. F.: Henoch's purpura based on food allergy. J. Allergy **12**, 579 (1941). — HANDLEY, D. A., N. S. PAINTER and M. R. P. HALL: Surgical treatment of duodenal ulceration in 2 haemophiliacs. Lancet **1961 I**, 482. — HANLON, D. G.: Some problems in the management and pathogenesis of idiopathic thrombocytopenic purpura. Proc. Mayo Clin. **27**, 273 (1952). — HANSSON, H., F. LINELL, L. R. NILSSON, L. SÖDERHJELM u. E. UNDRITZ: Die Chediak-Steinbrinck-Anomalie in Nordschweden. Folia haemat. (Lpz.) N. F. **3**, 152 (1959). — HARDERS, H.: Makroglobulinämie Waldenström, Beitrag zur Entstehung der Symptome. Dtsch. med. Wschr. **82**, 71 (1957). — Der Conjunctival-Kältetest. Eine Methode zum Studium „agglutinativer Kälteempfindlichkeit". Klin. Wschr. **36**, 74 (1958). — HARDISTY, R. M., and J. MARGOLIS: The role of Hageman factor in the initiation of blood coagulation. Brit. J. Haemat. **5**, 203 (1959). — HARDISTY, R. M., and J. L. PINNIGER: Congenital afibrinogenemia: further observations on the blood coagulation mechanism. Brit. J. Haemat. **2**, 139 (1956). — HARKAVY, J.: Vascular allergy. Pathogenesis of bronchial asthma with recurrent pulmonary infiltrations and eosinophilic polyserositis. Arch. intern. Med. **67**, 709 (1941). — Vascular allergy III. J. Allergy **14**, 507 (1943). — Cardio-vascular allergy. In: Progress in allergy, vol. III, p. 334. Basel: Karger 1952. — HARRINGTON, W. J.: Therapy of the purpuras (Symposium: The management of hematologic disorders). J. chron. Dis. **6**, 365 (1957). — HARRINGTON, W. J., V. MINNICH, J. W. HOLLINGSWORTH and C. V. MOORE: Demonstration of a thrombocytopenic factor in the blood of patients with thrombocytopenic purpura. J. Lab. clin. Med. **38**, 1 (1951/II). — HARRINGTON, W. J., C. SPRAGUE, V. MINNICH, C. V. MOORE, R. C. AULVIN and R. DUBACH: Immunologic mechanism in idiopathic and neonatal thrombocytopenic purpura. Ann. intern. Med. **38**, 433 (1953). — HARTERT, H.: Klinische Blutgerinnungsstudien mit der Thrombelastographie. Dtsch. Arch. klin. Med. **199**, 284 (1952). —

HARTMANN, J. R., and L. K. DIAMOND: Natural history of 73 patients with hemophilia and related hemorrhagic diseases. Amer. J. Dis. Child. **90**, 594 (1955). — HASSELBACK, R., R. B. MARION and J. W. THOMAS: Congenital hypofibrinogenemia in five members of a family. Canad. med. Ass. J. 88, 19 (1963). — HAYHOE, F. G. Y.: Thrombocytopenic purpura. Med. Press No 6139, 5 (1957). — HAYNES, H. A., u. A. P. ORMOND: Thrombopenische Purpura durch Bi-Arsphenamin-Sulfonat. J. Amer. med. Ass. **142**, 1066 (1950). — HEGGLIN, R.: Polyphile Reifestörung der Leucozyten und Thrombocyten. Arch. Klaus-Stift. Vererb.-Forsch. **20**, 1 (1945). — Differentialdiagnose innerer Krankheiten, 7. Aufl. Stuttgart: Georg Thieme 1960. — Persönliche Mitteilung 1962. — HEIJER, H., A. NILZÉN and E. SKOG: Drug reactions. Examination of a 5-year case series with special regard to evaluating the „thrombocytopenic" index. Acta derm.-venereol. (Stockh.) **40**, 35 (1960). — HEILMEYER, L.: Innere Medizin und Hautkrankheiten. Arch. Derm. Syph. (Berl.) **191**, 27 (1950). — HEILMEYER, L., u. H. BEGEMANN: Blut- und Blutkrankheiten. In: Handbuch der inneren Medizin, Bd. II. Berlin 1951. — HEILMEYER, L., u. L. WEISSBECKER: Funktion und Stoffwechsel der Schwermetalle. In: Handbuch der allgemeinen Pathologie (BÜCHNER-LETTERER-ROULET), Bd. IV/2. Springer 1957. — HEINI, P., u. I. KRAUS: Angeborene familiäre Gerinnungsstörung durch heparinartigen Hemmkörper. Klin. Wschr. **34**, 747 (1956). — HEINILD, S.: Purpura fulminans (streptococcal sepsis). Acta paediat. (Uppsala) **34**, 147 (1947). — HEINLEIN, H., W. VOLLAND u. K. VOGEL: Beitrag zur Nosologie und Pathogenese der Periarteriitis nodosa. Z. Kreisl.-Forsch. **50**, 849 (1961). — HELD, E.: Hämorrhagische Diathese mit Fibrinmangel in der Geburtshilfe. Schweiz. med. Wschr. **86**, 241 (1956). — HEMMELER, G.: Thrombopathie familiale. Schweiz. med. Wschr. 88, 1018 (1958). — HENNEMANN, H. H., u. B. WIESNER: Bedeutung und Interpretation des Tierversuchs zum Nachweis eines antithrombocytären Faktors bei „idiopathischer" thrombopenischer Purpura. Folia haemat. (Lpz.) **75**, 541 (1958). — HENOCH, E. H.: Über den Zusammenhang von Purpura und Intestinalstörungen. Klin. Wschr. **5**, 517 (1868). — Über eine eigentümliche Form von Purpura. Klin. Wschr. **11**, 641 (1874). — HENSTELL, H. H., and M. KLIGERMANN: Hyperglobulinaemic thrombohaemorrhagic diathesis. Nature (Lond.) **183**, 978 (1959). — HERMANSKY, F., et S. DEJMAL: Anticoagulant familial à activité antithromboplastique. Rev. Hémat. **14**, 12 (1959). — HERMANSKY, F., and P. PUDLAK: Albinism associated with hemorrhagic diathesis and unusual pigmented reticular cells in bone marrow: report of 2 cases with histochemical studies. Blood **14**, 162 (1959). — HERRMANN, W. P.: Immunoelektrophorese und ihre Anwendung in der Dermatologie. Arch. klin. exp. Derm. **212**, 88 (1960a). — Immunoelektrische Untersuchungen an Hautkrankheiten III. u. a. Purpuraformen. Arch. klin. exp. Derm. **212** (5), 452 (1960b). — HERZBERG, J. J., u. K. H. SCHULZ: Tuberkulöse Vasculitis unter dem Bilde einer Livedo racemosa. Hautarzt **7**, 442 (1956). — HESS, D.: Über die Ausreifungszeit der Thrombocyten. Diss. Zürich 1958. — HILL, J. M., and R. J. SPEER: Combined hemophilia and PTC-deficiency. Blood **10**, 357 (1955). — HIPPEL, E. VON: Angiomatosis. Albrecht v. Graefes Arch. Ophthal. **118**, 348 (1927). — HIRAMATSU, N.: Studies on „vitamin P" (Hesperidin). III. The effect of hesperidin upon experimental purpura in guinea pigs. Bibl. Sci. industr. Rep. **10**, 204 (1948). — HIRSCH, E. O., and E. DAMESHEK: Idiopathic thrombocytopenia. Review of 89 cases with particular reference to the differentiation and treatment of acute and chronic types. Arch. intern. Med. 88, 701 (1951). — HIRSCH, E. O., and F. H. GARDNER: The transfusion of human blood platelets. With a note on the transfusion of granulocytes. J. Lab. clin. Med. **39**, 556 (1952). — HITTMAIR, A.: Das Blutplättchen. Med. Welt **12**, 1091, 1128 (1938). — Bedeutung der Milz für Genese der Thrombopathien in „Hämorrhagische Diathesen". Internat. Symposium. Wien: Springer 1955, S. 33. — HITZIG, W. H.: Praktische und theoretische Ergebnisse neuerer Bluteiweißuntersuchungen. Schweiz. med. Wschr. **90**, 1449 (1960). — HITZIG, W. H., u. W. ZOLLINGER: Kongenitaler Faktor VII-Mangel: Familienuntersuchungen und physiologische Studien über Faktor VII. Helv. paediat. Acta **13**, 189 (1958). — HJORT, P. F.: Intermediate reactions in the coagulation of blood with tissue thromboplastin. Scand. J. clin. Lab. Invest. **9**, Suppl. 27 (1957). — HOAG, M. S., P. M. AGGELER and A. H. FOWELL: Disappearance rate of concentrated proconvertin extracts in congenital and acquired hypoproconvertinemia. J. clin. Invest. **39**, 554 (1960). — HODGSON, G. A., and F. F. HELLIER: Dermatitis caused by shirts in B.L.A. J. roy. Army med. Cps **87** (3), 110 (1946). — HOEFER, W.: Maligne Thrombopenie nach Lymphadenosis benigna cutis. Z. Haut- u. Geschl.-Kr. **17**, 368 (1954). — HÖRDER, W.: Isolierter Faktor V-Mangel, bedingt durch einen spezifischen Antikörper. Acta haemat. (Basel) **13**, 235 (1955). — Therapeutische Möglichkeiten bei hämorrhagischen Diathesen unter besonderer Berücksichtigung der Blutgerinnungsstörungen. Münch. med. Wschr. **1957**, 666. — Differentialdiagnose des kongenitalen Stuart-Faktor-Mangels. Klin. Wschr. **37**, 443 (1959). — HÖRDER, W., u. V. HIEMEYER: Die Diagnostik schwerer, mittelschwerer und leichter Formen der Haemophilie A. Dtsch. med. Wschr. **85**, 541 (1960). — HÖRDER, W., u. G. SOKAL: Inhibitorstudie bei familiärem Faktor V-Mangel. Acta haemat. (Basel) **14**, 65 (1955). — HOIGNÉ, R.: Über die Veränderungen von Blutgerinnungsfaktoren, Thrombocyten und Leukocyten im anaphylaktischen Schock, beim

Arthus-Phänomen und beim Sanarelli-Shwartzman-Phänomen. Diss. Zürich 1951. — Allergien gegen Nahrungsmittel. Mkurse ärztl. Fortbild. **10**, 551 (1960). — HOIGNÉ, R., P. FLÜCKIGER, J. FLÜCKIGER u. H. STORCK: Thrombocytentest „in vitro" bei medikamentösen Allergien. Int. Arch. Allergy **5**, 50 (1954). — HOIGNÉ, R., P. FLÜCKIGER J. FLÜCKIGER, H. STORCK u. F. KOLLER: Über die Bedeutung der Thrombocyten bei allergischen Vorgängen. Schweiz. med. Wschr. **84**, 1168 (1954). — HOIGNÉ, R., P. FLÜCKIGER, P. SCHMUZIGER and M. MUMENTHALER: The detection of the sensitizing substance in cases with acute thrombopenic purpura by new „in vitro" methods. Acta haemat. (Basel) **17**, 24 (1957). — HOIGNÉ, R., H. FREI u. H. STORCK: Über die Bedeutung der Thrombocyten bei allergischen Vorgängen. III. Mitt. Tierexperimentelle Untersuchungen zur Frage des Antikörpergehaltes der Thrombocyten. Schweiz. med. Wschr. **83**, 721 (1953). — HOIGNÉ, R., F. KOLLER u. H. STORCK: Die Beeinflussung des experimentellen Shwartzman-Phänomens durch ACTH. Dermatologica (Basel) **103**, 234 (1951). — HOIGNÉ, R., A. LOELIGER, L. MORANDI u. P. FLÜCKIGER: Thrombocytopenische Purpura bei drei Fällen von medikamentöser Allergie. Bull. schweiz. Akad. med. Wiss. **10**, 438 (1954). — HOIGNÉ, R., u. H. STORCK: Über die Bedeutung der Thrombocyten bei allergischen Vorgängen (II. Mitt. Thromb.-Agglutination im Pat.-Blut nach Zugabe von Allergen). Schweiz. med. Wschr. **83**, 31 (1953). — HOLEMANS, R., u. R. GROSS: Experimentelle Untersuchung der Fibrinolyse mittels Thrombelastographie. Acta haemat. (Basel) **26**, 110 (1961). — HOLST, A., u. TH. FRÖLICH: Skorbut. Norsk Mag. Laegevidensk. **68**, 721 (1907); **71**, 209 (1910). Z. Hyg. Infekt.-Kr. **72**, 1 (1912); **75**, 334 (1913). — HOLSTEIN, J.: Besondere Befunde von Blutungsfolgen im Röntgenbild der Hämophilie. Dtsch. Gesundh.-Wes. **16**, 1330 (1961). — HOLTER, H.: How things get into cells. Sci. Amer. 167, Sept. (1961). — HOLUB, K.: Hirnblutung und Blutgerinnungsstörung. Zbl. Chir. **87** (3), 121 (1962). — HOLZMANN, H., u. G. W. KORTING: Labiler Hypertonus und Manifestationsrhythmus einer chron.-thrombocytopenischen Purpura. Arch. klin. exp. Derm. **208**, 502 (1959). — HONG, R., W. K. SCHUBERT, E. V. PERRIN and C. D. WEST: Antibody deficiency syndrome associated with beta$_2$-macrobulinemia. J. Pediat. **61**, 831 (1962). — HOPE, R. E., L. G. MACNAMARA and R. MANGOLD: A virus-induced epizootic hemorrhagic disease of the Virginia white-tailed deer (Odocoileus virginianus). J. exp. Med. **111**, 155 (1960). — HORLER, R., and S. C. TRUELOVE: Chronic leg ulcers in nonthrombocytopenic purpura. Brit. med. J. **1955 I**, 633. — HOROWITZ, H. I., B. SHAPIRO and I. L. RUBIN: Athrombocytopenic purpura caused by chlorothiazide. N.Y. St. J. Med. **59** (6), 1117 (1959). — HORST, R. L. VAN DER: Purpura fulminans in a newborn baby. Arch. Dis. Childh. **37**, 194, 436 (1962). — HOUGIE, C.: A simple assay method for factor X (Stuart Prower Factor). Proc. Soc. exp. Biol. (N.Y.) **109**, 754 (1962). — HOUGIE, C., and J. B. GRAHAM: The blood clotting role and mode of inheritance of the Stuart factor, VIth Congr. int. Soc. Blood Transf. Boston 1956. — HSIA, D. Y. Y.: Inborn errors of metabolism. Chicago: Year Book Publ. 1959. — HUBLER, W. R., and E. W. NETHERTON: Cutaneous manifestations of monocytic leukemia. Arch. Derm. Syph. (Chic.) **50**, 70 (1947). — HUGUES, J.: Agglutination précoce des plaquettes au cours de la formation du clou hémostatique. Thrombos. Diathes. haemorrh. (Stuttg.) **3**, 177 (1959). — HUMBLE, G. J.: The mechanism of petechial hemorrhage formation. Blood **4**, 69 (1949). — HUMPHREY, I. H.: Mechanisms of Arthus reactions; role of polymorphonuclear leucocytes and other factors in reversed passive Arthus reactions in rabbits. Brit. J. exp. Path. **36**, 268, 285 (1955). — The immediate allergic and the Arthus phenomenon in immunopathology, p. 215. Basel: Benno Schwabe 1959. — HUNT, J. C., M. W. ANDERSON and D. G. HANLON: Hemorrhagic diathesis related to quinidine therapy. Proc. Mayo Clin. **33**, 87 (1958). — HUNTLEY, C. C., and S. C. DEES: Eczema associated with thrombocyteopenic purpura and purulent otitis media. Report of five fatal cases. Pediatrics **19**, 351 (1957). — HURIEZ, CL., F. DESMONS, P. AGACHE, M. BENOIT et J. P. DUPUIS: Discussion d'un aspect de purpura familial. Syndrome de Thomson? Arch. belges Derm. **17** (2), 161 (1961). — HURIEZ, CL., F. DESMONS et P. H. PELCÉ: Le purpura de la phénylbutazone (à propos de 4 observations). Bull. Soc. franç. Derm. Syph. **62**, 323 (1955). — HUTCHINSON, J.: A peculiar form of serpiginous and infective naevoid disease. Arch. Surg. (Lond.) **1**, 275 (1889). — A peculiar form of serpiginous disease. Arch. Surg. (Lond.) **2**, 71 (1890). — HY, R., et H. LAMOTTE: Sur un nouveau cas d'allergides nodulaires de Gougerot. Sem. Hôp. Paris **35**, 570 (1959).

IATRIDIS, S. G., and J. H. FERGUSON: Effect of surface and Hageman factor on the endogenous or spontaneous activation of the fibrinolytic system. Thrombos. Diathes. haemorrh. (Stuttg.) **6**, 411 (1961). — Active Hageman factor: a plasma lysokinase of the human fibrinolytic system. J. clin. Invest. **41**, 1277 (1962). — IIJIMA, S.: Die Gefäßreaktion des Kaninchenohrs bei Parallergie im intravitalen Photogramm. Beitr. path. Anat. **98**, 241 (1958). — Die Durchblutungsstörungen am Kaninchenohr bei allgemeiner und lokaler Anaphylaxie mit intravitalen Photogrammen. Beitr. path. Anat. **118**, 67 (1958). — IKKALA, E., and H. R. NEVANLINNA: Congenital deficiency of fibrin stabilising factor. Thrombos. Diathes. haemorrh. (Stuttg.) **7**, 567 (1962). — IKKALA, E., H. R. NEVANLINNA and K. A. SOLONEN: The treatment of hemophilia. Duodecim (Helsinki) **74**, 634 (1958). — Haemophilia. Scand. J. clin. Lab.

Invest. **12**, 1 (1960). — ILLIG, L.: Physiologie und Pathophysiologie des Capillarbettes. In: Angiologie von M. RATSCHOW, S. 124. Stuttgart: Georg Thieme 1959. — Störungen des Capillarkreislaufs: die spontane Blutstillung. In: Die terminale Strombahn. Berlin-Göttingen-Heidelberg: Springer 1961. — ILLIG, L., u. H. W. WEBER: Zur Entstehung, Benennung und Einteilung der örtlichen Kreislaufstörungen. Klin. Wschr. **36**, 183 (1958). — IMERSLUND, O.: Familiaere hemorragisk diateser med forlenget blødningstid. Nord. Med. **42**, 1191 (1949). — IMHOF, J. W., H. BAARS and M. C. VERLOOP: Clinical and haematological aspects of macroglobulinaemia Waldenström. Acta med. scand. **163**, 349 (1959). — INGLIS, J. A., and J. W. HALLIDAY: Thromboplastic activity of red cells. Nature (Lond.) **191**, 821 (1961). — INNELLA, F., and W. J. REDNER: Variations in prothrombin times caused by different thromboplastin reagents. Amer. J. clin. Path. **33**, 14 (1960). — ISLIKER, H.: Zur Chemie der Makroglobuline. Helv. med. Acta. **25**, 41 (1958). — ISRAEL, L., G. MATHÉ et J. BERNARD: Sur le syndrome de Schönlein-Henoch. Reproduction expérimentale par un immunosérum. 2. Test décelant le pouvoir capillarotoxique de l'immunosérum et du sérum de malades. Rev. franc. Étud. clin. biol. **1**, 57 (1956). — ISRAELS, M. C. G., H. LEMPERT and E. GILBERTSON: Hemophilia in a female. Lancet **1961 I**, 1375. — IVERSON, T., and P. BASTRUP-MADSEN: Congenital familial deficiency of factor V combined with deficiency in AHG. Brit. J. Haemat. **2**, 265 (1956).

JADASSOHN, W., et R. PAILLARD: Purpura de Schönlein-Henoch et purpura hyperglobulinémique. Dermatologica (Basel) **110**, 355 (1955). — JAKOB, J.: Blutungen bei Antikoagulantien-Therapie. Diss. Zürich 1953. — JAMES, D. H., and A. H. TUTTLE: Congenital hemangioma with thrombocytopenia. J. Pediat. **59**, 235 (1961). — JANSEN, L. H.: The so-called „dyskeratosis congenita". Dermatologica (Basel) **103**, 167 (1950). — JASPERS, K.: Allgemeine Psychopathologie, 6. Aufl. Berlin-Göttingen-Heidelberg: Springer 1953. — JASTREMSKI, B., and J. C. HOYT: Fulminating purpuric meningococcemia. U.S. Army Forces med. J. **3**, 769 (1952). — JENEY, A. VON, u. E. TÖRÖ: Die Wirkung der Askorbinsäure auf die Faserbildung in Fibroblastkulturen. Virchows Arch. path. Anat. **298** (1) (1938). — JENSEN, B.: Schönlein-Henoch-Purpura. 3 cases with fish or penicillin as antigen. Acta med. scand. **152**, 61 (1955). — JOBÉ, H.: Beitrag zur Behandlung von Kapillarbrüchigkeit mit Ascorbinsäure und Rutin. Praxis **43** (7) (1954). — JOHNSON, S. A., R. W. MONTO, J. L. MCKENNA and M. K. BUSCAGLIA: Conditions determining and products of prothrombin activation in serum. Amer. J. Physiol. **203**, 299 (1962). — JONES, J. H., C. R. RIZZA, R. M. HARDISTY, K. M. DORMANDY and J. C. MACPHERSON: Combined deficiency of factor V and factor VIII (antihaemophilic globulin). Brit. J. Haemat. **8**, 120 (1962). — JONES, T. G., K. L. G. GOLDSMITH and I. M. ANDERSON: Maternal and neonatal platelet antibodies in a case of congenital thrombocytopenia. Lancet **1961 II**, 1008. — JOSEPHSON, A. M., and R. LISKER: Demonstration of a circulating anticoagulant in PTA-deficiency. J. clin. Invest. **37**, 148 (1958). — JOSSO, F., O. PROU-WARTELLE et J. P. SOULIER: Etude d'un cas d'hypoprothrombinémie congénitale. Rev. Hémat. **2**, 647 (1962). — JUCKER, A.: Untersuchungen über die Resorption der Thrombokinase im Tierversuch bei subkutaner und i.m. Verabreichung. Diss. Bern 1960. — JÜRGENS, H.: Leukämie und Schwangerschaft. Zbl. Gynäk. **62**, 1886 (1938). — JÜRGENS, J.: Über die Ursache der Blutungsneigung bei der Makroglobulinaemie Waldenström. Verh. dtsch. Ges. inn. Med. **62**, 265 (1956). — JÜRGENS, J., u. F. K. BELLER: Klinische Methoden der Blutgerinnungsanalyse. Stuttgart: Georg Thieme 1960. — JÜRGENS, R.: Hämorrhagische Diathesen. Schweiz. med. Wschr. **79**, 817 (1949). — Pathophysiologie und Klinik der Thrombopathien. In: JÜRGENS u. DEUTSCH, Hämorrhagische Diathesen. Intern. Symposion. Wien: Springer 1955, S. 4. — Hereditäre Thrombopathien. 5. Kongr. Europ. Ges. Hämatol. 1955. Wien: Springer 1956, S. 396. — JÜRGENS, R., W. LEHMANN, O. WEGELIUS, A. E. ERIKSON u. E. HIEPLER: Mitteilung über den Mangel an AHG (Faktor VIII) bei der Aland-Thrombopathie. Thrombos. Diathes. haemorrh. (Stuttg.) **1**, 257 (1957). — JUNG, E. G.: A rapid quantitative assay of factor VIII (AHG) without the use of haemophilia A plasma. Thrombos. Diathes. haemorrh. (Stuttg.) **4**, 323 (1960). — The relative frequency of haemophilia A and B. Thrombos. Diathes. haemorrh. (Stuttg.) **4**, 331 (1960). — JUNG, E. G., u. F. DUCKERT: Wirkung von Plasmin (Fibrinolysin) auf die Gerinnungsfaktoren. Schweiz. med. Wschr. **90**, 1239 (1960). — JUNG, E. G., F. DUCKERT u. P. G. FRICK: Autoimmunes Antithromboplastin. Schweiz. med. Wschr. **91**, 419 (1961). — JUNG, H. D.: Schwere neosalvarsanbedingte thrombopenische Purpura unter dem Bilde des Morbus Werlhof, geheilt durch Periston N. Hautarzt **6**, 412 (1955).

KABAT, E. A., and H. LANDAU: A quantitative study of passive anaphylaxis in the guinea pig. J. Immunol. **44**, 69 (1942). — KÄMMERER, H., u. H. MICHEL: Allergische Diathese und allergische Erkrankungen. München: J. F. Bergmann 1956. — KAHN, I. S.: Henoch's purpura due to food allergy. J. Lab. clin. Med. **14**, 835 (1929). — KALINOWSKI, S. Z., and J. M. WALKER: Thrombocytopenic purpura in tuberculosis. Brit. J. Tuberc. **50**, 239 (1956). — KALKOFF, K. W.: Zur Unterscheidung verschiedener Purpuraformen auf Grund morphologischer Kriterien mit besonderer Berücksichtigung der Purpura pigmentosa progressiva.

Münch. med. Wschr. **101**, 14 (1959). — Hämorrhagien der Haut und ihre Bedeutung für die Differentialdiagnose von Blutungskrankheiten. In: Fortschritte praktischer Dermatologie und Venerologie, Bd. 4, S. 179. Berlin-Göttingen-Heidelberg: Springer 1962. — KANZOW, U.: Die nosologische Stellung der Makroglobulinämie Waldenström. 5. Kongr. Europ. Ges. Hämat. 1956, S. 633. — KANZOW, U., G. FRANKEN u. F. KUHN: Differenzierung der Paraproteine beim Plasmazytom und der Makroglobulinämie Waldenström. Dtsch. med. Wschr. **86**, 2437 (1961). — KAPLAN, E.: Congenital und neonatal thrombocytopenic purpura. J. Pediat. **54**, 644 (1959). — KAPPELER, R., A. KREBS u. G. RIVA: Klinik der Makroglobulinämie Waldenström. Helv. med. Acta **25**, 54 (1958). — KARLSON, P.: Kurzes Lehrbuch der Biochemie für Mediziner und Naturwissenschaftler, S. 56. Stuttgart: Georg Thieme 1962. — KARSNER, H. T., and A. R. MARITZ: Pathologic histology of the Shwartzman phenomenon with interpretative comments. J. exp. Med. **60**, 37 (1934). — KASABACH, H. H., and K. K. MERRITT: Capillary hemangioma with extensive purpura. Amer. J. Dis. Child. **1**, 1063 (1940). — KATSURA, H.: Untersuchungen über die experimentelle Purpura hemorrhagica beim Meerschweinchen, verursacht durch Hämangioendotheliotoxin. Trans. Jap. path. Soc. **14**, 152 (1924). — KAULLA, K. N. VON, u. E. VON KAULLA: Spontane Schwankungen der Gerinnbarkeit menschlichen Blutes in vivo. Med. Welt **1961**, 1850. — KAUNITZ, H., D. C. MALINS and D. MCKAY: Studies of the generalized Shwartzman reaction produced by diet. II. Feeding of fractions of oxidized cod liver oil. J. exp. Med. **115** (6), 1127 (1962). — KAYE, B. M., and F. X. DUFAULT: Idiopathic thrombocytopenic purpura and pregnancy. Obstet. and Gynec. **9**, 228 (1957). — KAYE, B. M., J. L. GRAZIANO and B. V. REANEY: New adjunctive therapy in purpura in the female. Amer. J. Obstet. Gynec. **82**, 1221 (1961). — KAZNELSON, P.: Verschwinden der hämorrhagischen Diathese bei einem Fall von essentieller Thrombopenie nach Milzexstirpation. Wien. klin. Wschr. **29**, 1051 (1916). — KEINING, E.: Auswirkungen peripherer Durchblutungsstörungen auf das klinische Bild der Kälteschädigungen und das Verhalten infektiöser Hautprozesse. Derm. Wschr. **125**, 543 (1952). — KELLER, F.: Vitamin K und seine klinische Bedeutung. Leipzig: Georg Thieme 1941 u. Helv. med. Acta **11**, 55 (1944). — KENDALL, A. G., L. LÖWENSTEIN and R. O. MORGEN: The hemorrhagic diathesis in renal disease (with special reference to acute uremia). Canad. med. Ass. J. **85**, 405 (1961). — KIENLE, F.: Intravitale Knochenmarkuntersuchungen durch Sternalpunktion bei essentieller Thrombopenie (M. Werlhof). Folia haemat. (Lpz.) **66**, 299 (1942). — KILDEBERG, P.: Aldrich-Syndrome. Pediatrics **27**, 362 (1961). — KINDERMANN, A.: Vasculäres Allergid nach Butalidon und Gefahren kombinierter Anwendung mit Athrombon (Phenylindandion). Derm. Wschr. **143**, 172 (1961). — KINGSLEY, C. S.: Familial factor V deficiency, the pattern of heredity. Quart. J. Med. **23**, 323 (1954). — KINNEY, V. R., A. M. OLSEN, N. G. G. HEPPER and E. G. HARRISON jr.: Wegener's granulomatosis. Report of 2 cases and brief review. Arch. intern. Med. **108**, 269 (1961). — KINT, A.: Les manifestations cutanées de la maladie de Kahler. Arch. belges Derm. **17**, 148 (1961). — KIRCHMAIER, H.: Thrombopenie unter Doriden-Medikation. Med. Klin. **1958 II**, 1683. — KISSMEYER-NIELSEN, F.: Thrombocytopenic purpura following quinine medication. Acta med. scand. **154**, 289 (1956). — KLEINMANS, M.: Pseudo-hémophilie par anticoagulant. Nouv. Rev. franç. Hémat. **1**, 527 (1961). — KLEINSORGE, H., u. G. KLUMBIES: Psychogene Hautreaktionen. Wiss. Z. Univ. Jena **4** (1955). — KLIMA, R.: Zur Pathophysiologie und Klinik hämorrhagischer Diathesen ohne Gerinnungsstörungen in „Hämorrhagische Diathesen“. Intern. Symposium. Wien: Springer 1955. — KLINGMÜLLER, G., A. LEINBROCK u. U. LAUMANNS: Pemphigus vulgaris mit Hemmkörperhämophilie. Hautarzt **7**, 200 (1956). — KLUG, H.: Über die Ursache der Teleangiektasien bei Lebercirrhose und Morbus Osler. Wien. Z. inn. Med. **30** (1949). — KNEPPER, R.: Über die Lokalisierung der experimentellen allergischen Hyperergie. Virchows Arch. path. Anat. **296**, 364 (1936). — KNOTH, W., u. W. MEYHÖFER: Beitrag zum Formenkreis der Periarteriitis nodosa und zur Bewertung der Riesenzellen bei Gefäßerkrankungen. Dermatologica (Basel) **119**, 1 (1959). — KÖNIG, Dr.: Purpura fulminans bei einem 19monatigen Kinde. Z. Kinderheilk. **32**, 282 (1922). — KOLLER, F.: Vitamin K und seine klinische Bedeutung, Leipzig: Georg Thieme 1941. — Die Klinik der hämorrhagischen Diathesen. Verh. dtsch. Ges. inn. Med. 58. Kongr. 1952, S. 508. — Is hemophilia a nosologic entity? Blood **9**, 286 (1954). — Klinik und Therapie der plasmatisch bedingten hämorrhagischen Diathesen. In: Hämorrhagische Diathese. Internat. Kongr. Wien: Springer 1955. — Der heutige Stand der Gerinnungsforschung. Thrombos. Diathes. haemorrh. (Stuttg.) **2**, 407 (1958a). — Importance of coagulopathia for genetics in general. Proc. 7th Internat. Congr. Soc. Hemat. Rom 1958b, Pensiero scientifico, S. 170. — Das Verhalten der Gerinnungsfaktoren in vitro und in vivo. Proc. 7. Congr. Internat. Soc. Blood transf. 1958c, Basel: Karger, S. 731. — Die Pathogenese der Thrombose und ihre therapeutische Konsequenzen. Dtsch. med. Wschr. **86**, 1793 (1961a). — La conception actuelle de la coagulation du sang. J. Physiol. (Paris) **53**, 131 (1961b). — KOLLER, F., u. Y. BOUNAMEAUX: Hämorrhagische Diathese nach Splen ektomie. Bull. schweiz. Akad. med. Wiss. **12**, 248 (1956). — KOLLER, F., C. GASSER, G. KRÜSI u. G. DE MURALT: Purpura fulminans nach Scharlach mit Faktor V-Mangel und Antithrom binüberschuß. Acta haemat. (Basel) **4**, 33 (1950). — KOLLER, F., G. KRÜSI u. P. LUCHSINGER: Über eine besondere Form der hämorrhagischen Diathese. Schweiz. med. Wschr. **80**, 1101 (1950). — KOLLER, F., A. LOELIGER and F. DUCKERT: Experiments on a new clotting factor (factor VII). Acta haemat. (Basel) **6**, 1 (1951). — KOLLER, F., A. LOELIGER, F. DUCKERT u. H. HU-WANG: Über einen neuen Gerinnungsfaktor (Faktor VII) und seine klinische Bedeutung. Dtsch. med. Wschr. **72**, 528 (1952). — KORNFELD, M.: Mikroangiopathia thrombotica (Thrombotische thrombocytopenische Purpura). Med. Klin. **53** (II), 1375 (1958). — KORSAN-BENGTSEN, K., P. F. HJORT and J. YGGE: Acquired factor X deficiency in a patient with amyloidosis. Thrombos. Diathes. haemorrh. (Stuttg.) **7**, 558 (1962). — KORTING, G. W.: Fehlbildungen der Haut (Ehlers-Danlos cutis laxa). In: Handbuch der Haut- und Geschlechtskrankheiten, Erg.-Bd. III/1, S. 413. Berlin-Göttingen-Heidelberg: Springer 1963. — KORTING, G. W., u. W. ADAM: Purpura Schönlein und Lebercirrhose in ihrer Abgrenzung von der Purpura hyperglobulinaemica. Derm. Wschr. **131**, 121 (1955). — KORTING, G. W., F. K. BELLER u. G. KÖPPEL: Schönlein-artiges Exanthem mit eigentümlicher Störung der Blutkuchenretraktion. Arch. klin. exp. Derm. **205**, 389 (1957). — KORTING, G. W., u. G. BREHM: Purpura hyperglobulinaemica mit positivem Coombs-Test. Arch. klin. exp. Derm. **202**, 449 (1956). — KORTING, G. W., u. H. EISSNER: Beitrag zur teleangiektatischen und purpurischen Erscheinungsformen des Erythema centrifugum anulare (Typ Gougerot & Patte). Derm. Wschr. **138**, 854 (1958). — KOSAKA, S., S. YAMADA, J. TERASHIMA, A. BEPPU, S. MAEGAWE, K. IZUCHI and M. ISOMURA: A family of haemorrhagic diathesis with combined deficiency of AHG and PTC. Res. Pap. blood coagul. Jap. (1960). — KOSZEWSKI, B. J., and T. F. HUBBARD: Congenital anaemia in hereditary ectodermal dysplasia. Arch. Derm. **74**, 159 (1956). — KRAMAR, J.: Stress and capillary resistence (Capillar fragility). Amer. J. Physiol. **175**, 69 (1953). — KRESBACH, H.: Postgrippöse Vasculitis „allergica“ unter dem Bild der Purpura necroticans mit Nierenbeteiligung. Arch. klin. exp. Derm. **209**, 30 (1959). — KRIVIT, W., and R. A. GOOD: Aldrich's syndrome (thrombocytopenia, eczema and infection in infants). Amer. J. Dis. Child. **97**, 137 (1959). — KRÖBER, K. H.: Purpura haemorrhagica als Nebenerscheinung bei der INH-Medikation. Tuberk.-Arzt **9**, 394 (1955). — KROGH, A., and G. A. HARROP: Studies on the physiology of capillaries. J. Physiol. (Lond.) **125**, 54 (1921). — KRÜGER, H.: Das Trisymptom von Gougerot im Rahmen der allergischen Vasculitis. Arch. klin. exp. Derm. **213**, 496 (1961). — KRUG, K., u. P. WELLER: Beitrag zur Diagnostik und therapeutischen Beeinflußbarkeit von Thrombocytenantikörpern bei idiopathisch-thrombopenischer Purpura. Folia haemat. (Lpz.) **77**, 79 (1960). — KRUIZINGA, E. E.: Adalin-Toxicodermie unter dem Bilde einer Dermatitis „lichenoïde purpurique et pigmentée“ (Gougerot-Blum). Ned. T. Geneesk **1950**, 1258. — KÜMMERLE, H. P., A. SENN, P. RENTCHNICK u. N. GOOSSENS: Klinik und Therapie der Nebenwirkungen. Stuttgart: Georg Thieme 1960. — KÜNZER, W., u. B. KÄMMERER: Zur Erstmanifestation der Hämophilie im Kindesalter. Münch. med. Wschr. **104**, (II), 2381 (1962). — KUGELMASS, I. N.: Thrombocytopenic purpura induced by pertussis toxin in allergic children. J. Amer. med. Ass. **107**, 2120 (1936). — KUHN, E.: Bemerkung zur Arbeit von G. W. KORTING u. G. BREHM über Purpura hyperglobulinaemica mit positivem Coombs-Test. Arch. klin. exp. Derm. **203**, 368 (1956). — KUPFER, H. G., B. L. HANNA and D. R. KINNE: Congenital factor VII deficiency with normal Stuart activity. Blood **15**, 146 (1960). — KUTSCHERA-AICHBERGEN, H.: Beitrag zum Waterhouse-Friderichsen-Syndrom. Z. Kinderheilk. **4**, 380 (1959).

LABHART, A.: Die Nebennierenrinde. In: Klinik der inneren Sekretion, S. 349. Berlin-Göttingen-Heidelberg: Springer 1957. — LA CHAPELLE, A. DE, E. IKKALA and H. R. NEVANLINNA: Haemophia A in a girl. Lancet **1961 II**, 578. — LAKI, K., and L. LORAND: On the solubility of fibrin clots. Science **108**, 280 (1948). — The clotting of fibrinogen. Sci. Amer. **206**, 60 (März 1962). — LANDBECK, G., u. P. HUATAVIKUL: Über die Thrombocytenfaktor 3-Aktivitätsminderung bei der Thrombopathie. Klin. Wschr. **37**, 227 (1959). — Zum Thema „Klinik und Therapie der Mastocytose“. Arch. klin. exp. Derm. **213**, 651 (1961). — LANDSBERGER, M.: Ein Fall von Kuhmilchintoleranz beim Säugling mit Purpura. Z. Kinderheilk. **39**, 569 (1925). — LAPIÈRE, S., MME. MATHUS et MME. JIJAKLI: Les dysglobulinémies en dermatologie. Laval méd. **34**, 675 (1963). — LARGIADÈR, F.: Haemophilieprobleme in Stomato- und Laryngologie. Pract. oto-rhino-laryng. (Basel) **24**, 239 (1962). — LARRIEU, M. J., J. CAEN, J. C. LELONG et J. BERNARD: Maladie de Glanzmann. Etude clin., biol. et pathogénique à propos de 5 observations. Nouv. Rev. franç. Hémat. **1** (5), 662 (1961). — LARRIEU, M. J., et J. P. SOULIER: Déficit en facteur antihémophilique A chez une fille, associé à un trouble du saignement. Rev. Hémat. 8, 361 (1953). — LASCH, H. G., H. HARTERT, K. SCHIMPF u. H. H. SESSNER: Über hepatogene Blutungen. Dtsch. Arch. klin. Med. **203**, 52 (1956). — LATALLO, Z., S. NIEWIAROWSKI and I. SABLINSKI: Studies on hemophilia in Poland. Pol. Tyg. lek. **14**, 3 (1959). — LAURELL, A. B., and I. M. NILSSON: Hypergammaglobulinemia, circulating anticoagulant and biologic false Wassermann-reaction. J. Lab. clin. Med. **49**, 694 (1957). — LAWRENZE, H. SH.: Cellular and humoral aspects of the hypersensitive states. New Yrok: Hoepner-Harper Books 1959. — LAZAROU, P.:

Prothrombine et les troubles hémorrhagiques chez les tuberculeux (à propos de 997 malades). Acta tuberc. scand. **39** (40), 251 (1960/61). — LECOMTE, J., et Y. BOUNAMEAUX: Action des antihistaminiques de synthèse et des anesthésiques locaux sur le purpura cutané provoqué par l'huile de croton. Acta allerg. (Kbh.) **9**, 27 (1955). — LECOMTE, J., Y. BOUNAMEAUX et H. VAN CAUWENBERGE: Etude du purpura cutané provoqué par l'huile de croton. Rev. belge Path. **27**, 195 (1960). — LE COULANT, P., L. TEXIER et J. MALEVILLE: Dermite purpurique et pigmentée papuloïde et réticulée, lentement extensive et généralisée (à propos de 2 cas). Ann. Derm. Syph. (Paris) **87**, 493 (1960). — LEDINGHAM, J. C.: The experimental production of purpura in animals by the introduction of anti-blood-platelet-sera. Lancet **1914I**, 1673. — LEDINGHAM, J. C., and S. P. BEDSON: Experimental purpura. Lancet **1915I**, 311. — LEE, L.: Reticuloendothelial clearance of circulating fibrin in the pathogenesis of the generalized Shwartzman reaction. J. exp. Med. **115**, 1065 (1962). — LEE, R. E., D. GOEBEL and L. A. FULTON: Anatomical and functional changes in the peripheral vascular system during certain induced increase in vascular fragility. Ann. N.Y. Acad. Sci. **61**, 665 (1955). — LEHMANN, W.: Bemerkung zur Genetik der haemorrhagischen Diathesen, S. 114. Wien: Springer 1955. — Zur Frage der Nomenklatur bei hämophilieähnlichen hämorrhagischen Diathesen. Medizinische **1958**, 598. — LENGGENHAGER, K.: Eine neue einfachste Plättchenzählmethode. Schweiz. med. Wschr. **1936**, 1289. — LEÖVEY, A., u. K. VEZEKÉNYI: Gemeinsames Vorkommen von Morbus Schamberg. Purpura anularis und einer Koagulationsanomalie. Derm. Wschr. **141**, 37 (1960). — LEPOW, H., L. RUBENSTEIN, F. WOLL and H. GREISMAN: A spontaneously precipitable protein in human sera, with particular reference to the diagnosis of polyarteriitis nodosa. Amer. J. Med. **7**, 310 (1949). — LEPPS, E.: Silicone surface and blood clotting. Canad. J. Med. Tuberc. **11**, 64 (1949). — LERNER, A. B., C. P. BARNUM and C. J. WATSON: Studies of cryoglobulins; spontaneous precipitation of proteins from serum at 5°C in various disease states. Amer. J. med. Sci. **214**, 416 (1947). — LETTERER, E.: Die allergische-hyperergische Entzündung. In: Handbuch der allgemeinen Pathologie, VII/1, S. 497, Berlin-Göttingen-Heidelberg: Springer 1956. — Die Morphologie der allergischen Reaktionen. Ber. 61. Zusammenkunft Dtsch. Ophthal.-Ges. 1957. — LEWIS, F. J. W., and F. NOUR-ELDIN: Factor IX in intravascular and extravascular blood coagulation. Blood **20**, 41 (1962). — LEWIS, J. H.: Coagulation defects. J. Amer. med. Ass. **178**, 1014 (1961). — LEWIS, J. H., and J. H. FERGUSON: Hypoproaccelerinemia. Blood **10**, 351 (1955). — LEWIS, J. H., J. H. FERGUSON and T. ARENDS: Hemorrhagic disease with circulating inhibitors of blood clotting. Blood **11**, 849 (1956). — LEYPOLD, F., u. M. CARNIEL: Hautnekrosen als Komplikationen bei Behandlungen mit Antikoagulantien. Münch. med. Wschr. **103**, 1675 (1961). — LIENHARD, G.: Polycythaemia vera (Histopathol. Untersuchungen der Gehirngefäße. 2 Beobachtungen). Diss. Basel 1962. — LINDAU, A.: Zur Frage der Angiomatosis retinae und ihrer Hirnkomplikationen. Acta ophthal. (Kbh.) **4**, 193 (1927). — LINDBERG, K.: Ein Beitrag zur Kenntnis der Periarteriitis nodosa. Acta med. scand. **76**, 183 (1931). — Über eine subkutane Form der Periarteriitis nodosa mit langwierigem Verlauf. Acta med. scand. **77**, 455 (1932). — LINDEBOOM, G. A.: Purpura hyperglobulinemica. Dermatologica (Basel) **96**, 337 (1948). — LINDEMAYR, W.: Purpura als Symptom erhöhter Lichtempfindlichkeit. Hautarzt **12**, 174 (1961). — LINKE, A.: Primäre und secundäre Dysproteinämie mit Purpura- und Raynaud-Syndrom. Arch. Derm. Syph. (Berl.) **191**, 123 (1950). — LINZBACH, A. J.: Pathol. Anatomie der Blutgefäße. In: Angiologie v. M. RATSCHOW, S. 140. Stuttgart: Georg Thieme 1959. — LISSIA, G.: Porpora cronica recidivante da focus tonsillar in splenectomizzata: guarigione dopo tonsillectomia. Minerva derm. **31**, 115 (1956). — LITTLE, R.: Purpura fulminans treated successfully with anticoagulation. J. Amer. med. Ass. **169**, 36 (1959). — LÖHR, G. W., H. D. WALLER u. R. GROSS: Beziehungen zwischen Plättchenstoffwechsel und Retraktion des Blutgerinnsels. Dtsch. med. Wschr. **86**, 897 (1961). — LOELIGER, A.: Fibrinogenmangel mit hämorrhagischer Diathese bei einem metastasierendem Melanom. Schweiz. med. Wschr. **87**, 1588 (1957). — LOELIGER, A., and E. J. J. ALSBACH: Prothrombin as co-factor in the circulating anticoagulant in systemic lupus erythematosus. Thrombos. Diathes. haemorrh. (Stuttg.) **3**, 237 (1959). — LOELIGER, A., and A. HENSON: Coagulation studies in a case of Hageman-Trait. Thrombos. Diathes. haemorrh. (Stuttg.) **5**, 187 (1960). — LOELIGER, A., and J. F. PH. HERS: Chronic antithrombinemia with hemorrhagic diathesis in a case of rheumatoid arthritis with hypergammaglobulinemia. Thrombos. Diathes. haemorrh. (Stuttg.) **1**, 499 (1957). — LOEWENTHAL, L. J. A.: Itching purpura. Brit. J. Derm. **66**, 95 (1954). — LOEWY, A. G., and J. T. EDSALL: Studies on the formation of urea-insoluble fibrin. J. biol. Chem. **211**, 829 (1954). — LORAND, L.: Interaction of thrombin and fibrinogen. Physiol. Rev. **34**, 742 (1954). — LORBER, J., and J. L. EMERY: Thrombotic thrombocytopenic purpura. Proc. roy. Soc. Med. **52**, 301 (1959). — LOZNER, E. L.: Differential diagnosis, pathogenesis and treatment of the thrombocytopenic purpuras. Amer. J. Med. **14**, 459 (1953). — The thrombocytopenic purpuras. Bull. N. Y. Acad. Med. **30**, 184 (1954). — LÜLLMANN, H.: Die Nebenwirkungen von Phenylbutazon. Dtsch. med. Wschr. **87**, 30 (1962). — LÜSCHER, E.: Die physiologische Bedeutung der Thrombocyten. Schweiz. med. Wschr. **56**, 345 (1956a). — A dialysable factor from plasma responsible for the „viscous metamorphosis“ of blood platelets. Its role in clot retraction and haemostasis. Experientia (Basel) 12, 268 (1956b). — LÜSCHER, E., u. A. LABHART: Blutgerinnungsstörung durch β_1-Globuline. Zur Kenntnis der Gerinnungsstörungen durch körpereigene Antikoagulantien. Schweiz. med. Wschr. **79**, 598 (1949). — LÜSCHER, E. F.: Biochemische Eigenschaften und physiologische Bedeutung der Blutplättchen. Schweiz. med. Wschr. **89**, 1012 (1959). — The significance of the blood platelets in hemostasis. Proc. 8th Congr. Europ. Soc. Haem. Vienna 1961, Bd. 2, S. 355. — Thrombocytenfaktoren. In: Erbliche Stoffwechselfaktoren, herausgeg. von F. LINNEWEH. München-Berlin: Urban & Schwarzenberg 1962. — LUTZ, R., and G. P. FULTON: The use of the hamster cheek pouch for the study of vascular changes at the microscopic level. Anat. Rec. **120**, 293 (1954).

MACAIGNE, M., et P. NICAUD: La périartérite noueuse (Maladie de Kussmaul) à forme chronique. Presse méd. **1932**, 665. — MACFARLANE, R. G.: A boy with no fibrinogen. Lancet **1938 I**, 309. — MACFARLANE, R. G., P. C. MALLAM, L. J. WILLS, E. BIDWELL, R. BIGGS, G. J. FRAENKEL, G. E. HONEY and K. B. TAYLOR: Surgery in hemophilia. Lancet **1957 II**, 251. — MACHER, E., u. E. VOGELL: Elektronenmikroskopische Untersuchungen an Hautkapillaren. Dermatologica (Basel) **124**, 110 (1962). — MACWHINNEY jr., J. B., J. T. PACKER, G. MILLER and R. B. GREENDYKE: Thrombotic purpura in childhood. Blood **19**, 181 (1962). — MAHON, R., J. MOULINIER, G. CANTORNÉ et G. LASSALLE: Purpura habituel du nouveau-né par incompatibilité foeto-maternelle antiplaquettaire. Gynéc. et Obstét. **56**, 517 (1957). — MAJOCCHI, D.: Sopra una dermatosi telangiectode non ancora descritta „Purpura annularis“. G. ital. Mal. vener. **31**, 263 (1896). — Purpura annularis teleangiectodes. Arch. Derm. Syph. (Berl.) **43**, 447 (1898). — MAJSKY, A., u. R. ZIKOVA: Eine neue Methode für den Nachweis von Thrombocytenagglutininen (Schüttelmethode mit Hilfe formalinisierter Thrombocyten). Z. ges. inn. Med. **15**, 276 (1960). — MALI, J. W. H., K. E. MALTEN u. F. C. J. VAN NEER: Die holländische Margarine-Krankheit. (Ein Erythem des 9. Tages.) Hautarzt **13**, 152 (1162). — MANWARING, W. H., R. C. CHILCOTE and V. M. HOSEPIAN: Anaphylactic reactions in isolated canine organs. J. Immunol. **8**, 233 (1923a). — Capillary permeability in anaphylaxis. J. Amer. med. Ass. **80**, 303 (1923b). — MARCHAL, G.: Diskussionsbemerkung. Sang **30**, 350 (1959). — MARCHAL, G., G. BILSKI-PASQUIER, M. SAMAMA et M. E. LEROUX: Sur un cas de maladie de Willebrand vasculaire pure. Sang **30**, 26 (1959). — MARCHAL, G., G. DUHAMEL, M. LEROUX, J. CHENDEROVITCH et G. GOGLIN: Deux cas de splénomégalie myéloïde avec thrombocythémie hémorragipare (Action du myléran. Intérêt des thrombo-élastogrammes). Sang **28**, 245 (1957). — MARCHAL, G., et M. E. LEROUX: Les désordres hémorragiques en odontologie. Intérêt de leur étude par une méthode nouvelle, la thrombo-dynamographie. Rev. franç. Odonto-stomat. No **3**, Mars (1958). — MARCHAL, G., M. E. LEROUX et M. SAMAMA: Les anomalies thrombo-dynamographiques dans les leucémies myéloïdes. Sang **29**, 265 (1958). — La thrombodynamographie dans les syndromes hémorrhagiques. Algérie méd. **63**, 1 (1959). — MARGOLIUS, A., D. P. JACKSON and O. D. RATNOFF: Circulating anticoagulants. A study of 40 cases. Medicine (Baltimore) **40**, 145 (1961). — MARINO, M. F.: Recherches sur les plaquettes du sang. C. R. Soc. Biol. (Paris) **58**, 194 (1905). — MARMONT, A., and S. GIACCA: A technical improvement of direct platelet counting by phase contrast microscopy. A special „thin-bottom“ counting chamber. Acta haemat. (Basel) **17**, 169 (1957). — MARMONT, A., A. PALMIERI, e ST. GIACCA: Sulle modificazioni quantitative indotte della somministrazione endovenosa di eparina sulla piastrinemia capillare e venosa dell'uomo. Arch. E. Maragliano Pat. Clin. **9**, 281 (1954). — MARS, G., F. GIANOTTI et M. CORONELLI: Considérations sur l'étiologie et la pathogénie du purpura sénile de Bateman, en particulier son rapport avec la vitamine E. Presse méd. **1957**, 2146. — MARX, R.: Zum Problem der Existenz mehrerer, im Serum nach der Blutgerinnung restierender Faktoren der Blutthrombokinasebildung. Klin. Wschr. **23**, 139 (1955). — MARX, R., u. G. FRUHMANN: Dominante, milde Hämophilie AB mit verlängerter Blutungszeit, eine Untergruppe der Purpuras. Klin. Wschr. **36**, 1109 (1958). — MARX, R., u. G. JEAN: Studien zur Pathogenese der Thrombasthenie Glanzmann-Naegeli. Klin. Wschr. **40**, 942 (1962). — MASON, R. G., E. J. HOCUTT, R. H. WAGNER and K. M. BRINKHOUS: Evolution and decay of platelet agglutinating activity in normal and pathologic human plasma. J. Lab. clin. Med. **59**, 645 (1962). — MASSON, G. M. C., A. MIKASA and H. YASUDA: Experimental vascular disease elicited by aldosterone and renin. Endocrinology **71**, 505 (1962). — MASURE, R.: Les inhibiteurs normaux et pathologiques de la coagulation sanguine. Paris: Masson & Cie 1960. — MATHÉ, G.: Syndrome de Schönlein-Henoch (purpura rhumatoïde ou purpura inflammatoire aigu). Rev. Prat. (Paris) **1954**, 1899. — MATIS, P., u. R. GROSS: Über die tagesperiodischen Untersuchungen der Thrombocyten und ihren Einfluß auf Retraktion des Blutkuchens. Schweiz. med. Wschr. **81**, 1043 (1951). — MAUER, A. M., W. DE VAUX and M. E. LAHEY: Neonatal and maternal thrombocytopenic purpura due to quinine. Pediatrics **19**, 84 (1957). — MAUPIN, B.: Les plaquettes sanguines de l'homme. Paris: Masson & Cie. 1954. — MAUPIN, B., J. MOULLEC et P. KHERUMIAN: Afibrinogénémie congénitale. 8. Kongr. Europ. Soc. Haemat. Wien 1961. — MAY, R.: Leucocytäre Einschlüsse, kasuistische Mitteilung. Dtsch. Arch. klin. Med. **96**, 1 (1909). — MCCARTHY, J. T., and

B. MAHER KESTEN: The problem of allergic cutaneous vasculitis. Ann. Allergy **17**, 519 (1959). — MCCLUSKEY, R. T., and B. BENACERRAF: Localization of colloidal substance in vascular endothelium. A mechanism of tissue damage. II. Experimental serum-sickness with acute glomerulonephritis induced passively in mice by antigen-antibody complexes in antigen excess. Amer. J. Path. **35**, 283 (1959). — MCCOMBS, R. P.: The clinical differentiation of „allergic" vasculitis from periarteritis nodosa. Int. Arch. Allergy **12**, 98 (1958). — MCCORMACK, P., D. J. O'BRIEN and R. A. M. OLIVER: Two cases of thrombohaemolytic thrombocytopenic purpura associated with changes in red cell morphology. J. clin. Path. **16**, 436 (1963). — MCFARLANE, A. S., A. DOVEY, G. B. SLACK and S. C. PAPASTAMATIS: An unusual case of hyperglobulinaemia. J. Path. Bact. **64**, 335 (1952). — MCGOVERN, J. J., and A. G. STEINBERG: Antihemophilic factor deficiency in the female. J. Lab. clin. Med. **51**, 286 (1958). — MCKAY, D. G., and F. W. ROWE: The effect on the arterial vascular system of bacterial endotoxin in the generalized Shwartzman reaction. Lab. Invest. **9**, 117 (1960). — MCKAY, D. G., and T. C. WONG: Studies of the generalized Shwartzman reaction produced by diet. I. Pathology. J. exp. Med. **115**, 1117 (1962). — MCKENZIE, A. W., J. H. O. EARLE, E. LOCKEY and G. B. MITCHELL-HEGGS: Essential cryoglobulinemia. Brit. J. Derm. **73**, 22 (1960). — MCKUSICK, V. A.: On the X chromosome of man. Quart. Rev. Biol. **17**, 69 (1962). — MCMILLAN, C. W., L. K. DIAMOND and L. K. SURGENOR: Treatment of classic hemophilia: the use of fibrinogen rich in F. VIII for hemorrhage and for surgery. New Engl. J. Med. **265**, 224, 277, 430 (1962). — MEACHAM, G. C., J. L. ORBISON, R. W. HEINLE, H. J. STEELE and J. A. SCHÄFER: Thrombotic, thrombocytopenic purpura, a disseminated disease of arterioles. Blood **6**, 706 (1951). — MEINDERSMA, E. I., and S. I. DE VRIES: Thrombocytopenic purpura after smallpox vaccination. Brit. med. J. **1962I**, 226. — MELLMAN, W. J., J. J. WOLMAN, H. A. WURZEL, P. S. MOORHEAD and D. H. QUALLS: A chromosomal female with hemophilia A. Blood **17**, 719 (1961). — MÉNACHE, D.: Action des macroglobulines de la maladie de Waldenström sur la coagulation. Etude in vitro. Sang **31**, 529 (1960). — MENNEN, F. R.: Immunologic experiments with platelets of human blood. J. infect. Dis. **31**, 455 (1922). — MENZI, P.: ACTH- und Cortisontherapie bei der Purpura Schönlein-Henoch. Ann. paediat. (Basel) **190**, 94 (1958). — MERSKEY, G.: The occurrence of hemophilia in the human female. Quart. J. Med. **20**, 299 (1951). — MERSKEY, G., and G. MACFARLANE: The female carrier of hemophilia. Lancet **1951I**, 487. — METTLER, N. E., L. G. MACNAMARA and R. E. SHOPE: The propagation of the virus of epizootic hemorrhagic disease of deer in newborn mice and HeLa cells. J. exp. Med. **116**, 665 (1962). — METTLER, R.: Suppression of local tissue reaction by nitrogen mustard, benzol and X-rays. Proc. Soc. Med. Biol. **69**, 247 (1948). — METZ, W.: Die geweblichen Reaktionserscheinungen an der Gefäßwand bei hyperergischen Zuständen und deren Beziehung zur Periarteriitis nodosa. Beitr. path. Anat. **88**, 17 (1932). — MEYERS, M. C.: Results of treatment in 71 patients with idiopathic thrombocytopenic purpura. Amer. J. med. Sci. **242**, 295 (1961). — MEYLER, L.: Schädliche Wirkungen von Arzneimitteln. Wien: Springer 1956. — Side effects of drugs. Amsterdam: Excerpta med. Foundation 1958. — MIALARET, J., J. CAEN, M. J. LARRIEU, J. CHOMÉ et M. JULIEN: Traitement chirurgical des purpuras thrombopéniques et des thrombocytopénies. Ann. Chir. **16**, 1331 (1962). — MICHAEL, S. R., I. L. VURAL, F. A. BASSEN and L. SCHAEFER: The hematologic aspects of disseminated (systemic) lupus erythematosus. Blood **6**, 1054 (1951). — MICHON, P., A. LARCAN et F. STREIFF: Etude clinique de la macroglobulinémie de Waldenström. Sang **31**, 369 (1960). — MIEDZINSKI, F., and I. GOLEBIOWSKA: Is angioma serpiginosum a nosologic unit? Przegl. derm. **6**, 105 (1956) [Polnisch mit engl. Zus.fass.]. — MIESCHER, G.: Über kutane Formen der Periarteriitis nodosa. Dermatologica (Basel) **92**, 225 (1946). — Über aleukozytäre hämorrhagische Phänomene. Schweiz. med. Wschr. **77**, 706 (1947). — Über vasculäre Allergide. Int. Arch. Allergy **8**, 32 (1956). — Abgrenzung des allergischen und toxischen Geschehens in morphologischer und funktioneller Sicht. Arch. klin. exp. Derm. **213**, 297 (1961). — MIESCHER, P.: Immunophagocytose des éléments cellulaires dans le sang. Schweiz. med. Wschr. **1953**, 216. — Immunothrombopenien. In: Hämorrhagische Diathesen, p. 37. Internat. Symposium Wien. Springer 1955. — Zur Immunologie vasculärer Entzündungen aus dem Formenkreis der Schönlein-Henochschen Purpura. Helv. med. Acta **24**, 405 (1957). — Die Rolle der Milz in der Hämatologie. Med. Welt **1960** (1)a, 7. — Autosensibilisierung. Dtsch. med. Wschr. **85**, 706 (1960b). — MIESCHER, P., A. REYMOND et O. RITTER: Le rôle de l'allergie bactérienne dans la pathogénèse de certaines vasculites. Schweiz. med. Wschr. **86**, 799 (1956). — MIESCHER, P., et A. VANOTTI: Leuco- et thrombopénie par „auto-anticorps". Bull. schweiz. Akad. med. Wiss. **10**, 85 (1954). — MIESCHER, P., A. VANOTTI, S. CRUCHAUD u. G. HEMMELER: Die Pathogenese der essentiellen Thrombocytopenie. Helv. med. Acta **19**, 434 (1952). — MIESCHER, P., u. K. O. VORLÄNDER: Immunpathologie in Klinik und Forschung. Stuttgart: Georg Thieme 1957 (2. Aufl. 1961). — MILLER, S. P.: Congenital deficiency of proconvertin. A clinical and laboratory report. Blood **14**, 1322 (1959). — MILLS, ST. D.: Purpura in childhood. (Observations in 187 cases.) J. Pediat. **49**, 306 (1956). — MILLS, ST. D., and R. K. WINKELMANN: Eczema, thrombocytopenic purpura and recurring infections. (Report of 4 families.)

Arch. Derm. **79**, 466 (1959). — MINOT, G. R.: Pathologic hemorrhage. Med. Clin. N. Amer. **1**, 1103 (1918). — A familial hemorrhagic condition associated with prolongation of the bleeding time. Amer. J. med. Sci. **175**, 301 (1928). — MOESCHLIN, S.: Physiopathologie des Hypersplenismus. Helv. med. Acta **23**, 416 (1956). — Die Auto-Immunerkrankungen (Autoaggresionskrankheiten). Acta haemat. (Basel) **18**, 13 (1957). — Exogen bedingte toxische Veränderungen des Knochenmarks. Schweiz. med. Wschr. **1962** (50), 35. — MONTAGNA, W.: The structure and function of skin, 2nd. edit. New York: Acad. Press 1962. — MONTAGNA, W., and R. A. ELLIS: Blood vessels and circulation. In: Advances in biology of the skin, vol. II. New York: Pergamon Press 1961. — MONTGOMERY, H., P. A. O'LEARY and N. W. BARKER: Nodular vascular diseases of the legs: erythema nodosum and allied conditions (175 cases). J. Amer. med. Ass. **128**, 334—338 (1945). — MOON, V. A.: The pathology and mechanism of anaphylaxis. Ann. intern. Med. **12**, 205 (1938). — MOOR-JANKOWSKI, I. K., H. J. HUSER, S. ROSIN, G. TRUOG, M. SCHNEEBERGER u. M. GEIGER: Haemophilie B. Basel: S. Karger 1958. — MOORE, D. H., and H. RUSKA: The fine structure of capillaries and small arteries. J. biophys. biochem. Cytol. **3**, 457 (1957). — MOORE, M. J., W. H. STRICKLAND and R. W. PRICHARD: Sprue with bleeding from hypoprothrombinemia. Arch. intern. Med. **97**, 814 (1956). — MORAWITZ, P.: Beiträge zur Kenntnis der Blutgerinnung. Dtsch. Arch. klin. Med. **79**, 128, 432 (1904). — MORAWITZ, P.: Haemorrhagische Diathesen. Verh. dtsch. path. Ges. **25**, 32 (1930). — MORGAN, M. C., and J. J. SZAFIR: Separation of platelets from whole blood by the use of silicone liquids. Blood **18**, 89 (1961). — MORITA, H., and M. KAGAMI: Congenital afibrinogenemia (1st case in Japan). Acta haemat. (Basel) **17**, 19 (1957). — MORRIS, M. B.: Thrombocytopenic purpura in the newborn. Arch. Dis. Childh. **29**, 75 (1954). — MOSCHCOWITZ, E.: An acute febrile pleiochromic anemia with hyaline thrombosis of the terminal arterioles and capillaries. Arch. intern. Med. **36**, 89 (1925). — MOULINIER, J.: Technique de la réaction de consommation d'antiglobuline. Rev. franç. clin. Biol. **1**, 355 (1956). — Iso-immunisation maternelle antiplaquettaire et purpura néonatal. Le système de groupe plaquettaire „duzo". Trans. 6. Congr. Europ. Soc. Haemat. 1957. Basel: S. Karger 1958, 2. Teil, S. 817. — MOULINIER, J., et X. SERVANTIE: Détection par le test de consommation d'antiglobuline de l'antigène D sur les plaquettes des individus Rh. Vox Sang. (Basel) **3**, 277 (1958). — MÜLLER, O.: Die feinsten Blutgefäße des Menschen. Stuttgart: Ferdinand Enke 1939. — MÜLLER, R.: Über die Purpura hyperglobulinaemica Waldenström. Z. klin. Med. **155**, 359 (1958). — MÜLLER-BERGHAUS, G., H. J. KRECKE u. H. G. LASCH: Thrombelastographische Untersuchungen zum Gerinnselaufbau. Klin. Wschr. **41**, 216 (1963). — MULZER, P., u. R. HABERMANN: Adalinexantheme unter dem Bilde der Purpura Majocchi. Z. ges. Neurol. Psychiat. **128**, H. 1—4 (1930). — MURRAY, M.: Vasculokinase, a clotting substance from arteries. Amer. J. clin. Path. **36**, 500 (1961). — MUSTARD, J. F., W. BASSER, G. HEDGARDT, D. SECORD, H. C. ROWSELL and H. G. DOWNIE: A comparison of the effect of serum and plasma transfusions on the clotting defect in canine haemophilia B. Brit. J. Haemat. **8**, 36 (1962). — MUSTARD, J. F., H. C. ROSWELL, G. A. ROBINSON, T. D. HOEKSEMA and H. E. DOWNIE: Canine hemophilia B. Brit. J. Haemat. **6**, 259 (1960). — MUSTARD, J. P., D. SECORD, T. D. HOEKSEMA, H. G. DOWNIE and H. C. ROWSELL: Canine factor VII deficiency. Brit. J. Haemat. **8**, 43 (1962).

NAEGELI, O.: Blutkrankheiten und Blutdiagnostik. Berlin 1931. — NAGLER, A. L., and B. W. ZWEIFACH: Pathogenesis of experimental shock. II. Absence of endotoxin activity in blood of rabbits subjected to graded hemorrhage. J. exp. Med. **114**, 195 (1961). — NAJEAN, Y.: Etude de la survie des plaquettes marquées au radio-chrome au cours du purpura thrombopénique. Bull. Soc. Méd. Paris, IV. Sér. **77**, 388 (1961). — NAPP, J. H.: Endokrines System. In: Klinik und Therapie der Nebenwirkungen von KÜMMERLE et al. Stuttgart: Georg Thieme 1960. — NASH, W.: Thrombocytopenic purpura following administration of gantrisin. N.Y. St. J. Med. **56**, 2114 (1956). — NEALE, A. V.: Thrombocytopenic purpura. Med. Press No 6045, 245 (1955). — NELKEN, D., N. GILBOA-GARBER and J. GUREVITCH: Studies on the osmotic fragility of human blood platelets. Acta haemat. (Basel) **26**, 75 (1961). — NELKEN, D., J. GUREVITCH and N. GILBOA-GARBER: Direct antiglobulin-consumption test for detection of immune antibody. Lancet **1961 I**, 742. — NELSON, M. G., and E. S. MITCHELL: Pseudo-tumor of bone in haemophilia. Acta haemat. (Basel) **28**, 137 (1962). — NESBITT, R. D., and J. B. RICHMOND: Hemophilia in a negro. J. Pediat. **34**, 315 (1949). — NEUSS, O.: Das Granuloma gangraenescens (Wegenersche Granulomatose), „missing link" zwischen Kollagenosen und Retikuloendotheliosen sowie entzündlichen und echten Geschwülsten. Z. Laryng. Rhin. **39**, 731 (1961). — NEVANLINNA, H. R., E. IKKALA and P. KUOPIO: Von Willebrand's disease. Acta haemat. (Basel) **27**, 65 (1962). — NICOLA, P. DE: 5. Congr. Hémat. Paris 1954, p. 168. — Die Bedeutung der Fibrinolyse für die Entstehung der hämorrhagischen Diathesen. In: Hämorrhagische Diathese. Internat. Symp. Wien: Springer 1955. — Differentialdiagnose der Gerinnungsstörungen. Ergebn. inn. Med. Kinderheilk. **94**, 310 (1955). — Der diagnostische Wert der Thrombelastographie. Triangel (Basel, Sandoz), Dez. (1959). — NICOLAU, S. G., u. S. TEODORESCU: Experimentelle Untersuchungen über die „vasculäre Allergie". Arch. klin. exp. Derm. **210**, 269 (1960a). — Recherches expérimentales sur le pouvoir dit „capillaro-toxique" exercé chez le cobaye par les sérums provenant de malades atteints de certaines dermatoses allergiques. Presse méd. **68**, 2336 (1960b). — NICOLAU, S. G., S. TEODORESCU u. A. BADANOIU: Besondere klinische Aspekte der von Staphylokokken hervorgerufenen allergischen Reaktionen. Derm.-Vener. (Buc.) **1958**, 481. — NIESSING, K., u. H. ROLLHÄUSER: Über den submikroskopischen Bau des Grundhäutchens der Hirnkapillaren. Z. Zellforsch. **39**, 431 (1954). — NILSSON, I., S. BERGMAN, J. REITALU and J. WALDENSTRÖM: Hemophilia A in a girl with male sex-chromatin pattern. Lancet **1959 I**, 264. — NILSSON, I., M. BLOMBÄCK u. B. BLOMBÄCK: Von Willebrand's disease in Sweden. Acta med. scand. **164**, 263 (1959). — Von Willebrand's disease with special reference to a plasmatic factor necessary for hemostasis. Proc. 8th. Congr. Europ. Soc. Haemat. Wien 1961, vol. II, p. 354. — NILSSON, I. M., M. BLOMBÄCK and I. v. FRANKEN: On an inherited autosomal hemorrhagic diathesis with AHG-deficiency and prolonged bleeding time. Acta med. scand. **159**, 35 (1957). — NILSSON, I., M. BLOMBÄCK, E. JORPES, B. BLOMBÄCK and S. A. JOHANSSON: Von Willebrand's disease and its correction with human plasma fraction I—0. Acta med. scand. **159**, 179 (1957). — NILSSON, I., M. BLOMBÄCK and O. RAMGREN: Hemophilia in Sweden. Coagulation studies. Acta med. scand. **170**, 665 (1961). — NILSSON, I., M. BLOMBÄCK, O. RAMGREN and I. v. FRANKEN: II. Carriers of haemophilia A & B. Acta med. scand. **171**, 223 (1962). — NILSSON, I., M. BLOMBÄCK, A. THILEN and I. v. FRANKEN: Carriers of hemophilia. Acta med. scand. **165**, 357 (1959). — NILZÉN, A.: The thrombocyte index following injection of tuberculin in sarcoidosis. Acta derm.-venereol. (Stockh.) **39**, 333 (1959). — NÖDL, F.: Purpura bei essentieller Kryoglobulinämie. Arch. klin. exp. Derm. **210**, 76 (1960). — NORDÖY, S.: Macroglobulinemia Waldenström. A case with unusual findings. Acta med. scand. **172**, 315 (1962). — NORDQVIST, P., G. CRAMER and P. BJÖRNTORP: Thrombocytopenia during chlorothiazide treatment. Lancet **1959 II**, 271. — NORKIN, S., and J. WIENER: Henoch-Schönlein-syndrome. Review of pathology and report of 2 cases. Amer. J. clin. Path. **33**, 55 (1960). — NOSSEL, H. L., R. K. ARCHER and R. G. MACFARLANE: Equine haemophilia. Report of a case and its response to multiple infusions of heterospecific AHG. Brit. J. Haemat. 8, 335 (1962). — NOUR-ELDIN, F., and J. F. WILKINSON: Factor VII deficiency with Christmas disease in one family. Lancet **1959 I**, 1173. — NOVER, A., u. G. BERNEAUD-KÖTZ: Experimentelle Untersuchungen über die Permeabilität der Bindehautgefäße, zugleich Beitrag über die Entstehung von Blutungen bei Paraproteinämien. Albrecht v. Graefes Arch. Ophthal. **159**, 582 (1958). — NUSSBAUM, M., and W. DAMESHEK: Transient hemolytic and thrombocytopenic episode (acute transient thrombohemolytic thrombocytopenic purpura) with probable meningococcemia. N. Engl. J. Med. **256**, 448 (1957).

OBERMAYER, M.: Psychocutaneous medicine. Springfield (Ill.): Ch. C. Thomas 1955. — O'BRIEN, J. R.: Un inhibiteur de la maladie de Christmas. Rev. Hémat. **12**, 294 (1957). — ODLAND, G. F.: The fine structure of the interrelationship of cells in the human epidermis. J. biophys. biochem. Cytol. **4**, 529 (1958). — A submicroscopic granular component in human epidermis. J. invest. Derm. **34**, 11 (1960). — OERI, J., M. MATTER, H. ISENSCHMID, F. HAUSER u. F. KOLLER: Angeborener Mangel an Faktor V, verbunden mit echter Hämophilie A bei zwei Brüdern. Med. Probl. Paediat. **1**, 575 (1954). — OKANA, K., and S. KAWAKAMI: Study of appearance of the platelets in the tissues in experimental purpura in guinea pigs. J. Osaka med. Soc. **37**, 2291 (1938). — ORBANEJA, J. G., u. J. R. PUCHOL: Über die Systematik der cutanen nekrotisierenden Gefäßerkrankungen. Hautarzt **11**, 453 (1960). — OREO, G. A. DE: Wegener's granulomatosis. Arch. Derm. **81**, 169 (1960). — ORR, F. R.: Haemorrhage in myxoedema coma. Lancet **1962 II**, 1012. — OSGOOD, ED. E., R. D. KOLER and M. E. HUGHES: Differential diagnosis and treatment of hemorrhagic diseases. Arch. intern. Med. **94**, 955 (1954). — OSKI, F. A., J. L. NAIMAN, D. M. ALLEN and L. K. DIAMOND: Leukocytic inclusions — Döhle bodies — associated with platelet abnormality. (The May-Hegglin anomaly.) Blood **20**, 657 (1962). — OSLER, W.: On multiple hereditary telangiectases with recurring haemorrhages. Quart. J. Med. **1**, 53 (1907). — OSTEN, W.: Thrombocytenzählung unter Verwendung von Sequestrennatrium- und hypotoner Kokainlösung. Röntgen- u. Lab.-Prax. **12**, 91 (1959a). — Aufgaben der Thrombocyten bei der Blutgerinnung. Thrombocytär bedingte haemorrhagische Diathesen. Ärztl. Wschr. **14**, 346 (1959b). — OSWALD, W.: Die Beeinflussung des experimentellen Shwartzman-Phänomens durch Stoffe mit Vitamin K-Wirkung. Z. Immun.-Forsch. **113**, 227 (1956). — OVARY, Z., and O. G. BIER: Quantitative studies on passive cutaneous anaphylaxis in the guinea pig and its relationship to the Arthus-phenomenon. J. Immunol. **71**, 6 (1953). — OWEN, W. W.: Die Wirkung von Dethyrona auf den Cholesterinspiegel im menschlichen Blut. Méd. et Hyg. (Genève) **19**, 462 (1961). — OWREN, P.: The coagulation of blood. Investigation on a new clotting factor. Acta med. scand. **194**, Suppl. (1947). (First publ. 1944.) — Parahaemophilia, haemorrhagic diathesis due to absence of a previously unknown clotting factor. Lancet **1947 I**, 446 und Acta med. scand., Suppl. 194 (1947). — OZER, F. L., W. E. TRUAX, D. C. MIESCH and W. C. LEVIN: Primary hemorrhagic thrombocythemia. Amer. J. Med. **28**, 807 (1960).

PADER, E., and H. GROSSMAN: Thrombocytopenic purpura in infectious mononucleosis. N.Y. St. J. Med. **56**, 1905 (1956). — PAGE, A. R., H. BENDERES, J. WARNER and R. A. GOOD:

The Chediak-Higashi-syndrome. Blood **20**, 330 (1962). — Page, I. H.: Serotonin (5-Hydroxytryptamine). Physiol. Rev. **34**, 563 (1954). — Palmerio, C., S. C. Ming, E. Frank and J. Fine: The role of the sympathetic nervous system in the generalized Shwartzman reaction. J. exp. Med. **115** (3), 609 (1962). — Pappenheimer, J. R.: Passage of molecules through capillary walls. Physiol. Rev. **33**, 387 (1953). — Pavlovsky, A., y H. Castellanos: Purpuras catameniales. Clin. lat. (Torino) **3**, 88 (1953). — Pavlovsky, A., A. Martinez-Canaveri, N. Quirno y F. Etchegoyen: Pseudohemofilia producida por un anticoagulante. Sangre (Santiago) **1**, 394 (1956). — Peck, S.: Pigmented purpuric lichenoid dermatitis (Gougerot). Arch. Derm. **38**, 506 (1938). — Pegum, J. S.: Purpuric lichenoid dermatitis. Brit. J. Derm. **69**, 97 (1957). — Peters, G. A., R. W. Moskowitz, L. E. Prickman and H. M. Carryer: Fatal necrotizing angiitis associated with hypersensitivity to penicillin and iodides. Report of a case. J. Allergy **31**, 455 (1960). — Peters, J.: Psychogene Stigmatisation. Rotterdam 1934. Zit. Schleyer 1948. — Petersen, W. F., and S. A. Levinson: The role of the endothelium in canine anaphylactic shock. J. Immunol. **8**, 349 (1923). — Peterson jr., O. R., and E. Larson jr.: Thrombopenic purpura in pregnancy. Obstet. Gynec. **4**, 454 (1954). — Petrides, P.: Neuzeitliche Gesichtspunkte der Therapie allergischer Knochenmarkschäden. Fortschr. Med. **71**, 329 (1953). — Medikamentöse Blutschäden. Folia haemat. (Lpz.), N.F. **1**, 280 (1957). — Pfeiffer, E. F., W. Spielmann u. H. Ditschuneit: Die klinische Bedeutung des Nachweises von Antikörpern gegen Thrombocyten bei thrombopenischer Purpura. Dtsch. med. Wschr. **1956**, 735. — Pfleger, L.: Zur Pathogenese unklarer Purpuraformen (Purpura Majocchi, Morbus Schamberg, Dermatitis Gougerot-Blum, Angioma serpiginosum). Arch. Derm. Syph. (Berl.) **197**, 187 (1954). — Pieper, G. R., S. Perry and J. Burroughs: Surgical intervention in hemophilia. J. Amer. med. Ass. **170**, 33 (1959). — Pierini, D. O., et J. Abulafia: Manifestations cutanées du syndrome de Chediak-Higashi. Arch. argent. Derm. **8**, 23 (1958). — Pinniger, J. L., and R. B. Franks: Hemophilia in a female. Lancet **1951 II**, 82. — Pinniger, J. L., and F. T. G. Prunty: Some observations on the blood clotting mechanism. Brit. J. exp. Path. **27**, 200 (1946). — Piomelli, S., M. Stefanini and R. H. Mele: Attempts at experimental production of acute vascular (anaphylactoid) purpura. Int. Arch. Allergy **21** (2), 65 (1962). — Pitney, W. R., and B. J. Arnold: Laboratory findings in families of patients suffering from v. Willebrand's disease. Brit. J. Haemat. **6**, 81 (1960). — Piyaratn, P.: Pathology of Thailand epidemic hemorrhagic fever. Amer. J. trop. Med. Hyg. **10**, 767 (1961). — Pohle, F. J., E. B. Cohen and W. Madison: Variations in blood platelets in allergic individuals following the ingestion of test foods. J. Lab. clin. Med. **32**, 1395 (1947). — Pola, V., u. J. Svojitka: Klassische Haemophilie bei Frauen. Folia haemat. (Lpz.) **75**, 43 (1957). — Pollak, F.: Zur Klinik der Stigmatisationen. Z. ges. Neurol. Psychiat. **162**, 606 (1938). — Pool, J. G., R. Desai and M. Kropatkin: Severe congenital hypoprothrombinemia in a negro boy. Thrombos. Diathes. haemorrh. (Stuttg.) **8**, 235 (1962). — Portwich, F.: Periarteriitis nodosa (Kussmaulsche Krankheit). Ergebn. inn. Med. Kinderheilk. **12**, 428 (1959). — Portwich, F., u. H. Maron: Tödlich verlaufene allergische Thrombopenie nach Grippeprophylaxe mit Merfen (Phenylhydrargyrum boricum). Ärztl. Wschr. **14**, 65 (1959). — Post, C. R., G. J. H. den Ottolander and P. G. Hoorweg: A familial form of idiopathic hypoprothrombinemia. Ned. T. Geneesk. **100**, 1981 (1956). — Powell, M.: Clinical manifestations of epidemic hemorrhagic fever. J. Amer. med. Ass. **151** (15), 1261 (1953). — Pratesi, G., e A. Rizzuto: Su i fattori etiopatogenetici della sindrome di Schönlein-Henoch. Rass. Fisiopat. clin. ter. **28**, 252 (1956). — Prentice, A. I. D.: A case of congenital afibrinogenemia. Lancet **1951 I**, 211. — Pribilla, W.: Purpura Henoch-Schönlein. Ärztl. Wschr. **1951**, 1044. — Proppe, A.: Osler's teleangiectasia haemorrhagica hereditaria. Derm. Wschr. **106**, 233 (1938). — Prosser-Thomas, E. W., and A. Rook: Pigmented purpuric lichenoid dermatitis of Gougerot and Blum. Brit. J. Derm. **61**, 21 (1949). — Puchol, J. R.: Histopatologia de las angéitis cutaneas (Monographie, Consejo superior de investigacions cientificas). Madrid 1962.

Quattrin, N.: Haemorrhagische Diathesen. Bemerkung in Jürgens u. Deutsch, S. 148. Wien: Springer 1955. — Le malattie emorragiche nella medicina pratica e sociale. Arch. Med. mutual. (Roma), Ed. Istituto naz. per l'assicurazione contro le malattie (1957). — The constitutional haemorrhagic diseases with mixed haemostatic defects. Acta med. scand. **163**, 403 (1959). — Quattrin, N., G. Bile, E. Dini e V. Ventruto: Crioglobulinemie e macroglobulinemie. Minerva med. **52** (75), 3197 (1961). — Quattrin, N., E. Dini and P. Piccoli: On the differentialdiagnosis and pathogenesis of the purpura with hypergammaglobulinemia or macroglobulinemia. Acta. med. scand. (Stockh.) **156**, 25 (1956). — Quick, A. J.: The prothrombin in hemophilia and in obstructive jaundice. J. biol. Chem. **109**, 523 (1935). — Hemorrhagic diseases. Philadelphia: Lea & Febiger 1957. — Hereditary bleeding diseases. J. Amer. med. Ass. **178**, 941 (1961 a). — The diagnosis of common hereditary hemorrhagic diseases. Ann. intern. Med. **55**, 201 (1961 b). Quick, A. J., and C. V. Hussey: Hyperheparinemia, report of a case. Amer. J. med. Sci. **234**, 251 (1957). — Haemophilia-like states in girl. Lancet **1958 I**, 1294. — Comparison of thrombotest with the one-stage prothrombin time. New Engl. J. Med. **265**, 1286 (1962). — Quick, A. J.,

A. V. Pisciotta and C. V. Hussey: Congenital hyprothrombinemic states. Arch. intern. Med. **95**, 2 (1955). — Quick, A. J., and M. Stefanini: Action of plasma thromboplastinogen and evidence of an inhibitor. Proc. Soc. exp. Biol. (N.Y.) **67**, 111 (1948).

Rabe, F., u. E. Salamon: Über Faserstoffmangel im Blut bei einem Fall von Haemophilie. Dtsch. Arch. klin. Med. **132**, 240 (1920). — Rabiner, S. F., and N. Kretschmer: The Stuart-Prower-Factor. Brit. J. Haemat. **7**, 99 (1961). — Raccuglia, G., and J. Neel: Congenital vascular defect associated with platelet abnormality and AHG deficiency. Blood **15**, 80 (1960). — Raccuglia, G., and C. J. D. Zarafonetis: Platelets and pharmacologic compounds in radiation induced hemorrhagic diathesis. Amer. J. med. Sci. **244**, 152 (1962). — Racine, A., R. Claisses, B. Weit et D. Durnesin: Tuberculose aigüe granulique et purpura. Presse méd. **60**, 193 (1952). — Radhakishun, K. S.: Een geval van congenitale idiopatische hypoprothrombinemie. Ned. T. Geneesk. **102**, 712 (1958). — Radl, H., u. K. Hekele: Purpura fulminans im Anschluß an Varizellen. Arch. Kinderheilk. **155**, 43 (1957). — Raffel, S.: Immunity, 2. Aufl., S. 560. New York: Appelton 1961. — Rak, K., u. K. Waltner: Über einen Fall von kongenitaler Hypoproconvertinämie (Faktor VII-Mangel). Thrombos. Diathes. haemorrh. (Stuttg.) **4**, 418 (1959). — Ràk, R., u. J. Kovacs: Die sog. Hämophilie C (PTA-Mangel), Rosenthal-Syndrom. Med. Welt **45**, 2349 (1961). — Rambert, P., J. Canivet, M. Tissier et J. Quichaud: Purpura fulminans infectieux (Syndrome de Waterhouse-Friderichsen). Bull. Soc. méd. Hôp. Paris **75**, 275 (1959). — Ramgren, O.: Haemophilia in Sweden. (Symptomatology with special reference to differences between haemophilia A and B.) Acta med. scand. **171**, 237 (1962). — Randall, S. J., R. R. Kierland and H. Montgomery: Pigmented purpuric eruptions. Arch. Derm. Syph. (Chic.) **64**, 177 (1951). — Randerath, E.: Die Bedeutung der allergischen Pathogenese bei der Arteriitis. Verh. dtsch. Ges. inn. Med. **60**, 359 (1954). — Rapaport, S. I., S. B. Ames and B. J. Duvall: A plasma coagulation defect in systemic lupus erythematosus arising from hypoprothrombinemia combined with antiprothrombinase activity. Blood **15**, 212 (1960). — Rapaport, S. I., and F. J. Moore: Anti-hemophilic globulin levels in carriers of hemophilia A. J. clin. Invest. **39**, 1619 (1960). — Rapaport, S. I., R. R. Proctor, M. J. Patch and M. Yettra: The mode of inheritance of PTA-deficiency. Blood **18**, 149 (1961). — Ratnoff, O. D.: A familial trait characterized by deficiency of a clot-promoting fraction of plasma. J. Lab. clin. Med. **44**, 915 (1954). — Ratschow, M.: Angiologie. Stuttgart: Georg Thieme 1959. — Rausen, A. R., A. Cruchaud, C. W. McMillan and D. Gitlin: A study of fibrinogen turnover in classical hemophilia and congenital afibrinogenemia. Blood **18** (6), 710 (1961). — Rechenberg, H. K. v.: Therapie der perakuten Meningokokkensepsis (Syndrom von Waterhouse-Friderichsen). Helv. med. Acta **20**, 381 (1953). — Zur Frage der Terminologie der perakuten Meningokokkeninfektion, perakuten Meningokokkensepsis, Meningitis epidemica maligna Waterhouse-Friderichsen. Schweiz. med. Wschr. **85**, 502 (1955). — Rees, H. M., and E. E. Ecker: An improved method for counting blood platelets. J. Amer. med. Ass. **80**, 621 (1923). — Regan, W. D.: The acquired hemorrhagic diathesis of pregnancy (7 cases). J. Indian. med. Ass. **50**, 984 (1957). — Régniers, P., R. J. Wieme, Ch. Wunderly and P. Burtin: A propos d'un cas de macroglobulinémie (M. de Waldenström) présentant quelques aspects histologiques et biochimiques remarquables. Schweiz. med. Wschr. **1956**, 1140. — Reichstein, T., A. Grüssner u. R. Oppenauer: Ascorbinsäure. Helv. chim. Acta. **16**, 561, 1019 (1933); **17**, 311, 510 (1934). — Reid, W. O., A. v. Somlyo, A. P. v. Somlyo and R. Ph. Custer: Role of the platelets in fibrinolysis. With a sensitive test for fibrinolytic activity. Amer. J. clin. Path. **37** (6), 561 (1962). — Reilly, J., E. Rivalier, A. Compagnon et R. Laplane: Hémorrhagie, lésions vasculaires et lymphatiques du tube digestif déterminées par l'injection périsplanchnique de substances toxiques diverses. C. R. Soc. Biol. (Paris) **116**, 24 (1934). — Renkin, E. M., u. J. R. Pappenheimer: Wasserdurchlässigkeit und Permeabilität der Capillarwände. Ergebn. Physiol. **49**, 59 (1957). — Revol, L.: Les thrombocytémies hémorragiques (la myélose hyperthrombocytaire). Sem. Hôp. Paris **38**, 2743 (1962). — Reymond, A., u. P. Miescher: Rezidivierende Vasculitis auf dem Boden einer bakteriellen Allergie (Beitrag zur Frage der allergischen Mikrobide). Verh. dtsch. Ges. inn. Med. 60. Kongr. 1954. — Rich, A. R.: The role of the hypersensitivity in periarteriitis nodosa. Bull. Johns Hopk. Hosp. **71**, 123 (1942). — Rich, A. R., and J. E. Gregory: The experimental demonstration that periarteriitis nodosa is a manifestation of hypersensitivity. Bull. Johns Hopk. Hosp. **72**, 65 (1943); **73**, 239 (1943). — Further experimental cardiac lesions of the rheumatic type produced by anaphylactic sensitivity. Bull. Johns Hopk. Hosp. **75**, 115 (1944). — Richter, W.: Teleangiectasia haemorrhagica hereditaria (Osler) in Verbindung mit Basedow amyotrophischer Enteralsclerose und Ulcus trophicum am Unterschenkel. Zbl. Haut- u. Geschl.-Kr. **43**, 616 (1933). — Rimbaud, P., P. Izarn, J. Ravoire et F. Duntze: Purpura thrombocytopénique essentiel (Effet de la splénectomie). Bull. Soc. franç. Derm. Syph. **66**, 534 (1959). — Rivera, A. M., and F. C. Biehusen: Aldrich's syndrom. J. Pediat. **57**, 86 (1960). — Roberts, G. F.: Thrombocytopenic purpura with thyrotoxicosis. Lancet **1948 I**, 65. — Robinow, M., and W. A. Newton jr.: Recurrent pannicular hemorrhages. A fatal disease related to thrombotic thrombocytopenic purpura. J. Dis. Child. **96**, 71 (1958). — ROBSON, H. N., and J. J. G. DUTHIE: Capillary resistance and adrenocortical activity. Brit. med. J. **1950 II**, 971; **1952 I**, 994. — RODER, H.: Rheumatische Purpura necroticans bei Kryoglobulinämie. Z. Haut- u. Geschl.-Kr. **30** (5), 148 (1961). — RODRIGUEZ-ERDMANN, F., u. H. C. LASCH: Quantitative und qualitative Störungen der Thrombocyten nach Injektion hochmolekularer Polymere. (Beitrag zum Sanarelli-Shwartzman-Phänomen.) Thrombos. Diathes. haemorrh. (Stuttg.) **6**, 518 (1961). — RÖCKL, H., H. BORCHERS u. F. SCHRÖPF: Lymphoretikulose der Haut mit Makroglobulinämie als Sonderform der Makroglobulinämie Waldenström? Hautarzt **13**, 491 (1962). — ROGERS jr., J. V., and A. E. ROBERTO: Circumscribed pulmonary lesions in periarteriitis nodosa and Wegener's granulomatosis. Amer. J. Roentgenol. **76**, 88 (1956). — ROLLHÄUSER, H.: Die Morphologie der Kapillaren. In: M. RATSCHOW, Angiologie, S. 73. Stuttgart: Georg Thieme 1959. — ROOS, J.: Blood coagulation as a continuous process. Thrombos. Diathes. haemorrh. (Stuttg.) **1**, 471 (1957). — ROOS, J., C. VAN ARKEL, M. C. VERLOOP and F. L. J. JORDAN: A "new" family with Stuart-Prower deficiency. Thrombos. Diathes. haemorrh. (Stuttg.) **3**, 59 (1959). — ROSCAM, J.: Leucémies, états hémorragipares et hérédité. C. R. Congr. franç. Méd., 36e Session 1947. Paris: Masson & Cie. 1949, p. 33. — ROSENTHAL, N.: The course and treatment of thrombopenic purpura. J. Amer. med. Ass. **112**, 101 (1939). — ROSENTHAL, R. L., O. H. DRESKIN and N. ROSENTHAL: New hemophilia-like disease caused by deficiency of a third plasma thromboplastin factor. Proc. Soc. exp. Biol. (N.Y.) **82**, 171 (1953). — ROTHBARD, S., and R. F. WATSON: Antigenicity of rat collagen. Distribution of antibody to rat collagen injected into rats. J. exp. Med. **116** (3), 337 (1962). — RUITER, M.: A case of allergic cutaneous vasculitis (Arteriolitis allergica). Brit. J. Derm. **65**, 77 (1953). — Some further observations on allergic cutaneous arteriolitis. Brit. J. Derm. **66**, 174 (1954). — Purpura rheumatica: A type of allergic cutaneous arteriolitis. Brit. J. Derm. **68**, 16 (1956). — Über die sog. Arteriolitis (Vasculitis) allergica cutis. Hautarzt **8**, 293 (1957a). — Clinical and histological features of „allergic" necrotising angitides with predominantly cutaneous localisation. Acta derm.-venereol. (Stockh.) Proc. 11th Intern. Congr. Derm. **11**, 172 (1957b). — The so-called cutaneous type of periarteriitis nodosa. Brit. J. Derm. **70**, 102 (1958). — Some histopathological aspects of vascular allergy. Int. Arch. Allergy **17**, 157 (1960). — Possible connection between an abnormal plasma fraction (HPF) and vascular fibrinoid in arteriolitis (vasculitis) allergica cutis. J. invest. Derm. **38** (3), 117 (1962). — RUITER, M., u. F. H. OSWALD: Weitere Beiträge zur Kenntnis der Arteriolitis (Vasculitis) „allergica" cutis (Purp. Schönlein, leukoklastische Mikrobide, anaphylaktoide Purp., maladie trisymptomatique de Gougerot, allergides nodulaires dermiques usw.). Hautarzt **14** (1), 6 (1963). — RUITER, M., A. W. M. POMPEN u. H. J. G. WYERS: Granulomatöse Panvaskulitiden mit ausschließlich kutan-subkutaner Lokalisierung. Dermatologica (Basel) **97**, 257 (1948). — RUMPEL, T.: Unsere bisherigen Erfahrungen mit dem Ehrkirchschen Präparat „606". Dtsch. med. Wschr. **36**, 2286 (1910). — RUSTAD, R. C.: Pinocytosis. Sci. Amer. **204**, 121 (Apr. 1961).

SACHS, O.: Über eine noch nicht beschriebene Purpuraform nach Genuß von Sardellenbutter. Arch. Derm. Syph. (Berl.) **123**, 835 (1916). — SACK, W. TH.: Psyche und Haut. In: JADASSOHNs Handbuch der Haut- und Geschlechtskrankheiten, Bd. IV/2. Berlin: Springer 1933. — SAILER, S., u. R. HINRICHS: Isolierter, kongenitaler Faktor-V-Mangel als Ursache einer hämorrhagischen Diathese. Wien. Z. inn. Med. **40**, 10 (1959). — SALTZSTEIN, S. L.: Phospholipid accumulation in histocytes of splenic pulp associated with thrombocytopenic purpura. Blood **18** (1), 73 (1961). — SAMARQ, P. R.: Anatomic pathologique de la maladie de Waldenström. Sang **31**, 473 (1960). — SAMUELS, P. B., B. M. SAMUELS and D. WEBSTER: New technics in study of venous endothelium. Lab. Invest. **1**, 50 (1952). — SANARELLI, G.: Experimental Cholera. Ann. Inst. Pasteur **38**, 11 (1924). — SANCHEZ-MEDAL, L., and E. REYNOSO: Anaphylactoid purpura (Henoch-Schönlein's syndrome). Clinical study of 45 cases. Rev. inst. Clin. **7**, 293 (1955). — SAUNDERS, R. L., DE C. H. J. LAWRENCE and D. A. MACIVER: Microradiographic studies of the vascular patterns in muscle and skin. In: X-Ray microscopy and microradiography, p. 539. New York: Academic Press 1957. — SCHÄFER, K. H., u. K. FISCHER: Thrombocytär bedingte hämorrhagische Diathesen. Dtsch. med. Wschr. **83**, 695 (1958). — SCHÄFER, K. H., G. LANDBECK u. K. FISCHER: Neue Erkenntnisse auf dem Gebiet der thrombocytär bedingten hämorrhagischen Diathesen (Thrombocytopathien). Dtsch. med. Wschr. **85**, 781 (1960). — SCHAMBERG, J.: A peculiar progressive pigmentary disease of the skin. Brit. J. Derm. **13**, 1 (1901). — SCHATZMANN, H. J.: Tödliche thrombocytopenische Purpura bei Benzolvergiftung. Schweiz. med. Wschr. **1955**, 1123. — SCHEIDEGGER, J. J., R. WEBER u. A. HÄSSIG: Zur Antigenstruktur der Makroglobuline beim Morbus Waldenström. Helv. med. Acta **25**, 25 (1958). — SCHEN, R. J., and M. RABINOVITZ: Thrombocytopenic purpura due to quinidine. Brit. med. J. **1958 II**, 1502. — SCHIMKE, K.: Beobachtung eines Gamma-Plasmozytoms mit plasmatischer Gerinnungsstörung. Dtsch. med. Wschr. **88**, 75 (1963). — SCHLEYER, F.: Die Stigmatisation mit den Blutmalen. Hannover 1948. — SCHMENGLER, F. E., u. H. ESSER: Zur Pathogenese der Purpura hyperglobulinaemica. Klin. Wschr. **30**, 30 (1952). — SCHMIDT, A.: Die Blutlehre. Leipzig 1892. — SCHNEIDER, CH. L.: Fibrination and defibrination. In: Physiologie und Pathologie der Blutgerinnung der Gestationsperiode. Stuttgart: Schattauer 1957. — SCHOCH, A.: Neue Ergebnisse in Klinik und Pathologie der Hautblutungen. Schweiz. med. Wschr. **70**, Nr 2 u. 3 (1940). — Klinische und hämatologische Beobachtungen bei Purpura Majocchi. Schweiz. med. Wschr. **71**, 653 (1941). — SCHÖNLEIN, J. L.: Allgemeine und specielle Pathologie. Würzburger Vorlesungen 1828—1932. — SCHOLER, H., H. IMHOF u. M. SCHNÖS: Beobachtungen an einem weiteren Träger der Hegglin'schen Anomalie der Granulozyten und Blutplättchen. Schweiz. med. Wschr. **90**, 1269 (1960). — SCHOOP, W.: Physiologie und Pathophysiologie der peripheren Durchblutung (Gefäßtonus). In: Angiologie v. M. RATSCHOW, S. 83. Stuttgart: Georg Thieme 1959. — SCHREIBER, M.: Ein Fall von erworbener Afibrinogenämie und hämorrhagischer Diathese bei akuter Myelose. Wien. klin. Wschr. **72**, 339 (1960). — SCHREINER, H. E.: Die Therapie von Hautkrankheiten mit NNR-Hormone. Zbl. Haut- u. Geschl.-Kr. **104**, 89 (1959). — SCHULMAN, I., C. H. SMITH and R. E. ANDO: Congenital thrombocytopenic purpura. Observations on three infants born of a non-affected mother. Amer. J. Dis. Child. **88**, 784 (1954). — SCHULTE, W., u. H. MAUNZ: Methode zur fortlaufenden Bestimmung der Retraktionskraft, Retraktionszeit und Haftfähigkeit des Blutkuchens. Dtsch. med. Wschr. **86**, 2233 (1961). — SCHULTZ, E. W.: Platelet deficiency, a factor in diminished coagulability of the blood in anaphylaxis. Proc. Soc. exp. Biol. (N.Y.) **22**, 343 (1924). — SCHULZ, H., u. E. HIEPLER: Über die Lokalisierung von gerinnungsphysiologischen Aktivitäten in submikroskopischen Strukturen der Thrombocyten. Klin. Wschr. **37**, 273 (1959). — SCHULZ, H., u. J. WEDELL: Elektronenmikroskopische Untersuchungen zur Frage der Fettphagocytose und des Fetttransportes durch Thrombocyten. Klin. Wschr. **40**, 1114 (1962). — SCHULZ, K. H., and M. JÄNNER: Vasculitis allergica mit Thrombocytopenie durch Thalidomid. Allergie u. Asthma **9**, 226 (1963). — SCHUPPENER, H. J.: Die Pigmentpurpura, ein Beitrag zu ihrem morphologischen Erscheinungsbild. Derm. Wschr. **130**, 803 (1954). — SCHWAB, P. J., and J. L. FAHEY: Treatment of Waldenströms macroglobulinemia by plasmapheresis. New Engl. J. Med. **263**, 574 (1960). — SCHWARZ, M.: Morbus Wiskott-Aldrich. Vermutung einer verspäteten Reifung der Gammaglobuline. Diskussions bemerkung in Ann. Paediat. **196**, 254 (1961). — SCOTT, D. G.: An immuno-histological study of connective tissue. Ann. rheum. Dis. **18**, 207 (1959). — SCOTT, J. S., and J. G. READER: Recurrent blood coagulation failure in pregnancy with birth of a live child. Brit. med. J. **1962 I**, 153. — SEIBERT, R. H., A. MARGOLIUS and O. D. RATNOFF: Observation on hemophilia, para hemophilia and coexistent hemophilia and parahemophilia. J. Lab. clin. Med. **52**, 449 (1958). — SESSNER, H. H., G. S. SCHÜTTERLE, W. REMMELE, V. LEHMANN u. H. G. LASCH: Allgemeine hämorrhagische Diathese und vasculäre Fibrinabscheidungen im sekundären Stadium der experimentellen Fettembolie. Med. Welt **1962** (40), 2105—2108. — SHAINOFF, J. R. and I. H. PAGE: Significance of cryoprofibrin in fibrinogenfibrin conversion. J. exp. Med. **116** (5), 687 (1962). — SHARNOFF, J. G.: Thrombotic thrombocytopenic purpura (Report of 3 cases). Amer. J. Med. **23**, 740 (1957). — SHAW, S.: Haemorrhagic thrombocythaemia (2 cases treated by radioactive phosphorus). Brit. med. J. **1961 I**, 1437. — SHECHTER, F. R., H. N. RASANSKY and H. LORZ: Hemorrhagic thrombocythemia. Amer. J. Gastroent. **38**, 569 (1962). — SHERRY, S., A. P. FLETCHER and N. ALKJAERSIG: Fibrinolysis and fibrinolytic activity in man. Physiol. Rev. **39**, 343 (1959). — SHMERLING, D. H., E. JUNG u. F. DUCKERT: Eine neue familiäre Koagulopathie infolge Mangels an fibrinstabilisierendem Faktor. Helv. paediat. Acta **15**, 471 (1960). — SHMUSHKOVICH, J., and E. DAVIS: Thrombocytopenic skin purpura following treatment with Trinitrin. Brit. J. Derm. **67**, 299 (1955). — SHORE, P. A., A. PLETSCHER, E. G. TOMICH, R. KUNTZMANN and B. B. BRODIE: Release of blood platelet serotonin by reserpine and lack of effect on bleeding time. Pharmacol. exp. Ther. **117**, 323 (1956). — SHULMAN, I., C. H. SMITH, M. ERLANDSON, E. FORT and R. E. LEE: Vascular hemophilia. Pediatrics **18**, 347 (1956). — SHULMAN, N. R.: Immunoreactions involving platelets. IV. Studies on pathogenicity of thrombocytopenia in drug purp. using test dosis of quinidine in sensitized individuals. Their implications in idiopathic thrombocytopenic purpura. J. exp. Med. **107**, 711 (1958). — SHULMAN, N. R., R. H. ASTER, H. A. PEARSON and M. C. HILLER: Immunoreaction involving platelets. VI. Reactions of maternal isoantibodies responsible for neonatal purpura. Differentiation of a second platelet antigen system. J. clin. Invest. Med. **41** (5), 1059 (1962). — SHUSTER, B., and H. SCARBOROUGH: Senile purpura. Quart. J. Med. **30**, 117 (1961). — SHWARTZMAN, G.: Studies on bacillus typhosus toxic substances. 1. Phenomenon of local skin reactivity to bacterial typhosus culture filtrate. J. exp. Med. **48** (12), 47 (1928). — Phenomenon of local skin reaction to bacterial filtrates. Elicitation of local reactivity by way of the vascular system. J. exp. Med. **62**, 621 (1935). — SIEGEL, B. M., I. A. FRIEDMAN, S. KESSLER and S. O. SCHWARTZ: Thrombohemolytic thrombocytopenic purpura with lupus erythematosus. Ann. intern. Med. **47**, 1022 (1957). — SIEGENTHALER, W. G., P. SCHMUZIGER u. R. KUONI: Die Klinik der Gefäßerkrankungen mit besonderer Berücksichtigung derjenigen des rheumatischen Formenkreises. Medizinische **43/44**, 3 (1959). — SIEMS, O. H., u. J. G. RAUSCH-STROOMANN: Sjögren-Syndrom und Purpura hyperglobulinaemica Waldenström. Ärztl. Wschr. **1955**, 647. — SIGG, A., A. CLAUSS, H. PESTALOZZI u. F. KOLLER: Steigerung der Antikoagulantienwirkung durch Butazolidin.

V. Kongr. Europ. Soc. Haemat. Freiburg i. Br. 1955, S. 465. — SIGUIER, F., C. BÉTOURNÉ, P. GODEAU et P. LEBORGNE: Grand lupus érythemateux aigu survenant an décours d'une splénectomie pour purpura thrombopénique d'allure essentielle. Bull. Soc. méd. Hôp. Paris **77**, (1), 159 (1961). — SILVA, C. C. DE, and R. S. THANABALASUNDARAM: Congenital afibrinogenemia. Brit. med. J. **1951 II**, 86. — SILVERSTEIN, M. N., and F. J. HECK: Acquired haemolytic anaemia and associated thrombopenic purpura with special reference to Evans-syndrome. Proc. Mayo Clin. **37**, 122 (1962). — SIMON, C.: Des stigmates cutanées des mystiques. Zbl. Haut- u. Geschl.-Kr. **82**, 178 (1953). — SIMPSON, N. E., and R. BIGGS: The inheritance of Christmas factor. Brit. J. Haemat. **8** (3), 191 (1962). — SINISCALCO, M., L. BERNINI u. B. LATTE: Koppelung von Glucose-6-Phosphatdehydrogenase-Defizit, Farbblindheit und Haemophilie. 2. Int. Kongr. Humangenetik Rom 1961. — SIQUEIRA, M., and O. G. BIER: Hemorrhagic reactions at sites of passive cutaneous anaphylaxis in guinea pig after intravenous inoculation of unrelated immune complex. Proc. Soc. exp. Biol. (N.Y.) **107**, 779 (1961). — SIQUEIRA, M., and R. A. NELSON jr.: Platelet agglutination by immune complexes and its possible role in hypersensitivity. J. Immunol. **86** (5), 516 (1961). — SISE, H. S., J. GAUTHIER, R. BECKER and J. BOLGER: Blood coagulation factors in total body irradiation. Blood **18**, 702 (1961). — SJØLIN, K.: Classical hemophilia and Christmas factor deficiency as simultaneous defects. Acta med. scand. **159**, 7 (1957). — Hemophilia disease in Denmark. Oxford: Blackwell Sci. publ. 1960 (Traduction). — SLADKI, E., A. WIERZBOWSKA u. H. E. SCHULTZE: Fall einer Dyspragia cryoglobulinaemica abdominalis intermittens im Verlauf einer sog. essentiellen Cryoglobulinämie. Klin. Wschr. **37**, 712 (1959). — SLEPYAN, A. H.: (Diskussionsbemerkungen zu M. SPENCER.) Pigmented purpuric lichenoid dermatosis (Gougerot and Blum). Arch. Derm. **63**, 646 (1951). — SLOCUMB, C. H., H. F. POLLEY and L. E. WARD: Diagnosis, treatment and prevention of chronic hypercortisonism in patients with rheumatoid arthritis. Ann. intern. Med. **46**, 86 (1957). — SMITH, C. C., P. M. ZEEK and J. MCGUIRE: Periarteriitis nodosa in experimental hypertensive rats and dogs. Amer. J. Path. **20**, 721 (1944). — SMITH, J. L., and M. I. LINEBACK: Hereditary hemorrhagic teleangiektasia. (Nine cases in one negro family, with special reference to hepatic lesions.) Amer. J. Med. **17**, 41 (1954). — SMITH, M. D., D. A. SMITH and M. FLETCHER: Haemorrhage associated with thrombocytopenic in megaloblastic anaemia. Brit. med. J. **1962 I**, 982. — SMITH, R., and T. H. BERTRAM: Purpura with intense abdominal pain as a late complication of scarlet fever. Canad. med. Ass. J. **16**, 555 (1926). — SMITH, R., TH. RODMAN and B. H. PASTOR: A comparative study of prothrombinopenic anticoagulant drugs; Bishydroxycoumarin, Diphenadione, Anisindione and Acenacoumarol. J. Amer. med. Ass. **174**, 1917 (1960). — SMYTH, CH. J., and O. B. GUM: Vasculitis, mast cells and the collagen diseases. Arthr. and Rheum. **4**, 1 (1961). — SNEDDON, I. B.: Purpuric eruption with particular reference to external contact causes. Proc. 10th Internat. Congr. Dermatol., London 1952. 1953, p. 296. — Purpura as seen by the dermatologist. Acta derm.-venereol. (Stockh.), **37**, 296 (1957). — SNYMAN, H. W., u. A. P. MCDONALD: Onyalai. Med. Klin. **1956**, 676. — SOKAL, G.: Etude morphologique des plaquettes sanguines et de la métamorphose visqueuse au moyen d'antisérums fluorescents antifibrinogènes et antiplaquettes. Acta haemat. (Basel) **28**, 313 (1962). — SOLOMON, A., and J. L. FAHEY: Plasmapheresis therapy in macroglobulinemia. Ann. intern. Med. **58**, 789 (1963). — SONNECK, H. J.: Über einen besonderen Fall von Obstallergie unter dem Bild einer thrombopenischen Purpura. Dtsch. Gesundh.-Wes. **1957**, 196. — SOULIER, J. P., CH. BLATRIX, O. PROU-WARTELLE et A. VIGNAL: Préparation d'une fraction sérique riche en convertine (VII), F. Stuart (X) et F. antihémophilique B (IX). Fraction CSB. Etude expérimentale chez le lapin. Nouv. Rev. franç. Hémat. **2**, 27 (1962). — SOULIER, J. P., M. I. D. LARRIEU, J. DUBRISAY et D. MAHOUDIAU: Etude biologique de deux cas d'afribrinogénémie congénitale. Rév. Hémat. **10**, 689 (1955). — SOULIER, J. P., and M. J. LARRIEU: Differentiation of hemophilia invo 2 groups. New. Engl. J. Med. **249**, 547 (1953). — SOULIER, J. P., and O. PROU-WARTELLE: New data on Hageman factor and PTA. Brit. J. Haemat. **6**, 88 (1960). — SOULIER, J. P., O. WARTELLE and D. MÉNACHÉ: Hageman trait and PTA deficiency; the role of contact of blood with glass. Brit. J. Haemat. **5**, 121 (1959). — SPAET, TH. H.: Microscopic studies on blood vessels of rats with experimental purpura. Amer. J. Physiol. **170**, 33 (1952a). — Vascular factors in the pathogenesis of hemorrhagic syndromes. Blood **7**, 641 (1952b). — SPAET, TH. H., ST. BAUER and S. MELAMED: Hemorrhagic thrombocythemia. A blood coagulation disorder. Arch. intern. Med. **98**, 377 (1956). — SPANOUDIS, S., F. EICHBAUM and G. ROSENFELD: Inhibition of the local Shwartzman-reaction by dicumarol. J. Immunol. **75**, 167 (1955). — SPENCER, M. C.: Pigmented purpuric lichenoid dermatitis (Gougerot and Blum). Arch. Derm. **63**, 645 (1951). — SPIELMANN, W., A. GATHOF, W. FRITZSCHE u. E. F. PFEIFFER: Über die Bedeutung der serologischen Reaktionen bei allergisch-medikamentös bedingten Thrombopenien, dargestellt an einem Fall von Chinidinpurpura. Acta haemat. (Basel) **17**, 287 (1957). — SPIER, H. W., u. R. MARX: Zur Kasuistik der dermatite lichénoide purpurique et pigmentée Gougerot-Blum. Hautarzt **4**, 436 (1953). — SQUIER, TH. L., and F. W. MADISON: Thrombocytopenic purpura due to food allergy. J. Allergy **8**, 143 (1936/37). — STAMM, H.: Einführung in die Klinik der Fibrinolyse. Basel: S. Karger 1961. — STAUBESAND, J.: Eigenarten des Gefäßmusters bei räumlicher und bei flächenhafter Ausbreitung der arteriellen Strombahn in Organen. Verh. dtsch. Ges. Kreisl.-Forsch. 1956 S. 263, Darmstadt: Steinkopff. — Anatomie der Blutgefäße. I. Funktionelle Morphologie der Arterien, Venen und arterio-venösen Anastomosen. In: Angiologie von M. RATSCHOW. Stuttgart: Georg Thieme 1959. — STAUDE, W.: Das Waterhouse-Friderichsen-Syndrom in einer Gruppenerkrankung. Dtsch. Gesundh.-Wes. **15**, 2410 (1960). — STECHER, G., H. WOLFERS u. P. NETTESHEIM: Polycythaemia vera. Dtsch. med. Wschr. **86**, 1861 (1961). — STECKER, H., E. T. YIN u. F. DUCKERT: Neue Beobachtungen bei einer hämorrhagischen Diathese. Schweiz. med. Wschr. **92**, 1365 (1962). — STEFAN, H.: Hypofibrinogenämie und Fibrinolyse als Blutungsursache beim Prostatakarzinom. Z. Urol. **52**, 735 (1959). — STEFANINI, M., and J. B. CHATTERJEA: Rate of platelet survival in thrombocytopenic purpura. J. clin. Invest. **30**, 676 (1951). — STEFANINI, M., J. B. CHATTERJEA and E. ADELSON: Immunological aspects of idiopathic thrombopenic purpura. J. clin. Invest. **31**, 665 (1952). — STEFANINI, M., J. B. CHATTERJEA, W. DAMESHEK, L. ZANNOS u. E. PEREZ-SANTIAGO: II. The effect of transfusion of platelet-rich polycythemic blood on the platelets and hemostatic function in „idiopathic" and „secondary" thrombocytopenic purpura. Blood **7**, 53 (1952). — STEFANINI, M., and W. DAMESHEK: Idiopathic thrombocytopenic purpura. Lancet **1953 II**, 209. — The hemorrhagic disorders. A clinical and therapeutic approach, 2nd ed. New York: Grune & Stratton 1962. — STEFANINI, M., W. DAMESHEK, J. B. CHATTERJEA, E. ADELSON and I. B. MEDNICOFF: Observations on the properties and mechanism of action of a potent platelet agglutinine detected in the serum of a patient with idiopathic thrombocyto penic purpura. Blood 8, 26 (1953). — STEFANINI, M., and I. B. MEDNICOFF: Zit. The hemorrhagic disorders. New York: Grune & Stratton 1955. — STEFANINI, M., S. PIOMELLI and R. MELE: Immunohematologic disorders in childhood. Int. Arch. Allergy **15**, 16 (1959). — STEFANINI, M., S. PIOMELLI, R. MELE, J. T. OSTROSKI and W. P. COLPOYS: Acute vascular purpura following immunization with Asiatic influenza vaccine. N. Engl. J. Med. **259**, 9 (1958). — STEFANINI, M., C. A. ROY, L. ZANNOS u. W. DAMESHEK: Therapeutic effect of ACTH in a case of Schönlein-Henoch purpura. J. Amer. med. Ass. **144**, 1372 (1950). — STEFANOVIC, S.: Hémophilie A chez une fillette. Sang **30**, 858 (1959). — STEFENELLI, N., H. TULZER u. F. WEWALKA: Hautnekrosen als Nebenwirkung der Therapie mit Antikoagulantien. Thrombos. Diathes. haemorrh. (Stuttg.) **5**, 136 (1960). — STEFFEN, C.: Weitere Untersuchungen und Überblick über die verschiedenen immunologisch bedingten Formen der hämorrhagischen Diathesen. Wien. Z. inn. Med. **37**, 452 (1956). — Isolierung von Thrombocytenautoantikörpern und Untersuchung über die passiv übertragbare thrombopenische Wirkung der Eluate im Tierversuch. Int. Arch. Allergy **13**, 348 (1958). — STEIGLEDER, G. K.: Die hämorrhagisch-pigmentären Dermatosen — ein Syndrom oder eine selbständige Erkrankung? Hautarzt **4**, 520 (1953). — STEINHARDT, M. J., and G. S. FISHER: Cold urticaria and purpura as allergic aspects of cryoglobulinemia. J. Allergy **24**, 335 (1954). — STEINKAMP, R., C. V. MOORE and W. G. DOUBECK: Thrombocytopenic purpura caused by hypersensitivity to quinine. J. Lab. clin. Med. **45**, 18 (1955). — STENDER, H. ST., u. O. ELBERT: Über das Verhalten einiger Blutgerinnungsfaktoren nach einer Ganzbestrahlung mit großen Strahlendosen. Strahlentherapie **90**, 625 (1953). — STENING, S. E. L.: Congenital or neonata thrombocytopenic purpura. Med. J. Austr. **1953 II**, 210. — STEPHENS, J. H., and H. L. FRED: Petechiae associated with systemic fat embolism. Arch. Derm. **86**, 515 (1962). — STETSON jr., CH. A.: The nature of the blood vessel damage in the Shwartzman phenomenon. J. clin. Invest. **30** (I), 676 (1951a). — Studies on the mechanism of the Shwartzman-phenomenon: Certain factors involved in the production of the local hemorrhagic necrosis. J. exp. Med. **93**, 489 (1951b). — (Shwartzman phenomenon): Similarities between reactions to endotoxins and certain reactions of bacterial allergy. J. exp. Med. **101**, 421 (1955). — STETSON jr., CH. A., and R. A. GOOD: (Shwartzman phenomenon): Evidence for the participation of polymorphonuclear leucocytes. J. exp. Med. **93**, 49 (1951). — STICH, W.: Hämatopoetisches System. In: Klinik und Therapie der Nebenwirkungen von P. KÜMMERLE u. a. Stuttgart: Georg Thieme 1960. — STÖCKLI, A.: Hautnekrosen bei Coumarin-Medikation. Praxis **51**, 1308 (1962). — STOEGER, R.: Morbus maculosus Werlhof (Essentielle Thrombopenie). Hippokrates (Stuttg.) **13**, 751 (1942). — STORCK, H.: Purpura rheumatica (Demonstrationen). Dermatologica (Basel) **100**, 387 (1950). — Haut- und Schleimhautveränderungen bei Erkrankungen des haematopoetischen Systems. Augsburger Fortbild. prakt. Med., 6. Vortragsreihe (1951a). — Über hämorrhagische Phänomene in der Dermatologie. Dermatologica (Basel) **102**, 197 (1951b). — Index thrombopénique dans les états allergiques. Sem. Hôp. Paris **1955**, 1897. — Hämorrhagische Phänomene in der Dermatologie. Arch. Derm. Syph. (Berl.) **200**, 257 (1955). — Purpura anularis teleangiectodes Majocchi. Dermatologica (Basel) **118**, 316 (1959). — STORCK, H., P. BIGLIARDI, H. BRENN u. R. HOIGNÉ: Über die Bedeutung der Thrombocyten bei allergischen Vorgängen. I. Thrombo cytenabfall in vivo nach Allergenexposition. Schweiz. med. Wschr. **1953**, 692. — STORCK, H., u. R. HOIGNÉ: Thrombocyten und Serologie bei medikamentösen Hautallergien. Dermatologica (Basel) **112**, 405 (1956). — Plaquettes et sérologie au cours de l'allergie cutanée médicamenteuse. Sem. Hôp. Paris (Path.-Biol.) **33**, 333 (1957). — STORCK, H., R. HOIGNÉ u. F. KOLLER: Thrombocytenabfall als Hilfsmittel zur Allergendiagnose. I. Internat. Allergiekongr., S. 739. Zürich: S. Karger 739. — Thrombocytes in allergic reactions. Arch. int. Allergy **6**, 372 (1955). — STORMORKEN, H., R. SVENKERUD, P. SLAGSVOLD, H. LIE and J. LUNDEVALL: Thrombocytopenic bleeding in young pigs due to maternal isoimmunization. Nature (Lond.) No 4885, 1116 (1963). — STRAUB, W., and F. DUCKERT: The formation of the extrinsic prothrombin activator. Thrombos. Diathes. haemorrh. (Stuttg.) **5**, 402 (1961). — STRAUSS, L., J. CHURG and F. G. ZAK: Cutaneous lesions of allergic granulomatosis. A histopathologic study. J. invest. Derm. **17**, 349 (1951). — STUART, A. E.: Thrombotic thrombocytopenic purpura. A hyperergic microangiopathy. Lancet **1956 I**, 473. — STUBER, H. W.: Das Syndrom Haemangiom, thrombopenische Purpura und Anämie im Säuglingsalter. Helv. paediat. Acta, Ser. C. **11**, 194 (1956). — STÜTTGEN, G.: Beitrag zur Pathogenese der salvarsanbedingten Purpura. Hautarzt **2**, 211 (1951). — Zur Entstehung bullös-vesiculös-hämorrhagischer Exantheme in der Haut. Arch. klin. exp. Derm. **201**, 311 (1955). — Purpura fulminans. Sitzgs.-Bericht Vereinigg Düsseldorfer Dermatologen (1955). Zbl. Haut- u. Geschl.-Kr. **93**, 64 (1955/56). — Hämorrhagische Ekzeme und intestinale Purpura (Henoch-Schönlein). Hautarzt **10**, 159 (1959). — STÜTTGEN, G., CH. BERGHAUS u. H. BRÜSTER: Megalothrombocyten bei Lupus erythematodes. Derm. Wschr. **145**, 164 (1962). — SÜNDER, L.: Über die zentrale Genese symmetrischer Hautblutungen bei Purpura fulminans. Dtsch. med. Wschr. **69**, 597 (1943). — SWAIMAN, K., M. SCHAFFHAUSEN and W. KRIVIT: Thrombotic thrombocytic purpura (Report of an unusual clinical case and Chr. 31-red cell survival study). J. Pediat. **60** (6), 823 (1962). — SYMMERS, W. ST.: The occurrence of angiitis and of other generalized diseases of connective tissues as a consequence of the administration of drugs (with a note on drug allergy as a cause of thrombotic purpura). Proc. roy. Soc. Med. **55**, (I), 120 (1962). — SYMON, W. E., R. J. ROHN and W. H. BOND: Some observations on hyperglobulinemic purpura (Waldenström). Amer. J. med. Sci. **234**, 160 (1957). — SZENT-GYÖRGY, A. v.: Ascorbinsäure. Biochem. J. **22**, 1387 (1928); **26**, 865 (1932).

TAMPONI, M.: Dimostrazione di un „fattore piastrinolitico in un caso di porpora trombocitopenica in corso di eritemato-viscerite maligna. Minerva derm. **33**, 473 (1958). — TATTERSALL, R. N., and R. SEVILLE: Senile Purpura. Quart. J. Med. **74**, 151 (1950). — TAYLOR, K., and R. BIGGS: A mildly affected female hemophiliac. Brit. med. J. **1957 I**, 1494. — TAYLOR, M.: The response of capillary endothelium to changes in intravascular pressure, as seen in the rabbits chamber. Aust. J. exp. Biol. med. Sci. **31**, 533 (1953). — TEICHMANN, K.: Beobachtungen über Stoffaustausch im Kapillargebiet mit Hilfe der intravitalen Fluoreszenzmikroskopie. Z. ges. exp. Med. **110**, 732 (1942). — TELFER, T. P., K. W. DENSON and D. R. WRIGHT: A „new" coagulation defect. Brit. J. Haemat. **2**, 308 (1956). — TÉMIME, P.: A propos d'une dermo-épidermite purpuracée et eczematoïde générale. Ann. Derm. Syph. (Paris) **81**, 152 (1954). — TEPPER, P. A., J. G. CELLARIUS, W. S. PASCHKOWA u. A. A. SJURIN: Über das pathologische Wesen der Schönlein'schen Krankheit. Z. ges. inn. Med. **12**, 987 (1957). — THIES, H. A., u. J. OERI: Antikoagulantien in der Chirurgie. Basel: Benno Schwabe 1960. — THOMAS, J. W., D. M. WHITELAW and W. H. PERRY: The hemophilic syndrome. Canad. med. Ass. J. **79**, 100 (1958). — THOMAS, L.: The Shwartzman-phenomenon and other reactions produced by the endotoxins of gram negative bacteria. In: Immunopathology. Trans. Internat. Kongr. Basel 1958. Basel: Benno Schwabe & Co. 1959, p. 325. — THOMAS, L., J. BRUNSON and R. T. SMITH: VI. Production of the Shwartzman reaction by the synergetic action of endotoxin with 3 synthetic acidic polymers (sodium polyanethol sulfonate, dextran sulfate and sodium polyvinyl alcohol sulfonate). J. exp. Med. **102**, 249 (1955). — THOMAS, L., F. W. DENNY jr. and J. FLOYD: III. Lesions of the myocardium and coronary arteries accompanying the Shwartzman reaction in rabbits prepared by infection with group A streptococci. J. exp. Med. **97** (1953). — THOMAS, L., and R. A. GOOD: The effect of cortisone on the Shwartzman reaction. J. exp. Med. **95**, 409 (1952a). — Studies on the generalized Shwartzman reaction. General observations. J. exp. Med. **96**, 605 (1952b). — THOMAS, L., R. T. SMITH and R. v. KORFF: (Shwartzman reaction): The role of fibrinogen in the deposition of fibrinoid after combined injections of endotoxin and synthetic acidic polymer. J. exp. Med. **102**, 263 (1955). — THOMAS, L., B. W. ZWEIFACH and B. BENACERRAF: Mechanisms of the production of tissue damage and shock by endotoxins. Trans. Ass. Amer. Phycns **70**, 54 (1957). — THOMSEN, O.: A method for direct count of the blood platelets in the blood. Acta med. scand. **53**, 507 (1919). — TIDY, H. L.: Hunterian oration on the haemorrhagic diathesis and angiostaxis. Lancet **1926 II**, 221, 365. — TISCHENDORF, W., u. F. HARTMANN: Makroglobulinämie (Waldenström) mit gleichzeitiger Hyperplasie der Gewebsmastzellen. Acta haemat. (Basel) **4**, 374 (1950). — TOBIN jr., J. R., and I. A. FRIEDMAN: Platelet transfusion with use of blood in plastic bags from routine storage. J. Amer. med. Ass. **172**, 100 (1960). — TOCANTINS, L. M.: The coagulation of blood, 2nd. edit. New York and London: Grune & Stratton 1962. — TOCANTINS, L. M., and H. L. STEWART: Experimental thrombopenic purpura. Amer. J. Path. **15**, 1 (1939). — TOMSI, FR., and J. CANDOVA: Splenic thrombocytopenic purpura in

Hodgkin's disease. Vnitřini Lek. 1, 819 (1955) u. Zbl. Haut- u. Geschl.-Kr. 97, 184 (1957). — TOURAINE, A.: Le purpura annulaire télangiectasique de Majocchi et ses parentés (les capillarites ectasiantes). Presse méd. 65, 934 (1949). — Le purpura télangiectasique arciforme. Ann. Derm. Syph. (Paris) 10, 5 (1950). — TSCHERMAK-SEYSENEGG, A. v.: Physiologische Grundlagen der Stigmatisation. Pontif. Acad. Sci. Comment. 2, 13 (1938). — TUBIANA, M., et M. BOIRON: Le traitement des thrombocytémies par le phosphore radio-actif. Sang 28, 291 (1957). — TULLIS, J. L.: Platelet antibody tests in the diagnosis of purpura. New Engl. J. Med. 249, 591 (1953). — TURIN, R. D., S. MANDEL and L. HORNSTEIN: Fulminating purpura with gangrene of lower extremity necessitating amputation. J. Pediat. 54, 206 (1959). — TZANCK, A., J. P. SOULIER et CH. BLATRIX: Deux nouvelles observations de syndrome hémorragique avec présence d'un anticoagulant circulant. Rev. Hémat. 4, 502 (1949).

UEHLINGER, E.: Über eine Blutgerinnungsstörung bei Dysproteinämie (Beitrag zur Kenntnis der körpereigenen Antikoagulantia). Helv. med. Acta H. 16, Ser. A (1949). — ULUTIN, O. N., and M. KARACA: A study on the pathogenesis of thrombopathia using the „platelet osmotic resistance test". Brit. J. Haemat. 5, 302 (1959). — UNDRITZ, E.: Die Chediak-Steinbrinck-Anomalie oder erblich-konstitutionelle Riesengranulation. Schweiz. med. Wschr. 88, 996 (1958). — Morphology and genetics in hereditary constitutional anomalies of leucocytes. Acta haemat. (Basel) 24, 59 (1960). — UNNA, G. P.: Über Purpura senilis. Wien. med. Presse 36, 1499 (1895). — URBAN, J.: Übernatur und Medizin. Ref. Innsbruck 1946 (Zusammenfassung bei SCHLEYER).

VENHO, E. V.: Pharmakologische Untersuchungen über die Toxicität und die Antagonisten der synthetischen Antikoagulantien. Ann. Med. exp. Fenn., Suppl. 6 (1959). — VEREL, D., S. J. MAZURKIE, E. K. BLACKBURN, J. L. EMERY, S. VARADI and L. WOLMAN: Thrombocytopenia in congenital heart disease. Brit. Heart. J. 24 (1), 92 (1962). — VERHEIJ, P., and M. C. VERLOOP: Acute thrombopenic purpura as a complication of infectious mononucleosis. Ned. T. Geneesk 103, 1115 (1959). — VERSCHUER, O. v.: Genetik des Menschen. München u. Berlin: Urban & Schwarzenberg 1959. — VERSTRAETE, M., and J. VANDENBROUKE: Combined antihemophilic globulin and Christmas factor deficiency in hemophilia. Lancet 1955 I, 869. — VEST, M.: Der Einfluß von Naphthohydrochinonderivaten auf Erythrocytenabbau und -regeneration bei Frühgeburten und auf das Glucuronidbildungsvermögen der Leber in vitro. Schweiz. med. Wschr. 88, 969 (1958). — VILANOVA, X., R. CASTILLO and J. PINOL-AGUARDE: Mastocytosis with coagulation defect induced by biopsy. Arch. Derm. 84, 603 (1961). — VILANOVA, X., J. PINO et A. R. MUREAU: Eczematid-like purpura. Bull. Soc. franç. Derm. Syph. 63, 448 (1956). — VILMAR, G.: Beitrag zur Kenntnis der „Dermatite lichénoïde purpurique et pigmentée". Arch. Derm. Syph. (Berl.) 186, 476 (1948). — VOISIN, G. A., and F. TOULLET: Modifications of capillary permeability in immunological reactions mediated through cells. Ciba Found. Symp. Cellular aspects of immunity 1960. — VORLÄNDER, K. O.: Auto-Antikörper und Pathogenität. Dtsch. med. Wschr. 87, 887 (1962). — VOSS, D., and BJ. A. WAALER: Congenital hypoproconvertinemia (Report on 12 cases with total and 19 cases with partial deficiency). Thrombos. Diathes. haemorrh. (Stuttg.) 3, 375 (1959). — VRIES, S. I. DE, M. T. BOSMAN and C. M. SMIERS: Deficiency of anti-haemophilic globulin in women, associated with a prolonged bleeding time. Acta haemat. (Basel) 21, 206 (1959). — VRIES, S. I. DE, T. ROSENBERG, S. KOCHWA and J. H. BOSS: Precipitating anti-fibrinogen antibody appearing after fibrinogen infusion in a patient with congenital afibrinogenemia. Amer. J. Med. 30, 486 (1961). — VUILLE, J. C.: Zur Frage der Thrombocythaemia haemorrhagica. (Thrombelastogramm und Retraktion des Blutgerinnsels bei Anreicherung normaler Plättchen in vitro.) Diss. Bern 1960. — VUKOBRATOVIČ, S.: Manifestations allergiques provoquées par les médicaments. Acta allerg. (Kbh.), Suppl. 5, 68 (1958).

WAKSMAN, B. H.: Cell lysis and related phenomena in hypersensitive reactions, including immunohematologic diseases. In: P. KALLOS, Progress in Allergy, Bd. V, p. 349. Basel: S. Karger 1958. — WAKSMAN, B. H., u. P. MIESCHER: In vivo-Auswirkung von Antigen-Antikörper-Reaktionen. In: P. MIESCHER u. K. O. VORLÄNDER, Immunpathologie in Klinik und Forschung. Stuttgart: Georg Thieme 1961. — WALDENSTRÖM, J.: Clinical methods for the detection of hyperproteinemia and their practical diagnostic value. A contribution to the study of the „essentially" increased erythrocyte sedimentation. Nord. Med. 20, 2288 (1943). — Incipient myelomatosis or „essential" hyperglobulinemia with fibrinogenopenia—a new syndrome. Acta med. scand. 117, 216 (1944). — Zwei interessante Syndrome mit Hyperglobulinämie. Schweiz. med. Wschr. 38, 927 (1948). — Purpura hyperglobulinaemia und verwandte Zustände. Verh. dtsch. Ges. inn. Med. 58, 557 (1952). — Three new cases of purpura hyperglobulinemica. A study in long-lasting benign increase in serum globulin. Acta med. scand., Suppl. 266—269, 931 (1952). — Die Makroglobulinämie. Ergebn. inn. Med. Kinderheilk. 9, 586 (1958). — WALLER, H. D., G. W. LÖHR, F. GRIGNANI u. R. GROSS: Über den Energiestoffwechsel normaler menschlicher Thrombocyten. Thrombos. Diathes. haemorrh. (Stuttg.) 3, 520 (1959). — WALTHER, H.: Ein kasuistischer Beitrag zur erworbenen Fibrinogenopenie. Z. ges. inn. Med. 21, 1007 (1959). — WASSMUTH, D. R., H. E. HAMILTON and R. F. SHEETS: May-Hegglin anomaly. Hereditary affection of granulocytes and platelets. J. Amer. med. Ass. **183**, 737 (1963). — WATRIN, J., P. MICHON, J. BEUREY, J. M. MOUGEOLLE et E. REMIGY: Purpura idiopathique aigu: particularités hématologiques. Bull. Soc. franç. Derm. Syph. **62**, 105 (1955). — WATSON, R. F., S, ROTHBARD and P. VANEMEE: The antigenicity of rat collagen. J. exp. Med. **99**, 535 (1954). — WATSON-WILLIAMS, E. J., A. I. S. MACPHERSON and Sir STANLEY-DAVIDSON: The treatment of idiopathic thrombocytopenic purpura. A review of 93 cases. Lancet **1958 II**, 221. — WEBB, A. T., F. L. MEYER and E. R. LONSER: Hemorrhagic thrombocythemia. Arch. intern. Med. **111**, 280 (1963). — WEDDEL, G.: Studies related to the mechanism of common sensibility. In: Advances in Biology of skin, vol. 1 (W. MONTAGNA). New York: Pergamon Press 1960. — WEGENER, F.: Über eine eigenartige rhinogene Granulomatose. Beitr. path. Anat. **102**, 36 (1939). — WEICKER, H., u. P. BIGLIARDI: A-Avitaminose und Thrombocytenzahl. Z. Kinderheilk. **72**, 532 (1953). — WEIGLE, W. O., C. G. COCHRANE and F. J. DIXON: Anaphylactogenic properties of soluble antigen-antibody complexes in the guinea pig and rabbit. J. Immunol. **85**, 469 (1960). — WEIGLE, W. O., and F. J. DIXON: Relationship of circulating antigen-antibody complexes antigen, elimination and complement fixation in serum disease. Proc. Soc. exp. Biol. (N.Y.) **99**, 226 (1958). — Immunopathologie entzündlicher Organerkrankungen. In: MIESCHER u. VORLAENDER, Immunpathologie in Klinik und Forschung. Stuttgart: Georg Thieme 1961. — WEINREICH, J.: Die diagnostische und klinische Abgrenzung von Makroglobulinaemie (Waldenström) und Purpura hyperglobulinaemica (Waldenström). Münch. med. Wschr. **1955**, 1988. — Neuere Untersuchungsergebnisse zur Frage des „Hypersplenismus". Med. Klin. **58**, 81 (1963). — WEINTRAUB, R. M., L. PECHET and B. ALEXANDER: Rapid diagnosis of drug-induced thrombocytopenic purpura. (3 cases: Quinine, Quinidine, Dilantin.) J. Amer. med. Ass. **180**, 528 (1962). — WEISE, H. J.: Zur Klinik der Waldenström'schen Krankheitssyndrome. Med. Klin. **56**, 426 (1961). — WEISS, H. J., J. DEMIS, M. L. ELGART and W. H. CROSBY: Treatment of two cases of hyperglobulinemic purpura with thioguanine. New Engl. J. Med. **268**, 753 (1963). — WELLMAN, F. C.: Brief conspectus of the tropical diseases common in the Highlands of West Central Africa. J. trop. Med. Hyg. **11**, 119 (1904). — WHITBY, L. E. H., and C. J. C. BRITTON: Disorders of the blood, 8th edit. London: Churchill 1957. — WHITTACKER, D. L., D. L. COPELAND and J. B. GRAHAM: Linkage of colour blindness to hemophilia A and B. Amer. J. hum. Genet. **14**, 149 (1962). — WIEL, TH. W. M. VAN DE, H. VAN DE WIEL-DORFMEYER and J. J. VAN LOGHEM: Studies on platelet antibodies in man. Vox Sang. (Basel) **6**, 641 (1961). — WILBRANDT, W.: Die Permeabilität der Zelle. Ergebn. Physiol. **40**, 204 (1938). — WILBRANDT, W., E. F. LÜSCHER u. H. ASPER: Physiologie der Zell- und Kapillarpermeabilität. Helv. med. Acta **13**, 141 (1946). — Der Einfluß von Thrombocytenprotein auf die Permeabilität der Blutkapillaren. Helv. physiol. pharmacol. Acta **14**c, 81 (1956). — WILE, S. A., and PH. STURGEON: Thrombotic thrombocytopenic purpura. Review of the subject with report of 3 cases in children. Pediatrics **17**, 882 (1956). — WILHELM, D. L.: Serum globulins as mediators of pathologic changes of capillar permeability. Proc. roy. Soc. Med. **49**, 575 (1956). — WILKINSON, J. F., and K. E. BARRETT: The management and treatment of haemophilia. Practitioner 188, 194 (1962). — WILKINSON, J. F., F. NOUR-ELDIN, M. C. G. ISRAEL and K. E. BARRETT: Haemophilia syndromes. Lancet **1961 II**, 947. — WILLEBRAND, E. A. v.: Über hereditäre Pseudohaemophilie. Acta med. scand. **76**, 521 (1926). — WILLEBRAND, E. A. v., u. R. JÜRGENS: Über ein neues vererbbares Blutungsübel: die konstitutionelle Thrombopathie. Dtsch. Arch. klin. Med. **175**, 453 (1931). — WILLI, H.: Innenkörperbildung durch wasserlösliches Vitamin K-Präparat. Schweiz. med. Wschr. **86**, 1453 (1956). — WILSON, C. J., and M. E. HAGGARD: Giant vascular tumors and thrombocytopenia. Arch. Derm. **81**, 432 (1960). — WINER, L. H., D. H. KLING and G. H. LEVIN: Ecchymosis in arthritis patients on prolonged corticosteroids. A histologic study. Arch. Derm. **86**, 654 (1962). — WINKELMANN, R. K.: Clinical and pathological findings in the skin in anaphylactoid purpura (allergic angiitis). Proc. Mayo Clin. **33**, 277 (1958). — Nerve endings in normal and pathologic skin. Springfield (Ill.): Ch. C. Thomas 1960. — WINKELMANN, R. K., u. H. MONTGOMERY: Über die cutane Periarteriitis nodosa. Hautarzt **11**, 82 (1960). — WINTERSTEIN, W.: Zur Biochemie der Gerinnungsfaktoren. In: Hämorrhagische Diathesen, Internat. Symposium Wien, S. 151. Wien: Springer 1955. — WINTROBE, M. M.: Clinical hematology, 9. edit. Philadelphia: Lea & Febiger 1951. — WISHART, C., C. A. SMITH, G. E. HONEY and K. B. TAYLOR: Dental extraction in hemophilia. Lancet **1957 I**, 363. — WISKOTT, A.: Familiärer, angeborener Morbus Werlhofii? Mschr. Kinderheilk. **68**, 212 (1937). — WITTE, S.: Die hämatologischen Befunde bei der experimentellen thrombocytopenischen Purpura. 5. Kongr. Europ. Ges. Hämat. **1956**, S. 799. — Über Beziehungen zwischen Blutgerinnung und Kapillarpermeabilität. Fol. haemat. (Lpz.), N. F. **1**, 320 (1957). — Die Steigerung der Kapillarpermeabilität durch Blutgerinnungsstörungen. Thrombos. Diathes. haemorrh. (Stuttg.) **2**, 146 (1958). — Über den Gefäßfaktor bei Blutungen und Blutungskrankheiten. Med. Welt **1960** (1), 718. — Die Wundheilung bei haemorrhagischen Diathesen. Proc. 8. Congr. Europ. Soc. Haemat. Wien 1961, Bd. II, S. 350. — WITTE, S., u.

Th. Schricker: Experimentelle Untersuchungen über das Verhalten der Thrombocyten im Kreislauf. Klin. Wschr. **36**, 1119 (1958). — Witte, S., Th. Schricker u. D. Bressel: Über die Wirkung der Plasmafraktion I auf den hämorrhagischen Gefäßfaktor. Klin. Wschr. **35**, 953 (1957). — Witte, S., u. K. Wilmes: Die Wirkung von Rutin bei der experimentellen thrombopenischen Purpura der Ratte. Acta haemat. **7**, 89 (1952). — Wiznitzer, T., F. B. Schweinburg, N. Atkins and J. Fine: On the relation of the size of the intraintestinal pool of endotoxin to the development of irreversibility in hemorrhagic shock. J. exp. Med. **112**, 1167 (1960). — Wolter, R., et H. Loeb: Deux cas de purpura fulminans septicémique traités par l'hydrocortisone intraveineuse. Acta paediat. belg. **10**, 130 (1956). — Wright, H. P.: The sources of blood platelets and their adhesiveness in experimental thrombocytosis. J. Path. **56**, 151 (1944). — Wright, I. S.: Nomenclature of blood clotting factors. Acceptance by the internat. Committee on nomenclature of 4 factors. Thrombos. Diathes. haemorrh. (Stuttg.) **3**, 435 (1959). — Wright, I. S., F. Koller and F. Streuli: Thrombolytic activity and related phenomena. Trans. Conf. Internat. Comm. Blood clotting factors. Princeton 1960. — Wuhrmann, F., u. Ch. Wunderly: Die Bluteiweißkörper des Menschen. Basel: Benno Schwabe & Co. 1947. — Wurzel, H. A.: Incidence of various coagulation defects and their association with different diseases. Amer. J. med. Sci. **241**, 625 (1961).

Zahnd, G., et A. Rohner: Paramyloidose purpurique dans un cas de myélome atypique. Schweiz. med. Wschr. **89**, 155 (1959). — Zeek, P. M.: Periarteritis nodosa: a critical review. Amer. J. clin. Path. **2**, 777 (1952). — Periarteritis nodosa and other forms of necrotizing angiitis. New Engl. J. Med. **248**, 764 (1953). — Ziff, M.: Genetics, hypersensitivity and the connective tissue disease. Amer. J. Med. **30**, 1 (1961). — Zollinger, H. U.: Die pathologische Anatomie der Makroglobulinämie Waldenström. Helv. med. Acta **25**, 153 (1958). — Zollinger, W.: Dissertation (in Vorbereitung). — Zollinger, W., u. W. H. Hitzig: Über den Erbgang bei kongenitalem Faktor VII-Mangel. Helv. med. Acta **25**, 475 (1958). — Erworbene Hypofibrinogenämie bei Paraleukoblastenleukämie mit Kälteagglutininämie im Kindesalter. Schweiz. med. Wschr. **89**, 1032 (1959). — Zucker, M. B.: Blood platelets. Sci. Amer. **204**, 58 (Jan. 1961). — Zucker, M. B., and J. Borelli: Relationship of some blood clotting factors to serotonin release from washed platelets. J. appl. Physiol. **7**, 432 (1955). — Zucker, M. B., A. B. Ley and K. Mayer: Studies on platelet life span and platelet deposits by use of DFP 32. J. Lab. clin. Med. **58**, 405 (1961). — Zukschwerdt, L., u. H. A. Thies: Antikoagulantien in der Humanmedizin. Bericht 3. Hamburg. Symp. Blutgerinnung 1961. — Zweifach, B. W.: Pathophysiology of the blood vascular barrier. Angiology **13**, 345 (1962)

Fremdkörpergranulome

Von

Hans Kuske-Bern

Mit 7 Abbildungen (davon 1 farbige)

A. Einleitung

1. Allgemeines

Auf Fremdkörperreize sind sowohl klinisch als auch histologisch ganz verschiedenartige Antworten möglich, weil zu dem rein mechanischen Insult auch toxische Wirkungen und sogar allergisierende Faktoren hinzukommen können. Die klassische Granulomatose, Entzündung mit Vorherrschen der Epitheloiden und mit Riesenzellenbildung, steht als besondere Form der Abwehr noch immer im Zentrum des Fragenkomplexes. Doch wäre es falsch, das Kapitel über Fremdkörper und Haut als längst abgeschlossen und kaum mehr ergänzungsbedürftig zu betrachten. Die seinerzeitige Bearbeitung und Zusammenstellung von POLLAND bildet eine sehr wertvolle Grundlage. In der Zwischenzeit sind aber neue Tatsachen hinzugekommen, die wir in Sonderabschnitten berücksichtigen müssen. So drängt sich vor allem je ein Kapitel über das Beryllium- und Zirkonium-Granulom auf. Ferner müssen die gerade in jüngster Zeit oft erörterten Zusammenhänge zwischen silikotischen oder Narbengranulomen und der Sarkoidosis als Allgemeinkrankheit eingehender besprochen werden.

Weitere notwendig gewordene Ergänzungen sind kurze Abschnitte über die Chrysiasis und die Eisenspeicherkrankheit — Abschnitte, welche sich, ohne prinzipiell neue Ausblicke zu eröffnen, dem bisherigen Wissen über die Argyrose anfügen lassen.

Die verschiedenen Kapitel der Arbeit von POLLAND werden nur soweit durch neuere Einzelbeobachtungen ergänzt, als diese über das bis jetzt Bekannte hinausgehen oder sonst praktisches oder theoretisches Interesse beanspruchen dürfen.

Je nachdem, welche Definition man für den ,,Fremdkörper" anwendet, kann das Problem Fremdkörper und Haut enger gefaßt oder breiter entwickelt werden. Im engeren und strengeren Sinne verstehen wir darunter einen unbelebten, gewebefremden, meist traumatisch eingedrungenen Körper. Die klassische Definition bezieht sich also hauptsächlich auf figurierte feste Stoffe, wie Kristalle, Stacheln, Splitter, Fäden usw. Man kann aber auch Flüssigkeiten in die Fremdkörper-Definition aufnehmen. Sofern diese flüssigen Substanzen nämlich nicht diffundieren und nur schwer resorbiert werden können, sind sie in ihrer Wirkung den gewöhnlichen Fremdkörpern gleichzusetzen. Als Beispiele seien die mineralischen Öle und Fette angeführt. In Ausnahmefällen können sogar Gase Fremdkörperreaktionen auslösen. So sind Embolien von schwer resorbierbaren Gasen in den Lymphgefäßen des Darmes beobachtet worden, welche zu feingeweblichen Veränderungen führten, die mit der Fremdkörperreaktion identisch sind (Lymphopneumatose cystique de Masson). Von der Haut ist allerdings nichts Ähnliches bekannt.

In der Regel wird es sich beim Fremdkörper um eine von außen in den Organismus eingedrungene Substanz handeln. Aber auch hier darf die Definition nicht zu eng gefaßt werden, denn es gibt auch endogen entstehende Fremdkörper, so z.B. Gewebeteile, die durch ein Trauma in eine neue Umgebung versetzt worden sind (Epithelcyste). Auch Zellen und Gewebe, die nicht mehr am normalen Stoffwechsel teilhaben und auf diese Weise chemisch verändert wurden, wirken in der Folge wie Fremdkörper (LANG).

Abweichende Reaktionsbilder entstehen immer dann, wenn vom Fremdkörper zusätzlich eine toxische Wirkung ausgeht. Meistens bildet sich daraufhin eher eine banale Entzündung mit Einschmelzung und Ausstoßen der eingedrungenen Substanzen aus. Im französischen Schrifttum wird deshalb streng zwischen einer toxischen und einer rein xenischen Reaktion unterschieden. (Xenische Reaktion wäre gleichbedeutend mit Fremdkörperreaktion, abgeleitet von Xenos = fremd [WORINGER 1936].) Die erwähnten Besonderheiten der Fremdkörper — ihre Natur, Größe, aber auch Art und Weise, sowie Tiefe des Eindringens, ob absichtlich oder zufällig, ob therapeutisch oder akzidentiell, ob endogen oder exogen — könnten als Unterlage für eine Einteilung des Kapitels verwendet werden. Wir möchten jedoch auf eine allzu systematische Gliederung des Stoffes verzichten und nach einem allgemeinen, vorwiegend die pathologische Anatomie und die Pathogenese behandelnden Abschnitt in einem speziellen Teil, in lockerer Folge, einzelne wichtige Kapitel besprechen.

2. Pathologische Anatomie und Genese der Fremdkörperreaktion

Über die pathologisch-anatomischen Gewebeveränderungen, die nach Eindringen eines Fremdkörpers auftreten können, besteht ein sehr ausgedehntes, kaum mehr zu übersehendes Schrifttum. Man ist der Frage seit jeher nicht nur durch sorgfältige klinische und histologische Einzelbeobachtung nachgegangen, sondern sie gab auch immer wieder Anlaß zu diesbezüglichen experimentellen Arbeiten. Darüber eingehend zu berichten ist unmöglich, müßten wir doch sowohl auf sehr frühe und doch immer noch aktuelle, wertvolle Beiträge von F. MARCHAND, von BAYER u.a. aus dem vorigen Jahrhundert, wie auch auf eine ganze Kette von Bearbeitern bis in die allerjüngste Zeit hinweisen. Mit Vorteil wendet man sich, um den unbedingt erforderlichen Überblick zu erhalten, an monographische Bearbeitungen wie diejenige von F. WORINGER, oder an Handbuchbeiträge aus den letzten Jahren, etwa an den Abschnitt von F. C. ROULET, die infektiösen spezifischen Granulome, in Springers Handbuch der allgemeinen Pathologie, 1956. Hier soll nur auf einige Fragen kurz eingegangen werden.

Der zentrale, wichtige, immer wieder beobachtete Typus der Fremdkörperreaktion mit epitheloidzellig-riesenzelligem Granulom hat wegen seiner Ähnlichkeit mit gewissen infektiösen, spezifischen Granulomen am meisten Interesse gefunden.

WEISS beschrieb 1876 Riesenzellen und Epitheloide, die sich um Fremdkörper bilden. Die experimentelle Forschung setzte ein mit Hipolythe MARTIN, der beweisen konnte, daß durch unbelebte Substanzen Pseudotuberkulosen entstehen. Das Granulationsgewebe oder Granulom ist eine morphologische Reaktion des Blutes und des Gewebes, durch welche der Organismus ganz allgemein eine Noxe — einen Infektionskeim oder ein Toxin usw. — bekämpft. Bei mikrobiell bedingten Entzündungen überwiegen exsudative, vasculäre Symptome. Bei der Fremdkörperreaktion überwiegen mehr die lokalen zelligen Reaktionen. Das Volumen des Fremdkörpers spielt für die zu erwartende Antwort nur eine untergeordnete Rolle, nicht aber seine Oberfläche und seine Resistenz gegenüber den

Einflüssen von Säften, Enzymen usw. Stark toxische Eigenschaften eines Fremdkörpers können die Granulombildung direkt verhindern und ausschalten. Es kommt zu einer Nekrose und zur Demarkation und Ausstoßung ohne eine typische Fremdkörperreaktion. Gute Beispiele dafür sind die Tintenstiftnekrose oder der Terpentinöl-Fixationsabsceß. Natürlich ist oft mit Fremdkörpern zu rechnen, die gleichzeitig toxische Eigenschaften aufweisen, daneben aber auch nicht resorbierbar sind. In einem solchen Falle folgen sich eine toxische akute Primärphase und eine chronische granulomatöse Sekundärphase. Ähnliches gilt für alle Fälle, bei

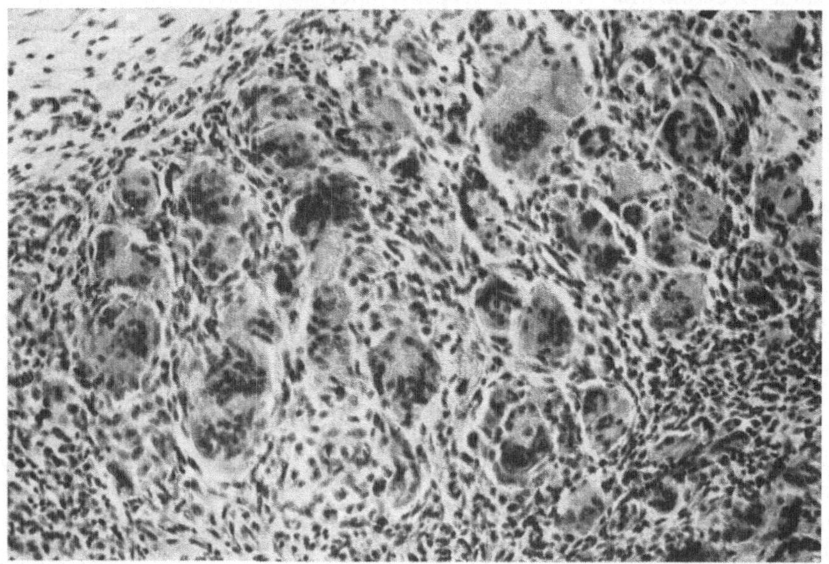

Abb. 1. Zahlreiche Fremdkörperriesenzellen in der Umgebung einer Epithelcyste

denen gleichzeitig mit dem Eindringen des Fremdkörpers eine bakterielle Infektion erfolgt.

Einen interessanten Sonderfall stellen die Epithelcysten dar, die so lange vom Gewebe toleriert werden, als sie intakt bleiben und durch Stoffwechselprodukte mit dem umgebenden Bindegewebe im Austausch leben. Sterben sie ab, so werden sie wie Fremdkörper behandelt. Es gibt Beispiele von ganz besonders schöner Fremdkörperriesenzellbildung gerade um Cystenwandteile herum (Abb. 1). Dabei zeigt sich oft, ähnlich wie in Implantationsexperimenten, daß die cutane Seite der Wand noch weiter toleriert wird, nicht aber die epidermale Seite.

Die pathologisch-anatomische Fremdkörperreaktion kann auf eine relativ einfache Formel gebracht werden. Es ist vorwiegend das reticulo-endotheliale System, das sich daran beteiligt. Nach Woringer kann man drei Stadien unterscheiden:

1. Das Blutstadium — Diapedese oder Infiltratphase mit leukocytärer Reaktion.
2. Das Gewebestadium — die histiocytäre Reaktion.
3. Das Narbenstadium — die Sklerose als Endausgang.

Die Frühphase mit Diapedese und Infiltration des Gewebes mit zelligen Elementen aus dem Blut ist — wie schon erwähnt — stark von der Toxicität der Fremdkörper abhängig und darum unterschiedlich ausgeprägt. Oft dauert sie nur wenige Tage und macht dann der zweiten, zelligen Phase Platz. Oft werden diese diskreten histopathologischen Erscheinungen auch übersehen, denn es handelt sich ja lediglich um Gefäßerweiterungen mit Vermehrung der Leukocyten in den Randzonen, um etwas Ödem, um wenige Leukocyten und einige Lymphocyten, die die Gefäße verlassen und in die Umgebung des Fremdkörpers einwandern. Kleinste Fremdkörper werden von Leukocyten phagocytiert. Dabei wird oft beobachtet, daß die phagocytierenden Zellen bald absterben. Der drohende Zelltod ist erkennbar am acidophilen und wenig transparenten Protoplasma und an der einsetzenden Kernpyknose. Später verlieren die Kerne die Färbbarkeit, das Protoplasma wird in Granulationen aufgelöst, und die Fremdkörper werden durch diesen Untergang der phagocytierenden weißen Blutzelle erneut freigesetzt. Der Zustrom von Leukocyten kann anhalten, er wird aber meist geringer, und die in der Zwischenzeit in Gang gekommene histiocytäre Gewebereaktion der zweiten Phase wird vorherrschen oder allein weiterbestehen.

Dieses zweite, relativ charakteristische Stadium der Fremdkörperreaktion beruht auf der Mobilisierung lokaler reticulo-endothelialer Elemente. Während sie im Ruhestadium nur schwer von einem Fibroblasten zu unterscheiden sind, bekommen diese Gewebehistiocyten nach Reizung besondere neue Eigenschaften. Der Kern wird größer, unregelmäßig rundlich, das Chromatin bleibt aber relativ fein verteilt und ohne Nucleolen; das Protoplasma wird deutlicher erkennbar als in der Ruhephase, man glaubt bei unregelmäßigen ungenauen Zellgrenzen Ausläufer zu erkennen, die mit benachbarten Zellen anastomosieren. Die Auffassung, es handle sich um ein ausgedehntes syncytiales Gewebe, dessen einzelne Elemente allerdings auf den ersten Blick isoliert erscheinen, hat lange vorgeherrscht. Elektronenmikroskopische Untersuchungen sprechen allerdings eher dafür, daß immer scharfe Zellgrenzen erhalten bleiben.

Die Histiocyten betätigen sich als Makrophagen. Wegen dieser phagocytierenden Eigenschaften sind sie seit langem bekannt und mit verschiedenen Namen belegt worden: Clasmatocyt (Ranvier), Adventitiazelle (Marchand), Histiocyt (Kiyono u. Nakanoin), Polyblast (Maximow). Je nach der als Reiz wirkenden Ursache scheint der Histiocyt noch besondere Spezialformen anzunehmen; die Epitheloidzelle, die Typhuszelle, sogar die Plasmazelle und der Mastocyt, vielleicht auch die Gewebeeosinophilen gelten als solche besonderen Abkömmlinge des gereizten Histiocyten.

Um einen Fremdkörper herum proliferieren die Histiocyten; oft umgeben sie kleine Partikel völlig; sind die Fremdkörper zu groß, so klebt eine histiocytäre Zelle an die andere, und so entsteht die Fremdkörperriesenzelle. Daß sich diese besondere Riesenzelle von Gewebehistiocyten ableiten läßt, wird mit weitgehender Übereinstimmung angenommen. Die Entstehungsweise allerdings wird noch immer diskutiert. Ernsthaft in Betracht kommen zwei Erklärungen, nämlich: die schon erwähnte Auffassung, daß die Riesenzellen entweder durch Fusion von Histiocyten entstehen (Maximow, Kiyono), eine Theorie, der sich auch Woringer anschließt, oder die Erklärung durch Knospung der Kerne ohne Teilung des Protoplasmas (Weigert, Herxheimer, Kreibich). Amitotische Teilungsfiguren sind nun allerdings sehr selten anzutreffen, was die zweite Erklärung etwas weniger wahrscheinlich macht.

Die Fremdkörperriesenzelle hat sehr große Ähnlichkeit mit der Langhansschen Riesenzelle. Man findet oft Exemplare mit 10—50 Kernen. Diese sind an der Grenze von Endo- und Exoplasma in Ring-, Kranz- oder Hufeisenform aufgereiht. Besonders wenn die Kerne peripher und regelmäßig angeordnet sind, findet man im Zentrum der Zelle eine Anhäufung von Centrosomen. Neben dem Typus der Langhansschen Riesenzelle mit kranzförmig angeordneten Kernen und acidophilem transparentem Plasma findet man auch den anderen Typus mit unregelmäßiger Anhäufung der Kerne im Zentrum und dunklem amphophilem Plasma (Abb. 2a u. b). Übergänge zwischen diesen beiden Zellformen sind häufig, und deshalb ist die Annahme, die Zellen mit unregelmäßigen Kernhaufen seien

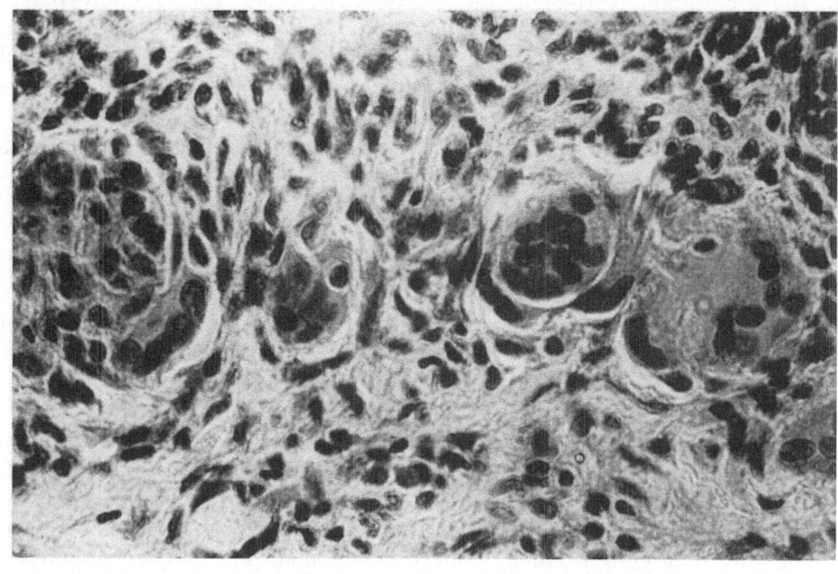

a

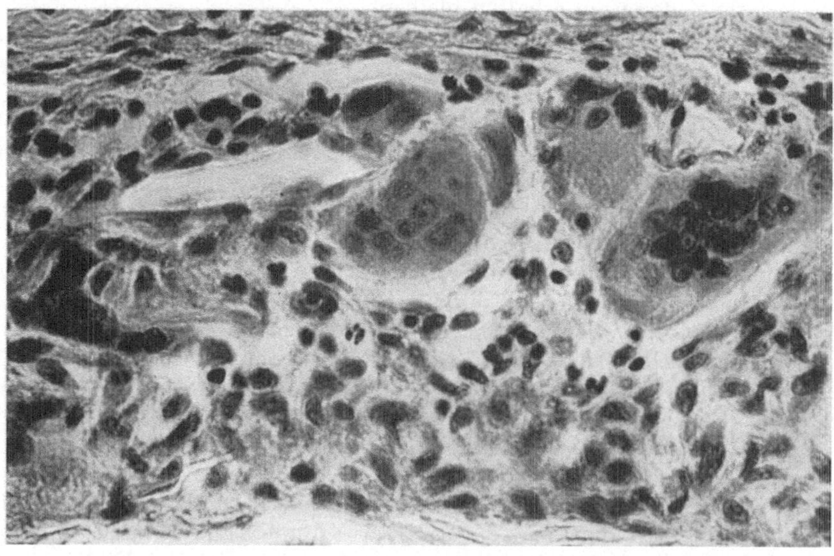

b

Abb. 2 a u. b. a Fremdkörperriesenzellen von verschiedenem Typus. b Fremdkörperriesenzellen an Cholesterinkristall angelagert (im Präparat herausgelöst)

lediglich Degenerationsformen, glaubhaft. Sicher behält die Riesenzelle die phagocytären Eigenschaften der Histiocyten, sicher ist sie imstande, mit dem Protoplasma Fremdkörper zu umschließen. Eine eigentliche Wanderfähigkeit besitzt sie wohl kaum. Als Einschlüsse findet man Leukocyten, zerstörte Lymphocyten, nekrotisches Zellmaterial usw. (Abb. 3).

Strahlige Einschlüsse in den Riesenzellen sind seit langem beobachtet worden; sie werden verschieden gedeutet. Vermutlich sind auch sie ein Degenerationsprodukt, am ehesten albuminoide Substanzen, die im Zellinnern auskristalliert sind.

Die Zahl der Riesenzellen bei der Fremdkörperreaktion steht in Abhängigkeit von der Resorbierbarkeit und von der Größe der Fremdkörper. Je schwieriger die Resorption, desto häufiger die Fremdkörperriesenzellen, je kleiner die Partikel, desto seltener Riesenzellen (Beispiel Tuschepartikel der Tatauierungen). Im Bereich des Granuloms gehen die elastischen Fasern zugrunde, während sich um das Granulom herum die Fibroblasten häufen und einen Abkapselungsprozeß vorbereiten, indem vermehrt kollagene Fasern gebildet werden.

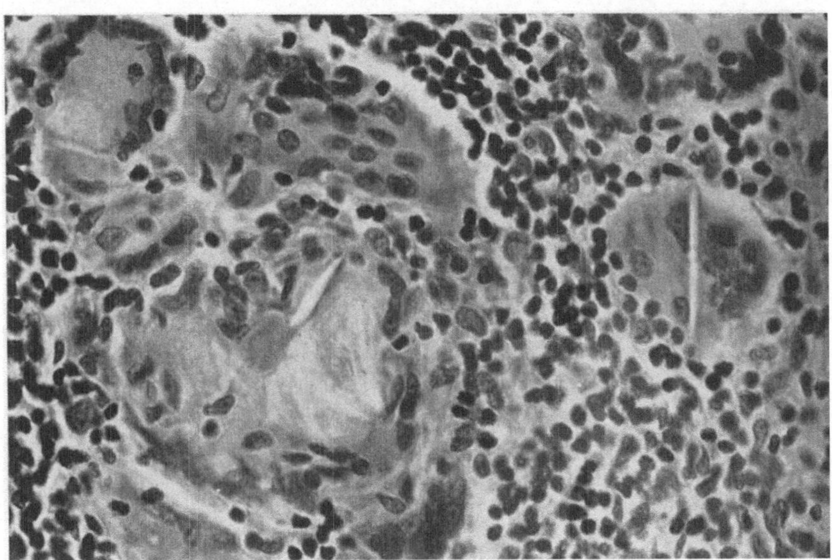

Abb. 3. Riesenzellen mit spaltförmigen Lücken (ausgelaugte Kristalle)

Besonders in den Fällen mit völlig unresorbierbaren Fremdkörpern nimm dieser sklerosierende Prozeß (die fibröse Abkapselung) ständig zu. Im Endzustand bekommt man dann den Eindruck, der Fremdkörper sei, vom Gewebe toleriert, ohne Abwehrreaktion aufgenommen worden. Tatsächlich aber ist er — anschließend an eine entzündliche Phase — durch eine isolierende Kapselhülle aus faserigem Bindegewebe vom Gewebe abgetrennt.

Neben diesen drei oft aufeinanderfolgenden Phasen der Abwehrreaktion unterscheidet Woringer drei besondere Typen der pathologisch-anatomischen Fremdkörperreaktion und legt sie seiner Einteilung des klinischen Stoffes zugrunde, nämlich:

a) Eine rein histiocytäre Reaktion als Antwort auf das Eindringen kleinster Partikel (Beispiel Tätowierung).

b) Die klassische granulomatöse Fremdkörperreaktion. Hier ist der Fremdkörper in der Regel größer als ein Histiocyt, hier finden wir die typische Antwort des Gewebes mit epitheloid- und riesenzelligem Granulom; später die Fibrose mit Abkapselung (Beispiel: Glassplitter, Silicium-Kristalle usw.).

c) Die polycystische Reaktion. Diese Gewebe-Reaktion finden wir als Antwort auf das Eindringen von körperfremden Fetten oder auch als Reaktion auf die Umwandlung von körpereigenem Fett bei der sog. Fettgewebsnekrose. Die Fetttropfen werden dabei aufgeteilt, in Cysten umgewandelt und von Histiocyten durchwuchert. Hier fehlen die Riesenzellen normalerweise ganz. Als Besonderheit finden sich aber in Leukocyten und histiocytären Makrophagen Fetteinschlüsse. Vermutlich sind die Histiocyten mit einem fettverdauenden Ferment ausgerüstet, das ihnen den Abbau von vegetabilen und tierischen Fetten erlaubt. In 3—4 Monaten sind solche injizierte Öle völlig resorbiert. Wenn ausnahmsweise mikrocystische Reaktionen auftreten, so sind sie vermutlich auf Verunreinigungen zurückzuführen.

Auf eine interessante histologische Abwehrreaktion gegen in die Haut eingebrachte Staphylokokken wurde kürzlich von HOPKINS, WELD und HUBER auf-

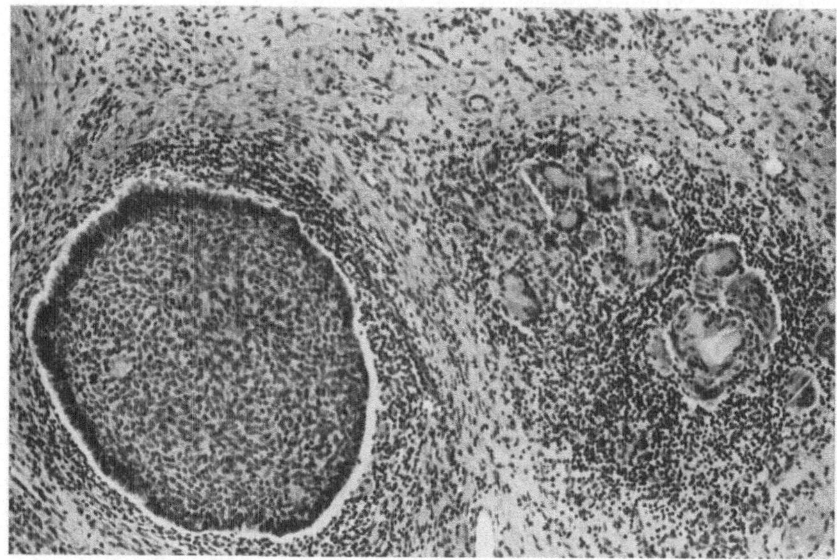

Abb. 4. Fremdkörperreaktion in der Nähe eines Basalzellcarcinoms

merksam gemacht. Es scheint, daß sich besonders abgetötete Keime in Kaninchenversuchen ähnlich wie Fremdkörper verhielten. Allerdings wurden die eingespritzten abgetöteten Staphylokokken bei sensibilisierten Tieren nicht mit einer granulomatösen Reaktion bekämpft, sondern sie wurden von einer Epithelwand, ausgehend vom Follikelepithel, umwachsen und als Cyste nachher ausgestoßen. Ferner entwickelten sich Horncysten und komedonenartige Follikelpfröpfe. Wenn sich diese Beobachtungen und ihre Interpretation bestätigen sollten, so wäre darin ein interessanter Abwehrmechanismus gefunden, welcher auch klinische Befunde, vor allem die sog. kalten Staphylokokken- und Talgretentionsabscesse bei der Acne profunda, oder die epidermale Sequestration beim Kolloidmilium auf eine völlig neue Weise erklären könnte. Zu der klassischen Fremdkörperreaktion bestehen allerdings nur sehr lockere Beziehungen. Trotzdem seien diese Befunde hier angeführt, weil sie vielleicht doch beweisen, daß eine allzu vereinfachende Auffassung über die Abwehrmöglichkeiten der Haut gegenüber Fremdkörpern und Fremdstoffen nicht zutreffen dürfte.

Am Schlusse dieses einleitenden, allgemeinen Kapitels sei noch darauf hingewiesen, daß der histologischen Fremdkörperreaktion auch bei vielen anderen Krankheitsbildern eine besondere Bedeutung zukommt. Als Beispiel erwähne ich die Granulome mit Fremdkörperriesenzellen, die man oft in der Umgebung infiltrativ wachsender oder degenerierter bösartiger Tumoren finden kann (Abb. 4).

Auch die Granulomatosis disciformis Miescher, eine scheibenförmige, degenerative Veränderung der Haut, die meist an den Unterschenkeln lokalisiert angetroffen wird, wurde von einzelnen Autoren als eine Fremdkörperreaktion eigenartiger Prägung aufgefaßt (WORINGER u. ULLMO).

B. Spezieller Teil

I. Unfallbedingte und gewerbliche Fremdkörperschädigungen

1. Das silicotische Narbengranulom

Im Anschluß an Verletzungen der Haut kommt es häufig zum Einheilen von kleinen Fremdkörpern. Am auffälligsten sind immer die banalen traumatischen Tätowierungen mit Kohle-, mit Asphalt- oder Teerpartikeln, weil dadurch bleibende, blauschwarze Verfärbungen zurückbleiben, wie wir sie auch sehr gut als Folge von Sprengunfällen mit Schwarzpulver kennen. Die dunklen Fremdkörperkörner schimmern, wie bei der gewollten Schmucktätowierung, blau durch das trübe Medium der darüberliegenden Hornschicht durch. Wie bei der Entfernung von Tätowierungen sieht man sich auch hier vor ein relativ schwierig zu lösendes kosmetisches Problem gestellt. Es ist deshalb außerordentlich wichtig, daß man bei derartigen Unfällen gleich zu Beginn der Behandlung möglichst alle in die Wunde geratenen Fremdkörperpartikel peinlich genau heraussucht (CARRIE).

Die bei Unfällen auf sandigen Wegen oder mit feinem Schotter gekiesten Plätzen und Straßen als Fremdkörper in die Wunden eindringenden Quarzteilchen sind oft sehr klein und viel weniger gut erkennbar. Sie werden darum übersehen und gelangen vorerst unbemerkt und fast reaktionslos zur Einheilung. Das Fremdkörpermaterial, d. h. seine chemische Beschaffenheit, dürfte dabei ausschlaggebend sein, denn nur so können wir verstehen, daß Kohle, Asphalt, Tuscheteilchen, praktisch immer reaktionslos einheilen, Silicatpartikel hingegen relativ oft zum typischen, silicotischen Fremdkörpergranulom Anlaß geben.

a) Beziehungen des silicotischen Narbengranuloms zum Morbus Besnier-Boeck-Schaumann

Beim silicotischen Narbengranulom ist eine lange Latenzzeit zwischen Verletzung mit Eindringen des siliciumhaltigen Fremdkörpers und der Ausbildung einer granulomatösen Reaktion besonders charakteristisch und von vielen Autoren immer wieder hervorgehoben worden (MIESCHER u. OTT; LÖFGREN, SNELLMAN u. NORDENSTAM). Sie wird mit einigen Monaten bis vielen Jahren angegeben. Diesem langen Zeitraum muß eine besondere Bedeutung beigemessen werden. Er spielt auch in den verschiedenen Deutungen der Beziehungen zum Morbus Boeck eine gewisse Rolle. Sehr viele Erklärungen für diese große Zeitspanne sind denkbar.

In erster Linie müssen wir in den siliciumhaltigen Fremdkörperteilchen eine nicht resorbierbare oder doch nur in geringsten Mengen in Lösung gehende chemische Substanz sehen. Die lange Latenz bis zum Erscheinen reaktiver Veränderungen läßt sich vielleicht mit chemischen Vorgängen, die sozusagen im Zeitlupentempo ablaufen, erklären. Andere Autoren deuten die granulomatöse Reaktion als Antwort auf piezoelektrische Vorgänge um die Siliciumkristalle herum (EVANS und ZEIT). Bei mechanischen Einflüssen wie Zug und Druck sollen um die asymmetrischen Kristalle elektrische Spannungen entstehen, die ihrerseits die

Ursache für die granulomatöse Entzündung abgeben. Dieser Erklärungsversuch scheint etwas kompliziert und gesucht, besonders wenn man bedenkt, daß die epitheloidzellig-riesenzellige Abwehrreaktion im Grunde genommen eine ganz allgemeine und auf die verschiedensten Reize hin einsetzende Gewebeantwort darstellt.

Bei sehr vielen silicotischen Granulationsgeschwülsten scheint nun im histologischen Bilde die Fremdkörperriesenzelle stark zurückzutreten. Damit ist eine frappante Ähnlichkeit des pathologisch-anatomischen Gewebsbildes mit der Sarkoidose gegeben (Abb. 5). Man spricht darum oft auch statt von granulomatöser von sarkoidaler Reaktion um solche kleinste und dem Untersucher viel-

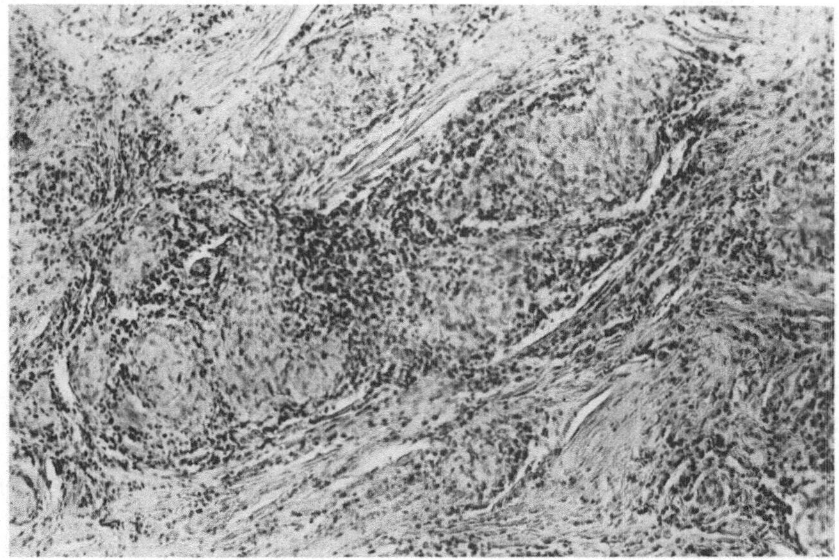

Abb. 5. Epitheloidzelliges (sarkoidales) Fremdkörpergranulom

leicht auch oft entgehende Fremdkörper herum. Der Fremdkörpernachweis kann tatsächlich schwierig sein. Im polarisierten Licht allerdings sind die doppelbrechenden Siliciumkristalle und -partikel auf dunklem Grunde aufleuchtend gut sichtbar. Bei allen Beobachtungen, die histologisch schwer zu interpretieren sind, sollte diese Untersuchungstechnik angewandt werden. Sie ist auch darum besonders wichtig, weil in gewissen Fällen Kristallstrukturen in granulomatösem Gewebe gefunden werden, die als körpereigene Substanzen, am plausibelsten als Polypeptid-Kristalle, gedeutet werden müssen; diese zeigen, im Polarisationsmikroskop betrachtet, keine Doppelbrechung.

Genauso schwierig wie die ätiologische Bestimmung eines infektiösen Granulationsgewebes (man denke an das Beispiel der histologischen Differentialdiagnose zwischen Tuberkulose, Lepra, Lues III, seltenen Mykosen) kann also auch die ätiologische Deutung einer Boeck-artigen oder sarkoidalen Gewebsreaktion sein. Beim Beryllium- und Zirkoniumgranulom sind die histologischen Analogien zur Sarkoidose ebenfalls besonders auffällig, wie wir in späteren Abschnitten sehen werden. Die Schwierigkeiten werden immer dann besonders groß, wenn noch klinische Anhaltspunkte für das tatsächliche Vorliegen einer Boeckschen Sarkoidosis beim Patienten vorhanden sind (Röntgenbild der Lunge, Ostitis multiplex [JÜNGLING]). Hier öffnet sich nur natürlich ein weites Feld für spekulative Erklärungen, für Kombinationen und Wechselwirkungen zwischen Fremdkörpergranulom und Sarkoidosis. Weil die nosologische Stellung der Boeckschen Krankheit noch immer umstritten ist und weil sich die Anerkennung der Sarkoidosis als besondere Verlaufsform der Tuberkulose nur schwer durchsetzt, wird das hier angedeutete Problem der Differenzierung im Einzelfall evtl. unlösbar. Auf einige strittige Punkte soll noch speziell eingegangen werden, da sie im jüngsten Schrifttum oft Erwähnung finden (Miescher und Ott, Degos und Carteaud).

In erster Linie muß darauf hingewiesen werden, daß die Sarkoidose tatsächlich eine Affinität zu Narben hat. Es ist bekannt, daß sich Läsionen der Boeckschen Krankheit oft in Operationsnarben, unter anderem auch nach Iridektomie, ansiedeln. Die Narbe wäre also als locus minoris resistentiae aufzufassen (Löfgren, Snellman und Nordenstam). In Einzelfällen kann man die Mitwirkung von Fremdkörpern mit aller Sicherheit ausschließen (Narbe nach Varicellen, Narbe nach reiner Quetschung durch Hammerschlag). In anderen Fällen (bei Narben nach Straßenverletzungen) mag das Eindringen von Quarzpartikeln oder — nach Operationen — das Einheilen von Talkteilchen, herrührend von den Operationshandschuhen, eine Rolle spielen. In der Narbe oder dem Narbengranulom muß man einen Realisationsfaktor sehen, der besonders bei Sarkoidose mit Generalisierungstendenz wichtig werden kann (Funk) und der das häufige Zusammentreffen von Morbus Boeck und sarkoidaler Narbenreaktion erklären könnte. Bei genauer Untersuchung soll man in 5—10% der Sarkoidosefälle Narbenefflorescenzen finden können (Löfgren). In diesem Zusammenhang sei auch eine Arbeit von Miescher und Ott erwähnt, die sich mit der Rolle des Traumas bei der Entstehung der Boeckschen Krankheit beschäftigt. Diesen Autoren gelang der Nachweis, daß bei 4 von total 28 Kranken mit Morbus-Besnier-Boeck-Schaumann die ersten Manifestationen der Erkrankung in Narbenregionen auftraten, und zwar einige Wochen, 2, 3 oder 9 Jahre nach der Hautverletzung. Ähnlich wie Degos und Carteaud vermuten Miescher und Ott, daß es sich kaum um ein zufälliges Zusammentreffen, auch nicht nur um eine traumatische Lokalisation im Sinne des locus minoris resistentiae handle, sondern es werden tiefere kausale Beziehungen zwischen Trauma und Morbus Boeck angenommen. Degos ist 1959 in einem zusammenfassenden Artikel im Hautarzt nochmals auf die beiden Beobachtungen zurückgekommen, die ihn veranlassen, an diese eigenartigen Zusammenhänge zwischen silicotischem Narbengranulom und Morbus Besnier-Boeck-Schaumann zu denken. Die verschiedenen Erklärungsmöglichkeiten werden dort diskutiert.

Wir wollen aber doch nochmals festhalten, daß nicht nur das silicotische Narbengranulom, sondern auch die Berylliosis und das Zirkoniumgranulom histologisch mit Sarkoidosis verwechselt werden können. Wenn der Fremdkörpernachweis eindeutig gelingt, so wird man in der Regel an der Diagnose sarkoidale Fremdkörperreaktion festhalten und nur in Ausnahmefällen eine Kombination von silicotischem Granulom und Morbus Boeck annehmen, dann nämlich, wenn die Lungenröntgenbilder, der progrediente Verlauf, das Befallensein von Drüsen, der negative Ausfall der Tuberkulinreaktion übereinstimmend dafür sprechen. Übrigens haben wir durchaus kein neues und besonders aktuelles Problem vor uns. Es darf daran erinnert werden, daß schon H. Martin 1888 über „Pseudotuberculose expérimentale" berichtet hat oder daß E. Kruckmann 1895 Untersuchungen über Fremdkörpertuberkulose und Fremdkörperriesenzellen mitteilte.

b) Schwimmbad-Granulome

Wiederholt ist das epidemieartige Auftreten von lupusähnlichen Granulomen im Anschluß an Hautverletzungen in künstlichen Schwimmbädern beschrieben worden. Neben der Infektion durch einen abgeschwächten Tuberkelbacillus

(Hellerström) oder durch das Mycobacterium balnei (Linell und Nordén) wurden in solchen Fällen auch die silicotischen Granulome in die Differentialdiagnose einbezogen.

2. Hauterscheinungen verursacht durch Beryllium

Wiederholt sind berufliche Erkrankungen durch Beryllium beschrieben worden, so vor allem nach Inhalation von Berylliumstaub und -dämpfen auftretende schwer verlaufende Pneumokoniosen. In solchen Fällen wurden z.T. gleichzeitig auch Hauterscheinungen gesehen. Sarkoidartige Fremdkörpergranulome der Haut und der Subcutis dagegen treten häufiger dann auf, wenn Berylliumteilchen bei einem Trauma unmittelbar in bzw. durch die Haut eindringen können.

Das Beryllium wird für die Herstellung von Fluorescenzröhren verwendet. Außerdem findet es Anwendung in der Metallurgie, in der keramischen Industrie, beim Bau von Präzisionsinstrumenten und Teilen von Radioapparaten. Wegen seiner besonderen Qualitäten wird es für bestimmte Leichtmetallegierungen bevorzugt, welchen es erhöhte Dauerhaftigkeit, antimagnetische und elektrizitätsleitende Eigenschaften vermittelt. Beryllium wurde deshalb im zweiten Weltkrieg sehr viel gebraucht; es galt direkt als „strategisches Metall“ (Leclerq). Beryllium (Be) ist zweiwertig und wird im periodischen System in die Gruppe der Erdalkalimetalle eingeordnet. Es ist das leichteste aller Metalle und kommt meistens als Doppelsalz, als Aluminium- und Beryllium-Silicat natürlich vor. Bei der Reindarstellung aus Erzen sind höchste Schmelztemperaturen erforderlich. Dabei entwickeln sich toxische Dämpfe.

Die breiteste Verwendung findet das Beryllium in der Leuchtröhrenindustrie. Als Beryllium-Silicat, als Phosphorsalz mit Zink und Mangan vermengt, gelangt es in die Leuchtstoffgemische. Neuerdings wird darnach getrachtet, das Beryllium nur noch in möglichst niederen Konzentrationen anzuwenden, etwa durch Reduktion von 5% auf 2% und 0,5%, oder man sucht es ganz durch weniger toxische Verbindungen zu ersetzen. Parallel mit der Lichtreklame haben die Fluorescenzröhren einen enormen Aufschwung genommen. Nachdem sie nun auch noch für die Raumbeleuchtung weitgehend herangezogen werden, sind ihrer Verwendung im täglichen Leben gar keine Grenzen mehr gesetzt. Damit mehren sich natürlich in der Industrie und auch dort, wo die Fertigprodukte Verwendung finden, die Möglichkeiten von Berylliumschädigungen.

Die Berylliumerkrankung der Lunge muß hier wenigstens kurz gestreift werden, weil immer wieder Vergleiche zwischen den Erscheinungen an der Lunge und der Haut gezogen werden, ferner, weil Fälle mit gleichzeitigem Lungen- und Hautbefall bekannt sind. Die Luftwege werden durch Inhalation von Berylliumstaub geschädigt. Es entsteht eine Lungenerkrankung mit eigenartigen Zügen. Der ganze Respirationstrakt kann akut oder chronisch geschädigt werden. Rhino-Pharyngitis, Tracheobronchitis und Bronchopneumonien wurden gesehen, wenn saure Berylliumverbindungen, Sulfate und Fluoride die Luftwege treffen. Besonders häufig aber sind die mehr chronisch verlaufenden Pneumokoniosen, die meistens primär-chronisch auftreten und sich nur selten sekundär aus akuten Lungenschäden entwickeln. Es handelt sich um eine Lungen-Granulomatose mit sehr ernster Prognose, rechnet man doch mit einer Mortalität von 20—25%, mit 40—45% dauernder völliger Arbeitsunfähigkeit und mit etwa 15% Kranken, die noch teilweise arbeitsfähig bleiben, während nur ungefähr 10% völlig ausheilen sollen (Midana).

Neben diesen bedenklichen Allgemeinerkrankungen — die aber weniger als 3% der Exponierten betreffen — sind die Berylliumschäden der Haut viel weniger schwer. Man unterscheidet nach Grier, Nash und Freiman und nach Dutra vier verschiedene Formen:

a) Akute Kontaktdermatitis,
b) Hautgeschwüre,
c) Hautgranulome,
d) Granulome der Subcutis.

a) Kontaktdermatitis durch Beryllium

Sie wird bei Arbeitern beobachtet, die mit löslichen Beryllium-Salzen zu tun haben, besonders mit Be-Fluoriden oder -Sulfaten. Offenbar tritt sie schon sehr bald, wenige Tage nach dem ersten Kontakt auf, so daß man eher obligat toxische Reaktionen bei Individuen mit niederen Schwellenwerten vermuten möchte, während ein allergischer Sensibilisierungsmechanismus weniger in Frage zu kommen scheint. Es handelt sich um papulo-vesiculöse Veränderungen, die anderen Berufsdermatosen gleichzusetzen sind und in diesem Kapitel nicht besprochen werden. CURTIS ist der Auffassung, daß Berylliumionen als Haptene wirksam seien, daß somit auch hier ein ekzem-allergischer Sensibilisierungsvorgang angenommen werden müsse.

b) Beryllium-Hautgeschwüre

Bei Beryllium-Arbeitern werden uncharakteristische Hautgeschwüre gesehen, wenn Kristalle von löslichen Berylliumsalzen durch Mikrotraumen in die Haut gelangen. Eine Heilung erfolgt erst, wenn die Kristalle entweder chirurgisch entfernt worden sind oder nachdem sie spontan durch eitrige Einschmelzung der Umgebung ausgestoßen wurden. Somit gilt die gleiche Gesetzmäßigkeit wie für andere Fremdkörper: nur indifferente können einheilen; differente, besonders lösliche hingegen verursachen eine kräftige Abwehrreaktion mit geschwürigem Zerfall und Elimination.

c) Cutanes Beryllium-Granulom

Solche Granulome sollen spontan bei Kranken auftreten, die an einer chronischen Berylliumgranulomatose der Lungen leiden. Histologisch findet man in der Lunge und an der Haut den gleichen Typus einer epitheloidzellig-granulomatösen Entzündung. Makroskopisch werden die Hauterscheinungen als kleine gerötete Papeln von 1—3 mm Durchmesser beschrieben, die an den oberen Extremitäten sitzen. Auf die besonders lange Latenzzeit zwischen Exposition und Auftreten der Schädigung wird für diese Fälle speziell hingewiesen. In einer Beobachtung von PYRE und OATWAY erkrankte ein Arbeiter, der ungefähr $^1/_2$ Jahr lang mit einer Flüssigkeit Kontakt hatte, welche Berylliumoxyd enthielt, erst 5 Jahre später an der charakteristischen Lungen- und Hautgranulomatose. Die Pathogenese der Hautveränderungen erscheint in diesen Beobachtungen recht dunkel. Vieles erinnert an die oft erst nach Jahren auftretenden granulomatösen Entzündungen, die bei Zinnobertätowierungen infolge langsam erfolgter Sensibilisierung des Organismus gesehen wurden (ULLMANN 1903, ARNING). Wir werden auf ähnliche Beobachtungen auch im Abschnitt über das Zirkonium-Granulom noch zu sprechen kommen.

d) Das cutan-subcutane Berylliumgranulom

Beobachtungen über diesen Typus der Berylliumhautschädigung sind in den letzten Jahren auffallend häufig geworden. Es handelt sich fast immer um die Folgen einer Verletzung mit Leuchtröhrensplittern. Die Innenseite der meisten Fluorescenzröhren ist mit einer Leuchtmasse bestrichen, die ungefähr 2% Beryllumsalze enthält. Letztere gelangt durch das Trauma in die Haut oder in die Subcutis. Solche Verletzungen treten vor allem bei Arbeitern der Leuchtröhrenindustrie auf, dann bei Elektrikern, welche die Röhren handhaben, und schließlich recht oft auch bei Kindern, die mit ausgedienten Röhren auf Schuttablagerungsplätzen spielen. Besonders in der amerikanischen Literatur ist eine ganze Reihe durchaus ähnlicher Beobachtungen veröffentlicht worden (GRIER, NASH und

Freiman; Coakley, Shapiro und Robertson; Nichol und Dominguez; Dutra; Neave, Frank und Tolmach). Daneben sind europäische Fälle in der Minderzahl (Midana; Bolgert und Busser), obwohl auch in Europa die Leuchtröhrenindustrie im letzten Jahrzehnt einen enormen Aufschwung genommen hat. Die Verwendung von Beryllium für die Herstellung von Lampen ist nach Allen neuerdings in Amerika gesetzlich verboten worden.

Die Hautveränderungen nach Verletzungen mit berylliumhaltigem Material entwickeln sich oft nach komplikationsloser Wundheilung und nach einer durchaus normalen Narbenbildung erst nach Monaten oder Jahren. In anderen Fällen deuten schon früh auftretende keloidartige, hypertrophische, gerötete und pigmentierte Narben an, daß der Heilungsprozeß gestört wurde. Anschließend entwickelt sich schleichend und ohne subjektive Beschwerden das subcutane Granulom. Die Hauterscheinungen sind gekennzeichnet durch cutan-subcutane Knotenbildungen ohne charakteristische Besonderheiten. Die akzidentell-traumatische Anamnese muß den Verdacht auf die chemische Ursache lenken, der klinische Befund allein würde kaum für eine Diagnose genügen. Immerhin wird die sorgfältige histopathologische Untersuchung in erster Linie an ein Fremdkörpergranulom denken lassen, denn man findet Epitheloidzellen, Histiocyten, Lymphocyten und Monocyten, ferner Fremdkörperriesenzellen und Zonen mit Nekrosen. Im Protoplasma der Riesenzellen sind kleine Fremdkörper mit hohem Brechungsindex nachgewiesen worden (Dutra). Das histologische Bild als Ganzes kann wechseln, indem bald mehr rein epitheloidzelliges Granulationsgewebe überwiegt, bald mehr nekrotische Zonen im Zentrum der Granulationsherde gefunden werden. Die Differentialdiagnose ist jedenfalls nicht einfach, und es ist immer wieder darauf hingewiesen worden, daß besonders auffällige Parallelen zum Bild der Besnier-Boeck-Schaumannschen Erkrankung, zur Tuberkulose oder Lues vorliegen können. In der Tat wird man in den Abbildungen von Lungen-Berylliosis und bei einzelnen Hautgranulomen zwingend an die epitheloidzellige Granulomatose oder an Tuberkulose erinnert.

Es kann aber keinem Zweifel unterliegen, daß die granulomatöse Reaktion eine direkte Folge des Eindringens von Beryllium in die Haut sein muß. Auch für die sog. spontan auftretenden kleinpapulösen cutanen Granulome der Arme bei Lungen-Berylliosis müssen wir annehmen, das Beryllium sei Monate oder Jahre zuvor durch kleinste Verletzungen in das Corium eingedrungen. Wir fassen sie somit als nur scheinbar spontan entstanden auf. Als beweisendes Argument für den direkten Zusammenhang zwischen Beryllium und Granulom wäre der spektrographische (Leclerq) Nachweis des Metalls in der Haut nach der Methode von Cholak und Hubbard (Dutra) anzuführen.

Dutra ist in sehr eingehenden Versuchen der Frage nachgegangen, ob das Beryllium an sich, ob seine verschiedenen Salze oder ob die beigemengten Silicate für die Granulombildung ausschlaggebend seien bzw. ob sie im Tierversuch und am Menschen differenzierbare histologische Reaktionen lieferten. Seine Ergebnisse können dahin zusammengefaßt werden, daß physikalisch-chemische Unterschiede, wie z.B. die Teilchengröße des auslösenden Materials, eine wichtige Rolle spielen. Wahrscheinlich haben wir es nicht mit einer reinen Fremdkörperreaktion zu tun, sondern minimale Mengen gelöster Substanz scheinen für die Besonderheiten der granulomatösen Bildungen verantwortlich zu sein. In den meisten Arbeiten fehlen leider Angaben über eine evtl. allergische Überempfindlichkeit gegenüber Beryllium-Salzen. A priori hätte man auch gar keinen Grund für die Annahme eines allergischen Mechanismus in der Pathogenese; merkwürdig sind allerdings die oft ungewöhnlich langen Latenzzeiten. Die neueste Entwicklung unserer Auffassungen über das Zirkonium-Granulom, ferner die sehr alten Beobachtungen über verruköse Granulationen in der Nähe von Zinnobertätowierungen bei Hg-Idiosynkrasie lassen aber doch solche Untersuchungen — und zwar Läppchenproben und intracutane Testungen — als wünschbar erscheinen.

Bei den Berylliumschäden der Haut haben wir es somit auf der einen Seite mit wichtigen Berufskrankheiten zu tun, bei denen vor allem noch die definitive pathogenetische Abklärung der sog. spontan auftretenden cutanen Granulome im Verlauf von Lungenberylliosis aussteht.

Die akzidentell-traumatischen Beryllium-Granulome interessieren uns als besondere Verlaufstypen von Fremdkörperreaktionen. Auf die problematischen Beziehungen zwischen solchen Granulomen und der Besnier-Boeck-Schaumannschen Krankheit ist im Abschnitt über die silicotischen Granulome näher eingegangen worden (Degos, Miescher und Ott). Beryllium-Granulome sind naturgemäß relativ seltene Vorkommnisse und stellen im Gegensatz zur Lungen-Berylliosis als Berufskrankheit weder prophylaktisch noch therapeutisch besondere Probleme. Das Beryllium-Granulom der Haut und der Subcutis wird in der Regel chirurgisch angegangen mit der Absicht, die verbleibenden Fremdkörper und das Fremdkörper-Granulom zu beseitigen. Bei kleinen Granulomen kann auch eine Elektrokoagulation genügen, um die pathologischen Veränderungen zu beseitigen und eine glatte Vernarbung einzuleiten.

3. Asbestknötchen oder Asbestwarzen

Das Eindringen von Asbestnadeln in die Haut löst eigenartige Reaktionen aus, die 1930 von Dewirtz zum ersten Mal beschrieben worden sind. Dieser russische Autor fand bei fast allen in den Asbestklüften mit dem Abbau des faserigen Gesteines beschäftigten Arbeitern warzenartige Papeln an den Beugeseiten der Finger oder an den Handflächen. Auch in den asbestverarbeitenden Betrieben wird die berufliche Schädigung häufig angetroffen. Wird viel Asbest verarbeitet, so steigen die Prozentzahlen der Befallenen. Dabei scheint auch die Qualität des verarbeiteten Materials eine große Rolle zu spielen. So hat Amosit, ein Isoliermaterial, das sich vom gewöhnlichen Asbest durch seine stärkeren Fasern unterscheidet, bei Werftarbeitern in über 50% zu Hautreaktionen geführt (Alden und Howell). Auch Dewirtz erwähnt in seiner Arbeit zwei Varianten von Asbest, eine serpentinförmige oder chrysolitische ($Mg_3\ H_4\ Si_2\ O_9$) und eine hornblendenartige ($(Mg_3\ Ca\ Si_2\ O_3)_4$), von denen die erstere im Asbestbetrieb die Hauptrolle spiele. Große Asbestvorkommen seien selten. Nur Canada, Südafrika (Rhodesien) und Rußland (in den östlichen Abhängen des Uralgebirges) verfügen über abbauwürdige Lagerstätten.

Die Hautveränderungen werden als nicht entzündliche, teils rundliche, teils polygonale Knötchen mit rauher Oberfläche beschrieben. Die Ausmaße schwanken von Hirsekorn- bis Erbsgröße je nach dem Alter der Veränderungen. Der Sitz ist immer derselbe: die Reaktionen halten sich an die Beugeseiten der Finger und an die Hohlhand. Ausnahmsweise findet man Asbestwarzen auch an den Fußsohlen, wenn Arbeiter im Sommer mit bloßen Füßen gehen. Bei Anfängern und bei Personen mit Handschweiß scheinen die Asbestknötchen besonders häufig vorzukommen. Wahrscheinlich spielt die Dicke und Festigkeit der Hornschicht eine Rolle. Die Arbeiter spüren in der Regel einen stechenden Schmerz nach dem Eindringen eines Splitters. Die Extraktion gelingt meist nicht. Die Beschwerden verschwinden ziemlich rasch. Nach ungefähr 10 Tagen kommt es aber an der betreffenden Stelle zur Ausbildung eines langsam wachsenden und verhornenden Knötchens. Auf dem Röntgenbild gelingt der Fremdkörpernachweis nicht. Eine Rückbildung kann erst erfolgen, wenn der Kristall herausgezogen oder ausgestoßen worden ist. Dann aber platten sich die Knötchen ab, und sie verschwinden völlig ohne Spuren zu hinterlassen.

Die *histologischen* Veränderungen sind charakterisiert durch eine starke Verdickung der Epidermis mit Hyperkeratose. Es liegt eine fast ausschließlich epidermale Papelbildung vor. Übereinstimmend wird darauf hingewiesen, daß im Corium entzündliche Veränderungen völlig oder fast völlig fehlen. Die Hyperkeratose ist immer sehr stark ausgeprägt. Man findet in der Hornschicht Fäserchen und Schollen von Asbestkristallen, die sich in der Hämatoxylin-Eosin-Färbung violett darstellen. Die Acanthose ist stark ausgebildet, die Intercellularspalten sind oft verbreitert. Es finden sich in den tieferen Epidermisschichten viele Mitosen. Dewirtz beschreibt Riesenzellen in der Epidermis(!), die an Fremdkörperriesenzellen erinnern. In ihrer Umgebung konnten aber keine Asbestteilchen nachgewiesen werden. In der Lederhaut fand er unmittelbar unter der Epithelschicht Zeichen von chronischer Entzündung in Form von Sklerose und kompakten lymphoiden Zellinfiltraten. Die hyperplastischen Reaktionserscheinungen lassen sich somit als vorwiegend einfache Epithelwucherung zusammenfassen, bei der keine Atypien auftreten. Es handle sich um eine Proliferation „nach oben", die zur Elimination der Asbestteilchen führe. Dewirtz schließt seine Betrachtungen mit dem Satz: „Wir haben also einen neuen Stoff vor uns, welcher nicht nur klinisch und gewerbehygienisch, sondern auch theoretisch interessant ist, insofern als er uns neues Material für die Beurteilung der Reaktion des Epithelgewebes liefert."

Aus anderen Beschreibungen (Alden und Howell) geht hervor, daß diese Berufsschäden im allgemeinen während der ersten 3—4 Monate nach Aufnahme der Asbestarbeit beobachtet werden. Eine Prophylaxe soll nur wenig nützen. Einzelne Arbeiter suchen unmittelbar nach dem Eindringen den Fremdkörper mit einer Pinzette zu entfernen und damit der papulös-verrukösen Reaktion zuvorzukommen. Die Asbestwarzen haben keine Beziehungen zur Lungenasbestose; es sind reine lokale Fremdkörperreaktionen, wobei die Besonderheit offenbar darin zu liegen scheint, daß die Asbestfasern und -kristalle nur relativ oberflächlich bis in die Epidermis eindringen und normalerweise nicht bis ins Corium gelangen können. Die charakteristische Reaktion spielt sich denn auch weitgehend epidermal ab als akanthotische Wucherung und warzige Hyperkeratose, während im Corium nur sehr unbedeutende entzündliche Veränderungen beschrieben werden.

4. Hautschädigungen durch Glasfasern (Glasseide und Glaswolle)

Glasfasern werden hauptsächlich zur Wärme- oder Schall-Isolation verwendet. Sie gewinnen in verschiedenen gewerblichen oder industriellen Betrieben zunehmende Bedeutung. Die Hautschädigungen, die mit derartigem Isoliermaterial entstehen können, sind harmlos und bei den meisten Betroffenen eher eintönig und übereinstimmend. Es handelt sich um kleine, disseminierte, meistens follikulär angeordnete Knötchen mit Lieblingslokalisation in den Interdigitalräumen der Hände, an den Handgelenken sowie an den Beugeseiten der Arme. Bei speziellen Expositionsbedingungen und sehr massivem Kontakt können sie auch am Hals und am Stamm auftreten, vor allem, wenn der Glasfaserstaub Gelegenheit bekommt, unter die Kleider und die Leibwäsche einzudringen. Die betroffenen Leute klagen über Stechen oder über einen Juckreiz, der sich unter Umständen äußerst lästig und quälend bemerkbar macht. Aus der *Anamnese* geht meistens hervor, daß der Juckreiz und die Hautläsionen schon nach dem allerersten Kontakt auftreten, daß sie rasch wieder verschwinden, wenn die Arbeiten mit dem Isoliermaterial abgeschlossen sind oder wenn Arbeitspausen, z.B. über das

Wochenende, eintreten. Die Vermutung liegt deshalb nahe, es handle sich um Schädigungen ohne Beteiligung eines allergischen Sensibilisierungsvorganges und ohne kompliziertere Pathogenese.

Tatsächlich konnten durch experimentelle Expositionen die gleichen Läsionen fast ausnahmslos bei allen daraufhin untersuchten Personen erzeugt werden (Leder). Bei einfachster Versuchsanordnung, nämlich durch Einstreuen fein zerriebener Glasfasern unter die Hemdärmel und Zubinden der Ärmel über Nacht, entstanden die pruriginösen, papulösen Läsionen schon nach dem ersten Kontakt, allerdings in verschieden starker Ausprägung. Die spontane Heilung erfolgte ausnahmslos nach 1—5 Tagen. Der Einstreuversuch scheint im übrigen zur Reproduktion besonders gut geeignet zu sein, während gewöhnliche Läppchenproben oder Einreiben des Glasstaubes nicht mit der gleichen Regelmäßigkeit positive Resultate ergeben, wie wir selber zusammen mit Bandi bei Kontrollversuchen zur Wirkung von Zimmerlindenblättern feststellen konnten.

Die histologischen Veränderungen sind bei gewerblichen Fällen und bei experimentell erzeugten Läsionen übereinstimmend. Die Glassplitter lassen sich entweder in Follikeltaschen nachweisen, oder sie durchstechen die Epidermis und dringen direkt bis ins subepitheliale Corium vor. In der Umgebung der lädierten Partie findet sich eine nur schwach ausgebildete reaktive Entzündung mit einem geringen, vorwiegend aus Lymphocyten zusammengesetzten zelligen Infiltrat. In der Arbeit von Leder wird nur ein Fall erwähnt, bei dem histologisch besondere, von der Regel abweichende Verhältnisse angetroffen wurden, in Form einer intraepidermalen Blasenbildung, bei der auch ein Splitterchen nachgewiesen werden konnte. Im Blaseninhalt fanden sich vorwiegend Leukocyten, was auf eine Pustelbildung hinwies, in der unmittelbaren Umgebung aber fanden sich spongiotische Veränderungen, d.h. ein ekzematoider Reaktionstypus. In einem anderen Falle zeigten sich im Einstreuversuch wie im Läppchentest bei einem Ekzematiker mit Ulcus cruris und chronischem Unterschenkelekzem schon klinisch ausgesprochen ekzemähnliche Veränderungen. Die sofort histologisch untersuchte Epidermis wies klassische spongiotische Reaktionen auf neben Splitterläsionen, und zwar z.T. unabhängig voneinander rein mechanische Reaktionen und spongiotische Bläschenbildung. Besonders wichtig ist die Feststellung, daß sich dieses Phänomen bei der gleichen Versuchsperson schon 14 Tage später trotz gleicher Bedingungen nicht mehr reproduzieren ließ. Der Einstreuversuch erzeugte banale Läsionen, d.h. obligate Splitterreaktionen, und der Läppchentest war diesmal negativ. Leder denkt an einen Zusammenhang mit dem sog. *Kogoj*-Effekt, wie er bei hämatogener experimenteller Pilzinfektion als Lokalisationsphänomen nach mechanischem Insult beobachtet wird. Er betont aber, daß die Erklärung schwierig ist, weil der ekzematöse Streuvorgang überhaupt noch relativ wenig abgeklärt sei. Ferner blieben Reaktionen auch bei solchen Ekzematikern aus, welche sich in einem Schubstadium befanden. Hier anschließend muß eine neuere Arbeit von Saipt über Glaswolle-Schädigungen kurz Erwähnung finden, da sie auf den ersten Blick in völligem Widerspruch zu den gewerbeärztlichen und experimentellen Feststellungen von Leder steht.

Die klinischen und die histologischen Befunde fallen bei Saipt derart aus dem Rahmen des sonst Beschriebenen und immer wieder Reproduzierbaren, daß ernste Zweifel an der Deutung auftauchen. Die Läsionen, die in dieser Arbeit abgebildet wurden, sind viel weniger diskret, weil viel stärker entzündlich als die gewöhnlichen Glaswolle-Reaktionen. Man möchte eher an ein Erythema exsudativum multiforme denken. Auch die Abbildung der histologischen Veränderungen mit Bläschenbildung und offenbar eindeutig fibrinösem Exsudat erinnert in allererster Linie an diese Diagnose. Die erwähnte Arbeit darf darum meiner Ansicht nach nur mit Vorbehalt in das Kapitel „Fremdkörper der Haut" aufgenommen werden. Die Widersprüche verschwinden aber, wenn wir annehmen, es handle sich um das zufällige Zusammentreffen von Erythema exsudativum multiforme und Exposition mit Glaswolle. Tatsächlich sind ja dann später beim gleichen Patienten nach neuerlichen Kontakten nur noch die banalen, diskreten Glassplitterreaktionen aufgetreten, was ebenfalls erlaubt, den ersten Schub als isomorphen Reizeffekt im Verlaufe eines multiformen Erythems aufzufassen.

Mit den hier erwähnten gewerblichen Hautschädigungen durch Isoliermaterial aus Glaswolle wird immer wieder zu rechnen sein, obwohl neuerdings weniger reizende Modifikationen verwendet werden, nämlich Matten, die nach außen durch Baumwoll- oder Cellulose-Watte abgeschirmt sind, ferner Isolierplatten, die die Glaswolle im Innern enthalten.

Schädigungen durch Glasfasern als Bestandteile von Wäsche- und Kleiderstoffen scheinen nur ganz ausnahmsweise vorgekommen zu sein. Derartige Beobachtungen liegen einer Mitteilung von SCHWARTZ zugrunde. Der Autor berichtet über das Auftreten von juckenden Hautausschlägen, die auf die Beimischung von Glaswolle zu Kleiderstoffen zurückgeführt werden konnten. Man mußte die betreffenden Gewebe und die daraus verarbeiteten Konfektionskleidungsstücke behördlich wieder einziehen lassen.

5. Haar-Granulome

Die Fremdkörpergranulome, die durch Eindringen von Haaren in die Haut entstehen können, bilden eine kleine Gruppe für sich. Die erste Beobachtung wurde 1915 von LAUENER aus der Berner Klinik mitgeteilt. Bei einem Melker war an einem Finger durch das Eindringen von Kuhhaaren eine Granulationsgeschwulst entstanden. Vermutlich waren die Fremdkörper durch Rhagaden in die Haut hineingelangt. Ähnliche Beobachtungen wurden in der Folge von EILERS, BECKER, OPPENHEIM, KITTINGER, BETTMANN, GOTTRON und HALTER mitgeteilt. GOTTRON schlug die Bezeichnung Melkergranulationsknoten vor und wies auf die Verwechslungsmöglichkeiten mit anderen Berufserkrankungen der Melker hin. Zweifellos sind solche Haar-Granulome bei Landwirten außerordentlich selten, sie spielen nur eine ganz untergeordnete Rolle. RÖCKL und MÜLLER haben hingegen 1957 in einer Arbeit „Granulome und Fisteln durch Haare" darauf hingewiesen, daß offenbar im Friseurberuf ähnliche Veränderungen viel häufiger vorkommen. Sie werden im ausländischen Schrifttum unter verschiedenen Bezeichnungen, als „interdigital pilonidal sinus", als „barbers disease" oder als „hair bearing sinus" usw., beschrieben. Eine pathogenetische Beziehung zu den Sacraldermoiden, die oft ebenfalls als „pilonidal sinus" bezeichnet werden, liegt natürlich nicht vor. Die Fisteln an den Schwimmhäuten der Coiffeure sind nicht als Mißbildungen zu erklären, sondern sie entstehen sekundär aus kleinen Granulationsgeschwülstchen, aus denen die Haare wieder ausgestoßen werden. Es resultieren fistelartige eingezogene Narben, in die sich dann erneut Haare einbohren können.

Der 2. und 3. Interdigitalraum scheinen stark bevorzugt zu werden; dabei dürfte, wie für den Sitz der Erosio interdigitalis oidiomycetica im 3. Interdigitalraum, die starke Maceration der Epidermis an dieser Stelle von ausschlaggebender Bedeutung sein.

Die histologische Untersuchung im von RÖCKL und MÜLLER beschriebenen Falle ergab ein scharf abgegrenztes Granulationsgewebe, das durch zwei mit Epithel ausgekleidete Fistelgänge mit der Hautoberfläche in Verbindung stand. Neben Fibroblasten und Riesenzellen vom Fremdkörpertyp werden herdförmige Ansammlungen von Neutrophilen, nekrotische Massen und Kerntrümmer beschrieben. Wie schon bei LAUENER und GOTTRON geschildert, fanden sich auch hier zusätzlich nesterförmig angeordnete Herde von Plasmazellen.

6. Fremdkörpergranulome durch Kakteenstacheln

Fremdkörpergranulome, verursacht durch Kakteenstacheln, kommen nur selten zur Beobachtung (WINER und ZEILENGA). Es sind nicht die groben Abwehrstacheln, sondern vielmehr die feinen Glochidien, welche leicht in die Haut eindringen können. Sie sind so scharf und fein, daß sie die Epidermis glatt durchstechen; außerdem lösen sie sich leicht von der Pflanze ab. Unmittelbar nach dem Eindringen verspürt der Patient Schmerzen, und es entwickelt sich in einigen Tagen eine Schwellung, die 2—3 Wochen bestehen bleibt. Anschließend entwickeln sich um die eingedrungenen Stacheln herum leicht erhabene, entzündliche Papeln von 2—4 mm Durchmesser oder etwas größere flache Plaques mit einem dunkelroten Rand und einer weißlich oder rosa gefärbten inneren Zone. Diese Elemente werden mit kleinen Efflorescenzen des Granuloma anulare verglichen.

Die beobachteten histologischen Veränderungen waren außerordentlich charakteristisch. In der Cutis fanden sich zahlreiche Herde von Epitheloidzellen, umgeben von Riesenzellen, welche scharf begrenzte, helle, ovale Räume enthielten. Bei verschiedenen Färbungen (MALLORY und HOTCHKISS-McMANUS) waren diese hellen Zonen in den Riesenzellen gefärbt, blau wie kollagen oder leuchtend rot wie ein Polysaccharid. Man konnte mit den genannten Färbungen Spicula von 5—10 μ Durchmesser und 50 μ Länge erkennen.

Die Kaktusstacheln wurden $3^1/_2$ Monate nach dem Eindringen spontan ausgestoßen. Es entstand eine lokale Nekrose und ein klinisch warzenartiges Bild, wenn die ausgestoßenen Massen das Stratum corneum erreichten.

7. Fremdkörpergranulome durch Stacheln von Süßwasserschwämmen

Einen besonderen Typus von Fremdkörperreaktion stellt die Berufskrankheit dar, die bei Theiß-Fischern in der Gegend von Szeged beschrieben worden ist (SZENTKIRALYI). In Tümpeln, Weihern und Gruben, die längs dem Flußlauf des Tisca seit der Durchführung einer Stromregulierung nach dem sog. chinesischen System entstanden waren, bildet sich nach den Hochwasserperioden eine interessante Lebensgemeinschaft von Mikro- und Makro-Flora und -Fauna aus. Die Fischerei ist in diesen Gewässern frei, sie wird mit reusenartigen Fanggeräten durchgeführt. Die Fischer waten dabei oft bis zum Bauch im Wasser und ziehen sich leicht ein heftig juckendes Hautleiden zu, das überall dort auftritt, wo die Haut mit dem Wasser in Berührung gekommen ist. Die Hauterscheinungen treten erst einige Tage später auf; es handelt sich um zerstreute rote Flecken, die sich in derbe stecknadelkopf- bis erbsgroße Papeln umwandeln. Wegen des heftigen Juckens werden diese Papeln meist aufgekratzt oder sogar mit den Taschenmessern abgeschabt, was am ehesten zum Aufhören des Juckreizes beitragen soll. Nach ungefähr einer Woche heilen die Papeln ab, indem sie Pigmentflecke zurücklassen. Nach neuerlicher Exposition in den Wassergruben und -tümpeln treten an anderen Hautstellen wieder neue Elemente auf. Die Fischer suchen sich durch das Tragen alter Leinwandhosen vor der Erkrankung zu schützen. Auch wissen sie, daß vor allem der längere Aufenthalt im Wasser gefährlich wird, sobald nämlich größere Mengen von Schlamm aufgewühlt worden sind. Auch Jäger und Sportangler wurden hin und wieder von der Krankheit befallen, wenn sie im stehenden Wasser der Teiche herumwaten; im offenen Flußlauf hingegen kann man sich die Erkrankung nicht zuziehen.

Die Ursache der Erkrankung war relativ einfach aufzufinden. Zuerst wurde an das Eindringen tierischer Organismen, an Wassermilben, an Plankton usw. gedacht, denn eine gewisse Analogie zur Cercarien-Dermatitis ist unverkennbar.

Immerhin beginnt der Juckreiz nach dem Eindringen von Cercarien meist sofort oder doch schon nach wenigen Stunden.

Bei der histologischen Untersuchung einer frischen Efflorescenz fand man einen feinen, spitzen, durchsichtigen Fremdkörper, der sich in die oberen Schichten der Epidermis eingebohrt hatte. Es stellte sich dann heraus, daß dieser Fremdkörper ein Stück eines Stachels des Süßwasserschwammes war. Diese kieselsäure- und kalkhaltigen Stacheln oder Spicula sind an beiden Enden spitzig, sie bilden das Gerüst des Schwammes. Es dürfte sich bei den Schädigungen durch das Eindringen der Schwammstacheln um eine rein mechanische Wirkung handeln; sie sind gleichzusetzen den Glaswollschäden oder den Dermatosen, die bei Jutearbeitern auftreten.

Den Zoologen sind übrigens diese Schädigungen bekannt. Sie wurden auch schon beobachtet, wenn Kolonien von Süßwasserschwämmen wie ein richtiger Schwamm zum Waschen verwendet wurden. Durch das massenhafte Eindringen von Spicula entstanden mehr flächenhafte Entzündungen, ebenso wenn experimentell ein Stückchen einer Süßwasserschwamm-Kolonie in die Haut eingerieben wurde.

8. Schädigungen durch Hochdruckfettpressen

Beim Arbeiten mit Hochdruckfettpressen sind Unfälle mitgeteilt worden, die in das Kapitel der traumatischen Fremdkörpergranulome aufgenommen werden müssen. Der Fettstrahl dringt in die Haut ein und verursacht vorerst eine kleine Wunde und eine Entzündung. Der kleine Defekt heilt zu; aber Wochen später kann sich an der betreffenden Stelle wieder eine Öffnung bilden, aus der sich in einem fistelnden Prozeß Sekret und wahrscheinlich unresorbierbare Fetttröpfchen entleeren. Das Personal, das mit solchen Hochdruckfettpressen arbeitet, scheint die Zwischenfälle gut zu kennen. Da sie offenbar meist spontan heilen, sind in der dermatologischen Literatur nur wenige Mitteilungen zu finden (COBURN, „Grease Gun Granuloma“). Der Unfallhergang erinnert an die Technik der Serieninjektion von Medikamenten ohne Nadel, wie sie in Amerika entwickelt worden ist, Europa aber gar nie erreicht hat (LARRICK und THOMPSON).

II. Fremdkörpergranulome durch Cosmetica, Medikamente und Medikamententräger

1. Vaselinome und Paraffinome

Vaselinome und Paraffinome sind spezielle Formen der entzündlichen, hyperplastischen Fremdkörpertumoren. Mineralöle, d.h. nicht resorbierbare (höhere) Kohlenwasserstoffe spielen bei ihnen die Rolle des Fremdkörpers. Klinisch haben diese Krankheitsbilder eine gewisse Ähnlichkeit zu Tumoren oder Neoplasmen, besonders, wenn sich auch in Lymphgefäßen oder -drüsen „Metastasen“ ausbilden. Daneben gibt es auch ölige Fremdkörper, die eine akute entzündliche, oft auch eitrige Reaktion auslösen. Musterbeispiele für solche Fälle wären der Bismutabsceß oder der Fixationsabsceß nach Injektion von Terpentinöl, wie er als unspezifische Reizkörpertherapie vor Zeiten üblich war.

Wie bereits erwähnt, spielen die Resorbierbarkeit und das Tempo, mit dem eine Assimilation erfolgen kann, eine bedeutende Rolle. Animalische und vegetabile Öle werden sehr langsam resorbiert. Trotzdem verursachen sie meist keine Komplikationen. Vaselinöl und Paraffin hingegen werden nur äußerst schwer oder überhaupt nicht resorbiert. Gerade deshalb wurden sie seinerzeit für kosmetische reparative Eingriffe oft verwendet.

Die Nachteile solcher Paraffinöl-Injektionen im Gesicht oder in die Brüste zeigten sich jedoch schon bald nach Einführung der Methode. Sie waren derart, daß das Verfahren völlig diskreditiert wurde und heute wohl kaum noch irgendwo angewandt wird.

Bis zum Auftreten der Komplikation verstreicht normalerweise immer eine lange Latenzzeit. Sie ist nur ausnahmsweise kurz (14 Tage nach MOOK und WANDER). Viel häufiger beträgt sie 3 Monate bis einige Jahre.

Das klinische Bild ist ziemlich übereinstimmend. Anfänglich tritt eine knotige Induration im subcutanen Fettgewebe auf. Diese ist vorerst verschieblich, dann aber kommt es meist zu einem Verwachsen mit der darunterliegenden Fascie oder mit der Cutis, oder mit beiden. Allmählich greift der Prozeß also über die Injektionsstelle hinaus. Bei der Palpation werden unregelmäßige Konturen getastet. Später kann eine ziemlich einheitliche, bretthart Induration entstehen. Oft ist diese Fremdkörperreaktion gar nicht druckempfindlich. In anderen Fällen ist ein dumpfer oder auch ausstrahlender Schmerz vorhanden. Eine Spontanheilung ist kaum möglich. Hingegen wird oft ein stationärer Zustand, der dem Patienten wenig Beschwerden verursacht, erreicht. Es sind aber auch andere Verlaufsarten möglich: vor allem akutere, entzündliche Schübe mit Rötung, Überwärmung und Schmerz. Es kann zur Absceßbildung kommen, an die sich nach Perforation wieder chronisch fistelnde Prozesse anschließen. In solchen Fällen lassen sich im sterilen Eiter meist Fetttröpfchen nachweisen.

Die Differentialdiagnose zu malignen Tumoren kann sich — wie schon erwähnt — dann stellen, wenn rosenkranzartige Lymphangitis und Drüsenvaselinome auftreten (FAVRE und CIVATTE). Im übrigen sollte die Diagnose nicht schwierig sein, sofern die Anamnese bekannt ist. Auf die Analogien und Verwechslungsmöglichkeiten mit syphilitischen Gummen, Bindegewebstumoren, Darier-Roussyschem Sarkoid, Tuberkulose, lipophagem Granulom sei hingewiesen.

Der histologische Aufbau dieser Geschwülste, die sich als weißlich-gelbe Massen präsentieren, ist charakterisiert durch zahlreiche kleine Hohlräume, aus denen evtl. eine ölige Flüssigkeit abfließt oder abgestrichen werden kann. Im Mikroskop erkennt man ein fibröses Gewebe mit dichter Zellinfiltration, das zahlreiche Cysten enthält. Diese histologischen Veränderungen, nämlich ein kleincystisches Fremdkörpergranulom, sind beinahe pathognomonisch. Die Durchmesser der Hohlräume sind verschieden, etwa stecknadelkopfgroß oder kleiner. WORINGER vergleicht sie mit den Löchern eines Gruyère-Käses.

Will man die Fettsubstanzen nachweisen, muß man sich einer Gefrierschnittmethode bedienen, beim gewöhnlichen Einbetten würden sie herausgelöst. Als Auskleidung der Cysten findet man abgeplattete Zellen, daneben mehrkernige Riesenzellen vom Fremdkörpertypus. Fibrocyten, Makrophagen oder sklerosiertes Bindegewebe bilden konzentrische Schichten um die Cystenhöhlen herum. Die ursprünglichen Ölmassen können dermaßen aufgeteilt werden, daß nur noch das entzündliche Gewebe mit seinen Lymphocyten und Histiocyten auffällt; es entstehen pseudotuberkulöse Knötchen mit Riesenzellen, Epitheloidzellen und Lymphocyten.

Die „Metastasen" erklärt man sich so, daß Makrophagen, mit aufgenommenen Öltröpfchen beladen, abwandern. Sie geben dann Anlaß zu neuen Fremdkörperreaktionen entlang den Lymphgefäßen und in den Lymphdrüsen (FAVRE und CIVATTE). GOUGEROT und DESAUX haben 1930 darauf hingewiesen, daß solche Oleome ein Eigenleben besitzen. Sie sollen tuberkulöser Natur sein. Man kommt also offenbar leicht zu ähnlichen Überlegungen, wie sie beim silicotischen Granulom auch immer wieder gemacht werden.

Es bleibt schwierig zu erklären, warum nur Einzelindividuen in der beschriebenen Weise auf solche Injektionen reagieren. Es sind Ausnahmefälle, für deren Reaktionsweise wir eine Erklärung finden sollten. Eine Sensibilisation wurde bisher nicht festgestellt. Man erklärte die Erscheinung darum als individuelle Prädisposition bei geschwächten Personen. Zweifellos müssen wir aber auch nach den chemischen Eigenschaften der eingespritzten Flüssigkeiten fragen; ihre Reinheit kann von ausschlaggebender Bedeutung sein. Daneben ist offenbar auch der Schmelzpunkt sehr wichtig. Er muß sich zwischen 43° und 46° bewegen, will man keine unangenehmen Reaktionen in Kauf nehmen.

Die Verhältnisse beim Menschen konnten auch in experimentellen Versuchen am Affen (Weidman und Jefferies) und beim Hund (Gildeeren) nachgeahmt werden. Die histologischen Reaktionen konnten dabei genau verfolgt werden. Nach der Diapedese von Leukocyten entwickelten sich die Phasen mit mikrocystischem Fremdkörpergranulom, gefolgt von der Sklerose.

2. Die Zirkoniumgranulome der Achselhöhlen

Vor wenigen Jahren trat in den Vereinigten Staaten von Amerika ein neues, wohlumrissenes Krankheitsbild auf, dessen Ursache auch bald aufgedeckt werden konnte: Nach Anwendung desodorierender Stifte zeigten sich in den Achselhöhlen papulöse, histologisch granulomatöse, entzündliche Reaktionen. Die ersten Mitteilungen stammen von Weber et al. 1956, Rubin et al. 1956, Weber und Neuhauser 1957, Rubin 1957. Ihnen folgten dann zahlreiche klinische Demonstrationen anläßlich von Tagungen, ferner zusammenfassende Arbeiten von Sheard u. Mitarb. und schließlich von Shelley und Hurley, denen wir wichtige und interessante Aufschlüsse über die Ätiologie und Pathogenese der Zirkoniumgranulome verdanken.

Die anamnestischen Angaben waren in solchen Fällen übereinstimmend gleich. Seit kürzerer oder längerer Zeit verwendeten die erkrankten Personen einen neuen zirkoniumhaltigen Stift als Desodorans in den Achselhöhlen. Meistens wurden gleichzeitig auch die Achselhaare rasiert. Die charakteristischen Hautläsionen zeigten sich in der Regel nach mehrwöchigem Gebrauche des Cosmeticums. Es handelte sich um rote, oft auch etwas pigmentierte, dichtstehende Papeln (Abb. 6). Oft waren sie länglich, so daß der Eindruck entstand, kleine Kratzer oder Schnittverletzungen beim Rasieren hätten das Eindringen einer schädigenden Noxe erleichtert. Erst die Biopsie und histologische Untersuchung gestatten die definitive Diagnose. Es wird ein epitheloidzelliger granulomatöser Prozeß gefunden, der von allen Untersuchern als außerordentlich sarkoidähnlich beschrieben wird.

Auch wenn der zirkoniumhaltige Stift nicht mehr weiter angewandt wird, besteht das Granulom wochen- und monatelang fort. Es bildet sich nur sehr langsam wieder zurück. Subjektive Symptome, wie Juckreiz und Schmerz, fehlen.

Das Krankheitsbild ist selten, es wurde trotz millionenfacher Anwendung dieser speziellen desodorierenden Stifte nur in einer sehr beschränkten Anzahl von Fällen gesehen. Shelley und Hurley konnten in einer meisterhaften Studie beweisen, daß es sich um eine besondere Form von allergischer Reaktion auf Zirkoniumionen handelt. Ohne Zweifel werden die Ergebnisse, die man aus dem genauen experimentellen Studium des Zirkoniumgranuloms ableiten konnte, auch allgemein medizinisch von großer Bedeutung sein, so für die Erklärung von Pneumokoniosen, möglicherweise aber auch von granulomatösen Prozessen bei Lepra, Tuberkulose, Boeck usw. Von den Ergebnissen Shelleys und Hurleys seien hier nur die wichtigsten kurz festgehalten. Es handelt sich beim Zirkoniumgranulom nicht, wie man eigentlich erwarten könnte, um ein einfaches Fremdkörpergranulom. Weder chemisch noch spektrographisch ist der Nachweis von Zirkonium in den granulomatösen Läsionen gelungen. Darum hat man an andere auslösende Ursachen gedacht, vor allem an Stearate, an Beimengungen wie Silicon u.a.

Es gelang nun aber beim Menschen experimentell, unter streng gewählten Versuchsbedingungen, mit einem handelsüblichen desodorierenden Stift, der während längerer Zeit jeden Morgen eingerieben wurde, Zirkoniumgranulome auszulösen.

Unter sonst genau gleichen Bedingungen wurde in der einen Axilla der etwa 5% zirkoniumhaltige geruchbindende Stift, in der anderen Axilla ein sonst gleich zusammengesetzter Stift ohne Zirkonium verwendet. Jeden 2. Tag wurden zusätzlich die Haare rasiert. Die Stifte wurden jeden Morgen 5 min lang kräftig eingerieben. Andere Cosmetica, Seifen, Puder usw., durften von den Versuchspersonen nicht verwendet werden. Nach verschiedenen Intervallen wurden aus beiden Achselhöhlen Biopsien entnommen und in Serienschnitten durchuntersucht.

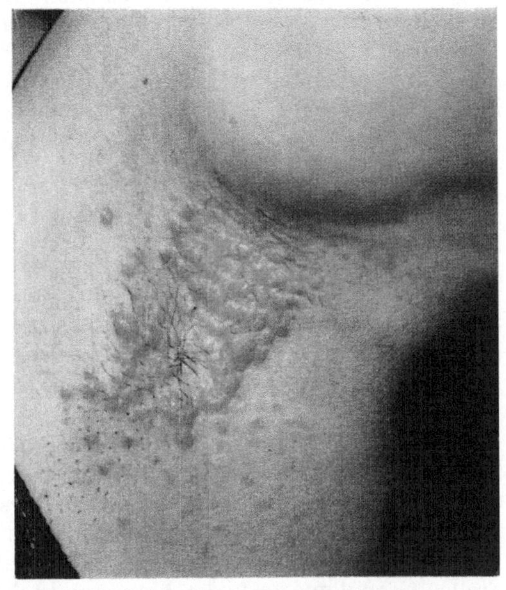

Abb. 6. Zirkoniumgranulom der Achselhöhlen. [Aus Shelley u. Hurley, Brit. J. Derm. **70**, 75 (1958)]

Von den 30 Versuchspersonen erkrankte eine an einem klinisch und histologisch typischen axillären Zirkoniumgranulom, während bei drei anderen Personen lediglich unspezifische, rasch vorübergehende entzündliche papulöse Reaktionen auftraten. In einer weiteren Versuchsserie trat wieder ein typischer Fall auf.

Gewöhnliche Läppchenproben mit dem zirkoniumhaltigen desodorierenden Stift waren bei den zwei Individuen, bei denen experimentell Granulome ausgelöst worden waren, negativ. Hingegen waren intradermale Proben mit stark verdünnten Lösungen von Natrium-Zirkoniumlactat bei beiden positiv, bei sämtlichen Kontrollen aber negativ. Im einen Fall waren Konzentrationen von 1:10000 und höhere, im anderen Fall 1:1000 und höhere positiv. Die spezifische Überempfindlichkeit bezieht sich auf das Element Zirkonium und nicht auf ein besonderes Salz. Injektionen von Zirkoniumchlorid und Zirkoniumnitrat bewirkten ebenfalls ein Granulom an der Injektionsstelle. Kontrollen mit Berylliumsulfat und kolloidem Silicat ergaben weder bei den Überempfindlichen noch bei den übrigen Versuchspersonen irgendwelche Reaktionen. Nach 10 Tagen und nach 4 Wochen waren an den Teststellen granulomatöse Infiltrate auch histologisch nachweisbar. Eine passive Übertragung der Zirkoniumüberempfindlichkeit mit Serum der Probanden war nicht möglich. Der Nachweis der Antigen-Antikörperreaktion in vitro mißlang ebenfalls, weil Zirkonium die Serumeiweiße in allen Proben ausfällte. Die klassischen Präcipitin- und Agglutininreaktionen in den Seren sind deshalb hier nicht brauchbar.

Nach diesen experimentellen Vorarbeiten konnten Shelley und Hurley ihre Auffassung auch an klinisch beobachteten Fällen belegen. Bei vier Patienten im Krankengut der Autoren waren Zirkoniumgranulome in den Achselhöhlen nach

Gebrauch des Antischweißmittels aufgetreten. Alle vier erwiesen sich als zirkoniumüberempfindlich, indem sich bei ihnen nach intradermaler Injektion von 0,2 cm³ verdünnter Natrium-Zirkoniumlactat-Lösung 1:10000 und 1:1000 späte allergische Reaktionen in der Form von epitheloidzelligen Granulomen ausbildeten. Intradermale Kontrollreaktionen mit Berylliumsulfat 10^{-3} und Siliciumdioxyd 10^{-3} waren auch bei diesen zirkoniumüberempfindlichen Patienten negativ.

Bei dieser Testung sollte sich die entzündliche Papel erst nach einer Latenzperiode von mehreren Tagen ausbilden; frühere unspezifische Reaktionen sind möglich; histologische Kontrollen zwischen der 3. und 6. Woche müssen aber beweisen, daß eine granulomatöse Entzündung vorliegt. Es ist hervorzuheben, daß schon unvorstellbar kleine Mengen von Zirkonium bei solchen überempfindlichen Personen granulomauslösend wirken. Es genügten nämlich 2×10^{-7} g von Natrium-Zirkoniumlactat, um eine, wenn auch kleine, so doch deutlich sichtbare Papel entstehen zu lassen.

Es scheint sich hier um den Prototyp eines allergischen Granuloms zu handeln. Die Patienten werden erst durch den fortgesetzten Gebrauch überempfindlich. Durch Epitheldefekte, durch kleine Verletzungen, durch intertriginöse oder andere banal entzündliche Mikroläsionen dringen kleine Mengen in die Cutis ein und führen dann nach erfolgter Sensibilisierung bei neuer Zufuhr zu allergischen granulomatösen Epitheloidzellenreaktionen. Die einmal erworbene Empfindlichkeit bleibt offenbar sehr lange bestehen. Auch nach 2 Jahren war sie noch nachweisbar.

Die Erkrankung wird hier bei den Fremdkörperreaktionen abgehandelt, weil zweifellos Analogien zu bekannten Fremdkörpergranulomen angenommen werden dürfen. Sicher müssen wir im Entstehungsmechanismus ein lokales Eindringen von Zirkonium transepidermal in die Cutis fordern. In der Folge wird aber die ganze Hautdecke überempfindlich; es wäre also denkbar, daß sich auch an anderen Stellen Granulome ausbilden könnten. In den Achselhöhlen sind die Entstehungsbedingungen lediglich besonders günstig. Zirkonium wird in den Vereinigten Staaten auch in Salben zur Behandlung von Kontaktdermatitis verwendet. Es gilt mit Recht als ein Metall von ganz besonders geringer Toxicität. In der zirkoniumverarbeitenden Industrie sind denn auch kaum je Berufsekzeme beobachtet worden. Auch eine „Zirconiosis" analog zur Beryllium-Pneumokoniose ist bisher noch nicht beschrieben worden.

Den beim Studium und bei der pathogenetischen Abklärung der Zirkonium-Granulome erarbeiteten neuen Erkenntnissen darf man große allgemeine Bedeutung beimessen. Sie werden möglicherweise unsere bisherigen Deutungen verschiedener granulomatöser Prozesse umstürzen. SHELLEY schließt darum einen Aufsatz mit den Worten: „In der Allergieforschung ist eine neue Front entstanden."

3. Talk-Granulome

Im neueren, und zwar hauptsächlich im chirurgischen Schrifttum ist mehr und mehr von Talkgranulomen die Rede (OLIVIER et al. 1951; JOHNSON, HÜBNER, HABERICH, GATTERMANN, MACHER, THOMPSON, RÖSSLE, SAXEN, STACHER, SEELIG et al., BYRON und WELCH, FIENBERG, GERMAN u. MCKEE, GRIECO, KLEMM). Sie treten sowohl nach Operationen in der Bauchhöhle als auch nach chirurgischen Eingriffen in Hautnarben auf. Man vermutet die Ursache im Talk (Magnesium-Silicat), mit dem die Gummihandschuhe vor der Sterilisation behandelt werden. In Kaninchenversuchen kann man leicht Fremdkörpergranulome erzeugen, indem man Talk in die Bauchhöhle des Versuchstieres einstreut. Einen sehr guten Überblick über das vorliegende Fremdkörperproblem vermittelt die Arbeit von SEELIG, VERDA u. KIDD. Es ist offenbar so, daß durch unvorsichtiges Umgehen mit talkgepuderten Operationshandschuhen sehr viel mehr Unheil angerichtet wird, als man gemeinhin annimmt. Die zitierten Autoren warnen denn auch vor dieser Komplikation nach chirurgischen Eingriffen im Abdomen, weil sie zu sehr schweren Darmverwachsungen führen können. Sie weisen einen interessanten Weg zur Vermeidung der Zwischenfälle. Von allen Pudersubstanzen, welche die Autoren als Ersatz für Talkpuder geprüft und z.T.experimentell am Kaninchen- oder Rattenperitoneum daraufhin getestet haben, bewährte sich einzig Kaliumbitartrat, das gleichzeitig bakteriostatisch auf Coli und Staphylococcus aureus wirke.

Die Talkgranulome in Hautnarben haben nun allerdings nicht die gleiche allgemeinmedizinische und prognostische Bedeutung wie diese vorerwähnten Nebenerscheinungen nach Operationen in der Peritonealhöhle oder im Pleuraraum. Immerhin wird ab und zu auf derartige Narbengranulome auch von dermatologischer Seite hingewiesen (MACHER). Vermutlich entstehen sie häufiger durch absichtliches Einstreuen von Wundpudern in akzidentelle oder chirurgische Hautwunden und nicht wie die Talkgranulome nach Bauchoperationen schon durch die relativ kleinen Mengen von Talk, die nach Platzen oder Anstechen eines Operationshandschuhes aus den Fingerlingen in die serösen Höhlen austreten können.

a) Lycopodium-Granulome

Ganz ähnliche Beobachtungen wurden von Lycopodiumsporen mitgeteilt (CLINE, ERB), welche von den Handschuhen der Chirurgen in die Operationswunden gelangten und Anlaß zu Fisteln und Verwachsungen gaben (ANTOPOL und ROBBINS). Als interessante historische Reminiszenz sei erwähnt, daß H. MARTIN (1881) mit Lycopodiumsporen „experimentelle Tuberkulose" — heute würden wir sagen „sarkoidale Fremdkörperreaktionen" — ausgelöst hat.

b) Granulome nach Verwendung von Wundpudern

In diesem Zusammenhang darf erwähnt werden, daß es eine Zeitlang üblich war, entweder sulfonamidhaltige Wundpuder oder desinfizierende Puder, die Antibiotica enthielten, bei der chirurgischen Wundversorgung zu verwenden. Man hoffte so Infektionen bei traumatisch entstandenen Verwundungen besser zu verhüten. Es hat sich aber gezeigt, daß dadurch recht oft die normale Wundheilung eher gestört wurde. In einzelnen Fällen kam es zu ausgedehnten, kissenartigen Granulomen in der Subcutis. Abb. 7a u. b zeigt eine solche Granulationsgeschwulst, die klinisch etwas an Tuberkulose erinnert. Sie entstand nach chirurgischer Wundversorgung mit Naht. Weil am Handrücken nicht ausreichend excidiert werden konnte, war prophylaktisch Penicillin-Streptomycin-Puder eingestreut worden. Im histologischen Bild ist eine deutliche Fremdkörperreaktion zu erkennen. Man findet in den Riesenzellen phagocytierte Partikel, die als Reste des Wundpuders angesprochen werden müssen.

Im chirurgischen Schrifttum ist in den vergangenen Jahren wiederholt zu diesem Problem Stellung genommen worden (CARTON, SCHMUZIGER). Eine ganze Reihe von Autoren lehnt das prophylaktische Einstreuen von Wundpudern völlig ab. Man hat den Eindruck, diese Methode werde über kurz oder lang wieder ganz verlassen werden. Selbst völlig resorbierbare Sulfonamid- oder Antibioticapulver scheinen die Wundheilung empfindlich zu stören. Sie sind darum abzulehnen und höchstens für den Gebrauch an Oberflächen zulässig. Sehr oft enthalten solche

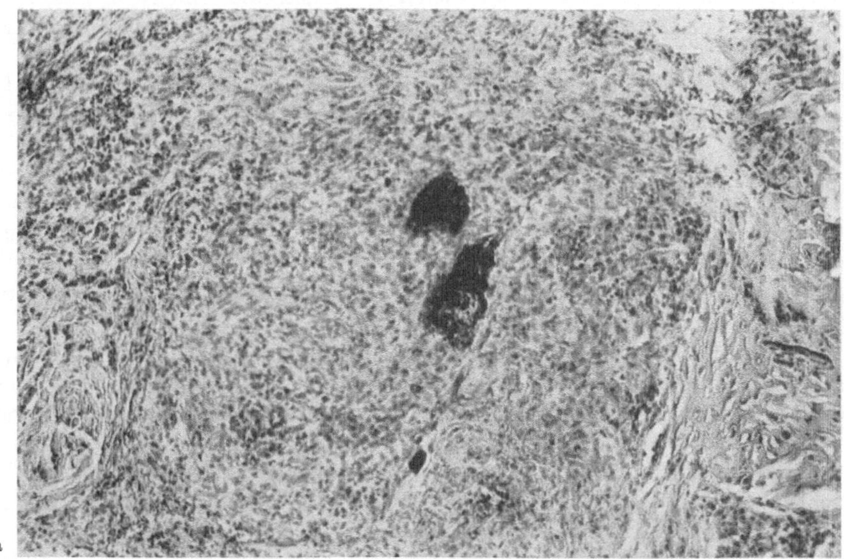

a

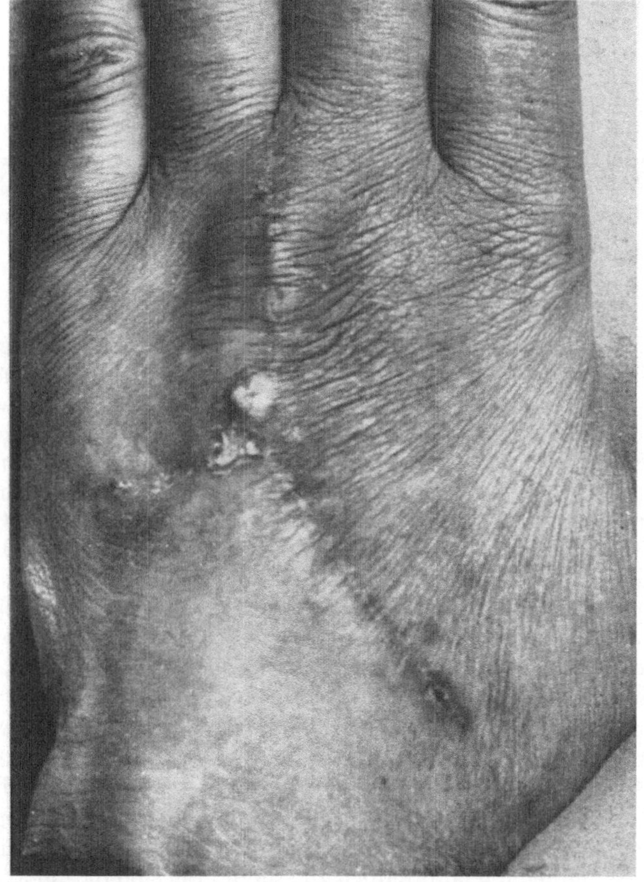

b

Abb. 7a u. b. Fremdkörpergranulom durch Wundpuder

Wundpuder auch Zusätze von Talk, so daß man annehmen muß, ein Teil der beobachteten Granulome seien als Fremdkörperreaktionen gegen unresorbierbare Talkpartikel zu deuten (CARTON).

4. Chrysiasis, Auriasis

Während die Geschichte der Argyrie als einer Komplikation der Behandlung mit Silbersalzen sehr weit, nämlich mindestens bis ins 18. Jahrhundert, zurückreicht, sind Beobachtungen über Goldimprägnationen der Haut viel jüngeren Datums. Darum fehlt selbst im Artikel von POLLAND noch ein entsprechender Abschnitt. In der Therapie spielten Goldverbindungen zeitweise eine bedeutende Rolle, und zwar bei den Indikationen: Tuberkulose, chronischer Gelenkrheumatismus, Lupus erythematodes und Asthma bronchiale. Die jüngste Entwicklung hat diese Medikamentgruppe allerdings wieder stark in den Hintergrund gedrängt.

Am häufigsten wurden komplexe Auroverbindungen (mit einwertigem Gold) benützt, nämlich Verbindungen vom Typus des Krysolgan, des Solganal (Aurothioglucose) und des Sanocrysins (Natriumaurothiosulfat). Im Organismus verhalten sich die Goldverbindungen ähnlich wie die Salze der meisten schweren Metalle; ihre Ausscheidung erfolgt langsam, zur Hauptsache mit dem Urin. Gold wird aber sehr lange im Körper zurückgehalten. Noch 2 Jahre nach Abschluß von Goldkuren ließ es sich im Urin und in den Faeces nachweisen. Bei den Goldkuren kam es in nahezu einem Drittel der Fälle zu toxischen Nebenwirkungen; vor allem zu Nephritis, Stomatitis, evtl. Colitis. Auch die schweren allergischen Hauterscheinungen, die häufig bis zur generalisierten exfoliierenden Erythrodermie fortschritten, waren gefürchtet. Die uns hier beschäftigende *Chrysiasis*, eine gräuliche Verfärbung der Haut an den lichtexponierten Stellen, ist hingegen als eine relativ sehr seltene Komplikation der Goldbehandlung zu werten. Man hat sie besonders bei über lange Zeit fortgesetzten oder bei häufig wiederholten Kuren beobachtet.

HANSBORG hat 1928 den ersten Fall von Goldablagerung unter dem Namen Chrysiasis beschrieben. Bei dieser ersten Beobachtung handelte es sich um eine 20jährige Kranke mit Lungentuberkulose, die mit 12,35 g Sanocrysin (Natriumaurothiosulfat) intravenös behandelt worden war. Auf elementares Gold umgerechnet, ergeben sich 4,62 g Au. Die Verfärbung zeigte sich erst 2 Jahre später. Sie erinnerte sehr stark an Argyrie und trat nur an den dem Lichte dauernd ausgesetzten Hautpartien stärker hervor. Die Patientin starb an ihrer Tuberkulose. Im Anschluß an die Sektion konnte auch in Nierengewebsstückchen, welche längere Zeit dem Licht ausgesetzt worden waren, histochemisch Gold nachgewiesen werden. Nach diesem ersten Bearbeiter wird das Gold also nicht nur in der Haut, sondern auch in inneren Organen abgelagert.

Ein zweiter Fall von Chrysiasis wurde von ZIMMERLI und LUTZ beschrieben. Wieder betraf es eine Lungenkranke, die mit Sanocrysin behandelt worden war. Am 10. Tag ihrer ersten Goldkur machte sie eine flüchtige erythematöse Dermatitis durch (vermutlich ein „exanthème du 9ème jour"), die schnell und ohne eine Pigmentierung zurückzulassen, wieder abklang. Die Verfärbung durch Goldeinlagerung trat dann erst ein Jahr nach Beginn der Goldbehandlung und nach Abschluß der dritten Kur in Erscheinung.

In der Folge wurden aus verschiedenen Ländern einzelne Beobachtungen von Chrysiasis veröffentlicht, so unter anderen 1939 der erste Fall aus Deutschland durch KOCHS. Das klinische Bild wird in allen Publikationen übereinstimmend geschildert. Die bläulichgraue Verfärbung wirkt eigenartig auf den Beobachter. Der Farbton ist so auffällig, daß er im französischen Schrifttum gerne, aber zu Unrecht, als Chrysocyanose beschrieben wird. Befallen werden nur die gewöhnlich dem Licht ausgesetzten Hautpartien, Gesicht, Hals, Hände, evtl. Vorderarme. Die Grenzen, besonders am Halsausschnitt, sind oft sehr scharf. Ausgespart bleiben die tiefsten Punkte von Hautfalten und -fältchen, also die vom Licht geschützten Streifen. Histologisch findet sich das Gold als feinste amorphe Teilchen im Corium zum größten Teil extracellulär eingelagert. Spezielle

Untersuchungstechniken wie Auflichtmikroskopie oder Untersuchung im Dunkelfeld nach der Leuchtbildmethode von E. HOFFMANN am ungefärbten Schnitt lassen die Verteilung der Einlagerungen besonders gut erkennen. Man findet sie in den obersten Coriumschichten am dichtesten, oft zu einem zusammenhängenden subepithelialen Saum angehäuft. Es sind also histologisch Analogien zur Argyrie vorhanden, allerdings bestehen auch kennzeichnende Abweichungen. Winzige goldglänzende Körnchen sind wenigstens stellenweise auch noch in der Basalzellenschicht nachweisbar, in höheren Epidermisschichten findet sich noch etwas Gold diffus verteilt. [Silber wurde hingegen nie in der Epidermis und ihren Anhangsgebilden nachgewiesen (ZOON)]. Mit den obersten lebenden Zellagen soll die Goldablagerung aufhören. Hornschicht und Haare sind spektrographisch untersucht und frei von Gold befunden worden. Auch die subcutanen Gewebsschichten bleiben fast völlig frei von Goldniederschlägen. In den Haarwurzelscheiden und in bindegewebigen Zellen des Haarbalges findet sich hingegen wieder besonders reichlich Gold in amorpher Anordnung, ebenso im perifollikulären Gewebe und in den Schweißdrüsen.

Außerordentlich wichtig ist die Feststellung, daß wir auch in Hautpartien, die makroskopisch keine Verfärbung aufweisen, also an den bedeckten, nicht dem Lichte ausgesetzten Körperstellen des Rumpfes, reichliche Mengen von Goldeinlagerungen finden können. Der subepitheliale Saum mag etwas weniger stark ausgeprägt sein, im übrigen ist aber der histologische Befund der gleiche. Auch Untersuchungen mit der Emissionsspektralanalyse, wie sie KOCHS mitgeteilt hat, bestätigen und ergänzen die geschilderten feingeweblichen Besonderheiten der Goldeinlagerung. Dabei war in Nägeln, in veraschten Haaren Gold nicht nachweisbar, wohl aber im Stuhl, im Urin und im Venenblut, hingegen nicht im Schweiß der betreffenden Patientin. Mit der Emissionsspektralanalyse wurde auch in einem Kontrollfall, bei einem Patienten, der ebenfalls Goldkuren durchgemacht hatte, bei dem aber keine Chrysiasis aufgetreten war, Gold in der Haut nachgewiesen. Man könnte in einem solchen Fall von einer latenten Chrysiasis sprechen. Sämtliche manifest Erkrankten hatten übrigens das Gold durch intravenöse Injektionen zugeführt erhalten. Dabei war die Dosierung in den früheren Jahren zum Teil erheblich höher als heute (ROBERT: 15,29 g Gold in 8 Jahren). Man wird also in Zukunft eher mit weniger neuen Fällen zu rechnen haben, dies um so mehr, als zwei früher wichtige Indikationsgebiete, Hauttuberkulose und Erythematodes, durch die moderne Weiterentwicklung therapeutischer Möglichkeiten wesentlich eingeengt worden sind. In der inneren Medizin und auch in der Dermatologie verbleiben natürlich immer noch Anwendungsgebiete für die Goldbehandlung. Sowohl beim primär chronischen Gelenkrheumatismus als beim Bronchialasthma besteht übrigens die Tendenz, die Dosierung evtl. bis an die Grenze toxischer Reaktionen voranzutreiben, noch weiter zu Recht. Damit bleibt die Möglichkeit, daß fernerhin Erkrankungen an Chrysiasis auftreten werden.

Eine einmal ausgebildete Chrysiasis ist therapeutisch schwer zu beeinflussen. Durch ständige geringe Ausscheidung von Gold im Stuhl und im Urin ist ein allmählicher spontaner Rückgang der Verfärbung denkbar. Es sind Versuche mit Dimercaprol (BAL) zur Mobilisierung der Golddepots, ferner mit sog. Ionenaustauschern gemacht worden. Sämtliche toxischen Nebenwirkungen der Goldbehandlung sollen mit Dimercaprol als Schwermetall-Antidot behoben werden können (DAVISON, COHEN et al., RAGAN und BOOTS). Über günstige Beeinflussung von Chrysiasis sind mir keine Mitteilungen bekannt. Bei den eigenen Beobachtungen von Chrysiasis wurde keine entsprechende Behandlung versucht, da es sich um Insassen von Pflegeheimen handelte, bei welchen die Verfärbung auch kosmetisch nicht störend wirkte.

III. Die Eisenspeicherkrankheit — Hämochromatose

Die Eisenspeicherkrankheit sei anschließend an die Ausführungen über Chrysiasis kurz erwähnt. Es bestehen insofern analoge Verhältnisse, als sich ebenfalls Schwermetalleinlagerungen in die Haut vorfinden. Die pathogenetischen Auffassungen über die Hämochromatose haben sich in den letzten Jahren grundlegend gewandelt. Während sie früher lediglich als Symptom bei verschiedenen internen Krankheiten angesehen wurde, glaubt man heute eher an eine scharf umschriebene nosologische Einheit. Die Hämochromatose wird jetzt als Resorptionsstörung aufgefaßt. Bei diesen Kranken nimmt der Darm wahllos alles zur Verfügung stehende Eisen auf. Die sonst normalerweise durch den Bedarf gesteuerte und kontrollierte Eisenaufnahme ist dadurch um ein Vielfaches erhöht. Als Folge der uneingeschränkten Resorption zirkuliert im Blut erhöhtes Serumeisen, ferner findet eine Einlagerung in die Leber, in das Pankreas, in die Nieren, in die Haut usw. statt. Besonders in der Leber und im Pankreas hat die Eisenspeicherung deletäre Wirkung, gibt sie doch den Anlaß zu einer Fibrose dieser Organe mit schweren Rückwirkungen auf ihren Stoffwechsel und ihre Funktionen (Pigmentcirrhose, Bronzediabetes, Syndrom von TROISSIER-HANOT-CHAUFFARD).

Für den Hautarzt ist die Erkrankung vor allem wichtig, weil er in solchen Fällen vom Internisten zur konsiliarischen Beurteilung des Hautkolorites zugezogen werden kann oder weil ihm bei Einsendung von Excisionen ab und zu die Frage nach der Möglichkeit einer Hämochromatose gestellt wird.

Das Wesentliche an den histologischen Veränderungen in der Haut ist der Nachweis von reichlich Eisen, und zwar frei im Corium und nicht nur an bestimmte Gewebsteile (wie apokrine Schweißdrüsen-Epithelien) gebunden. Es sollte — will man brauchbare Resultate erhalten — mit der Methode von TURNBULL, modifiziert nach HUECK, gearbeitet werden. Ferner sollte die Entnahmestelle bekannt sein (SOLTERMANN). Bei Internisten hat sich — vermutlich in Befolgung von Anregungen HEDINGERs — die Biopsie aus der Axillargegend eingebürgert. Hier ist aber immer damit zu rechnen, daß auch bei gesunden Individuen in apokrinen Schweißdrüsen Eisen bzw. Hämosiderin nachweisbar ist. Zur Beurteilung besser geeignet sind Biopsien aus dem Vorderarm und aus anderen Bezirken ohne apokrine Schweißdrüsen. Man soll sich aber bewußt bleiben, daß die Hauthistologie allein für die Annahme oder den Ausschluß der Diagnose Hämochromatose nicht ausschlaggebend sein darf. HEDINGER berichtet in seiner Zusammenstellung, daß zweimal der Verdacht auf Eisenspeicherkrankheit fallen gelassen worden sei, weil durch die Hautbiopsie kein Eisen im Gewebe nachgewiesen wurde. Die Sektion aber bestätigte die ursprüngliche Diagnose, und es fand sich in beiden Fällen eine schwere Hämochromatose innerer Organe.

IV. Die Tätowierung

Einige Mitteilungen berichten über dauerhafte kosmetisch störende Verfärbungen der Haut, welche im Anschluß an therapeutische Maßnahmen bei vesiculöser Kontaktdermatitis oder bei Verbrennungen auftraten. Es handelte sich um eine Art akzidenteller Tätowierung (jedenfalls um einen Vorgang, der der bekannten traumatischen Tätowierung und der lokalen Argyrose gleichgesetzt werden darf), heilten doch offenbar Metallniederschläge derart ein, daß sie als kleinste und indifferente Fremdkörperpartikelchen einen bleibenden schiefergrauen oder braunen Farbton verursachten. Solche unerwünschten Nebenwirkungen wurden nach der Behandlung von nässender Kontaktdermatitis mit 4%igen Ferrosulfat-Umschlägen beobachtet (REYNER; BECKER u. STENHOUSE), einem Procedere, das in Amerika für die Giftefeu-Ausschläge empfohlen wird. In anderen Fällen wurde zuerst Bleiacetat, dann Eisensulfat als Umschlagsflüssigkeit verwendet. Es entstanden ebenfalls intensiv braune, dauernde Verfärbungen (Weiss et al. 1941).

Ähnliche Veränderungen wurden im Anschluß an die Behandlung von Verbrennungswunden nach der Methode von Bettmann beobachtet. Nach Wundreinigung wird 5‰ Tanninlösung mit einem Spray aufgetragen und unmittelbar nachher zur Beschleunigung der Schorfbildung eine 10%ige Silbernitratlösung. Auch dadurch kann es zu einer Fremdkörpereinlagerung kommen, die als lokalisierte *Argyrosis* bezeichnet werden muß. In einem von Ayres geschilderten Fall kam es sogar wegen der kosmetischen Beeinträchtigung zu einer Schadenersatzklage gegen den behandelnden Arzt.

Im übrigen ist dem Kapitel über Tätowierungen kaum Wesentliches und Neues beizufügen. In vielen europäischen Ländern ist ja die Schmucktätowierung stark im Rückgang begriffen. Selbst in der französischen Fremdenlegion ist das Tätowieren verboten und unter Strafe gestellt worden. Nur einzelne Berufsarten scheinen noch hartnäckig an diesem Brauche festzuhalten, ferner auch die Angehörigen der Handels- und Kriegsmarine.

Über interessante kulturhistorische und ethnographische Probleme haben Schönfeld, Marchionini, Ohya und andere Autoren berichtet.

Versuche und Vorschläge, die Tätowierung in die Gruppenmedizin einzuführen, wie etwa zur dauernden Kennzeichnung der Blutgruppen, sind nicht zu einer international anerkannten Konvention gediehen (Urbach).

Besondere Erwähnung verdient hier noch eine Arbeit von Sulzberger und Tolmach über allergische Aufflammungs-Reaktionen in roten Tätowierungen (beobachtet 4 Tage nach intracutaner Injektion einer Influenza-Vaccine, die als Zusatz ein organisches Hg-Präparat enthielt). Das alte Problem der späten granulomatösen oder hyperkeratotischen Reaktion durch spezielle zur Tätowierung verwendete Farbstoffe oder „Pigmente" wird nochmals an Hand von neuen Beispielen aufgegriffen.

Im größeren Zusammenhang interessieren diese Einzelfälle, weil sie eben schon seit 1903, seit der Mitteilung von Ullmann, dargetan haben, daß es auch durch Chemikalien ausgelöste granulomatöse Entzündungen gibt, die auf einer allergischen Überempfindlichkeit beruhen. Von hier aus betrachtet, sind die neuen Befunde von Shelley und Hurley beim Zirkonium-Granulom (auf die in einem anderen Kapitel eingegangen wurde) eine Fortsetzung und Ergänzung unseres Wissens geworden. Während bei Allergie gegen Tätowierungsfarben Granulome und warzige Hyperkeratosen gesehen wurden, entstanden durch Zirkonium succulente Granulationsgeschwülstchen. Hier mag neben der chemischen Differenz der Haptene auch das besondere lokale Terrain der Achselhöhle eine Rolle spielen. Auf den Unterschied in bezug auf das Bestehen einer gleichzeitigen epidermalen ekzem-allergischen Überempfindlichkeit bei den verschiedenen Fällen sei hingewiesen, Unterschiede, die noch der Klärung bedürfen.

Eine weitere wertvolle Arbeit von Rostenberg, Brown u. Carlo über Tätowierungen sei speziell erwähnt, weil sie sich eingehend mit den verschiedenen Farbstoffen befaßt, die zur Erzeugung blauer, roter, grüner oder gelber Farbtöne verwendet werden. Falls sich eine derartige Frage zur Abklärung stellt, wird man mit Vorteil auf die erwähnte Arbeit zurückgreifen.

Auch im jüngeren Schrifttum wird ab und zu auf Übertragung von Infektionskrankheiten durch das Tätowieren hingewiesen (Smith, Schönfeld 1939). Unter solchen Mitteilungen gebührt der Arbeit von Porrit und Olsen eine Sonderstellung, wird doch über die gleichzeitige Übertragung von Lepra anläßlich einer

Tätowierung bei mehreren Schiffsleuten berichtet. Eine solche Einzelbeobachtung, bei der mit einiger Sicherheit auch die Inkubationszeit zwischen Einimpfung und Auftreten der ersten leprösen Hautläsionen bestimmbar ist, darf als einmaliges Kuriosum hier besonders hervorgehoben werden.

Schließlich muß auch die Frage nach der Behandlung oder Beseitigung von Tätowierungen kurz erwähnt werden. Wirklich neue Gesichtspunkte ergeben sich auch hier kaum. Mit der Einführung des hochtourigen Schleifens (SCHREUS) ist eine Weiterentwicklung des Kromayerschen Verfahrens mit rotierenden Instrumenten in die Hauttherapie eingeführt worden, das auch für die Beseitigung von Farbstoffpartikelchen aus der Haut Anwendung finden kann. Die Methode reiht sich anderen Verfahren an, die mit Ätzung, Elektrokoagulation usw. die Ausstoßung der Farbstoffpartikel anstreben. Auch sie kann nur zu einer kosmetisch mehr oder weniger befriedigenden Narbe führen und ist darum ähnlich wie die älteren Prozeduren zu bewerten.

Literatur

ALDEN, H. S., and W. M. HOWELL: The asbestos corn. Arch Derm. Syph. (Chic.) **49**. 312 (1944). — ALLEN, R. A.: A case of general Argyria. J. Amer. med. Ass. **47**, 1829 (1906). Zit. bei STILLIANS. — ANTOPOL, W.: Lycopodium granuloma. Arch. Path. **16**, 326 (1933), Zit. bei SEELIG et al. — ANTOPOL, W., and C. ROBBINS: Lycopodium granuloma resulting from use of anal suppositories. J. Amer. med. Ass. **109**, 1192 (1937). Zit. bei SEELIG et al. — ARNING, E.: Klinische und histologische Beobachtungen an Tätowierten. Arch. Derm. Syph. (Berl.) **123**, 225 (1916). — ARZT, L.: Campheröl-Hautinfiltrat. Arch. Derm. Syph. (Berl.) **133**, 67. Zit. in GANS-STEIGLEDER. — Fremdkörpergranulationsgewebe nach Fistelfüllung mit Jodoformglycerinbaryum. Wien. Dermatol. Ges., Sitzg v. 21. 11. 29. Zbl. Haut- u. Geschl.-Kr. **33**, 542 (1930). — Zur Differentialdiagnose granulomatöser Prozesse (Granulomatosis disciformis chronica progressiva, Nekrobiosis lipoidica diabeticorum, atypisches Tb-Granulom). Hautarzt **3**, 488 (1952). — Fremdkörpereinsprengung. Zbl. Haut- u. Geschl.-Kr. 88, 362 (1954). — Foreign body granulomas and Boeck's Sarcoid. J. invest. Derm. **24**, 155 (1955). — AYRES, S.: Localized argyria following treatment of burn with tannic acid and silver nitrate. Arch. Derm. Syph. (Chic.) **38**, 645 (1938). — AYRES, W. W., W. B. OBER and P. K. HAMILTON: Posttraumatic subcutaneous granulomas associated with a crystalline material. Amer. J. Path. **27**, 303 (1951).

BALLIN, D. B.: Cutaneous hypersensitivity to mercury from tattooing: Report of case. Arch. Derm. Syph. (Chic.) **27**, 292 (1933). — BAUER, F. K., B. CASSEN, E. YOUTCHEFF and L. SHOOP: Jet injections of radioisotopes. Amer. J. med. Sci. **225**, 374 (1953). — BAUER, TH., u. I. FLEISSIG: Zur Frage des Fremdkörpergranulationsgewebes. Virchows Arch. path. Anat. **217**, 1 (1914). — BAYER, H. v.: Fremdkörper im Organismus. Einheilung. Bruns' Beitr. klin. Chir. **58** (1908). Zit. bei LAUENER, Diss. Bern. — BECKER, S. W., and E. STENHOUSE: Permanent pigmentation following the application of ferrous sulfate for the treatment of Poison Ivy. Arch. Derm. Syph. (Chic.) **37**, 920 (1938). — BECKMANN, K.: Hämochromatose (Bronzediabetes). In: Handbuch der inneren Medizin, Bd. III/2, S. 857. Berlin-Göttingen-Heidelberg: Springer 1953. — BEERMAN, H.: Some aspects of berylliosis. Amer. J. med. Sci. **221**, 462 (1951). — BEISENHERZ: Sofortbehandlung von Schmutztätowierung. (III. Kongr. d. Dtsch. Ges. f. aesthet. Med.) Derm. Wschr. **139**, 389 (1959). — BERGEL, S.: Über künstliche Erzeugung verschiedenartiger Granulationsneubildungen und Zellwucherungen. Virchows Arch. path. Anat. **230**, 461 (1921). — BETHUNE, N.: Pleural poudrage. J. thorac. Surg. **4**, 251 (1935). Zit. bei SEELIG et al. — BETTMANN, S.: Melkerschwielen und eigenartige interdigitale fistelbildende Affektion. Zbl. Haut- u. Geschl.-Kr. **41**, 541 (1932). Zit. bei RÖCKL u. MÜLLER, Haargranulome. — BEZZOLA, C.: Sulla produzione sperimentale e sulla istogenesi di alcune neoformazioni inflammatorie a cellule giganti. Pathologica **4**, 55 (1912). Zit. bei SEELIG et al. — BIEBER, PH.: Argyrie cutanée. Bull. Soc. franç. Derm. Syph. **64**, 210 (1957). — BLASCHKO, A.: Über das Vorkommen von metallischem Silber in der Haut von Silberarbeitern. Mh. prakt. Derm. **5**, 197 (1886). Zit. bei GANS-STEIGLEDER. — BOLGERT, M., et F. BUSSER: Curieuse histoire d'une lésion cutanée provoquée par le béryllium (présentation de coupes). Bull. Soc. franç. Derm. Syph. **63**, 167 (1956). — BORCHARDT, H.: Über experimentelle Chrysosis bei Kaninchen und Hunden und ihren histochemischen Nachweis. Virchows Arch. path. Anat. **267**, 272 (1928). Zit. bei GANS-STEIGLEDER — BORK, K.: Zur Lehre von der allgemeinen Hämochromatose. Virchows Arch. path. Anat. **269**, 178 (1928). — BRAEUCHLI: Granulationsgeschwulst, hervorgerufen durch Glassplitter. Inaug.-Diss. Zürich

1897. — Brandt, R.: Sarcoid-like granuloma, foreign-body type. Central States Dermatol. Soc., Cincinnati, 19. 3. 1955. Arch. Derm. **72**, 479 (1955). — Brandt, R., and H. Plotnick: Multiple cutaneous and subcutaneous sarcoid-like foreign-body granulomas. Report of a case with a parallel course in the various sites. Arch. Derm. **74**, 128 (1956). — Büchmann, P., u. G. Schenz: Zur Diagnose der Hämochromatose. Dtsch. med. Wschr. **1948**, 634. — Byron, F. X., and C. S. Welch: Complication from use of glove powder (Talc nodules in surgical scars). Surgery **10**, 766 (1941).

Carrie, C.: Zur Behandlung von Fremdkörpereinsprengungen der Haut. Derm. Wschr. **139**, 390 (1959). — Carton, F.: Granulome sulfamidique. Gaz. méd. Picardie **265**, 11 (1957). Zit. in Ann. Derm. Syph. (Paris) **86**, 164 (1959). — Cascos, A.: Etude comparative des pigmentations métalliques, argyrose et chrysose. Ann. Derm. Syph. (Paris) **7**, 751 (1936). Zit. bei Gans-Steigleder. — Cass jr., J. W.: Spontaneous remission of chronic beryllium poisoning from fluorescent lamp manufacturing; report of case. Arch. industr. Hyg. **3**, 569 (1951). Zit. in Allen, Diseases of the skin. — Cattani, P.: Das Tatauieren. Basel: Benno Schwabe & Co. 1922. Zit. bei Gans-Steigleder. — Chambers, R., and C. G. Grand: The chemotactic reaction of leucocytes to foreign substance in tissue culture. J. cell. comp. Physiol. **8**, 1 (1936). Zit. bei Seelig et al. — Civatte, J.: Quelques problèmes posés par les granulomes silicotiques et les granulomes bérylliques cutanés. Sem. Hôp. Paris **1955**, 3757—3759. — Cline, J. W.: Lycopodium granuloma, an avoidable surgical complication. Calif. Med. **48**, 189 (1938). — Coakley, W. A., R. N. Shapiro and G. W. Robertson: Granuloma of the skin at site of Injury by a fluorescent bulb. J. Amer. med. Ass. **139**, 1147 (1949). — Coburn, J. C.: Grease gun granuloma. Brit. J. Derm. **68**, 308 (1956). — Cohen, A., Goldman and Dubbe: Dimerkrapol. J. Amer. med. Ass. **133**, 749 (1947). — Cormia, F. E., and Ch. Sheard jr.: Granuloma of axilla (Zirconium?) from deodorant stick. (Discussion.) Arch. Derm. **75**, 903 (1957). — Cornbleet and Popper: Arch. Derm. Syph. (Chic.) **47**, 637 (1943). — Paraffin oil in the tissues shows vivid turquoise fluorescence under Wood's light. Zit. in Sutton, Disease of the Skin, 1956, p. 196. — Counter, C. E., and L. H. Winer: Contact dermatitis, complicated by foreign-body granuloma formation. Arch. Derm. **75**, 761 (1957). — Cozen, L., and M. Fonda: Palm thorn injuries — difficulty in diagnosis of late sequelas. Calif. Med. **79**, 40 (1953). — Crossland, P. M.: Silica granuloma of the skin. Arch. Derm. Syph. (Chic.) **71**, 457 (1955). Zit. in Sutton, Diseases of the Skin, p. 200. — Currie, A. R., T. Gibson and A. L. Goodall: Interdigital sinuses of barbers-hands. Brit. J. Surg. **41**, 278 (1953). — Curtis, G. H.: Cutaneous hypersensitivity due to beryllium. Study of 13 cases. Arch. Derm. Syph. (Chic.) **64**, 470 (1951). Zit. in Sutton, Diseases of the skin.

Darabos, L.: Ein Fall von Tintenstiftnekrose. Dermatologica (Basel) **85**, 411 (1942). — Davison, R. A.: Dimerkaprol. Stanf. med. Bull. **5**, 37 (1947). Zit. in Møller, Pharmakologie. — Degos, R., et A. Carteaud: Granulome silicotique à type de sarcoidose. Discussion d'une maladie de Schaumann authentique. Bull. Soc. franç. Derm. Syph. **60**, 258 (1953). — Degos, R., u. J. Civatte: Das Silikosegranulom der Haut. Hautarzt **10**, 106 (1959). — Degos, R., J. Delort et J. Hewitt: Maladie de Schaumann posttraumatique (érythème sarcoidique). Aspect rappelant celui d'un granulome sarcoidique silicotique. Bull. Soc. franç. Derm. Syph. **60**, 412 (1953). — Degos, R., E. Lortat-Jacob, J. Civatte et C. Barre: Granulome silicotique et maladie de Besnier-Boeck-Schaumann (nouveau cas). Bull. Soc. franç. Derm. Syph. **63**, 325 (1956). — Desaulles, P., W. Schuler u. R. Meier: Unabhängigkeit der Bildung des Fremdkörpergranuloms und seiner Beeinflussung durch Compound E von der Hypophyse. Experientia (Basel) **7**, 188 (1951). — Vergleich der Wirkung des Aldosterons auf das Fremdkörpergranulom der Ratte mit derjenigen von Cortexon, Corticosteron, Cortison und Hydrocortison. Experientia (Basel) **11**, 68 (1955). — Dewirtz, A. P.: Asbestwarzen. Arch. Derm. Syph. (Berl.) **161**, 1 (1930). — Dohi, Sh.: Über Argyrie. Virchows Arch. path. Anat. **193**, 148 (1908). Zit. bei Gans-Steigleder. — Tätowierung und Syphilis. Arch. Derm. Syph. (Berl.) **96**, 1 (1909). Zit. bei Gans-Steigleder. — Dubreuilh, W., et A. Venot: Tumeur d'aspect sarcomateux causée par des corps étrangers multiples. Ann. Derm. Syph. (Paris) **1900**, 1062. — Duperrat, B.: Les fausses tumeurs cutanées à corps étrangers. Sem. Hôp. (Paris) **28**, 3067—3071 (1952). — Les granulomes silicotiques cutanés. Minerva derm. **29**, 150 (1954). — Duperrat, B., Schwartz u. Leger: Paraffininjektionen. Zit. bei Lutz, Dermatologica (Basel) **89**, 278 (1944). — Dupont, A.: Huilomes spontanés ou pathomimie? Bull. Soc. franç. Derm. Syph. **63**, 501 (1956). — Dutra, F. R.: Pneumonitis and granulomatosis peculiar to beryllium workers. Amer. J. Path. **24**, 1137 (1948). — Beryllium granulomas of the skin. Arch. Derm. Syph. (Chic.) **60**, 1140 (1949). — Experimental beryllium granulomas of the skin. Arch. industr. Hyg. **3**, 81 (1951).

Engle jr., R. L.: The association of iron-containing crystals with Schaumann bodies in the giant cells of sarcoid type. Amer. J. Path. **27**, 1023 (1951). — Epstein, E.: Silica granuloma of the skin. Arch. Derm. Syph. (Chic.) **71**, 24 (1955). — Epstein, E., B. Gerstl, M. Berk and J. P. Belber: Silica pregranuloma. Arch. Derm. Syph. (Chic.) **71**, 645 (1955). —

ERB, I. H.: Lycopodium granuloma. Surg. Gynec. Obstet. **60**, 40 (1935). — EVANS, S. M.: Tissue responses to physical forces: I. The pathogenesis of silicosis: a preliminary report. J. industr. Hyg. **30**, 353 (1948). — EVANS, S. M., and W. ZEIT: Tissue responses to physical forces: II. The response of connective tissue to piezo-electrically active crystals. J. Lab. clin. Med. **34**, 592 (1949). — III. The ability of galvanic current to stimulate fibrogenesis. J. Lab. clin. Med. **34**, 610 (1949).

FAVRE et CIVATTE: Le vaselinome ganglionnaire. Bull. Soc. Biol. **84**, 8 (1921). — FELDAKER, M., H. O. PERRY and D. G. HANLON: Dermatologic manifestations associated with cryoglobulinemia. Arch. Derm. **73**, 325 (1955). — FELKE: Fremdkörpergranulome unter dem Bild eines Morbus Boeck. Derm. Wschr. **132**, 971 (1955). — „*Fiberglas*": Queries and minor notes. J. Amer. med. Ass. **152**, 1290 (1953). — FIENBERG, R.: Talcum powder granuloma. Arch. Path. **24**, 36 (1937). Zit. bei SEELIG. — FISHER, A. A.: Nonsurgical treatment of cutaneous beryllium-granuloma. Arch. Derm. Syph. (Chic.) **68**, 214 (1953). — Beryllium granuloma and ulceration of fingers: rapid improvement with cortisone ointment. Arch. Derm. Syph. (Chic.) **67**, 523 (1953). — Beryllium granuloma of the ring finger. Arch. Derm Syph. (Chic.) **67**, 103 (1953). — FLECK, E. F.: Zur Differentialdiagnose und Behandlung des Berylliumgranuloms der Haut. Derm. Wschr. **129**, 649 (1954). — FLECK, F.: Zum Problem der Granulomatosis disciformis chronica et progressiva. Derm. Wschr. **127**, 541 (1953). — FLEGEL, H.: Zur Spezifität einiger tuberkuloid-granulomatöser Hautaffektionen. Arch. klin. exp. Derm. **205**, 112 (1957). — FUHS, H.: Zur Klinik der Fremdkörpertumoren. Derm. Z. **1928**, 183. — FUNK, C. F.: Morbus Besnier-Boeck-Schaumann. Die Sarkoidose. In: GOTTRON-SCHÖNFELD, Bd. II/2, S. 1200. — Zur Differentialdiagnose des sarkoiden Gewebsbildes. Hautarzt **3**, 472 (1952). — FUNK, D. FR.: Boeck'sches Sarkoid als Allgemeinerkrankung. Med. Mschr. **4**, 721 (1950). Zit. bei GANS-STEIGLEDER.

GAGER, L. T., and E. M. ELLISON: Generalized therapeutic Argyria. Int. Clin. **4**, 118 (1935). Zit. bei STILLIANS. — GAHLEN, W., u. N. KLÜCKEN: Über Fremdkörpergranulome und Morbus Besnier-Boeck. Arch. Derm. Syph. (Berl.) **194**, 121 (1952). — GALANTE, R.: Sul reperto delle cellule giganti nei vaselinomi. Contributo allo studio della genesi e del significato. Haematologica **6** (1925). Zit. bei GANS-STEIGLEDER. — GANS, O., u. G. K. STEIGLEDER: Fremdkörper. In: Histologie der Hautkrankheiten, Bd. 2, S. 152. Berlin-Göttingen-Heidelberg: Springer 1957. — GARDNER, L. U.: The similarity of the lesions produced by silica and by the tubercle bacillus. Amer. J. Path. **13**, 13 (1937). — GATTERMANN, E.: Beitrag zur Frage der Gewebsschädigung durch Talk. Zbl. Chir. **1951**, 1822. — GAUL, L. E., and A. H. STAUD: Clinical spectroscopy. J. Amer. med. Ass. **104**, 1387 (1935). — GEDIGK, P., u. W. PIOCH: Über die Bildung von organischen Substanzen in Siliciumdioxydgranulomen. Virchows Arch. path. Anat. **328**, 513 (1956). — GELDEREN, CHR. v.: Histologische Veränderungen im subcutanen Bindegewebe nach subcutaner Paraffininjektion. Virchows Arch. path. Anat. **257**, 805 (1925). — GERBER, H. R.: Tierexperimentelle Untersuchungen zur Frage der Epitheloidzellbildung im normalen und tuberkulösen Organismus unter besonderer Berücksichtigung der Tuberkulinallergie. Diss. Zürich. Arch. Derm. Syph. (Berl.) **205**, 628 (1958). — GERMAN, W. M.: Lupoid-sarcoid reaction induced by foreign body (silica). Amer. J. clin. Path. **10**, 245 (1940). — GERMAN, W., and MCKEE: Dusting powder granulomas following surgery. Surg. Gynec. Obstet. **76**, 501 (1943). — GERRIE, J., F. KENNEDY and S. L. RICHARDSON: Canad. med. Ass. J. **62**, 544 (1950). Ref. Zbl. Haut- u. Geschl.-Kr. **77**, 305 (1951/52). — GINSBURG, J. E., and L. A. BECKER: Silicon granuloma of skin due to traumatic sand inoculation. J. Amer. med. Ass. **147**, 751 (1951). — GLASS, E.: Klinisch-experimenteller Beitrag zu den Verletzungen durch Kakteenstacheln. Langenbecks Arch. klin. Chir. **145**, 658 (1927). — GÖTZ, H.: Zur Frage der Beziehungen zwischen der Granulomatosis disciformis chronica et progressiva (MIESCHER) und der Necrobiosis lipoidica diabeticorum. Hautarzt **7**, 156 1956). — GOTO, K.: Über experimentell erzeugte Fremdkörpergranulome an Sehnen, Gelenkkapseln und in der Haut. Path. Inst. Zürich/Krankheits-Forsch. **9**, 52 (1931). — GOTTRON, H. A.:Haarglanulome. Med. Klin. **30**, 330 (1934). Zit. in RÖCKL. — Granulomatosis (tuberculoides) pseudosclerodermiformis symmetrica chronica. Arch. Derm. Syph. (Berl.) **172**, 142 (1935). — Argyrie. Zit. bei LUTZ, Dermatologica (Basel) **85**, 367 (1942). — GOUGEROT, M..: Sarcoides par corps étrangers. Bull. Soc. franç. Derm. Syph. **41**, 1370 (1934). — GOUGEROT, H., et A. DESAUX: Deux observations de sarcoides hypodermiques par corps étranger (injection d'huile camphrée) démontrées tuberculeuses par la guérison au moyen de vaccins antituberculeux. Arch. derm.-syph. (Paris) **1930**, 482. Zit. nach WORINGER, Vaselinome et paraffinome. Nouvelle Pratique Dermat., vol. VI, p. 595. Paris: Masson & Cie. 1936. — GREEN, W. S., and L. UNDERWOOD jr.: Cutaneous beryllium granuloma? Arch. Derm. **74**, 562 (1956). — GRIECO, F.: Granuloma di licopodio e da talco in seguito a laparotomia. Arch. ital. Chir. **42**, 641 (1936). — GRIER, R. S., P. NASH and D. G. FREIMAN: Skin lesions in persons exposed to beryllium compounds. J. industr. Hyg. **30**, 228 (1948).

HAAS, W.: Zur Verletzung durch Phosphorgeschosse. Zbl. Chir. **45**, 792 (1918). — HABERICH, M.: Zur Frage der Fremdkörpergranulome des Peritoneums. Chirurg **22**, 252 (1951). —

Habermann, R.: Über Argyria cutis nach Silbersalvarsan und den Wert der Leuchtbildmethode E. Hoffmann für ihren Nachweis. Derm. Z. **40**, 65 (1924). — Halter, K.: Melkergranulationsknoten. Zbl. Haut u. Geschl.-Kr. **60**, 377 (1938). Zit. in Röckl u. Müller, Haargranulome. — Hamperl, H. Gewebereaktion („Fremdkörperreaktion") gegen Schleim und Urin. Nord Med. **41**, 66 u. engl. Zus.fass. 69 (1949). Ref. Zbl. Haut- u. Geschl.-Kr. **75**, 8 (1950/51). — Hamperl, H., u. K. W. Kalkoff: Knotenbildung der Haut mit intracellulärer Ablagerung von Eiweißkristallen. Hautarzt **4**, 418 (1953). Zit. bei Gans-Steigleder. — Hardy, H. L., and I. R. Tabershaw: Delayed chemical pneumonitis ocurring in workers exposed to beryllium compounds. J. indust. Hyg. **28**, 197 (1946). Zit. bei Neave, Frank and Tolmach. — Hare, P. J.: A case of occupational iron pigmentation of the skin. Brit. J. Derm. **63**, 63 (1951). — Harker, J. M., and D. Hunter: Occupational Argyria. Brit. J. Derm. **47**, 441 (1935). Zit. bei Stillians. — Hass, G. M.: Tissue reactions to natural oils and fractions thereof. Arch. Path. **26**, 956 (1938). Zit. in Sutton, Diseases of the Skin, 1956, p. 195. — Hedinger, Chr.: Zur Pathologie der Hämochromatose als Syndrom. Helv. med. Acta, Suppl. **32** (1953). — Heller: Über Hautveränderungen beim Diabète bronzé. Dtsch. med. Wschr. **1907 II**, 1216. — Hellerström, S., H. Ericsson and R. Lagerkrantz: Different types of swimming-pool infections caused by mycobacteria. Acta derm.-venereol. (Stockh.) **36**, 249 (1956). — Henschen, K.: Über subcutane Fremdkörpergeschwülste aus nicht resorbierten Campherölinjektionen (Ölgranulome). Zbl. allg. Path. path. Anat. **25**, 417 (1914). Zit. in Gans-Steigleder. — Herxheimer, G., u. W. Roth: Zur feineren Struktur und Genese der Epitheloidzellen und Riesenzellen des Tuberkels. Beitr. path. Anat. **61**, 1 (1916). — Hill, W. R., and H. Montgomery: Argyria. Arch. Derm. Syph. (Chic.) **44**, 588 (1941). — Hodara, M., Houloussi, Behdjet u. Sureya: Histologische Untersuchung und experimentelle Studie über die Pathogenese einer durch Gerstenpollen hervorgerufenen, juckenden, erythematös-vesikulösen Hauterkrankung. Derm. Wschr. **76**, 209 (1923). Zit. bei Gans-Steigleder. — Höfs, W.: Ein neues Gerät zur Beseitigung von Fremdkörpereinsprengungen und großen Naevi. Dtsch. Gesundh.-Wes. **1951**, 574. Ref. Zbl. Haut- u. Geschl.-Kr. **80**, 147 (1952). — Hopf, G., u. A. Winkler: Fremdkörpergranulome durch metallisches Quecksilber. Derm. Wschr. **136**, 1273 (1957). — Hopkins, J. G., J. T. Weld and W. M. Huber: Cyst formation, acneform lesions and hair growth following intradermal injection of staphylococci in sensitized rabbits. J. invest. Derm. **16**, 339 (1951). — Hübner, O.: Über Talkumgranulome der Haut nach chirurgischen Operationen. Zbl. Chir. **79**, 498 (1954). — Hyslop, F., E. D. Palmer, W. B. Alford, A. R. Monaco and L. T. Fairhall: The toxicology of Beryllium. Nat. Inst. Hlth Bull. **181**, United States Public Health service. Federal security Agency, 1943. Zit. bei Naeve, Frank, Tolmach.

Jahn: Über Argyrie. Beitr. path. Anat. **16**, 218 (1894). Zit. bei Gans-Steigleder. — Johnson, N.: Talcum powder granuloma. Aust. N. Z. J. Surg. **23**, 1 (1953). Ref. Zbl. Chir. **134**, 178 (1954). — Jordan, P., u. K. Wulf: Lupus miliaris mit Dissemination am Orte von Fremdkörpereinsprengungen in Haut und Bindehaut. Hautarzt **1**, 470 (1950). — Joseph, H. L., and H. Gifford: Barbers' interdigital pilonidal sinus. Arch. Derm. Syph. (Chic.) **70**, 616 (1954).

Kalkoff, K. W., u. E. Macher: Über Riesenzentrosphären und intra- sowie extracelluläre Einschlüsse in ihrer Bedeutung für den Morbus Boeck. Hautarzt **5**, 481 (1954). — Kanitz, H.: Über Argyrie der Haut. Arch. Derm. Syph. (Berl.) **94**, 49 (1909). Zit. bei Gans-Steigleder. — Kile, R. L.: Treatment of Lupus vulgaris by injections of starch. Arch. Derm. Syph. (Berl.) **39**, 471 (1939). Zit. bei Seelig et al. — Kittinger, A.: Das Panaritium der Melker. Zbl. Haut- u. Geschl.-Kr. **37**, 630 (1931). Zit. in Röckl u. Müller, Haargranulome. — Kino, F.: Über Argyria universalis. Frankfurt. Z. Path. **3**, 398 (1909). Zit. bei Gans-Steigleder. — Kiyono: Die vitale Karminspeicherung. Gustav Fischer 1914. Zit. in Woringer, Diss. — Klemm, C.: Fremdkörpergranulomatose des Peritoneums verursacht durch Talkpuder. Helv. chir. Acta **14**, 181 (1947). — Kobert, R.: Über Argyrie in Vergleich zur Siderose. Arch. Derm. Syph. (Berl.) **25**, 773 (1893). Zit. bei Stillians. — Kochs, A. G.: Zur Kenntnis der Chrysiasis. Arch. Derm. Syph. (Berl.) **178**, 330 (1939). — Kölsch, F.: Über gewerbliche, totale Argyrie. Münch. med. Wschr. **1912**, 304. Zit. bei Gans-Steigleder. — Die versicherungsmedizinische Bedeutung der beruflich verursachten Argyrie (Argyrose). Arch. Gewerbepath. Gewerbehyg. **14**, 594 (1956). Ref. Zbl. Haut- u. Geschl.-Kr. **97**, 178 (1957). — Kogoj, Fr.: Experimentelle Beiträge zur Lehre von den Dermatomykosen mit besonderer Berücksichtigung der Lokalisationsbestimmung hämatogener Infektionen. Arch. Derm. Syph. (Berl.) **150**, 333 (1926). — Kozikowski, E. S.: Granuloma of axillae (Zirconium ?). Arch. Derm. **75**, 892 (1957). — Kreibich, C.: Zur Genese der tuberkulösen Riesenzellen. Arch. Derm. Syph. (Berl.) **142**, 393 (1923). — Kronenberg, M. H.: Dust dangers exposed (dusting of rubber gloves with talc). Mod. Hosp. **49**, 84 (1937). Zit. bei Seelig et al. — Kruckmann: Über Fremdkörper-Tuberkulose und Fremdkörper-Riesenzellen. Virchows Arch. path. Anat. **138**, Suppl., 118 (1895). — Kumer, L.: Mechanische, chemische, thermisch und aktinische Schädigungen der Haut. In: Arzt-Ziehler, Hautkrankheiten, Bd. II, S. 71. Berlin u. Wien: Urban & Schwarzenberg 1935. — KUZELL, W. C., PILLSBURY u. GELLERT: Dimerkaprol. Stanf. med. Bull. **5**, 197 (1947). Zit. in MØLLER, Pharmakologie. Basel: Benno Schwabe & Co. 1953. — KVORNING, A. A.: Foreign-body granulomas in tattoo marks. Acta derm.-venereol. (Stockh.) **36**, 214 (1956). Ref. Zbl. Haut- u. Geschl.-Kr. **97**, 43 (1957). — KYRLE, J.: Über die tuberkuloiden Gewebsstrukturen der Haut. Arch. Derm. Syph. (Berl.) **125**, 481 (1918).

LACOURT: Réactions gigantocellulaires et tissulaires consécutives aux injections hypodermiques de corps étrangers. Thèse de Nancy, 1928. — LANG, F. J.: Lipophage Fremdkörpergranulome nach traumatischer Schädigung einer Epidermoid- und einer Dermoidcyste. Langenbecks Arch. klin. Chir. **165**, 450 (1931). — LANZA: Silicosis und Asbestosis, vol. 1. New York: Oxford University Press 1938. — LAPIÈRE, M. S.: Deux cas de granulomes périsilicotiques cutanés. Etiopathogénie et traitement. Bull. Soc. franç. Derm. Syph. **62**, 17 (1955). — LARRICK, L. E., and R. G. THOMPSON: The hypospray and its relation to dermatology. J. invest. Derm. **13**, 361 (1949). — LAUENER, P.: Über einen durch Kuhhaare hervorgerufenen Fremdkörpertumor bei einem Melker. Diss. Bern 1915. Derm. Wschr. **60**, 529 (1915). — LECLERQ, R.: Les granulomes cutanés dus au béryllium. Ann. Derm. Syph. (Paris) **78**, 589 (1951). — LEDER, M.: Untersuchungen über die Hautwirkung von Glasfasern (Glasseide, Glaswolle). Dermatologica (Basel) **91**, 138 (1945). — LEHMANN, HAROLD: Durch berylliumhaltige Fremdkörper ausgelöste Granulome vom Aufbau des Morbus Boeck. Hautarzt **7**, 173 (1956). — LENARTOWICZ, J., et B. JALOWY: Essais de production d'argyrie artificielle chez les animaux. Ann. Derm. Syph. (Paris) **1938**, 483. — LENDLE, L.: Argyrie (Fragekasten). Münch. med. Wschr. **1959**, 906. — LENORMANT, CH., et P. RAVAUT: Les tumeurs artificielles provoquées par les injections sous-cutanées d'huiles minérales. Ann. Derm. Syph. (Paris) **1926**, 601. — LEWANDOWSKY, F.: Tuberkulose-Immunität und Tuberkulide (experimentelle Studien). Arch. Derm. Syph. (Berl.) **123**, 1 (1916). — LEVE, I. A.: Granulomas of the axillae caused by deodorant. Arch. Derm. **75**, 765 (1957). — LICHTMAN: Surg. Gynec. Obstet. **83**, 531 (1946). Zit. in: SUTTON, Diseases of the skin, p. 200. — LIEBAU, H.: Zur Kasuistik der Hämochromatose. Med. Klin. **1950**, 44. — LIMOUSIN, H., et B. DUPERRAT: Granulome silicotique. Bull. Soc. franç. Derm. Syph. **58**, 455 (1951). — LINCOLN, C. S., and R. C. NORDSTROM: Pigment color in tattoo sections, identification by polarized light. Arch. Derm. **77**, 336 (1958). — LINELL, F., and A. NORDÉN: Mycobacterium balnei, a new acid-fast bacillus occurring in swimming pools and capable of producing skin lesions in humans. Acta tuberc. scand., Suppl. XXXIII (1954). — LIPSCHITZ, J. I.: Beryllium granuloma of the skin. S. Afr. med. J. **1951**, 509. Ref. Zbl. Haut- u. Geschl.-Kr. **82**, 164 (1953). — LISCH, K.: Chrysosis bulbi. Klin. Mbl. Augenheilk. **102**, 103 (1939). Zit. bei LUTZ, Dermatologica (Basel) **81**, 337 (1940). — LÖFGREN, S., B. SNELLMAN and H. NORDENSTAM: Foreign body granulomas and sarcoidosis; a clinical and histopathologic study. Acta chir. scand. **108**, 405 (1955). — LÖHE, H.: Ungewöhnlicher Fall von Fremdkörperschädigung. Derm. Wschr. **121**, 82 (1950). — LÖWY, J.: Über eine lokale Toxikose nach Verletzung mit Kakteenstacheln. Med. Klin. **22**, 290 (1926). — LUTON, P., J. CHAMPEIX et P. FAURE: La pneumoconiose par terre de diatomés dans les gisements français de Kieselguhr (étude clinique, radiologique, expérimentale). Arch. Mal. prof. **10**, 217 (1949). — LUTZ, W.: Dermatosen aus vorwiegend äußeren Ursachen. Dermatologica (Basel) **79**, 352, 356 (1939); **81**, 331, 336 (1940); **85**, 365, 367 (1942); **87**, 275, 276 (1943); **89**, 278, 283 (1944). — Durch externe physikalische und chemische Ursachen bedingte Dermatosen. Dermatologica (Basel) **95**, 126 (1948). — Glaswolledermatitis. In: Lehrbuch der Haut- und Geschlechtskrankheiten, S. 365. Basel: Karger 1951. — Hautveränderungen durch externe und interne Einflüsse. Dermatologica (Basel) **102**, 388 (1951).

MACHER, E.: Die Bedeutung des Talkumgranuloms in der Dermatologie. Hautarzt **4**, 529 (1953). — MADDEN, J. F.: Chronic inflammation in tattoo mark. Arch. Derm. Syph. (Chic.) **38**, 481 (1938). — MALI, J. W. H.: Granulomatosis disciformis chronica et progressiva (MIESCHER). A form of tuberculosis? Dermatologica (Basel) **101**, 84 (1950). — MALKINSON, F., and J. O. PRIESTLEY: Sarcoid reaction — foreign body granuloma? Arch. Derm. **74**, 687 (1956). — MARCHAND, E.: Bildungsweise der Riesenzellen um Fremdkörper. Virchows Arch. path. Anat. **93**, 518 (1883). — Einheilung von Fremdkörpern. Beitr. path. Anat. **4** (1888). — Untersuchungen über die Einheilung von Fremdkörpern. Beitr. path. Anat. **4**, 2 (1889). Zit. bei LAUENER, Diss. Bern. — Die Veränderungen der peritonealen Deckzellen nach Einführung kleiner Fremdkörper. Beitr. path. Anat. **69**, 1 (1921). — MARCHIONINI, A., u. R. SCHUHMACHERS-BRENDLER: Zur Entfernung von Tätowierungen. Scritti medici in onore di Franco Flarer. Minerva med. **1959**, 289. — MARTIN, H.: Nouvelles recherches sur la tuberculose spontanée et expérimentale des séreuses. Arch. Physiol., norm. path. **8**, 49 (1881). Zit. bei SEELIG et al. — Tuberculose des séreuses et du poumon. Pseudotuberculose expérimentale. Arch. Physiol. norm. Path. 1888. Zit. bei WORINGER, Diss. — MARTLAND, H. S., H. A. BRODKIN and H. S. MARTLAND jr.: Occupational beryllium poisoning in New Jersey. J. Med. Soc. N.J. **45**, 5 (1948). Zit. bei NEAVE, FRANK and TOLMACH. — MASON and ALLEN:

Indelible pencil injuries. Ann. Surg. **113**, 131 (1941). Zit. in Sutton, Diseases of the skin, 1956, p. 200. — Masson, P.: La lymphopneumatose kystique. Ann. Anat. path. **4**, 541 (1925). Zit. bei Woringer, Diss. — Maximow: Experimentelle Untersuchungen über die entzündliche Neubildung von Bindegewebe. Beitr. path. Anat. **5**, Suppl. (1902). — Maylahn, D. J.: Thorn-induced „tumors" of bone. J. Bone Jt Surg. A **34**, 386 (1952). — McAdams, G. B.: Granulomas caused by absorbable starch glove powder. Surgery **39**, 329 (1956). — McCormick: Talc granuloma of the eye following surgery for correction of muscle imbalance. Amer. J. Ophthal. **32**, 1252 (1949). Zit. in: Sutton, Diseases of the skin, p. 200. — McCormick, E. J., and T. L. Ramsey: Postoperative peritoneal granulomatous inflammation caused by magnesium silicate. J. Amer. med. Ass. **116**, 817 (1941). — Meier, R., u. P. Desaulles: Über die Entwicklung des Fremdkörpergranuloms in verschiedenen Organsystemen. Experientia (Basel) **12**, 197 (1957). — Meier, R., P. A. Desaulles u. P. Loustalot: Wirkung eines tumorhemmenden Stoffes, des Triäthylenmelanins, auf das Wachstum von Fremdkörpergranulom und Tumor. Experientia (Basel) **12**, 61 (1956). — Meier, R., P. Desaulles u. B. Schär: Über die Wirkungen von Mischungen eines antigenhaltigen Plasmas mit einem antikörperhaltigen Serum auf die Entwicklung des F emdkörpergranuloms. Experientia (Basel) **11**, 442 (1955). — Meier, R., W. Schuler u. P. Desaulles: Zur Frage des Mechanismus der Hemmung des Bindegewebswachstums durch Cortisone. Experientia (Basel) **6**, 469 (1950). — Mettler, M.: Badeverletzungen durch Polypen, Medusen und Quallen. Mitt. med. Abt. SUVA, Nr 39 (1959). — Meyer, G.: Bindegewebe und Fremdkörper. Virchows Arch. path. Anat. **271**, 317 (1929). Zit. bei Gans-Steigleder. — Michon, J., Murard et Martin: Le diagnostic des tumeurs consécutives aux injections d'huile camphrée. Lyon méd. **130**, 267 (1921). Zit. in Gans-Steigleder. — Midana, A.: Le manifestazioni cutanee della berilliosi. Minerva derm. **27**, 41 (1952). — Miescher, G., u. M. Leder: Granulomatosis disciformis chronica et progressiva (Atypische Tuberkulose). Dermatologica (Basel) **97**, 25 (1948). — Miescher, G., e F. Ott: Granuloma cicatriziale e Morbus Boeck. Scritti medici in onore di Franco Flarer. Minerva med. **1959**, 305. — Miller, J. W., and R. R. Sayers: The physiological response of the peritoneal tissue to dusts introduced as foreign bodies. Publ. Hlth Rep. (Wash.) **49**, 80 (1934). — Moncorps, C.: Über die Beseitigung ausgedehnter Fremdkörpereinsprengungen mittels kombinierten Fräs-Ätzverfahrens. Münch. med. Wschr. **1942 I**, 587. — Mook, W. H., and W. G. Wander: Camphorated oil tumores. J. Amer. med. Ass. **73**, 1340 (1919). Arch. Derm. Syph. (Chic.) **1**, 304 (1920). Zit. in Sutton, Diseases of the skin, 1956. — Müller, O.: Über einen Fall von Hautgeschwulstbildungen auf dem Boden einer Tätowierung. Derm. Wschr. **106**, 6 (1938). — Müller, P.: Beitrag zur experimentellen Berylliose. Schweiz. Z. allg. Path. **15**, 354 (1952). — Muscatello, G.: Über den Bau und das Aufsaugungsvermögen des Peritoneums. Virchows Arch. path. Anat. **142**, 327 (1895). — Myers, C. N.: Argyria and its relation to silver therapy. Amer. J. Syph. **7**, 125 (1923). Zit. bei Gans-Steigleder.

Neave, H. J., S. B. Frank and J. A. Tolmach: Cutaneous granuloma following laceration by fluorescent light bulbs. Arch. Derm. Syph. (Chic.) **61**, 401 (1950). — Newcomer, V. D.: Sclerosing lipogranuloma Vs. foreign body lipogranuloma. Arch. Derm. Syph. (Chic.) **69**, 383 (1953). — Nichol, A. D., and Rafael Dominguez: Cutaneous granuloma from accidental contamination with beryllium phosphors. J. Amer. med. Ass. **140**, 855 (1949). — Nimpfer, Th.: Fremdkörpereinsprengungen in die Haut als berufliche Schädigung bei Installateuren. Derm. Z. **66**, 313 (1933). — Nonclerq, M. E.: Détatouage d'une victime d'accident du travail. Bull. Soc. franç. Derm. Syph. **61**, 250 (1954). — Nørgaard, O.: Investigations with radioactive Ag into the resorption of silver through human skin. Acta derm.-venereol. (Stockh.) **34**, 415 (1954). — Norris, R. P., and F. J. McEwen: Exogenous hemochromatosis following multiple blood transfusions. J. Amer. med. Ass. **143**, 740 (1950). — Novy jr., F. G.: Generalized mercurial (Cinnabar) reaction following tattooing. Arch. Derm. Syph. (Chic.) **49**, 172 (1944).

Obermayer, M. E., and M. Hassen: Sarcoidosis with sacroidal reaction in tattoo. Arch. Derm. Syph. (Chic.) **71**, 766 (1955). — Ohya, Z.: Etude sur le tatouage au Japon. Scritti medici in onore di Franco Flarer. Minerva med. **1959**, 477. — Olivier, Cl., I. Bertrand et G. Cerbonnet: Le granulome postopératoire au talc. Mém. Acad. Chir. **77**, 769 (1951). — Olivier, H., P. Morand et R. Brun: Considérations à propos des granulomes cutanés de l'amiante. Arch. Mal. prof. **10**, 516 (1949). — Oppenheim, M.: Riesenzellentumoren nach subkutaner Einspritzung eines Arsen-Eisenpräparates. Arch. Derm. Syph. (Berl.) **116**, 439 (1913). — Zur Ätiologie des Boeck'schen Sarkoides (Lupoids). Arch. Derm. Syph. (Berl.) **138**, 326 (1922). — Interdigitale Hautbrückenbildung durch Kuhhaare (Melker). Zbl. Haut- u. Geschl.-Kr. **37**, 425 (1931). — Ordstrand, H. S. van: Current concepts of beryllium poisoning. Ann. intern. Med. **35**, 1203 (1951). — Ordstrand, H. S. van, R. Hughes, J. M. De Nardi and M. G. Carmody: Beryllium poisoning. J. Amer. med. Ass. **129**, 1084 (1945). Zit. bei Neave, Frank and Tolmach. — Orfuss, A. J.: Granulomatous dermatitis of the axillae. Arch. Derm. **77**, 748 (1958). — Owen, M. A.: Peritoneal response to glove powder containing talc. Tex. St. J. Med. **32**, 482 (1936). Zit. bei Seelig et al.

PELLIER: Über den histologischen Befund der Gewebe nach Einspritzung von Oleum cinereum. Ann. Derm. Syph. (Paris) **1909**. Ref. Mh. prakt. Derm. **49**, 66 (1909). — PERGENS, E.: Argyrosis der Conjunctiva bei Protargolgebrauch. Klin. Mbl. Augenheilk. **38**, 256 (1900). Zit. bei STILLIANS. — PETRIDES, P., u. H. WILD: Zur Klinik der Hämochromatose. Klin. Wschr. **1948**, 521. — PHILPOTT, O. S., A. R. WOODBURNE and J. A. PHILPOT jr.: Deep foreign body granulomata. A reaction to penicillin. Arch. Derm. Syph. (Chic.) **69**, 494 (1954). — PINKUS, H., and I. BOTVINICK: Deodorant stick eruption (zirconium granuloma) of axillae. Arch. Derm. **75**, 756 (1957). — PODWYSSOZKI, W. v.: Zur Frage über die formativen Reize (Riesenzellengranulome durch Kieselguhr hervorgerufen). Beitr. path. Anat. **47**, 270 (1910). — POLEMANN, G.: Zur Wirkung des Cortison auf das experimentelle Quarzgranulom der Maus. Arch. Derm. Syph. (Berl.) **193**, 257 (1951). — POLEMANN, G., u. G. JOHN: Über die Toxizität des Berylliums und seiner Verbindungen. Zbl. Arbeitsmed. **3**, 168 (1953). — Das Beryllium und seine Toxikologie. Berufsdermatosen **2**, 179 (1954). — POLICARD, A., et A. COLLET: Images au microscope électronique des rapports entre cellules conjonctives et formations collagènes. Bull. Soc. franç. Derm. Syph. **64**, 529 (1957). — PORRITT, R. J., and R. E. OLSEN: Two simultaneous cases of leprosy developing in tattoos. Amer. J. Path. **23**, 805 (1947). — PRIOR, J., H. RUSTAD and G. CRONK: Pathological changes associated with desodorant preparations containing sodium zirconium lactate: an experimental study. J. invest. Derm. **29**, 449 (1957). — PYRE, J., and W. H. OATWAY jr.: Beryllium granulomatosis. Ariz. Med. **4**, 21 (1947).

RAGAN, C., and R. H. BOOTS: Treatment of gold dermatides; use of BAL (2—3, Dimercaptopropanol). J. Amer. med. Ass. **133**, 752 (1947). — RAMSEY, T. L.: Magnesium silicate granuloma. Amer. J. clin. Path. **12**, 553 (1942). — RAMSEY, T. L., and F. M. DOUGLAS: Granulomatous inflammation produced by foreign body irritants. J. Int. Coll. Surg. **3**, 3 (1940). Zit. bei SEELIG et al. — REES, R. B., and J. H. BENNETT: Granuloma following swimming pool abrasion. J. Amer. med. Ass. **152**, 1606 (1953). — REFVEM, O.: I. Chronic granulomas in the alimentary tract caused by minute mineral praticles. II. ,,Boeck's disease" and occurrence of minute mineral particles. Acta path. microbiol. scand. **25**, 118 (1948). — The pathogenesis of Boeck's disease (Sarcoidosis). Acta med. scand., Suppl. **294**, 1 (1954). — REYNER, C. E.: Pigmentation following the use of iron salts. Arch. Derm. Syph. (Chic.) **40**, 380 (1939). — RIECKE, E.: Das Tatauierungswesen im heutigen Europa. Jena 1925. .Zit in GANS-STEIGLEDER. — RIZZUTI, A. B.: Beryllium granulomas of anterior ocular structures. N.Y. St. J. Med. **51**, 1065 (1951). Zit. in ALLEN, Diseases of the skin. — ROBBINS, J. J., and W. F. LYONS: Beryllium granulomatosis, report of case showing response to cortisone. Ann. intern. Med. **38**, 120 (1953). Zit. in ALLEN, Diseases of the skin. — ROBERT, P.: Auriasis. XXVII. Tagg Schweiz. Ges. Derm. Dermatologica (Basel) **92**, 271 (1946). — RÖCKL, H., u. E. MÜLLER: Granulome und Fisteln durch Haare. Derm. Wschr. **136**, 912 (1957). — RÖSSLE, R.: Über die chronische Entzündung von Geweben durch Talk infolge ärztlicher Maßnahmen. Ärztl. Wschr. **1950**, 233. Zit. in GANS-STEIGLEDER. — ROSTENBERG jr., A., R. A. BROWN and M. R. CARLO: Discussion of Tattoo Reactions with report of a case showing a reaction to a green color. Arch. Derm. Syph. (Chic.) **62**, 540 (1950). — ROTH, H.: Über Fremdkörpertuberkulose des Bauchfells. Frankfurt. Z. Path. **29**, 59 (1923). — ROULET, F. C.: Die infektiösen ,,spezifischen Granulome". In: Handbuch der allgemeinen Pathologie, Bd. VII/1, S. 465. Berlin-Göttingen-Heidelberg: Springer 1956. — RUBIN, L.: Case for diagnosis. Arch. Derm. **75**, 598 (1957). — RUBIN, L., A. H. SLEPYAN, L. F. WEBER and I. NEUHAUSER: Granulomas of the axillas caused by deodorants. J. Amer. med. Ass. **162**, 953 (1956).

SABIN: Reactions to fractions isolated from tubercle bacilli. Physiol. Rev. **12**, 141 (1932). Zit. in SUTTON, Diseases of the skin. — SABIN, F. R., C. A. DOAN and C. E. FORKNER: J. exp. Med. **52**, Suppl. 3, p. 1. Zit. bei SHELLEY and HURLEY 1958. — SAIPT, O.: Zu den Glaswollschäden der Haut. Hautarzt **4**, 175 (1953). — SAKURANE, K.: Über das Schicksal subkutan injizierter Substanzen, insbesondere von Paraffin. Arch. Derm. **80**, 401 (1906). — SARANAC, Symposium on the Beryllium problem. J. Amer. med. Ass. **137**, 648 (1948). — SARKANY, I. (for Dr. C. D. CALNAN): Deodorant granuloma of the axillae. Brit. J. Derm. **70**, 259 (1958). — SAUNDERS, TH. S.: Granulomas of the axillae caused by deodorants. Arch. Derm. **76**, 619 (1957). — SAVITSCH, E. DE: Granuloma resulting from penetration of talcum powder; report of case. Med. Ann. D. C. **9**, 169 (1940). Zit. in SUTTON, Diseases of the skin, p. 200. — SAXEN, A., and P. I. TUOVINES: Experimental and clinical observations on granulomas caused by talc and some other substances. Acta chir. scand. **96**, 130. — SCHLÄPPI, V.: Un cas d'argyrose professionnelle de l'oeil. Ref. Schweiz. med. Wschr. **1959**, 387. — SCHLIENGER, F.: Zur Kenntnis der medikamentösen Lipogranulome. Dermatologica (Basel) **98**, 289 (1949). — SCHMIDT, K.: Beitrag zur Differentialdiagnose der Hämochromatose. Klin. Wschr. **1949**, 566. — SCHMIDT, O. E. L.: Chrysiasis. Arch. Derm. Syph. (Chic.) **44**, 446 (1941). — SCHMUZIGER, P., u. OBWEGESER: Erfahrungen mit Implantaten am Zürcher Zahnärztl. Inst. Méd. et Hyg. No 395, 10. 5. 1958. — SCHÖNFELD, W.: Dermatologische und volkstümliche Nachlese zu Tätowierungen. Derm. Wschr. **109**, 1255 (1939). — Brandmarken und

Tätowierungen als Erkennungs- und Strafzeichen bei europäischen Völkern. Derm. Wschr. **113**, 1037 (1941). — Einige medizinische Tätowierfolgen. Hautarzt **2**, 208 (1951). — Körperbemalen, Brandmarken, Tätowieren in Europa. Beweggründe und Bildgut. Hautarzt **4**, 169 (1953). — SCHREUS, TH.: Hochtouriges Schleifen der Haut. Arch. Derm. Syph. (Berl.) **191**, 678 (1950). — SCHWARTZ, L.: Dermatitis from glass fabrics. Arch. Derm. Syph. (Chic.) **55**, 258 (1947). — SCHWARTZ, W. F., and H. N. COLE: Arch. Derm. Syph. (Chic.) **37**, 872 (1938). Zit. bei LUTZ, Dermatologica (Basel) **79**, 352 (1939). — SCOTT, M. J.: Cutaneous reactions to embedded extraneous hair. Arch. Derm. **76**, 39 (1957). — SEELIG, M. G., D. J. VERDA and F. H. KIDD: The talcum powder problem in surgery and its solution. J. Amer. med. Ass. **123** 950 (1943). — SEIFERT, E.: Zur Behandlung der Fadenfistel. Münch. med. Wschr. **1959** 824. — SHATTOCK, S. G.: Pseudotuberculoma silicoticum of the lip. Proc. roy. Soc. Med. (Sect. Path.) **10**, 6 (1916). — SHEARD jr., C., F. E. CORMIA, S. C. ATKINSON and E. L. WORTHINGTON: Granulomatous reactions to deodorant sticks. J. Amer. med. Ass. **164**, 1085 (1957). — SHELLEY, W. B., and H. J. HURLEY: The allergic origin of zirconium deodorant granulomas. Brit. J. Derm. **70**, 75 (1958). — SHELLEY, W. B., H. J. HURLEY, R. L. MAYOCK, H. P. CLOSE and R. T. CATHCART: Preliminary and short report: Intradermal tests with metals and other inorganic elements in sarcoidosis and anthraco-silicosis. J. invest. Derm. **31**, 301 (1958). — SILVERMANN, S. B., and C. C. ERICKSON: Subcutaneous beryllium granuloma. Arch. Path. **50**, 63. Zit. bei LUTZ, Dermatologica (Basel) **102**, 388 (1951). — SILVESTRE, P., et E. WITZIG: L'effacement des tatouages. Praxis **41**, 790 (1952). — SMITH, B. F.: Occurrence of hepatitis in recently tattooed service personnel. J. Amer. med. Ass. **144**, 1074. Zit. bei LUTZ, Dermatologica (Basel) **102**, 388 (1951). — SNEDDON, I. B.: Berylliosis. Proc. roy. Soc. Med. **48**, 175 (1955). — SOLTERMANN, W.: Die Bedeutung des Eisennachweises in der Haut für die Diagnose einer Hämochromatose unter besonderer Berücksichtigung der Axillargegend und der apokrinen Schweißdrüsen. Dermatologica (Basel) **112**, 355 (1956). — SOMMERVILLE, J., et J. A. MILNE: Pseudo-tuberculoma silicoticum. Brit. J. Derm. **62**, 105 (1950). — SPIEGEL, L.: A discoloration of the skin and mucous membrane resembling Argyria, following the use of bismuth and silver arsphenamine. Arch. Derm. Syph. (Chic.) **23**, 266 (1931). — STACHER, A.: Talc granuloma. Wien. klin. Wschr. **1954**, 313. — STILLIANS, A.: Argyria. Arch. Derm. Syph. (Chic.) **35**, 67 (1937). — STRÄTER, R.: Beitrag zur Lehre von der Hämochromatose und ihren Beziehungen zur allgemeinen Hämosiderose. Virchows Arch. path. Anat. **218**, H. 1. — SULZBERGER, M. B.: Tattoo dermatitis (Sensitivity to Cinnabar?). Arch. Derm. Syph. (Chic.) **36**, 1265 (1937). — SULZBERGER, M. B., and R. L. BAER: The effects of fiberglas on animal and human skin: experimental investigation. Industr. Med. Surg. **11**, 482 (1942). — SULZBERGER, M. B., A. KANOF and R. L. BAER: Complications following tattooing: Sensitization and desensitization to mercury; report of case. U.S. nav. med. Bull. **43**, 889 (1944). — SULZBERGER, M. B., u. J. A. TOLMACH: Allergische Aufflammungs-Reaktionen in roten Tätowierungen. Hautarzt **10**, 110 (1959). — SUSSET, Mme V.: Le granulome silicotique de la peau. Thèse, Paris 1953. — SUTTON, R. L.: Paraffinoma (Oelgranuloma). In: Diseases of the skin, p. 196. St. Louis: C. V. Mosby Comp. 1956. — SWEET, R. D.: Sarcoidosis following injury. Brit. J. Derm. **62**, 324 (1950). — SWINNY, B.: Generalized chronic dermatitis due to tattoo: report of case. Ann. Allergy **4**, 295 (1946). — SZENTKIRÁLYI, S. v.: Dermatitis artificialis durch Engelhaare. Derm. Wschr. **93**, 1302 (1931). — Über eine durch Süßwasserschwämme verursachte Hauterkrankung der Tisza-(Theiß)-Fischer. Derm. Wschr. **104**, 602 (1937).

TAPPEINER, S.: Zur Klinik und Histologie der Granulomatosis disciformis chronica et progressiva (MIESCHER) (Atypisches Sarkoid). Arch. Derm. Syph. (Berl.) **194**, 341 (1952). — Krankendemonstration: Fremdkörpergranulom unter dem Bilde eines Boeck'schen Sarkoids. Ver. Österr. Derm. Ges., 26. 9. 1957. Derm. Wschr. **138**, 1165 (1958). Hautarzt **10**, 188 (1959). — TELLER, H., u. M. KLINGBEIL: Fremdkörpergranulome und Reaktionen, hervorgerufen durch pflanzliche, insbesondere Rosen-Dornen. Z. Haut- u. Geschl.-Kr. **25**, 211 (1958). — THIERS, H., et J. FAYOLLE: Granuloma à corps étrangers. Difficultés thérapeu-Aiques. Bull. Soc. franç. Derm, Syph. **62**, 82 (1955), — TOMPSON, S. A.: Development of cardiopericardial adhesions following use of talc. Proc. Soc. exp. Biol. N.Y. **40**, 260 (1939). — TOLMACH, J. A., and S. B. FRANK: Granuloma of the skin with tubercle formation following swimming pool injury. J. Amer. med. Ass. **151**, 724 (1953). — TOLMAN, M., and S. MOSCHELLA: Axillary granuloma due to underarm deodorant. Arch. Derm. **77**, 469 (1958).

ULLMANN, J.: Über eigentümliche Geschwulstbildung in einer Tätowierungsmarke. Mh. prakt. Derm. **37**, 49 (1903). — UNGAR, J.: (1955), in Ciba Foundation Symposium on experimental tuberculosis. Edit. by G. E. W. WOLSTENHOLME and M. P. CAMERON, Boston, p. 68. Zit. bei SHELLEY and HURLEY, 1958. — UNNA, P. G.: Die Wirkung des Höllensteins. Derm. Wschr. **63**, 915, 941, 971, 1032 (1916). Zit. bei GANS-STEIGLEDER. — UNNA, P.: Quecksilberüberempfindlichkeit und Tätowierung. Arch. Derm. Syph. (Berl.) **160**, 153 (1930). Zit. L. H. WINER, Arch. Derm. Syph. (Chic.) **38**, 481 (1938). — URBACH, E.: Feststellung von vorausgegangenen Tierseruminjektionen durch international zu regelnde Tätowierungen. Klin. Wschr. **1936**, 2012. — URBACH, E., u. M. STEINER: Gerstenstaubidiosynkrasie, ein

Beitrag zur physikalischen Allergie der Haut. Arch. Derm. Syph. (Berl.) **153**, 772 (1927). — UTEAU et J. BOUGET: Danger des blessures par les épines. Bull. Soc. Chirurgie Paris **20**, 715 (1928).

VONKENNEL, J., u. M. FIEBIG: Fremdkörpereinlagerungen. In: Kosmetisch störende Erkrankungen der Haut; Handbuch von GOTTRON-SCHÖNFELD, Bd. II/1, S. 288. Stuttgart: Georg Thieme 1958. — VULCAN, P., and ST. TANASESCU: Asbestos granulomas and warts. Derm.-Vener. (Buc.) **3**, 21 (1958).

WAISMAN, M., and R. G. OLIVETT: Pilonidal sinus of the hand. Arch. Derm. Syph (Chic.) **66**, 466 (1952). — WARIS, W.: Barbers' disease. Industr. Med. Surg. **22**, 111 (1953). Ref. J. Amer. med. Ass. **152**, 1466 (1953). — WEBER, L., and I. NEUHAUSER: Tuberculide? Arch. Derm. **75**, 597 (1957). — WEBER, L., L. RUBIN, A. H. SLEPYAN and H. SHELLOW: Granuloma of axillas. J. Amer. med. Ass. **162**, 65 (1956). — WEED, L. A., and J. L. GROVES: Surgical gloves and wound infections. Surg. Gynec. Obstet. **75**, 661 (1942). Zit. bei SEELIG et al. — WEIDMANN et JEFFERIES: Experimental production of paraffin oil tumors in monkeys. Arch. Derm. Syph. (Chic.) **7**, 209 (1923). — WEISS: Über Bildung und Bedeutung der Riesenzellen und über epithelähnliche Zellen, welche um Fremdkörper im Organismus sich bilden. Virchows Arch. path. Anat. **68** (1876). — WEISS; Arch. Derm. Syph. (Chic.) **43**, 650 (1941). Zit. bei LUTZ, Dermatologica (Basel) **85**, 365 (1942). — WELANDER, E.: Noch einige Worte über die Elimination des Quecksilbers nach der Injektion schwerlöslicher Quecksilberpräparate. Arch. Derm. Syph. (Berl.) **96**, 163 (1909). — WELLS, G. C., and W. N. GOLDSMITH: Tuberculous or silicotic granulomata. Brit. J. Derm. **62**, 325 (1950). — WEYBRECHT, H.: Allgemeine Argyrosis. Derm. Wschr. **127**, 494 (1953). Zit. bei GANS-STEIGLEDER. — WINER, L. H., and R. H. ZEILENGA: Cactus granulomas of the skin. Report of a case. Arch. Derm. **72**, 566 (1955). — WORINGER, FR.: Les granulomes à corps étrangers de la peau. Strasbourg, Diss., 1929. — Vaselinome et paraffinome. In: Nouvelle pratique dermatologique, Bd. VI, p. 591. Paris: Masson & Cie. 1936. — Granulomatose disciforme chronique et progressive de MIESCHER? Bull. Soc. franç. Derm. Syph. **63**, 282 (1956). — WORINGER, FR., et A. ULLMO: Granulomatosis disciformis chronica et progressiva MIESCHER. Ann. Derm. Syph. (Paris) **84**, 22 (1957).

ZELONY, A.: Unusual case of dermatitis factitia. Arch. Derm. **78**, 398 (1958). — ZIEGLER, E.: Ein Fall von konnatalem Ovarialteratom mit Fremdkörpergranulationstumoren im Peritoneum bei einem Kinde. Helv. chir. Acta **14**, 202 (1947). — ZIELER, K.: Experimentelle Untersuchungen über tuberkulöse Veränderungen an der Haut ohne Mitwirkung von Tuberkelbacillen. Münch. med. Wschr. **1908**, 1685. — ZIMMERLI, E., u. W. LUTZ: Eine eigenartige Form von Pigmentierung nach Goldbehandlung. Arch. Derm. Syph. (Berl.) **157**, 523 (1929). — ZOON, J. J.: Über histologische Befunde bei Argyria cutis. Derm. Z. **70**, 125 (1935). — *Ohne Autor:* Rubber gloves in surgery, editorial. Brit. J. Surg. **30**, 283 (1943). Zit. bei SEELIG et al.

Lupus erythematodes discoides

By

Frances Pascher-Brooklyn (N.Y.)

With 15 Figures in the Text

Introduction

Approximately three decades have gone by since the subject of lupus erythematodes discoides was explored by VEIEL. The apparent relationship of this form of lupus erythematodes to the systemic disease was not questioned at the time. Consequently certain phases of lupus erythematodes discoides were discussed from the point of view of lupus erythematodes as a whole rather than with reference to any of its forms. Although the consensus at present is that these two conditions are linked, there are differences in opinion as to the nature of the bond. Data and views pertaining to this relationship shall therefore be discussed in detail. Lupus erythematodes discoides will be discussed not only as an entity but will also be compared and contrasted with systemic lupus erythematosus.

Some advances have been made in past thirty years. One can now say unequivocally that tuberculosis is not the cause of lupus erythematodes and that lupus vulgaris erythematodes [tumidus (LELOIR)] is a tuberculoderm and not a transition or mixed form of lupus erythematodes and tuberculosis. Chilblain lupus (HUTCHINSON) although rare is nevertheless distinct from lupus pernio which is now recognized as a form of sarcoidosis.

The major strides have been in therapy and management of the disorder. Scarification, cauterization and all forms of irradiation have been abandoned. Thus erysipelas and iatrogenic disfigurement resulting from these modalities have been eliminated. It may very well be too, that the incidence of scars, and squamous cell epithelioma in lupus erythematodes lesions will be reduced or become negligible because these procedures are no longer employed. Antimalarial therapy, despite some limitations and side effects is acknowledged to be a definite advance in the suppression of the disease.

1. Terminology

a) Synonymous Terms

Discoid lupus erythematosus, chronic discoid lupus erythematosus, erythematodes discoides, lupus erythematodes chronicus and lupus erythematodes discoides are presently used most often to identify the dermatosis. Erythematosus has been retained despite the fact that it has been pointed out repeatedly (ROST, GOLD) that this is etymologically incorrect. For that matter ROST has suggested that the term lupus be dropped since it has been shown that tuberculosis has no pathogenetic relationship to lupus erythematodes discoides. He thought erythematodes discoides chronicus would be more appropriate and this suggestion has been accepted by some.

b) Disseminated Lupus Erythematodes

Lupus erythematodes discoides and discoid lupus erythematosus are nevertheless used most often whether one has reference to the fixed (localized) type or the widespread (generalized) form of the disorder. Lupus erythematodes disseminatus or chronic disseminated lupus erythematosus was used almost exclusively in the past for the latter form. In recent years disseminated has taken on a different meaning. When used by American and English writers it designates the systemic disease rather than discoid lupus erythematosus. Thus systemic lupus erythematosus and disseminated lupus erythematosus are used interchangeably and synonymously (Jessar et al.; Harvey et al.; Kusniruk). The adjectives, widespread or generalized, have been substituted for disseminated with reference to the discoid form of the disease. The tendency likewise has been to drop the arbitrary subdivision of acute and subacute disseminated lupus erythematosus and to refer to them as systemic lupus erythematosus.

2. Classification

a) Forms of Lupus Erythematodes discoides

Most authorities recognize two principal forms: α) Localized or fixed type, β) Generalized or widespread (chronic disseminated lupus erythematosus of earlier classifications) (O'Leary; Kierland).

α) Localized Form. There is some difference of opinion as to the boundary line for the localized type. Some would limit the lesions to the head and face (Montgomery and McCreight; Dubois and Martel) others to the head and neck (O'Leary; Rothfield et al.) while others permit extension of the eruption to the upper chest (Haserick and Kellum). All agree the lesions may be symmetrically or asymmetrically distributed over these areas and that they may vary considerably in number, size and depth.

β) Generalized or Widespread Cutaneous Form. The lesions are distributed symmetrically as a rule over the head, neck, chest, back and upper extremities. Two types of lesions may be seen in this form: discoid lesions as in Group I and ill-defined superficial erythematosus macular scaly or telangiectatic lesions as seen in systemic lupus erythematosus. These superficial lesions may persist as such, fade without apparent sequelae or they many evolve as well marginated infiltrated violaceous plaques with keratotic plugs.

b) Concepts of the Generalized Form

There is considerable difference of opinion as to whether or not this form is asymptomatic as far as systemic or visceral manifestations are concerned. Some maintain it is (O'Leary; Cohen and Cadman) others differ (Montgomery and McCreight; Dubois and Martel). One may question also whether patients with constitutional or visceral symptoms should be placed in this category or should be classified as systemic lupus erythematosus (Cannon and Curtis). While certain signs and symptoms are accepted by some as compatible with the diagnosis of generalized discoid lupus erythematosus, they are rejected by others. Some maintain as long as discoid lesions are present, regardless of other findings, the condition should be classified as discoid disease (Rothfield and coauthors).

As O'Leary and Cannon and Curtis among others have pointed out it is not always possible to fit a particular case into a particular category. The author is inclined to agree with those who maintain that at times generalized discoid lupus erythematosus may be associated with mild or vague symptoms e.g. malaise, joint pains, transitory episodes of low grade fever (VEIEL) and/or certain laboratory features e.g. mild leukopenia (WILSON and JORDAN; MARTEN and BLACKBURN) or an elevated sedimentation rate (COCHRANE), and to exclude cases with bouts of unexplained fever, progressive weight loss and/or related renal, cardiac or pulmonary involvement. It would seem proper to classify the latter as examples of the systemic disease.

3. Relationship of Lupus Erythematodes Discoides to Systemic Lupus Erythematosus

Whether or not lupus erythematodes discoides is related to systemic lupus erythematosus has given rise to much speculation and disputation. A few observers (CECIL and LOEB; MICHELSON) have taken the position that we are dealing with two different diseases. Most authors think both are variants of the same basic disorder (GOLD; BECKETT and LEWIS; CROSS; BRAVERMAN et al.) and some even maintain that the division into discoid and systemic forms is artificial (HARVEY et al.) and that lupus erythematodes discoides is either potentially systemic or in fact a systemic disease (DUBOIS and MARTEL; LAWLER and LUMPKIN). The question is of more than academic interest, since it has a direct bearing on prognosis and management. If it can be shown lupus erythematodes discoides is systemic or potentially systemic it would mean that the possibility of dissemination has to be borne in mind at all times and that certain preventative measures cannot be ignored (ALLENDE).

a) General Considerations

In support of the unity of the two conditions are 1. the occurrence of lupus erythematodes discoides and systemic lupus erythematosus among members of the same family (BECKETT and LEWIS; BUCHHOLTZ), 2. examples of the transformation of the discoid form to systemic form or vice versa (JESSAR et al.; WILSON and JORDAN; ZIFF et al.; GANOR and SAGHER), 3. see-sawing in some instances from lupus erythematodes discoides to the systemic disease and back again, 4. the demonstrability of all gradations of severity (GOLD and GOWING; MARTEN and BLACKBURN; COHEN and CADMAN) from cases with torpid lesions that may persist almost unchanged for decades to the rapidly fatal systemic form, 5. the predilection of the eruption in both the discoid and systemic disease for the areas exposed to light, 6. the "butterfly" or "bat-wing" ("vespertilio") configuration of the eruption common to both conditions, 7. the indistinguishable features of early lesions common to both (MONTGOMERY) and 8. the presence of discoid lesions in cases that are systemic from the start (SCOTT and REES).

Among the significant differences between the two conditions are the relatively asymptomatic character of the discoid forms, the relatively benign course of the disease as far as the patient's general health is concerned, and the much smaller ratio of female cases 2 or less than 2:1 (ALLENDE; GOLD) in discoid lupus erythematodes versus 4 or 5:1 (HARVEY) in the systemic disease.

b) Transformation and Transmutations of Lupus Erythematodes Discoides to Systemic Lupus Erythematosus

α) Incidence. Estimates vary considerably as to the frequency with which conversion of the discoid disease to systemic disease takes place. CANNON and CURTIS observed this change in 1/126 cases, ALLENDE in 6/110, STORCK in 10/137,

Lamb and Young in 12/120, Dubois in 2/62, Cohen and Cadman in 1/9, Tumulty in 3/105, Scott and Rees in 10/30. Varying periods of time from 18 months to eight years or longer (Scott and Rees; Larson) may elapse before systemic involvement becomes manifest. Intervals as long as 25 years (Shearn and Pirofsky) and 41 years (Brunsting et al.) may elapse before the change takes place.

β) Localized Versus Widespread Form. Haserick is of the opinion that conversion to the systemic form is more likely in the presence of widespread erythematosus lesions than in the localized form. Scott and Rees on the other hand found the transition took place in eight of their localized cases and in six with generalized lesions.

γ) Case Histories of systemic lupus erythematosus subjects disclosed discoid lesions had been present at one time in 6/34 (Shearn and Pirofsky) and 9/112 cases (Brunsting et al.) in 20—25% of cases in at least three different series (Jessar et al.; Wilson and Jordan; Ziff et al.); in 6% of acute disseminated lupus erythematosus, 17% of subacute disseminated lupus erythematosus and in 30% of chronic disseminated lupus erythematosus (Montgomery and McCreight). In a review of the subject which includes some of the papers quoted, Allende found 77/558 or 13.8% had had discoid lesions.

δ) Systemic Lupus Erythematosus to Lupus Erythematodes Discoides. Ganor and Sagher point out that there are relatively few documented reports on the change from systemic lupus erythematosus to the chronic discoid type. They cited two cases of their own (one which was problematic) and culled a few from the literature. It is difficult to say in such instances, as these authors point out, whether the systemic disease actually has changed to lupus erythematodes discoides or whether chronic discoid lesions have made their appearance in systemic cases. The latter is not a rare occurrence (Carr and Levine). Haserick (1955) for example noted nine instances in a group of 126 patients with systemic lupus erythematosus. Four cases of systemic lupus erythematosus in which discoid lesions appeared during the first year of the systemic illness were observed also by Scott and Rees.

ε) Dissenting Views. Rose and Pillsbury maintain such an occurrence is rare and it is Michelson's (1954) opinion that although the change exists it is "extremely rare and rarely needs to be considered". He goes on to say that when it does occur, the various explanations for the transmutation given e.g. exposure to sunlight, frost, surgical procedures are not valid. Reiches' poll likewise shows that 600/1200 dermatologists had never seen an example of the transition from the discoid to the systemic form. Reiches himself however did see (as did many of the others who answered his questionnaire) three such cases. Andrews who feels acute disseminated lupus erythematosus (systemic lupus erythematosus) bears little kinship to the discoid type, acknowledges that some cases do develop from the discoid type and that discoid lupus erythematosus may be the only sign of the systemic disease.

c) Clinical and Laboratory Findings[1]

α) Incidence of Systemic Manifestations. Utilizing "broad" criteria, and to some minds including the author's criteria far too broad, Dubois and Martel found evidence of systemic involvement in almost all (96% of 41) cases of discoid lupus erythematosus. On the other hand, Scott and Rees who applied "strict"

[1] A detailed discussion of clinical and laboratory findings will be found in sections (5) and (8) respectively.

criteria in their cases found signs and/or symptoms of systemic involvement in only 12% of 102 cases. Regrettably these "strict" criteria were not recorded. Presumably a positive lupus erythematodes test, abnormal serum protein patterns, and the concurrence of two or more symptoms associated with the systemic disorder e.g. a transitory "butterfly" erythema, purpura, plueral or pericardial pain, nephrotic syndrome, arthritis or arthralgia, had to be present. Most observers would agree with these "strict" criteria with the exception perhaps of arthritis and arthralgia. The significance of the latter has to be evaluated in view of the high incidence of these symptoms among controls.

β) Histologic Findings. The findings of lupus erythematodes discoides are considered distinctive and unlike those of acute and subacute lupus erythematodes (systemic lupus erythematosus). Nevertheless it has been Montgomery's experience that histologic transitions from acute to chronic discoid lupus erythematosus may at times be seen in the same section. Moreover, he found that at times it is possible for a biopsy of a cutaneous lesion in the systemic lupus erythematosus to disclose features associated with discoid lesions and conversely in cases in which the course and most of lesions conformed to the discoid type to find changes comparable to those with acute lupus erythematodes. Although histochemical studies (Stoughton and Wells; Johnson) show more similarities than differences the results are nevertheless inconclusive.

γ) Hematologic Data. Leukopenia (Wilson and Jordan; Marten and Blackburn) elevated sedimentation rate (Cochrane), hyperglobulinemia (Walker and Benditt) electrophoretic (Walker and Benditt) and immunoelectrophoretic (Herrmann and Schulz) patterns similar to those found in systemic lupus erythematosus have also been reported in discoid lupus erythematosus. These changes however are more striking and consistent in the systemic form.

The lupus erythematodes test is positive in approximately 5% of cases of chronic discoid lupus erythematosus as compared with an average incidence of 74% in systemic lupus erythematosus. The latter figure is based on the results obtained by the following investigators: 80% (Braunsteiner), 67% (Suksta and Conley), 68% (Dubois) and 82% (Harvey et al.).

Similarly a chronic biologic false positive serologic reaction for syphilis is found in approximately 4% of cases of chronic discoid lupus erythematosus as compared with an estimated incidence of positive reactions in about 15% (Miller et al.; Rein and Kostant; Montgomery and McCreight) to approximately 1/3 of systemic lupus erythematosus cases (Braverman et al.). It is interesting to note also that the incidence of chronic biologic false positive reactions in discoid lupus erythematosus is about the same as it is among relatives of systemic lupus erythematosus subjects [3.5% (Siegel et al.)].

δ) Summary. The data appears to support the hypothesis that lupus erythematodes discoides and systemic lupus erythematosus are interrelated. Additional material and comparisons pertinent to this question will be found in other sections. They were omitted here to avoid unwarranted duplication or because inconclusive or conflicting results were obtained with particular studies. Despite transitions, transmutations and some laboratory features in common one must not lose sight of the fact that in the majority of instances lupus erythematodes discoides and systemic lupus erythematosus are separable clinical entities. The discoid disease is essentially a dermatologic condition whereas systemic lupus erythematosus tends to involve more than one system or different systems at different times. Discoid lupus erythematosus moreover is a chronic disease which persists in most instances with little change except for remissions that can usually be brought about by adequate treatment. Systemic lupus erathematosus, on the other hand, shows a more variable course that may be fulminating or may last for years with exacerbations and remissions associated with varying degrees of disability.

4. Etiology

In the past few decades interest has centered about the etiologic and predisposing factors pertinent to systemic lupus erythematosus rather than lupus erythematodes discoides. If one accepts the essential unity of these conditions it would follow that the theories and hypothesis advanced for the systemic disease would apply to the discoid form as well (GOLD and GOWING; HARVEY et al.; PASCHER 1959).

Incidence

Most articles deal with lupus erythematodes as a disease rather than with its individual forms. Statistics pertaining solely to lupus erythematodes discoides are not readily available.

α) General Considerations. The discoid form appears to be more common that the systemic form (GOLD; MARTEN and BLACKBURN; KADYROVA). This could very well vary, however, with who is reporting the clinical material. Some internists rarely see the discoid form whereas some dermatologists (REICHES) rarely see the systemic form. GOLD (1960) found that the number of new cases of discoid lupus erythematosus in recent years corresponded closely to the incidence reported by RADCLIFFE-CROCKER 50 years before.

LOCALIZED (fixed) lupus erythematodes discoides in turn appears to be more prevalent than the widespread or generalized form. This is substantiated by a number of papers. KADRYROVA found 70 patients with the localized variety as compared with 44 examples of the "disseminated" form. In MARTEN and BLACKBURN's paper the ratio of discoid to systemic cases was 11 to 1.

β) Age, Sex, Race. The largest incidence is among individuals in their thirties or forties. It is rather unusual to find the condition in persons under fifteen (Gold 1960; KADYROVA). MCCUISTION and SCHOCH reported a case in a white infant who presented at birth clinical as well as histologic features of discoid lupus erythematosus. Regression of the process was evident by three months of age and there were no residua except slight atrophy at five months of age. The mother of this baby developed systemic lupus erythematosus eleven months after the child was born. Discoid lupus erythematosus in a newborn of a negro mother with systemic lupus erythematosus during pregnancy was reported by EPSTEIN and LITT.

Women are affected more often than men. The ratio of females to males has been given as approximately 2:1 (ALLENDE), 1.7:1 (ROTHFIELD et al.), 1.5:1 (GOLD 1960) compared to a 5:1 ratio in the systemic form in a large series gathered by HARVEY et al. It has also been noted that among Moroccans the men are far more prone than the women to the fixed, scarring form (BOLLIER et PELBOIS). COHEN and CADMAN however are of the opinion that lupus erythematodes discoides is distributed equally between the sexes.

It has been shown that systemic lupus erythematosus occurs at least as often among negroes as whites in the United States (JESSAR et al.). Whether the discoid form is more or less prevalent among negroes is not ascertainable at this time. REISS in his discussion of a case of discoid lupus erythematosus in a Chinese made the point that lupus erythematodes was almost non-existent in China and that he saw only a few cases of the discoid type over a period of 19 years. KESTEN found discoid lupus erythematosus to be three times as common in persons with fair complexions than in brunettes.

γ) Familial Incidence. It is rare for more than one member of a family to have lupus erythematodes discoides. BECKETT and LEWIS gathered 40 familial cases occurring during 1901—1959 in which the majority had the discoid form. BUCHHOLZ reported an unusual example of three members with chronic discoid lupus erythematosus in one family and SHAW, in a discussion of this presentation cited an example of three brothers with the same disorder. There are also two reports of erythematodes chronicus in identical female twins (VON GRUENHAGEN; STEAGALL et al.). In the latter, in my opinion, the clinical picture in one of the sisters was that of systemic lupus erythematosus rather than discoid lupus erythematosus.

Although it is not common for lupus erythematodes discoides and systemic lupus erythematosus to occur in the same family, their number is too large to be coincidental (ROTHFIELD et al.; BECKETT and LEWIS; BRAVERMAN et al.; ZEISLER and BLUEFARB). The author can recall a patient with lupus erythematodes discoides of the scalp whose niece developed lupus erythematodes profundus. In another family, one of two sisters had lupus erythematodes discoides while the other died of systemic lupus erythematosus. One may assume many similar examples have gone unrecorded. One should also point out there are families in which the systemic form alone appears to be prevalent (CALLOMON; BRUNJES et al.).

The familial incidence, although not great, together with a consistently higher percentage of significant laboratory features e.g. dysproteinemia, hypergammaglobulinemia and antinuclear serum factors among relatives of lupus erythematodes patients as compared with controls (SIEGEL et al.; HOLMAN and DEICHER; ROTHFIELD et al.) suggests the possibility of an inherited predisposition to the disease. The preponderance of female cases, moreover, leads to the supposition that a genetic predisposition, if present, may be sex linked. However, as has been pointed out by SIEGEL et al. the possibility of common environmental factors cannot be excluded.

δ) Season and Climate. The response to climate and season does not appear to be consistent. Exacerbations in the spring and summer are more common than in fall and winter according to KADYROVA. WEBER on the other hand found that onset as well as healing were independent of season. Low temperatrues were found to have an adverse effect in 2/66 persons with the localized form and in 1/6 with the disseminated form of lupus erythematodes (MARTEN and BLACKBURN). GOLD (1960) found heat was aggravating more often than cold.

ε) Sunlight. KESTEN and KIERLAND believe lupus erythematodes subjects are more sensitive to light than normal individuals and GARZÓN et al. are inclined to be rather emphatic about the matter. In their opinion, sunlight, vascular lability and local tissue susceptability account for the localization of the lesions. MICHELSON (1952), STORCK and BERZUPS, as well as WEBER on the other hand find no evidence of photosensitivity.

Statistics although sparse indicate exposure to sunlight may be pathogenetic. In a group of 77 patients with unequivocal discoid lupus erythematosus, SCOTT and REES found the onset in 24 was associated with exposure to light and 47 were reactivated by further exposure. MARTEN and BLACKBURN likewise noted that the lesions were aggravated by sunlight in 41/66 patients with the localized form and 4/6 with the generalized form of the disease.

There is a paucity of experimental evidence on the subject. KESTEN and SLATKIN were able to reproduce typical clinical lesions in two patients with discoid lupus erythematosus by repeated applications of three to four times the minimal erythema dose with an action spectrum of 3900 Å. A Kromayer lamp was the source of light in these experiments. GARZÓN et al. likewise were able to reproduce clinical and histologic features of lupus erythematodes with repeated exposures to ultraviolet light for two to four minutes intervals. They found, moreover, this reaction could be blocked to some extent by the application of an antiactinic cream containing antipyrine. BETTLEY and PAGE noted that the average minimal erythema dose of ultraviolet light in lupus erythematodes subjects was about half that for normal individuals, and SAPPUPO found a shortening of the latency of the erythema.

QUIROGA and MOM on the other hand were able to reproduce cutaneous lesions in human subjects only in rare instances by irradiation with ultraviolet light. MAGNUS and ROTTIER independently found that lupus erythematodes subjects who appeared to be sensitive to sunlight did not appear to react to any specific light band. HARBER et al. used four T-12, 20-watt Westinghouse fluorescent sunlamp tubes giving an emission between 2750 Å and 3300 Å, as the light source in their studies. They could demonstrate no significant difference between the erythema threshhold or the magnitude of erythema response in 24 hours in 16 patients with polymorphous light eruptions, 20 normal volunteers and in six patients with chronic discoid lupus erythematosus.

Interpretation. Sunlight appears to play a role in the distribution of the eruption in lupus erythematodes discoides and in the activation of lesions in some cases. The way in which this is effected however remains obscure. A Koebner-like phenomenon or a possible phototoxic effect of sunlight have also been entertained as plausible explanations (McCHESNEY et al.). Experiments conducted thus far have failed to disclose clear cut evidence of photosensitivity. Future investigators may be more successful.

ζ) Trauma. Various forms of trauma have been linked with discoid lesions (KERN and SCHIFF). These include burns from mustard gas (KING-SMITH), chemical burns (SPENCER), thermal burns, sunburn, frostbite, direct blows, gunshot wounds, lacerations, tatooing, lipbiting, skin planing and roentgen rays. The consensus is that sunburn too may be followed by dissemination of the lesions or conversion of discoid lupus erythematosus to the systemic form.

η) Infection. In 1931, it was still held, although with reservations, that tuberculosis was of etiologic significance (VEIEL). Lupus vulgaris erythematodes (LELOIR) was considered a form of lupus erythematodes rather than a tuberculoderm. There is no longer any doubt that this condition is unrelated to discoid lupus erythematosus and that tubercle bacilli have no more than a fortituitous association with lupus erythematodes. Nevertheless, the matter is still being pursued by some investigators (KADYROVA; SIPOS and JÁKSO; NAGY and LÖVEY).

Foci of infection or chronic infections of various types have also been incriminated (GARZÓN et al.) as possible etiologic factors in discoid lupus erythematosus. Here again there is no evidence that the association is more than coincidental.

ϑ) Hormones and Deranged Metabolism. Whether or not female sex hormones play a role in this disease has been considered because of the greater incidence among women (Suschevskaya-Dmitrevskaya). No corroborative evidence has come forth.

Defective metabolism of the flavonoids including riboflavine has been mentioned by BRAVERMAN, JOHNSON and LERNER as a possibility. The similarity in chemical structure of the flavinoids to some of the antimalarials and the therapeutic benefits with the latter led to this hypothesis.

5. Localization and Clinical Forms

a) Areas of Predilection

The predilection for the areas exposed to the elements is well known. TRAMIER's cogitations on the subject make fascinating reading. He feels that the distribution and configuration of the lesions of the face in particular, correspond to those areas where there are no underlying muscles and the skin is in almost direct contact with the skeleton. The same is true of the vertex, mastoid region, zygomatic area, ears, bridge of the nose and dorsal aspect of the fingers in proximity to the insertion of the tendons. The absence of underlying protective muscle and the consequent "lack of nourishment", to his mind are far more important than external and internal factors emphasized by other writers.

b) Typical Forms

Two principal forms have been recognized: A. the localized or fixed form and B. the widespread or generalized form (chronic disseminated lupus erythematosus of earlier classification). Both forms have been described in great detail by VEIEL.

α) The boundary line between the **localized (fixed)** and **generalized (widespread)** forms of discoid lupus erythematosus is a rather arbitrary one. In the localized form the lesions are generally confined to the face, scalp and ears. When typical discoid lesions are also found on the neck and/or the chest, the distribution may still be regarded by some (HASERICK and KELLUM) as compatible with the localized rather than with the widespread (disseminate) form. Characteristically, discoid lesions are well marginated, somewhat infiltrated, a violaceous red topped by keratotic plugs and scales. The end stage is usually an atrophic depigmented scar surrounded by hyperpigmentation.

β) In the **widespread or generalized** form similar but generally smaller discoid plaques are found symmetrically distributed over the extensor aspect of upper extremities, upper chest and back as well as over the head and neck. Lesions may appear in lesser numbers on any part of the body. Dispersed among the discoid plaques one usually finds poorly defined superficial somewhat scaly erythematous lesions that lead to superficial atrophy and scarring.

γ) **"Butterfly" Erythema.** Well defined erythema symmetrically distributed over the bridge of the nose and malar eminences may be a feature of both forms, but is more often associated with the widerspread or generalized type. The erythema takes on a "butterfly" ("bat-wing" or "vespertilio") configuration also known as érytheme centrifuge (BIETT), erytheme centrifuge symmetrique (BROCQ). The "butterfly" usually persists and in time atrophy and altered pigmentation follow. Symmetrical erythema with the same pattern but less well defined may also be a manifestation of the systemic disease. In acute systemic lupus erythematosus this configurate erythema tends to fluctuate in degree and may wane without atrophy or scarring. In less acute cases (subacute disseminated lupus erythematosus of early classifications) there is also a tendency toward atrophy and scarring with altered pigmentation as seen in the discoid form. Some obsevers (LELIS) however maintain érytheme centrifuge generally connotes systemic involvement and consequently should not be considered a manifestation of the chronic discoid form.

c) Unusual Forms

α) **Chilblain Lupus of Hutchinson.** In 1931 (VEIEL) there was still doubt as to the propriety of including chilblain lupus as a manifestation of discoid lupus erythematosus. In this rare form, the lesions are most conscpicuous over the tip of the nose and ears but are otherwise typical. A case reported by GARB was associated with cryoglobulinemia which may have been a factor in the localization.

β) Telangiectatic Lupus Erythematodes (Crocker) according to VEIEL is characterized by exquisitely symmetrical, sharply circumscribed red areas on both cheeks "corresponding exactly in size and circumference to the red spots clowns paint on their faces". The author has seen only a single example of lupus erythematodes telangiectaticum of the localized discoid type in the course of thirty years of dermatologic practise. In the latter there were two plaques on the face,

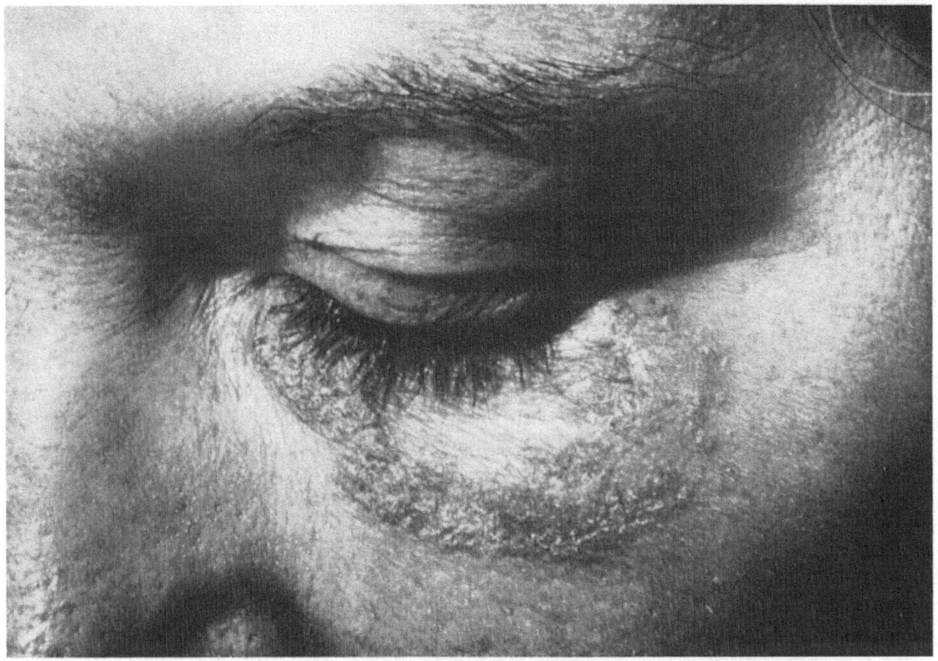

Fig. 1. An example of the acute localized edematous type of lupus erythematodes discoides described by MICHELSON. The lesion is edematous, erythematous, sharply circumscribed and disc-like

one over the right malar area and the other over the left side of the jaw. The lesions were associated with poikiloderma (CIVATTE) and telangiectases of the skin of the chest. Telangiectasia it should be pointed out is not an uncommon component of lupus erythematodes lesions in widespread eruptions or in systemic lupus erythematosus.

γ) Acute Localized Edematous Type. MICHELSON described an acute localized edematous form in which he found an erythematous, sharply circumscribed disc that felt like "an elastic node". An example of such a lesion is seen in Fig. 1. In a relatively short time, the lesion shrank leaving a superficial red spot with a central depression. The end result may be a typical discoid lesion or it may heal without a trace.

δ) Bullous Discoid Lupus Erythematodes appears to be especially rare. In the discussion of BLOOM's case (1956), COSTELLO recalled having seen an example of this form. Another case was brought to my attention by ORFUSS. In his patient vesicular and bullous lesions continued to recur over a period of 14 years in a plaque with a "butterfly" distribution. KOGOJ's patient showed signs of systemic involvement.

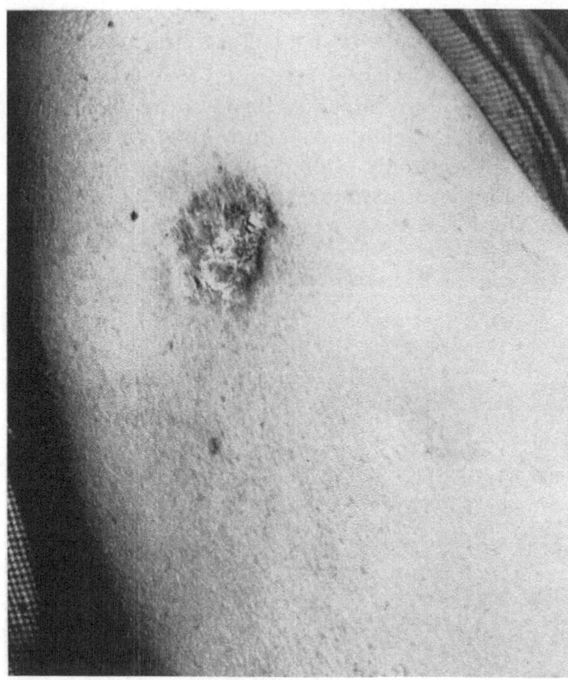

Fig. 2. Lupus erythematodes profundus of the deltoid area in a 31 year old woman. The proximal lesion is deep seated, retracted, covered by adherent scales. Below there is an atrophic area that marks the site of a resorbed subcutaneous nodule

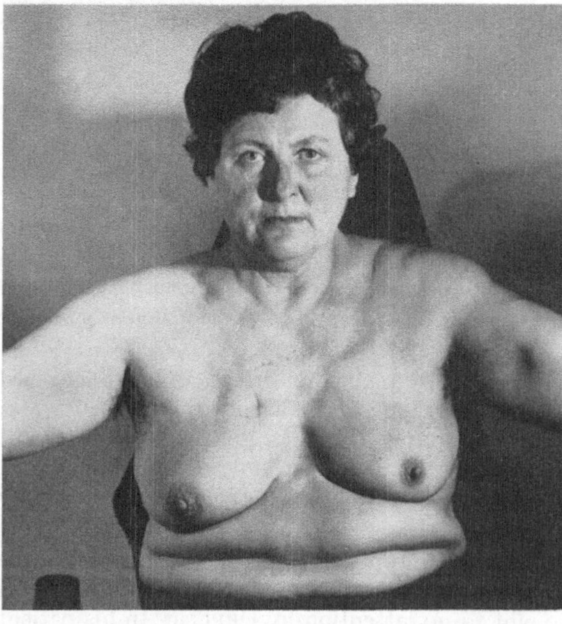

Fig. 3. Irregular, linear and rounded depressed scars of varying size and shape are the end result of healed subcutaneous lesions on the chest, shoulders and arms in a case of lupus erythematodes profundus (Courtesy Drs. C. G. SCHIRREN and D. EGGERT). [Fig. 3—5: Arch. klin. exp. Derm. **216**, 541 (1963)]

ε) Lupus Erythematodes Profundus (Kaposi-Irgang). It is difficult to categorize this rare form of lupus erythematodes properly because one may find signs and symptoms of the systemic form as well as features of lupus erythematodes discoides, either concurrently or at different times. One finds subcutaneous nodules involving the hypoderm combined with indurated discoid plaques in the skin. The nodules may vary in size and number and they are usually firm, sometimes tender. It is possible for the lesions to resolve without any apparent trace, or they may surface to involve the overlying skin. Cup-like or retracted scars of varying size and depth may ensue. The configuration and distribution of the sears are portrayed in Figs. 2—5. The cases presented in these illustrations have bean published in detail (PASCHER et al.; SCHIRREN and EGGERT). The plaques may be independent of the nodules or they may be combined with them. At times it is possible to demonstrate the histologic features of discoid lupus erythematosus over the nodules even when the skin appears normal. The areas of predilection are the face, deltoid region, the buttocks and the thighs. PASCHER, SIMS and PENSKY reported a case in 1955 and reviewed the literature at that time. A number of reports have appeared since (GUIMARES; OLSSON; NELSON).

ζ) Lupus Erythematodes Hypertrophicus et Profundus. Lupus erythematodes hypertrophicus et profundus (BECHET) should not be confused with lupus erythematodes profundus (KAPOSI-IRGANG). The former is really a variant of discoid lupus erythematosus in which one finds verrucous and hyperkeratotic lesions that heal with cribriform scarring particularly over the chin and in the circumoral area. Involvement of the hypoderm was not demonstrated in BECHET's cases. PECK also reported a case of lupus erythematodes hypertrophicus et profundus. In my opinion lupus erythematodes profundus (KAPOSI-IRGANG) would have been the proper designation for PECK's case. IRGANG (1958) also reported a case of lupus erythematodes papularis and nodularis which he felt was related to lupus erythematodes hypertrophicus et profundus (BECHET). This is confusing for lupus erythematodes nodularis once thougth to be a form of lupus erythematodes, has been shown since to be a tuberculoderm.

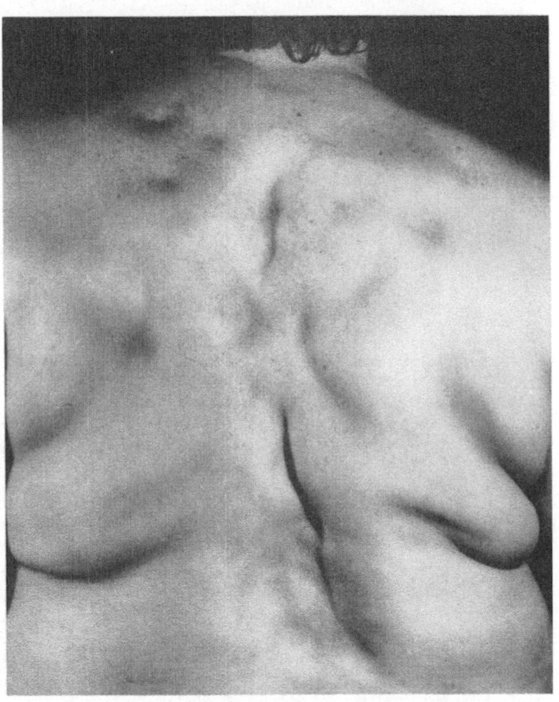

Fig. 4. Many deep, irregular, retracted scars mark the site of healed subcutaneous lesions on the back in a case of lupus erythematodes profundus (Courtesy Drs. C. G. SCHIRREN and D. EGGERT)

η) Miscellaneous Variants are sometimes seen e.g. psoriasiform lupus erythematodes (this variant is seen in Fig. 6), lupus erythematodes hypertrophicus (LESSER), acne rosacea-like (lupus erythemato acneique-Hardy), lichen-planus-like lesions and annular lesions (an example of annular configuration is seen in Fig. 7) (VEIEL). Psoriasis and lupus erythematodes discoides may on rare occasions be found concomitantly (SCHUPPENER and BORNS).

d) Unusual Localizations

α) Fingers and Finger-Nails. Discoid lesions may be found over the palms and dorsa of the hands in the widely disseminated form (VEIEL). Perniosis (chilblains) was noted in 25/77 or in 31% of patients by SCOTT and REES. There were no features of systemic lupus erythematodes nor evidence of RAYNAUD's phenomenon, however, in this group. Whether or not the finding of the latter would militate against the diagnosis of discoid lupus erythematosus is debatable (SCOTT and REES). The author is in accord with those who maintain the phenomenon is indicative of systemic involvement.

Changes in the nails appear to be most rare. Perusal of the literature disclosed one example (YOUNG). The nails were markedly thickened resembling bird's claws, lusterless, discolored with shallow longitudinal fissures. From the description it is difficult to say however whether this was a case of generalized discoid or systemic lupus erythematosus.

β) Mucous Membranes. Involvement of the mucous membranes with the exception of the lips as VEIEL has shown, is quite rare in lupus erythematodes dis-

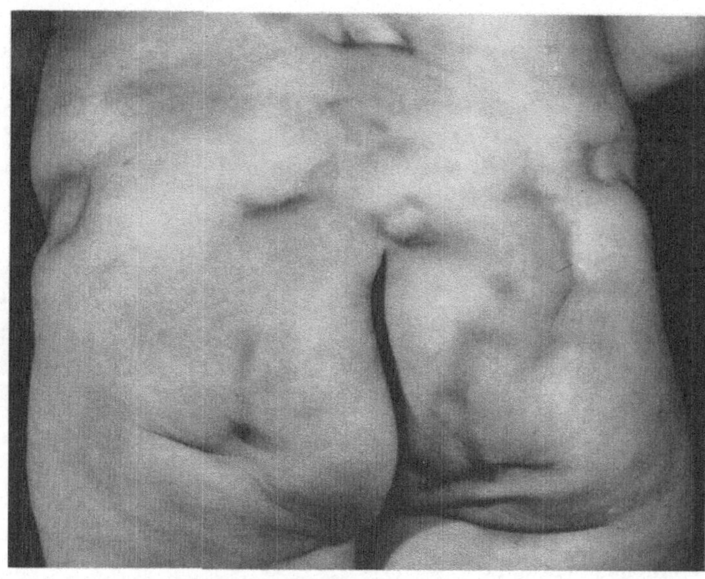

Fig. 5. Many deep, retracted scars are the end-stage of subcutaneous lesions on the buttocks in a case of lupus erythematodes profundus (Courtesy Drs. C. G. Schirren and D. Eggert)

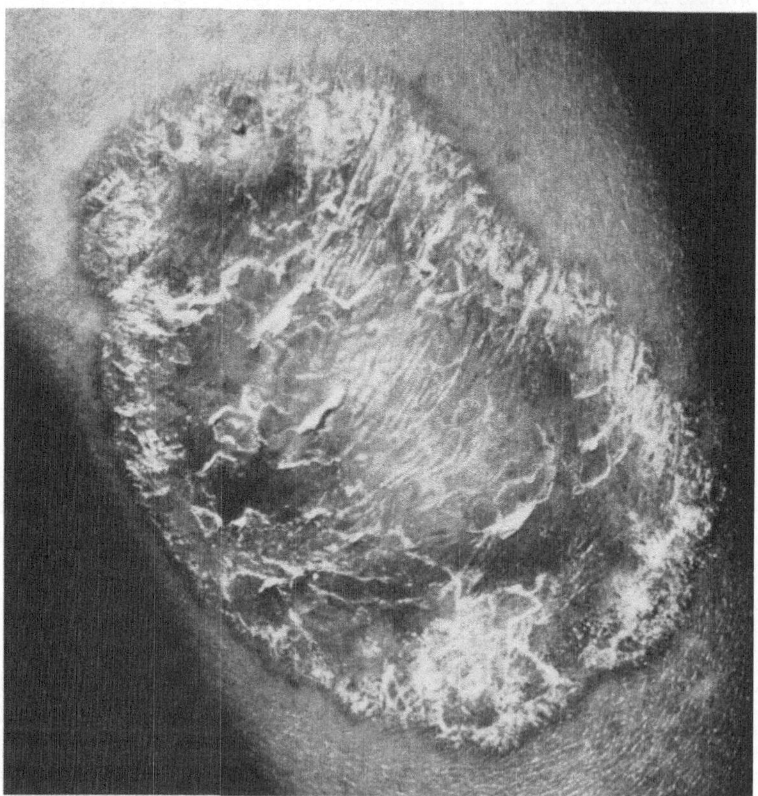

Fig. 6. Lupus erythematodes discoides with a psoriasiform appearance in a 41 year old woman. Symmetrically distributed sharply marginated plaques of erythema, infiltration and scaling have been present for four years. Courtesy of Dr. Arthur B. Hyman

coides (an example of lupus erythematodes chronicus of the vermilion border of the upper lip is seen in Fig. 8). Lesions were found in the oral mucosal in 5/70 cases by KADYROVA and in 4/72 by MARTEN and BLACKBURN. In one of these four the possibility of a reaction to quinacrine could not be excluded. In no instance were the changes specific. Linear streaks or plaques resembling lichen planus or leukoplakia as well as marginated ulcers have been described (THOMA and GOLDMAN; DE GRACIANSKY and BOULLE).

γ) Eyelids and Conjunctiva. KLAUDER and DELONG judge this localization to be most rare. They reviewed the literature in 1932 and described three cases of their own. KLAUDER finally found two more cases after twenty-seven years. The report by VILANOVA et al. is of particular interest because a histologic as well as clinical study was made of the lesions of the conjunctiva. The microscopic features parelled those of the glabrous skin except for the lack of keratinization. The lesions moreover, responded quite favorably to chloroquine phosphate.

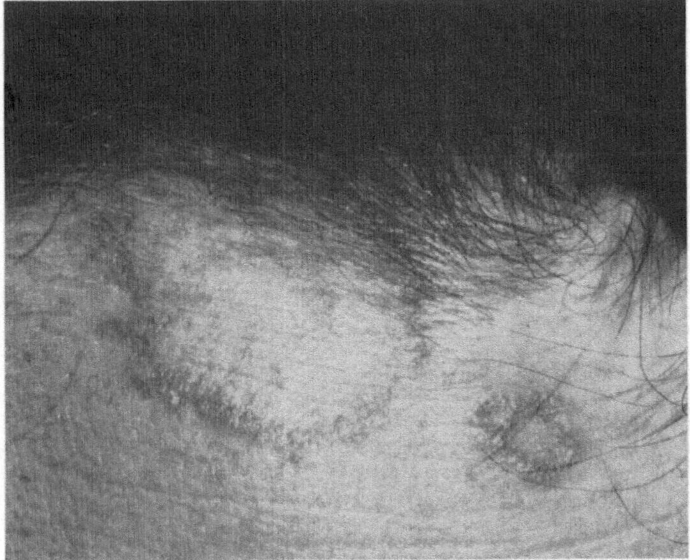

Fig. 7. Lupus erythematodes discoides with an annular configuration of four years duration in a 29 year old woman. The border is raised, somewhat infiltrated, dull red in color with adherent scales. Superficial atrophy and hypopigmentation are found within the border

6. Symptoms

Lupus erythematodes discoides is generally asymptomatic. Patients may complain at times of itching, burning or tenderness of the lesions. The majority feel well and seem to be able to carry out a full program of work. Whether or not lupus erythematodes discoides may be accompanied by systemic manifestations is questioned.

α) Fever. All patients were afebrile in one group of 72 (MARTEN and BLACKBURN) and in another series of 77 (SCOTT and REES). JADASSOHN on the other hand noted that low grade fever was manifested particularly in the course of the dissemination of the cutaneous lesions in the generalized form. MONTGOMERY and McCREIGHT also noted pyrexia in 5% of 80 cases of chronic disseminated lupus erythematodes. A second group of 23 patients in their study, however, proved afebrile.

β) Loss of Weight. MARTEN and BLACKBURN found 17/72 patients gained weight whereas only 5/72 lost weight. Weight loss was noted by ROTHFIELD and co-workers in 11/65 cases of discoid lupus erythematosus. Antimalarial therapy with its attendant anorexia and/or other gastrointestinal symptoms may have been responsible for the weight loss in some of their cases.

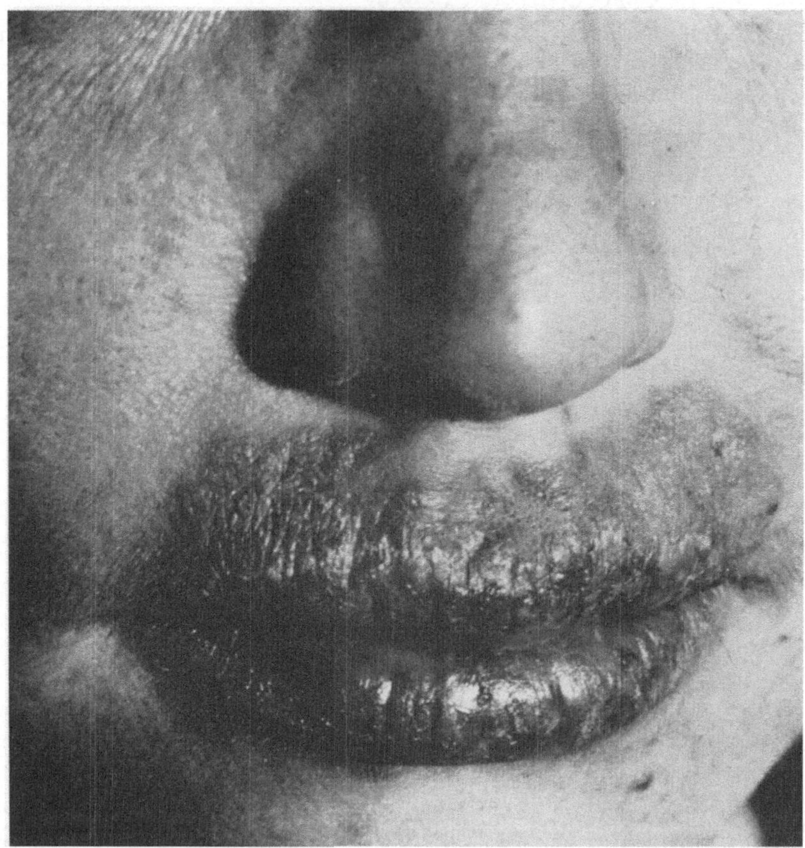

Fig. 8. Lupus erythematodes discoides of three months duration of the upper lip including the vermilion border in a 31 year old woman. Edematous well defined plaques are also present over the malar area. The patient was first seen by the author when she was eight years old. During the intervening years there were recurrent episodes of erythema perstans solare (Lamb) that healed without sequelae

γ) Fatigue. Increased fatiguability was mentioned by ALLENDE and by DUBOIS and MARTEL. In a comparative study (ROTHFIELD et al.), whereas 3/65 controls complained of fatigue, 19/65 patients with discoid lupus erythematosus complained of this symptom. Antimalarial therapy may have been a contributory factor in some instances.

δ) Arthritis, Arthralgia and Myalgia. These symptoms were recorded in 7/61 (GOLD 1960), 5/77 (SCOTT and REES), 15/72 (MARTEN and BLACKBURN), 25/65 (ROTHFIELD et al.) cases of discoid lupus erythematosus. The incidence is impressive until one compares the statistics for matched controls. As many as 20/65 patients in one series (ROTHFIELD et al.) and 18/142 in another (SIEGEL et al.) had the same complaints.

ε) Miscellaneous Symptoms. Lymphadenopathy was noted in 37% of KADYROVA's cases and in 3/11 by DUBOIS and MARTEL. In the former series there were an unusually large number of generalized cases and in the latter there were one or two with signs and symptoms suggestive of systemic lupus erythematosus. There was no palpable enlargement of the nodes on the other hand in a group of 77 patients with discoid lupus erythematosus (SCOTT and REES). Nor was this symptom mentioned in two other comprehensive papers (MONTGOMERY and McCREIGHT; MARTEN and BLACKBURN).

ζ) Interpretation. It would seem low grade fever is found at times in patients with the diagnosis of discoid lupus erythematosus, at least in the generalized form. Weight loss that is neither striking nor progressive likewise may be associated with this dermatosis. Since fatiguability, arthritis, arthralgia and myalgia are rather prevalent among matched controls these symptoms may or may not be relevant.

7. Complications

Disfiguring scars to the point of mutilation are possible (HOLLANDER and KRUGH). Permanent alopecia often marks the site of scalp lesions.

α) Skin Cancer is an uncommon complication. In a recent survey, 160 cases of squamous cell epithelioma were collected by ANDREEV and co-workers. They added two examples, an epithelioma in an active lupus erythematodes lesion and another in an old sclerotic lesion. To these one may also add a number of cases that were overlooked (JACOBSON and ANNAMUNTHODO; HOLTZMAN; SKLARZ). A hitherto unreported example of discoid lupus erythematosus of the lip complicated by squamous cell epithelioma has been presented by the author (see Fig. 9).

The carcinoma is usually of the squamous cell type (SCHWARZ). JACOBSON and ANNAMUNTHODO and SKLARZ each reported a case of keratoacanthoma which later proved to be a squamous cell carcinoma. Knowing the difficulty in making the correct differential diagnosis at times between prickle cell epithelioma and keratoacanthoma, one is tempted to suggest these lesions may have been epitheliomas to begin with.

Undoubtedly the inflammatory process and the subsequent atrophy and scarring all have a part in the development of these epitheliomas. One must bear in mind however that the face and the lower lip in particular are areas of predilection for carcinoma of the squamous cell type. Treatment of lupus erythematodes in the past by scarification or by various forms of irradiation may have been contributory. UHLMANN and SCHAMBYE found that in a group of 107 cases, about 1/3 had received roentgen therapy, radium or actinic radiation. MONTGOMERY feels the incidence of epitheliomatous degeneration is smaller in lupus erythematodes discoides than in lupus vulgaris.

β) Pregnancy. Generally it is thought pregnancy does not influence the course of lupus erythematodes discoides. MARTEN and BLACKBURN found however that although 5/9 cases were not affected and three improved, one was aggravated. CRAWFORD and LEEPER also reported a case of chronic discoid that grew worse and two that disseminated during pregnancy. In one of the latter a severe sunburn antedated the dissemination.

8. Laboratory Findings

a) Histopathology

α) Lupus Erythematodes Discoides. A detailed description of the histologic changes with excellent photomicrographs has been presented by VEIEL. The features of lupus erythematodes discoides (MONTGOMERY) may be summarized as follows: relative and absolute hyperkeratosis of varying degrees independent of the cutaneous appendages; keratotic plugging of the follicular orifices and sweat ducts; preservation or thickening of the granular layer; acanthosis with adjacent areas of atrophy of the prickle cell layer; liquefaction necrosis of the basal cell layer; perivascular lymphocytic infiltration chiefly about the dermal

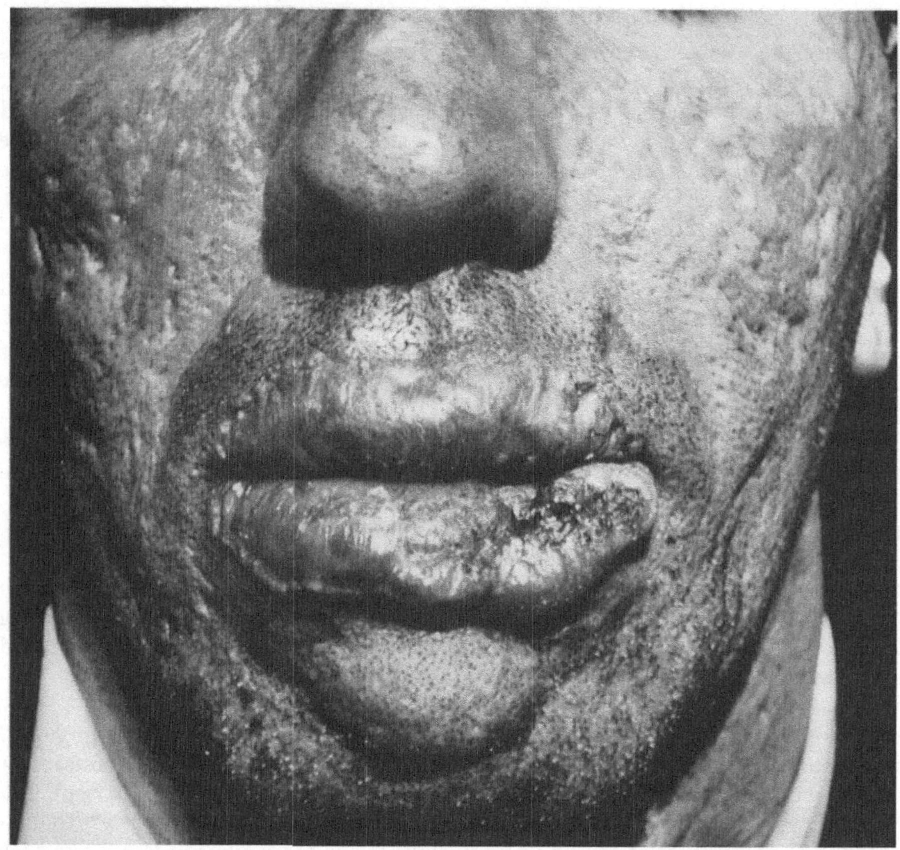

Fig. 9. Lupus erythematodes discoides of the lower lip complicated by a squamous cell epithelioma in a 37 year old man. The epithelioma appeared after lupus erythematodes discoides had been present for ten years. Courtesy of DR. ANDREW G. FRANKS

appendages; dilatation of the superficial capillaries and lymphatics; edematous changes in the cutis and destruction of the elastic tissue where the infiltration occurs; a varying number of chromatophores laden with melanin; absence of proliferative or obliterative changes in the walls of the deeper vessels. MONTGOMERY has shown also that typical features of lupus erythematodes discoides may not be present in early lesions and that several weeks may elapse before a diagnostic pattern appears. He found moreover, that it is possible for a specimen from a relatively active lesion to show histologic changes of acute lupus erythematodes when the most of the lesions and the course of the disease are those of chronic discoid lupus erythematosus. The converse may also be true. MCCREIGHT and MONTGOMERY were impressed by the minor changes in the collagen and the paucity of fibrinoid degeneration in the walls of the vessels in lupus erythematodes discoides as is true of the systemic disease.

Changes in the Fat. Prior to our study (PASCHER, SIMS and PENSKY) it was taught that the histopathologic process in lupus erythematodes was limited to the epidermis and cutis. PAUTRIER claimed that the pathologic process in discoid lupus erythematosus sometimes extends to the deepest portions of the cutis "just licking the fat", leaving the subcutaneous tissue otherwise undisturbed. We found a sparse to moderate involvement of the fat in 28/100 specimens (Fig. 10 and 11). A cellular infiltration made up principally of lymphocytes and histocytes, mild collagenization and edema of the vessel walls were the major features.

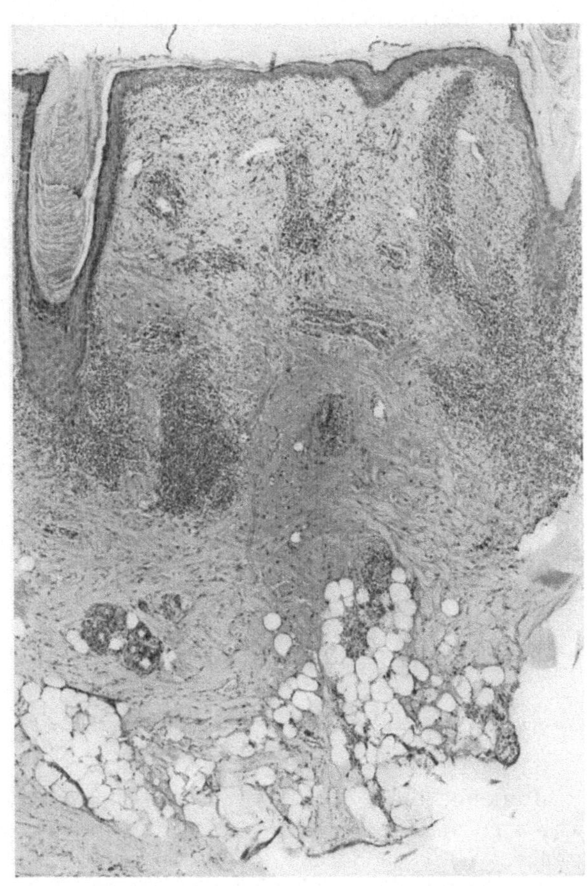

Fig. 10[1]. The reaction in the fat is graded as sparse in a typical case of lupus er thematodes discoides. Collections of lymphocytes and wande-:.ng connective tissue cells are seen in the septa (63 ×)

β) Lupus Erythematodes Profundus. The major changes are in the deep corium and fat (see Figs. 12—15). The overlying epidermis and cutis may not be involved. More often, however, typical features of lupus erythematodes discoides are present even in the absence of visible lesions. Detailed descriptions of these histologic changes — have been recorded in the papers by PASCHER et al. and by SCHIRREN and EGGERT. The inflammatory changes in the fat may be analogous to those seen in acute or subacute lupus erythematodes in which case one would find fibrinoid degeneration and or necrosis of the collagen in the deep cutis and hypoderm as well as obliterative and destructive changes in the vessel walls and collagenization of the fat (SILVA and PORTUGAL; COSTA and JUNQUEIRA). Or one may find inflammatory rather than destructive changes in the walls of the vessels together with a predominantly lymphocytic infiltrate among the fat cells and in the septa (Fig. 13 and 15) (IRGANG 1940; ARNOLD). The latter findings differ only quantitatively from those seen in chronic discoid lupus erythematosus. Combinations of destructive and inflammatory features are also possible (GUIMARES).

---

[1] The photomiergrophes Figs. 11—13 were published in the J. invest. Derm. **25, 34** (1959). The author is indebted to WILLIAMS and WILKINS for their permission to reproduce them.

b) Histochemical Studies

Have been carried out by a number of investigators. STOUGHTON and WELLS used the Hotchkiss-McManus technic [periodic-acid Schiff (PAS) stain] for polysaccharides in 18 cases of discoid lupus erythematosus and in eight cases of systemic lupus erythematosus. They found similar changes in the amount and distribution of the polysaccharides in both forms of lupus erythematodes. Alterations in the appearance of this material, interpreted as "disintegration" were seen only in the systemic form.

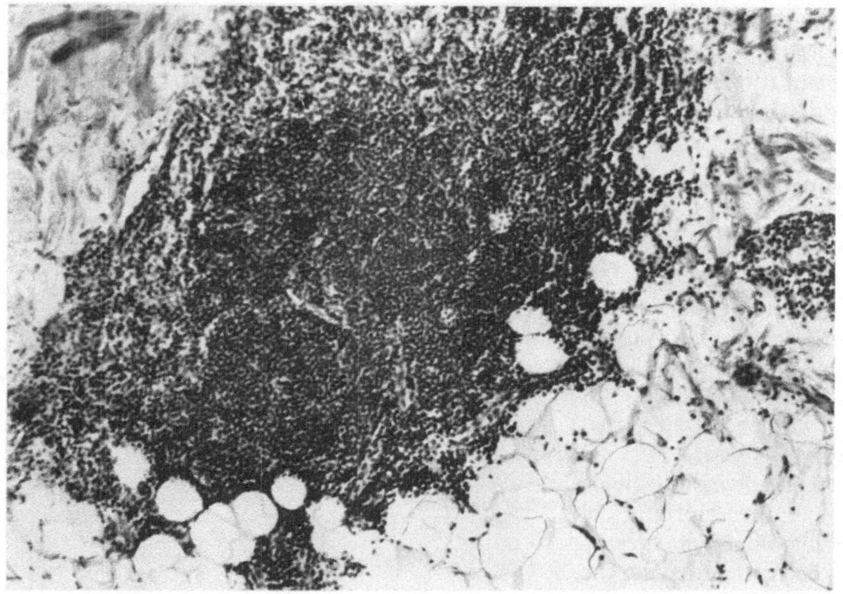

Fig. 11. The reaction in the fat wis graded as moderate in a typical case of chronic discoid lupus erythematodes. The cellular reaction consists of collections of small round and wandering connective tissue cells throughout the fat (185.5 ×)

JOHNSON found collodial iron, toluidine blue with a p_H of 3 and acian blue with a p_H of 2.7—3 far superior to PAS in the investigation of the ground substance[1]. With the former, only quantitative changes were seen. This increase in the amount of ground substance was present in all forms of lupus erythematodes but more consistently and to a greater extent in the acute, subacute and profundus types than in discoid lupus erythematosus. In JOHNSON's opinion this is not a specific change but one of the ways tissue may react to injury.

STORCK likewise mentioned changes with toluidine blue which were regarded as indicative of "pathologic modifications in the synthesis of mucopolysaccharides in chronic lupus erythematodes". He described "red bodies", i.e. intracellular hyaline bodies in the skin of systemic lupus erythematosus which were formed, he thought, from altered lymphocytic and fibroblastic nuclei, probably identical with hematoxylin bodies and the inclusions of lupus erythematodes cells. Focal destructive changes of connective tissue in clinically normal skin as well as affected skin in chronic lupus erythematodes were noted by RAKHMANOV and IVANOV. They considered this involvement of unaffected skin indicative of a systemic process.

[1] According to FLEISCHMAJER, whereas neutral polysaccharides take the PAS stain acid mucopolysaccharides stain with colloidan iron, toluidine and acian blue.

c) Hematologic Findings

α) Blood Count. A more than negligible incidence of leucopenia (less than 4000 leukocytes/ml.) has been noted by a number of observers (Gold 1960; Cohen and Cadman; Marten and Blackburn; Braverman et al.). Gold (1960) had the impression that anemia was not uncommon; a mild hypo-or normchronic anemia was recorded in 5/66 cases by Marten and Blackburn. Scott and Rees on the other hand found no evidence of anemia or leukopenia in 77 cases of chronic discoid lupus erythematosus. The discrepancy may be due to the fact that the

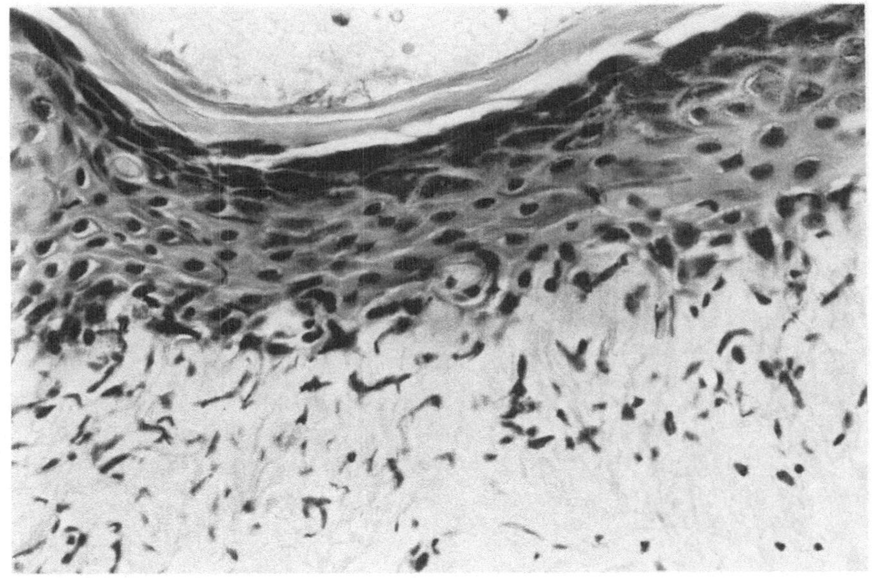

Fig. 12. Hyperkeratinization, liquefaction of the basal cell layer and subepidermal edema are evident overlying the reaction in the fat in lupus erythematodes profundus (see Fig. 13) (498 ×)

latter used 3000 leukocytes/ml. as the lower limit of normal. In evaluating these deviations one should not lose sight of the possible effect of chemotherapeutic agents used in the treatment of the disorder and or possible unrelated causes. Arndt reported a reticulohistiocytosis in the peripheral blood in most of his cases, a finding that has not been mentioned or confirmed by other observers.

β) Erythrocyte Sedimentation Rate (E.S.R.). The rate may be elevated in about $^1/_3$ or $^1/_2$ of the cases but as a rule not to an impressive degree. Cochrane felt that readings of 30 mm./hr. or more (Westergen method) portended refractoriness to treatment or a poor prognosis.

γ) Serum Proteins. There has been considerable interest in the comparative findings of this component of the blood in the discoid and systemic forms. Whereas Walker and Benditt found an elevation in the total proteins with an inversion of the A/G ration in 4/14 cases of chronic discoid lupus erythematosus; Marten and Blackburn found no such change in six patients. A rise in the serum globulin above 3.7 mg-% was also noted in 7/15 cases (Bennett, Osment and Holley). Dubois and Martel reported an increased concentration of this protein in 95% of cases but it should be noted they used 2.5 mg-% as the norm, a value lower than usual.

Electrophoretic studies according to Walker and Benditt showed changes in chronic discoid lupus erythematosus similar to the systemic form, differing only in degree. A study of 16 cases by another group (Bennett, Osment and Holley) disclosed changes that were interpretated as "subtle immunopathologic manifestations which were strongly suggestive of the systemic disease". Paper chromatography (Chórazak) likewise disclosed similar abnormal patterns in both conditions but more consistently in systemic lupus erythematosus. Utilizing the immunoelectrophoretic technic Herrmann and Schulz found the same pattern in acute lupus erythematodes as in chronic discoid lupus erythematosus, namely an elevation in the alpha 1 and alpha 2 glycoproteins, beta 2 and gamma globulin

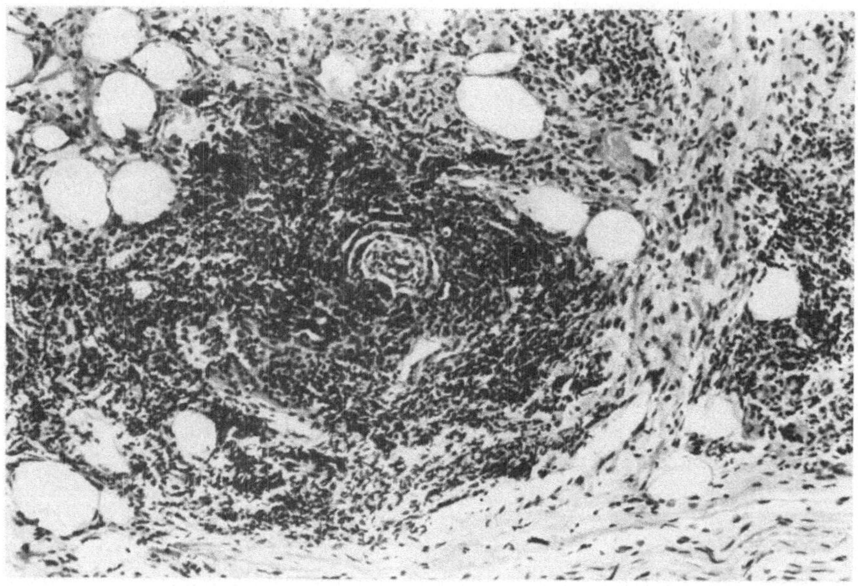

Fig. 13. The deep corium and fat is the seat of a pronounced inflammatory reaction in lupus erythematodes profundus (see Figs. 2 and 12). There is a diffuse and perivascular infiltrate made up of small round cells, connective tissue cells and an occasional polymorphonuclear leukocyte. There is also a pronounced vasculitis and perivasculitis. The walls of the blood vessels show edema and proliferative changes with narrowing of the lumen (185.5 ×)

and a decrease in beta 1 and albumin concentrations. Immunoelectrophoresis differes from electrophoresis in that antigens or antibodies may influence the magnitude of the precipitate as well as the concentration of the respective proteins. The zinc turbidity test as an indicator of increased globulins was used by Rothfield and associates. They found a rise above 10 Kunkel units in 7/25 cases of chronic discoid lupus erythematosus as compared with 2/65 controls.

Chórazak found a cryoglobulinemia in 48/72 cases of discoid lupus erythematosus. Gentele et al. could not demonstrate any such change. The discrepancy may be explained by differences in technic and by what is regarded as a significant concentration of this abnormal protein. Lerner and Watson have shown that traces of this abnormal globulin may be found in normal individuals and that concentrations under 25 mg.-% are generally not clinically significant. Cryoglobulinemia, one may add, is likewise an uncommon finding in the systemic form (Feldaker et al.).

Interpretation. If a large enough number of discoid lupus erythematosus cases is studied it appears some will show a significant rise in total globulins and/or gamma ("immune") globulin, among other changes in the electrophoretic pattern. Since these changes are similar albeit not as distinct or as constant as in the systemic form they suggest a common immuno-pathologic basis for the two conditions.

δ) Chronic Biologic False Positive (C.B.F.P.) Reactions. The incidence of false positive serologic tests for syphilis in lupus erythematodes discoides varies considerably with different reports. The number and sensitivity of tests employed, the times repeated, the size of the group investigated and the criteria for the diagnosis of generalized (disseminated) lupus erythematodes versus systemic lupus erythematosus could account for this variance. The statistics are as follows: 0/12 (MARTEN and BLACKBURN), 0/77 (SCOTT and REES), 1/15 (BENNETT, OSMENT and HOLLEY), 4/38 (DUBOIS and MARTEL), 3/65 (ROTHFIELD and associates). This makes a total of 9/207 or 4%. REIN and KONSTANT reported 15% positives in chronic localized discoid lupus erythematosus and 18% in chronic disseminate lupus erythematodes, results parallel to those of MONTGOMERY and MCCREIGHT. Since the number of patients tested was not given in either of the papers they were not included in ascertaining the average. There also isolated reports of chronic biologic false positive reactions (MILLER et al.). In one group of controls 1/65 (ROTHFIELD et al.) gave a chronic biologic false positive reaction and in another 0/142 (SIEGEL et al.).

ε) Lupus Erythematodes-Test. Negative results in lupus erythematodes discoides were reported in three different papers totaling 119 cases (COHEN and CADMAN; SCOTT and REES; PETERSON and GOKCEN). A low incidence of positive reactions was found by others; 9/112 (BRUNSTING et al.), 3/65 (ROTHFIELD et al.), 2/15 (BENNETT et al.), in one of the latter there were symptoms suggestive of systemic lupus erythematosus; 11/66

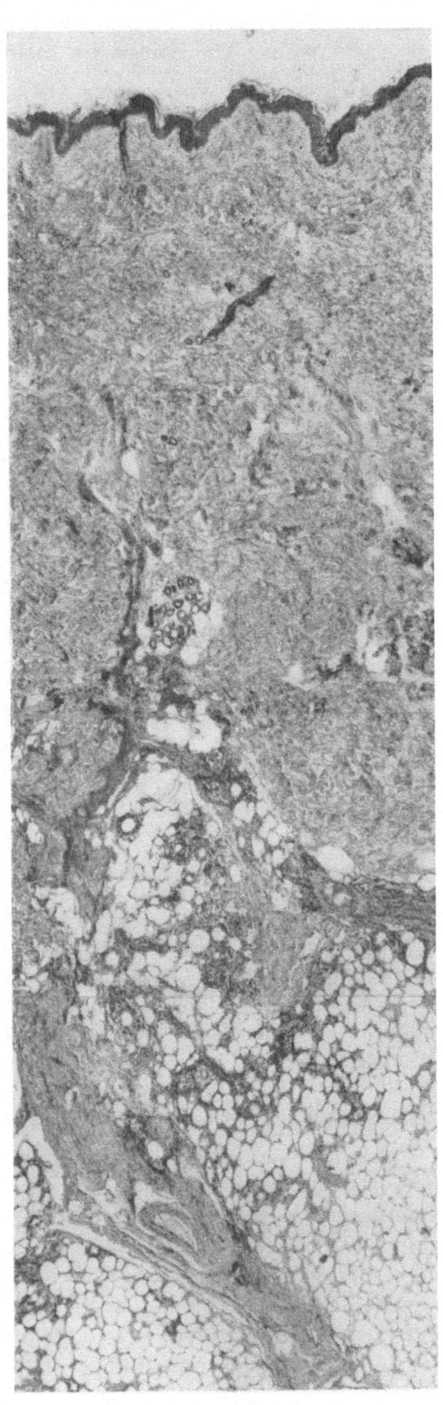

Fig. 14. This is a histologic section of a subcutaneous nodule located on the arm in the patient presented in Figs. 3—5. Except for livid erythema, there was no evidence of involvement of the overlying skin. Nevertheless hyperkeratinization and follicular plugging are seen in the epidermis and a sparse perivascular infiltrate in the cutis. A striking infiltrate composed of lymphocytes and histiocytes and marked thickening of the vessel walls with narrowing the lumen are seen in the subcutaneous tissue (Courtesy Drs. E. G. SCHIRREN and D. EGGERT)

(MARTEN and BLACKBURN) 3/38 (DUBOIS and MARTEL); 3/105 (PASCHER et al.). In two of the latter there were also symptoms suggestive of systemic lupus erythematosus. The composite incidence is 33/575 or 5%.

ζ) Fluorescent Antinuclear Antibodies. A search for these antibodies in lupus erythematodes discoides has been made by two independent groups of investigators in the past year. One group, WEIR et al., found antinuclear antibodies in 13 % of a series of 71 cases of chronic discoid lupus erythematosus while PETERSON and GOKCEN found a positive reaction in 28/34 (82%) patients tested. Technical

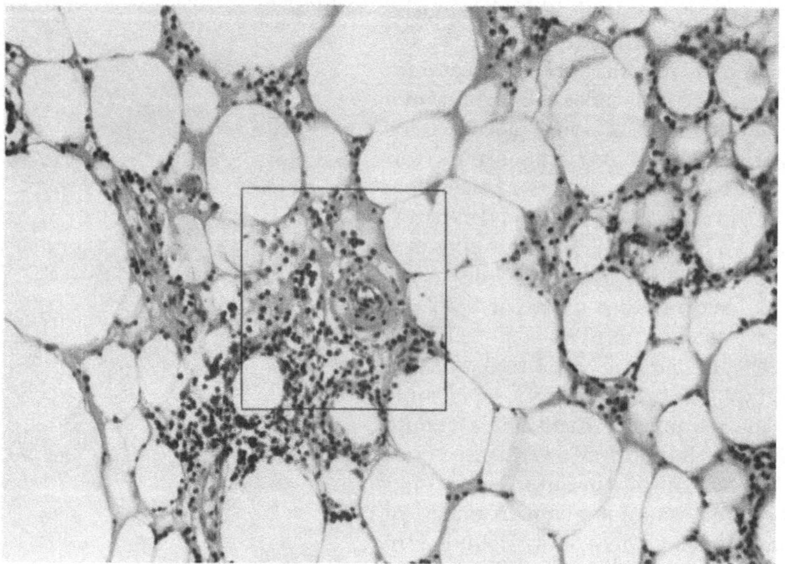

Fig. 15. Almost total obliteration of a vessel is found in an infiltrated area of the fat in Fig. 14

differences are probably responsible for the disparity in the results. It should be noted that positive fluorescence may at times be obtained in random sera (SIEGEL et al.) and not uncommonly in patients with rheumatoid arthritis (WIDELOCK et al.). Although this reaction is regarded as a sensitive indicator of the autoimmune process, it is not as specific as the lupus erythematodes test (WIDELOCK et al.).

d) Skin Test with Suspension of Homologous and Autologous Leukocytes

A delayed hypersensitive reaction to an intradermal suspension of leukocytes in systemic lupus erythematosus was first demonstrated by FRIEDMAN et al. and confirmed by BENNETT and HOLLEY. This test was later evaluated in subjects with a variety of conditions including chronic discoid lupus erythematosus and in controls (TROMOVITCH and MARCH). Ten out of 31 patients with discoid lupus erythematosus gave positive reactions. However a high incidence of positivity was also found in atopics, in leukemia and lymphoma, a lesser incidence in a variety of unrelated dermatoses and an occasionall positive among controls.

e) Miscellaneous Procedures

Objective signs of renal disease have been noted on rare occasions (SCOTT and REES; MONTGOMERY and MCCREIGHT; BENNETT et al.). The possibility of fortuitous involvement has to be considered in view of the duration of the disease and the age of many of the patients. Among the rare examples cited one could also take exception to the classification of some as discoid lupus erythematosus.

In the course of an electromyographic study O'LEARY et al. found 2/4 patients with generalized discoid lupus erythematosus who showed a pattern similar to systemic lupus erythematosus.

f) Capillary Microscopy

LAWLER and LUMPKIN as well as DAVIS and LAWLER before them demonstrated a marked decrease in the number of capillaries, 50% or more, in the unaffected as well as the affected skin of the forearm in patients with chronic discoid lupus erythematosus. "Damage" to small vessels in their opinion was equally severe in both forms of lupus erythematodes and at times marked even in the absence of lesions.

g) Plethysmography of Digital Blood Flow

HUFF et al. found abnormalities indicative of a defective circulation in 11 cases of chronic discoid lupus erythematosus and in 1 case of chronic disseminated lupus erythematosus. Since similar changes were noted in individuals with arteriosclerosis, hypertension and pseudoxanthoma elasticum, the findings cannot be considered specific. Moreover, FARBER and his associates were not able to demonstrate any alteration in the digital blood flow rates either under normal conditions or in response to local ischemia in subjects with discoid or systemic lupus erythematosus.

9. Course and Prognosis

The clinical manifestations of lupus erythematodes discoides, whether one refers to the fixed or generalized form, usually remain localized to the skin. It is estimated that approximately 5—10% of discoid cases may convert to the systemic form either spontaneously or more often following excessive exposure to sun or cold. In such instances it is possible for the systemic disease to revert back to the discoid form. According to JADASSOHN the chances of this favorable turn taking place are better than if the condition had been one of systemic lupus erythematosus from the beginning. Whether or not patients with the generalized form of lupus erythematodes discoides are more prone to develop systemic lupus erythematosus than those with the localized type remains unsettled.

Lupus erythematodes discoides may persist for decades. Spontaneous remissions are possible; more often they are brought about by appropriate therapy. Such an induced remission may last five years or longer (SCOTT and REES). The dermatosis is generally compatible with good health and most patients go through life without developing systemic manifestations. Nevertheless, many clinicians feel the prognosis should be guarded and that the danger of dissemination should always be borne in mind. COCHRANE may be correct in believing a high erythrocyte sedimentation rate is indicative of impending dissemination. WILSON and JORDAN are more inclined to consider leukopenia a danger signal.

Fixed lesions tend to go on to atrophy, scarring and unsightly depigmentation or hyperpigmentation. When the scalp is involved a cicatrizing alopecia may ensue (LAYMON). The outcome, to a certain if not large extent depends on adequate treatment.

10. Diagnosis

The diagnosis can readily be made on clinical grounds in most instances. Doubtful cases can sometimes be resolved by careful inspection of the scalp where a typical plaque is readily concealed by hair. At times it may be difficult to categorize a particular case as discoid lupus erythematosus or systemic lupus erythematosus because of transitions between the two. Absence of significant general or visceral symptoms, a negative lupus erythematodes test, a negative serologic test for syphilis, serum protein values within normal limits, a normal blood count and negative findings on urinalysis would mitigate against systemic involvement. Since it may take several weeks for the characteristic histologic picture of discoid lupus erythematosus to develop, biopsy of an early lesion is not always helpful (Montgomery).

11. Differential Diagnosis

The conditions to be entertained in the differential diagnosis depend on the number and character of the lesions, their localizations and distribution.

a) Chronic Polymorphous Light Eruptions

Papular and eczematous reactions are not likely to be confused with lupus erythematodes discoides. Plaque-like reactions referred to as the erythematoid type (Wolf), or as erythema perstans solare (Lamb) or erythematodes-like photodermatosis (Keining) on the other hand may simulate lupus erythematodes discoides. Light eruptions are much more likely to be strictly seasonal in occurrence, appearing in the spring and healing spontaneously in the fall. They can be elicted as a rule by an adequate exposure to sunlight and the covered areas are spared. Lupus erythematodes-like light eruptions moreover appear as circumscribed areas of edema with loose, lamellar scales that involute without permanent sequelae (Weber). Lupus erythematodes discoides on the other hand, may appear or heal independent of season and its course is not necessarily influenced by sun-light. Discoid lesions furthermore are at times found on covered areas of the body. Moreover, induration, adherent scales, follicular plugs and permanent sequelae are characteristic of lupus erythematodes discoides. Cahn et al. pointed out that light sensitivity of the polymorphic type may be the prodromal stage of lupus erythematodes. The author can cite a case in which photosensitivity antedated the development of discoid lupus erythematosus by 13 years (Fig. 8). The consensus is that the histologic picture of an early discoid lesion and an erythematodes-like photodermatitis is indistinguishable.

b) Lymphocytic Infiltration of the Skin (Jessner-Kanof)

In contradistinction to discoid lupus erythematosus these lesions are smooth and show no follicular plugging. As they expand they tend to clear in the center without sequelae. Although well circumscribed, the plaques of infiltration are irregular in shape rather than disc-like. Lymphocytic infiltrations may heal spontaneously and they have been known to respond to a wide variety of agents e.g. penicillin, arsenicals, sulfapyridine, roentgen radiation and antimalarials (Jessner and Kanof). The histologic picture in lymphocytic infiltration is of a non-specific type that may be seen in a variety of dermatoses (Gottlieb and Winkelmann) in contrast to discoid lesions which have a characteristic histologic pattern.

c) Cicatrizing Alopecias of the Scalp

Lichen plano-pilaris, folliculitis decalvans, pseudopalade of BROCQ and favus have to be considered (LAYMON). Follicular hyperkeratosis tends to be irregular and patchy in lichen planopilaris, more regular or rounded in lupus erythematodes discoides. Inspection of the mucous membranes and glabrous skin will often disclose corroborative evidence of one or the other diagnosis. Folliculitis decalvans is characterized by the presence of follicular pustules at the periphery of a circumscribed area of expanding alopecia. FAVUS may be distinguished by a search for achorion Schoenleini. Involvement of the nails, not uncommon in favus, is most uncommon in lupus erythematodes discoides. Tinea tonsurans may also be confused with discoid lupus erythematosus of the scalp (HOWELL et al.).

d) Congenital Teleangiectatic Erythema Resembling Lupus Erythematodes in Dwarfs (Bloom's Syndrome)

This is a rare disorder characterized by telangiectatic lesions over the nose and malar areas, photosensitivity and dwarfism (KATZENELLENBOGEN and LARON). Some of the cases were mistaken for lupus erythematodes until BLOOM recognized the congenital nature of the disorder. Awareness of this syndrome should be sufficient to make the diagnosis clear.

e) Subcutaneous Nodules

Subcutaneous nodules in rheumatic fever and rheumatoid arthritis are usually distributed over the extensor aspect of the elbow and knee joints. In lupus erythematodes profundus they are found over the deltoid regions, thighs and buttocks. It is usually possible to demonstrate microscopic or macroscopic evidence of lupus erythematodes in the skin overlying the nodules or discoid lesions elsewhere on the body or scalp in discoid lupus erythematosus.

f) Relapsing Febrile Non-Suppurative Panniculitis (WEBER-CHRISTIAN)

Large shallow or deeper cup-like scars attributable to the inflammatory changes in the fat are features of both lupus erythematodes profundus and WEBER-CHRISTIAN's disease. The scars are symmetrically distributed in the latter and irregularly scattered in the former. Typical discoid lesions of the glabrous skin or the scalp and histologic features of lupus erythematodes can usually be demonstrated in the skin overlying the panniculitis in lupus erythematodes profundus.

g) Miscellaneous Conditions

Acne rosacea, seborrheic dermatitis, psoriasis, Boeck sarcoid, superficial basal cell epithelioma and actinic dermatitis may at times be simulated, depending on whether the discoid lesions are single or multiple, typical or atypical. The fact that the term seborrheic congestiva (HEBRA) was used at one time for lupus erythematodes shows how well seborrheic dermatitis may be mimiked. In some cases a biopsy will make the differential diagnosis clear. In others a period of observation may be necessary.

12. Treatment

a) General Management

Patients should be cautioned against overexposure to sunlight and cold. Titanium dioxide added to a shake lotion or a cream and/or para-aminobenzoic acid in concentrations of 10—15% in alcohol, petrolatum or a water-soluble cream make effective sunscreens. Surgical procedures can usually be carried out with impunity and pregnancy rarely has an adverse effect on the course of the lesions.

b) Antimalarials

The consensus is that the antimalarials, despite some limitations and side effects are the drugs of choice for chronic discoid lupus erythematosus (MERWIN and WINKELMANN; Medical Letter on Drugs and Therapeutics). Chloroquine phosphate (aralen, nivaquine B, sonoquine, resochin, resoquine, 'SN-7618') and hydroxchloroquine sulfate (plaquenil-Winthrop) are generally well tolerated and the most widely used. Antimalarials suppress but do not cure the disease. The relapse rate however is high upon discontinuance of these agents (MERWIN and WINKELMANN) and toxic effects are far from negligible. Despite these drawbacks they nevertheless surpass gold salts, arsenic and bismuth.

Some patients respond better to one antimalarial than another or they may respond differently at different times to the same drug. Some physicians favor the continuance of a minimal effective maintenace dose whereas others discontinue the drug a month or two after suppression has been achieved. The latter practice appears preferable since maintenance therapy does not insure against a relapse. Moreover, it has been shown that the effects may be cumulative (Medical Letter). It is estimated blood and tissue levels reach a peak about four months after therapy has been initiated and may persist for weeks and months after therapy has been stopped (Medical Letter 1960). Whether or not antimalarials in combination e.g. triquin (WINTHROP) a mixture of quinacrine, chloroquine and hydroxychloroquine have a synergistic effect or a reduced potential for evoking undesirable effects, since a smaller amound of each drug than is otherwise used is still uncerain (TYE et al.).

α) The Mode of Action is unknown despite more than three decades of use. Light filtration, inhibition of antibody formation and a non-specific anti-inflammatory effect are among the hypotheses proposed. It is now generally accepted that these drugs do not act as sun-screens. DUBOIS (1954) has shown that adequate concentrations of quinacrine can block the lupus erythematodes phenomemon in vitro. This may be related to the fact that quinacrine prevents the absorption of the lupus erythematodes serum factor by the leukocytes (HOLMAN and KUNKEL). Hydralazine (apresoline) on the other hand, which bears some resemblence to quinacrine in chemical structure may elicit the lupus erythematodes syndrome including a positive lupus erythematodes test (PERRY and SCHROEDER). Thus it appears drugs with a quinolone structure are in some way related or connected with the "autoimmune process" which is held by many to day to be the pathogenetic mechanism in systemic lupus erythematosus. Only time and continued research can clarify the situation. There is no doubt that the 4-aminoquinolines have an antiphlogistic effect but through what channels this action is mediated remains obscure.

β) Side Effects (MERWIN and WINKELMANN; MEYLER; Medical Letter). Anorexia, nausea, vomiting, loss of weight, dizziness, palpitation and tinnitus are among the general reactions common to all. These symptoms subside when the drugs are discontinued. Fever and an elevated sedimentation rate have also been linked with quinacrine (atabrine, mepacrine). Arthralgia, myalgia and amenorrhoea have followed the use of amodiaquine (camoquine, flavoquine, camoquinal, SN-'10—751').

The *cutaneous* side-effects are diverse. Disturbances in pigmentation resulting in yellow, brown, gray and blue-gray discoloration of the skin, oral mucosa, nails and subungual tissues are common to all the antimalarials (MAGUIRE; DUPERRAT and GOETSCHEL; FORMAN). The cause of the melanosis is not entirely clear. Loss of pigment with the development of blond or white hairs is not unusual after approximately three months of chloroquine therapy. A wide variety of inflammatory reactions e.g. morbilliform, urticarial, erythema-multiforme-like reactions also have been described. More serious reactions, e.g. exfoliative dermatitis, alopecia and lichenoid dermatitis with anhidrosis have attended the administration of quinacrine.

Hematopoietic. Leukopenia may follow the administration of any of the antimalarials. Agranulocytosis, aplastic anemia, pancytopenia, thrombocytopenic purpura have been reported following the administration of quinacrine and amodiaquine (MEYLER, MERWIN and WINKELMANN; PERRY et al.). MAGUIRE found that the administration of 10 mg. of prednisolone together with amodiaquine prevented a marked leukopenia that previously accompanied the use of this drug. At least one case of thrombocytopenic purpura due to chloroquine has also been reported (MEYLER). The author can recall a case of acute hemolytic anemia early in the course of chloroquine therapy.

Hepatitis has been attributed to quinacrine (MEYLER; MERWIN and WINKELMANN). Acute porphyria and porphyrinuria have followed the administration of chloroquine (DAVIS and VAN DER PLOEG; LINDEN et al.; MARSDEN). Paradoxically there is a report of a case of porphyria cutanea tarda successfully treated with chloroquine.

Ocular Effects. Diplopia, blurring of vision, colored halos about lights, corneal opacities are reversable symptoms that may be elicited by these drugs (MERWIN and WINKELMANN; MEYLER). *The dreaded although uncommon complication is retinopathy* (MERWIN and WINKELMANN; Medical Letter, MEYLER). Most cases have occurred after chloroquine 0.5—0.75 gm. has been taken daily for a year or more (Medical Letter). Hydroxychloroquine sulfate has thus far been incriminated in only one case. Since the latter has not been used as widely or as long as chloroquine phosphate, it is too early to say it is safer (Medical Letter).

The signs of retinal damage are impaired central vision (pericentral scotomas), peripheral constriction of the visual fields, marked attenuation of the retinal vessels, pigmentary changes of the macula and peripheral pigmentary change. Twenty-seven cases have been reported to date. *Loss if vision is irreversible and may be progressive* even after the drug is discontinued (HOBBS et al.; OKUN et al.; J. L. SMITH). Ophthalmological examination is therefore considered mandatory before treatment is started and at periodic intervals during the course of treatment (Medical Letter), since *Chloroquine Retinopathy may be Asymptomatic Until Loss of Vision Sets in.*

γ) Contraindications to Antimalarial Therapy. Hepatic disease, alcoholism and psoriasis are the major conditions to be considered (SCHOCH). Since the antimalarials are potentially hepatotoxic and high concentrations of the drug have been demonstrated in the livers of experimental animals (GOODMAN and GILMAN), these drugs should be administered with caution if at all in the presence of impaired liver function. The reasoning is the same for alcoholism because of its deleterious effect on hepatic tissue. The danger of exfoliative dermatitis as a consequence of antimalarial therapy in psoriasis is well documented (MERWIN and WINKELMANN).

δ) Mode of Administration. The average dose is two or three tablets orally daily of the selected antimalarial, but individual requirements may vary. Intralesional injections of chloroquine dihydrochloride 50 mg./ml. (WINTHROP) are generally reserved for resistant plaques. A detailed account of the technic used is available (PELZIG et al.). The latter found that injections of this drug were followed in several hours by slight to considerable swelling depending on the size or activity of the lesion. In no instance was there any lasting untoward effect. The response however was not uniform; some lesions resolved, others improved considerably but some were unchanged. EVERETT and COFFEY also found intradermal chloroquine an effective remedy.

ε) Antimalarials Compared with Corticosteroids. Antimalarials are generally more effective than the corticosteroids. The consensus is corticosteroid therapy if used at all should be reserved for cases of generalized or widespread chronic discoid lupus erythematosus that prove refractory to antimalarial therapy or for patients who tolerate antimalarial therapy poorly. The combination of chloroquine and steroids has been recommended for resistant lesions (ALEXANDER and COWAN).

A number of observers have found the intralesional injection of triamcinolone more effective than chloroquine administered in this manner (FERGUSON-SMITH; ROWELL). Approximately 0.1 cc of 10 mg./ml. per centimeter of affected skin is injected with a fine hypodermic needle and tuberculin syringe. This may be repeated a number of times at weekly intervals.

ζ) Chloroquine Compared with Gold Salts. CRISSEY and MURRAY compared the effectiveness of chloroquine orally with gold sodium thiosulfate intravenously. They found the recurrence rate to be much higher with chloroquine but this was off-set by the superior rate of action of chloroquine in bringing about suppression and by the ease of administration.

c) Treatment with Heavy Metals

Prior to the development of antimalarial therapy, the heavy metals, gold (VEIEL) and bismuth salts in particular, were formost in the dermotologist's armamentarium. Gold sodium thiosulfate, Solganol B, bismuth subsalicylate and bismuth sodium triglycollamate (Bistrimate) were the preparations of choice (PASCHER et al.; SAWICKY; PASCHER). It might be well not to lose sight entirely of these preparations lest adverse effects still unknown come to the fore with long term antimalarial therapy. It should be remembered that the danger of irreversible retinopathy eventuating in partial or total blindness was not appreciated until the antimalarials had been used extensively for ten years or more.

d) Miscellaneous

Pantothenic acid combined with Vitamin E, nicotinic acid, sodium para-amino-benzoate, oxyphenarsine, triple sulfonamides, antibiotics have been advocated by some but have been found wanting by most.

e) Surgical Procedures and Cauterizing Agents

An attempt has been made to remove the scars resulting from chronic discoid lupus erythematosus by plastic surgery but the results generally have been unsatisfactory (CORNBLETT et al.; CHARGIN). Solid carbon dioxide is sometimes used to reduce residual foci of infiltration. This modality has been replaced to a great extent by intralesional therapy with triamcinolone or chloroquine.

References

ALEXANDER, S., and M. A. COWAN: The treatment of chronic discoid lupus erythematosus with a combination of antimalarial and corticosteroid drugs. Brit. J. Derm. **73**, 359 (1961). — ALLENDE, M. F.: Lupus erythematosus, discoid and systemic: One disease. Postgrad. Med. **20**, 254 (1956). — ANDREEV, V., R. RAITSCHEV and A. STOJANOV: Lupus erythematodes und Krebs der Haut. Derm. Wschr. **144**, 823 (1961). — ANDREWS, G. C.: Diseases of the skin, 4th ed. Philadelphia: W. B. Saunders Company 1954. — ARNDT, H.: Blutbildveränderungen beim Lupus erythematodes, insbesondere der chronischen Form. Z. ges. inn. Med. **14**, 280 (1959). — ARNOLD jr., H. L.: Lupus erythematosus profundus (Kaposi-Irgang). Arch. Derm. Syph. (Chic.) **57**, 196 (1948).

BECHET, P. E.: Lupus erythematosus hypertrophicus et profundus. Arch. Derm. Syph. (Chic.) **45**, 33 (1942). — Lupus erythematosus hypertrophicus et profundus. A further attempt to elucidate its status. Arch. Derm. Syph. (Chic.) **61**, 495 (1950). — BECKETT, A. G., and J. G. LEWIS: Familial lupus erythematosus: A report of two cases. Brit. J. Derm. **71**, 360 (1959). — BENNETT, J. C., and H. L. HOLLEY: Intradermal sensitivity in systemic lupus erythematosus. Arthr. and Rheum. **4**, 64 (1961). — BENNETT, J. C., L. S. OSMENT and H. L. HOLLEY: Immunologic manifestations of a group of patients with a diagnosis of discoid lupus Erythematosus. Arthr. and Rheum. **4**, 490 (1961). — BETTLEY, F. R., and F. PAGE: The effect of mepacrine on light sensitivity in lupus erythematosus. Brit. J. Derm. **66**, 287 (1954). — BLOOM, D.: Congenital telangiectatic erythema resembling lupus erythematosus in dwarfs. J. Dis. Child. 88, 754 (1954). — Lupus erythematosus bullosus. Arch. Derm. **73**, 290 (1956). — BOLLIER, R., et F. PELBOIS: Aspects du lupus érythémateux au maroc, Etude de 274 cas. Bull. Soc. franç. Derm. Syph. **68**/2, 274 (1961). — BRAUNSTEINER, H.: The physiology and pathology of leukocytes. Translated by D. ZUCKER-FRANKLIN, chap. XIII by P. MIESCHER, p. 244. New York and London: Grune & Stratton 1962. — BRAVERMAN, I., M. L. T. JOHNSON, A. B. LERNER, A. ELBERT and H. S. M. UHL: Recognition and management of lupus erythematosus. Lippincot's Medical Science (Philad.) **9**, 749 (1961). — BRUNJES, S., K. ZIKE and R. JULIAN: Familial systemic lupus erythematosus. A review of the literature with a report of 10 additional cases in four families. Amer. J. Med. **30**, 529 (1961). — BRUNSTING, L. A., J. M. STICKNEY, G. L. PEASE and W. B. REED: The clinical significance of the lupus erythematosus clot test. Arch. Derm. **73**, 307 (1956). — BUCHHOLZ, A. M.: Chronic discoid lupus erythematosus occuring in three out of five members of one family. Arch. Derm. **78**, 281 (1958).

CAHN, M. M., E. J. LEVY, B. SHAFFER and H. BEERMAN: Lupus erythematosus and polymorphous light eruptions. J. invest. Derm. **21**, 375 (1953). — CALLOMON, F. T.: Neuere Arbeiten des amerikanischen Schrifttums. III. Lupus erythematodes. Hautarzt **9**, 433 (1958). — CANNON, E. F., and A. C. CURTIS: A survey of lupus erythematosus in the University of Michigan Hospital Since 1918. Arch. Derm. **78**, 196 (1958). — CARR, R. D., and R. LEVINE: Systemic lupus erythematosus of long duration. Arch. Derm. **81**, 427 (1960). — CECIL, R. L., and R. F. LOEB: A textbook of medicine, section on disseminated lupus erythematosus by GEORGE BAEHR, Philadelphia, 9th ed., p. 495. London: W. B. Saunders Company 1955. — CHARGIN, L.: Recurrence of lupus erythematosus in grafted skin. Arch. Derm. Syph. (Chic.) **61**, 532 (1950). — CHÓRAZAK, T.: Cryoglobulins in chronic lupus erythematosus. Acta derm.-venereol. (Stockh.) **38**, 322 (1958). — COCHRANE, T.: Early prognosis in Lupus erythematosus discoides. Arch. Derm. Syph. (Chic.) **63**, 323 (1951). — COHEN, H., and E. F. B. CADMAN: Natural history of lupus erythematosus and its modification by cortisone and corticotropin. Lancet **1953 II**, 305. — CORNBLETT, T., J. BARSKY and L. HOIT: Discoid lupus erythematosus scars treated by plastic surgery. Arch. Derm. **74**, 219 (1956). — COSTA, O. G., and M. A. JUNQUEIRA: Lupus erythemateux de Kaposi-Irgang. Ann. Derm. Syph. (Paris) **82**, 144 (1955). — CRAWFORD, G. M., and R. W. LEEPER: Diseases of the skin in pregnancy. Arch. Derm. Syph. (Chic.) **61**, 753 (1950). — CRISSEY, J. T., and P. F. MURRAY: A comparison of chloroquine and gold in the treatment of lupus erythematosus. Arch. Derm. **74**, 69 (1956). — CROSS, R. J.: Systemic lupus erythematosus combined Staff Clinic, discussion by D. LARSON. Amer. J. Med. **28**, 416 (1960).

DAVIS, M. J., and J. C. LAWLER: The capillary circulation of the skin. Arch. Derm. **77**, 690 (1958). — DAVIS, M. J., and D. E. VAN DER PLOEG: Acute porphyria and coproporphyrinuria following chloroquine therapy. Arch. Derm. **75**, 796 (1957). — DUBOIS, E. L.: Effect of the lupus erythematodes cell test on the clinical picture of systemic lupus erythematosus. Ann. intern. Med. **38**, 1265 (1953). — Simplified method for lupus erythematodes cell test. Arch. intern. Med. **92**, 168 (1953). — Quinacrine (atabrine) in treatment of systemic and discoid lupus erythematosus. Arch. intern. Med. **94**, 131 (1954). — DUBOIS, E. L., and S. MARTEL: Discoid lupus erythematosus, an analysis of its systemic manifestations. Ann. intern. Med. **44**, 482 (1956). — DUPERRAT, B., et G. GOETSCHEL: Pigmentation flavoquinique. Bull. Soc. franç. Derm. Syph. **66**, 151 (1959).

EPSTEIN, H. C., and J. Z. LITT: Discoid lupus erythematosus in a new born infant. New Engl. J. Med. **265**, 1106 (1961). — EVERETT, M. A., and C. M. COFFEY: Intradermal administration of chloroquine. Arch. Derm. **83**, 977 (1961).

FARBER, E., A. MORECI and R. SAGE: Digital blood flow rates in lupus erythematosus. Arch. Derm. **79**, 340 (1959). — FELDAKER, M., H. O. PERRY and D. G. HANLON: Dermatologic manifestations associated with cryoglobulinemia. Arch. Derm. **73**, 325 (1956). — FLEISCHMAJER, RAOL.: Personal communication. — FORMAN, L.: Discoid lupus erythematosus; pigmentation of nail beds following administration of amodiaquine hydrochloride. Proc. roy. Soc. Med. **53**, 563 (1960). — FRIEDMAN, E., W. BARDA, J. MERRILL and C. HANAN: Delayed cutaneous hypersensitivity to leukocytes in disseminated lupus erythematosus. New Engl. J. Med. **262**, 486 (1960).

GANOR, S., and F. SAGHER: Systemic lupus erythematoses changing to the chronic discoid type. Dermatologica (Basel) **125**, 81 (1962). — GARB, J.: Lupus erythematosus disseminatus with cryoglobulinemia. Arch. Derm. **78**, 772 (1958). — GARZÓN, R., L. FERRARI y C. CANCIO: Contribucion al estudio experimental del Lupus eritematos. Rev. argent. Dermatosif. **33**, 106 (1949). — GENTELE, H., B. LAGERHOLM and A. LODIN: Cryoglobulins in chronic discoid lupus erythematosus. Acta derm.-venereol. (Stockh.) **39**, 207 (1959). — GOLD, S.: Lupus erythematosus. Postgrad. med. J. **27**, 577 (1951). — Progress in the understanding of lupus erythematosus. Brit. J. Derm. **72**, 231 (1960). — GOLD, S. C., and W. F. GOWING: Systemic lupus erythematosus. A clinical and pathologic study. Quart. J. Med. **22**, 457 (1953). — GOODMAN, L. S., and A. GILMAN: The pharmacological basis of therapeutics, 2nd ed. New York: Macmillan, publisher 1956. — GOTTLIEB, B., and R. K. WINKELMANN: Lymphocytic infiltration of skin. Arch. Derm. **86**, 626 (1962). — GRACIANSKY, P. DE, and S. BOULLE: Color atlas of dermatology. Translation and adaptation by M. B. SULZBERGER and S. DOBKEVITCH-MORRELL. Chicago: Year Book Publishers 1955. — GRUENHAGEN, H. V.: Erythematodes chronicus bei eineiigen Zwillingen. Derm. Wschr. **126**, 1089 (1952). — GUIMARES, N. A.: Contribucion al estudio de las lesiones hypodermicas del lupus eritematoso. Hospital (Rio de J.) **55** (1), 43 (1959).

HARBER, L. C., R. M. HOLLOWAY and M. MORAGNE: Polymorphous light eruptions-office diagnosis and management. N.Y. St. J. Med. (in press). — HARVEY, A. M.: Auto-immune disease and the chronic biologic false positive test for syphilis. J. Amer. med. Ass. **182**, 513 (1962). — HARVEY, A. M., L. E. SHULMAN, P. A. TUMULTY, C. L. CONLEY and E. H. SCHOENRICH: Systemic lupus erythematosus. Review of the literature and chemical analysis of 138 cases. Medicine (Baltimore) **33**, 291 (1954). — HASERICK, J. R.: Modern concepts of Systemic lupus erythematosus. J. chron. Dis. **1**, 317 (1955). — Personal communication. — HASERICK, J. R., and R. E. KELLUM: Primer for patients with lupus erythematosus. Dept. of Derm., Cleveland Clinic Foundation, Cleveland, Ohio 1962. — HERRMANN, W. P., and K. H. SCHULZ: Immunoelectrophoretic studies of patients with skin diseases. II. Lupus erythematosus, dermatomyositis, scleroderma. Arch. klin. exp. Derm. **212**, 246 (1961). — HOBBS, H. E., A. SORSBY and A. FREEDMAN: Retinopathy following chloroquine therapy. Lancet **1959 II**, 478. — HOLLANDER, L., and F. J. KRUGH: Spontaneous absorption of ear lobes in discoid lupus erythematosus. Arch. Derm. Syph. (Chic.) **62**, 142 (1950). — HOLMAN, H. R., and H. R. DEICHER: The reaction of lupus erythematosus (L.E.) cell factor with deoxyribonucleoprotein of the cell nucleus. J. clin. Invest. **38**, 2059 (1959). — HOLMAN, H. R., and H. G. KUNKEL: Affinity between the lupus erythematosus serum factor and cell nuclei and nucleoprotein. Science **126**, 162 (1957). — HOLTZMAN, I. N.: Chronic discoid lupus erythematosus complicated by superimposed squamous cell epithelioma. Arch. Derm. Syph. (Chic.) **68**, 209 (1953). — HOWELL, J. B., J. W. WILSON and M. R. CARO: Tinea capitis caused by trichophyton tonsuraus. Arch. Derm. Syph. (Chic.) **65**, 194 (1952). — HUFF, S. E., H. L. TAYLOR and A. KEYS: Observations on the peripheral blood in chronic discoid lupus erythematosus. J. invest. Derm. **14**, 21 (1950).

IRGANG, S.: Lupus erythematosus profundus. Report of an example with clinical resemblance to Darier-Roussy sarcoid. Arch. Derm. Syph. (Chic.) **42**, 97 (1940). — Lupus erythematosus papularis and nodularis. Dermatologica (Basel) **119** (2), 79 (1958).

JACOBSON, F. W., and H. ANNAMUNTHODO: Squamous cell carcinoma arising in discoid lupus erythematosus. Dermatologica (Basel) **117**, 455 (1958). — JADASSOHN, J.: Cited by VEIEL. Lupus erythematodes (Cazenave). In: Handbuch der Haut- und Geschlechts-Krankheiten, Bd. X/1, S. 687. Berlin: Springer 1931. — JESSAR, R. A., R. W. LAMONT-HAVERS and C. RAGAN: Natural history of lupus erythematosus disseminatus. Ann. intern. Med. **38**, 717 (1953). — JESSNER, M., and N. B. KANOF: Lymphocytic infiltration of the skin. Arch. Derm. Syph. (Chic.) **68**, 447 (1953). — JOHNSON, WAYNE C.: Personal communication.

KADYROVA, M. M.: Kronicheskaia aritematoznaia volchanka po dannym Kliniki Kozhnykh i Venericheskikh Bolezney I Leningradskogo Meditsinskogo Instituta. Vestn. Derm. Vener. **32** (2), 80 (1958). — KATZENELLENBOGEN, I., and Z. LARON: A contribution to Bloom's syndrome. Arch. Derm. **82**, 609 (1960). — KERN, A. B., and B. L. SCHIFF: Discoid lupus erythematosus following trauma: Report of case and analysis of questionnaire. Arch. Derm. **75**, 685 (1957). — KESTEN, B. M.: Photosensitivity in various dermatoses. Lupus erythematosus, urticaria due to light and polymorphic light eruptions. Arch. Derm. **74**, 40 (1956). — KESTEN, B. M., and M. SLATKIN: Diseases related to light sensitivity. Arch. Derm. Syph. (Chic.) **67**, 284 (1953). — KIERLAND, R. R.: Classification and cutaneous manifestations of lupus erythematodes. Proc. Mayo Clin. **15**, 675 (1940). — KING-SMITH, D.: External irritation as a factor in the causation of lupus erythematosus discoides. Arch. Derm. Syph. (Chic.) **14**, 547 (1926). — KLAUDER, J. V.: The interrelationship of some cutaneous and ocular diseases. Arch. Derm. **80**, 515 (1959). — KLAUDER, J. V., and P. DELONG: Lupus erythematosus of the conjunctiva, eyelids and lid margins. Arch. Ophthal. **7**, 856 (1932). — KOGOJ, F.: Bullous variety of discoid lupus erythematosus. Dermatologica (Basel) **117**, 325 (1958). — KUSNIRUK, W.: Systemic involvement in chronic lupus erythematosus. Canad. med. Ass. J. **76**, 184 (1957).

LAMB, J. H., C. J. YOUNG and C. KEATY: Therapy of chronic and acute lupus erythematosus. Postgrad. Med. **10**, 182 (1951). — LARSON, D. L.: Systemic lupus erythematosus, 1st ed. Boston: Little, Brown, publisher 1962. — LAWLER, J. C., and L. R. LUMPKIN: Cutaneous capillary changes in lupus erythematosus. Arch. Derm. **83**, 636 (1961). — LAYMON, C. W.: Lesions of the scalp in certain scalp dermatoses. A histologic study. Arch. Derm. Syph. (Chic.) **62**, 181 (1950). — LELIS, I. I.: K voprosu o khronicheskoy forme sistomoy krasnoy volchanki i tsentrobezhnoy eritemy. Vestn. Derm. Vener. **36**/**1**, 13 (1962). — LERNER, A. B., and C. J. WATSON: Studies on cryoglobulins. Unusual purpura associated with high concentration and cryoglobulin. Amer. J. med. Sci. **214**, 510 (1947). — LINDEN, I. H., C. G. STEFFEN, V. D. NEWCOME and M. CHAPMAN: Development of porphyria during chloroquine therapy for chronic discoid lupus erythematosus. Calif. Med. **81**, 235 (1954). — LONDON, I. D.: Porphyria cutanea tarda. Report of a case successfully treated with chloroquine. Arch. Derm. **75**, 712 (1957).

MAGNUS, I.: Cited by S. GOLD, Progress in the understanding of lupus erythematosus. Brit. J. Derm. **72**, 231 (1960). — MAGUIRE, A.: Amodiaquine hydrochloride in the treatment of chronic discoid lupus erythematosus. Lancet **1962** (I), 665. — Amodiaquine hydrochloride. Corneal deposits and pigmented palate and nails after treatment of chronic discoid lupus erythematosus. Lancet **1962** (I), 667. — MARSDEN, C. W.: Porphyria during chloroquine therapy. Brit. J. Derm. **71**, 223 (1959). — MARTEN, R. H., and E. K. BLACKBURN: Lupus erythematosus. Clinical and hematologic studies in 77 cases. Arch. Derm. **73**, 1 (1956). — MCCHESNEY, E. W., F. C. NACHOD and M. L. TAINTER: Rationale for the treatment of lupus erythematosus with antimalarials. J. invest. Derm. **29**, 97 (1957). — MCCREIGHT, W. G., and H. MONTGOMERY: Cutaneous change in lupus erythematosus. Arch. Derm. Syph. (Chic.) **61**, 1 (1950). — MCCUISTION, C. H., and E. P. SCHOCH: Possible discoid lupus erythematosus in a newborn infant. Report of a case with subsequent development of acute systemic lupus erythematosus in the mother. Arch. Derm. Syph. (Chic.) **70**, 782 (1954). — *Medical Letter on Drugs and Therapeutics:* Aralen, and plaquenil, published by Drug and Therapeutic Information, New York **4**, 6 (1960). — Aralen, plaquenil and retinopathy, published by Drug and Therapeutic Information, New York **4**, 103 (1962). — MERWIN, C. F., and R. K. WINKELMANN: Antimalarial drugs in the therapy of lupus erythematosus. Proc. Mayo Clin. **37**, 253 (1962). — MEYLER, L.: Side effects of drugs, unwanted effects of drugs as reported in the Medical Literature of the World. Amsterdam-London-New York: The Excerpta Medica Foundation 1960. — MICHELSON, H. E.: The boundaries of dermatology. Arch. Derm. Syph. (Chic.) **65**, 1 (1952). — Review and appraisal of present knowledge concerning lupus erythematosus. Arch. Derm. Syph. (Chic.) **69**, 694 (1954). — MILLER, J. L., M. BRODEY and J. H. HILL: Studies on the significance of biologic false positive reactions. J. Amer. med. Ass. **164**, 1461 (1957). — MONTGOMERY, H.: Pathology of lupus erythematosus. J. invest. Derm. **2**, 343 (1939). — MONTGOMERY, H., and W. G. MCCREIGHT: Disseminated lupus erythematosus. Arch. Derm. Syph. (Chic.) **60**, 356 (1949).

NAGY, E., u. A. LÖVEY: A Lupus erythematosus es tuberculosis kapcsolata. Bőrgyőgy. vener. Szle **12**, 241 (1958). — NELSON, C. T.: Chronic discoid lupus erythematosus with lupus erythematodes profundus, possible involvement of the parotid gland. Arch. Derm. **78**, 814 (1957).

OKUN, E., P. GOURAS, H. BERNSTEIN and L. VON SALLMANN: Chloroquine retinopathy. Arch. Ophthal. **69**, 59 (1963). — O'LEARY, P. A.: Disseminated lupus erythematosus. Minn. Med. **17**, 637 (1934). — O'LEARY, P. A., E. A. LAMBERT and G. P. SAYRE: Muscle studies in cutaneous disease. J. invest. Derm. **24**, 301 (1955). — OLSSON, K.: Lupus erythematosus profundus (Kaposi-Irgang). Acta derm.-venereol. (Stockh.) **37**, 306 (1957). — ORFUSS, A. J.: Lupus erythematosus in a Chinese. Discussed by F. REISS. Arch. Derm. Syph. (Chic.) **67**, 219 (1953). — Personal communication.

PASCHER, F.: Treatment of lupus erythematosus with calciferol, antibiotics and gold preparations. Arch. Derm. Syph. (Chic.) **61**, 909 (1950). — Lupus erythematosus. Med. Clin.

N. Amer. **43**, 917 (1959). — Pascher, F., A. Borota and B. Davis: Pitfalls in interpretation of lupus erythematosus preparations. J. invest. Derm. **24**, 311 (1955). — Pascher, F., H. H. Sawicky, M. G. Silverberg and R. Emmett: Assay I: Bistrimate for lupus erythematosus, lichen planus and other dermatoses. J. invest. Derm. **10**, 441 (1948). — Pascher, F., C. F. Sims and N. Pensky: Lupus erythematosus profundus (Kaposi-Irgang). Report of a case including a comparative study of the histopathology with that of chronic discoid lupus erythematosus. J. invest. Derm. **25**, 347 (1955). — Pautrier, L. M.: A propos du Pseudo-Lupus erythemateux profond (Kaposi-Irgang). Ann. Derm. Syph. (Paris) **80**, 233 (1953). — Peck, S. M.: Cosmetic repair (surgical) of lupus erythematosus hypertrophicus et profundus. Arch. Derm. Syph. (Chic.) **60**, 839 (1949). — Pelzig, A., V. H. Witten and M. B. Sulzberger: Chloroquine for chronic discoid lupus erythematosus (intralesional injections). Arch. Derm. **83**, 146 (1961). — Perry, H. M., and H. A. Schroeder: Syndrome simulating collagen disease caused by hydralazine (apresoline). J. Amer. med. Ass. **154**, 670 (1954). — Perry, H. O., L. G. Bartholomew and D. G. Hanlon: Nearly fatal reaction to amodiaquine. J. Amer. med. Ass. **179**, 599 (1962). — Peterson, W. C., and M. Gokcen: Antinuclear factor in chronic discoid lupus erythematosus. Arch. Derm. **86**, 783 (1962). — Prunièras, M., and H. Montgomery: Histopathology of cutaneous lesions in systemic lupus erythematodes. Arch. Derm. **74**, 177 (1956).

Quiroga, M. I., y A. M. Mom: Fotosensibilizacion en el Lupus eritematoso experimental. Rev. argent. Dermatosif. **31**, 386 (1947).

Rakhmanov, V. A., i O. L. Ivanov: Gistokhimicheskie issledovaniia soedinitelnoy tkani kozhi pri khronicheskoy krasnoy volchanke. Vestn. Derm. Vener. **36** (7), 23 (1962). — Reiches, A. J.: The lupus erythematosus syndrome. The relationship of discoid lupus erythematosus (cutaneous) to systemic (disseminated) lupus erythematosus. Ann. intern. Med. **46/2**, 678 (1957). — Rein, C. R., and G. H. Kostant: Lupus erythematosus: Serological and chemical aspects. Arch. Derm. Syph. (Chic.) **61**, 898 (1950). — Rose, E., and D. M. Pillsbury: Acute disseminated lupus erythematosus. — A systemic disease. Ann. intern. Med. **12**, 951 (1939). — Rost, G. A.: Zur Pathogenese und Terminologie des Erythematodes. Münch. med. Wschr. **100**, 1021 (1958). — Rothfield, N., C. H. March, P. Meischer and C. McEwen: Chronic discoid lupus erythematosus. A Study 665 patients and 65 controls. New Engl. J. Med. **269**, 1155 (1963). — Rottier, P. B.: Cited by S. Gold, Progress in the understanding of lupus erythematosus. Brit. J. Derm. **72**, 321 (1960). — Rowell, N. R.: Treatment of chronic discoid lupus erythematosus with intralesional triamcinolone. Brit. J. Derm. **74**, 354 (1962).

Sapuppo: Cited by R. Gross, The Koebner phenomenon in its relationship to photosensibility. Arch. Derm. **74**, 43 (1956). — Sawicky H. H.: Therapy of lupus erythematosus. Bismuth sodium triglycollamate, sodium paraaminobenzoate and the tocopherols (Vitamin E). Arch. Derm. Syph. (Chic.) **61**, 909 (1950). — Schirren, C. G., and D. Eggert: Beitrag zum Erythemodes Profundus (Kaposi-Irgang). Arch. klin. exp. Derm. **5**, 216, 541 (1963). — Schoch jr., E. P.: Antimalarial drugs in lupus erythematosus and light sensitive eruptions. Tex. St. J. Med. **54**, 349 (1958). — Schuppener, H. J., and A. Borns: Simultaneous occurience of psoriasis vulgaris and lupus erythematosus. Derm. Wschr. **142**, 976 (1960). — Schwarz, J.: Carcinomentstehung in Lupus erythematodes chronicus. Z. Haut- u. Geschl.-Kr. **14**, 187 (1953). — Scott, A., and E. G. Rees: The relationship of systemic lupus erythematosus and discoid lupus erythematosus. A clinical and hematologic study. Arch. Derm. **79**, 422 (1959). — Shearn, M. A., and B. Pirofsky: Disseminated lupus erythematosus. Analysis of 34 cases. Arch. intern. Med. **90**, 790 (1952). — Siegel, M., S. L. Lee, D. Widelock, E. B. Reilly, G. J. Wise, S. B. Zingale and H. T. Fuerst: The epidemology of systemic lupus erythematosus: Preliminary results in New York City. J. chron. Dis. **15**, 131 (1962). — Silva, R. E., and H. Portugal: Cas de lupus erythemateux profond. Ann. Derm. Syph. (Paris) **82**, 34 (1955). — Sipos, K., u. G. Jákso: Untersuchungen über die tuberkularische Uhrempfindlichkeit beim Erythematodes chronicus. Derm. Wschr. **144**, 829 (1961). — Sklarz, E.: Tumorbildung auf Lupus Erythematodes. Z. Haut- u. Geschl.-Kr. **19**, 321 (1955). — Smith, J. F.: Intralesional triamcinolone as an adjunct to antimalarial drugs in the treatment of chronic discoid lupus erythematosus. Brit. J. Derm. **74**, 350 (1962). — Smith, J. L.: Chloroquine macular degeneration. Arch. Ophthal. **68**, 186 (1962). — Spencer, G. A.: Lupus erythematosus following burns from hydrochloric acid. Arch. Derm. Syph. (Chic.) **64**, 215 (1951). — Steagall, R. W., H. T. Ash and L. B. Fentanes: Familial lupus erythematosus. Arch. Derm. **85**, 394 (1962). — Storck, H.: Übersicht über Klinik, Pathogenese und Therapie des Lupus erythematodes. Schweiz. med. Wschr. **87** (2), 1057 (1957). — Storck, H., and S. Berzups: Über Lupus erythematodes unter besonderer Berücksichtigung des Übergangs von lokalisierten in generalisierte Formen. Dermatologica (Basel) **124**, 142 (1962). — Stoughton, R., and G. Wells: Histochemical study on polysaccharides in normal and diseased skin. J. invest. Derm. **14**, 37 (1950). — Suksta, A., and C. L. Conley: Some observations on lupus erythematodes cell. J. Lab. clin.

Med. **37**, 597 (1951). — Suschevskaya-Dmitrevskaya, K. K.: K etiologić i patogenezu krasnoi volchanki. Vestn. Derm. Vener. **32**, 21 (1958).

Thoma, K. H., and H. M. Goldman: Oral pathology, 5th ed. St. Louis: C. V. Mosby Comp. 1960. — Tramier, G.: Apropos des localisations du lupus érythemateux chronique et, en particulier, de la topographie au « Vespertilio ». Bull. Soc. franç. Derm. Syph. **65**, 144 (1958). — Tromovitch, T. A., and C. March: Intradermal tests with autologous white blood cells in chronic discoid lupus erythematosus, systemic lupus erythematosus and control subjects. J. invest. Derm. **37**, 345 (1961). — Tumulty, P. A.: The clinical course of systemic lupus erythematosus. J. Amer. med. Ass. **156**, 949 (1954). — Tye, N. J., H. White, B. Appel and B. Ansell: Lupus erythematosus treated with combination of quinacrine, hydroxychloroquine and chloroquine. New Engl. J. Med. **260**, 63 (1959).

Uhlmann, E., and G. Schambye: Lupus erythematosus and carcinom. Arch. Derm. Syph. (Berl.) **170**, 500 (1934).

Veiel, F.: Lupus erythematodes (Cazenave). In: Handbuch der Haut- und Geschlechtskrankheiten, Bd. X/1, S. 687. Berlin: Springer 1931. — Vilanova, X., C. Cardenal and J. M. Copdevila: Chronischer Lupus erythematodes der Conjunctiva. Dermatologica (Basel) **113**, 226 (1956).

Walker, S. A., and E. P. Benditt: The serum proteins in diseases of connective tissue; an electrophoretic study. J. invest. Derm. **14**, 113 (1950). — Weber, G.: Zur Klinik und Differentialdiagnose der Erythematodes-ähnlichen Lichtdermatose. Hautarzt **9**, 400 (1958). — Weir, D. M., E. J. Halborow and G. D. Johnson: A clinical study of serum antinuclear factors. Brit. med. J. **1961I**, 933. — Weiss, R., and S. Swift: The significance of a positive lupus erythematodes phenomen. Arch. Derm. **72**, 103 (1955). — Widelock, D., G. Gilbert, M. Siegel and S. Lee: Fluorescent antibody procedure for lupus erythematosus: Comparative use of nucleated erythrocytes and calf thymus cells. Amer. J. publ. Hlth **51**, 829 (1961). — Wilson, A. P., and J. W. Jordan: Relationship of chronic discoid and disseminated lupus erythematosus. N.Y. St. J. Med. **50**, 2449 (1950).

Young, K. L.: Lupus erythematosus with unusual changes in the fingertips and nails. Acta derm.-venereol. (Stockh.) **16**, 365 (1935).

Zeisler, E. P., and S. M. Bluefarb: Association of lupus erythematosus and thyrotoxicosis in brother and sister. Arch. Derm. Syph. (Chic.) **49**, 111 (1954). — Ziff, M., P. Esserman and C. McEwen: Observations on the course and treatment of systemic lupus erythematosus. Arthr. and Rheum. **1**, 332 (1958).

Der viscerale Lupus erythematodes*

Von

Peter A. Miescher, Robert T. McCluskey,**

Naomi F. Rothfield und Annatina Miescher-New York

Mit 14 Abbildungen (davon 7 farbige)

Definition

Als visceraler Erythematodes wird eine nicht infektiöse, nicht neoplastische, in Schüben verlaufende, generalisierte entzündliche Erkrankung unbekannter Ätiologie mit genetisch determinierter Prädisposition benannt, die praktisch jedes Organ befallen kann, und die mit einer Reihe abnormaler immunologischer Vorgänge einhergeht. Die klinischen Manifestationen sind mannigfaltig; folgende Symptome werden in den meisten Fällen festgestellt: intermittierendes Fieber, Arthritis, weniger regelmäßig nephritische Zeichen und Hauteruptionen. Im Blut treten im Verlauf der Krankheit antinucleare Sarumantikörper auf. Eine Vielfalt weiterer autoimmunitärer Vorgänge kommen vor, meistens ohne Organ- und Species-Spezifität. Pathologisch-anatomisch sind die sog. hämatoxyphilen Körperchen (alteriertes Nucleoprotein) pathognomonisch. Andere Gewebsveränderungen („wireloop" Nephritis, vasculäre „onion skin lesions", atypische verruköse Endokarditis, fibrinoide Degeneration) sind charakteristisch, ohne für den visceralen Lupus erythematodes pathognomonisch zu sein.

1. Geschichtliche Daten

In Hebras „Hautkrankheiten" (1845) findet sich die erste eindeutige Beschreibung der für den cutanen Lupus erythematodes typischen und später von Cazenave entsprechend benannter Hautläsionen. Hebra unterschied zwei Formen, die von Kaposi als discoider und disseminierter Lupus erythematodes bezeichnet wurden. Neben dieser „cutanen" Form der Krankheit beschrieb Kaposi 1872 erstmals eine mit Fieber und toxischen Manifestationen einhergehende Form, die er „Erysipelas perstans faciei" nannte. Die Beziehung dieser generalisierten Krankheit zum cutanen Lupus erythematodes wurde von Osler postuliert. Bemerkenswerterweise erwähnte Osler bereits maligne viscerale Verlaufsformen dieser Krankheit, die ohne Hauteruptionen verliefen (1895). Jadassohn beschrieb im Handbuch der Hautkrankheiten treffend die viscerale Verlaufsform des Lupus erythematodes unter besonderer Würdigung folgender Lokalisationen: Gelenke, seröse Häute, Niere, Schleimhäute.

In den folgenden 20 Jahren wurde der visceralen Verlaufsform des Lupus erythematodes wenig Beachtung geschenkt. Dann erschienen wieder verschiedene bemerkenswerte klinische und pathologische Beiträge (Goeckerman 1923, Grishman 1963, Keefer 1924, Libman und Sacks 1924): 1924 beschrieben Libman und Sacks vier Fälle von nicht-bakterieller Endokarditis, wobei zwei Patienten gleichzeitig typische Lupus erythematodes-Hauteruptionen aufwiesen. Diese

* Mit Unterstützung des National Institutes of Health, Grants No. A-3777 und A-4819.

** Health Research Council Career Scientist of the City of New York.

Form der Herzklappenentzündung wurde darauf von vielen Autoren zu Unrecht als für den visceralen Erythematodes pathognomonisch betrachtet; mit „Libman-Sacks-Syndrom“ wurde dann die viscerale Verlaufsform des Lupus erythematodes schlechthin bezeichnet. Von diesem Irrtum haben sich die meisten Autoren heute wieder freigemacht (VOLKMANN). BAEHR, KLEMPERER und SCHIFRIN berichteten *1935* über 23 Fälle von visceralem Lupus erythematodes und gaben die bis dahin beste Beschreibung der klinischen Symptomatologie und der pathologisch anatomischen Veränderungen der Krankheit. KLEMPERER und seine Mitarbeiter (1941) suchten für die vielfältigen Veränderungen einen gemeinsamen Nenner und glaubten, diesen im Zwischengewebe gefunden zu haben. Unter dem Namen „collagen disease“ faßte KLEMPERER (1950) eine Reihe von Affektionen ungeklärter Pathogenese zusammen, womit ausgesagt sein sollte, daß es sich um Krankheiten mit Veränderungen im Zwischengewebe handle, die miteinander eine gewisse Ähnlichkeit aufweisen, auch wenn jede der einzelnen Krankheiten morphologische Eigenarten zeigen. Der Begriff der Kollagenose hat sich bei den Klinikern rasch verbreitet, da eine Anzahl verschiedener, z. T. schlecht definierter Affektionen damit bequem zusammengefaßt werden konnten. KLEMPERER hat jedoch speziell darauf aufmerksam gemacht, daß ein solcher differentialdiagnostischer Sammeltopf nicht darüber hinwegtäuschen darf, daß diese Kollagenosen ätiologisch und pathogenetisch verschieden seien. Mit „Kollagenosen“ wurde ein topographischer und nicht ein ätio-pathogenetischer Begriff geprägt.

KLEMPERER trug wesentlich zur Morphologie der Organveränderungen des visceralen Lupus erythematodes bei. Er beschrieb die charakteristischen Veränderungen der Nierenglomeruli, ferner die für die Krankheit pathognomonischen hämatoxyphilen Körperchen (KLEMPERER u. Mitarb. 1941, 1948, 1950). Es konnte später gezeigt werden, daß diese Hämatoxylin-Körperchen den im Lupus erythematodes- (L. E.-) Zell-Phänomen vorkommenden Kernveränderungen entsprechen (KLEMPERER u. Mitarb. 1950).

Mit der Beschreibung des Lupus erythematodes-Zellphänomens durch HARGRAVES u. Mitarb. (1952) begann eine neue Phase in der Erforschung des visceralen Erythematodes. Nachdem zunächst vermutet wurde (INDERBITZIN 1953, 1954, KURNICK 1956, KURNICK u. Mitarb. 1952a u. b, 1953), daß es sich um den Ausdruck einer biochemischen metabolischen Störung handle, konnte später MIESCHER den Nachweis erbringen, daß das L.E.-Phänomen durch einen Serumfaktor ausgelöst wird, der alle Eigenschaften eines Autoantikörpers gegen Nucleoprotein besitzt (MIESCHER u. FAUCONNET 1954a u. b). Die daraufhin einsetzende immunopathologische Forschung hat eine erstaunliche Fülle von autoimmunitären Vorgängen aufgedeckt, die zur Vermutung führten, daß dem visceralen Lupus erythematodes eine Störung des immunologisch kompetenten Systems zugrunde liege, oder zumindest, daß der viscerale Lupus erythematodes mit einer derartigen Störung einhergehe.

In den letzten Jahren haben genetische Studien weiter zum Verständnis des visceralen Lupus erythematodes beigetragen (LEONHARD 1957, FUDENBERG u. Mitarb. 1962). Folgende Veränderungen bzw. Affektionen wurden gehäuft in bestimmten Familien angetroffen: Agammaglobulinämie, Hypergammaglobulinämie, visceraler Lupus erythematodes, primär chronische Polyarthritis. Der gemeinsame Nenner dieser Affektionen scheint in einer Störung des Antikörperbildenden Systems zu liegen. Die Verhältnisse sind aber dadurch noch weiter kompliziert, daß der cutane Lupus erythematodes, der zweifellos mit dem visceralen Lupus erythematodes nahe verwandt ist und in der obigen Liste mit aufgeführt werden muß, nur gelegentlich immunologische Störungen aufweist und nicht ohne weiteres unter diesem gemeinsamen Nenner angeführt werden kann.

2. Alters-, Geschlechts- und Rassen-Verteilung. Morbidität

Die meisten Neuerkrankungen an visceralem Lupus erythematodes erfolgen im dritten Dezennium (20—30 Jahre) (Harvey u. Mitarb. 1954, Dubois 1956b, Dörner u. Mitarb. 1961, Siegenthaler u. Hegglin 1956, Rothfield u. Mitarb. 1961). Die Krankheit kann jedoch in jedem Alter beginnen. Unser jüngster Patient war 15 Monate alt, der älteste 81 Jahre. Der viscerale Lupus erythematodes ist bei Frauen wesentlich häufiger als bei Männern, 75—85% aller Erkrankungen befallen das weibliche Geschlecht (Harvey u. Mitarb. 1954, Baehr u. Mitarb. 1935, Dubois 1956b, Rothfield u. Mitarb., Montgomery u. McCreight 1949, Dörner u. Mitarb. 1961). Dieses Verteilungsbild ist nicht auf das geschlechtsreife Alter beschränkt. Unter unseren eigenen zehn Fällen von Kindern unter 10 Jahren befinden sich acht Mädchen. Eine Rassenabhängigkeit wurde nicht festgestellt. Die Erkrankung kommt bei der kaukasischen, mongolischen und schwarzen Rasse vor.

In einer gemischten Bevölkerung muß, vorsichtig geschätzt, mit einer Neuerkrankung jährlich je 100000 Einwohner oder einer Erkrankung je 10000 Einwohner bei einer durchschnittlichen Krankheitsdauer von 10 Jahren gerechnet werden (Siegel u. Mitarb.).

3. Familiäres Vorkommen

Leonhard (1957) faßte die Literatur über familiäres Vorkommen von visceralem und cutanem Erythematodes bis 1957 zusammen und berichtete über eine eigene Beobachtung einer Familie mit 14 Kindern mit auffallender Häufigkeit von Hypergammaglobulinämie (acht Patienten). Drei der hypergammaglobulinämischen Geschwister (alles Mädchen) erkrankten an visceralem Lupus erythematodes. Leonhard vermutete, daß eine genetische Störung in der Gammaglobulinproduktion vorliege. Spätere Berichte bestätigten diese Vermutung (Fudenberg u. Mitarb. 1962, Hogg 1957, Morteo u. Mitarb. 1961).

Interessanterweise kommen bei Familienangehörigen der gleichen Sippschaft nicht nur eine Über-, sondern auch eine Unterproduktion der Gammaglobuline vor (Good u. Mitarb. 1963). Folgende Krankheiten bzw. Symptome scheinen mit dieser genetischen Reaktionslage in Zusammenhang zu stehen: Hypo- bzw. Agammaglobulinämie, visceraler Lupus erythematodes, cutaner Erythematodes, primär chronische Polyarthritis, Sjögrens Syndrom, generalisierte Sklerodermie. Folgende Serumbefunde werden gehäuft bei Angehörigen entsprechender Familien gefunden: Vermehrung oder Verminderung von Serum-Gammaglobulin, Rheumafaktor, falsch positive Wassermannsche Reaktion, antinucleare Reaktionen. Es ist bemerkenswert, daß der cutane Erythematodes an sich nicht mit einer Störung der Gammaglobuline einherzugehen scheint, was darauf hinweist, daß die somatische Folge der genetischen Störung nicht auf die Gammaglobulin-Produktion limitiert sein kann (Epstein u. Litt 1961, McCuistion u. Schoch 1954, Steagall u. Mitarb. 1962). Der dem cutanen Erythematodes zugrunde liegende Krankheitsmechanismus ist noch vollständig unbekannt. Die Erforschung der Pathogenese dieser Affektion dürfte weitere wertvolle Aufschlüsse über die Erfolgsmechanismen der genetischen Störung geben.

4. Disponierende Faktoren

Eine Anzahl äußerer Einflüsse, physikalischer und psychischer Natur, wurden als Faktoren beschrieben, die den Ausbruch eines visceralen Lupus erythematodes begünstigen.

An erster Stelle ist Sonnenbestrahlung zu nennen, deren Einfluß auf die Hauteruptionen außer Zweifel steht. Ob tatsächlich die viscerale Aktivität eines Erythematodes durch Sonnenbestrahlung verstärkt oder ausgelöst werden kann, ist nicht bewiesen, wenn auch Einzelbeobachtungen dafür sprechen.

Infekte wurden beschrieben, ohne daß Beweise dafür vorliegen. Es sei hier erwähnt, daß massive, mit Gewebszerstörung einhergehende Infekte zur Bildung antinuclearer Faktoren führen können (eigene Beobachtungen).

Medikamentöse Überempfindlichkeiten werden ebenfalls als auslösendes Element für eine viscerale Lupus erythematodes-Erkrankung angeführt (Gold 1951, Ruppli u. Vossen 1957, Shulman u. Harvey 1960, Ayvazian u. Badger 1948, Miescher u. Jackson 1962, Dustan u. Mitarb. 1954, Perry u. Schroeder 1954, Honey 1956). Heftige allergische Reaktionen gehen oft mit einem positiven Pseudo-L.E.-Phänomen einher (Miescher 1959). Selten kommt es zu einem typischen L.E.-Zellphänomen, und noch seltener treten klinische Symptome auf, die denjenigen des visceralen Lupus erythematodes gleichen. Das Hydralazin-Syndrom (Dustan u. Mitarb. 1954, Perry u. Schroeder 1954) ist in dieser Hinsicht besonders bekannt, wobei hier nicht feststeht, ob es sich um eine medikamentöse Reaktion bei Patienten mit latentem visceralen Lupus erythematodes handelt.

Slocumb (1953) vermutet, daß plötzliches Absetzen der Steroid-Behandlung bei Patienten mit primär chronischer Polyarthritis Krankheitszeichen und serologische Reaktionen eines visceralen Lupus erythematodes auslösen können. Da plötzlicher Entzug von Corticosteroiden bei Patienten mit visceralem Lupus erythematodes einen akuten Schub der Erkrankung auslösen kann, vermuten Harvey u. Mitarb., daß bei diesen Patienten von vornherein eine viscerale Lupus erythematodes-Erkrankung vorlag, die durch den Steroidentzug nur aktiviert wurde.

Emotionelle Faktoren mögen ebenfalls einen Einfluß auf eine „latente Erythematodes-Erkrankung“ haben. Eine unserer Patientinnen erkrankte unmittelbar nach schwerem psychischem Trauma an einem perakuten visceralen Lupus erythematodes mit cerebraler und renaler Symptomatologie. Diese Erkrankung erfolgte „aus voller Gesundheit heraus“, während die Patientin sich auf der Flucht von zu Hause befand.

Die beschriebenen Faktoren kommen nicht nur als die Krankheit auslösendes Element in Frage; sie mögen auch einen Einfluß auf den Verlauf eines schon manifesten visceralen Lupus erythematodes haben. In dieser Beziehung sei noch besonders auf die *Schwangerschaft* eingegangen.

Die vereinzelten Berichte über die gegenseitige Beeinflussung von Schwangerschaft und visceralem Lupus erythematodes stimmen darin überein, daß in der ersten Schwangerschaftshälfte und in den ersten 2 Monaten nach Geburt des Kindes Exacerbationen des visceralen Lupus erythematodes gehäuft auftreten (Friedman u. Rutherford 1956, Garsenstein u. Mitarb. 1962). Die Lebenserwartung der Patientinnen scheint jedoch dadurch nicht beeinflußt zu werden. Garsenstein u. Mitarb. berichten über eine erhöhte intrauterine Sterblichkeit des Kindes und über eine Neigung zu Frühgeburten bei Patientinnen mit visceralem Lupus erythematodes.

5. Ätiologie und Pathogenese des visceralen Lupus erythematodes

Die Ätiologie des visceralen Lupus erythematodes ist ungeklärt. Wohl steht fest, daß die Erkrankung auf dem Boden einer genetischen Disposition entsteht, doch herrscht Ungewißheit über die Faktoren, die die eigentliche Krankheit auslösen. Im speziellen ist es nicht bekannt, ob die auslösenden Ursachen immunologischer oder nicht immunologischer Natur sind. Beim cutanen discoiden Erythematodes gehören immunologische Phänomene eher zur Ausnahme (ROTHFIELD u. Mitarb. 1963, ROWELL 1962) und bei Anerkennung der engen Beziehungen dieser Hauterkrankung zum visceralen Lupus erythematodes (WILSON u. JORDAN 1959) muß mit der Möglichkeit gerechnet werden, daß sich auch der viscerale Lupus erythematodes zunächst auf nicht-immunologischer Ebene abspielt. Die Hypothese ist z.B. vorgeschlagen worden, daß die genetisch vererbte Diathese in einer Permeabilitätsstörung intracellulärer Organellen liege, speziell der Lysosome (LEWIS THOMAS), und daß jede Einwirkung auf die enzymreichen Lysosome die Krankheit in Gang bringen können (z.B. intensive Sonnenbestrahlung, Endotoxin usw.). Unter dem Gesichtswinkel dieser Hypothese wären dann die immunologischen Phänomene als Folge der intracellulären Permeabilitätsstörung aufzufassen.

Die Tatsache, daß medikamentöse Überempfindlichkeitsreaktionen das Krankheitsbild (klinisch und serologisch) eines visceralen Lupus erythematodes vortäuschen können, hat zur Vermutung geführt, daß derartige Reaktionen bei entsprechender genetischer Konstitution einen visceralen Lupus erythematodes auszulösen vermögen.

Die genetisch verankerte Störung scheint vor allem in einer Diathese zur Autoantikörperbildung zu liegen (CALLENDER und RACE 1946). Das schließt die Möglichkeit nicht aus, daß diese Diathese bereits sekundärer Natur sei, z.B. auf Grund der oben genannten intracellulären Permeabilitätsstörung. Ob die Krankheitszeichen Folge der Autosensibilisierung oder Folge primär nicht immunologischer entzündlicher Vorgänge darstellt, ist unbekannt.

In jüngster Zeit ist vermutet worden (GOOD u. Mitarb. 1963), daß die Thymusdrüse Sitz der dem visceralen Lupus erythematodes zugrunde liegenden genetischen Störung sei. Die Bedeutung dieses Organs für die Ausbildung des immunitären Systems steht heute außer Zweifel (MOFFAT u. Mitarb. 1950). In der Myasthenia gravis wurde schon früher auf die Bedeutung des Thymus hingewiesen (CASTLEMAN u. NORRIS 1949). Auf Grund neuerer Untersuchungen (WHITE und MARSHALL 1962) ist es gerechtfertigt, die Myasthenia gravis zu den Autoimmun-Erkrankungen par excellence zu zählen, wobei die übergeordnete immunologische Störung im Thymus liegen mag. Interessanterweise werden bei der Myasthenia gravis nicht nur Serumkörper gegen Muskelgewebe gefunden, sondern in 30% der Fälle können auch antinucleare Faktoren nachgewiesen werden (STURGILL und STRAUSS). Es steht zur Diskussion, ob der Myasthenia gravis eine analoge genetische Störung zugrunde liege wie dem visceralen Lupus erythematodes. Die Rolle der Thymusdrüse wäre bei beiden Krankheiten darin zu sehen, daß dieses immunologisch übergeordnete Organ in seiner regulierenden bzw. dirigierenden Funktion versagt unter Ausbildung von Zell-Kloni, die nicht zwischen „hetero-" und „autologem" Antigen unterscheiden können („forbidden clones" nach BURNET). Es käme damit zu einer der „Runt-Disease" analogen Auseinandersetzung zwischen den immunologisch aktiven Zellen des „forbidden clone" und dem „Wirtsorganismus" (s. auch SIMONSEN 1962). Diese Überlegungen sind vorerst rein theoretischer Art, haben sich aber bereits fruchtbar auf den Gang der experimentellen Forschung ausgewirkt.

Im folgenden seien die einzelnen immunologischen Phänomene hinsichtlich ihrer pathogenetischen Bedeutung besprochen.

Antinucleare Faktoren kommen wahrscheinlich im Verlauf jeder visceralen Lupus erythematodes-Erkrankung vor (FALLET 1960, FRIOU 1958, HARGRAVES u. Mitarb. 1952, HASERICK 1951, LEE u. Mitarb. 1950, LEONI 1954, MIESCHER 1957, ROTHFIELD u. Mitarb., SCHULTEN u. Mitarb. 1962, SELIGMANN 1961). Es konnte aber gezeigt werden, daß diese Faktoren nicht an den Zellkern lebender Zellen gelangen können (MIESCHER u. FAUCONNET 1954). Das durch Nucleoprotein-Antikörper ausgelöste L.E.-Phänomen betrifft die Phagocytose von Zellkernen bereits geschädigter Zellen. Während Antikörper gegen Nucleoprotein zur Bildung des L.E.-Zell-Phänomens unerläßlich sind (HOLMAN u. KUNKEL 1957, HOLMAN u. DEICHER 1959, MIESCHER u. FAUCONNET 1954, SPIEGELBERG), scheinen Antikörper gegen Desoxyribonucleinsäure und gegen Histon die Morphologie der L.E.-Zellen zu beeinflussen (SPIEGELBERG).

Die antinuclearen Faktoren kommen nicht als direkt cytotoxische Noxe in Frage. Passiv übertragen, lösen sie keine Krankheitssymptome aus (Transfusionen von Erythematodes-Blut an Drittpersonen; Übertragung der Antikörper diatransplacental von Müttern auf den kindlichen Organismus (BERLYNE u. Mitarb. 1957, BRIDGE u. FOLEY 1954, OUDSTEN u. Mitarb. 1958). Die hämatoxyphilen Körperchen sind zweifellos Folge der Einwirkung antinuclearer Serumkörper auf Zellkerne im Gewebe (GODMAN u. Mitarb. 1958), doch dürften sie wahrscheinlich als eine Nebenerscheinung in der Pathogenese des visceralen Lupus erythematodes aufgefaßt werden. Als Quelle für die hämatoxyphilen Körperchen kommen nur abgestorbene Zellen in Frage. Trotz ihrer ausgesprochenen Spezifität für den visceralen Lupus erythematodes kommt ihnen keine große praktische diagnostische Bedeutung zu, da ihr Nachweis nur sehr selten gelingt (ROTHFIELD u. Mitarb. 1963). Ihre Bildung kann leicht verstanden werden durch die Einwirkung antinuclearer Faktoren auf bloßgelegte Zellkerne, d.h. auf bereits devitalisierte Zellbestandteile. In analoger Weise kommt es auch zu eigentlicher L.E.-Zellbildung in Pleuraexsudaten (VAN DOORMAAL u. SCHREUDER 1950) oder ganz allgemein unter Bedingungen, bei welchen Zellen in Gegenwart von Nucleoprotein-Antikörpern und phagocytären mobilen Zellen untergehen (SEAMAN u. CHRISTERSON 1952, WILSON u. Mitarb. 1961, JASINSKI u. Mitarb. 1953). Auf die mögliche Rolle antinuclearer Antikörper in der Bildung zirkulierender Antigen-Antikörper-Komplexe werden wir später eingehen.

Autoantikörper gegen die verschiedenen Blutzell-Elemente können pathogen sein. Ob die Pathogenität vom Serumtiter oder von der Natur der Antikörper abhängt, ist noch unbestimmt.

Immunhämolytische Anämie (DUBOIS 1952, ETCHEVERRY u. Mitarb. 1951, GORDON u. Mitarb. 1955, PISCIOTTA u. Mitarb. 1951, ZOUTENDDYK 1951) kann durch nicht komplementbindende 7 S-Antikörper bedingt sein. Komplementbindende antierythrocytäre Antikörper kommen aber häufiger vor (LEDDY u. Mitarb.). Leukocytäre Autoantikörper können bei vielen Patienten mit visceralem Lupus erythematodes nachgewiesen werden (MIESCHER u. Mitarb. 1964, STEFFEN, VAN LOGHEM u. Mitarb. 1957, GOUDSMITH u. VAN LOGHEM 1953). Sehr wahrscheinlich ist die bei ungefähr einem Drittel der Erythematodes-Patienten vorkommende Leukopenie mit myeloischer Knochenmarkhyperplasie Folge der Autoantikörpereinwirkung auf die Leukocyten. Gegen Thrombocyten gerichtete Autoantikörper (DAUSSET 1956, DAUSSET u. Mitarb. 1961, MIESCHER 1959, MUELLER u. RADOJICIC 1956) kommen ebenfalls als komplementbindende und nichtkomplementbindende Antikörper vor (SELIGMANN 1958). Im ersten Fall wird nur sehr wenig Komplement fixiert. Es ist möglich, daß der Erfolg der Splenektomie im Falle einer Autoimmunthrombopenie davon abhängt, ob Komplement gebunden wird oder nicht. Bei einem unserer Patienten mit visceralem Lupus erythematodes und Immunothrombopenie mit einem im direkten Antiglobulinkonsumtionstest nachgewiesenen Plättchenautoantikörper war der Erfolg der Splenektomie nur bescheiden, d. h. die Thrombocyten stiegen nach der Operation nur langsam von 5000 auf 90000 je mm^3 an (nach 2 Wochen). Es konnte gezeigt werden, daß es sich um einen Komplement-fixierenden antithrombocytären Antikörper handelte. Zirkulierende Antikoagulantien, die wahrscheinlich Autoantikörper gegen Gerinnungsfaktoren darstellen, können vermutlich eine hämorrhagische Diathese bedingen oder zumindest eine bestehende verstärken (Hitzig u. Mitarb. 1951, Frick 1955, Loeliger 1959).

Die organ-aspezifischen anticytoplasmatischen Faktoren haben keine cytotoxischen Eigenschaften. Sie mögen für die Bildung pathogener Antigen-Antikörper-Komplexe in Frage kommen.

Antikörper gegen Thyreoglobulin sind wahrscheinlich ohne pathogene Bedeutung. Diese Antikörper werden beim visceralen Lupus erythematodes meist nur mit niedrigem Titer nachgewiesen. Antikörper gegen Leber- und Nierenparenchym wurden als pathogenetische Faktoren für Läsionen in den entsprechenden Organen postuliert. Bis jetzt sind aber Leber- und Nieren-spezifische Autoantikörper nicht mit Sicherheit nachgewiesen worden, d.h. als solche bezeichnete Serumfaktoren wurden nicht auf ihre Organspezifität hin untersucht. Nachdem heute anticytoplasmatische organ-nicht-spezifische Antikörper häufig bei Patienten mit visceralem Lupus erythematodes festgestellt werden, sind sog. Nieren- oder Leber-spezifische Antikörper durch diesen Befund in Frage gestellt.

Es wurde wiederholt postuliert, daß Immunreaktionen vom Spätreaktionstypus in der Pathogenese des visceralen Lupus erythematodes eine Rolle spielen. Der Leukocyten-Hauttest (Friedmann u. Mitarb. 1960) wird als Hinweis für das Bestehen einer Autoimmunisierung vom Spätreaktionstypus angeführt. Jedoch ist der Mechanismus dieser Reaktion nicht abgeklärt. Die Tatsache, daß gelegentlich auch eine gesunde Kontrollperson einen positiven Hauttest mit autologen Leukocyten aufweist, läßt an der Annahme, daß es sich hier um eine Reaktion von pathogener Bedeutung handelt, Zweifel aufkommen.

Eine Anzahl von Befunden lassen vermuten, daß *Antigen-Antikörper-Komplexe* eine maßgebende Rolle in der Pathogenese des visceralen Lupus erythematodes spielen. Der viscerale Lupus erythematodes kann als eine vasculäre Erkrankung verschiedener Organlokalisation angesehen werden, wobei die Gefäßveränderungen folgendermaßen charakterisiert sind: Entzündliche Veränderungen der Gefäßwand mit Neigung zu fibrinoider Degeneration, ferner mit Ablagerung von Eiweiß, das auf Grund von Immunofluorescenzstudien Gammaglobulin und Komplement enthält (Lachmann u. Mitarb. 1962, Mellors u. Mitarb., Muller-Eberhard 1962). Das Vorhandensein von Fibrin ist noch umstritten (Gitlin u. Mitarb. 1957, Vasquez u. Dixon 1960, Vassalli u. Mitarb.). Diese Veränderungen sind in den Nierenglomeruli besonders ausgesprochen. Die Ablagerung der Eiweißstoffe findet hier in einem Bereich statt, der den polymorphkernigen Leukocyten schwer zugänglich ist. Aus diesem Grund sind die Veränderungen wahrscheinlich nicht oder nur unvollkommen reversibel. In der experimentellen chronischen Serumkrankheit konnte gezeigt werden, daß in der Niere lokalisierte Antigen-Antikörper-Komplexe nach Sistieren der Antigenzufuhr praktisch nicht verschwinden (Dixon 1962). Dies würde auch erklären, warum die Erythematodes-Glomerulitis therapeutisch kaum beeinflußt werden kann. Mit der Behandlung dürften nur die akut entzündlichen Reaktionen in der Niere gedämpft werden; ferner wird gehofft, daß die Verabreichung von Steroiden die Ablagerung weiterer Eiweißkomplexe in der Niere verhindere. In der Milz kommt es zu Gefäßveränderungen, die als „onion-skin-lesion“ bezeichnet werden. In anderen Organen sind die Gefäßveränderungen meist weniger ausgesprochen und scheinen auch reversibel zu sein. Die vasculäre Pathologie der Nieren gleicht in frappanter Weise derjenigen der experimentellen chronischen Serumkrankheit des Kaninchens (Dixon 1962). Bei Patienten mit renaler Beteiligung ist zudem der Serumkomplementspiegel meist stark erniedrigt, ferner können hochtitrige Autoantikörper nachgewiesen werden, was die Vermutung bestärkt, daß zirkulierende Antigen-Antikörper-Komplexe pathogenetisch im Spiel sind. Alle bisherigen Versuche zur Aufdeckung von Gewebsstoffen, die als Antigen für die Komplexe in Frage kommen, haben fehlgeschlagen. Insbesondere konnte in den Ablagerungen zwischen Basalmembran und Fußprozessen der Nierenglomeruli mit einer Ausnahme kein Kernmaterial nachgewiesen werden. BROWN u. Mitarb. (1963) berichteten über einen Fall von Erythematodes-Nephritis mit Nachweis von Feulgen-positivem Material in den Ablagerungen der Glomeruli-Schlingen. Es ist möglich, daß eine Vielzahl von Autoantigenen am Zustandekommen von Immun-Komplexen beteiligt ist, was die Schwierigkeit des Antigen-Nachweises verständlich machen würde. Für die Pathogenität immunologischer Komplexe dürfte die relative Zusammensetzung und die Beteiligung von Komplement wichtiger sein als die Natur des oder der Antigene.

6. Pathologisch-anatomische Veränderungen

Eine Vielfalt von Gewebsveränderungen verschiedener Intensität und wechselnder Lokalisation werden bei Patienten mit visceralem Lupus erythematodes gefunden. Die in den meisten Beschreibungen hervorgehobenen typischen Befunde wie fibrinoide Degeneration (KLINGE 1933) und hämatoxyphile Körperchen treten zurück gegenüber uncharakteristischen, oft geringgradigen Veränderungen. Als fibrinoide Degeneration wird eine mit Aufquellung und Homogenisierung verbundene Alteration der Intercellularsubstanz bezeichnet. Der fibrinoiden Degeneration wurde lange Zeit eine hochgradige Spezifität zugesprochen. Heut wissen wir, daß Vorgänge verschiedenster Natur zum morphologischen Korrelae der fibrinoiden Degeneration führen können, wobei die histochemische Zusamment setzung von Fall zu Fall verschieden sein kann (v. ALBERTINI u. ALB 1947, DIXON 1961). Das „Fibrinoid" des visceralen Lupus erythematodes enthält auf Grund immuno-histochemischer Untersuchungen Gammaglobulin und Komplement (LACHMANN u. Mitarb. 1962, MELLORS u. Mitarb., MULLER-EBERHARD 1962), was für eine immunologische Entstehungsweise spricht. Fibrin wurde von einigen Forschern ebenfalls gefunden (GITLIN u. Mitarb. 1957, VASSALLI u. Mitarb.), von anderen dagegen nicht (VASQUEZ u. DIXON 1960). Die Beteiligung von Fibrin bzw. Gerinnungsfaktoren mag von sekundären entzündlichen Vorgängen abhängen. Fibrinoid kann in praktisch allen Geweben von Erythematodes-Patienten gefunden werden.

Die sog. Hämatoxylin-Körperchen stellen wohl das einzige wirklich „spezifische" anatomopathologische Substrat des visceralen Lupus erythematodes dar. Es handelt sich um homogene Massen, die sich mit Hämatoxylin purpurig färben lassen und im frischen Stadium Feulgen-positiv sind. Ältere hämatoxyphile Körperchen verlieren die Feulgen-Färbbarkeit und werden PAS-positiv (POLLACK 1959). Die Größe dieser Körperchen schwankt von 5—20 μ Durchmesser. Sie kommen dadurch zustande, daß durch Zelluntergang freigewordene Zellkerne durch antinucleare Antikörper zur Quellung und Homogenisierung gebracht werden. Je nachdem, ob einer oder mehrere Zellkerne an ihrer Bildung beteiligt sind, sind sie kleiner oder größer. Früher waren die Hämatoxylin-Körperchen ein häufiger Befund; sie wurden hauptsächlich in Herzklappen-Vegetationen, in alterierten Lymphknoten und in veränderten Nierenglomeruli gefunden (KLEMPERER u. Mitarb. 1941). Heute werden sie nur noch selten beobachtet, wohl zufolge der intensiven Steroidbehandlung der Erythematodes-Patienten. Gelegentlich werden sie noch in einer Nieren- oder Hautbiopsie nachgewiesen, doch handelt es sich hier mehr um die Ausnahme als die Regel. In unserem eigenen Material zahlreicher Biopsien und Autopsien wurden in den letzten 3 Jahren überhaupt keine hämatoxyphilen Körperchen mehr gefunden.

Intensive und typische Gewebsläsionen finden sich am häufigsten in der Niere (MUEHRCKE u. Mitarb. 1955, POLLACK u. Mitarb. 1958, VERNIER u. Mitarb. 1958), besonders in bioptisch erhaltenem Gewebe von frisch erkrankten Patienten mit klinisch manifester Nierenbeteiligung. Es handelt sich hier in der Regel um eine fokale Erkrankung der Glomeruli („*fokale Glomerulitis*", s. Abb. 1). Gewöhnlich weist nur ein Teil eines einzelnen Glomerulus Läsionen auf. In diesem Bereich des befallenen Glomerulus sind die Endothelien und die intercapillaren Zellen geschwollen, z.T. mit proliferativer Tendenz (MUEHRCKE u. Mitarb. 1957, ROTHFIELD u. Mitarb. 1963). Das Capillarlumen erscheint verengt oder gar obliteriert. In der Regel besteht auch eine neutrophile leukocytäre Infiltration in diesem Bereich. Herdförmige Nekrosen kommen häufig vor, mit Untergang der normalen Glomerulus-Struktur, Karyorrhexis und mit Anhäufung von Material, das dem Fibrin ähnlich sieht (s. Abb. 2). Sogenannte „wire loop-lesions" kommen gelegentlich zur Beobachtung: diese Veränderungen können definiert werden als fokale Verdickung (Fibrinoid) von Capillarschlingen. Die Verdickungen bestehen aus einem leuchtend eosinophilen, PAS-positivem Material, das alle färberischen Eigenschaften von Fibrin hat. Der Begriff der „wireloop lesion" hat zu einer gewissen Verwirrung geführt, da einige Autoren darunter auch Verdickungen von glomerulären Capillarschlingen verstehen, die durch eine solche der Basalmembran zustande kommt und folglich die färberischen Eigenschaften der Basalmembran aufweist. Adhäsionen glomerulärer Schlingen an die Bowmansche Kapsel mit periglomerulären Infiltraten von Lymphocyten, Plasmazellen und Eosinophilen stellen auch einen charakteristischen Befund der akuten fokalen Erythematodes-Glomerulitis dar. Hämatoxylin-Körperchen wurden von einigen Autoren häufig (MUEHRCKE u. Mitarb. 1957), von anderen selten oder überhaupt nicht in bioptischem Material gefunden (ROTHFIELD u. Mitarb. 1963).

Wenn die meisten der genannten Veränderungen vorliegen, kann die Diagnose eines visceralen Lupus erythematodes praktisch mit Sicherheit gestellt werden. Es muß aber betont werden, daß keine einzige der erwähnten Veränderungen, mit Ausnahme der selten gefundenen Hämatoxylin-Körperchen, für den visceralen Lupus erythematodes pathognomonisch sind. „Wire loop lesions" sind wohl recht charakteristisch, können aber auch bei anderen Krankheiten vorkommen, z.B. bei der akuten Glomerulonephritis. Auf Grund elektronenoptischer Untersuchung besteht die „wire loop lesion" vor allem in Ablagerungen eines optisch dichten Materials, das in Schollen zwischen Endothelzellen und Basalmembran zu finden ist (FARQUHAR u. Mitarb. 1957). VASSALI u. Mitarb. konnten eine analoge Läsion beim Kaninchen reproduzieren durch Injektion von Agentien, die zu einer intravasculären Gerinnung führen. Die daraus resultierenden Ablagerungen in den Glomeruli wiesen alle Zwischenformen von Fibrin und „Fibrinoid" auf. Das Fibrinoid der Kaninchen ist also aus dem Fibrin durch Degradationsvorgänge entstanden. Daß das Fibrinoid der „wire loop lesion" in analoger Weise zustande kommt, ist zumindest möglich. Wir haben schon erwähnt, daß das Fibrinoid Gammaglobulin und Komplement (LACHMANN u. Mitarb. 1962, MELLORS u. Mitarb., MULLER-EBERHARD 1962), d.h. also, daß es wahrscheinlich Antigen-Antikörper-Komplexe enthält. In diesem Zusammenhang sei erwähnt, daß Antigen-Antikörper-Komplexe Gerinnungsvorgänge auslösen können. GITLIN u. Mitarb. (1957) haben denn auch Fibrin in der „wire loop lesion" nachweisen können, jedoch steht diesem Bericht derjenige von VASQUEZ und DIXON (1960) entgegen mit fehlendem Fibrinnachweis.

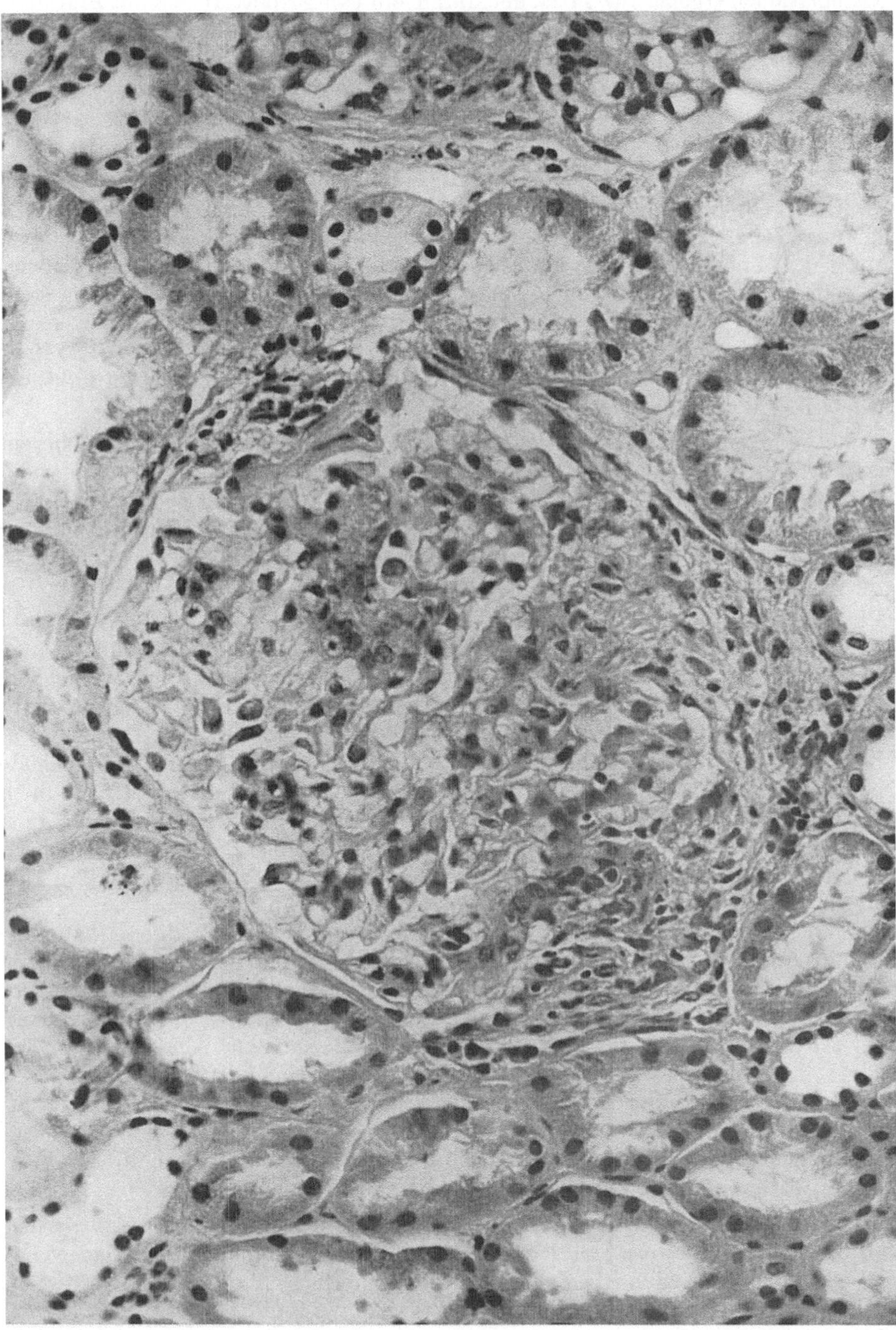

Abb. 1. Nierenbiopsie bei einer Patientin mit floridem visceralem Lupus erythematodes mit Nierenbeteiligung. Der Glomerulus zeigt Foci mit Schwellung und Proliferation von Zellen, diskreter neutrophiler Infiltration und Karyorrhexis. Es bestehen ferner Adhäsionen im Bereich der Bowmanschen Kapsel

Elektronenoptische Studien haben weitere Besonderheiten der Erythematodes-Nierenläsionen ergeben: Die Basalmembran kann aufgesplittert sein mit Fibrinoid-Ablagerungen zwischen den einzelnen Schichten. Fibrinoid wird auch zwischen den Capillaren gefunden oder auf der epithelialen Seite der Basalmembran. Die Basalmembran selbst kann wesentlich verdickt sein; ferner werden Basalmembran-artiges Material oder kollagene Fasern in den intercapillären Bezirken gefunden (Grishman u. Mitarb. 1963).

Während in den befallenen Glomeruli Gammaglobulin und Komplement nachgewiesen werden kann (Mellors u. Mitarb., Vasquez u. Dixon 1960, Lachmann u. Mitarb. 1962, Muller-Eberhard 1962), gelang es in der Regel nicht, das als Antigen in Frage kommende Material in den Läsionen aufzudecken. Der eigentliche Beweis, daß Immunkomplexe die glomerulären Läsionen verursachen, steht damit immer noch aus. Es sei noch erwähnt, daß die Zellkerne in Bezirken von Gewebsläsionen nie mit Gammaglobulin überzogen sind (Burkholder 1963, Beutner u. Mitarb. 1962), ein weiterer Hinweis, daß die antinuclearen Faktoren nicht in vitale Zellen eindringen.

Bei wenigen Patienten mit visceralem Lupus erythematodes sind die Nierenveränderungen erheblich diffuser und gleichen der „subakuten Glomerulonephritis". Oft werden dabei die oben beschriebenen charakteristischen Eigenheiten vermißt. Es handelt sich bei dieser diffusen Form der Nierenbeteiligung gewöhnlich um eine rasch progrediente Nierenerkrankung, die schließlich in eine terminale Urämie übergeht (Muehrcke u. Mitarb. 1957, Rothfield u. Mitarb. 1963).

Die Niere kann nicht nur im glomerulären Anteil befallen sein, sondern auch im übrigen vasculären System. Fokale Arteriitis, gekennzeichnet durch fibrinoide Nekrosen kleiner Arterien, wird gelegentlich in der Niere gefunden, weniger häufig in anderen Organen wie Myokard, Leber, Pankreas, Milz (Klemperer u. Mitarb. 1941). In der Frühphase der fokalen Arteriitis erkennt man subintimale Niederschläge von Fibrinoid, die allmählich an Dicke zunehmen, um schließlich die ganze Gefäßwandung einzunehmen. Es entsteht dann eine perivasculäre entzündliche Reaktion. Diese fokale Arteriitis gleicht der Polyarteriitis nodosa, jedoch kommt es nur ganz selten beim visceralen Lupus erythematodes zu entsprechend schweren und disseminierten arteriellen Veränderungen.

Eine Sonderform der fokalen Arteriitis sind wahrscheinlich die Gefäßveränderungen in Milz- und Lymphknoten mit konzentrischer periarterieller Fibrose (onion-skin lesion). Oft ist die periarterielle fibröse Reaktion nur sehr geringgradig. Venöse Läsionen wurden beim visceralen Lupus erythematodes beschrieben, sind aber selten; sie bestehen in subendothelialen fibrinoiden Ablagerungen mit endothelialer Proliferation. Die Herzklappen können ebenfalls befallen sein unter Ausbildung von Vegetationen. In der eigentlichen Klappe kommt es zu Entzündungsherden mit fibrinoidem Material. Die Vegetationen bestehen aus dichtem fibrinartigem Material; sie können Hämatoxylin-Körperchen enthalten (Klemperer u. Mitarb. 1941, Grishman u. Mitarb. 1963, Gross 1940).

Die Synovia der Gelenke kann folgende Veränderungen aufweisen: Ablagerung von fibrinartigem Material an der Oberfläche oder innerhalb des Synoviagewebes mit Untergang von Synovia-Zellen und geringgradige entzündliche Reaktionen (Cruickshank 1958).

Pleura und Perikard weisen gelegentlich ähnliche Läsionen auf mit Ablagerung von Fibrinoid mit chronischen Entzündungsherden und Fibrose. Diese Veränderungen sind nicht für den visceralen Lupus erythematodes spezifisch (Klemperer u. Mitarb. 1941).

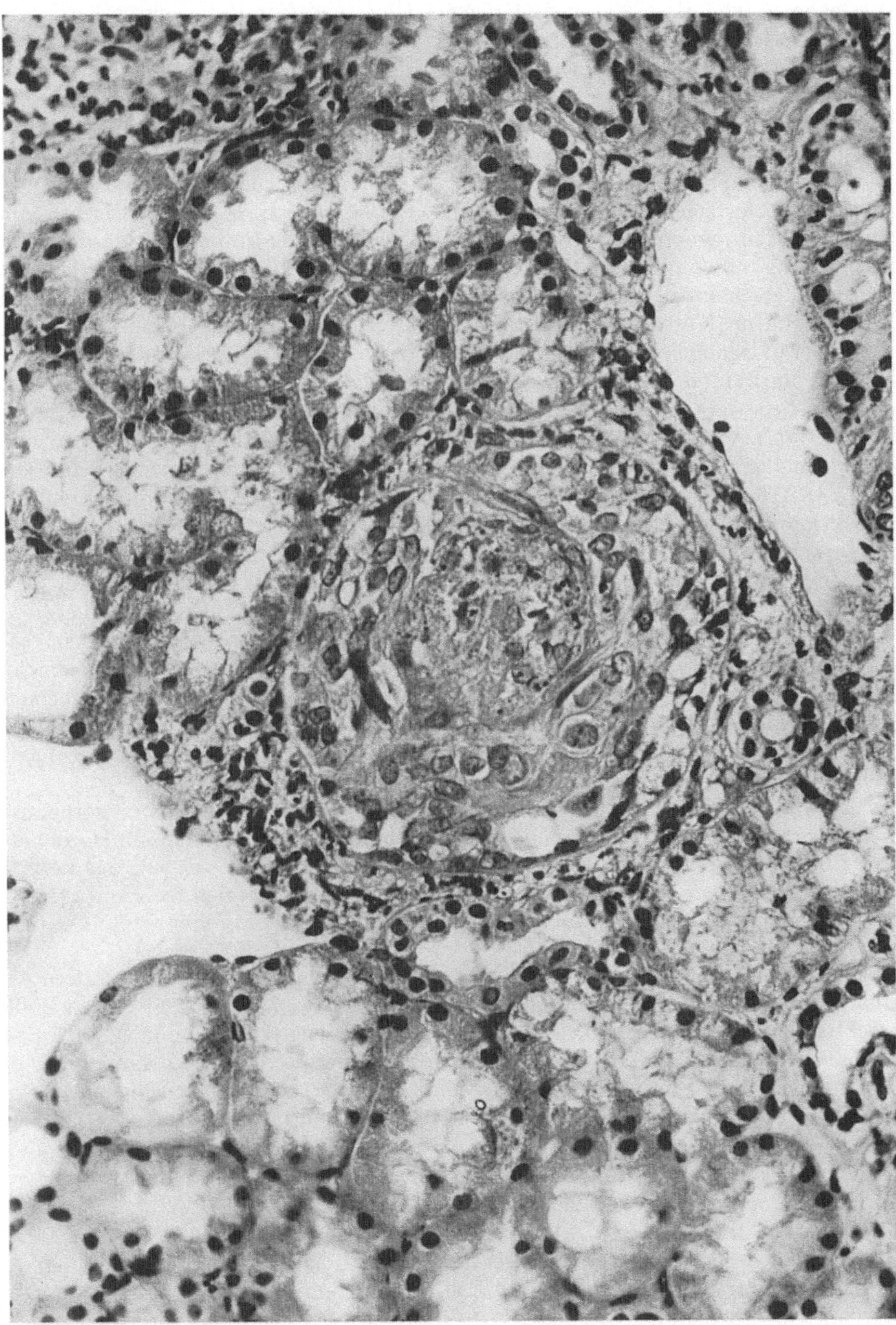

Abb. 2. Nierenbiopsie bei einer Patientin mit aktiver, schwerer Nierenbeteiligung im aktiven Stadium der Krankheit. Der tangential geschnittene Glomerulus zeigt Nekrose von Glomerulus-Schlingen mit Ansammlung von körnigem, eosinophilen Material und Kernresten. Der Nekroseherd ist umgeben von proliferierenden Epithelien. Beachte die akute periglomerulitische Reaktion

Lymphknoten zeigen gelegentlich entzündliche Veränderungen mit Ödem, Vermehrung von Histiocyten und Plasmazellen, herdförmigen Nekroseherdchen, in denen oft Hämatoxylin-Körperchen gefunden werden (Fox u. Rosahn 1943, Klemperer u. Mitarb. 1941).

Die Leber ist meist frei von Veränderungen. Mit der Fluorescenzantihumanglobulin-Reaktion wurde bei einigen Patienten Gammaglobulin in den Kupfferschen Zellen nachgewiesen, was als Phagocytose von Antigen-Antikörper-Komplexen aufgefaßt werden könnte (Beutner u. Mitarb. 1962, Cooper 1961).

Der histologische Befund von Hautläsionen ist oft recht charakteristisch, wenn auch nicht pathognomonisch. Die Epidermis erscheint verdünnt, mit verwaschener Begrenzung zufolge ödematöser Durchtränkung der Basalschicht (s. Abb. 3). Fibrinoid erscheint in den äußeren Coriumschichten, unter Verlust der kollagenen Grundstruktur (Klemperer u. Mitarb. 1941). Elektronenoptisch konnten dagegen keine Veränderungen der kollagenen Fasern festgestellt werden. Das Gewebe kann leicht von Lymphocyten und polymorphkernigen Leukocyten infiltriert sein. Gelegentlich werden einige der oben beschriebenen vasculären Läsionen beobachtet. Ferner wurde eine erhebliche Dilatation der Capillaren beschrieben mit unregelmäßigen Windungen und Verzweigungen des Capillarnetzes (Smith u. Kurban 1962). Diese Veränderungen unterscheiden sich deutlich von denjenigen des chronischen discoiden Lupus erythematodes; diese zeichnen sich aus durch Hyperkeratose und durch alternierende Zonen von Atrophie und Hyperplasie der Epidermis, ferner durch follikuläre Keratinpfropfbildung, leichte mononucleäre Infiltration um kleine Gefäße und um die Haut-Adnexe (s. Abb. 4). Letztere Gebilde (Talgdrüsen, Schweißdrüsen) können in fortgeschrittenen Stadien verlorengehen. Nekrotisierende Arteriitis und fibrinoide Veränderungen gehören nicht zum Bild des chronischen discoiden Lupus erythematodes. In Übergangsformen (z.B. bei Patienten mit discoidem Erythematodes und gleichzeitig bestehendem visceralen Lupus erythematodes) können die oben beschriebenen Veränderungen neben denjenigen des discoiden Erythematodes vorliegen.

Es wurden schließlich granulomatöse Veränderungen beschrieben, vornehmlich in serösen Häuten, Lungen und Lymphknoten. Es handelt sich um Herdchen mit fibrinoid-nekrotischem Zentrum und epitheloiden Zellen, die um das nekrotische Zentrum angeordnet sind. Die epitheloiden Zellen können mehrkernig sein. In solchen Herden wurden auch Hämatoxylin-Körperchen beobachtet (Pollak 1959).

Zusammenfassend können eine Reihe von Gewebsveränderungen bei Patienten mit visceralem Lupus erythematodes nachgewiesen werden,mit von Fall zu Fall wechselndem Verteilungsbild. Die morphologische Vielgestalt kann mit der Hypothese verstanden werden, daß Antigen-Antikörper-Komplexe zusammen mit Komplement und Fibrin am Zustandekommen der vasculären Läsionen verantwortlich sind, wobei zusätzliche, u. U. unspezifische Faktoren die Lokalisation der Ablagerungen dieser Komplexe bedingen dürften. Läsionen ähnlicher Verteilung konnten an der Maus durch intravenöse Injektion löslicher Antigen-Antikörper-Komplexe reproduziert werden (McCluskey u. Mitarb. 1960, 1962). N. Cooper (New York University, N.Y.) konnte kürzlich Gammaglobulin in den Kupfferschen Zellen der Leber immunofluorescenztechnisch nachweisen, was als Phagocytose von Immunkomplexen durch das reticulo-endotheliale System gedeutet werden kann (persönliche Mitteilung). Fibrinoides Material mag die Ablagerung der Immunkomplexe begleiten, da bekannterweise Gerinnungsvorgänge durch Immunkomplexe ausgelöst werden können. Für eigentlich cytotoxische Vorgänge (anticytoplasmatische Antikörper, antinucleare Antikörper) liegen keine histomorphologischen Anhaltspunkte vor.

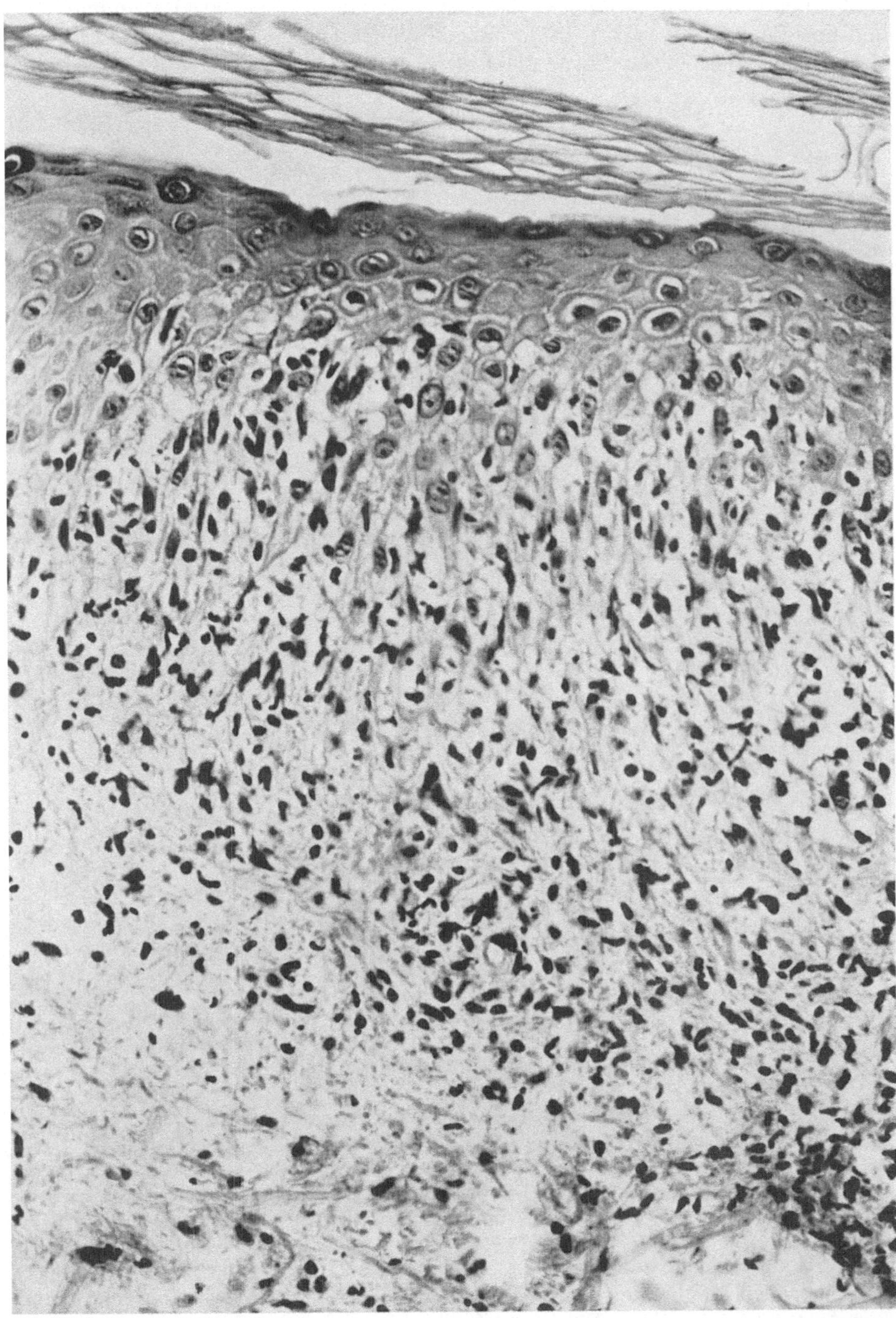

Abb. 3. Hautbiopsie einer floriden Hauteruption bei einer Patientin mit akutem visceralem Erythematodes. Starke ödematöse Durchtränkung der Epidermis und der oberen Dermis-Schicht mit Ruptur der Basalschicht. Entzündliche Infiltration mit mononuclearen Zellelementen

7. Klinische Manifestationen

Früher wurde angenommen, daß der viscerale Erythematodes obligat akut und hochfieberhaft verläuft, in der Regel mit letalem Ausgang. Heute trifft das sicher nicht mehr zu, und zwar nicht etwa deshalb, weil sich das Krankheitsbild

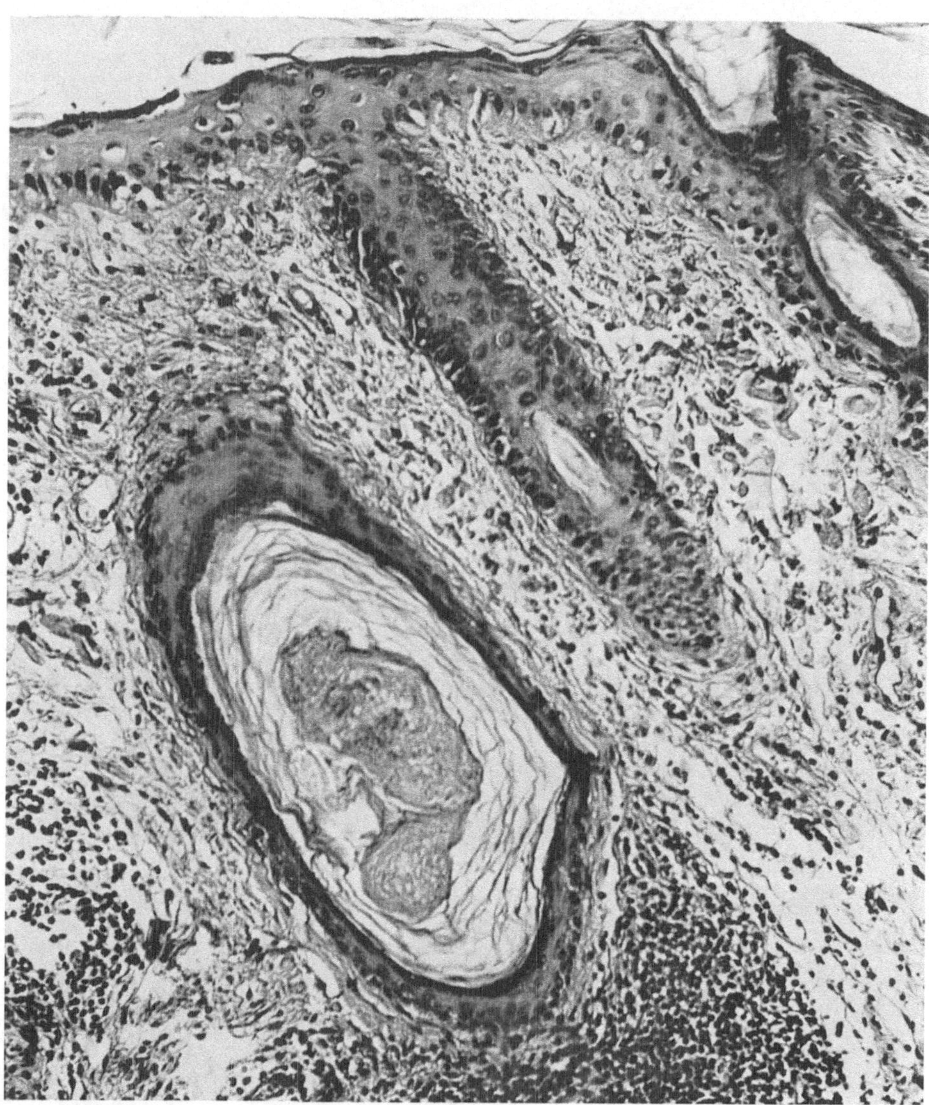

Abb. 4. Hautbiopsie eines Patienten mit chronischem discoidem Lupus erythematodes. Die charakteristischen Veränderungen bestehen in Hyperkeratosis, Keratinpfropfen und in einer lymphocytären Infiltration

im Laufe der Zeit geändert hat, sondern vielmehr auf Grund der viel besseren diagnostischen Möglichkeiten, die Verlaufsformen erkennen lassen, welche früher dem Arzt entgangen sind. Der akute Beginn des visceralen Lupus erythematodes gehört heute zu den Ausnahmen. Von den 127 Patienten, die wir in den letzten 3 Jahren am Bellevue Medical Center beobachten konnten, zeigten nur 37 eine akut fieberhafte Ersterkrankung. Häufiger beginnt die Krankheit oligosymptomatisch mit Zeichen allgemeiner Abgeschlagenheit, Inappetenz und Gewichtsabnahme. Diese Phase kann von kurzer Dauer sein oder Monate bis Jahre dauern. Je nach der Natur der ersten Symptome wurden bei unseren 127 New Yorker Fällen als erstes Krankheitszeichen angegeben:

Arthritis	64	Pleuritis	2
Hauteruption	33	Psychose	2
Fieber	9	Halsschmerzen	2
epileptische Anfälle	5	„Blutarmut“	2
Müdigkeit	3	Nierenkrankheit	1
Husten	3	Purpura	1

Acht Patienten (ein Mann und sieben Frauen) hatten während 2—31 Jahren vor Beginn des visceralen Lupus erythematodes einen einwandfrei festgestellten chronischen discoiden Lupus erythematodes (6% aller Patienten). 9% der Patienten wiesen während mehreren Jahren den charakteristischen Verlauf einer primär chronischen Polyarthritis auf, ohne daß retrospektiv die Krankheit schon früher als visceraler Lupus erythematodes hätte bezeichnet werden können.

Im folgenden sei auf die einzelnen Symptome näher eingegangen (s. auch Tabelle 1):

Allgemeinsymptome wie Müdigkeit, Inappetenz, Gewichtsverlust fehlen wohl nie, werden aber von den Patienten nicht immer zugegeben. Fieber kommt wahrscheinlich auch bei allen Patienten während meistens kurzer Zeit vor, wird aber nicht immer gemessen. In Zweifelsfällen ist den Kranken zu empfehlen, die Temperatur zu Hause zu messen und aufzuschreiben.

Hautmanifestationen werden in ungefähr $^3/_4$ aller Fälle angetroffen. Die sog. Schmetterlingseruption (erythematöse Eruption beider Wangen und Nasenrücken, s. Abb. 5) trat bei 40% unserer Fälle auf. Für den chronischen cutanen Lupus erythematodes charakteristische Hautveränderungen wurde in 16% beobachtet. Eine Anzahl weiterer Hauterscheinungen kommen regelmäßig bei einzelnen Erythematodes-Patienten vor: Haarausfall (Abb. 6), maculo-papulo-erythematöse Eruption (Abb. 7), Urticaria, lokalisierte passagere Ödeme, vor allem an Extremitäten und im Gesicht, Purpura (vasculäre auf Grund einer Vaskulitis und thrombopenische), bullöse (Abb. 8), aber auch ulceröse Eruptionen, Fingernägelveränderungen in Form eines Erythems der Nagelbasis. In ungefähr $^1/_5$ der Patienten besteht ein Zusammenhang zwischen Sonnenbestrahlung und Auftreten einer Hauteruption.

Die meisten Hautläsionen heilen narbenfrei. Gelegentlich treten Depigmentationen oder Hyperpigmentationen an der Stelle der Hautläsionen auf. Die für den chronischen discoiden Erythematodes charakteristischen Eruptionen heilen entsprechend unter Narbenbildung. Teleangiektasien werden nicht selten an Stelle des Erythems nach dessen Abheilung gefunden.

Sonnenbelichtete Hautstellen werden fast ausnahmslos befallen, und nur selten tritt anderswo eine Eruption auf.

Schleimhautläsionen werden häufig beobachtet, wenn man sie sucht. Es handelt sich meist um rote Verdickungen, oft mit einer Erosion oder einem kleinen Ulcus im Zentrum. Diese Eruptionen kommen vorzugsweise an Lippen (Abb. 9) und an der Mundschleimhaut (Abb. 10) vor.

Gelenksymptome stellen die häufigste Organmanifestation des visceralen Lupus erythematodes dar. Es handelt sich um Schwellungen verschiedener Gelenke, vorwiegend der Hand und Finger, weniger häufig der Gelenke an den unteren Extremitäten, mit Überwärmung und Schmerzen bei passiver und aktiver Bewegung. Die Veränderungen können denjenigen der primär chronischen Polyarthritis ähnlich sein. Deformitäten werden häufiger beobachtet als allgemein angenommen wird. Sie sind jedoch meist nur leichter Art und erreichen nie die extremen Grade der primär chronischen Polyarthritis.

Tabelle 1. *Prozentuale Häufung verschiedener klinischer Manifestationen*

	Autoren und Anzahl Patienten					
	Eigene Fälle	HARVEY u. Mitarb.	DUBOIS	JESSAR u. Mitarb.	SHEARN u. PIROFSKY	MIESCHER u. VORLAENDER
Anzahl der Patienten	127	105	520	44	34	100
1. Allgemeine Symptome:						
Gewichtsverlust	60	71	51,3	100	74	95
Fieber	97	86	83,6	95	100	91
2. Haut:						
Alle Formen	72	85	71,5	68	91	76
Schmetterlingserythem	40	39	56,7			48
Discoide Erythematodes-Eruption	16					
Urticaria	16					
Bullöse Eruption	6		6,9			
Purpura	12	9	19,8		15	
Durch Sonnenbestrahlung ausgelöste Eruption	22	11	32,7		58	
Schleimhauteruption		14	9,1	18		
Veränderungen an Nägel	9					
3. Gelenk:						
Alle Formen	81	90	91,9	77	86	85
Transitorische Arthritis	40					
Chronische Arthritis ohne Deformitäten	20					
Chronisch-deformierte Arthritis	20	27	26,3		12	39
4. Nieren:						
Alle Formen	61	65	46,1	70	62	67
Nephritis	55					
Nephrose	6		23,0			
Nierenbefall mit Hypertonie	15	14		18	32	
Urämie		11	18,0			
5. Herz:						
Alle Formen	54	52		70		61
Tachykardie	54					
Kardiomegalie	30	15	15,7	34		
Auskultatorischer Befund (Geräusch)	32	44	21,3	55	71	
Herzinsuffizienz	10	8	5,0		21	
Pathologisches Elektrokardiogramm	56		35,1			
6. Seröse Membranen:						
Alle Formen	56					40
Perikarditis	15	45	30,5	23	18	
Pleuritis	39	57	45,0	39	24	
Peritonitis	13	0	11,3		15	
7. Lungen:						
„Atypische Infiltrate“	15	22	0,9	20		45
8. Leber:						
Vergrößerung	35	32	23,2	29	44	
Ikterus	6	3	3,8		12	
9. Milz:						
Vergrößerung	21	15	9,0	27	41	48
10. Lymphknoten:						
Vergrößerung	48	58	58,6	37	68	

Tabelle 1. (Fortsetzung)

	Autoren und Anzahl Patienten					
	Eigene Fälle	Harvey u. Mitarb.	Dubois	Jessar u. Mitarb.	Shearn u. Pirofski	Miescher u. Vorländer
11. Gastrointestinale Symptome:						
Alle Formen	25	10	53,2	22	35	23
12. Schilddrüse:						
Vergrößerung	3					
13. Parotis:						
Vergrößerung	5					
14. Periphere Gefäße:						
Alle Formen	20					29
Raynaudsches Syndrom	15	10	18,4	16	6	
Thrombophlebitis . .	16					
15. Zentralnervensystem:						
Alle Formen	44		25,5			18
Psychose	22,5	19	12,1	9		21
Konvulsive Anfälle . .	10	17	13,8	7	15	
16. Peripheres Nervensystem:						
Alle Formen	14		11,7			16
17. Augen:						
Alle Formen	15	30		20	28	
„Cytoid bodies" . . .	8	25	9,6			
Hypertonieveränderungen . . .	5					
Hämorrhagie			10,5			
Conjunctivitis	14	5	10,3			

Nierensymptome leichter Art werden häufig beobachtet (Muehrcke u. Mitarb. 1955, Pollack u. Mitarb. 1958, Stevens u. Knowles 1962, Vernier u. Mitarb. 1958, Yamauchi u. Mitarb. 1962). Mehr als die Hälfte der Patienten weisen einen pathologischen Nierenbefund auf. Harnstoffretention ist im Anfangsstadium der Krankheit selten, jedoch kommt es bei $^1/_5$—$^1/_4$ der Fälle im späteren Verlauf dazu. Proteinurie stellt das leichteste Zeichen dar und ist kein Grund zu spezieller Besorgnis, wenn nicht gleichzeitig Erythrurie und Cylindrurie bestehen. Mikrohämaturie deutet bereits auf eine schwere Nierenbeteiligung hin, ebenso Cylindrurie (meist handelt es sich um die fokale Erythematodes-Glomerulitis). Bei ungefähr $^1/_4$ der Patienten mit initialen Nierensymptomen kommt es zu einer „renalen Verlaufsform" des visceralen Lupus erythematodes mit Ausgang in Urämie. Dies ist eine ziemlich hohe Patientenquote, doch kann nicht gesagt werden, daß die Niereninsuffizienz die häufigste Todesursache sei. Von unseren 127 New Yorker Patienten sind 25 nach 3jähriger Beobachtung gestorben. Todesursache war nur in sechs Fällen Urämie (in acht war der Tod nicht renal bedingt, in neun Fällen verlief eine interkurrente Infektion tödlich, einmal kam es zu einer Lungenembolie und einmal zu einer cerebralen Blutung).

Zu einem nephrotischen Syndrom ist es bei 6% unserer Fälle gekommen. Eine renale Hypertonie wird in einer Häufigkeit von 10—20% angetroffen.

Nierenbeteiligung bedeutet nicht unbedingt eine ernste Prognose. Bei vielen Patienten bleiben die Befunde jahrelang stationär oder normalisieren sich. Im Einzelfall ist es schwierig, ja meist unmöglich, den weiteren Verlauf der renalen Affektion vorauszusehen. Fälle mit leichtem Nierenbefund gehen mitunter ganz plötzlich in eine renale Insuffizienz über, währenddem andere Fälle mit scheinbar ernster Nierenbeteiligung einen günstigeren Verlauf nehmen.

Bei Proteinurie kann u.U. das L.E.-Phänomen durch den Urin ausgelöst werden (KORTING u. SCHMITZ 1952).

Kardiale Symptome. Die Häufigkeit der kardialen Beteiligung ist schwierig einzuschätzen. Viele Patienten klagen lediglich über ein leichtes Oppressionsgefühl über der linken Brustgegend und weisen eine Tendenz zu Tachykardie auf. Wenn gleichzeitig ein Galopprhythmus auskultiert wird, dürfte am Vorliegen einer Myokarditis nicht mehr gezweifelt werden. Herzgeräusche werden weniger häufig angetroffen. Bei sorgfältiger und wiederholter Untersuchung der Patienten wird nicht selten im Verlauf der Krankheit eine Vergrößerung des Herzens festgestellt, meist als Folge einer Myokarditis oder Perikarditis. Bei ungefähr einem Zehntel aller Patienten werden eindeutige Zeichen einer Herzinsuffizienz als Folge der Erythematodes-Erkrankung gefunden.

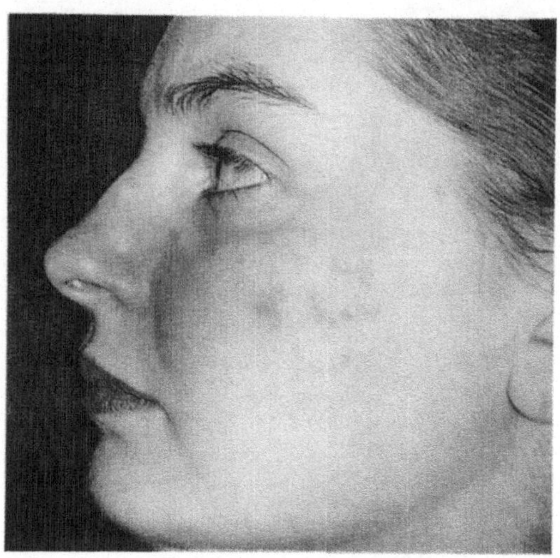

Abb. 5. „Butterfly"-Eruption über Nasenrücken und Wangen

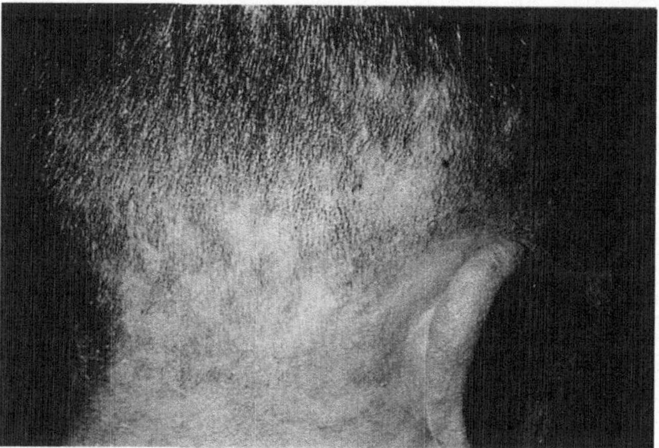

Abb. 6. Alopecia mit maculo-papulo-erythematöser Eruption an Kopf

Veränderungen im Elektrokardiogramm werden mit verschiedener Häufigkeit angegeben. Sie bestehen in Verbreiterung des QRS-Komplexes, evtl. mit Aufsplitterung, oder in Verlängerung des PQ-Intervalles oder in Störungen der Nachschwankung, überhöhte ST-Segmente, negative T-Wellen.

Die *serösen Häute* gehören ebenfalls zu den Prädilektions-Lokalisationen des visceralen Lupus erythematodes. Nach den meisten Mitteilungen sind die Pleuren an erster Stelle befallen, an zweiter das Perikard und am wenigsten häufig das Peritoneum. In der Regel liegt nur geringgradiges Exsudat vor, große Ergüsse sind selten.

Die *pulmonale Lokalisation* des visceralen Lupus erythematodes ist wohl häufiger als gewöhnlich angenommen wird. HARVEY u. Mitarb. haben besonders auf die „Lupus-Pneumonitis" hingewiesen. Da Lungenkomplikationen unspezifischer Art nicht selten im Verlauf der Krankheit angetroffen werden, wurde den „spezifischen" Lupus erythematodes-Veränderungen zuwenig Aufmerksamkeit geschenkt. Umgekehrt kann die „spezifische" Natur einer Lungenveränderung im Einzelfall meist nicht mit Sicherheit als solche erkannt werden.

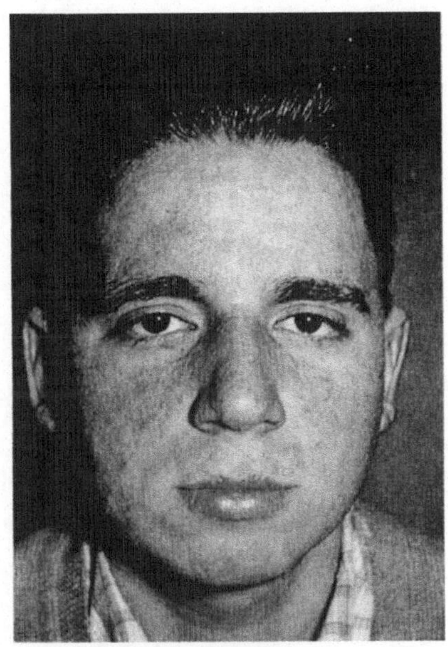

Abb. 7. Konfluierende maculo-papulo-erythematöse Hauteruption an Hautstellen, die dem Sonnenlicht ausgesetzt sind

Die pulmonale Lokalisation des visceralen Lupus erythematodes führt zu „interstitiellen" Parenchymveränderungen. Die perkussorischen und auskultatorischen Zeichen sind meist gering und unauffällig. Röntgenologisch bestehen kleinfleckige, evtl. streifige, über mehr oder weniger ausgedehnte Lungenbezirke sich erstreckende Verschattungen. Dyspnoe und Neigung zu Cyanose wird gelegentlich beobachtet und dürfte auf Störungen des Gasaustausches infolge der interstitiellen Veränderungen oder durch streifenförmige Atelektasen bedingt sein.

Die Tatsache, daß die Lungen Sitz eigentlicher Erythematodes-Veränderungen sein können, darf aber nicht darüber hinwegtäuschen, daß unspezifische bakterielle und auch tuberkulöse Komplikationen immer wieder im Verlauf einer visceralen Lupus erythematodes-Erkrankung auftreten. Besonders gefürchtet sind tuberkulöse Infektionen, welche im Schatten der allgemeinen Steroid-Behandlung zu einer disseminierten, letal endenden Tuberkulose führen können.

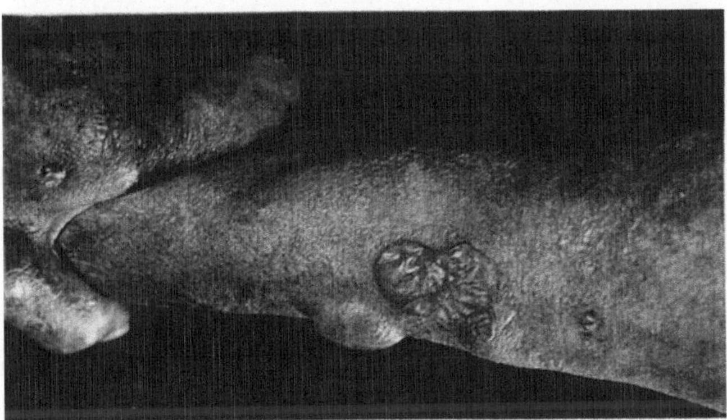

Abb. 8. Bullöse Hautläsionen

Die *Leber* steht selten im Zentrum des Krankheitsgeschehens. Eine leichte Lebervergrößerung wird wohl in ungefähr einem Drittel der Fälle gefunden, jedoch in der Regel ohne Beeinträchtigung der Leberfunktion. Ikterus ist ein wenig häufiges Symptom und meist Folge einer unspezifischen Komplikation, wie Hepatitis, oder Folge einer hämolytischen Anämie.

In den letzten Jahren wurde ein Syndrom als „lupoide Hepatitis“ beschrieben, das durch eine chronische Leberentzündung mit vorwiegend plasmacellulärer Reaktion („Plasmazell-Hepatitis“), eine massive Hypergammaglobulinämie und häufig durch einen positiven L.E.-Zelltest gekennzeichnet ist, und das vor allem bei jungen Frauen angetroffen wird (Bearn u. Mitarb. 1956, Fallet 1960, Gray u. Mitarb. 1958, Holman u. Tomasi 1960; Kayhoe u. Mitarb. 1960, Kunkel u. Mitarb. 1951, Mackay u. Mitarb. 1956). Trotzdem die lupoide Hepatitis eine gewisse Ähnlichkeit mit dem visceralen Lupus erythematodes hat, unterscheidet sie sich in vielen Zügen von ihr, so daß heute allgemein angenommen wird, daß

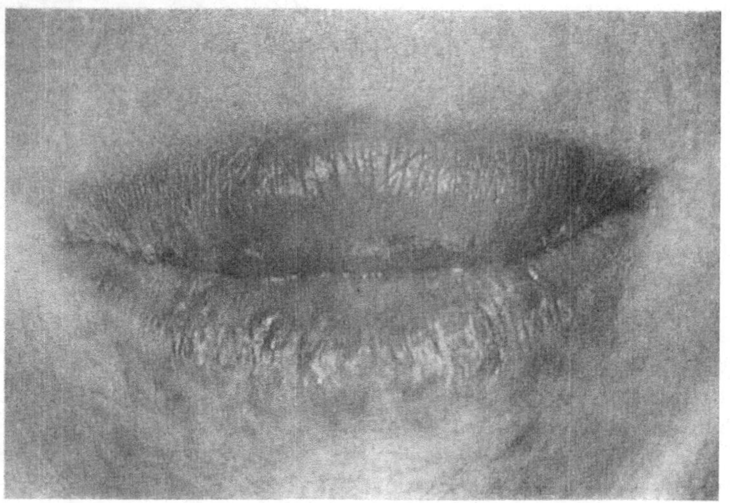

Abb. 9. Maculo-erythematöse Eruption an Lippe

es sich um verschiedenartige Affektionen handelt. Insbesondere wird bei der lupoiden Hepatitis die für den visceralen Lupus erythematodes charakteristische disseminierte Symptomatologie vermißt, und im speziellen fehlen die charakteristischen Nierenveränderungen sowie die Hautläsionen. Äußerst selten werden beide Krankheitsbilder gleichzeitig beobachtet (nach unserer Erfahrung in weniger als 1% aller Erythematodes-Patienten).

Bei anderen Leberleiden kommt es sehr selten zur L.E.-Zellbildung (Heller u. Mitarb. 1956).

Milz und *Lymphknoten* sind oft vergrößert. Die Häufigkeit ist je nach Alter verschieden. Unter 10 Jahren wird selten eine Lymphknoten- oder Milzvergrößerung vermißt. Im zweiten Lebensjahrzehnt nimmt die Reaktivität des reticuloendothelialen Systems rasch ab, um ein Plateau zu erreichen, das erst in fortgeschrittenem Alter weiter sinkt. Entsprechend nimmt die Beteiligung dieser Organe am Krankheitsgeschehen des visceralen Erythematodes mit zunehmendem Alter ab. Bei Patienten über 50 Jahren wird die Milz nur noch ausnahmsweise palpiert, und meist besteht auch keine Vergrößerung der Lymphknoten bei solchen älteren Patienten.

Gastrointestinale Symptome sind in der Regel unspezifischer Art. Selten dominieren sie das klinische Bild. In einem unserer Fälle war ein rezidivierender Subileus Leitsymptom der Krankheit. Ähnliche Fälle wurden beschrieben (Bruce 1959, Dörner u. Mitarb. 1961). Die Differentialdiagnose gegenüber anderen Ursachen eines akuten Abdomen kann dann sehr schwierig sein.

Die *Schilddrüse* erscheint selten vergrößert. In nur einem unserer Fälle lag mit großer Wahrscheinlichkeit eine eigentliche Thyreoiditis vor. Das gleichzeitige Bestehen einer chronischen, lymphocytären Thyreoiditis und eines visceralen Lupus erythematodes ist selten.

Vergrößerung der *Parotis-Drüsen* stellt wohl eine unspezifische Komplikation dar, meist in der terminalen Phase der Erkrankung.

Die *peripheren Gefäße* können auf verschiedene Art befallen sein. Perivasculäre Entzündung kleinster Hautgefäße führt zum Bild der vasculären Purpura. Die Histologie kann derjenigen der Schönlein-Henochschen Purpura gleichen. Thrombophlebitiden kleinerer Venen mit exquisit chronischem Verlauf kommen gelegentlich vor und dürften ebenfalls eine spezifische Erythematodes-Manifestation darstellen. Schließlich wird das Raynaudsche Syndrom nicht selten beobachtet, wobei die Pathogenese dieser vasculären Manifestation nicht klar ist. Selten besteht gleichzeitig eine Kryoglobulinämie, die als Ursache eines Raynaudschen Syndrom in Frage kommt.

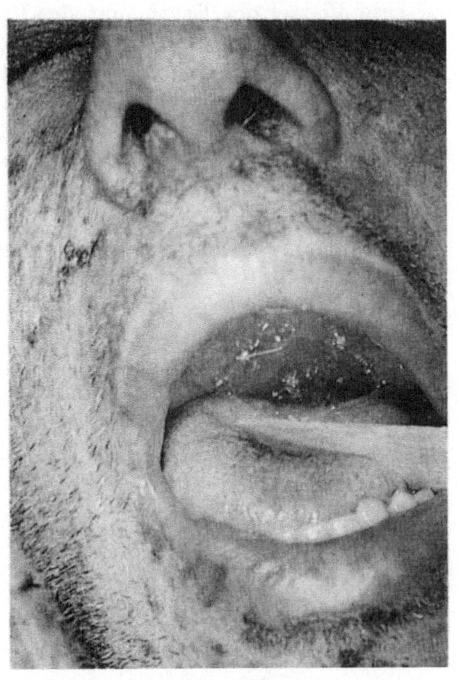

Abb. 10. Ulceröse Schleimhautläsion (mit Pfeil bezeichnet)

Das *zentrale Nervensystem* ist gelegentlich Sitz spezifischer Erythematodes-Veränderungen (Vaskulitiden). Die Symptomatologie ist entweder durch psychotische Veränderungen des Charakters gekennzeichnet (O'Connor 1959) oder durch zentrale motorische Symptome (Konvulsionen, athetotische motorische Störungen, selten sensible Störungen). Das Zusammentreffen der Diagnosen Epilepsie und primär chronische Polyarthritis ist äußerst verdächtig auf das Bestehen eines visceralen Erythematodes. In vereinzelten Fällen scheint dieser Symptomenkomplex durch eine Hydantoin-Überempfindlichkeit ausgelöst zu sein (Dustan u. Mitarb. 1954, Ruppli u. Vossen 1957). Wir konnten 1952 einen Fall von Hydantoin-Überempfindlichkeit mit positivem Pseudo-L.E.-Zellphänomen beobachten, bei welchem nach Absetzen von Hydantoin alle Überempfindlichkeitssymptome verschwanden (Miescher u. Delacretaz 1953). Nachdem heute fest steht, daß auch andere medikamentöse Überempfindlichkeitszustände das Krankheitsbild eines visceralen Lupus erythematodes nachahmen können (Hydralazin [Erickson u. Mitarb. 1956, Henn u. Mitarb. 1955, Perry u. Schroeder 1954, Shearn u. Pirofsky 1952], Chlorpromazin [Miescher u. Jackson 1962]), muß bei Epileptikern mit positivem L.E.-Zellphänomen an diese differentialdiagnostischen Möglichkeiten gedacht werden.

Aseptische Meningitis mit Eiweiß- und Zellvermehrung im Liquor kommt vor. Die Zellvermehrung beträgt maximal einige Hundert Zellen. Die Art der Zellen ist uncharakteristisch; es kann sich um vorwiegend polymorphnucleare oder mononucleare Elemente handeln.

Periphere neurologische Symptome sind seltener (ungefähr $^1/_6$ der Patienten) und bestehen in leichten Paresen und Neuritiden.

Augensymptome werden in $^1/_5$ der Erythematodes-Patienten beobachtet. Am häufigsten sind kleine, umschriebene, weißliche Herde im Augenhintergrund („cytoid bodies"), seltener Blutungen und Papillenödem. Conjunctivitis ist meist ein Begleitsymptom einer Hauteruption in diesem Bereich.

8. Blutveränderungen

Drei Viertel der Erythematodes-Patienten weisen eine normocytäre, normochrome Anämie mittleren Grades auf (Hämoglobin weniger als 12 g-%). In ungefähr 5% liegt eine eigentliche hämolytische Anämie mit hoher Reticulocytose und positivem Coombs-Test vor (Dubois 1956, Etcheverry u. Mitarb. 1951, Harvey u. Mitarb. 1954, Leddy u. Mitarb., Marmont 1951, Michael u. Mitarb. 1951, Pisciotta u. Mitarb. 1951, Zoutendyk 1951). In diesen Fällen ist die Milz fast immer erheblich vergrößert.

Eine leichte Leukopenie wurde schon lange als häufiger Befund eines visceralen Lupus erythematodes beschrieben (Harvey u. Mitarb. 1954, Dörner u. Mitarb. 1961). Zwei Drittel der Fälle weisen eine Leukocytenzahl von weniger als 5000 auf. Eine hohe Leukocytenzahl läßt einen Sekundärinfekt vermuten. Meist besteht eine geringgradige Linksverschiebung.

Die Blutplättchen sind in einem Drittel der Fälle auf weniger als 150000 vermindert. Eine eigentliche thrombopenische Purpura mit Thrombocytenzahlen unter 50000 kommt in weniger als 5% vor. Die thrombopenische Purpura weist alle Charakterzüge der idiopathischen chronischen thrombopenischen Form auf. Ist die Thrombopenie Vorläufer des visceralen Lupus erythematodes, kann sie bei Fehlen anderer Zeichen als idiopathische Thrombopenie diagnostiziert werden. Meist ist die Blutsenkung jedoch erhöht, und bei positivem Nachweis antinuclearer Antikörper kann schon früh die Diagnose eines visceralen Lupus erythematodes gestellt werden (Dameshek u. Reeves 1956, Rabinowitz u. Dameshek 1960).

Knochenmarksausstriche sind wenig charakteristisch für den visceralen Lupus erythematodes. Meist liegt eine leichte Vermehrung der Plasmazellen vor. Im Falle einer hämolytischen Anämie besteht eine reaktive Erythropoese, im Falle einer Leukopenie meist eine myeloische Hyperplasie, bei Verminderung der Blutplättchen sind die Megakaryocyten fast immer vermehrt mit Vorherrschen unreifer, scharf begrenzter Zellformen. Feinere cytologische Studien werden gegenwärtig von Burkhard an der Münchener Medizinischen Klinik vorgenommen. Es scheint, daß das Knochenmark Sitz tiefergreifender Störungen ist, als bisher angenommen wurde.

In weniger als 5% der Fälle liegt eine Gerinnungsstörung vor (Hitzig u. Mitarb. 1951, Laurell u. Nilsson 1957, Lee u. Sanders 1955, Loeliger 1959), die in einer Hemmung der Thromboplastinaktivität besteht und durch zirkulierende Antikoagulantien gegen Faktoren der ersten Gerinnungsphase bedingt ist. Eine milde hämorrhagische Diathese kann deren Folge sein (Epistaxis, Menorrhagie, leichtes Auftreten von Ekchymosen). Bei Integrität der Blutplättchen und der Gefäße besteht eine normale Blutungszeit, und der Rumpel-Leedesche Test fällt negativ aus.

Die Plasmaproteine sind in der Regel gestört; im akuten, entzündlichen Stadium besteht eine Vermehrung der α_2- und γ-Globuline, später, bei Sistieren der akut entzündlichen Erscheinungen, verschwindet die α_2-Vermehrung. Die γ-Globuline bleiben meistens verändert, auch nach Abklingen eines Schubes (Selig-

MANN u. HANAU 1958). β_{1c}-Globulin kann ebenfalls vermindert sein als Ausdruck der Komplementverminderung (MORSE u. Mitarb. 1961). Selten besteht eine Hypogammaglobulinämie (WEINSTOCK u. LEE 1960).

Die Serumlabilitätsproben geben meistens ein pathologisches Resultat: in über 90% der Fälle ist die Erythrocytensedimentation mäßig bis sehr stark beschleunigt. Ebenso häufig ist das C-reaktive Protein vermehrt. Kephalin-Flokkulation und Thymoltrübungstest sind in wechselndem Ausmaß positiv. Kryoglobuline werden nicht selten gefunden (CHRISTIAN u. Mitarb. 1963).

Eine Reaktion mit Paratoluensulfonsäure wurde als spezifischer Test für den beschrieben visceralen Lupus erythematodes (JANBON u. Mitarb. 1959, JONES und THOMPSON 1958). Es stellte sich aber heraus, daß damit nur eine Vermehrung von Gammaglobulin nachgewiesen wird, und die Reaktion somit zur Gruppe der unspezifischen Serumlabilitätsproben gehört (JANBON u. Mitarb. 1959).

Serumkomplement ist bei Patienten mit visceralem Lupus erythematodes häufig erniedrigt, besonders in akuten Stadien und bei Nierenbeteiligung (MORSE u. Mitarb. 1961, TOWNES u. Mitarb. 1962).

9. Immunologische Veränderungen

Keine Krankheit weist eine größere Vielfalt autoimmunitärer Reaktionen auf als der viscerale Erythematodes. Eine Anzahl dieser Phänomene haben diagnostische Bedeutung, andere sind vorerst nur von theoretischem Interesse.

a) Antinucleare Reaktionen

Eine Reihe von Antikörpern gegen die verschiedenen Kernbestandteile sind im Serum von Erythematodes-Patienten nachgewiesen worden (BARBU u. Mitarb. 1960, CEPELLINI u. Mitarb. 1957, DEICHER u. Mitarb. 1959, HOLBOROW u. Mitarb. 1957, KUNKEL u. Mitarb. 1960, MIESCHER u. FAUCONNET 1954, MIESCHER u. STRAESSLE 1957). Bis jetzt ist keine klinisch eindeutige Erythematodes-Erkrankung mit Fehlen antinuclearer Faktoren während der ganzen Dauer der Erkrankung beobachtet worden. Diese Faktoren scheinen also obligat zum Krankheitsbild des visceralen Lupus erythematodes zu gehören, wobei damit nicht gesagt sei, daß sie zu jeder Zeit vorliegen müssen. Bei anderen Affektionen kommen solche Antikörper sehr viel weniger häufig vor, und bei keiner anderen Krankheit stellen sie einen regelmäßigen Befund dar. Es wird deshalb vermutet, daß den antinuclearen Faktoren eine wesentliche Rolle in der Pathogenese des visceralen Lupus erythematodes zukomme. Aus dem gleichen Grund haben sie eine große Bedeutung für die Diagnostik.

Entsprechend dem Kernsubstrat, mit welchem die antinuclearen Faktoren reagieren, können folgende Antikörper unterschieden werden: 1. gegen Nucleoprotein; 2. gegen Histon; 3. gegen Desoxyribonucleinsäure; 4. gegen einen chemisch noch nicht determinierten Kernbestandteil im Nucleolus (wahrscheinlich Ribonucleoprotein); 5. gegen eine leicht eluierbare Substanz (wahrscheinlich ein Glykoprotein).

Gegen *Nucleoprotein* gerichtete Antikörper haben die größte Bedeutung erlangt, da diese an Leukocyten ein morphologisch charakteristisches Phänomen induzieren, das sog. L.E.-Zellphänomen. 1948 beschrieben HARGRAVES, RICHMOND und MORTON im Knochenmark von Patienten, die an einem visceralen Lupus erythematodes litten, eine eigenartige Zelle, die sie in der Folge L.E.-Zelle nannten. Es handelt sich um eine phagocytäre Zelle (polymorphkerniger Leukocyt, meistens Neutrophile, sehr selten Eosinophile und Basophile, gelegentlich Monocyten) mit einem Zellkern, der durch eine große Einschlußmasse an die

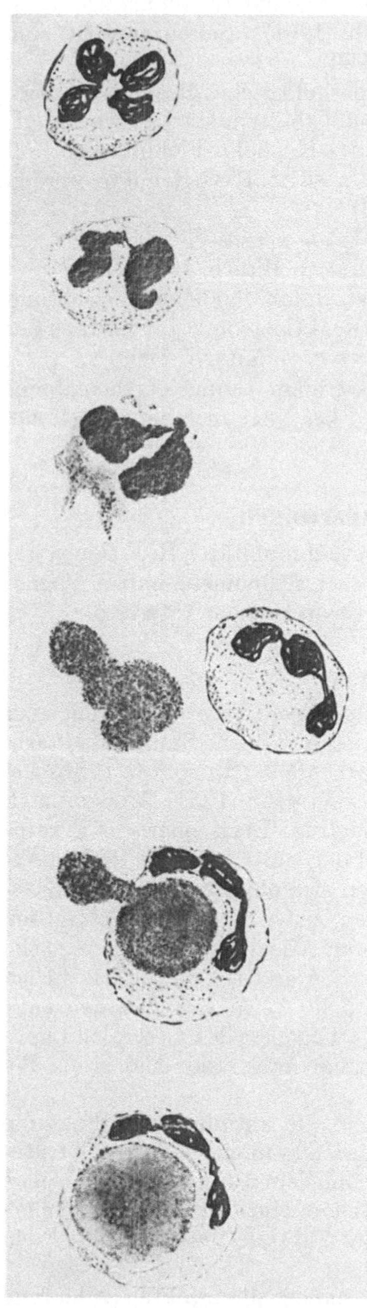

Abb. 11a–f. Schematische Darstellung des L.E.-Zellphänomens (gezeichnet von A. Miescher). Das erste Stadium (b, c) besteht in einer leichten Schwellung und Homogenisierung des Zellkernes in Zellen mit beschädigtem Cytoplasma (Schädigung des Cytoplasmas ist Vorbedingung für das Eindringen des L.E.-Faktors in das Zellinnere). Das zweite Stadium ist durch freie, charakteristisch veränderte Kernkörper gekennzeichnet (d). Das dritte Stadium besteht in der Phagocytose dieser alterierten Kernmassen (e,f)

Peripherie gedrückt erscheint. Die Einschlußmasse ist Feulgen-positiv, d.h. sie enthält Desoxyribonucleinsäure und erweist sich als mehr oder weniger homogene Masse polychromatischen Charakters (Hargraves u. Mitarb. 1948, 1949, 1952, Godman 1959). Währenddem ursprünglich angenommen wurde, daß es sich um das Resultat einer biochemischen Störung handelt (Haserick u. Bortz 1951, Inderbitzin 1953, 1954, Kurnick u. Mitarb. 1952a und b, 1953, Kurnick 1956), konnte später bewiesen werden, daß es sich um die Phagocytose von Kernmaterial handelt, ausgelöst durch den sog. L.E.-Zellfaktor, der alle Eigenschaften eines gegen Nucleoprotein gerichteten Antikörpers besitzt (Miescher u. Mitarb. 1953, 1954, 1960, Miescher u. Fauconnet 1954a und b, Miescher u. Holländer 1955, Miescher 1955, 1957a, b, 1959, Holman u. Kunkel 1957). Der für die L.E.-Zellbildung verantwortliche Faktor ist ein Gammaglobulin mit der Sedimentationskonstante von 7 Svedberg-Einheiten (Haserick u. Bortz 1950, Miescher u. Mitarb. 1954, Fallet u. Mitarb. 1959), das unter Beteiligung von Komplement zur Phagocytose von Kernmaterial führt. Daneben gibt es andere Antikörper gegen Nucleoprotein, die nicht zur L.E.-Zellbildung führen (eigene Beobachtungen). In einem Fall lag ein hochtitriger 19 S-Antikörper gegen Nucleoprotein vor, der Komplement fixierte, jedoch ohne daß L.E.-Zellen gebildet wurden. Damit sei jedoch nicht gefolgert, daß jeder 19 S-Antikörper gegen Nucleoprotein außerstande sei, nucleophagocytäre Phänomene auszulösen.

Der L.E.-Zellfaktor kann den Zellkern einer vitalen Zelle nicht erreichen (Miescher u. Fauconnet 1954, Rapp 1962, Scheffer 1961). Erst wenn die Zelle durch Alter oder anderswie alteriert ist (Abb. 11b), dringt der Antikörper bis zum Zellkern vor und erzeugt folgende Veränderungen: Der Zellkern schwillt an (wahrscheinlich durch Aufnahme von Wasser neben Aufnahme von Protein (Godman u. Mitarb. 1958, Godman u. Deitch 1957), verliert seine Chromatinstruktur und seine färberischen Eigenschaften. Die starke Basophilie des Zellkernes beruht auf dem sauren Charakter der Nucleinsäure. Die Reaktion des Nucleoproteins mit dem Antikörper führt zur Maskierung freier saurer Valenzen (GODMAN u. Mitarb. 1958, GODMAN u. DEITCH 1957, GODMAN 1959). Derart veränderte Zellkerne verlieren deshalb einen Teil ihrer Basophilie und erscheinen metachromatisch. Diese färberischen Eigenschaften der geschwollenen Zellkerne sind diagnostisch wichtig zur Abgrenzung des L.E.-Zellphänomens gegenüber anderen nucleophagocytären Reaktionen. Die bis jetzt beschriebenen Kernveränderungen können sich unter teilweiser Erhaltung des Cytoplasmas der Zellen abspielen. Jedoch verlieren die Zellen bald das Cytoplasma, wodurch die veränderten Zellkerne isoliert in Erscheinung treten (Abb. 11c, d und Abb. 12a). Sie werden dann „L.E.-Körperchen" genannt oder im Gewebe auf Grund ihrer besonderen färberischen Eigenschaften

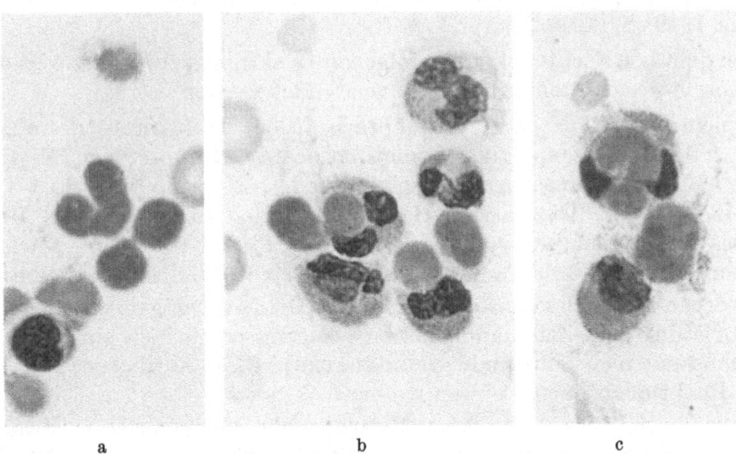

Abb. 12a—c. Positives L.E.-Zellphänomen. a Freie alterierte Kernkörper. b Beginnende Phagocytose der alterierten Kernkörper. c L.E.-Zelle. Daneben alterierter Kern eines polymorphkernigen Leukocyten mit Resten von Cytoplasma

„hämatoxyphile Körperchen" (KLEMPERER u. Mitarb. 1941, 1950). Derart veränderte Zellkerne werden durch phagocytierende Zellen in Gegenwart von Komplement aufgenommen, unter Bildung der L.E.-Zellen (Abb. 11e, f und Abb. 12b, c). L.E.-Zellen werden äußerst selten im direkten Blutausstrich gefunden (CHOMET u. Mitarb. 1953). Zu ihrem Nachweis muß Blut in vitro inkubiert werden.

Eine Vielzahl von Methoden wurde beschrieben zum Nachweis des L.E.-Zellphänomens (BARNES u. Mitarb. 1950, BERMAN u. Mitarb. 1950, BERTRAND 1952, GONYEA u. Mitarb. 1950, HARGRAVES u. Mitarb. 1949, HASERICK u. BORTZ 1949, HASERICK 1954, LEE 1951, MAGATH u. WINKLE 1952, MILLER 1961, SNAPPER u. NATHAN 1955, WEISBERGER u. Mitarb. 1952, ZINKHAM u. CONLEY 1956). Die Technik nach ZIMMER und HARGRAVES (1952) hat den Vorteil der Einfachheit bei gleichzeitiger großer Empfindlichkeit:

10 ml Blut werden ohne Verwendung eines gerinnungshemmenden Stoffes durch Venenpunktion entnommen und unter sterilen Bedingungen während 90 min in einem Inkubator bei 37°C bebrütet. Darauf wird das Serum vom Blutkuchen getrennt (ohne Zentrifugation) und der Blutkuchen durch ein feines metallenes Teesieb getrieben. Der Blutkuchensaft wird mit einer feinen Glaspipette in ein Hämatokritröhrchen (z.B. nach WINTROBE) gebracht und während 10 min mit 2800 Touren je Minute zentrifugiert. Anschließend wird das Röhrchen während 8 min im Wasserbad bei 37°C inkubiert, damit die durch die vorgängige Manipulation freigelegten Zellkerne durch den L.E.-Faktor opsonisiert und von noch lebenden Phagocyten aufgenommen werden können. Nach sorgfältigem Entfernen des Serums wird die graue Leukocytenschicht mit einer Pasteur-Pipette aspiriert und auf einem Objektträger ausgestrichen. Nach May-Grünwald-Giemsascher Färbung wird das Präparat mikroskopisch untersucht.

Da die polymorphkernigen Leukocyten die lädierbarsten Blutzellen darstellen, sind vor allem sie Sitz der beschriebenen Kernveränderungen und liefern daher das meiste Kernsubstrat für die Reaktion mit dem L.E.-Faktor. Gleichzeitig stellen diese Zellen aber auch die aktivsten Phagocyten dar. Seltener werden die alterierten Kernmassen in Monocyten, Eosinophilen oder gar Basophilen gefunden (Aisenberg 1959, Holman u. Kunkel 1957, Lee u. Mitarb. 1951, Marmont 1952, 1953, Robineaux 1959, Rohn u. Bond 1952, Suksta u. Conley 1951, Sundberg u. Lick 1949, Verloop 1954).

Die Reaktivität des L.E.-Zellfaktors ist ohne Organ- und ohne Species-Spezifität, d.h. Zellkerne jeglicher Organ- und Species-Herkunft werden durch den L.E.-Faktor opsonisiert (Berman u. Mitarb. 1950, Haserick u. Bortz 1949, Miescher 1959, Spiegelberg).

Neben dem L.E.-Zelltest können folgende Reaktionen zum Nachweis der gegen Nucleoprotein gerichteten Antikörper verwendet werden:

Komplementfixation (Barbu u. Mitarb. 1960, Holborow u. Weir 1959, Scalettar 1960), Latexpartikel-Agglutinationstest (Christian u. Mitarb. 1958, Miescher 1959), Fluorescenzantikörpermethode („Nucleoprotein-spot-Technik") (Friou 1957, 1958). Die passive Hämagglutination (nach Boyden 1951) gibt unzuverlässige Ergebnisse wegen der schlechten Fixierbarkeit von Nucleoprotein auf Erythrocyten, die mit Tanninsäure behandelt worden sind (Miescher 1959).

Antikörper gegen *Desoxyribonucleinsäure* (DNS) vermögen wahrscheinlich die Morphologie des L.E.-Zellphänomens zu beeinflussen, jedoch sind sie allein zur L.E.-Zellbildung nicht imstande (Spiegelberg). Diese Antikörper können durch folgende Reaktionen nachgewiesen werden:

Komplementfixation (Barbu u. Mitarb. 1960, Ceppellini u. Mitarb. 1957, Jokinen u. Mäkitalo 1960, Kayhoe u. Mitarb. 1960, Pearson u. Mitarb. 1958), Latexpartikel-Agglutinationstest (Miescher 1959), Bentonitpartikel-Agglutinationstest (Bozicevich u. Mitarb. 1960, Kayhoe u. Mitarb. 1960).

Weniger empfindlich sind Präcipitationsreaktionen (Ceppellini u. Mitarb. 1957, Deicher u. Mitarb. 1959, 1960, Seligmann 1958, 1959). Unregelmäßige Ergebnisse werden mit der passiven Hämagglutinationsmethode erhalten (Jokinen u. Mäkitalo 1960, Lee u. Epstein 1960, Mäkitalo u. Jokinen 1958).

Die serologische Spezifität der Antikörper gegen DNS wurde in den letzten Jahren durch zwei Forschergruppen neu bearbeitet.

Levine u. Mitarb. (Levine 1962, Stollar u. Mitarb. 1962a und b) machten die Beobachtung, daß Alkali-Behandlung von T_2-Bakteriophag die Antigenität erheblich verstärkt. Antikörper, welche durch Immunisierung mit derart vorbehandelten Bakteriophagen erhalten wurden, reagieren viel stärker mit denaturierter Bacteriophag-DNS (Einzelhelix) als mit der Doppelhelix strukturierten nativen DNS (Levine u. Mitarb. 1960). Die Autoren untersuchten darauf DNS-Antikörper von Erythematodes-Patienten. Es zeigte sich, daß die meisten Seren viel stärker mit denaturierter (Einzelhelix) DNS reagieren (Stollar u. Mitarb. 1962a und b). Hemmreaktionen ergeben eine Reaktivität, die je nach Serum verschieden war (Stollar u. Levine 1963). Mit einzelnen Seren war Polythymidin-Säure am wirkungsvollsten, mit anderen Seren Desoxyadenylsäure. Mit einem Serum hemmte Theobromin die DNS-Reaktivität am stärksten. Diese Ergebnisse lassen die Frage aufkommen, ob die Reaktion von Erythematodes-Serum mit DNS nur eine Kreuzreaktion darstellt. Auch Chloroquin erwies sich als starker Inhibitor, jedoch auf Grund eines verschiedenen Mechanismus. Chloroquin reagiert mit DNS und verhindert so dessen Reaktivität mit entsprechenden Antikörpern.

BUTLER u. Mitarb. wiesen einen experimentellen Weg zur Gewinnung von Antikörpern gegen DNS: 6-Trichloromethyl-Purin, das leicht durch Bindung an Aminogruppen an Eiweiß gebunden werden kann, wurde an bovines Serumalbumin gekoppelt, zur Immunisierung von Kaninchen verwendet. Die regelmäßig entstehenden Antikörper reagierten gut mit aufgespaltener DNS, dagegen nicht mit der Doppelhelix-strukturierten DNS (BUTLER u. Mitarb. 1962).

Antikörper gegen Histon (HOLMAN u. Mitarb. 1959, KUNKEL u. Mitarb. 1960) vermögen allein das L.E.-Zellphänomen nicht auszulösen, dagegen können sie es modifizieren (SPIEGELBERG). Mit Histon absorbiertes L.E.-Serum führt zur Bildung von L.E.-Zellen mit folgenden Merkmalen: Die phagocytierte Kernmasse hat die ursprüngliche Kernbasophilie weitgehend erhalten. Ferner liegt sie nicht in homogener, sondern in körniger Form vor, oft unter Ausbildung eines dunklen Randes. Es besteht Grund zur Annahme, daß Antikörper gegen DNS und gegen Histon an der morphologischen Eigenheit des L.E.-Zellphänomens maßgebend beteiligt sind. Jedes individuelle L.E.-Serum führt nämlich zu einem L.E.-Zellphänomen mit einer Anzahl von morphologischen Eigenheiten, die von Patient zu Patient beträchtlich wechseln können.

Der Antikörpernachweis gegen Histon wird selten zu diagnostischen Zwecken verwendet. Kommerziell erhältliches Histon ist meist mehr oder weniger denaturiert, weshalb die Ergebnisse mit verschiedenen Histonpräparaten schwer miteinander verglichen werden können. Ferner sind Histonpräparate meist erheblich antikomplementär. Diese Eigenschaft kann allerdings durch Entfernung der unlöslichen Histonpartikelchen mittels Zentrifugation eliminiert werden.

Neben den erwähnten Techniken zum Nachweis von Reaktionen gegen spezifische Kernbestandteile wurden zwei Methoden entwickelt, die ganze Zellkerne als Substrat für die Reaktion verwenden: 1. Der Antiglobulinkonsumptionstest mit isolierten Zellkernen als Substrat (MIESCHER 1955, 1957). 2. Fluorescenzantikörpermethode (BECK u. Mitarb. 1962, CALABRESI 1959, CRAWFORD u. Mitarb. 1959, FRIOU 1958, HALL u. Mitarb., HOLBOROW u. Mitarb. 1957, RAPP 1962).

Der von STEFFEN (1962) ausgearbeitete Antiglobulinkonsumptionstest hat sich zum Nachweis antinuclearer Reaktionen unter Verwendung isolierter Zellkerne sehr bewährt (MIESCHER 1955, DÖRNER u. Mitarb. 1961). Wenn der Test mit der nötigen Sorgfalt durchgeführt wird (es handelt sich um ein technisch heikles Procedere), ist er von diagnostischer Bedeutung, da er mit großer Empfindlichkeit antinucleare Antikörper aufdeckt (s. Abb. 13).

Die Fluorescenzantikörpermethode hat sich ebenfalls als sehr empfindlich zum Nachweis antinuclearer Faktoren erwiesen. In der Hand eines ungeübten Beobachters kommt es jedoch leicht zu falschen Ergebnissen, meist in der Form falsch-positiver Tests, die den Kliniker irreführen können. Die Fluorescenzantikörpermethode erlaubt, verschiedene Formen der Kernreaktion zu unterscheiden (BECK 1961, BECK u. Mitarb. 1962, ROWELL 1962): Homogene Fluorescenz der Kerne tritt auf, wenn Antikörper gegen Desoxynucleoprotein vorliegen. Weniger häufig erscheint eine feinpunktierte Fluorescenz. Diese „gesprenkelte Fluorescenz" scheint durch Reaktion eines Serumfaktors mit einem in physiologischer Kochsalzlösung löslichen Kernbestandteil bedingt zu sein (Glykoprotein). Schließlich ist eine weitere Form der Kernfluorescenz beschrieben, die auf den Nucleolus beschränkt ist (Ribonucleinsäure ?). Liegen gleichzeitig mehrere Formen der Kernreaktion vor, kann die Aufdeckung der „gesprenkelten" und der „Nucleolus"-Fluorescenz schwierig sein. Verdünnung des Patientenserums erlaubt in einem Teil der Fälle mehrere Reaktionen nachzuweisen. Ferner kann die gesprenkelte oder nucleoläre Fluorescenz nach Absorption des Erythematodes-Serums mit Nucleoprotein in Erscheinung treten.

Der Leukocyten-Aggregations-Hemmtest (Lee 1958) beruht wahrscheinlich auch auf antinuclearen Reaktionen. Leukocyten agglomerieren im Moment ihres

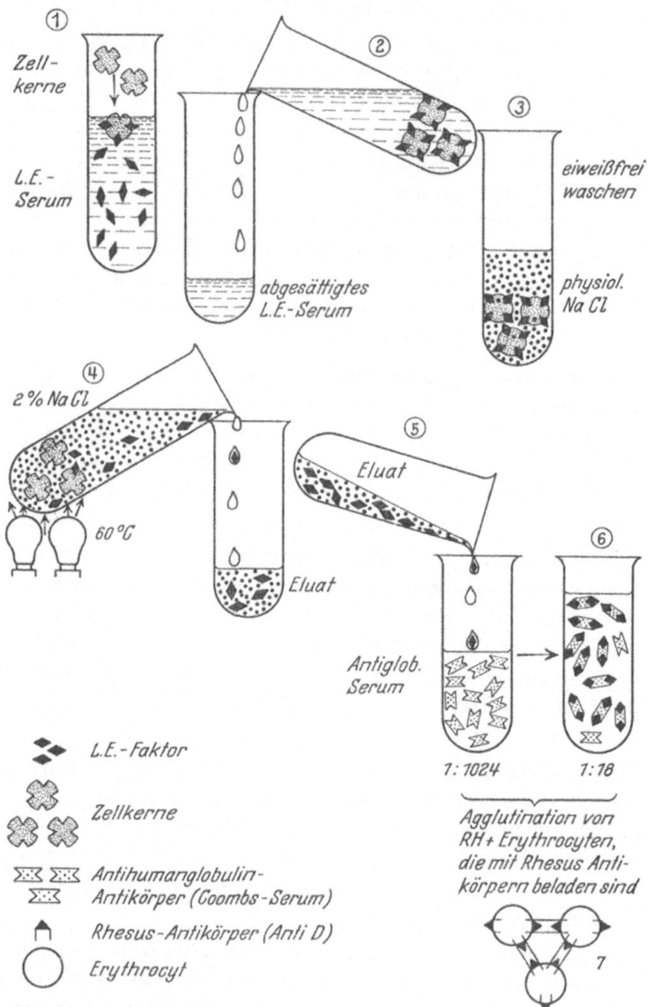

Abb. 13. Schematische Darstellung des Antiglobulin-Konsumptionstests. 1: Fixation antinuclearer Immunglobuline auf isolierte Zellkerne. 2 und 3: Waschen der „sensibilisierten" Zellkerne in physiologischer Kochsalzlösung. 4: Elution der antinuclearen Globuline durch 2% Kochsalzlösung bei 60°C. 5 und 6: Titration des Eluats mit Antihumanglobulinserum. Titerbestimmung des Antihumanglobulinserums erfolgt durch Agglutination von Rh^+-Erythrocyten, welche mit inkompletten Antikörpern beladen sind

beginnenden Zerfalles, wahrscheinlich durch Fusion von freiwerdendem Nucleoprotein bzw. Nucleinsäure. Diese unspezifische Aggregation wird durch L.E.-Serum gehemmt.

Auf experimentelle antinucleare Antikörper kann in diesem Rahmen nicht eingegangen werden (Bardawil u. Mitarb. 1958, Capelli 1952a und b, Deicher u. Heide 1962, Finch u. Mitarb. 1953, Miescher 1953, Miescher u. Mitarb. 1953, 1954, Zimmermann u. Mitarb. 1953).

b) Übrige Immunreaktionen

In 5—10% aller SLE-Patienten ist der direkte Coombs-Test positiv, und zwar meist in Form der Antikomplement-Reaktion, weniger häufig der Antihumangammaglobulinreaktion, selten in der kombinierten Form. Eine immunhämolytische Anämie besteht nur in der Hälfte der Patienten mit positivem Coombs-Test (DUBOIS 1956, ETCHEVERRY u. Mitarb. 1951, HARVEY u. Mitarb. 1954, LEDDY u. Mitarb., MARMONT 1951, MICHAEL u. Mitarb. 1951, PISCIOTTA u. Mitarb. 1951, ZOUTENDYK 1951).

Leukocytenspezifische Antikörper werden am besten mit dem direkten Antiglobulinkonsumptionstest erfaßt (DAUSSET u. COLOMBANI 1961, MIESCHER u. Mitarb. 1964, VAN LOGHEM u. Mitarb. 1957). In $^4/_5$ der Fälle ist dieser Test positiv. Eine wesentlich kleinere Anzahl von Patienten dürfte tatsächlich eine Autoimmunleukopenie aufweisen mit peripherer Leukopenie und zentraler myeloider Hyperplasie.

Bei Patienten mit aktiver SLE-Erkrankung, die nicht unter Steroid-Therapie stehen, wird oft eine Verminderung der Redox-Aktivität der Leukocyten gefunden (CHAUDHURI und MARTIN 1953, COOPER u. Mitarb. 1959). Durch das Serum dieser Patienten kann die Redox-Aktivität normaler Leukocyten ebenfalls vermindert werden. Bis jetzt sind keine Versuche durchgeführt worden zur näheren serologischen Abklärung dieses Phänomens. Es ist möglich, daß antileukocytäre Antikörper dafür verantwortlich sind.

Die Wanderungsgeschwindigkeit von Leukocyten im elektrischen Feld wird wohl auch durch Antikörper, die mit der Zelloberfläche reagieren, beeinflußt (CHAUDHURI u. MARTIN 1953, RUHENSTROTH-BAUER 1961).

Antithrombocytäre Antikörper (HARRINGTON u. Mitarb. 1956, MIESCHER u. FAUCONNET 1954, MIESCHER u. Mitarb. 1964, MUELLER u. RADOJICIC 1956, SELIGMANN 1958) werden am besten im direkten Antiglobulinkonsumptionstest mit patienteneigenen Blutplättchen nachgewiesen (DAUSSET u. Mitarb. 1961, MIESCHER u. Mitarb.). Dieser Serumfaktor ist vom antileukocytären Antikörper verschieden (DAUSSET u. Mitarb. 1961, MUELLER u. RADOJICIC 1956). Er kommt in ungefähr $^4/_5$ der Fälle vor. Eine Autoimmunthrombopenie mit peripherer Thrombocytopenie und zentraler Vermehrung der Megakaryocyten dürfte in der Hälfte dieser Fälle vorliegen (DAUSSET u. Mitarb. 1961, DAMESHEK u. REEVES 1956, MIESCHER 1959, STEFFEN 1962).

Gerinnungshemmende Faktoren werden in verschiedenen Gerinnungstests aufgedeckt (CONLEY 1952, CONLEY u. HARTMANN 1952, GORDON u. Mitarb. 1955, HITZIG u. Mitarb. 1951, LAURELL u. NILSSON 1957, LEE und SANDERS 1955, LEY u. Mitarb. 1951, LOELIGER 1959). Sie sind dadurch charakterisiert, daß sie im Normalblut den Gerinnungsablauf hemmen, d.h. der Gerinnungsdefekt beruht nicht auf einem Mangel an einem Gerinnungsfaktor, sondern auf dem Vorhandensein eines Hemmfaktors, der sich in der Gammaglobulinfraktion befindet und wahrscheinlich einen Autoantikörper darstellt. Vermutlich gibt es verschiedene derartige Antikörper. Hemmfaktoren gegen die erste Phase der Gerinnung und solche, die später einwirken, wurden beobachtet. So wurden Faktoren gegen PTC (Faktor IX), gegen Plättchenphospholipid und gegen Thromboplastin beschrieben, sowie gegen die zweite Gerinnungsphase (wahrscheinlich gegen Prothrombin (LOELIGER 1959).

Die „falsch positive“ Wassermannsche Reaktion ist eine weitere, für die Diagnostik wichtige Autoimmunreaktion. In allen Syphilis-Seroreaktionen, in welchen „Cardiolipin“ als Antigen figuriert, wird nicht ein spezifischer Antikörper gegen Treponema pallidum, sondern ein „Autoantikörper“ erfaßt, der besonders häufig bei syphilitischen Patienten gebildet wird, ferner bei einer Anzahl von Patienten mit verschiedenen Affektionen (HARVEY u. Mitarb. 1954, MOORE u. LUTZ 1955, KOSTANT 1956, PAYNE 1894, REIN u. KOSTANT 1950, ULLMAN 1928, ZIFF u. Mitarb. 1958).

Es handelt sich um eine Reaktion gegen ein Phospholipid, das aus fast allen Organen mit Alkohol oder Aceton extrahiert werden kann und das keine Species-Spezifität aufweist. Alle Syphilis-Reaktionen, die als Antigen dieses Phospholipid enthalten, sind geeignet, diesen bei 10—20% von Patienten mit visceralem Lupus erythematodes vorkommenden Antikörper aufzudecken. Zur Abgrenzung gegen entsprechende, bei syphilitischer Infektion vorkommende Autoantikörper müssen Seroreaktionen mit Treponema-Antigen durchgeführt werden (NELSON u. Mitarb. 1949).

Der sog. *Rheumafaktor* findet sich bei ungefähr $^1/_3$ der visceralen Erythematodes-Patienten (FALLET u. Mitarb. 1959, GOSLINGS u. Mitarb. 1961, KIEVITS u. Mitarb. 1956, MARMONT 1959, PIERCE u. Mitarb. 1959). Es handelt sich um ein 19 S-Immunglobulin, welches gegen aggregiertes 7 S-Immunglobulin gerichtet ist. Dieser Faktor vermag wahrscheinlich nicht mit unverändertem Gammaglobulin zu reagieren. Nachdem 7 S-Immunglobulin mit dem entsprechenden Antigen in Reaktion getreten, oder durch physikalische Eingriffe (z.B. Erhitzen) aggregiert worden ist, wird es gegenüber dem Rheumafaktor reaktionsfähig. Es handelt sich also sehr wahrscheinlich um einen Antikörper, dessen Bildung durch zirkulierende Antigen-Antikörper-Komplexe ausgelöst worden ist (ABRUZZO u. CHRISTIAN 1961). Ursprünglich wurden sensibilisierte, nicht agglutinierte Schaferythrocyten zu dessen Nachweis verwendet. Heute liegt eine Vielzahl von Methoden vor, von welchen sich in erster Linie der Latex-Agglutinationstest für das Routine-Laboratorium durchgesetzt hat (SINGER u. PLOTZ 1956). Besonders empfindliche Reaktionen, wie der Schaferythrocyten-Agglutinationshemmtest (ZIFF u. Mitarb.), sind zu heikel, um in einem Routine-Laboratorium durchgeführt zu werden.

Eine Reihe weiterer autoimmunitärer Phänomene wurden beim visceralen Lupus erythematodes beobachtet. In 20% der Fälle liegen niedrig-titrige Antikörper gegen Thyreoglobulin vor (DÖRNER u. Mitarb. 1961). Eine Thyreoiditis ist jedoch beim visceralen Lupus erythematodes selten. Leberspezifische Antikörper sowie nierenspezifische Antikörper wurden wiederholt beschrieben (GAJDUSEK 1958, MACKAY u. GAJDUSEK 1958, VORLAENDER 1955). Auf Grund neuerer Untersuchungen dürfte es sich aber nicht um leberspezifische Antikörper, sondern um organunspezifische anticytoplasmatische Serumfaktoren handeln (KUNKEL u. Mitarb. 1960, WIEDERMANN u. Mitarb. 1964). Wahrscheinlich handelt es sich um verschiedene Antikörper, die mit cytoplasmatischen Antigenen reagieren. Absorptionsversuche mit Fraktionen, die mit den verschiedenen corpusculären Cytoplasmabestandteilen angereichert sind, haben zu Ergebnissen geführt, die das Bestehen von mindestens vier verschiedenen Antikörpern vermuten lassen (Antikörper gegen Antigene, die in den Lysosomen, Mitochondrien, Mikrosomen lokalisiert sind; ferner Antikörper gegen lösliche cytoplasmatische Antigene) (WIEDERMANN u. Mitarb. 1964). Die mit diesen Antikörpern reagierenden cytoplasmatischen Antigene finden sich in Zellen verschiedener Organherkunft; ja, es besteht auch keine Species-Spezifität. Cytoplasmatische Fraktionen, welche aus Leukocyten gewonnen wurden, reagieren ebenfalls mit diesen Antikörpern. Mit intakten Leukocyten kommt es zu keiner Reaktion, da es sich um intracelluläre Antigene handelt, die nicht an der Zelloberfläche vertreten sind. Die schon erwähnten Leukocyten-spezifischen Antikörper sind von den hier erwähnten anticytoplasmatischen Faktoren verschieden. Im Gegensatz zu ihnen reagieren sie mit der Leukocytenoberfläche und weisen eine leukocytäre Spezifität auf. Tabelle 2 orientiert über die Reaktionsfähigkeit von Leukocyten gegenüber einer Reihe von Auto- und Isoantikörpern.

Tabelle 2. *Immunologische Reaktionen mit Leukocyten*

	Leukocyten-spezifität	Lokalisation der antigenen Determinanten		
		Zelloberfläche	intracytoplasmatisch	Zellkern
Leukocytäre Autoantikörper . .	+	+	?	—
Leukocytäre Isoantikörper . . .	—(?)	+	?	—
Cytoplasmatische Autoantikörper	—	—	+	—
Nucleare Autoantikörper	—	—	—	+

Eine Reihe weiterer, immunologisch schlecht definierter, „organ-spezifischer" Immunreaktionen wurden auf Grund von Ergebnissen beschrieben, welche mit Organsubstraten als Antigen in verschiedenen Tests erzielt wurden (STEFFEN 1962). In Ermangelung einer weiteren immunologischen Abklärung über die Spezifität dieser Reaktionen müssen diese Resultate mit Vorsicht aufgenommen werden.

Schließlich sei noch die sog. „Buffy coat"-Hautreaktion genannt. Autologes heparinisiertes Blut wird scharf zentrifugiert zur Gewinnung der leukocyten- und thrombocytenreichen Schicht (buffy coat). 0,1 ml dieser Schicht wird intracutan gespritzt. 8—24 Std später entsteht bei den meisten Patienten mit visceralem Lupus erythematodes eine Hautreaktion, die einer Tuberkulinreaktion ähnelt. Die Spezifität der Reaktion ist recht gering. Es handelt sich um eine immunologisch nicht näher definierte Reaktion; es ist nicht einmal erwiesen, ob es sich überhaupt um ein immunologisches Phänomen handelt.

10. Diagnose und Differentialdiagnose

Mehr als $^2/_3$ aller Erythematodes-Erkrankungen beginnen schleichend, während die primär akute Verlaufsform zur Ausnahme geworden ist. Bei einem Drittel bis zur Hälfte der Fälle besteht das erste klinische Symptom in Gelenkbeschwerden (BOCK 1956, DÖRNER u. Mitarb. 1961, HARVEY u. Mitarb. 1954, TUMULTY 1949, 1954). 10—20% der Patienten werden mit der Diagnose eines Status febrilis hospitalisiert. Hauteruptionen stellen in 20—25% der Fälle das erste Symptom dar. Diese Feststellungen sind für die Differentialdiagnose wichtig. Es geht daraus hervor, daß entgegen früherer Annahmen nicht mit einem akuten Krankheitsbeginn gerechnet werden muß und daß die Krankheit oft oligosymptomatisch beginnt.

Die Symptomatologie des visceralen Lupus erythematodes wurde in Tabelle 1 in 17 Systeme eingeteilt. Wenn dazu noch Blut als 18. System gerechnet wird (Thrombopenie, Anämie oder Leukopenie) und die Patienten nach Anzahl von Systemerkrankungen gruppiert werden, ergibt sich für unsere Patienten das in Abb. 14 aufgezeichnete Verteilungsbild. Daraus geht hervor, daß bei $^1/_4$ der Patienten nur 3—4 der 18 Systeme beteiligt sind. Unter dieser Einschränkung gilt das Postulat, daß zur Diagnosestellung des visceralen Lupus erythematodes der Nachweis erbracht werden muß, daß es sich um eine Multisystemerkrankung handelt. Dabei spielen zwei Faktoren in der Bewertung der Symptome eine Rolle. Erstens sind gewisse Einzelsymptome besonders wichtig, zweitens gibt es charakteristische Symptomkonstellationen.

Im Falle einer Multisystemerkrankung kommt „Erythematodes"-Hautveränderungen eine große Bedeutung zu. Sowohl die für den discoiden Haut-Erythematodes charakteristischen Läsionen als auch der akute Erythematodes-

Ausschlag der Wangen (sog. Schmetterlingseruptionen), erlauben dann mit großer Wahrscheinlichkeit die Diagnose eines visceralen Lupus erythematodes zu stellen. Ferner kommt der Gelenkbeteiligung eine große Wichtigkeit zu, vor allem wenn das Bild einer frischen primär-chronischen Polyarthritis vorliegt.

Folgende Symptomkonstellationen sind weiterhin sehr verdächtig auf das Vorliegen eines visceralen Lupus erythematodes: Gelenkbeteiligung und Pleuritis. Gelenkbefall und Nierenbeteiligung. Polyarthritis und Herzbeteiligung. Polyarthritis und Zentralnervensystem- und/oder Nierenbeteiligung. Herz- und Nierenbeteiligung.

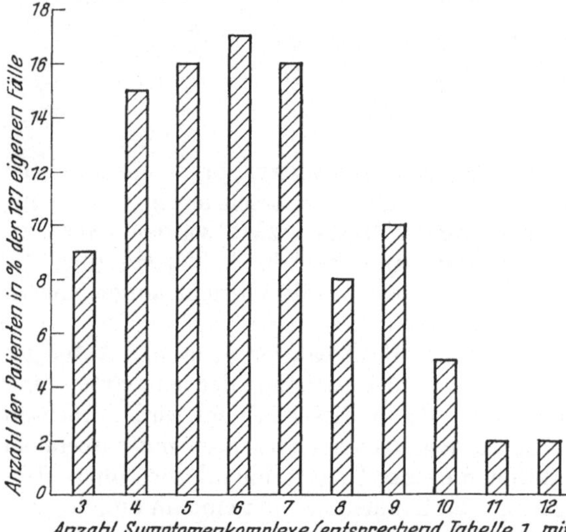

Abb. 14. Prozentuale Verteilung von 127 eigenen Erythematodes-Patienten nach Anzahl von Organen, die klinisch durch die viscerale Lupus erythematodes-Erkrankung betroffen sind

In bezug auf die Laboratoriumsergebnisse ist zunächst hervorzuheben, daß 98,5 % unserer Fälle eine Blutsenkung von 20 mm oder mehr (Westergreen) aufwiesen. Eine Vermehrung der Gammaglobuline wird in über 80% der Fälle beobachtet.

Der Rheumafaktor ist in ungefähr $^1/_3$ der Fälle vorhanden und hat eine diagnostische Bedeutung insofern, als er für das Vorliegen einer Erkrankung spricht, bei welcher während langer Zeit Antigen-Antikörper-Komplexe im Blut zirkulieren, oder die mit einer genetisch determinierten Störung der Immunglobulin-Produktion einhergeht.

Eine falsch positive Lues-Serologie ist bei klinischem Verdacht auf visceralem Lupus erythematodes ein wichtiger Befund zugunsten dieser Diagnose.

Außerordentlich wichtig ist der Nachweis antinuclearer Faktoren. Bei wiederholtem Suchen darnach werden sie wohl nie vermißt, so daß der wiederholt negative Ausfall antinucleärer Reaktionen die Diagnose eines visceralen Lupus erythematodes außerordentlich fragwürdig erscheinen läßt. Seltene Ursachen eines „falsch-negativen" L.E.-Zelltestes sind: Mangel an Komplement (FORMIJNE u. VAN SOEREN 1958), mangelhafte Leukocyten. Das Verhalten antinuclearer Faktoren im Verlauf der Erkrankung geht deutlich aus folgender Aufstellung hervor, in welcher die Ergebnisse des Antiglobulinkonsumptionstestes mit isolierten Zellkernen bei Erythematodes-Patienten (64 Patienten) zu verschiedenen Zeitpunkten der Erkrankung gegeben sind:

Tabelle 3. *Ausmaß der Antiglobilinkonsumption in der Elutionstechnik mit Zellkernen als Substrat bei Patienten mit aktiver und klinisch inaktiver Erythematodes-Erkrankung*

	Positivität des Antiglobulinkonsumptionstestes						
	3+	4+	5+	6+	7+	8+	%+(3–8+)
70 Kontrollpersonen	0	0	0	0	0	0	
24 Erythematodes-Patienten in inaktiver Phase der Erkrankung (Remission)	9	3	2	0	1	0	59%
40 Erythematodes-Patienten in aktiver Phase der Erkrankung	5	17	2	8	5	1	97%

Bei Nachweis antinuclearer Faktoren kommen, abgesehen von einer Erythematodes-Erkrankung, folgende Affektionen in Betracht:

1. Positives L.E.-Zellphänomen (BERTRAND 1952, DÖRNER u. Mitarb. 1961, FALLET 1960, FALLET u. Mitarb. 1959, HASERICK 1954, JACOBS 1955, MARMONT 1951, 1955 und 1959, OGRYZLO u. SMYTHE 1957, RASPONI 1955, SHULMAN und HARVEY 1960, STEVENS u. Mitarb. 1963, WALSH u. EGUN 1952, WALSH u. ZIMMERMANN 1953, WEISS u. SWIFT 1955). Primär-chronische Polyarthritis (in 5—10% der Fälle), generalisierte Sklerodermie (ungefähr 25%), Dermatomyositis (ungefähr 25%), Plasmazell-Hepatitis (FISCHER 1962, HOLMAN u. TOMASI 1960, MACKAY u. Mitarb. 1956), medikamentöse Überempfindlichkeitsreaktionen, selten in Form des eigentlichen L.E.-Zellphänomens (bei Hydralazin- [COMENS 1956, HENN u. Mitarb. 1955], Hydantoin- [MIESCHER u. DELACRÉTAZ 1953, RUPPLI u. VOSSEN 1957], Chlorpromazin-Medikation [MIESCHER u. JACKSON 1962]), häufiger in Form des sog. Pseudo-L.E.-Zellphänomens (DELACRÉTAZ u. Mitarb. 1954, HELLER u. ZIMMERMANN 1956, MARMONT 1955), das folgendermaßen charakterisiert ist: Phagocytose von Zellkernen, die ihre Chromatinstruktur noch weitgehend erhalten und kaum die typische Kernbasophilie verloren haben. Intracelluläre Kernveränderung bei polymorphkernigen Leukocyten in Form der Kernschwellung, Verlust der Chromatinstruktur und der Basophilie werden nicht beobachtet; ebenso werden freie „L.E.-Körperchen" vermißt.

2. Antiglobulinkonsumptionstest mit Zellkernen (DÖRNER u. Mitarb. 1961, FALLET 1960). Primär-chronische Polyarthritis (in 20—25% der Fälle), generalisierte Sklerodermie (etwa 50%), Dermatomyositis (ungefähr 39%), discoider cutaner Erythematodes (5—10%), medikamentöse Überempfindlichkeitsreaktionen, nekrotisierende bakterielle Erkrankungen, nekrotisierende Malignome, SJOEGRENs Syndrom.

3. Fluorescenzantikörpermethode (FRIOU 1957, FRIOU 1958, HOLBOROW u. Mitarb. 1957). Primär-chronische Polyarthritis (20—25%), generalisierte Sklerodermie (vorwiegend nucleolare Fluorescenz), discoider cutaner Erythematodes (24% homogene Kernfluorescenz + 10% gesprenkelte Fluorescenz (BECK u. Mitarb. 1962, ROWELL u. BECK 1962), SJOEGRENs Syndrom (hauptsächlich gesprenkelte Fluorescenz (BLOCH 1963).

4. Serologische Reaktionen mit Nucleoprotein (Komplementfixation, Reaktion mit Latex-Partikel) haben ähnliche diagnostische Bedeutung wie das L.E.-Phänomen. In wenigen Fällen besteht Diskordanz beider Reaktionen (BARDAWIL u. Mitarb. 1958, HOLBOROW u. WEIR 1959, LEE u. EPSTEIN 1960, SCALETTAR u. Mitarb. 1960).

5. Reaktionen mit Desoxyribonucleinsäure (BARBU u. Mitarb. 1960, HOLMAN u. DEICHER 1959, JOKINEN u. MÄKITALO 1960, KAYHOE u. Mitarb. 1960, MIESCHER u. STRAESSLE 1957, PEARSON u. Mitarb. 1958, SELIGMANN 1959) haben mehr theoretische als praktische Bedeutung. Diese Reaktion ist allgemein nur in Fällen mit heftiger Erythematodes-Erkrankung positiv, d.h. in Fällen ohne besondere diagnostische Schwierigkeiten. Positive Reaktionen kommen bei anderen Krankheiten selten vor (primär-chronische Polyarthritis: $\sim$2%).

Die Differentialdiagnose zwischen primär-chronischer Polyarthritis, visceralem Erythematodes und discoidem cutanem Erythematodes verdient besondere Erwähnung.

Die primär-chronische Polyarthritis ist, oberflächlich gesehen, eine Krankheit, die sich nur an den Gelenken manifestiert, mit mehr oder weniger heftiger Reaktion von seiten des reticuloendothelialen Systems. Bei genauerer histologischer Betrachtung kann allerdings auch die primär-chronische Polyarthritis als eine mehr generalisierte Affektion bezeichnet werden. Zunächst schien der L.E.-Zelltest entscheidend in der Abgrenzung der primär-chronischen Polyarthritis vom visceralen Erythematodes, auch bei Fehlen klinischer Zeichen eines visceralen Lupus erythematodes. Bald mußte diese Auffassung fallen gelassen werden, da es sich herausstellte, daß in 7—10% von eindeutigen primär-chronischen Polyarthritis-Erkrankungen ein positives L.E.-Zellphänomen auftreten kann (DÖRNER u. Mitarb. 1961, FALLET u. Mitarb. 1959, KIEVITS u. Mitarb. 1956, MIESCHER 1959, ZIFF u. Mitarb. 1958).

Sorgfältige Nachuntersuchungen dieser Patienten ergab, daß der weitere Verlauf der Krankheit nach diesem Befund nicht vom Verlauf anderer primär-chronischer Polyarthritis-Fälle abwich. Nur ein kleiner Teil dieser Patienten dürfte in eigentlichen visceralen Lupus erythematodes übergehen. Es liegen aber eine Anzahl von Beobachtungen vor über eigentliche Erythematodes-Erkrankungen bei Patienten, die jahrelang an einer primär-chronischen Polyarthritis mit negativen L.E.-Zellphänomenen gelitten hatten. Dieser Krankheitsverlauf dürfte in etwas weniger als 1% der primärchronischen Polyarthritis-Fälle vorkommen. Ebensowenig wie ein positiver L.E.-Zelltest eine primär-chronische Polyarthritis ausschließt, entscheiden andere serologische Tests zum Nachweis antinuclearer Serumfaktoren, ob eine primärchronische Polyarthritis oder ein visceraler Lupus erythematodes vorliegt. In der Differentialdiagnose zwischen primär-chronischer Polyarthritis und visceralem Lupus erythematodes müssen klinische und serologische Befunde gleichermaßen verwertet werden. Bei manifestem Befall verschiedener Organe neben der Gelenkaffektion und bei Nachweis antinuclearer Antikörper kann, auch bei jahrelang bestehender primär-chronischer Polyarthritis, ein visceraler Lupus erythematodes diagnostiziert werden, d.h. es ist eine dem visceralen Lupus erythematodes angemessene Behandlung indiziert.

Der cutane Erythematodes wurde bald als eine vom visceralen Lupus erythematodes grundverschiedene Krankheit aufgefaßt und überhaupt nicht als differentialdiagnostisches Problem erwähnt, bald als eine dem visceralen Lupus erythematodes identische Erkrankung leichteren Grades unter diesem Gesichtspunkt diskutiert. Neuere Untersuchungen haben bewiesen, daß enge Zusammenhänge zwischen cutanem und visceralem Erythematodes bestehen, allerdings ohne daß damit die Identität beider Erkrankungen bewiesen wäre (ROTHFIELD u. Mitarb. 1963, ROWELL u. BECK 1962).

Im Gegensatz zur primär-chronischen Polyarthritis haben antinucleäre und andere autoimmunitäre Erscheinungen wesentliche diagnostische Bedeutung bei Patienten mit cutanem Erythematodes. Zunächst sei daran erinnert, daß die für den cutanen Erythematodes typischen Hautveränderungen bei 16% der Patienten mit visceralem Lupus erythematodes zur Beobachtung kommen und geradezu für die Diagnose eines visceralen Lupus erythematodes ausschlaggebend sein können bei Vorliegen einer fieberhaften Erkrankung mit Befall verschiedener Organsysteme. Bei Patienten mit länger bestehendem cutanen Erythematodes muß bei positivem Ausfall antinuclearer Reaktionen sehr mit der Möglichkeit gerechnet werden, daß ein visceraler Lupus erythematodes vorliege oder entstehe. Solche Fälle unterscheiden sich in der Regel nicht nur serologisch, sondern auch klinisch von denjenigen mit unkompliziertem cutanem Erythematodes, z.B. in Form einer Thrombopenie, eines ungeklärten Status febrilis usw. Vorzugsweise werden weibliche Patienten von dieser „malignen“ Entwicklung betroffen. So waren bei unseren Fällen von cutanem Erythematodes 63% weiblich und 37% männlich. Bei Berücksichtigung der Tatsache, daß die Geschlechtsverteilung von Patienten mit Übergang in visceralen Erythematodes derjenigen aller visceralen Lupus erythematodes-Patienten gleichkommt (85% weibliche Patienten), ergibt sich bei einer visceralen Lupus erythematodes-Erkrankungsquote von 3,5% aller

Patienten mit cutanem Erythematodes eine Aussicht von 4,5% für weibliche und eine solche von 2% für männliche Patienten, um im späteren Verlauf der cutanen Affektion an einem visceralen Lupus erythematodes zu erkranken.

Die Differentialdiagnose zur Plasmazell-Hepatitis („lupoide Hepatitis") (BEARN u. Mitarb. 1956, GRAY u. Mitarb. 1958, KAYHOE u. Mitarb. 1960, KUNKEL u. Mitarb. 1951, MACKAY u. Mitarb. 1956) dürfte meist nicht schwer fallen, da diese Affektion außer der Leber in der Regel keine anderen Organe manifest befällt. Erkrankt eine junge Frau an einer schleichend verlaufenden Gelbsucht, zunächst ohne wesentliche subjektive Krankheitszeichen, jedoch mit progredient zunehmender Hypergammaglobulinämie, und zeigt die Leberbiopsie eine plasmacelluläre Hepatitis, so kann die Diagnose einer lupoiden Hepatitis auch bei positivem L.E.-Zellphänomen gestellt werden. Diese Krankheit ist ja geradezu durch das Vorhandensein antinuclearer Antikörper gekennzeichnet (mit oder ohne positivem L.E.-Zellphänomen). Wir haben schon erwähnt, daß diese Form der Leberbeteiligung beim visceralen Erythematodes, wenn überhaupt, so zumindest außerordentlich selten vorkommt. Wegen der guten Ansprechbarkeit der lupoiden Hepatitis auf 6-Mercaptopurin-Behandlung ist die exakte Diagnosestellung dieser Affektion praktisch wichtig.

Es seien noch zwei Krankheiten erwähnt, deren mögliche Beziehung zum visceralen Lupus erythematodes diskutiert wurde: die thrombotische thrombopenische Purpura und die DNS (Desoxyribonucleinsäure)-empfindliche hämorrhagische Eruption.

Die thrombotische thrombopenische Purpura ist gekennzeichnet durch ein mit Erythrocytenfragmentation einhergehendes hämolytisches Syndrom, eine periphere Thrombopenie mit purpurischen Efflorescenzen, multiple Thrombosen kleiner Gefäße mit klinischen Zeichen, welche je nach Sitz der Thrombosen wechseln, jedoch fast immer in neurologischen Symptomen bestehen. Diese Affektion wird meist als Autoimmunkrankheit bezeichnet, doch fehlen objektive Grundlagen. Insbesondere sind der L.E.-Zelltest, die Antihumanglobulinreaktion mit Erythrocyten und der direkte Antiglobulinkonsumptionstest mit Blutplättchen in den meisten Fällen negativ. Die Pathogenese der hämolytischen thrombotischen Thrombopenie ist immer noch unbekannt (SINGER 1954).

Die hämorrhagische Eruption mit DNS-Reaktivität (LEVIN u. PINKUS 1961, SCHWARTZ u. Mitarb. 1962) ist gekennzeichnet durch spontan auftretende, schmerzhafte Schwellungen mit Ekchymosen an den Extremitäten. Ganz frische Läsionen (eine Stunde nach Auftreten der Schwellung) sind histologisch durch ein massives Ödem mit Extravasaten von Erythrocyten gekennzeichnet. Entzündliche Infiltrate fehlen in diesem Frühstadium. Später kommt es zu einer Vasculitis von Arteriolen des untersten Corium und der oberflächlichen Partien der Subcutis. Vorwiegend polymorphkernige Leukocyten beteiligen sich an der Entzündung. Interessanterweise findet man eine Anzahl Hämatoxylin-positiver Körperchen mit einem Durchmesser von 1—7 μ, welche sich als Feulgen-positiv erwiesen, d.h. Desoxyribonucleinsäure enthalten. In älteren Läsionen bestehen die cellulären Infiltrate vorwiegend aus Rundzellen. Die intradermale Injektion von kleinsten Mengen (0,005 γ) Desoxyribonucleinsäure reproduziert die spontan auftretende Läsion. Nur die Haut der Extremitäten erwies sich als reaktiv. Im Serum der zwei bisher beobachteten Patienten konnte kein Serumkörper gegen DNS nachgewiesen werden. Mit der Fluorescenzantikörper-Technik konnte kein Gammaglobulin in den Hautläsionen gezeigt werden. Die Pathogenese dieser Affektion ist noch unklar. Eine immunologische Genese steht zur Diskussion, kann aber auf Grund der vorliegenden Ergebnisse nicht als bewiesen gelten. Ein Zusammenhang mit dem visceralen Erythematodes scheint nicht zu bestehen.

Erwähnenswert ist, daß diese hämorrhagische Eruption mit DNS-Reaktivität sehr gut auf Chloroquin anspricht (LEVIN u. PINKUS 1961, SCHWARTZ u. Mitarb. 1962). Diese Feststellung ist bemerkenswert im Lichte der histologisch faßbaren Feulgen-positiven Hämatoxylin-Körperchen und der Hautreaktivität gegenüber DNS. Chloroquin weist bekanntlich eine große Affinität zu Nucleoprotein auf.

Differentialdiagnostisch müssen ferner bakterielle Erkrankungen in Erwägung gezogen werden. Dies gilt nicht nur für den Fall einer Neuerkrankung, sondern besonders auch für Fieberschübe im Verlaufe einer Erythematodes-Erkrankung. Wir haben verschiedene Fälle von septischen Komplikationen bei Erythematodes-Patienten gesehen, die zunächst als Exacerbation der Grundkrankheit fehldiagnostiziert wurden. Eine zu spät erkannte Sepsis oder disseminierte Tuberkulose kann für den Patienten verhängnisvoll sein. Gerade im Zeitalter der Steroidbehandlung von Patienten mit visceralem Lupus erythematodes ist besondere Sorgfalt in der Früherkennung bakterieller Komplikationen angebracht. Wenn im Moment eines neuen Fieberschubes der L.E.-Zelltest negativ ausfällt und der Serumtiter antinuclearer Antikörper gegenüber früher nicht ansteigt oder gar abfällt, besteht großer Verdacht, daß keine Erythematodes-Exacerbation, sondern eine bakterielle Erkrankung vorliegt.

11. Behandlung

Die Behandlung von Patienten mit visceralem Lupus erythematodes hat zum Ziel, die entzündlichen Phänomene so lange zu dämpfen, bis die Krankheit in eine „inaktive Phase" übergeht. Zu diesem Zweck werden antientzündliche Mittel verwendet (Steroide; wahrscheinlich antiinflammatorische Komponente von Antimetaboliten). Von der Annahme ausgehend, daß Immunreaktionen in der Pathogenese der Zell- und Gewebsläsionen eine wichtige Rolle spielen, wird therapeutisch versucht, die immunologische Reaktionsweise des Organismus zu dämpfen (Antimetabolite, Steroide). Schließlich wird versucht, die Ablagerung von Fibrinoid in den Nierenglomeruli im Falle einer renalen Beteiligung des Erythematodes durch Antikoagulantien zu verhindern. Wo die Antimalaria-Mittel in diesem Behandlungsschema einzureihen sind, d.h. ob es sich hier um eine antiinflammatorische Wirkung oder um eine direkte Kernwirkung handelt, oder um eine Hemmung der Antikörperbildung, ist unbekannt.

Schließlich müssen die Patienten ständig auf das Auftreten unspezifischer, infektiöser Komplikationen hin untersucht werden. Aus der Liste der Todesursachen geht nämlich hervor, daß infektiöse Komplikationen an erster Stelle stehen.

Ob der spontane Krankheitsverlauf durch die Behandlung beeinflußt wird, kann nicht bewiesen werden, da die Schwere der Krankheit keine großen Kontrollserien unbehandelter Patienten verantworten läßt. Es ist jedoch die Meinung der meisten Kliniker, welche über eine große Erfahrung auf diesem Gebiet verfügen, daß akute Schübe, die sonst letal verlaufen würden, durch Behandlung gemeistert werden können. Aus den Zahlen über die Mortalität des visceralen Lupus erythematodes geht hervor, daß die meisten Todesfälle in den ersten 5 Jahren der Erkrankung erfolgen. Gelingt es, den Patienten über diese erste Periode der Erkrankung hinüberzubringen, verbessern sich die weiteren Lebensaussichten wesentlich.

Glucosteroide haben sich zur Eindämmung der akut entzündlichen Erscheinungen bewährt (BAEHR u. Mitarb. 1950, DUBOIS 1956, ROBINSON 1962, SOFFER 1950). Am besten wird mit einer hohen Anfangsdosis begonnen, im Falle einer akuten schweren Erkrankung mit 60 mg Prednison täglich, oder evtl. mit einer

Dauerinfusion von 40 mg ACTH täglich. Ausnahmsweise werden höhere Prednisondosen empfohlen, so vor allem bei schwerer Nierenbeteiligung. Gewöhnlich können mit diesem Vorgehen die entzündlichen Erscheinungen in wenigen Wochen zum Verschwinden gebracht werden. Die Dosierung wird darauf vorsichtig vermindert, in dreitägigen Intervallen, nie mehr aber als um 5 mg, bis zu einer Tagesdosis von 20 mg. Diese Dosierung wird vorteilhaft mindestens 6 Monate weiter verabreicht. Anschließend empfiehlt es sich, eine Erhaltungsdosis von 7,5—15 mg täglich während 1—2 Jahre beizubehalten. Im Falle einer Verschlimmerung muß sofort die Dosis erhöht werden, ebenso im Falle eines interkurrenten Infektes, dann natürlich zusammen mit Antibioticagaben.

Antimalariamittel werden schon lange zur Behandlung des cutanen discoiden Erythematodes verwendet (MERWIN u. WINKELMANN 1962, ROBINSON 1962). In den letzten Jahren haben sie sich auch zur Behandlung des visceralen Lupus erythematodes nützlich erwiesen, wenn auch ihre Wirksamkeit relativ bescheiden ist (MULLINS u. Mitarb. 1955, 1956). Die Kernaffinität dieser Antimalariamittel ist bemerkenswert in bezug auf die Bedeutung antinucleärer Reaktionen für den visceralen Lupus erythematodes. Quinacrine hemmt das L.E.-Phänomen und auch DNS-Seroreaktionen (DUBOIS 1955, STOLLAR u. Mitarb. 1962). Antimalariamittel allein sollten nie zur Behandlung eines schweren Erythematodes-Schubes gegeben werden; dagegen hat die klinische Erfahrung gezeigt, daß die Verabreichung von Antimalariamitteln erlaubt, die Steroiddosierung zu vermindern. Ferner können diese Mittel mit oder an Stelle von Steroiden in Form einer Dauertherapie gegeben werden. Allerdings sind Nebenerscheinungen (von seiten des Magen-Darmtraktes oder oculäre Störungen) nicht selten und oft schwer genug, um das Absetzen der Antimalariamittel zu bedingen. Am häufigsten werden Chloroquin und Hydroxychloroquin verwendet. Die Dosierung ist individuell sehr verschieden (Chloroquin: 0,25—0,75 g täglich, Hydroxychloroquine: 0,4—1,2 g täglich). Der Wirkungsmechanismus dieser Mittel ist unbekannt.

Besonderer Erwähnung bedürfen die oculären Nebenwirkungen der Antimalariamittel (SALLMANN u. BERNSTEIN 1963). Relativ häufig (30—70% der mit Chloroquin oder Hydroxychloroquin behandelten Patienten) sind feine Niederschläge von Chloroquin oder metabolischer Produkte auf die Hornhaut. Oft wird diese *Keratopathie* gar nicht bemerkt. Gelegentlich kommt es zu Symptomen wie Halo-Bildung, Photophobie oder auch nur unklarer Sicht. Diese Keratopathie ist reversibel. Schwerwiegender ist die Chloroquin-Retinopathie, die bei ungefähr einem von 1000—2000 Patienten auftritt. Periphere Gesichtsausfälle, Schwierigkeit beim Lesen, Photophobie, entoptische Erscheinungen (Lichtblitze und Striche) deuten bereits auf eine schwere Störung hin, die in Pigmentdegenerationsherden mit Untergang der Sehzellen besteht. Wenn die Sehzellen einmal befallen sind, liegt eine irreversible, permanente Schädigung vor.

Chloroquin und verwandte Mittel weisen eine starke Gewebsaffinität auf (vor allem zu Zellkernen). Die Konzentration in Leber, Milz, Nieren und Lungen kann einige hundertmal größer sein als die Plasmakonzentration (SALLMANN u. BERNSTEIN 1963). Ferner ist Chloroquin sehr stark angereichert in Geweben, die Melanin enthalten (Iris, Chorioidea, Pigmentepithel der Retina). Die Bindung von Chloroquin an Melanin erklärt wahrscheinlich die Retinopathie. Gelegentlich auftretende Verfärbung von Haaren mag auf dem gleichen Prinzip beruhen.

In den letzten Jahren hat sich ein neuer Behandlungsweg durch die Einführung von Cytostatica eröffnet (SCHWARTZ und ANDRÉ 1962). 6-Mercaptopurin ist das zur Zeit wichtigste Mittel dieser Gruppe. Experimentell kann damit die Antikörperbildung und der Spätreaktionstypus bei verschiedenen Species verhindert oder gehemmt werden. Ferner können experimentelle Autoimmunkrankheiten verhindert oder schon bestehende erfolgreich damit behandelt werden (Spiegelberg u. Miescher 1963). Die klinische Erfahrung mit dieser Behandlung bei Patienten mit visceralem Lupus erythematodes ist noch ungenügend. Ursprünglich wurde eine zu hohe Dosierung gewählt mit Auftreten unangenehmer Nebenwirkung. Wir verabreichen 50 mg 6-Mercaptopurin zusammen mit 15 mg Prednison täglich. Bei dieser Dosierung sind keine unangenehmen Nebenwirkungen aufgetreten. Die klinische Aktivität der Krankheit ist bei allen Patienten mehr oder weniger zurückgegangen, das L.E.-Zellphänomen wurde bei zwei Kranken nach 4wöchiger Behandlung negativ. Eine Patientin nimmt bereits über ein Jahr 50 mg 6-Mercaptopurin täglich ein. Die Prednisonmedikation wurde nach 3 Monaten abgesetzt. Eine Patientin wurde nach 8, eine zweite nach 12 Monaten resistent gegenüber 6-Mercaptopurin. Bei einer Patientin wurde die Behandlung mit Erfolg durch Amethopterin (Methotrexate) weitergeführt.

Neuerdings hat Miescher eine Wirksamkeit von Amethopterin (Methotrexate) bei drei perakuten Verlaufsformen feststellen können, die derjenigen einer massiven Steroid-Medikation gleichkommt, dabei praktisch ohne Nebenwirkungen war. Die intravenöse Injektion von 100 mg Methotrexate führte innerhalb von 48 Std zu einer starken Verminderung oder Normalisierung der Körpertemperatur. Die klinische Symptomatologie besserte sich in allen drei Fällen rapid. Die Behandlung wurde zunächst durch intravenöse Verabreichung des Amethopterin weitergeführt in Form einer Injektion von 50 mg je Woche. Nach 2—3 Wochen wurde Amethopterin oral verabreicht, alternierend an einem Tag 5 mg, am anderen 2,5 mg (25 mg bzw. 27,5 mg wöchentliche Dosis). Bei der intravenösen Verabreichung wird eine maximale Blutkonzentration des Mittels erreicht mit raschem, exponentiellem Abfall zufolge renaler Ausscheidung. Das Mittel soll nicht in einer Tropfinfusion gegeben werden, da damit eine vollkommen verschiedene Verteilung von Amethopterin im Gewebe erreicht wird. In einer Tropfinfusion könnte die Verabreichung von 100 mg zu erheblichen toxischen Nebenwirkungen führen. Im Falle einer Niereninsuffizienz muß das Mittel mit großer Vorsicht gegeben werden, da es nicht zu einer gleich schnellen Eliminierung kommt. Durch die rasche intravenöse Injektion können höchste Konzentrationen von Amethopterin im blutnahen Gewebe erreicht werden. Die gegenüber Amethopterin sehr empfindliche Schleimhaut des intestinalen Tractus wird dabei geschont. Entsprechend kommt es nicht zu den sonst für die große Dosierung dieses Mittels bekannten Nebenerscheinungen. Die für die orale Verabreichung angegebene Dosierung liegt unter der toxischen Schwelle, d.h. die Behandlung kann ohne Gefahr über längere Zeit durchgeführt werden. Leukocyten, Thrombocyten und Leberfunktion müssen regelmäßig kontrolliert werden.

Von besonderem Interesse sind Patienten mit visceralem Erythematodes mit Immunocytopenie: Behandlung mit den beiden angeführten Antimetaboliten führt gelegentlich zunächst zu einer Verstärkung der Cytopenie (Thrombopenie, Leukopenie). In verschiedenen Fällen folgte nach merklicher Verminderung der Thrombocyten- bzw. Leukocytenzahl eine Normalisierung der Werte. Bei einer Patientin ging die Plättchenzahl in einer Woche von 50000 auf 20000, um dann rapid, innerhalb von 5 Tagen, auf 170000 zu steigen. Bei einer anderen Patientin kam es ohne initiales Absinken der Blutplättchen zu einem Anstieg von 110000 auf 280000. Ähnliche Verläufe der weißen Blutzellen wurden von uns beobachtet. Aus diesen Beobachtungen darf gefolgert werden, daß eine *Cytopenie mit Hyperplasie der entsprechenden Knochenmarksvorstufen* keine Kontraindikation gegen Behandlung mit Antimetaboliten darstellt. Es sei nochmals wiederholt, daß diese Mittel bei Patienten mit Nierenläsion mit großer Vorsicht verabreicht werden müssen wegen der gestörten Eliminierung der Antimetabolite.

Wegen der enzymatischen Adaptation des Organismus an die erwähnten Antimetaboliten empfehlen wir, eine Schaukeltherapie mit 3monatigem Wechsel vorzunehmen, z.B. 50 mg 6-Mercaptopurin + 10 mg Prednison täglich während 3 Monate, anschließend Methotrexate, 5 und 2,5 mg an alternierenden Tagen + täglich 10 mg Prednison. Nach weiteren 3 Monaten wird wieder zu 6-Mercaptopurin gewechselt. Bei ungenügender Wirksamkeit kann die Steroid-Dosierung erhöht werden.

Es ist anzunehmen, daß 6-Mercaptopurin und Methotrexate nicht nur auf dem Weg einer Unterdrückung von Antikörperbildung und/oder der cellulären Immunität wirkt, sondern auch durch antiinflammatorische Aktivität. Diese tritt erst nach ungefähr 2wöchiger Behandlung in Erscheinung und dürfte vielleicht in der Unterdrückung der Bildung für den Entzündungsvorgang wichtiger Enzyme eine Erklärung finden. Wenn 6-Mercaptopurin zur Behandlung verwendet wird (oder Methyl6-Mercaptopurin [„Imuran"]), muß mit einer mehrwöchigen Medikation zur Erreichung der vollen therapeutischen Wirkung gerechnet werden. Wenn 6-Mercaptopurin oder Methotrexate verschrieben wird, muß die Patientin darauf aufmerksam gemacht werden, daß im Falle einer Gravidität das Mittel sofort abgesetzt werden muß, da die Gefahr von Mißbildungen des kindlichen Organismus besteht. Noch besser ist dafür zu sorgen, daß unter keinen Umständen eine Schwangerschaft eintritt, z.B. durch Enovid- (oder Anovular)-Medikation.

Die renale Erkrankung des visceralen Lupus erythematodes bedarf noch einer besonderen Besprechung in bezug auf die Behandlung. Da einmal abgelagertes Fibrinoid in den Glomeruli nicht oder kaum mehr entfernt werden kann, muß versucht werden, weitere Niederschlagsbildung zwischen Basalmembran und Fußprozessen unter allen Umständen zu verhindern. Wahrscheinlich ist auch die Steroidbehandlung in dieser Hinsicht erfolgversprechend, da erfahrungsgemäß damit der Komplementspiegel günstig beeinflußt wird. Komplement wird bekanntlich in den Glomerulus-Schlingen entlang der Basalmembranen bei der Erythematodes-Glomerulitis gefunden. Die Serumkomplement-Verminderung darf deshalb wahrscheinlich als Indicator für die Niederschlagsbildung in den Glomerulus-Schlingen verwertet werden, sofern ein renaler Sitz der Erkrankung besteht. Durch die Steroidmedikation wird vor allem die initiale, akute entzündliche Phase (Glomerulitis) gedämpft, was sich bei Früherkrankungen durch einen raschen Abfall des Bluthamstoffes bemerkbar macht. Eine Verminderung der Harnstoffretention in fortgeschrittenen Stadien der Erkrankung ist dagegen nicht mehr zu erwarten. Dies ist ein weiterer Grund, warum die Früherfassung eines renalen Erythematodes so wichtig ist.

Unter der Behandlung von Erythematodes-Patienten nach den genannten Prinzipien gehen nicht nur die klinischen Zeichen der Krankheit zurück; auch die Immunreaktionen nehmen an Intensität ab. Bei Erniedrigung des Serumkomplementes steigt der Titer unter Steroidmedikation. Am schwersten sind die renalen Krankheitszeichen beeinflußbar. Auf Grund der pathologisch-anatomischen Besonderheiten ist dies auch verständlich. Im Tierexperiment konnte gezeigt werden, daß Niederschläge zwischen Basalmembran und „Fußprozessen", auch bei Sistieren der Einwirkung der Noxe, sich praktisch nicht mehr zurückbilden. Aus diesem Grund ist es wichtig, zu verhindern, daß sich irreparable Nierenläsionen bilden. Dieses Ziel kann erreicht werden, wenn die Patienten möglichst früh nach Beginn der Erkrankung behandelt werden und wenn die ärztliche Überwachung der Patienten in kurzen Intervallen über mehrere Jahre geschieht. Die Aktivität der Krankheit wird sorgfältig aus den klinischen und Laboratoriumsdaten eruiert. Bei Wiederauftreten von Aktivitätszeichen muß der Patient erneut behandelt werden.

12. Verlauf und Prognose

Der viscerale Lupus erythematodes gehört zu den „self perpetuating"-Krankheiten, d. h. ohne faßbare äußere Ursachen entstehen entzündliche Erscheinungen, die ebenso unberechenbar wieder abklingen können, um nach einiger Zeit wieder aufzuflackern. Dieser schubweise Verlauf weist zu Beginn der Erkrankung meist crescendo-Charakter auf. Todesfälle treten fast alle in den ersten 5 Jahren auf. Von 127 eigenen Patienten starben 24 in dieser Zeitspanne. Ein Patient starb im 9. Jahr der Erkrankung in urämischem Zustand. 78 Patienten sind noch am Leben, 24 konnten nicht weiter verfolgt werden. Nach Ablauf von 5 Jahren nimmt die Sterbequote stark ab. Der klinische Verlauf wird später gewöhnlich milder, und bei vielen Patienten liegen schließlich kaum noch aktive Krankheitszeichen eines visceralen Lupus erythematodes vor (sog. „ausgebrannte" Fälle). Die Krankheit weist also eine Prognose auf mit einer Überlebenschance von ungefähr 75%, während der ersten 5 Jahre. Ist diese Zeit ohne irreparable Organschäden überstanden, erscheint die Lebenserwartung wesentlich weniger durch den visceralen Lupus erythematodes beeinträchtigt zu sein.

Die Todesursache kann sehr unterschiedlich sein. Von den 24 Todesfällen unseres Patientengutes waren 8 der Aktivität der Krankheit zuzuschreiben (Tod im akuten Schub). 6 Patienten starben an Urämie, 2 an Gefäßkomplikationen (cerebrale Blutung, Lungenembolie) und 9 an den Folgen einer Sekundärinfektion. Letztere Todesursache dürfte zumindest klinisch der langen Steroid-Behandlung zuzuschreiben sein.

Literatur

ABRUZZO, J. L., and C. L. CHRISTIAN: The induction of a rheumatoid factor-like substance in rabbits. J. exp. Med. **114**, 791 (1961). — AISENBERG, A. C.: Studies on the mechanism of the lupus erythematosus phenomenon. J. clin. Invest. **38**, 325 (1959). — ALBERTINI, A. v., u. O. ALB: Über die atypische, verrucöse Endocarditis Libman-Sachs und ihre Beziehungen zum Lupus erythematodes acutus. Cardiologia (Basel) **12**, 133 (1947). — AYVAZIAN, L. F., and TH. L. BADGER: Disseminated lupus erythematosus occuring among student nurses. New Engl. J. Med. **239**, 565 (1948).

BAEHR, G., P. KLEMPERER, and A. SCHIFRIN: Diffuse diseases of the peripheral circulation (usually associated with lupus erythematosus and endocarditis). Trans. Ass. Amer. Phycns **50**, 139 (1935). — BAEHR, G., and L. J. SOFFER: Treatment of disseminated lupus erythematosus with cortisone and A.C.T.H. N.Y. Acad. Med. Bull. **26**, 229 (1950). — BARBIER, F.: La cellule L.E. est-elle spécifique pour le lupus érythémateux aigu disséminé? Acta med. scand. (Stockh.) **147**, 325 (1953). — BARBU, E., M. SELIGMANN et M. JOLY: Réactions entré des acides desoxyribonucléiques diversement dénaturés ou dégradés et les anticorps anti-acide desoxyribonucléique du sérum de malades atteints de lupus érythémateux disséminé. Ann. Inst. Pasteur **99**, 695 (1960). — BARDAWIL, W. A., B. L. TOY, and N. GALLINS: Hypersensitivity to histone, induced experimentally in rabbits. Lancet **1958 I**, 888. — BARDAWIL, W. A., B. L. TOY, N. GALLINS, and T. B. BAYLES: Disseminated lupus erythematosus, scleroderma and dermatomyositis asmanifestations of sensitivity to DNA-protein. Amer. J. Path. **34**, 607 (1958). — BARNES, S., T. W. MOFFATT, C. W. LANE, and R. S. WEISS: Studies on the L.E. phenomenon. Arch. Derm. **62**, 771 (1950). — BEARN, A. G., H. G. KUNKEL, and R. J. SLATER: The problem of chronic liver disease in young women. Amer. J. Med. **21**, 3 (1956). — BECK, J. S.: Variations in the morphological patterns of „autoimmune" nuclear fluorescence. Lancet **1961 I**, 1203. — BECK, J. S., J. R. ANDERSON, A. J. MCELHINNEY, and N. R. ROWELL: Antinucleolar antibodies. Lancet **1962 II**, 575. — BERLYNE, G. M., I. A. SHORT, and C. F. H. VICKERS: Placental transmission of the LE-factor. Report of two cases. Lancet **1957 II**, 273. — BERMAN, L., A. R. AXELROD, H. L. GOODMAN, and R. I. MCCLAUCHERY: So called lupus erythematosus inclusion phenomenon of bone marrow and blood. Amer. J. clin. Path. **20**, 403 (1950). — BERNSTEIN, S. I.: Corneal changes caused by antimalarials. Skin **2**, 86 (1963). — BERTRAND, L.: Les cellules de la lupo-érythémato-viscérite maligne. Presse méd. **1952**, 929. — BEUTNER, E. H., M. SULLIVAN, G. BARNES, and E. WITEBSKY: Studies of in vivo reactions of nuclear antibodies. Proc. IInd Symposium Immunopathology, p. 331. Basel: Benno Schwabe & Co. 1962. — BLOCH, K. J.: In: Immunological aspects of rheumatoid arthritis and SLE. Arthritis and Rheumatism **6**, 532 (1963). — BOCK, H. E.: Internistisch Beachtenswertes bei

Lupus erythematodes disseminatus. Ärztl. Wschr. **11**, 537 (1956). — BOYDEN, ST.: The adsorption of proteins on erythrocytes with tannic acid and subsequent hemagglutination by antiprotein-sera. J. exp. Med. **93**, 107 (1951). — BOZICEVICH, J., J. P. NASOU, and D. E. KAYHOE: Desoxyribonucleic acid — Bentonite flocculation test for lupus erythematosus. Proc. Soc. exp. Biol. (N.Y.) **103**, 636 (1960). — BRIDGE, R. G., and F. E. FOLEY: Placental transmission of the lupus erythematosus factor. J. med. Sci. **227**, 1 (1954). — BROWN, J. T., M. P. HUTT, J. F. REGER, and S. W. SMITH: Localization of „Fibrinoid" deposits in lupus nephritis: an electron microscopic demonstration of glomerular endothelial cell phagocytosis. Arthr. and Rheum. **6**, 599 (1963). — BRUCE, J.: Disseminated lupus erythematosus of the alimentary tract. Lancet **1959 I**, 795. — BURKHOLDER, P. M.: Complement fixation in diseased tissues. Amer. J. Path. **42**, 201 (1963). — BUTLER, V., S. BEISER, B. ERLANGER, S. TANENBAUM, S. COHEN, and A. BENDICH: Purine-specific antibodies which react with DNA. Proc. nat. Acad. Sci. (Wash.) **48**, 1957 (1962).

CALABRESI, P., E. A. EDWARDS, and R. F. SCHILLING: Fluorescent antiglobulin studies in leukopenic and related disorders. J. clin. Invest. **38**, 2091 (1959). — CALLENDER, S. T., and R. R. RACE: A serological and genetical study of multiple antibodies formed in response to blood transfusion by a patient with lupus erythematosus diffusus. Ann. Eugen. (Lond.) **13**, 102 (1946). — CAPELLI, E.: Primi riliev sul fenomeno dell'autoeritrofagocitosi in vitro. Raffranto col meccanismo formativo e tentativo d'interpretazione delle cosidette „cellule del lupus eritematose". Minerva derm. **27**, No 5 (1952a). — Basi teoriche e realizzazione sperimentale in vitro del „fenomeno del lupus eritematose" nel sangue di individui normali mediante un siero entireticulo-endotelio umano. Minerva derm. **27**, No 10 (1952b). — CASTLEMAN, B., and E. H. NORRIS: Pathology of thymus in myasthenia gravis. Medicine (Baltimore) **28**, 27 (1949). — CEPELLINI, R., E. POLLI, and F. A. CELEDA: DNA-reacting factor in serum of a patient with lupus erythematosus diffusus. Proc. Soc. exp. Biol. (N.Y.) **96**, 572 (1957). — CHAUDHURI, S. H., and S. P. MARTIN: The migration and oxidation-reduction activity of leukocytes from patients with acute disseminated lupus erythematosus. J. Lab. clin. Med. **41**, 108 (1953). — CHOMET, B., M. M. KIRSHEN, G. SCHAEFFER, and P. MUDRIK: The finding of the L.E.-cells in smears of untreated freshly drawn peripheral blood. Blood **8**, 1107 (1953).— CHRISTIAN, CH. L., W. B. HATFIELD, and P. H. CHASE: Cryoprecipitation of SLE sera. J. clin. Invest. **42**, 823 (1963). — CHRISTIAN, CH. L., R. MENDEZ-BRYAN, and D. L. LARSON: Latex agglutination test for disseminated lupus erythematosus. Proc. Soc. exp. Biol. (N.Y.) **98**, 820 (1958). — COBURN, A. F., and D. H. MOORE: The plasma proteins in disseminated lupus erythematosus. Bull. Johns Hopk. Hosp. **73**, 196 (1943). — COMENS, P.: Experimental hydralazine disease and its similarity to disseminated lupus erythematosus. J. Lab. clin. Med. **47**, 444 (1956). — CONLEY, L. E.: Disorders of the blood in disseminated lupus erythematosus. Amer. J. Med. **13**, 1 (1952). — CONLEY, L. E., and R. C. HARTMANN: A hemorrhagic disorder caused by circulating anticoagulant in patients with disseminated lupus erythematosus. J. clin. Invest. **31**, 621 (1952). — COOPER, C. D., W. R. FELTS, TH. MCP. BROWN, and R. H. WICHELHAUSEN: Determination of redox activity of leukocytes as a diagnostic aid in systemic lupus erythematosus. J. Lab. clin. Med. **53**, 457 (1959). — COOPER, N.: Persönliche Mitteilung 1961. — CRAWFORD, H. J., R. M. WOOD, and M. H. LESSOF: Detection of antibodies by fluorescent-spot technique. Lancet **1959 II**, 1173. — CRUICKSHANK, B.: Lesions of joints and tendon sheaths in systemic lupus erythematosus. Ann. rheum. Dis. **18**, 111 (1958).

DAMESHEK, W., and W. H. REEVES: Exacerbation of lupus erythematosus following splenectomy in „idiopathic" thrombocytopenic purpura and autoimmune hemolytic anemia. Amer. J. Med. **21**, 60 (1956). — DAUSSET, J.: Immuno-hématologie biologique et clinique. Paris: Flammarion 1956. — DAUSSET, J., J. COLOMBANI, and M. COLOMBANI: Study of leukopenias and thrombocytopenias by the direct antiglobulin consumption test on leukocytes and/or platelets. Blood **17**, 672 (1961). — DEICHER, H., u. G. HEIDE: Experimentelle antinukleäre Antikörper und Serumfaktoren des Lupus erythematodes visceralis. Dtsch. Internistenkongr. 1962. — DEICHER, H. R., H. R. HOLMAN, and H. G. KUNKEL: The precipitin reaction between DNA and a serum factor in systemic lupus erythematosus. J. exp. Med. **109**, 97 (1959). — Anticytoplasmic factors in sera of patients with SLE and certain other diseases. Arthr. and Rheum. **3**, 1 (1960). — DEICHER, H. R., H. R. HOLMAN, H. G. KUNKEL, and Z. OVARY: Passive cutaneous anaphylaxis reactions with a systemic lupus erythematosus serum factor and isolated DNA. J. Immunol. **48**, 106 (1960). — DELACRÉTAZ, J., TH. INDERBITZIN et P. MIESCHER: Les phénomènes pseudo L.E. Schweiz. med. Wschr. **1954**, 1103. — DITTRICH, H., u. E. FRÜHMANN: Untersuchungen zum Problem der experimentellen Bildung von L.E.-Zellen. Acta haemat. (Basel) **10**, 239 (1953). — DIXON, F.: Diskussion über die Zusammensetzung von Fibrinoid. In Proceedings II. Internat. Symposium Immunopathologie, p. 90. Basel: Benno Schwabe & Co. 1961. — DIXON, F. J.: Tissue injury produced by antigen-antibody complexes. Second Internat. Symposium Immunopathology, Benno Schwabe Publisher, 1962, p. 71. — DÖRNER, M., M. ENDERLIN, H. SPIEGELBERG u. P. MIESCHER: Klinik und Serologie des visceralen Erythematodes. Dtsch. med. Wschr. **86**, 374, 431

(1961). — DOORMAAL, T. A. J. VAN, u. J. T. R. SCHREUDER: Über die sog. Erythematodes-Zelle und deren Vorkommen in der Pleuraflüssigkeit. Dermatologica (Basel) **101**, 167 (1960). — DUBOIS, E. I.: Acquired hemolytic anemia as the presenting syndrome of lupus erythematosus disseminatus. Amer. J. Med. **12**, 197 (1952). — DUBOIS, E. L.: Effect of quinacrine upon L.E. phenomenon. Arch. Derm. **71**, 570 (1955). — Prednisone and prednisolone in the treatment of systemic lupus erythematosus. J. Amer. med. Ass. **161**, 427 (1956a). — Systemic lupus erythematosus: recent advances in its diagnosis and treatment. Ann. intern. Med. **45**, 163 (1956b). — Lupus erythematosus. Discoid and systemic. Blakiston Division. New York City (N.Y.): McGraw Hill Book Co. inc. (Im Druck.) — DUSTAN, H. P., A. C. CORCORAN, and R. HASERICK: Urinary sediment in acute diffuse lupus erythematosus: nature and response to treatment. Zit. nach E. L. DUBOIS, Ann. intern. Med. **45**, 163 (1956). — DUSTAN, H. P., R. D. TAYLOR, A. C. CORCORAN, I. H. PAGE: Rheumatic and febrile syndrome during prolonged hydralazine treatment. J. Amer. med. Ass. **154**, 23 (1954a). — Rheumatic febrile syndrome during prolonged hydralazine treatment. J. Amer. med. Ass. **154**, 23 (1954b).

EPSTEIN, H. C., and J. Z. LITT: Discoid lupus erythematosus in a newborn infant. New Engl. J. Med. **265**, 1106 (1961). — ERICKSON, J. G., E. A. HINES jr., J. L. PEASE, and L. A. BRUNSTING: Rheumatoid and lupus-erythematosus-like syndromes: complications of hydralazine therapy for hypertension. Arch. Derm. **74**, 640 (1956). — ETCHEVERRY, M. A., C. REUSSI, E. E. CAPALBO y J. A. PENALVER: Lupus eritematose disseminado agudo y anemia hemolitica adquirida con autoanticuerpos. Rev. Soc. argent. Hem. **3**, 325 (1951).

FALLET, G. H.: Sérologie du lupus érythémateux disséminé. Schweiz. med. Wschr. **90**, 73 (1960). — FALLET, G. H., J. COSPALLUTO et M. ZIFF: Etudes chromatographiques et électrophorétiques de facteur C. E. Erstes Internat. Symposium, Immunopathologie. BennoSchwabe & Co. 1959. S. 438. — FALLET, G. H., H. VASEY, E. MEYER et J. SPAHR: Les polyarthrites chroniques évolutives à cellules L.E. Rev. Rhum. **26**, 553 (1959). — FARQUHAR, M. G., R. L. VERNIER, and R. A. GOOD: An electron microscope study of the glomerulus in nephrosis, glomerulonephritis and lupus erythematosus. J. exp. Med. **106**, 649 (1957). — FINCH, S. C., J. F. ROSS, and F. G. EBAUGH: Immunologic mechanisms of leucocyte abnormalities. J. Lab. clin. Med. **42**, 555 (1953). — FISCHER, A.: The „lupoid hepatitis" syndrome, report of a case followed by serial liver biopsies. Ann. intern. Med. **57**, 988 (1962). — FORMIJNE, P., and F. VAN SOEREN: Negative L.E. cell phenomenon in ture systemic lupus erythematosus. Lancet **1958 II**, 1206. — FOX, R. A., P. D. ROSAHN: The lymph nodes in disseminated lupus erythematosus. Amer. J. Path. **19**, 73 (1943). — FREEDMAN, P., and A. S. MARKOWITZ: Isolation of antibody-like gamma globulin from lupus glomeruli. Brit. med. J. **1962 I**, 1175. — FRICK, P. G.: Acquired circulating anticoagulants in systemic „collagen disease". Blood **10**, 691 (1955). — FRIEDMAN, E. A., W. A. BARDAWIL, J. P. MERRILL, and C. HANAU: „Delayed" cutaneous hypersensitivity to leukocytes in disseminated lupus erythematosus. New Engl. J. Med. **262**, 486 (1960). — FRIEDMAN, E. A., and J. W. RUTHERFORD: Pregnancy in lupus erythematosus. Obstet. and Gynec. **8**, 601 (1956). — FRIOU, G. J.: Clinical application of lupus serum — nucleoprotein reaction using fluorescent antibody technique. J. clin. Invest. **36**, 890 (1957). — FRIOU, G. J.: The significance of the lupus erythematosus globulin reaction with nucleoprotein. Ann. intern. Med. **49**, 866 (1958). — FUDENBERG, H., J. L. GERMAN, and H. G. KUNKEL: The occurrence of rheumatoid factor and other abnormalities in families of patients with agammaglobulinemia. Arthr. and Rheum. **5**, 565 (1962).

GAJDUSEK, D. C.: An „autoimmune" reaction against human tissue antigens in certain acute and chronic diseases. Arch. intern. Med. **101**, 9 (1958). — GARSENSTEIN, M., V. E. POLLAK, and R. M. KARK: SLE and pregnancy. New Engl. J. Med. **267**, 165 (1962). — GASSER, C.: Die Pathogenese der essentiellen chronischen Granulocytopenie im Kindesalter auf Grund der Knochenmarksbefunde. Helv. paediat. Acta **7**, 428 (1952). — GASSER, C., u. M. R. VRITLEK: Essentielle chronische Granulocytopenie im Kindesalter. Schweiz. med. Wschr. **82**, 1122 (1952). — GERMAN, J. L.: Studies in the pathogenesis of lupus erythematosus. Experimental production of hematoxyphil bodies in the kidney. J. exp. Med. **108**, 179 (1958). — GITLIN, P., J. M. CRAIG, and C. A. JANEWAY: Studies on the nature of fibrinoid in the collagen diseases. Amer. J. Path. **33**, 55 (1957). — GODMAN, G. C.: The nature and pathogenetic significance of the L.E. cell phenomenon of SLE. J. Mt Sinai Hosp. **26**, 241 (1959). — GODMAN, G. C., and A. D. DEITCH: A cytochemical study of the L.E. bodies of systemic lupus erythematosus. I. Nucleic acids. J. exp. Med. **106**, 575 (1957). — GODMAN, G. C., A. D. DEITCH, and P. KLEMPERER: The composition of the L.E. and hematoxylin bodies of systemic L.E. Amer. J. Path. **34**, 1 (1958). — GOECKERMAN, W. H.: Lupus erythematosus as a systemic disease. J. Amer. med. Ass. **80**, 542 (1923). — GOLD, S.: Role of sulphonamides and penicillin in the pathogenesis of systemic lupus erythematosus. Lancet **1951 I**, 260. — GONYEA, L. M., R. A. KALLSEN, and A. A. MARLOW: The occurence of the L.E. cell in clotted blood. J. invest. Derm. **15**, 11 (1950). — GOOD, R. A., C. MARTINEZ, A. P. DALMASSO, B. W. PAPERMASTER, and A. E. GABRIELSEN: Studies on the role of the thymus in developmental biology, with a consideration of the association of thymus abnormalities and clinical disease. Third Internat. Symposium Immunopathology. Basel: Benno Schwabe & Co. 1963, p. 177. — GOODMAN, H. C., J. L. FAHEY, R. A. MALGREN, and G. BRECHER: Separation of factors in lupus erythematosus serum reacting with components of cell nuclei. Lancet **1959 II**, 382. — GORDON, C., C. MEACHAM, and A. S. WEISBERGER: Unusual manifestations of disseminated lupus erythematosus. Ann. intern. Med. **43**, 143 (1955). — GOSLINGS, J., J. H. KIEVITS, H. M. HAZEVOET, W. HIJMANS, and A. CATS: The significance of the L.E. cell phenomenon for the symptomatology and the prognosis of rheumatoid arthritis. Proc. Xth Congr. Internat. League against rheumatism. Rome: Minerva Med. 1961. — GOUDSMITH, R., and J. J. VAN LOGHEM: Studies on the occurence of leuco-antibodies. Vox Sang. (Basel) **3**, 3, 89 (1953). — GRAY, N., I. R. MACKAY, L. I. TAFT, S. WEIDEN, and I. J. WOOD: Hepatitis, colitis and lupus manifestation. Amer. J. dig. Dis. **3**, 481 (1958). — GRISHMAN, E., J. CHURG, W. MAUTNER, and Y. SUZUKI: Pathology of lupus nephritis. J. Mt Sinai Hosp. **30**, 117 (1963). — GROSS, L.: The cardiac lesions in Libman-Sacks disease with consideration of its relationship to acute diffuse lupus erythematosus. Amer. J. Path. **16**, 375 (1940).

HALL, A. P., W. A. BARDAWIL, TH. B. BAYLES, A. D. MEDNIS, and N. GALINS: The relations between the antinuclear, rheumatoid and L.E. cell factors in the systemic rheumatic diseases. New Engl. J. Med. **263**, 769 (1960). — HARGRAVES, M. M., H. RICHMOND, and R. MORTON: Presentation of two bone marrow elements: the „tart" cell and the „L.E." cell. Proc. Mayo Clin. **23**, 25 (1948). — Production in vitro of the L.E. cell phenomenon. Proc. Mayo Clin. **24**, 234 (1949). — The L.E. cell phenomenon. Proc. Mayo Clin. **27**, 419 (1952). — HARRINGTON, W. J., V. MINNICH, and G. ARIMURA: The autoimmune thrombocytopenias. Progr. Hemat. **1**, 166 (1956). — HARVEY, A. M., L. E. SHULMAN, PH. A. TUMULTY, C. L. CONLEY, and E. H. SCHOENRICH: Systemic lupus erythematosus. Review of the literature and clinical analysis of 138 cases. Medicine (Baltimore) **33**, 291 (1954). — HASERICK, H. R.: Plasma L.E. test in systemic lupus erythematosus. Study of twenty-three patients with positive L.E. test. J. Amer. med. Ass. **146**, 16 (1951). — Blood factor in lupus erythematosus. Modern trends in dermatology (Second serie s), ed. by R. M. B. MCKENNA. London: Butterworth & Co. 1954. — HASERICK, H. R., and D. W. BORTZ: Blood factor in acute disseminated lupus erythematosus. Induction of specific antibodies against L.E. factor. Blood **5**, 718 (1950). — Preliminary and short reports. Normal bone marrow inclusions phenomena induced by lupus erythematosus plasma. J. invest. Derm. **13**, 47 (1949). — Simulation of the lupus erythematosus phenomenon by materials of fungal origin. J. invest. Derm. **16**, 211 (1951). — HAUSER, W.: Lupus erythematodes acutus mit Begleitretikulose und mit Beteiligung von Retikulumzellen an der LE-Zellbildung. Med. Klin. **46**, 412 (1951). — HAUSER, W., u. F. GEIER: Chronischer Lupus erythematosus mit akuter Exacerbation und Manifestation am Zentralnervensystem. Nervenarzt **23**, 181 (1952). — HELLER, P., and H. J. ZIMMERMAN: Nucleophagocytosis. Studies on three hundred thirty-six patients. Arch. intern. Med. **97**, 403 (1956). — HELLER, P., H. J. ZIMMERMAN, S. ROZENGVAIG, and K. SINGER: The L.E.-cell phenomenon in chronic hepatic disease. New Engl. J. Med. **254**, 1160 (1956). — HENKIND, P., and N. F. ROTHFIELD: Ocular abnormalities in patients treated with synthetic antimalarial drugs. New Engl. J. Med. **269**, 433 (1963). — HENN, M. J., TH. W. PARKIN, M. M. HARGRAVES, and M. O. HOWARD: Acute systemic lupus erythematosus syndrome from hydralazine hydrochloride. Arch. intern. Med. **95**, 857 (1955). — HITZIG, W. H., A. LABHART u. E. UEHLINGER: Transitorische Hemmkörperhämophilie bei Rheumatismus. Helv. med. Acta **18**, 410 (1951). — HOGG, G. R.: Congenital, acute lupus erythematosus associated with subendocardial fibroelastosis: report of case. Amer. J. clin. Path. **28**, 648 (1957). — HOLBOROW, E. J., and D. M. WEIR: Histone, an essential component for the lupus erythematosus antinuclear reaction. Lancet **1959 I**, 809. — HOLBOROW, E. J., D. M. WEIR, and G. D. JOHNSON: A serum factor in lupus erythematosus with affinity for tissue nuclei. Brit. med. J. **1957 II**, 732. — HOLMAN, H. R.: In: Immunologic aspects of rheumatoid arthritis and SLE. Arthr. and Rheum. **6**, 538 (1963). — HOLMAN, H. R., and H. DEICHER: The reaction of the lupus erythematosus cell factor with deoxyribonucleoprotein of the cell nucleus. J. clin. Invest. **38**, 2059 (1959). — HOLMAN, H. R., H. DEICHER, and H. G. KUNKEL: The LE cell and the LE serum factor. Bull. N.Y. Acad. Med. **35**, 409 (1959). — HOLMAN, H. R., and H. G. KUNKEL: Affinity between the lupus erythematosus serum factor and cell nuclei and nucleoprotein. Science **126**, 162 (1957). — HOLMAN, H. R., and T. TOMASI: Lupoid hepatitis. Med. Clin. N. Amer. **44**, 633 (1960). — HONEY, M.: Systemic lupus erythematosus presenting with sulfonamide hypersensitivity reaction. Brit. med. J. **1956 II**, 1272.

INDERBITZIN, TH.: The experimental production of leukocytic changes in normal blood similar to L.E.-cells and morphologically identical with L.E.-cells. J. invest. Derm. **20**, 67 (1953). — Zum Problem der Deutung des L.E.-Zellphänomens. Acta haemat. (Basel) **12**, 268 (1954).

JACOBS, A. G.: A false-positive L.E. test. Ann. intern. Med. **42**, 1097 (1955). — JANBON, M., O. FLANDRE, and M. DAMON: Etude d'un test sérique à l'acide para-toluène-sulfonique:

son application à l'appréciation rapide du taux des gamma-globulines. Rev. franc. Étud. clin. biol. 4, 818 (1959). — JASINSKI, B., G. E. STIEFELK, M. MÄRKI u. F. WUHRMANN: Über ein dem L.E.-Phänomen ähnliches Zellbild im Cataridenblaseninhalt und seine Beziehungen zu den Gammaglobulinen. Klin. Wschr. **1953**, 252. — JESSAR, R. A., R. LAMONT-HAVERS, and C. RAGAN: Natural history of lupus erythematosus disseminatus. Ann. intern. Med. **38**, 717 (1953). — JOKINEN, E. J., and R. MÄKITALO: The occurence of the L.E. serum factor in patients with systemic lupus erythematosus detected with passive hemagglutination technique. Acta rheum. scand. **6**, 31 (1960). — JONES, K. K., and H. E. THOMPSON: Evaluation of simple precipitation test for systemic lupus erythematosus. J. Amer. med. Ass. **166**, 1424 (1958).

KAPOSI, M. K.: Neue Beiträge zur Kenntnis des Lupus erythematosus. Arch. Derm. Syph. (Berl.) 4, 36 (1872). — KAYHOE, D. E., J. P. NASOU, and J. BOZICEVICH: Clinical evaluation of the DNA bentonite flocculation test for SLE. New Engl. J. Med. **263**, 3 (1960). — KEEFER, C. S., and A. R. FELTY: Acute disseminated lupus erythematosus. Bull. Johns Hopk. Hosp. **35**, 294 (1924). — KIEVITS, J. H., J. GOSLINGS, H. R. E. SCHUIT, and W. HIJMANS: Rheumatoid arthritis and the positive L.E. cell phenomenon. Ann. rheum. Dis. **15**, 211 (1956). — KLEIN, E.: Lupus erythematodes visceralis sive disseminatus. Dtsch. med. Wschr. **1955**, 226. — KLEMPERER, P.: The concept of collagen diseases. Amer. J. Path. **26**, 505 (1950). — KLEMPERER, P., B. GUEFT, L. S. LEE, C. LEUCHTENBERGER, and K. W. POLLISTER: The pathogenesis of lupus erythematosus and allied conditions. Ann. intern. Med. **28**, 1 (1948). — Cytochemical changes of acute lupus erythematosus. Arch. Path. **49**, 503 (1950). — KLEMPERER, P., A. D. POLLAK, and G. BAEHR: Pathology of disseminated lupus erythematosus. Arch. Path. **32**, 569 (1941a). — Pathology of disseminated lupus erythematosus. Arch. Path. **32**, 569 (1941b). — KLINGE, F.: Der Rheumatismus; pathologisch-anatomische und experimentell-pathologische Tatsachen und ihre Auswertung für das ärztliche Rheumaproblem. Ergebn. allg. Path. path. Anat. **27**, 1 (1933). — KORTING, G. W., and R. SCHMITZ: Induktion des Lupus-erythematodes-Zellphänomens mittels Urins. Derm. Wschr. **125**, 174 (1952). — KOSTANT, G. H.: Biologically false positive reactions to serologic tests for syphilis. Bull. Wld Hlth Org. **14**, 235 (1956). — KUNKEL, H. G., E. H. AHRENS, W. J. EISENMENGER, A. M. BONGIOVANNI, and R. J. SLATER: Extreme hypergammaglobulinemia in young women with liver disease. J. clin. Invest. **30**, 654 (1951). — KUNKEL, H. G., H. R. HOLMAN, and H. R. G. DEICHER: Multiple „autoantibodies" to cell constituents in systemic lupus erythematosus. Ciba Foundation Symposium Cellular Aspects of Immunity. London: Churchill 1960, p. 429. — KURNICK, N. B.: A rational therapy of systemic lupus erythematosus. Arch. intern. Med. **97**, 562 (1956). — KURNICK, N. B., S. PARISER, L. I. SCHWARTZ, S. L. LEE, and W. IRVINE: Studies on desoxyribonuclease in systemic lupus erythematosus. Non participation of serum desoxyribonuclease in the L.E. phenomenon. J. clin. Invest. **31**, 1036 (1952a). — KURNICK, N. B., L. SCHWARTZ, S. PARISER, and S. LEE: A specific inhibitor form human desoxyribonuclease andan inhibitor of the L.E. phenomenon from leucocytes. J. clin. Invest. **32**, 193 (1953). — KURNICK, N. B., L. SCHWARTZ, S. PARISER, S. LEE, and W. IRVINE: The role of desoxyribonuclease and a nuclease inhibitor from leucocytesin the lupus erythematosus cell phenomenon. J. clin. Invest. **31**, 645 (1952b).

LACHMANN, P. J.: Quoted by H. KUNKEL. In: Immunologic aspects of rheumatoid arthritis and SLE. Arthr. and Rheum. **6**, 538 (1963). — LACHMANN, P. J., H. J. MUELLER-EBERHARD, H. G. KUNKEL, and F. PARONETTO: The localization of in vivo bound complement in tissue sections. J. exp. Med. **115**, 63 (1962). — LAURELL, A. B., and I. M. NILSSON: Hypergammaglobulinemia, circulating anticoagulant and biologic false positive Wassermann reaction. J. Lab. clin. Med. **49**, 694 (1957). — LEDDY, J. PL., R. W. HILL, S. N. SWISHER, and J. H. VAUGHAN: Observations on the immunochemical nature of red cell autosensitization. Proc. 3rd Internat. Symposium Immunopathology. Basel: Benno Schwabe & Co. (in print). — LEE, R. C., and W. V. EPSTEIN: Hemagglutination study of serum factors related to LE cell formation. Arthr. and Rheum. **3**, 41 (1960). — LEE, S. L.: A simple test for L.E. cells. Amer. J. clin. Path. **21**, 492 (1951). — Inhibition of leukocyte agglutination by serum from patients with SLE. A manifestation of the L.E. cell phenomenon. Blood **13**, 778 (1958). — LEE, S. L., S. R. MICHAEL, and I. L. VURAL: The lupus erythematosus cell. Bull. N.Y. Acad. Med. **26**, 266 (1950). — The L.E. cell. Clinical and chemical studies. Amer. J. Med. **10**, 446 (1951). — LEE, S. L., and M. SANDERS: A disorder of blood coagulation in systemic lupus erythematosus. J. clin. Invest. **34**, 1814 (1955). — LEONHARD, T.: Familial hypergammaglobulinemia and systemic lupus erythematosus. Lancet **1957 II**, 1200. — LEONI, A.: A proposito della specifità del fenomeno L.E. Minerva med. Acta **45**, 1 (1954). — LEVIN, M. B., and H. PINKUS: Autosensitivity to desoxyribonucleic acid. Report of case with inflammatory skin lesions controlled by chloroquine. New Engl. J. Med. **264**, 533 (1961). — LEVINE, L.: Determinants of specificity of proteins, nucleic acids and polypeptides. Fed. Proc. **21**, 711 (1962). — LEVINE, L., W. T. MURAKAMI, H. VAN VUNAKIS, and L. GROSSMAN: Specific antibodies to thermally denatured desoxyribonucleic acid of phage T4. Proc. nat. Acad. Sci. (Wash.) **46**, 1038 (1960). — LEY, A. G., G. G. READER, C. W. SORENSON, and R. S. OVERMAN: Idiopathic hypoprothrombinemia associated with hemorrhagic diatheses, and the effect of vitamin K. Blood **6**, 740 (1951). — LIBMAN, E., and B. SACKS: A hitherto undescribed form of valvular and mural endocarditis. Arch. intern. Med. **33**, 701 (1924). — LOELIGER, A.: Prothrombin as co-factor of the circulating anticoagulant in systemic lupus erythematosus. Thrombos. Diathes. haemorrh. (Stuttg.) **3**, 237 (1959). — LOGHEM, J. J. VAN, M. VAN DER HART, and H. BORSTEL: The occurrence of complete and incomplete white cell antibodies. Vox Sang. (Basel) **2**, 257 (1957).

MACKAY, I. R., and D. C. GAJDUSEK: An „autoimmune" reaction against human tissue antigens in certain acute and chronic diseases. II. Clinical aspects. Arch. intern. Med. **101**, 30 (1958). — MACKAY, I. R., L. I. TAFT, and D. C. COWLING: Lupoid hepatitis. Lancet **1956 II**, 1323. — MÄKITALO, R., and E. J. JOKINEN: Affinity of the L.E. factor for several commercial deoxyribonucleic acid preparations. Ann. Med. exp. Fenn. **36**, 309 (1958). — MAGATH, TH. B., and V. WINKLE: Technic for demonstrating L.E. cells in blood. Amer. J. clin. Path. **22**, 586 (1952). — MARMONT, A.: Le cosidette angiomesenchimopathie reattive diffuse. Correlazione al 52. Congr. Soc. Ital. Med. Int. Pozzi Roma 1951a. — Immunoematologia. Attualità in ematologia. Roma: Abruzzini Ed. 1951b. — Beobachtungen über das sogenannte L.E.-Phänomen. Schweiz. med. Wschr. **1952**, 1111. — Observations et remarques sur le phénomène L.E. C. r. VIIIe Congr. de dermatologistes et syphiligraphes de langue française Nancy-Vittel 1953. — Value and limitations of the L.E. cell test in the syndrome known as systemic lupus erythematosus without skin eruptions. Acta haemat. (Basel) **13**, 257 (1955). — Nucleolytic phagocytosis in systemic lupus erythematosus, rheumatoid arthritis and systemic scleroderma. 1. Internat. Symposium Immunopathologie Seslisberg. Benno Schwabe & Co. 1959, p. 479. — MARMONT, A., and M. PIUMA: Immagini L.E. simili e pseudofenomeni L.E. Boll. Soc. ital. Emat. **3**, 253 (1955). — MCCOMBS, R. P., and J. F. PATTERSON: Factors influencing course and prognosis of systemic lupus erythematosus. New Engl. J. Med. **260**, 1195 (1959). — MCCUISTION, C. H., and E. P. SCHOCH: Possible discoid lupus erythematosus in newborn infant: report of case with subsequent development of acute systemic lupus erythematosus in mother. Arch. Derm. **70**, 782 (1954). — MCCLUSKEY, R. T., B. BENACERRAF, J. POTTER, and F. MILLER: The pathologic effects of intravenously administered soluble antigen-antibody complexes. J. exp. Med. **111**, 181 (1960). — MCCLUSKEY, R. T., F. MILLER, and B. BENACERRAF: Passive acute glomerulonephritis induced by antigen-antibody complexes solubilized in hapten excess. Proc. Soc. exp. Biol. (N.Y.) **111**, 764 (1962). — MELLORS, R. C., L. F. ORTEGA, and H. R. HOLMAN: Role of gammaglobulins in pathogenesis of renal lesions in systemic lupus erythematosus and chronic membranous glomerulonephritis, with an observation on the lupus erythematosus cell reaction. J. exp. Med. **106**, 191 (1957). — MERWIN, CH. F., and R. K. WINKELMANN: Antimalarial drugs in the therapy of lupus erythematosus. Proc. Mayo Clin. **37**, 254 (1962). — MICHAEL, S. R., I. L. VURAL, F. A. BASSEN, and L. SCHAEFER: The hematologic aspects of disseminated lupus erythematosus. Blood **6**, 1059 (1951). — MIESCHER, P.: Immunophagocytose des éléments cellulaires dans le sang. Schweiz. med. Wschr. **1953**, 216. — Mise en évidence du facteur L.E. par la réaction de consommation d'antiglobuline. Vox Sang. (Basel) **5**, 116 (1955). — The antigenic constituents of the neutrophilic leukocyte with special reference to the L.E.-phenomenon. Vox Sang. (Basel) **2**, 145 (1957a). — Zur Serologie des L.E.-Phaenomens. Hautarzt **8**, 502 (1957b). — Étude experimentale sur l'evolution d'une infection intraoculaire au virus variolique en presence d'anticorps anti-uveaires. C. r. IIe Congr. Nat. Transfusion Sang. Bordeaux: Imp. Delmas 1958a, p. 461. — Le lupus erythemateux dissemine. Le phenomene L.E. et les seroreactions antisubstance nucleaires. Third Internat. Congr. of Allergy. Paris: Flammarion 1958b, p. 537. — Die Serologie des visceralen Erythematodes. Akt. Probl. Derm. **1**, 322 (1959). — MIESCHER, P., L. BARKER, I. VAINIO, and G. WIEDERMANN: Immune mechanisms of cell and tissue damage in SLE. Proc. Elkhard Symposium on Inflammation (1964). — MIESCHER, P., et J. DELACRÉTAZ: Démonstration d'un phénomène „L.E." positif dans deux cas d'hypersensibilité médicamenteuse. Schweiz. med. Wschr. **1953**, 356. — MIESCHER, P., et M. FAUCONNET: L'absorption du facteur „L.E." par des noyaux cellulaires isolés. Experientia (Basel) **10**, 252 (1954a). — Les constituants antigéniques du leucocyte polynucléaire et leur importance clinique. Schweiz. med. Wschr. **1954** b, 1036. — MIESCHER, P., M. FAUCONNET et TH. BÉRAUD: Immuno-nucléophagocytose expérimentale et phénomène L.E. J. exp. Med. Surg. **11**, 173 (1953). — MIESCHER, P., et L. HOLLÄNDER: Les hémopathies par „auto-anticorps". Rev. méd. Suisse rom. **75**, 398 (1955). — MIESCHER, P., L. HOLLÄNDER et A. HÄSSIG: Localisation des „autoanticorps" érythrocytaires et plaquettaires dans les fractions plasmatiques de Cohn. Internat. Kongr. Ges. für Bluttransfusion Paris 1954. — MIESCHER, P., u. F. W. JACKSON: Autoimmunitäre Phänomene im Verlauf von Arzneimittelallergien. Schweiz. med. Wschr. **92**, 384 (1962). — MIESCHER, P., A. MIESCHER et M. FAUCONNET: Immunophagocytose der Blutzellen in vitro. Dtsch. med. Wschr., Allergie-Beilage **1954**, 9. — MIESCHER, P., and R. STRAESSLE: New serological methods for the detection of the L.E. factor. Vox Sang. (Basel) **2**, 145 (1957). — MIESCHER, P., L. THOMAS, B. BENACERRAF, N. S. COOPER, E. FRANK-

LIN, and N. ROTHFIELD: The immunopathology of lupus erythematosus. Brit. J. Derm. 72, 221 (1960). — MIESCHER, P., u. K. O. VORLAENDER: Der viscerale Erythematodes. Immunopathologie in Klinik und Forschung, 2. Aufl., S. 501. Georg Thieme 1962. — MILLER, J. F. A. P.: Immunological function of the thymus. Lancet **1961 II**, 748. — MOFFAT, TH. W., S. S. BARNES, and R. S. WEISS: The induction of the L.E. cell in normal peripheral blood. J. invest. Derm. **14**, 153 (1950). — MONTGOMERY, H., and W. G. MCCREIGHT: Disseminated lupus erythematosus. Arch. Derm. **60**, 356 (1949). — MOORE, J. E., and W. B. LUTZ: The natural history of systemic lupus erythematosus; an approach to its study through biologic false positive reactions. J. chron. Dis. **1**, 297 (1955). — MOORE, J. E., and C. F. MOHR: The incidence and etiologic background of chronic false positive reactions in serologic tests for syphilis. Ann. intern. Med. **37**, 156 (1952). — MORSE, J. H., H. J. MULLER-EBERHARD, and H. G. KUNKEL: Depression of complement components in systemic lupus erythematosus and the effect of steroids. Arthr. and Rheum. **4**, 427 (1961). — MORTEO, O. G., E. C. FRANKLIN, C. MCEWEN, J. PHYTHYON, and M. TANNER: Studies of relatives of patients with systemic lupus erythematosus. Arthr. and Rheum. **4**, 356 (1961). — MUEHRCKE, R. C., R. M. KARK, C. L. PIRANI, and V. E. POLLAK: Lupus nephritis: a clinical and pathological study based on renal biopsies. Medicine (Baltimore) **36**, 1 (1957). — MUEHRCKE, R. C., R. M. KARK, C. PIRANI, V. E. POLLAK, and J. E. STECH: Histological evolution of lupus-nephritis. Ann. rheum. Dis. **14**, 371 (1955). — MUELLER, P., u. B. RADOJICIC: Leukocytenagglutination und thrombocytäre Antikörper bei akutem Lupus erythematosus. Klin. Wschr. **1956**, 577. — MULLER-EBERHARD, H. J.: Detection of in vivo bound complement in systemic lupus erythematosus. Proc. IInd Internat. Symposium Immunopathology. Benno Schwabe & Co. 1962, p. 326. — MULLINS, J. F., J. M. KIRK, and E. M. SHAPIRO: Chloroquin treatment of lupus erythematosus. Sth. med. J. (Bgham, Ala.) **48**, 732 (1955). — MULLINS, J. F., F. L. WATTS, and CH. WILSON: Plaquenil in the treatment of lupus erythematosus. J. Amer. med. Ass. **161**, 879 (1956).

NELSON, R. A., M. M. MAYER, J. A. DIENDRUCK, and J. T. EAGAN: The treponema-immobilizing test. J. exp. Med. **89**, 369 (1949).

O'CONNOR, J. F.: Psychoses associated with SLE. Ann. intern. Med. **51**, 526 (1959). — OGRYZLO, M. A., and H. A. SMYTHE: Systemic lupus erythematosus and syndromes possibly related. Pediatrics **19**, 1109 (1957). — OSBORNE, E. O., J. W. JORDAN, F. C. HOAK, and F. J. PSCHIERER: Nitrogen mustard therapy in cutaneous blastomatous disease. J. Amer. med. Ass. **135**, 1123 (1947). — OSLER, W.: On the visceral complications of erythema exudativum multiforme. Amer. J. med. Sci. **110**, 629 (1895). — OUDSTEN, S. A. VAN DEN, J. E. VAN LOGHEM, and H. DORFMEIJER: Difference in behaviour of the „Rose" factor and the L.E. factor in regard to placental transmission. Vox Sang. (Basel) **3**, 192 (1958).

PAYNE, J. F.: A post-graduate lecture on lupus erythematosus. Clin. J. **4**, 223 (1894). — PEARSON, C. M., CH. G. CRADDOCK, and N. SIMMONS: Complement fixation reactions with DNA and leukocyte material in SLE. J. Lab. clin. Med. **52**, 580 (1958). — PERRY, H. M., and H. A. SCHROEDER: Syndrome simulating collagen disease caused by hydralazine. J. Amer. med. Ass. **154**, 670 (1954). — PIERCE, F. L., R. IRBY, and E. C. TOONE: L.E. cells in patients with chronic rheumatoid arthritis. 2. Panameric. Congr. Rheumat. Dis. 1959. — PISCIOTTA, A. V., J. J. GILIBERTI, J. J. GREENWALT, and W. W. ENGSTROM: Acute hemolytic anemia in disseminated lupus erythematosus. Amer. J. clin. Path. **21**, 1138 (1951). — POLLACK, A. D.: Some observations on the pathology of systemic lupus erythematosus. J. Mt Sinai Hosp. **26**, 224 (1959). — POLLAK, V. E., C. L. PIRANI, R. C. MUEHRCKE, P. C. PULOS, P. C. KARK, and I. E. STECK: On renal involvement in systemic lupus erythematosus and other collagen diseases. Arthr. and Rheum. **1**, 204 (1958).

RABINOWITZ, Y., and W. DAMESHEK: Systemic lupus erythematosus after idiopathic thrombocytopenic purpura; a review. Ann. intern. Med. **52**, 1 (1960). — RAPP, F.: Localization of antinuclear factors from L.E. sera in tissue culture. J. Immunol. 88, 732 (1962). — RASPONI, L.: Sulla questione della specifita del fenomeno L.E. G. ital. Derm. **96**, 619 (1955). — REIN, C. R., and G. H. KONSTANT: Lupus erythematosus: serologic and chemical aspects. Arch. Derm. Syph. (Chic.) **61**, 898 (1950). — ROBINEAUX, R.: Étude microcinématographique en contraste de phase du mécanisme du phénomène L.E. 1. Internat. Symposium Immunopathologie. Benno Schwabe & Co. 1959, p. 416. — ROBINSON, W.: Management of systemic lupus erythematosus. Arthr. and Rheum. **5**, 521 (1962). — ROHN, R. J., and W. H. BOND: Some supravital observations on the L.E. phenomenon. Amer. J. Med. **12**, 422 (1952). — ROTHFIELD, N., R. T. MCCLUSKEY, and D. S. BALDWIN: Renal disease in systemic lupus erythematosus. New Engl. J. Med. **269**, 537 (1963). — ROTHFIELD, N., C. MARCH, and P. MIESCHER: Chronic discoid lupus erythematosus, a studi of 65 patients and 65 controls. New Engl. J. Med. **269**, 1155 (1963). — ROTHFIELD, N. F., J. M. PHYTHYON, C. MCEWEN, and P. MIESCHER: The role of antinuclear reactions in the diagnosis of systemic lupus erythemaeosus. A study of 53 cases. Arthr. and Rheum. **4**, 223 (1961). — ROWELL, N. R.: Lupus trythematosus cells in systemic sclerosis. Ann. rheum. Dis. **21**, 70 (1962). — ROWELL, N. R., and J. S. BECK: Immunological abnormalities in 120 patients with chronic discoid lupus erythematosus. Internat. Congr. Derm. Washington 1962. — RUHENSTROTH-BAUER, G., E. STRAUB, P. SACHTLEBEN u. G. F. FUHRMANN: Die elektrophoretische Beweglichkeit von Blutzellen beim Gesunden und bei Kranken. Münch. med. Wschr. **103**, 794 (1961). — RUPPLI, H., u. R. VOSSEN: Nebenwirkung der Hydantoinkörpertherapie unter dem Bilde eines visceralen Lupus erythematosus. Schweiz. med. Wschr. **83**, 1555 (1957).

SALLMANN, L. v., and H. N. BERNSTEIN: Adverse effects of chloroquine and related antimalarial drugs on ocular structures. Bull. rheum. Dis. **14**, 327 (1963). — SCALETTAR, R., D. M. MARCUS, L. A. SIMONTON, and L. H. MUSCHEL: The nucleoprotein complement fixation test in the diagnosis of systemic lupus erythematosus. New Engl. J. Med. **263**, 226 (1960). — SCHEFFER, E.: An investigation into the effect of lupus erythematosus serum on living cells. The finding of so-called „purple bodies". Konikl. Ned. Akad. Wetenschap. Proc., Ser. C **64**, 501 (1961). — SCHULTEN, H., H. H. HENNEMANN u. W. KUHN: Praktische Hinweise zur Diagnostik und Therapie des visceralen Erythematodes. Med. Welt **1962**, 993. — SCHWARTZ, R., and J. ANDRE: The chemical suppression of immunity. Proc. second Internat. Symposium Immunopathology. Benno Schwabe & Co. 1962, p. 385. — SCHWARTZ, R. S., F. B. LEWIS, and W. DAMESHEK: Hemorrhagic cutaneous anaphylaxis due to autosensitization to deoxyribonucleic acid. New Engl. J. Med. **267**, 1105 (1962). — SEAMAN, A. J., and J. W. CHRISTERSON: Demonstration of L.E. cells in pericardial fluid. Report of a case. J. Amer. med. Ass. **149**, 145 (1952). — SELIGMANN, M.: Études immunologiques sur le lupus érythémateux disséminé. Rev. franç. Étud. clin. biol. **3**, 358 (1958). — Études immunologiques sur le lupus érythémateux disséminé et les anticorps anti-acide désoxyribonucléique. 1. Internat. Symposium Immunopathologie. Benno Schwabe & Co. 1959, p. 402. — Données récentes sur le phénomène L.E. et sur les anticorps du lupus érythémateux disséminé. Presse med. **69**, 1643 (1961). — Immunologic aspects of rheumatoid arthritis and systemic lupus erythematosus; DNA antibodies. Arthr. and Rheum. **6**, 542 (1963). — SELIGMANN, M., et C. HANAU: Étude immunoelectrophoretique du serum des malades atteints de lupus erythemateux dissemine. Rev. Hémat. **13**, 239 (1958). — SHEARN, M. A., and B. PIROFSKY: Disseminated lupus erythematosus. Arch. intern. Med. **90**, 790 (1952). — SHULMAN, L. E., and A. M. HARVEY: The nature of drug induced systemic lupus erythematosus. Arthr. and Rheum. **3**, 464 (1960) — SIEGEL, M., S. L. LEE, M. GREENBERG, D. WIDELOCK, E. B. REILLY, G. J. WISE, S. B. ZINGALE, and H. T. FUERST: Epidemiological study on systemic lupus erythematosus. 1961 Annual Meeting Amer. Rheum. Ass. — SIEGENTHALER, W., u. R. HEGGLIN: Der viscerale Lupus erythematosus. Ergebn. inn. Med. Kinderheilk. **7**, 373 (1956). — SIMONSEN, M.: The mechanism of runt disease. Proc. second Internat. Symposium Immunopathology. Benno Schwabe & Co. 1962, p. 233. — SINGER, J. M., and C. M. PLOTZ: The latex fixation test. Amer. J. Med. **21**, 888 (1956). — SINGER, K.: Thrombotic thrombocytopenic purpura. In: Advanc. intern. Med. **6**, 195 (1954) (Chicago: Year Book Publisher, Inc., W. DOCK and I. SNAPPER, Edit.). — SLOCUMB, CH. H.: Rheumatic complaints during chronic hypercortisonism and syndromes during withdrawal of cortisone in rheumatic patients. Proc. Mayo Clin. **28**, 655 (1953). — SMITH, E. W., and A. KURBAN: Capillary alterations in lupus erythematosus. Bull. Johns Hopk. Hosp. **110**, 202 (1962). — SNAPPER, I., and D. NATHAN: The mechanism of the L.E. cell phenomenon, studied with a simplified test. Blood **10**, 718 (1955). — SOFFER, L. J., M. F. LEVITT, and G. BAEHR: Use of cortisone and A.C.T.H. in acute disseminated lupus erythematosus. Arch. intern. Med. **86**, 558 (1950). — SPIEGELBERG, H.: Die Rolle der antinukleären Antikörper beim Zustandekommen des L.E.-Phänomens. Haemat. Acta **24**, 230 (1960). — SPIEGELBERG, H. L., and P. A. MIESCHER: The effect of 6-mercaptopurine and methotrexate on experimental immune thyroiditis in guinea pigs. J. exp. Med. **118**, 869 (1963). — STEAGALL, R. W., H. T. ASH, and L. B. FENTANES: Familial lupus erythematosus (discoid lupus erythem. in identical twin females). Arch. Derm. **85**, 394 (1962). — STEFFEN, C.: Das Problem der Autoaggression. Wien. klin. Wschr. **44**, 865 (1956). — Die Bedeutung der Thrombocyten-Autoantikörper und Thrombocyten-Antigene für die Pathogenese der Immunothrombopenie. Proc. Eighth Congr. Europ. Soc. Haemat. S. Karger 1962a, p. 208. — Der Antiglobulin-Konsumptionstest. Seine theoretischen Grundlagen, Technik und Anwendungsbereiche. Klin. Wschr. **40**, 613 (1962b). — Grundriß der Immunopathologie. Stuttgart: Georg Thieme (im Druck). — STEVENS, M. B., H. ABBEY, and L. E. SHULMAN: The clinical significance of extracellular material in L.E.-cell preparations. New Engl. J. Med. **268**, 976 (1963). — STEVENS, M. B., and B. KNOWLES: Significance of urinary gamma globulin in lupus nephritis. New Engl. J. Med. **267**, 1159 (1962). — STOLLAR, D., and L. LEVINE: Antibodies to denatured DNA in lupus erythematosus serum. IV. Evidence for purine determinants in DNA. Arch. Biochem. **101**, 417 (1963). — STOLLAR, D., L. LEVINE, H. I. LEHRER, and V. VAN VUNAKIS: The antigenic determinants of denatured DNA reactive with lupus erythematosus serum. Proc. nat. Acad. Sci. (Wash.) **48**, 874 (1962b). — STOLLAR, D., L. LEVINE, and J. MARMUR: Antibodies to denatured deoxyribonucleic acid in L.E. serum. II. Characterization of antibodies in several sera. Biochim. biophys. Acta (Amst.) **61**, 7 (1962a). — Sturgill, B., A. Strauss, and R. Carpenter: Personal communication. — Suksta, A., and L. Conley: Some observations on the L.E. cell. J. Lab. clin. Med. **37**, 597 (1951). — Sundberg, R. D., and N. B. Lick: L.E. cells in the blood in acute disseminated lupus erythematosus. J. invest. Derm. **12**, 83 (1949).

Townes, A. S., C. R. Stewart, and A. G. Osler: Immunologic studies in systemic lupus erythematosus. Proc. 2nd. Internat. Symposium Immunopathology. Benno Schwabe & Co. 1962, p. 315. — Tumulty, P. A.: The clinical course of disseminated lupus erythematosus. Bull. Johns Hopk. Hosp. **85**, 47 (1949). — The clinical course of systemic lupus erythematosus. J. Amer. med. Ass. **156**, 947 (1954).

Ullman, K.: Über Lupus erythematodes. Wien. klin. Wschr. **41**, 1159 (1928).

Vasquez, J. J., and F. J. Dixon: Immunohistochemical analysis of lesions associated with fibrinoid change. Arch. Path. **66**, 504 (1960). — Vassalli, P., G. Simon, and C. Rouiller: (to be published). — Verloop, M. C.: Some observations concerning the L.E. phenomenon. Acta med. scand. **148**, 183 (1954). — Vernier, R. L., M. G. Farquhar, J. G. Brunson, and R. A. Good: Chronic renal disease in children. Amer. J. Dis. Child. **96**, 306 (1958). — Volkmann-Zehr, M. M.: Das sogenannte „Litman-Sackssche Syndrom". Helv. med. Acta **13**, Fasc. 5 (1946). — Vorlaender, K. O.: Das Auto-Immunisierungsproblem bei Nieren- und Lebererkrankungen in klinischer Sicht. Dtsch. Arch. klin. Med. **202**, 253 (1955). — Vorlaender, K. O., K. W. Fritz u. J. Ross: Serumproteine und Nierenerkrankung. Med. Welt **17**, 883 (1960). — Vorlaender, K. O., u. H. Nuessgens: Die Gefäßveränderungen beim visceralen Erythematodes und ihre immunologischen Grundlagen. Z. Immun.-Forsch. **114**, 353 (1957). — Vorsaender, S., K. O. Vorlaender u. H. Luechtrath: Versuche zur künstlichen Lokalisation eines Infektes auf die Rattenniere. Klin. Wschr. **1956**, 1069.

Walsh, J. R., and R. L. Egun: The reliability of the L.E. test. New Engl. J. Med. **246**, 775 (1952). — Walsh, J. R., and H. J. Zimmermann: The demonstration of the L.E. phenomenon in patients with penicillin hypersensitivity. Blood **8**, 65 (1953). — Weinstock, I., and S. L. Lee: Hypogammaglobulinemia in SLE. Amer. J. Dis. Child. **99**, 132 (1960). — Weisberger, A. S., G. C. Meacham, and R. Heinle: Simple method for demonstrating the L.E. phenomenon in peripheral blood. J. Lab. clin. Med. **39**, 480 (1952). — Weiss, R. S., and Sh. Swift: The significance of a positive L.E. phenomenon. Arch. Derm. **72**, 103 (1955). — White, R. G., and A. H. E. Marshall: The autoimmune response in myasthenia gravis. Lancet **1962 II**, 120. — Wiedermann, G., M. Doerner, and P. Miescher: Immunopathologie der Leber. Schweiz. med. Wschr. **1964** (in press). — Wilson, A. P., and J. W. Jordan: Relationship of chronic discoid and disseminated lupus erythematosus. N.Y. St. J. Med. **50**, 2449 (1959). — Wilson, R. M., R. R. Abbott, and D. K. Miller: The occurrence of L.E. cells and hematoxylin bodies in the naturally occurring cutaneous lesions of SLE. Amer. J. med. Sci. **241**, 73 (1961).

Yamauchi, H., P. Rooney, and J. Hopper: Nephrotic state as the chief manifesta ion of SLE. Ann. intern. Med. **57**, 981 (1962).

Zellman, H. E.: The incidence of positive serologic tests for syphilis in the collagen diseases. Amer. J. Syph. **36**, 163 (1952). — Ziff, M., P. Esserman, and C. McEwen: Observations on the course and treatment of systemic lupus erythematosus. Arthr. and Rheum. **1**, 332 (1958). — Zimmer, F. E., and M. M. Hargraves: The effect of blood coagulation on L.E. cell formation. Proc. Mayo Clin. **27**, 424 (1952). — Zimmermann, H. J., J. R. Walsh, and P. Heller: Production of nucleophagocytosis by rabbit antileukocytic serum. Blood **8**, 651 (1953). — Zinkham, W. H., and C. L. Conley: Some factors influencing the formation of L.E. cells. A method for enhancing L.E. cell production. Bull. Johns Hopk. Hosp. **98**, 102 (1956). — Zoutendyk, A.: Autoantibodies in the pathogenesis of disease. A preliminary study of autosensitization of red cells in various diseases. S. Afr. med. J. **25**, 665 (1951).

Dermatomyositis

By

Frances Pascher-Brooklyn (N.Y.)

With 10 Figures in the Text (2 in Colour)

1. History

WAGNER is credited with having been the first to describe the muscle disorder that is the subject of this chapter. In 1887 WAGNER introduced the term polymyositis for a rapidly fatal case associated with cutaneous manifestations. UNVERRICHT described similar cases, showing a preference for the term dermatomyositis to mark the association with cutaneous involvement and recognized that not all cases were fatal. HEPP in turn pointed out that the morbid changes in the muscles in the absence of skin lesions were the same as in their presence. Dermatomucomyositis was suggested by OPPENHEIM to draw attention to the involvement of the mucous membranes as well as the glabrous skin in many instances.

OPPENHEIM, PETGES and CLÉJAT soon recognized chronic forms accompanied by sclerodermatous changes, cutaneous atrophy and poikiloderma. Some years later PETGES and PETGES reviewed the subject of myositis with poikiloderma and reported two additional cases under the title of "Poikilodermatomyosite". In 1939 GUY et al. expressed the view that dermatomyositis and poikilodermatomyositis were variants of the same process, a view widely held today.

STERTZ and KANKELEIT in 1916 were the first to note the coexistence of polymyositis with visceral malignancy. The significance of these reports was not fully appreciated until BEZECNY reported two additional cases. It is now generally held that the association of dermatomyositis with malignancy is not coincidental, that it is usually seen in adults and that a malignant lymphoma or sarcoma as well as a visceral neoplasm may elicit the disease.

Whether or not dermatomyositis is a disease sui generis or one that is necessarily associated with a collagen disorder has given rise to much disputation. PFEIFFER it appears was the first to express the view that dermatomyositis may not be a primary myopathy but a dyscrasia secondary to an obscure affection of connective tissue. This controversial question remains unsettled and will be explored further in the sections on classification and pathogenesis.

The most notable advances in the past decade have been in the fields of electrodiagnosis and enzyme chemistry. Similarly despite the reservations of some, an impressive number of observers with wide experience are of the opinion that the availability of corticosteroids and adrenocorticotropin (ACTH) constitutes a major development in the management of dermatomyositis.

2. Terminology and Nosology

a) Terminology

Dermatomyositis has been defined by STEINER as an acute, subacute or chronic disease of unknown origin characterized by a gradual onset with vague and indefinite prodromata followed by edema, dermatitis and multiple muscle inflammation. It might be well however to modify the last phrase to read, "nonsuppurative inflammation of multiple groups of striated muscle".

According to WALTON and ADAMS *polymyositis* and *dermatomyositis* were used interchangeably by early writers. Later accounts, however, reflected some uncertainty as to the relationship between dermatomyositis and similar acute or chronic muscle diseases without cutaneous involvement. In recent years observers have been again inclined to use dermatomyositis and polymyositis synonymously. This is based largely on the fact that electrodiagnostic technics and enzyme studies as well as extensive histopathologic investigation have failed to disclose any essential difference in the nature of the morbid process, whether or not skin lesions are present.

Nevertheless the author is inclined to side with those who now draw the distinction between dermatomyositis and polymyositis. It does not seem appropriate to use the former in the absence of cutaneous findings. Secondly there are other variations in the clinical picture, albeit, not major ones, as PEARSON (1962) points out. Dermatomyositis tends to have a more acute onset than polymyositis, to run a more progressive course, to occur more commonly in children and to be associated with a malignant tumor in adults. Exceptions to this generalization, however, are by no means uncommon.

The term *neuromyositis* was introduced by SENATOR in 1893 for the combination of nerve and muscle lesions. WALTON and ADAMS and BRUYN and VAN BEUSEKOM find little justification for retaining the term. They regard the rare changes in the peripheral nerves as secondary to the surrounding inflamed muscular and subcutaneous tissues. BARRON and FINE on the other hand, feel neuromyositis is a variant of dermatomyositis. Recent studies by CÖERS and WOOLF and by VANDERMEIREN and COËRS with vital staining of the motor end plate support their view since degeneration characteristically confined to the terminal axons after they have emerged from the muscle bundles have been demonstrated in some cases of dermatomyositis. Some cases, moreover, exhibit clinical evidence of nerve involvement (LAPOVSKY).

b) Nosology

It is difficult to arrive at a satisfactory classification of dermatomyositis because of the vagaries of the clinical picture and the absence of pathognomonic pathologic, biochemical and/or electrodiagnostic features. Classifications taking into account all facets of this complex disorder have been offered by WALTON and ADAMS, GARCIN et al. and by EATON. The classification proposed below is limited to the dermatologic aspect of the disorder and is based on my clinical experience and an analysis of the literature.

DERMATOMYOSITIS

1. Primary (Idiopathic) — acute, subacute, chronic
   Acute
   Chronic
   Subacute > Sclerodermatomyositis, Poikilodermatomyositis
2. Dermatomyositis Combined or Associated with Collagen Disorders: systemic lupus erythematosus (S.L.E.), generalized scleroderma, polyarteritis nodosa or rheumatoid arthritis (viscero-cutaneous collagenoses of PAGEL and TREIP)
3. Dermatomyositis Associated with Malignancy

That a primary or idiopathic form of dermatomyositis more often seen in children occurs without confusing signs and symptoms of collagen disease can hardly be doubted (EVERETT and CURTIS; CHRISTIANSON et al.). Nevertheless some observers insist that dermatomyositis cannot be separated from collagen disorders (KAMPMEIER; DOMZALSKI and MORGAN; VIGLIOGLIA). There is little question, as many authors have emphasized that a close relationship between dermatomyositis and the collagen or connective tissue disorders exists. WALTON and ADAMS maintain the consensus is that many if not most cases of dermatomyositis (or polymyositis) are related to the collagen group. The resemblance to systemic lupus erythematosus, generalized scleroderma and rheumatoid arthritis in particular have been emphasized by LEINWAND et al.; DOWLING and GRIFFITHS; DOWLING; WINKELMANN; MARCUS and WOOLDRIDGE; PEARSON(1959). PAGEL and TREIP suggested the term "viscero-cutaneous collagenoses" for these overlapping syndromes. In such patients, ZIFF maintains the diagnosis of two or more of these diseases can be made simultaneously on the basis of clinical, histologic and serologic evidence. Transitional, intermediate and mixed forms are also possible. ADAMS, DENNY-BROWN and PEARSON on the other hand are inclined to distinguish between polymyositis, dermatomyositis and neuromyositis as a group and so-called interstitial (nodular) polymyositis, which they find in association with rheumatoid arthritis, rheumatic fever, scleroderma and lupus erythematosus disseminatus. According to the latter the histopathologic changes are largely parenchymatous in idiopathic dermatomyositis and principally in the endo-and perimysium i.e. interstitial, when associated with one of the collagen disorders.

A striking difference likewise between dermatomyositis (or polymyositis) per se and collagen diseases with or without dermatomyositis is the appreciable incidence of malignancy in the former and the no more than chance or coincidental association in the latter (HENSON et al.; FIRMAT and LIPSETT; SCHEUERMANN; ARUNDELL et al.; R. C. WILLIAMS). This is the consensus despite the experience of CHRISTIANSON, BRUNSTING and PERRY, namely that the incidence of malignancy was no higher in dermatomyositis than scleroderma. R. C. WILLIAMS and THIES are of the opinion that generally speaking the cutaneous manifestations are more florid when dermatomyositis is associated with malignancy than in the primary form, while the muscle involvement is about the same.

3. Etiology and Pathogenesis

The factors to be considered are somewhat different for the three subgroups of dermatomyositis. There has been considerable speculation as to the cause or causes of the primary (idiopathic) form of dermatomyositis. Many theories have been entertained, among them vitamin E deficiency, infective agents particularly streptococcal, physical agents and hormone imbalance. In a few instances the administration of a drug appeared to be related to the development of symptoms (HYMAN et al.; FALLET and PFENNINGER; BEICKERT and KÜHNE).

A plausible hypothesis proposed by KAMPMEIR to explain the association of dermatomyositis with one of the collagen diseases, is that the basic immunologic process in these conditions is the same but is variously manifested depending on the tissue involved. ZIFF's view is that a common genetic abnormality links the so called connective tissue diseases.

Recent studies in dermatomyositis associated with malignancy suggest a possible autoimmune mechanism. The pathways for the development of this reaction in striated muscles and data in support of this hypothesis are given by GRACE and DAO and by CURTIS, HECKAMAN and WHEELER.

Incidence

α) General. It is difficult to arrive at a reliable appraisal of the true incidence of dermatomyositis. Up to 1959 not more than 600 cases had been gathered by two different reviewers (DOMZALSKI and MORGAN; R. C. WILLIAMS). Since many cases undoubtedly have gone unreported, the condition may not be quite as rare as these papers would indicate. On the other hand the high estimate of BRUYN and VAN BEUSEKOM of "1:6500 in any population" is hard to understand.

Two large clinics in the United States averaged approximately one case a year over a 20 year period (EVERETT and CURTIS; CECIL and LOEB). At the Mayo Clinic (CHRISTIANSON, BRUNSTING and PERRY) however the census was six new cases a year, from 1916 to 1950, 17 new cases a year from 1950 to 1956 and a high of 25 patients in 1953. This impressive number may be explained by the fact that the latter clinic attracts diagnostic and therapeutic problems from all parts of the United States and abroad.

β) Geographic. Cases have been reported in all races around the globe (SUNDE; CABALLERO). Although most papers deal chiefly with white subjects, one can cite three negroes in the Johns Hopkins Hospital series (CECIL and LOEB), two in IRGANG's paper and one or two in many of the larger series. Dermatomyositis in an American Indian was noted in a paper by WHEELER et al.

γ) Age and Sex. The disease may occur at any age. It is most rare, however in infancy judging from the isolated case reports in this age group (DEMEL; CARLISLE and GOOD; WEDGWOOD et al.). The incidence appears to rise abruptly after three years of age reaching a peak from the fifth to the 15th year. There is a second peak from the 30th to the 50th year (BRUYN and VAN BEUSEKOM; PEARSON 1962). Although some observers are under the impression the disease is more prevalent in childhood, BRUYN and VAN BEUSEKOM maintain that not more than 20% of their patients were under the age of 15.

Authorities are rather divided as to whether or not the disease affects females more often than the male. Parity among children (SUNDE, WEDGWOOD et al.) and a 2:1 preponderance of adult females hold true for most recorded series (R. C. WILLIAMS and CHRISTIANSON et al.).

δ) Familial. It is most unusual for more than one member of a family to be affected. In a rare example (CHRISTIANSON et al.), dermatomyositis proved fatal in a 42-year old woman while in her sibling the disease was arrested. WEDGEWOOD and co-authors record an instance in which identical female twins developed the disease one year apart.

ε) Collagen Disease. It is not possible to assess how often dermatomyositis is associated with signs and symptoms of collagen disease. Nor will this statistic be ascertainable until the cause and pathogenesis of both disorders have been clarified. WALTON and ADAMS are of the opinion that many if not most cases are related to the so-called connective tissue diseases.

ζ) Malignancy. No clear example of an associated visceral malignancy has been found in childhood (CHRISTIANSON et al.; ARUNDELL et al.; R. C. WILLIAMS; CURTIS, BLAYLOCK and HARRELL). Perusal of the literature did disclose one case of dermatomyositis in a girl of eleven with a chromophobe adenoma (a benign tumor as a rule) of the hypophysis (SUNDE). Since the dermatosis improved considerably a year *before* the tumor was successfully removed, there probably was no causal relationship.

There are a few reports of an associated malignancy in individuals between 20 and 40 years of age (KANKELEIT; CURTIS, BLAYLOCK and HARRELL; LANE; SCHWARTZ; DUVERNE et PLATHEY; DOSTROVSKY and SAGHER) but the major incidence is in individuals over forty. Statistics vary considerably. ARUNDELL et al. found an incidence of 52.2% (12/23) patients over 40. SHEARD and KNOEPFLER found only one hidden malignant condition among 50 autopsies in patients between 40 and 70 years of age. Between these extremes are the reports by R. C. WILLIAMS who found an incidence of 15.3% based on a review of 590 cases, SCHUERMANN who cited 12.9% in a review of 356 cases and CHRISTIANSON et al. who found 26% (18/66) of cases associated with malignancy. There are also many isolated examples of the combination in the literature and one may assume, some if not many have gone unreported.

Judging from the aforementioned one may conclude there is more than a fortuitous association between malignancy and dermatomyositis. A mean of 14,4% by averaging R. C. WILLIAM's and SCHUERMANN's figures would suggest the correlation is rather high. SCHUERMANN believes malignant tumors occur five times as often in dermatomyositis as in the general population. In view of the outcome of a recent study by DORN and CUTLER of an expected incidence of one case of malignant disease in 100 in the general population over 40, SCHUERMANN's appraisal may prove too conservative.

Most often the tumor is a carcinoma of the stomach, breast, lung or genitourinary tract, although tumors of every organ have been described in association with it. A malignant lymphoma or leukemia was found in 9/92 malignancies in R. C. WILLIAM's series. Coexistance with sarcoma, multiple myeloma, plasmocytoma and other rare tumors e.g. dysgerminoma of the ovary (CORTES et al.) have been reported. Of particular interest to the dermatologist are the reports of dermatomyositis with an epithelioma of the vagina (R. C. WILLIAMS) and with a malignant melanoma (AMORETTI et al.).

4. Symptoms

The symptoms may be most variable and atypical clinical patterns may offer considerable difficulty in diagnosis. In the classical case, the combination of edema, a characteristic dermatitis and symmetrical muscle weakness, particularly of the proximal skeletal groups is diagnostic. All gradations of morbidity are possible from focal or diffuse involvement of a few skeletal groups to a severe generalized disorder including striated muscle of vital organs.

a) Onset and Prodromata

The onset may be acute strikingly suggestive of an infectious disease, or it may be insidious without demonstrable prodromata.

b) General Symptoms

A low grade to moderate intermittent or remittent fever, general fatigue, weakness, loss of weight and anorexia are more likely to be associated with the acute form. Weight loss may be negligible or it may be as much as forty pounds. Whereas EVERETT and CURTIS noted an absence of arthritis and arthralgia in their series, joint involvement of one type or another was mentioned as part of the syndrome by O'LEARY and WAISMAN. Muscle pains, it should be noted, may at times be mistaken for joint pains. PEARSON (1959) found mild arthritic or rheumatic features in 35/116 cases of polymyositis. BRUYN and VAN BEUSEKOM regarded the knee and elbow joints as the sites of predilection for these manifestations.

c) Skin and Appendages

α) Integument

The appearance of skin lesions may precede, coincide, or follow muscle involvement. There may or may not be any correlation between the degree of the muscular destruction and the extent of the eruption. PEARSON (1962) found typical cutaneous features in 40%, atypical features in 24%, and an absence of cutaneous manifestations, exclusive of RAYNAUD's phenomenon, in 26% of cases. Pruritus is inconspicuous unless there is an associated malignancy. Paresthesias including numbness and tingling were among the complaints in 9/40 patients reported by O'LEARY and WAISMAN.

αα) Early Phase. Patients may present a striking lachrymose expression. Edema and a lilac (heliotrope) hue limited to the eyelids and periorbital area are characteristic of dermatomyositis (see Fig. 1).. This violaceous puffiness may be transitory or persistent, may be localized to the lids and periorbital area or may extend to involve the rest of the face, neck, chest, particularly over manubrium, shoulders, back and extremities. At times the eruption is confined to areas exposed to light as demonstrata in Fig. 2. Sparing of the nose and perioral area has been emphasized by DE GRACIANSKY and BOULLE. Puffiness of the hands and feet is not unusual and fleeting erythema of the trunk may be missed unless the skin is inspected frequently. The edema of the trunk and limbs is usually of a brawny type and the areas involved are not necessarily related or limited to the skin over the affected muscles.

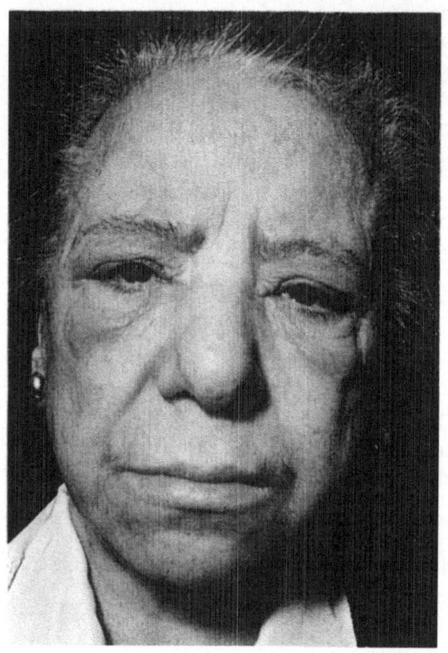

Fig. 1. Classical periorbital edema with a violaceous hue in a 68 year old woman with dermatomyositis secondary to an inoperable carcinoma of the cervix

The presence of ill defined violaceous plaques, particularly over the elbows, knees and small articulations of the hands is also typical. These plaques are generally present over the dorsal aspect rather than along the shaft of the fingers. Edema, purplish erythema, and telangiectasis of the finger-tips and periungual areas are not uncommon. Some of these features together with an erythematous eruption with a butterfly distribution over the face as seen in systemic lupus erythematosus without overt myositis is not unusual.

Within a few weeks or months the skin of the face and the plaques may become shiny, thinned, telangiectatic, irregularly atrophic with areas of hypo-or hyperpigmentation. The Heuck-Gottron phenomenon, namely the presence of small atrophic spots with telangiectases over the distal juxta-articular part of the middle or distal interphalangeal joints of the fingers is considered by BRUYN and VAN BEUSEKOM to be the most specific dermatologic change.

KEIL was of the opinion that although changes in and around the distal phalanges were fairly common in dermatomyositis there was another feature of even greater diagnostic significance. He described hyperkeratosis comprised of yellowish tissue projecting irregularly and unevenly for a short distance over the lunula from the proximal nail fold and occasionally from portions of the lateral nail fold.

A wide variety of non-specific eruptions have also been noted. These include vesicular and bullous lesions, exfoliative dermatitis, psoriatic lesions, macular and papular eruptions, erythema multiforme-like lesions, erythema nodosum, urticaria, ill-defined erythematous areas, purpuric eruptions, follicular keratosis, pityriasis rubra-like eruptions (CHRISTIANSON et al.) and vesicles of the ears and fingers (MINAZZI).

Photosensitivity is not unusual in dermatomyositis. This was a feature in 7/19 (37%) and 5/25 (20%) cases reported by EVERETT and CURTIS and WEDGWOOD et al. respectively, and in 4/20 cases of dermatomyositis with collagen disease (WALTON and ADAMS). As O'LEARY and WAISMAN pointed out, the predilection of the cutaneous lesions for areas exposed to light is highly suggestive of some mechanism involving photosensitivity. Occasionally one reads of a dramatic case in which striking symptoms followed within 24 hours after exposure to sunlight (GRACE and DAO).

Acrocyanosis and RAYNAUD's, a feature in about 20% of the cases will be discussed under cardiovascular manifestations.

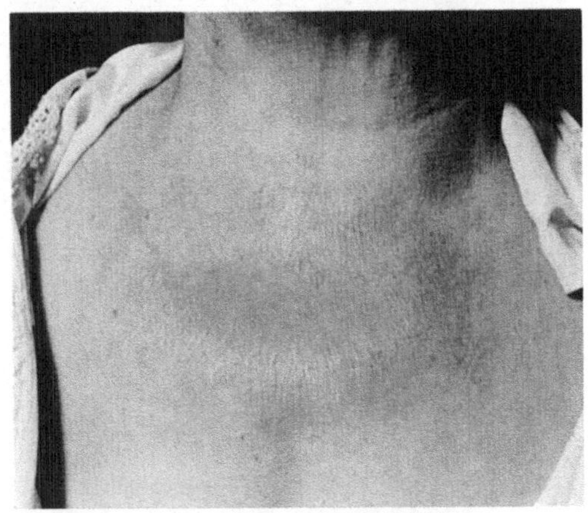

Fig. 2. Circumscribed ill-defined violaceous edema of the anterior chest wall accompanies the periorbital edema seen in Fig. 1. The skin otherwise is not involved

ββ) Late Phase. Although induration and sclerodermatous thickening of the skin, particularly of the face and distal parts of the extremities (sclerodermatomyositis) may be initial features, they are more often preceded by an edematous phase. The overlying skin may be tense, shiny, and either pale or erythematous. In time evidence of atrophy associated with telangiectases and a reticulated type of hyperpigmentation (poikilodermatomyositis) appears (see Figs. 3—6). Ultimately the cutaneous picture may be indistinguishable from poikiloderma atrophicans vasculare secondary to other causes (M. OPPENHEIM). In a group of 19 children EVERETT and CURTIS found induration and/or poikiloderma in 11 or 12, O'LEARY and WAISMAN in a group of 40 adults and children found four patients with increased pigmentation of the face, neck, extremities and portions of the trunk as the sole change, five with sclerodermatous changes as well as hyperpigmentation, seven with induration and thickening without alterations in the degree of pigmentation and poikiloderma atrophicans vasculare in a boy of six.

Deposits of calcium in the subcutaneous tissue, fascial planes, muscles and tendons may take the form of circumscribed pea sized nodules or stony hard plaques. At times these may be sufficiently extensive to be termed calcinosis universalis (CHRISTIANSON et al., MULLER et al., ZELGER). Calcinosis may appear within a few months after the onset or as late as five years (LUGT). According to WHEELER et al. the face and neck are almost always spared and there is a tendency for larger deposits to accumulate over the thighs, arms and trunk. They found also that on the whole there was a greater tendency for widespread large deposits to form rather than small circumscribed lesions as in scleroderma. This was not true of the cases described by O'LEARY and WAISMAN who had four patients with stony nodules on the fingers or in the proximity of the larger joints. There is a tendency moreover for an inflammatory reaction or slowly healing ulcers to set in around these calcareous deposits. Lime salts are sometimes extruded through these ulcerations. Osteoporosis, a consistent finding in advanced cases of dermatomyositis, may be particularly marked in patients with calcinosis.

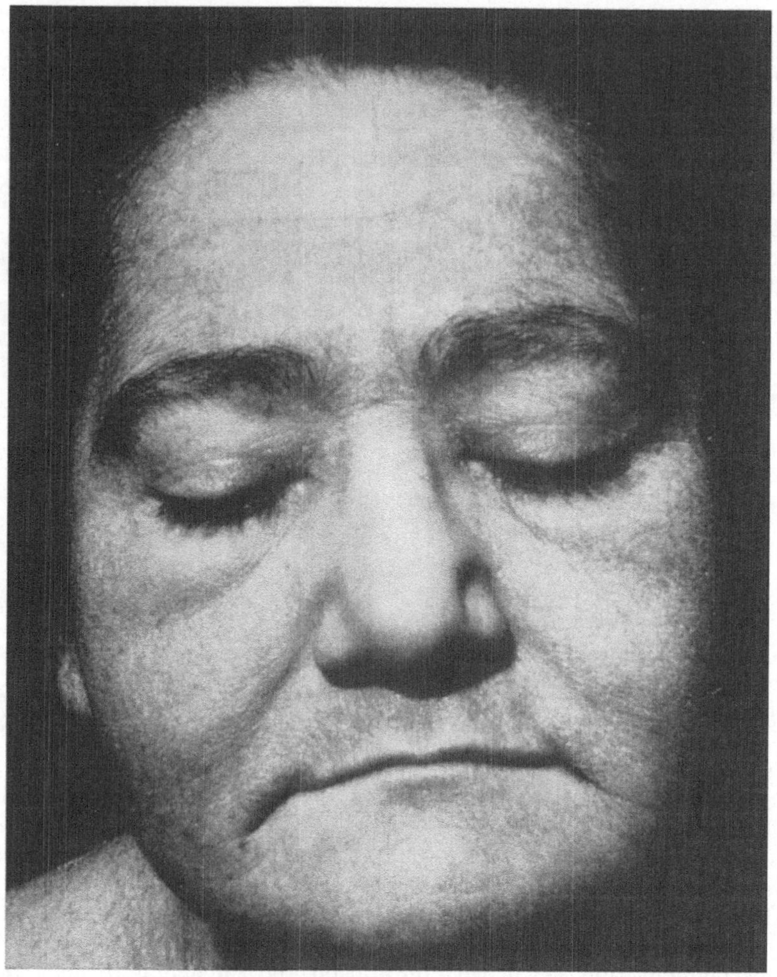

Fig. 3. Diffuse edema of the face and eyelids accompanied by redness and mottled hyperpigmentation in a 44 year old woman with dermatomyositis of one year's duration. The chest and extremities are also involved. See Fig. 4—6. (Courtesy Dr. MAX JESSNER)

β) Cutaneous Appendages

Alopecia of varying degrees has been noted in 3/19 children (EVERETT and CURTIS) and in 7/40 adults (O'LEARY and WAISMAN). Hyperidrosis mentioned in one paper was dismissed as inconsequential in another. An instance of pitted nails has also been described.

d) Mucous Membranes

Involvement of the mucous membranes was sufficiently striking in OPPENHEIM's cases for him to suggest the term dermatomucomyositis. One may find various combinations of redness, edema, dryness, atrophy and crusted erosions of the tongue, gums, and the buccal, pharyngeal and laryngeal mucosa. KEIL felt that the finding of small white or slightly yellow flat leukoplakia-like areas over the cheeks, tongue and palate was of diagnostic significance. WALTON and

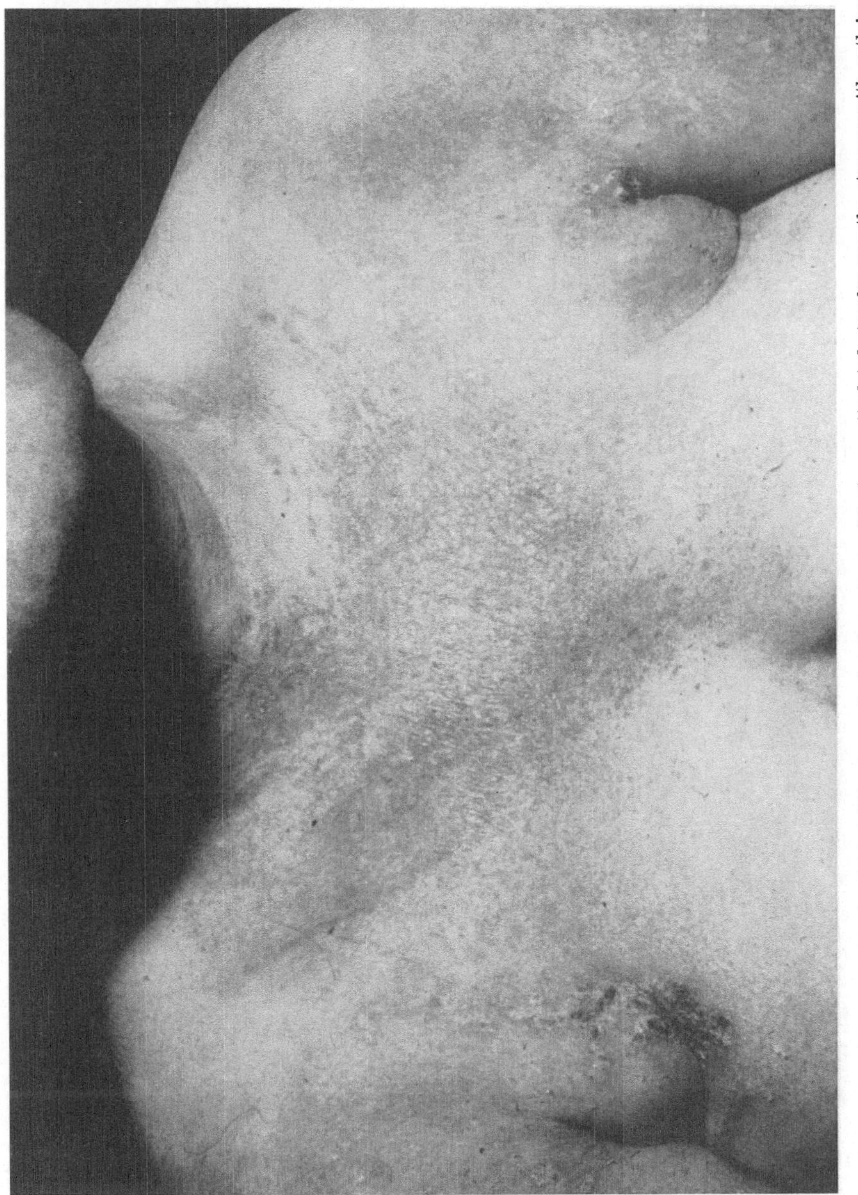

Fig. 4. The skin of the anterior chest wall in a case of sclerodermatomyositis shows reticulated atrophy over the sternum with outlying hyperpigmentation, erythema and scaling (Courtesy Dr. MAX JESSNER)

ADAMS likewise describe leukoplakia-like changes. Stomatitis was present in 9/40 of O'LEARY and WAISMAN's patients, 2/26 in series WEDGWOOD et al.

e) Musculature

Weakness and pain are the outstanding symptoms. Weakness due to symmetrical involvement of proximal skeletal muscle groups, e.g. shoulder and pelvic

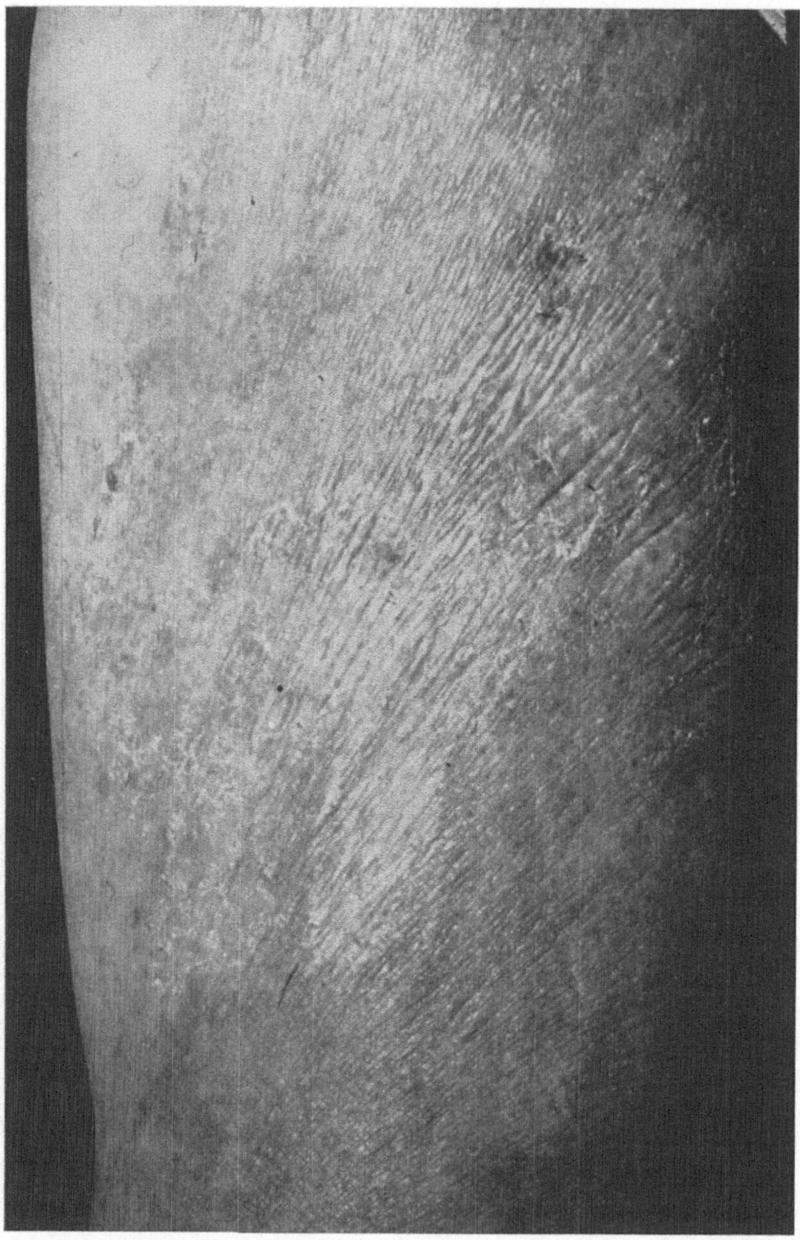

Fig. 5. The lateral aspect of the arm shows an ill-defined area of cutaneous atrophy surrounded by diffuse erythema, scaling, hyper- and depigmentation. These changes are symmetrically distributed over the thighs as well as the arms. Sclerodermatous changes characterized by brawny induration are also present, particularly over the distal portions of the extremities (Courtesy Dr. Max Jessner)

girdle, thighs and arms, in association with dysphonia and dysphagia is characteristic of dermatomyositis. The disorder is by no means limited to these groups and may involve any group of striated muscle. Pearson (1962) found the incidence to be as follows: proximal muscles of the lower extremities-97%, proximal muscles of the upper extremities-80%, flexors of the neck-63%, muscles of deglutition-60%, distal muscles of the extremities-42%, facial muscles-12%. The affection may also extend to cardiac muscle, muscles of respiration, diaphragmatic as well as intercostal, laryngeal, extraocular, and sphincter muscles. Weakness may develop slowly and insidiously over a period of months or it may be incapacitating within a matter of weeks.

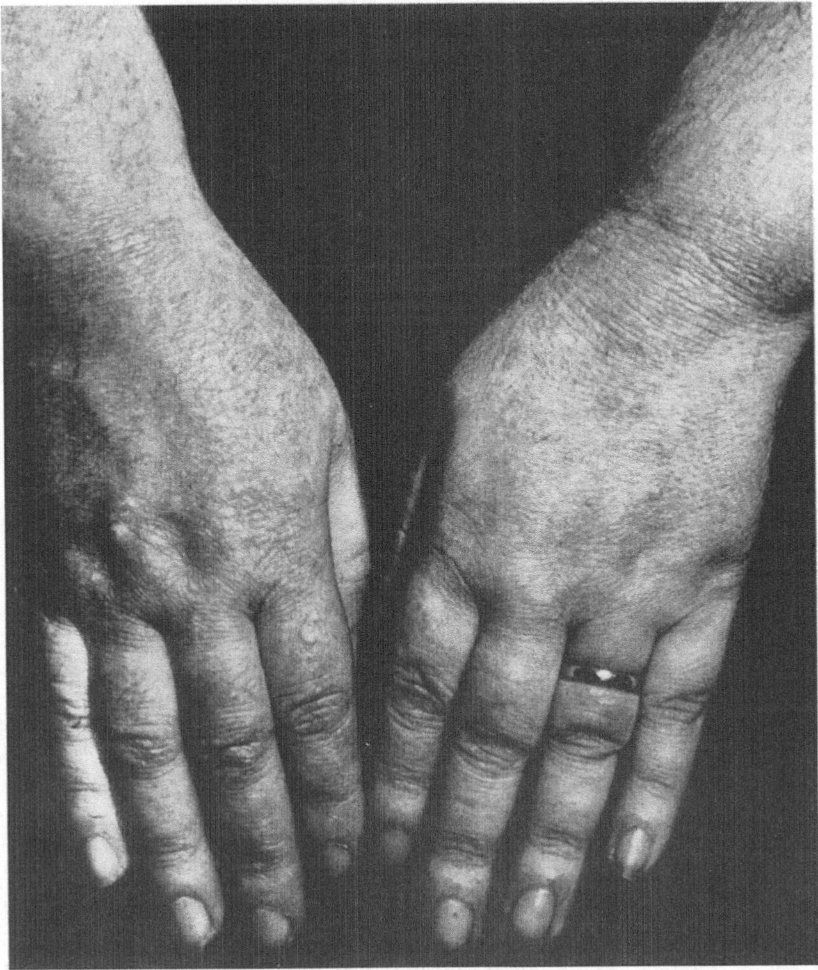

Fig. 6. The hands are edematous and the skin is somewhat erythematous and indurated in sclerodermatomyositis (Courtesy Dr. MAX JESSNER)

α) Early Phase. Pain or tenderness accompany the early phase, particularly in the acute forms of the disease. The intensity of these symptoms varies considerably and is related partially at least to the degree of edema. Patients have been known to cry out with pain and the author can recall one case of morphine addiction in a young woman who died of the disease within two years after the onset. If tenderness is not too exquisite one can palpate ill-defined swollen doughy areas within the muscles. Diffuse swelling with complete loss of muscle definition may ensue.

Weakness of the involved muscles may be overt or it may not be evident until the patient is asked to perform certain actions, e.g. to rise from a chair or to change from the supine to the sitting position, or to reach for an object. A good deal can be ascertained from the individual's gait which may be awkward, shuffling or unsteady. Running without tripping or falling may become impossible. Depending on the muscles involved there may also be head drop, difficulty in swallowing or breathing, hoarseness, diplopia and/or impaired sphincter control. Pearson has directed attention to the disparity between the early marked weakness and the minimal degree of muscle atrophy.

β) Late Phase. Wasting and/or fibrotic changes may be the end stage in chronic cases. The result may be partial or total invalidism, loss of tendon reflexes, paralyses, joint fixation, contractures and calcium deposits in the muscles.

f) Viscera and Special Organs

Visceral manifestations on the whole are uncommon in the primary (idiopathic) form of dermatomyositis. In the presence of collagen disease, depending on the degree and nature of the overlapping, there may be mixed or confusing clinical pictures. Sparing of the kidneys in the primary form is in sharp contrast to the high incidence of renal involvement in systemic lupus erythematosus and malignant scleroderma. It is most unusual to find casts or albumin in the urine. When associated with malignancy, the location and nature of the tumor may influence the symptomatology.

α) Cardiovascular System

A rapid pulse, disproportionately high for the degree of fever should arouse suspicion of cardiac involvement. Some objective evidence of cardiac participation was found in 9/40 in one series (O'LEARY and WAISMAN) and in 8/19 in another (EVERETT and CURTIS). Examination may disclose cardiac enlargement (O'LEARY and WAISMAN) but insufficiency (DOMZALSKI and MORGAN), pericarditis (EVERETT and CURTIS) and/or hypertension (BOYLAN and SOKOLOFF), appear to be most unusual.

αα) Electrocardiographic changes of a non-specificnature have been noted by a number of observers (O'LEARY and WAISMAN). TALBOTT and FERRANDIS found prolongation of the P-R, QRS, and Q-T intervals, minimal variations in the appearance of RS-T segments and T waves as well as slurring and notching of QRS deflections in multiple leads.

ββ) Raynaud's phenomenon may be a concomitant symptom (O'LEARY and WAISMAN) or it may precede the rest of the clinical picture by as long as four years (GARZON et al.). PEARSON (1962) found an incidence of 22 in 116 cases of polymyositis. On the whole, it is more likely to accompany sclerodermatous changes (WALTON and ADAMS). Conversely it may be instructive to point out that in a group of 45 cases of RAYNAUD's phenomenon, 32 were associated with scleroderma, two with systemic lupus erythematosus, one with dermatomyositis and the balance with other disorders (DE TAKATS and FOWLER).

γγ) Teleangiectasis of the nail beds, fingertips and periungual areas is not an uncommon finding. Capillary microscopy of the nail fold disclosed striking changes in one of SUNDE's cases but not in the other. He found the number of capillaries markedly reduced, markedly tortuous, with thin afferent and dilated efferent portions.

δδ) An example of **peripheral vascular disease** simulating thromboangitis obliterans has also been recorded by SILVERMAN and POWELL.

β) Gastrointestinal Tract

αα) Dysphagia is attributed largely by most observers to weakness of the hypopharyngeal muscles (DONOGHUE et al.; T. T. BUNIM). Diffuse oesophageal involvement may also be present. According to DONOGHUE et al. the pattern of esophageal mobility on roentgenographic examination in dermatomyositis may be indistinguishable from scleroderma.

ββ) Multiple ulcerations of the gastro-intestinal tract as well as ulcers of the duodenum and oesophagus were recognized as part of the intrinsic pathology of the disease prior to the advent of adrenocorticotrophin and corticosteroids (BOYLAN and SOKOLOFF). It is speculative at this time as to whether or not the incidence of ulceration is indeed greater since steroids have been used in the management of dermatomyositis. MALKINSON and ROTHMAN made an exhaustive study including detailed histologic examination of two cases in which the gastrointestinal tract was involved. BOYLAN and SOKOLOFF were of the opinion that the sclerotic changes in the small arteries and arterioles in their cases were important factors in the gastro-intestinal involvement. Ulceration may be accompanied by microscopic or gross hemorrhage, abdominal pain and occasionally by perforation with symptoms of an acute abdomen.

γ) Spleen, Liver and Lymph Nodes

In no instance has the enlargement of these organs been impressive. Slight or mild hepatomegaly was noted in some of the larger series in 4/19 (EVERETT and CURTIS), 5/40 (O'LEARY and WAISMAN) and 3/26 (WEDGWOOD et al.) cases respectively; slight splenomegaly in 8/40 (O'LEARY and WAISMAN) and 2/26 cases (WEDGWOOD et al.). Mild lymphadenopathy was mentioned in one paper in 3/40 patients (O'LEARY and WAISMAN).

δ) Eyes

In addition to listing conjunctivitis, iritis, ptosis, exophthalmos and paralysis of the extraocular muscles, BRUCE described three examples of what he considered to be an unusual form of retinitis associated with dermatomyositis. This was manifested by distension of the retinal veins, hemorrhage and ill-defined areas of grayish-yellow exudate of varying size, now known as "cotton-wool exudates", [cytoid bodies or "nodule dysorique" (LISMAN; THOMAS et al.)]. These findings have been confirmed by a number of authors. Some think these exudates are inflammatory, others see them as islands of degeneration secondary to inflammation. Time and study have shown moreover that these so-called cytoid bodies are not specific for they have been found in other collagen diseases and in a wide variety of unrelated conditions (WALSH).

ε) Miscellaneous Symptoms

Reports are extant on the association of dermatomyositis with pulmonary lesions (GOLDFISCHER and RUBIN; MILLS and MATTHEWS), orchitis (GARZÓN et al.), aplastic anemia (DUNCAN et al.), non-iatrogenic CUSHING's syndrome and SJOGREN's syndrome (BUNIM).

5. Special Features

a) Dermatomyositis in Childhood

On the whole the clinical picture and laboratory findings in children are the same as in adults. Abdominal pain, nausea, alternating episodes of constipation and diarrhea have been mentioned more often among the early symptoms. Two analyses direct attention to the earlier onset, higher incidence and greater degree of calcinosis in children (Christianson et al.; Muller et al.). Sclerodermatous changes, poikiloderma and osteoporosis likewise appear to be more prevalent (Everett and Curtis; O'Leary and Waisman).

b) Manifestation of Malignancy

Symptoms and signs of dermatomyositis may antedate or coincide with those of the tumor, or may not appear until several weeks or several years later (R. C. Williams; Dostrovsky and Sagher; Cortes et al.). R. C. Williams is of the opinion that generally speaking the cutaneous manifestations are more florid and better defined when associated with malignancy while the muscle involvement is about the same. He maintains moreover that intense pruritus, a feature of the combination is conspicuously absent in dermatomyositis without malignancy. In the experience of Arundell et al. distinct improvement in the dermatomyositis followed treatment of the cancer in 6/9 patients, and in three of these patients a subsequent exacerbation coincided with further progression of the neoplasia. Miehlke and Hollander on the other hand found no correlation with treatment of the neoplastic condition.

6. Diagnostic Procedures: Findings and Interpretation

a) Biopsy of Skin, Subcutaneous Tissue and Muscle

α) Skin and subcutaneous Tissue

The findings are non-specific and in most instances are those of a chronic dermatitis (Allen). Sclerodermatous lesions may show thickening of the collagen bundles, along with homogenization and sclerosis as in scleroderma. These changes are seen in Fig. 7. Lever is of the opinion that subacute lupus erythematosus may be simulated and that in poikilodermatomyositis the histologic changes in the skin are the same as in poikiloderma atrophicans vasculare secondary to other conditions. Dowling and Freudenthal maintain there are distinguishing features. A moderate to marked non-specific panniculitis according to Allen is fairly common and calcification in the areas of panniculitis is not unusual.

β) Muscle Biopsy

αα) Selection of the site for excision should be made with considerable care and an adequate specimen should be taken for study. Pearson (1962) recommends using an accessible muscle which is neither clinically strong nor very weak. Preliminary electromyographic study may be quite helpful in locating maximum pathology (O'Leary, Lambert and Sayre). Despite these precautions specimens may prove negative because of the focal nature of the degenerative and inflammatory changes.

ββ) The microscopic findings depend largely on the stage of the disease during which the sampling is made and the severity of the process. According to some observers (Adams, Denny-Brown and Pearson) the type of dermatomyositis (see classification), particularly whether or not there is an associated collagen disorder, may likewise influence the histologic picture.

The basic changes with many variations in degree and extent may be described under the headings: (A) an inflammatory reaction primarily involving the *interstitial tissue* and (B) degeneration and necrotization accompanied by inflammation and regeneration of the *muscle fibers*. Either (A) or (B) may dominate the histologic scene; more often they are admixed in varying proportions. In Figs. 8—10 the finding are essentially parenchymatous. Degeneration and atrophy are striking in the case of sclerodermatomyositis; inflammation and degeneration are conspicuous in the case of dermatomyositis.

According to ADAMS, DENNY-BROWN and PEARSON (1962), (A) is striking in cases associated with rheumatoid arthritis, rheumatic fever, scleroderma and systemic lupus erythematosus, and they refer to these changes as interstitial (nodular) polymyositis. WALTON and ADAMS, however, and it will be noted

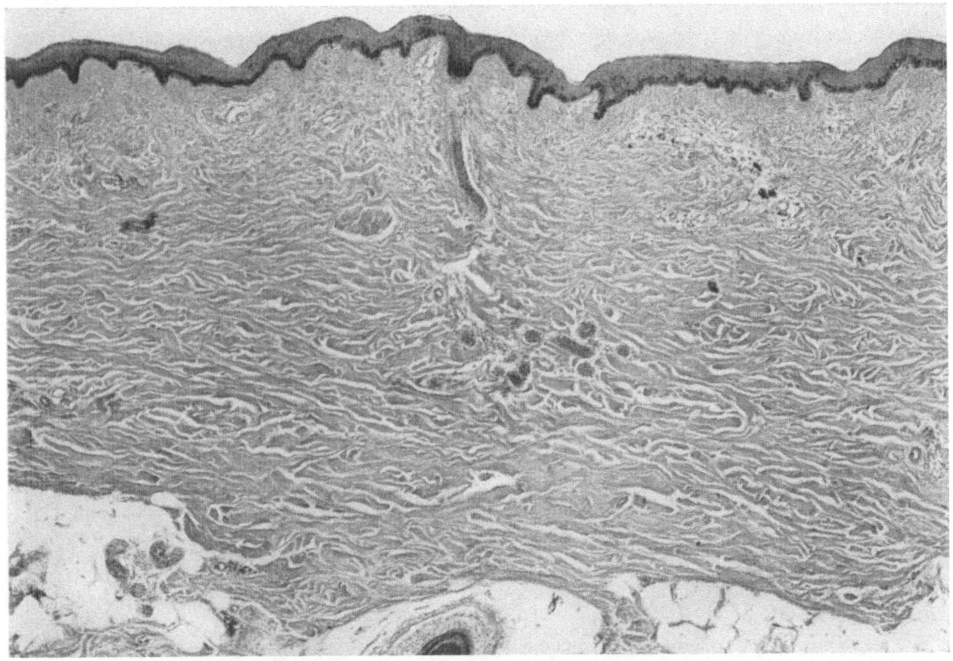

Fig. 7[1]. Section of skin in a case of sclerodermatomyositis: The epidermis is mildly irregular with short rete ridges and correspondingly short papillary bodies. The corium reveals sclerosis of the collagen bundles with few, if any, adnexae. The mid-corium presents a single cluster of sweat glands and part of a sweat duct may be seen to transverse the upper corium. A few scattered dilated vessels and a sparse cellular infiltration composed for the most part of lymphocytes and some histiocyles are noted in some areas (72.8×)

ADAMS is a co-author of both texts, do not draw a distinction between interstitial (nodular) polymositis and primary polymyositis or dermatomyositis. The principal features of (A) are collections of lymphocytes, plasma cells and histiocytes about the small vessels of the perimysium and endomysium, generally in the immediate vicinity of an area of degeneration of a muscle fiber. Diffuse or massive infiltration throughout the interstitial tissue, however, is not unusual. In chronic cases fibrosis replaces the infiltrative phase.

The principal features of (B) are: focal, granular and hyalin degeneration and necrosis of muscle fibers, cellular infiltration with histiocytes, plasma cells and lymphocytes about these areas of degeneration and necrosis, phagocytosis of muscle fibers, regeneration of muscle cells, extreme variation in the diameter of the muscle fibers, atrophy, replacement fibrosis or sclerosis in long-standing cases.

---

[1] To Figures 1—10: The author is indebted to Dr. IRVING SEIDMAN, Dep't of Pathology, University Hospital for the histologic Sections, to Dr. CHARLES F. SIMS ans Mrs. ELEANOR MORELAND of the New York Skin and Cancer Unit, New York University Medical School for the interpretation of the slides and the preparation of the photomicrographs in Figs. 7—10.

Madden noted varying degrees of nodular myositis with degenerative changes in dermatomyositis (12 biopsies in eight cases) as well as in lupus erythematosus (6/21 specimens in 19 cases). O'Leary et al. grouped their findings in dermatomyositis under five categories: 1. degenerative and regenerative changes limited to the parenchyma, 2. interstitial plus parenchymatous changes, 3. interstitial changes with insignificant findings in the muscle, 4. atrophy of the muscle with diffuse interstitial fibrosis and 5. granular degeneration of muscle fibers at the border of the fascicle or muscle tendon junction with minimal intrafascicular involvement.

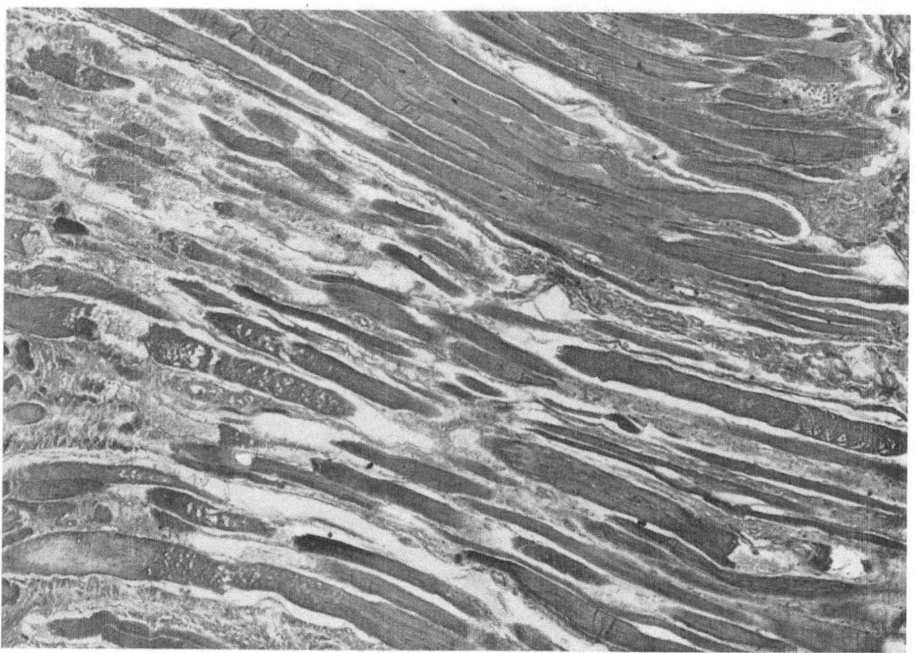

Fig. 8. Section of muscle underlying skin in Fig. 7: Some of the muscle fibers are relatively normal retaining visible striations. Others show edema, loss of continuity, cellular infiltration composed of lymphocytes, and granular degeneration. Total degeneration is also seen in some areas. Edema of the interstitial spaces is also present (72.8 ×)

Boylan and Sokoloff found the sclerotic changes in the small arteries and arterioles in their cases. They felt they could distinguish between these vascular changes and those accompanying polyarteritis nodosa.

γγ) Observers differ as to the **diagnostic value** of a muscle biopsy in dermatomyositis and pathologists do not always agree on the interpretation of the findings (Wallace et al., Greenfield et al.). Although one cannot point to pathognomonic features, when demonstrable the combination of inflammatory, degenerative and regenerative changes in the parenchyma in the same section is fairly characteristic.

δδ) Histochemical studies have been attempted. Utilizing the Hotchkiss-McManus method (periodic acid Schiff [PAS] stain) Stoughten and Wells were able to demonstrate remarkable alteration in the appearance of the polysaccharide material in dermatomyositis. Johnson on the other hand found an increased rather than an altered ground substance. The quantitative change was seen principally in muscle, between and replacing muscle fibers in involved areas. The discrepancy in the findings can be explained by the difference in stains employed.

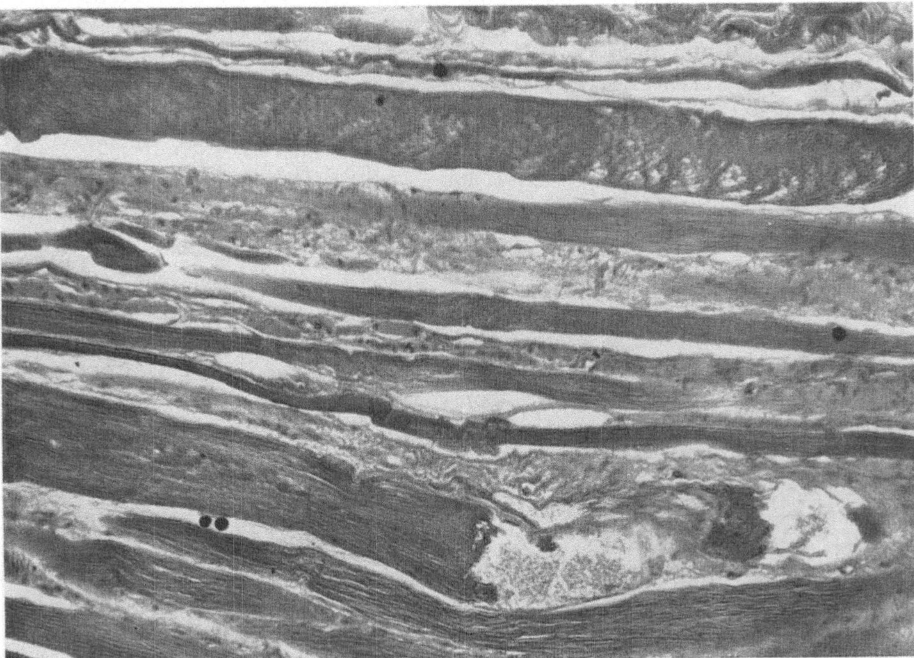

Fig. 9. Section of muscle underlying skin in Fig. 7: Atrophy and degeneration of the muscle fibers with small accumulations of sarcolemma nuclei are present. Some of the fibers are replaced by cellular infiltration, edema and fibrin strands (206 ×)

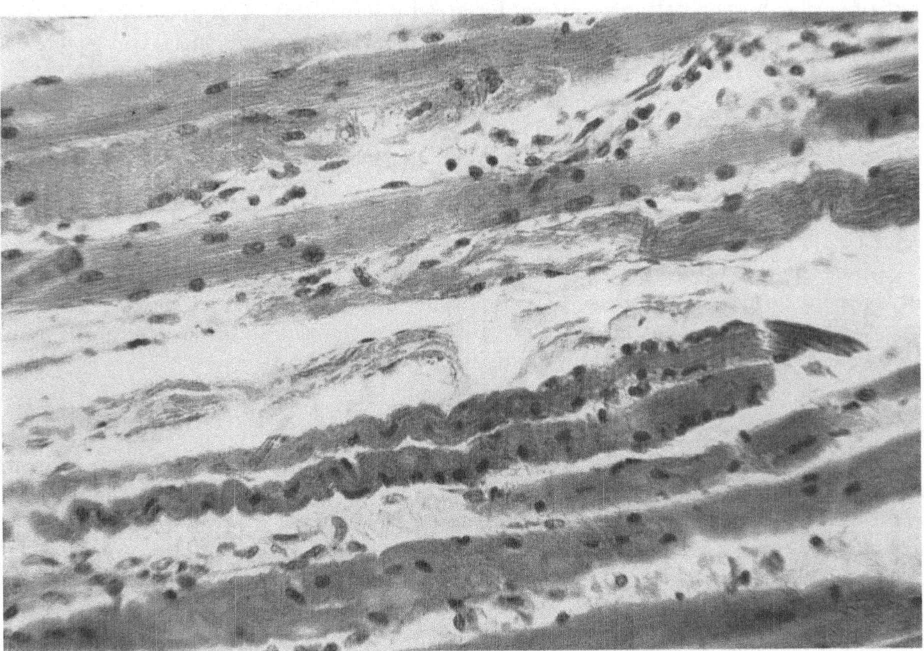

Fig. 10. Section of deltoid muscle in a case of dermatomyositis: Muscle fibers in varying stages of degeneration are seen. Undulation, fragmentation and areas of granular degeneration are present. Edema and focal infiltration made up of lymphocytes, macrophages and few neutrophiles are seen in the interstial spaces. Some relatively normal muscle fibers with visible striations are also present (415 ×)

JOHNSON used colloidal iron, alcian blue with a p_H of 2.7—3 and toluidine blue with a p_H of 3. In his opinion these agents are reliable indicators of hyaluronic acid, the major component of ground substance whereas PAS reacts the with neutral mucopolysaccharides, a minor component.

εε) Motor Point Biopsy may yield additional information. By this method it is possible to study the terminal intramuscular motor innervation [motor end plate (COËRS and WOOLF; VAN DER MEIREN and CÖERS)]. This technic which is still in the investigative phase must be practiced longer before conclusions can be drawn.

b) Electromyography

It is beyond the scope of this chapter to go into a detailed discussion of the applications and limitations of this procedure (O'LEARY et al.; LICHT; HEATHFIELD and WILLIAMS; D. WILLIAMS; Mayo Clinic Foundation, OESTER et al.; ROGOFF). The consensus is that electromyography is quite helpful in distinguishing between the primary myopathies, to which group polymyositis and dermatomyositis belong and diseases of the lower motor neuron. It is also considered to be of value in separating the myotonias from the other primary myopathies since the former have characteristic electrical features. Electromyographers are divided, however, as to whether or not it is possible to distinguish between polymyositis and dystrophic conditions. In polymyositis generally there is a greater tendency to fibrillation potentials.

The characteristic albeit non-specific features of the electromyogram in poly- and dermatomyositis are as follows: 1. extreme irritability on needle insertion, with trains of fine potentials persisting for longer periods than in other conditions. 2. the presence of fibrillation potentials at rest; 3. the presence of extremely narrow potentials, usually with a duration of no more than that of a fibrillation but of rather higher voltage (several hundred microvolts). 4. reduced interference pattern on moderate voluntary contractions. In neuromyositis the electrical pattern is frequently of a neuritic type (LAPOVSKY).

Electromyography appears to be of little help in differentiating between dermatomyositis and certain members of the collagen family. O'LEARY et al. found abnormal electrical activity similar to that in dermatomyositis in a few cases of systemic lupus erythematosus and scleroderma. In polyarteritis nodosa, on the other hand, the electromyogram in some cases, is the same as in polyneuritis.

Since degeneration may be only focal or spotty in dermatomyositis, electromyography is particularly useful in scanning the musculature to locate areas of maximum activity. Biopsies of such sites rather than at random are more likely to disclose significant histologic changes.

c) Enzyme Determinations

Elevated serum enzyme activity is attributed to the release of enzymes from damaged myofibrils and increased permeability of damaged muscle membrane. White found that patients with dermatomyositis showed a pronounced variation in serum enzyme activity, parallel to the severity and extent of the disease. The rise in serum aldolase (normal < 9.5 units/ml.) and lactic dehydrogenase (LDH) (normal 212—424 units/ml.) levels was more striking than glutamic-oxalacetic transaminase (SGOT) (normal < 32 units/ml.) and phosphohexose isomerase (PHI) (normal 40 units/ml.). VICKERS found a consistent elevation of SGOT and a correlation between the degree of activity of the myositis and the rise of SGOT titre.

It should be pointed out, however, that an elevation in the serum activity of these enzymes may be found as well in association with a number of unrelated conditions, e.g. muscular dystrophy, myocardial infarction, carcinomatosis and body injury (White; Aronson). The consensus nevertheless is that serum enzyme activity levels are more reliable measures of muscle damage than creatinuria.

d) Urinary Creatine and Creatinine Determination

According to many authorities the determination of creatine in the urine is the most practical method of demonstrating muscle deterioration. Under normal conditions no more than 200 mg./24 hrs. of creatine appears in the urine of men and 400 mg./24 hrs. or less in the urine of women, children or castrates (Domzalski and Morgan). Striking elevations as high as 3,220 mg./24 hrs. have been reported in dermatomyositis (Domzalski and Morgan). Creatinuria, however, may be found in a wide variety of conditions as in other myopathies, endocrinopathies, poliomyelitis and starvation.

α) Ratio of creatinine to creatine. The conversion of creatine to creatinine depends on the presence of physiologically active muscle and in a normal individual the ratio of creatinine to creatine in the urine is 5—10:1. In dermatomyositis and in the other conditions noted before, the creatinine/creatine ratio is reversed 1:5—10. By the same token the creatinine coefficient is also reduced for it measures the amount of creatinine excreted in terms of body weight in 24 hours (normal approximately 13 mg./kg. for newborns up to 18—32 mg./kg. for adults).

β) The creatine tolerance test which is considered by some to be more helpful, may be beyond the reach of the average clinical laboratory (Domzalski and Morgan). A normal patient will retain 70—80% of an oral test dose of 1.32 mg. of creatine hydrate. It is then excreted slowly into the urine as creatinine. If there is insufficient muscle, however, creatine cannot be stored, and it will spill over into the urine as such.

e) Miscellaneous Laboratory Findings

α) Blood Count. A polymorphonuclear leukocytosis with a relative lymphopenia has been noted in acute cases more frequently than other changes (Bruyn and van Beusekom). Whereas O'Leary and Waisman found a moderate eosinophilia in 11/40 patients, Noser recorded a monocytosis of 8% to 17%. A tendency to anemia has been observed in chronic cases (Bruyn and van Beusekom; O'Leary and Waisman).

β) Erythrocyte Sedimentation Rate. The erythrocyte sedimentation rate is elevated in acute cases.

γ) Serum-pyruvic acid. According to Bruyn and van Beusekom the concentration of this substance is normal in dermatomyositis. Minazzi who gives the normal value as 0.6—0.9 mg/100 ml. found a consistent increase.

δ) Electrophoresis. Bergouignan et al. considered dysprotinemia to be rare. A decrease in the serum albumin and an increase of the alpha 2- and gamma globulin fractions have been recorded in two studies (Bruyn and van Beusekom; Herrmann and Schulz). Garcin et al. found a reversal in the albumin/globulin ratio. Walker and Benditt on the other hand found no significant increase in the gamma globulin fraction, only a decrease in albumin and total protein levels. Interestingly enough Janeway et al., reported a case of dermatomyositis associated with agamma-globulinemia.

ε) Immunologic Procedures. A positive lupus erythematodes phenomenon was demonstrated in approximately 5% of cases by MIESCHER. Consistently negative lupus erythematodes tests on the other hand were reported by SCOTT and REES. These results are not necessarily contradictory. Differences in the nature of the dermatomyositis might account for the disparity (see classification). Serum complement levels were found to be reduced in active dermatomyositis but the significance of this finding could not be explained by WILLIAMS and LAW. Rheumatoid factor, nuclear fluorescence, antinuclear, anti DNA reacting gamma globulin have been demonstrated in some cases (BARDAWIL et al.). Curiously no exmples of chronic biologic false positive Wassermann reactions have been recorded.

ζ) Urinalysis. Albumin and casts have been found only on rare occasions.

7. Course and Prognosis

The disease may run an acute, subacute or chronic course in accordance with STEINER's definition. BRUYN and VAN BEUSEKOM also speak of cases with a slowly progressive or cyclic course with spontaneous exacerbations and remissions.

α) In the **acute form,** the progression of muscular weakness is rapid, reaching a peak in a matter of a few months or a year. Death may ensue within a few weeks or few months. Despite rapid progression, the disease is not always fatal, total recovery is at times possible in such instances. Most of the survivors of the acute phase however develop varying degrees of disability.

β) In the **subacute form** exacerbations and remissions are possible over a period of two or three years. The threat to life continues during this period because of involvement of vital musculature or intercurrent infection. Arrest of the active phase usually takes place within three years or may extend for a period of four or five years.

γ) Chronic form. Approximately $^1/_3$ of the cases follow a slowly progressive and insidious course. This is more apt to be true of older patients with polymyositis without skin or connective tissue (collagen disease) involvement. Varying degrees of morbidity and disability are found depending on the degree and extent of atrophy, contractures, calcinosis and osteoporosis.

δ) Mortality rate. Because of the paucity of statistics it is difficult to arrive at a mortality rate. The consensus is that prior to the advent of steroids approximately 60% of patients died of cardiorespiratory failure, inanition or intercurrent infection within the first two or three years. On the whole, the prognosis appears to be worse in the presence of florid skin changes and/or manifestations of collagen disease. Children and young adults with commensurate manifestations seem to fare somewhat better however than older individuals (WALTON and ADAMS). Generally speaking an acute onset is more likely to be followed by rapid progression and a serious outcome.

ε) Influence of corticosteroid therapy. Although a final evaluation of corticotrophin (ACTH) and corticosteroid therapy is not possible at this time, most observers are of the opinion that prognosis is ever so much better because of their availability. Dramatic arrest has been reported in acute cases and striking improvement in subacute cases.

ζ) Serum enzyme activity as an indicator. Evaluation of serum enzyme activity may serve as a useful objective indicator of the extent and activity of the disease (WHITE). An initial rise in the enzyme levels followed by a spontaneous decline in or a drop in response to corticosteroid therapy may be interpreted as favorable prognostic signs (PEARSON 1962, WHITE).

η) Influence of malignancy. The prognosis in cases associated with malignant disease is determined largely by the amenability of the tumor to treatment or extirpation. Curiously enough spontaneous improvement in the dermatomyositis or a remission induced by steroids has been noted occasionally even in the presence of a disseminating neoplasm.

8. Diagnosis

The diagnosis is not difficult in the classical case. It is based on the coexistence of typical cutaneous manifestation, symmetrical weakness of the proximal muscle groups with pain and tenderness along with the notable absence of important visceral changes. When the skin is not involved or the findings in this organ are minimal or equivocal, differentiation of polymyositis from other myopathies and neuropathies may not be simple.

In some cases, the extent and degree of connective tissue participation may be such as to make separation from some of the collagen disorders difficult. As the section on classification indicates dermatomyositis may be associated with one or another of the collagen disease (viscerocutaneous collagenoses of PAGEL and TRIEP). In adults, particularly in individuals over forty, the possibility of an associated malignancy must always be borne in mind and excluded by appropriate investigation.

Conclusive results are not to be expected from any single diagnostic procedure. Data gathered from histologic examination of muscle, electromyography, electrical conduction time, enzyme studies and creatine and creatinine determinations are often helpful.

9. Differential Diagnosis

The conditions that have to be considered in the differential diagnoses are almost unlimited depending largely on the presence or absence of cutaneous manifestations and on the distribution of muscular involvement. Some cases of dermatomyositis cannot be distinguished from systemic lupus erythematosus, generalized scleroderma and rheumatoid arthritis because of the overlap of clinical and histologic findings. As has been pointed out it may be correct to regard dermatomyositis associated with collagen disease as one form of the disorder (see classification).

a) Systemic Lupus erythematosus

Signs of visceral involvement, particularly renal and cardiac, would favor systemic lupus erythematosus. On the other hand, pain, tenderness and progressive symmetrical weakness of proximal muscle groups, periorbital or diffuse violaceous edema of the face, repeatedly negative lupus erythematodes tests would favor the diagnosis of dermatomyositis.

b) Generalized Scleroderma

While sclerosis, RAYNAUD's phenomenon, calcinosis and/or disturbances in pigmentation may be common to generalized scleroderma and dermatomyositis in the chronic phase of these disorders, the early cutaneous manifestations of dermatomyositis are not seen in scleroderma. Photosensitivity, a feature of some cases of dermatomyositis is not evident in scleroderma. While muscular weakness associated with severe pain and tenderness of proximal muscle groups is characteristic of the acute phase of dermatomyositis, stiffness with limitation of motion of the distal parts of the extremities predominate in scleroderma.

c) Polyarteritis nodosa

May resemble dermatomyositis because of muscle weakness due to polyneuritis in the former. Nephritis, hypertension, signs and symptoms, peripheral nerve of involvement commonly seen in polyarteritis nodosa are not features of dermatomyositis. Subcutaneous nodules along the vessels, ulcerations and purpura are the principal cutaneous manifestations of polyarteritis. In dermatomyositis one finds typical periorbital edema or a lachrymose facies. Considerable difficulty may be encountered in distinguishing between the polymyositic form of polyarteritis nodosa and polymyositis without cutaneous manifestations. The dissimilar electromyographic and histologic findings are useful in arriving at the correct diagnosis.

d) Trichinosis

The history of pork ingestion, chemosis as well as edema of the eyelids, conjunctival and subungual hemorrhages, photophobia, and a positive trichinella skin test (Bachman test) serve to distinguish the two diseases. According to WALLACE it is possible to demonstrate the larvae in muscle biopsies in about 1/5 cases of trichinosis.

e) Contact Dermatitis

Early cases of dermatomyositis may be mistaken for contact dermatitis, since the inflammatory reaction in the skin and the areas of predilection may be the same. Awareness of this pitfall and examination for the presence or absence of muscle involvement should suffice to clarify the situation.

f) Photodermatitis

Polymorphus light eruptions may mimic the cutaneous manifestations of dermatomyositis, particularly when the latter is associated with photosensitivity. The seasonal character of polymorphous light eruptions, the absence of morbidity other than the cutaneous manifestations and responsiveness to antimalarials should make the diagnosis clear.

g) Other Primary Myopathies

α) Progressive muscular dystrophy may mimic the chronic form of polymyositis because progressive weakness and wasting of the proximal muscles may occur in both diseases. A history or the presence of skin changes, RAYNAUD's phenomenon, dysphagia, muscle pain and tenderness, severe weakness of the neck muscles together with uneven progression of muscle symptoms would exclude muscular dystrophy. Some electromyographers claim they can distinguish between dystrophic and polymyositic patterns.

β) Myasthenia Gravis. Ptosis, diplopia and rapid fatigability upon sustained muscular effort that improves in striking fashion after prostigmine or rest is characteristic of this disease. These symptoms are rare in polymyositis and muscular wasting is much more marked in polymyositis. The so-called tensilon test, whereby 1—2 cc of edrophonium chloride (ROCHE) injected intraveously is followed by strengthening of the muscles is characteristic of myasthenia gravis (Mayo Clinic). Motor point biopsy may disclose a specific abnormality in myasthenia gravis (CÖERS and WOOLF).

h) Other Myopathies and Neuropathies

α) Steroid myopathy (R. S. WILLIAMS) may simulate the myopathy of dermato- and polymyositis or may conceivably be superimposed on these conditions.

Scattered areas of vacuolization and proliferation of the sarcolemmal nuclei as well as creatinuria are found. Interrogation relative to use of corticosteroids and/or adrenocorticotrophin should be routine in every case. An affirmative answer and/or signs and symptoms of iatrogenic CUSHING's syndrome would be most significant.

β) Myopathies secondary to hyperthyroidism, myxedema, sarcoidosis among other conditions must also be considered. Multiple disseminated tumors in muscles are possible in sarcoidosis (ADAMS, DENNY-BROWN and PEARSON).

γ) Neuropathies as seen in association with malignant tumors, alcoholism, vitamin deficiency, sarcoidoses, Guillain-Barre syndrome among other conditions have to be considered because of the attendant pain and weakness.

10. Treatment

α) Micellaneous measures. The foremost dangers during the first two or three years are severe dysphagia, respiratory failure and intercurrent infection. Prior to the advent of steroids and antibiotics, there was little of value in the doctor's armamentarium. Vitamin E, paraminobenzoic acid, iodized oil, EDTA (ethylene diaminetetracetic acid) are among the measure that have been used or recommended in the past with questionable success in some cases and none in others. The antimalarials are ineffective (WINKELMANN).

β) Corticosteroid therapy. WALTON and ADAMS are of the opinion "the advent of corticotrophin (ACTH) and cortisone has revolutionized the treatment of this group of disorders". Not all observers would agree. A study of published results indicates a marked variability in responsiveness (CARLISLE and GOOD; WEDGWOOD et al.; GARZON et al.; WEDGWOOD; BERGOUIGNAN et al.; OPPEL et al.; NARANJO y BORRERO; BARAN et CIVATTE). Some cases have proved refractory, in others the tendency to gastrointestinal ulcerations may have been enhanced.

Acute cases on the whole appear to be more responsive to steroids, but not uniformly so. WALTON and ADAMS have the impression that generally speaking cases that show a striking infiltration of muscle with inflammatory cells respond better. As one would expect, the response to steroid therapy is poor or transitory when malignancy coexists (PEARSON 1962). Despite the variability in responsiveness one may conclude these hormones are indicated during the active phase of the disease. Potential adverse effects (MEYLER; GILES et al.) must of course, be borne in mind, particularly the possibility of enhanced gastrointestinal ulceration and steroid myopathy (R. S. WILLIAMS).

Prednisone is generally regarded as the steroid of choice in dermatomyositis and the collagen diseases. Triamcinolone and dexamethasome are less desirable because of the greater likelihood of steroid myopathy. An initial daily dose of about 50—60 mg. of prednisone may be needed to check symptoms. Suppressive therapy with gradual reduction of the dose is continued until the activity subsides. This may be a matter of months or years. PEARSON (1962) found serial analyses of serum enzymes a helpful guide in determining dosage. VICKERS on the other hand objects to the use of serial estimations of SGOT because systemic steroids "may interfere in some way with either production or release of transaminase without actually influencing the underlying process".

γ) Salicylates and other analgesics. Acetylsalicylic acid (aspirin) and other salicylates are best for the relief of pain and tenderness which may be exquisite. Other analgesics may be needed. Codeine and other morphine derivaties should be eschewed. The author can recall a pitiful case of morphine addiction in a woman in her early thirties.

δ) **Physiotherapy** is generally withheld during the acute phase. Splints however may be used to lessen the discomfort from acutely inflamed muscles. At the proper time physical therapeutic measures including gentle massage, exercise and/or traction and other rehabilitative procedures should be instituted to prevent deformities and contractures.

ε) **Examination for malignancy.** A thorough search for a visceral malignancy or malignant lymphoma must be made in all individuals or over twenty. Repeated examinations at intervals may be necessary before an otherwise silent malignant tumor may be disclosed. Successful extirpation of such a tumor may be followed by a recovery.

References

Adams, R. D., D. Denny-Brown and C. M. Pearson: Diseases of muscle. A study in pathology, 2nd rev. edit. New York: Paul B. Hoeber 1962. — Allen, A. C.: The skin. A clinicopathologic treatise. St. Louis: C. V. Mosby Co. 1954. — Amoretti, A. R., F. Burgoa, P. Ravecca y R. Vignale: Melanoma en leucoderma y dermatomiositis. An. Fac. Med. Montevideo **46**, 77 (1961). — Aronson, S. M.: Enzyme determinations in neurologic and neuromuscular diseases of infancy and childhood. Pediat. Clin. N. Amer. **7** (3), 527 (1960). — Arundell, F. D., R. D. Wilkinson and J. R. Haserick: Dermatomyositis and malignant neoplasms in adults. A survey of twenty years' experience. Arch. Derm. **82**, 772 (1960).

Baran, L. R., et J. Civatte: Sur une Dermatomyosite aigue traitée par l'hydrocortisone intraveineuse et l'alpha-tocophéryl-quinone en solution alcoolique. Bull. Soc. franç. Derm. Syph. **66**/4, 600 (1959). — Bardawil, W. A., B. L. Toy, N. Galins and T. B. Bayles: Disseminated lupus erythematosus, scleroderma and dermatomyositis as manifestations of sensitization to DNA protein. I. An immunohistochemical approach. Amer. J. Path. **34**, 607 (1958). — Barron, K. D., and D. I. M. Fine: Neuromyositis. J. nerv. ment. Dis. **128**, 497 (1959). — Beickert, A., and W. Kühne: Dermatomyositis with immunoleucopenia due to phenthiozine. Schweiz. med. Wschr. **90**, 132 (1960). — Bergouignan, H. Leger, Mesnier et Force: Le problème des dysproteinémies dans les dermatomyosites. J. Méd. Bordeaux **137**, 1375 (1960). — Bezecny, R.: Dermatomyositis. Arch. Derm. Syph. (Berl.) **171**, 242 (1935). — Boylan, R. C., and L. Sokoloff: Vascular lesions in dermatomyositis. Arthr. and Rheum. **3**, 379 (1960). — Braunsteiner, H., and D. Zucker-Franklin (edit.): Physiology and pathology of leukocytes. In: P. Miescher, Antibodies directed against nuclei, chapt. 13. New York and London: Grune & Stratton 1962. — Bruce, G. M.: Retinitis in dermatomyositis. Trans. Amer. ophthal. Soc. (N.Y.) **36**, 282 (1938). — Bruyn, G. W., and G. Th. van Beusekom: Dermatomyositis. A survey of its present status. Psychiat. Neurol. Neurochir. (Amst.) **63**, 398 (1960). — Buchthal, F.: An introduction to electromyography. København: Gyldendal, Scandinavian University Books 1957. — Bunim, J. J.: A broader spectrum of Sjögren's syndrome and its pathogenetic implications. Ann. rheum. Dis. **20**, 1 (1961). — Bureau, Y., A. Jarry et H. Barrière: A propos de deux observations d'éruptions nécrotiques au cours de dermatomyosites. Bull. Soc. franç. Derm. Syph. **67** (2), 402 (1960).

Caballero, G. M.: Dermato-muco-miositis. Arch. Med. interna **1**, 114 (1935). — Carlisle, J. W., and R. A. Good: Dermatomyositis in childhood. Report of studies on 7 cases and a review of literature. J.-Lancet **79**, 266 (1959). — Cecil, R. L., and R. F. Loeb (edit.): A textbook of medicine. In: A. M. Harvey, Dermatomyositis, 10th edit., p. 465. Philadelphia and London: W. B. Saunders Co. 1959. — Christianson, H. B., L. A. Brunsting and H. O. Perry: Dermatomyositis, unusual features, complications and treatment. Arch. Derm. **74**, 581 (1956). — Coërs, C., et J. E. Desmedt: Mise en évidence d'une malformation caractéristique de la jonction neuromusculaire dans la myasthenie, corrélations histo- et physiopathologiques. Acta neurol. belg. **59**, 539 (1959). — Coërs, C., and A. L. Woolf: The innervation of muscle. A biopsy study. Springfield (Ill.): Ch. C. Thomas 1959. — Cortes, F. M., C. E. Morris and R. V. Hutter: Polymyositis, observations in three cases. Amer. J. med. Sci. **243**, 77 (1962). — Curtis, A. C., H. C. Blaylock and E. R. Harrell: Malignant lesions associated with dermatomyositis. J. Amer. med. Ass. **150**, 844 (1952). — Curtis, A. C., J. H. Heckaman and A. H. Wheeler: Study of the autoimmune reaction in dermatomyositis. J. Amer. med. Ass. **178**, 571 (1961).

Demel, V. C.: Di un caso di sclerema dei neonati a forma polimiositica. Arch. ital. Derm. **4**, 81 (1928). — Domzalski, C. A., and V. C. Morgan: Dermatomyositis: Diagnostic features and therapeutic pitfalls. Amer. J. Med. **19**, 370 (1955). — Donoghue, F. E., R. K. Winkelmann and H. J. Moersch: Esophageal defects in dermatomyositis. Ann. Otol. (St. Louis) **69**, 1139 (1960). — Dorn, H. F., and S. J. Cutler: Morbidity from cancer in the United States. Part I. Variation in incidence by age, sex, race, marital status, and geographic region. Public

Health Monograph No. 29, Public Health Service Publication No. 418, U.S. Dept. of Health, Education and Welfare, Public Health Service (Washington) 1955. — DOSTROVSKY, A., and F. SAGHER: Dermatomyositis and malignant tumour. Brit. J. Derm. 58, 52 (1946). — DOWLING, G. B.: Scleroderma and dermatomyositis. Brit. J. Derm. 67, 275 (1955). — DOWLING, G. B., and W. FREUDENTHAL: Dermatomyositis and poikiloderma atrophicans vascularis: A clinical and histological comparison. Brit. J. Derm. 50, 519 (1938). — DOWLING, G. B., and W. J. GRIFFITHS: Dermatomyositis and progressive scleroderma. Lancet **1939 I**, 1424. — DUNCAN, P. R., P. W. HARVEY and R. H. SEVILLE: Dermatomyositis presenting as aplastic anemia. Brit. J. Derm. 71, 344 (1959). — DUVERNE, J., et J. PLATHEY: Dermatomyosite et cancer. J. Méd. Lyon 38, 895 (1957).

EATON, L. M.: The perspective of neurology with regard to polymyositis, a study of 41 cases. Neurology (Minneap.) 4, 245 (1954). — EVERETT, M. A., and A. C. CURTIS: Dermatomyositis. A review of nineteen cases in adolescents and children. Arch. intern. Med. 100, 70 (1957).

FALLET, G., et A. PFENNINGER: Collagénose apparue sous traitement à la Mésantoine. Rev. méd. Suisse rom. 78, 790 (1958). — FIRMAT, J., and M. B. LIPSETT: Cancer and dermatomyositis. Cancer (Philad.) 11, 63 (1958).

GARCIN, R.: Considérations générales sur les maladies dites du collagène. Rev. neurol. 92, 419 (1955). — GARCIN, R., J. LAPRESLE, J. GRUNER et J. SCHERRER: Les polymyosites. Rev. neurol. 92, 465 (1955). — GARZÓN, R., M. OLMEDO DIAZ y L. FERRARIS: Dermatomiositis. A proposito de dos observaciones. Rev. Fac. Cienc. méd. Univ. Córdoba 17, 127 (1959). — GILES, C. L., G. L. MASON, I. F. DUFF and J. A. MCLEAN: The association of cataract formation and systemic corticosteroid therapy. J. Amer. med. Ass. 182, 719 (1962). — GOLDFISCHER, J., and E. H. RUBIN: Dermatomyositis with pulmonary lesions. Ann. intern. Med. 50, 194 (1959). — GRACE, J. T., and T. L. DAO: Dermatomyositis in cancer: A possible etiological mechanism. Cancer (Philad.) 12, 648 (1959). — GRACIANSKY, P., and S. BOULLE: Color atlas of dermatology, translation and adaptation by M. B. SULZBERGER and S. DOBKEVITCH-MORRILL, vol. 1. Chicago: Year Book Publ. 1955. — GREENFIELD, J. G., G. M. SHY, E. C. ALVORD and L. BERG: An atlas of muscle pathology in neuromuscular diseases. Edinburgh: E. & S. Livingstone, Ltd. 1957. — GUY, W. H., R. C. GRAUER and F. M. JACOB: Poikilodermatomyositis. Arch. Derm. Syph. (Chic.) 40, 867 (1939).

HEATHFIELD, K. W. G., and J. R. B. WILLIAMS: Diagnosis of polymyositis. Lancet **1960 I**, 1157. — HENSON, R. A., D. S. RUSSELL and M. WILKINSON: Carcinomatous neuropathy and myopathy. A clinical and pathological study. Brain 77, 82 (1954). — HEPP, R.: Über einen Fall von acuter parenchymatöser Myositis, welche Geschwülste bildete und Fluctuation vortäuschte. Berl. klin. Wschr. 24, 389 (1887). — HERRMANN, W. P., u. K. H. SCHULZ: Immunoelektrophoretische Untersuchungen an Hautkranken. II. Erythematodes, Dermatomyositis, Sklerodermie. Arch. klin. exp. Derm. 212, 233 (1961). — HYMAN, I., C. E. ARBESMAN and K. L. TERPLAN: Dermatomyositis following penicillin injections. Neurology (Minneap.) 6, 63 (1956).

IRGANG, S.: Dermatomyositis in the negro. A clinical and histologic study of the skin of two cases. Urol. cutan. Rev. (St. Louis) 46, 251 (1942).

JANEWAY, C. A., D. GITLIN, J. M. CRAIG and D. S. GRICE: "Collagen disease" in patients with congenital agammaglobulinemia. Trans. Ass. Amer. Phycns (Philad.) 69, 93 (1956). — JOHNSON, WAINE C.: Personal communication.

KAMPMEIER, R. H.: Collagen diseases — Unanswered questions on pathogenesis and etiology. Arch. Derm. 83, 466 (1961). — KANKELEIT: Über primäre nichteitrige Polymyositis. Dtsch. Arch. klin. Med. 120, 335 (1916). — KEIL, H.: The manifestations in the skin and mucous membranes in dermatomyositis, with special reference to the differential diagnosis from systemic lupus erythematosus. Ann. intern. Med. 16, 828 (1942). — KOVACS, L.: Dermatomyositis or rheumatism? Rheumatism 17, 86 (1961).

LANE, C. W.: Dermatomyositis. Sth. med. J. (Bgham, Ala.) 31, 287 (1938). — LAPOVSKY, ARTHUR J.: Personal communication. — LEINWAND, I., A. W. DURYEE and M. N. RICHTER: Scleroderma (based on a study of over 150 cases). Ann. intern. Med. 41, 1003 (1954). — LEVER, W. F.: Histopathology of the skin, 3rd edit. Philadelphia and Montreal: J. B. Lippincott Co. 1961. — LICHT, S.: Electrodiagnosis and electromyography, by D. HARRIMAN, 2nd edit., chapt. V. New Haven (Connecticut): Elizabeth Licht 1961. — LISMAN, J. V.: Dermatomyositis with retinopathy. Report of a case. Arch. Ophth., N.s. 37, 155 (1947). — LUGHT, L. V. D.: Dermatomyositis. Acta derm.-venereol. (Stockh.) 32, 27 (1952).

MADDEN, J. F., and I. M. KARON: Comparisons of muscle biopsies and bone marrow examinations in dermatomyositis and lupus erythematosus. Arch. Derm. Syph. (Chic.) 62, 192 (1950). — MALKINSON, F. D., and ST. ROTHMAN: Changes in the gastrointestinal tract in scleroderma and other diffuse connective tissue diseases. Amer. J. Gastroent. 26, 414 (1956). — MARCUS, M. D., and W. E. WOOLDRIDGE: Poikilodermatomyositis (Poikiloderma vasculare atrophicans). Report of a case exhibiting features of panniculitis, scleroderma, periarteritis nodosa and calcinosis cutis. Arch. Deım. Syph. (Chic.) **62**, 131 (1950). — *Mayo Clinic* and *Mayo Foundation* (Sections of Neurology): Clinical Examinations in Neurology. Philadelphia and London: W. B. Saunders Co. 1956. — MEIREN, L. VAN DER, et C. CÖERS: Contribution a la clinique, l'histologie et l'electrophysiologie de la dermatomyosite (Etude de cinq cas). Arch. belges Derm. **16** (1), 142 (1960). — MEYLER, L.: Side effects of drugs, chapt. XIX, Hormones, 3rd edit. Amsterdam-London-New York: Excerpta med. Foundation 1960. — MIEHLKE, K., and J. L. HOLLANDER: The cardiac involvement of dermatomyositis. Abstracts of papers presented at the second Pan-American Congress on Rheumatic Diseases, Washington and Bethesda, 1959. A. I. R. Arch. inter-amer. Rheum. (Rio de J.) **2**, 251 (1959). — MILLS, E. S., and W. H. MATHEWS: Interstitial pneumonitis in dermatomyositis. J. Amer. med. Ass. **160**, 1467 (1956). — MINAZZI, M.: Contributo allo studio della dermatomiosite. Neurone (Mantova) **6** (2), 183 (1958). — MOSER, K.: Myalgie und Myositis. In: Handbuch der Neurologie, Bd. IX, S. 5, bearb. von O. BUMKE u. O. FOESTER. Berlin: Springer 1935. — MULLER, S. A., R. K. WINKELMANN and L. A. BRUNSTING: Calcinosis in dermatomyositis. Observations on course of disease in children and adults. Arch. Derm. **79**, 669 (1959).

NARANJO, V. A., y R. J. BORRERO: Dermatomiositis, presentación de cuarto nuevos casos. Antioquia méd. **10**, 425 (1960).

OESTER, Y. T., A. A. RODRIGUEZ and J. J. FUDEMA: Electromyographic findings in dermatomyositis. Arch. Derm. **76**, 91 (1957). — O'LEARY, P. A., E. H. LAMBERT and G. P. SAYRE: Muscle studies in cutaneous disease. J. invest. Derm. **24**, 301 (1955). — O'LEARY, P. A., and M. WAISMAN: Dermatomyositis; a study of forty cases. Arch. Derm. Syph. (Chic.) **41**, 1001 (1940). — OPPEL, T. W., C. COKER and A. T. MILHORAT: Effect of pituitary adrenocorticotropin (ACTH) in Dermatomyositis. Ann. intern. Med. **32**, 318 (1950). — OPPENHEIM, H.: Zur Dermatomyositis. Berl. klin. Wschr. **36**, 805 (1899). — Über die Polymyositis. Berl. klin. Wschr. **40**, 381 (1903). — Poikilodermia vascularis atrophicans (Jacobi). In: Handbuch der Haut- und Geschlechtskrankheiten von J. JADASSOHN, Vol. 8/2, S. 635. Berlin: Springer 1931.

PAGEL, W., and C. S. TREIP: Viscero-cutaneous collagenosis. A study of the intermediate forms of dermatomyositis, scleroderma, and disseminated lupus erythematosus. J. clin. Path. 8, 1 (1955). — PEARSON, C. M.: Rheumatic manifestations of polymyositis and dermatomyositis. Arthr. and Rheum. **2**, 127 (1959). — Polymyositis and dermatomyositis. Bull. rheum. Dis. **12**, 268 (1962). — PETGES, G., et C. CLÉJAT: Sclérose atrophique de la peau et myosite généralisée. Ann. Derm. Syph. (Paris) **7**, 550 (1906). — PETGES, G., and A. PETGES: Poikilodermatomyosite dans la jeunesse et l'enfance. Ann. Derm. Syph. (Paris) **1**, 441 (1930). — PFEIFFER, R.: Die Polymyositis resp. Dermatomyositis acuta. Zbl. allg. Path. path. Anat. **7**, 81 (1896). — PUCHOL, J. R., y A. CARBALLIDO: La actividad transaminasica del suero en la dermatomiositis. Act. dermo-sifiliogr. (Madr.) **49** (8), 528 (1958).

ROGOFF, J. B.: Clinical electromyography, usefulness in differentiating myopathies from neuropathies. N.Y. St. J. Med. **60**, 512 (1960).

SCHUERMANN, H.: Maligne Tumoren bei Dermatomyositis und progressiver Sklerodermie. Arch. Derm. Syph. (Berl.) **192**, 575 (1951). — SCHWARTZ, G., E. GREVILLIOT et L. GERY: Essai provisoire de classification des granulomatoses malignes. Apropos d'un cas de reticulogranulomatose maligne à prédominance cutanée et musculaire („dermatomyosite"), avec état leucémique terminal. Bull. Soc. franç. Derm. Syph. **44** (7), 1498 (1937). — SCOTT, A., and E. G. REES: The relationship of systemic lupus erythematosus and discoid lupus erythematosus. A clinical and hematological study. Arch. Derm. **79**, 422 (1959). — SENATOR, H.: Über acute Polymyositis und Neuromyositis. Dtsch. med. Wschr. **19**, 933 (1893). — SHEARD, C., and P. T. KNOEPFLER: Dermatomyositis and the incidence of associated malignancy. Arch. Derm. **75**, 224 (1957). — SILVERMAN, J. J., and V. E. POWELL: Peripheral vascular changes in dermatomyositis. Amer. Heart J. **30**, 441 (1945). — STEINER, W. R.: Dermatomyositis, with report of a case which presented a rare muscle anomaly but once described in man. J. exp. Med. **6**, 407 (1901—1905). — Dermatomyositis, with report of two cases. J. Amer. med. Ass. **78**, 271 (1922). — STERTZ, G.: Polymyositis. Berl. klin. Wschr. **53**, 489 (1916). — STOUGHTON, R., and G. WELLS: A histochemical study in polysaccharides in normal and diseased skin. J. invest. Derm. **14**, 37 (1950). — SUNDE, H.: Dermatomyositis in children. Acta paediat. (Uppsala) **37**, 287 (1949).

TAKATS, G. DE, and E. F. FOWLER: Raynaud's phenomenon. J. Amer. med. Ass. **179**, 1 (1962). — TALBOTT, J. H., and R. MOLERES FERRANDIS: Collagen diseases. New York: Grune & Stratton 1956. — THIES, W.: Beitrag zur Frage Dermatomyositis und Neoplasma. Derm. Wschr. **135**, 292 (1957). — THOMAS, C., J. CORDIER et A. DUPREZ: Manifestations ophthalmoscopiques des dermatomyosites. Bull. Soc. franç. Derm. Syph. **66** (3), 349 (1959).

UNVERRICHT, H.: Polymyositis acuta progressiva. Z. klin. Med. **12**, 533 (1887). — Dermatomyositis acuta. Dtsch. med. Wschr. **17**, 41 (1891).

VICKERS, C. F. H.: Serum transaminase estimations in the differential diagnosis of collagen disease. Brit. J. Derm. **73**, 185 (1961). — VIGLIOGLIA, P. A.: Dermatomiositis. Día méd. **33**, 2781 (1961).

WAGNER, E.: Fall einer seltenen Muskelkrankheit. Arch. Heilk. **4**, 282 (1863). — Ein Fall von acuter Polymyositis. Dtsch. Arch. klin. Med. **40**, 241 (1887). — WALKER, S. A., and E. P. BENDITT: The serum proteins in diseases of connective tissue. An electrophoretic study. J. invest. Derm. **14**, 113 (1950). — WALLACE, S. L., R. LATTES and C. RAGEN: Diagnostic significance of the muscle biopsy. Amer. J. Med. **25**, 600 (1958). — WALSH, F. B.: Clinical neuro-ophthalmology, 2nd edit. Baltimore: Williams & Wilkins Co. 1957. — WALTON, J. N., and R. D. ADAMS: Polymyositis. Edinburgh and London: E. & S. Livingstone, Ltd. 1958. — WEDGWOOD, R. J. P.: Discussion on paper by H. M. ROBERTS and L. A. BRUNSTING on, Dermatomyositis in childhood: Summary of 40 cases. In: Year Book of Pediatrics, p. 411. Chicago: Year Book Publ. 1955/56. — WEDGWOOD, R. J. P., C. D. COOK and J. COHEN: Dermatomyositis. Report of 26 cases in children with discussion of endocrine therapy in thirteen. Pediactrics **12**, 447 (1953). — WHEELER, C. E., A. C. CURTIS, E. P. CAWLEY, R. H. GREKIN and B. ZHEUTLIN: Soft tissue calcification with special reference to its occurrence in the "collagen diseases". Ann. intern. Med. **36**, 1050 (1952). — WHITE, L. P.: Serum enzymes. Variations of activity in disease of muscles. Calif. Med. **90**, 1 (1959). — WILLIAMS, D. (edit.): Modern trends in neurology, 2nd series. New York: Paul B. Hoeber 1957. — WILLIAMS, P. C., and D. H. LAW: Serum complement in connective tissue disorders. J. Lab. clin. Med. **52**, 273 (1958). — WILLIAMS, R. C.: Dermatomyositis and malignancy: A review of the literature. Ann. intern. Med. **50**, 1174 (1959). — WILLIAMS, R. S.: Triamcinolone myopathy. Lancet **1959I**, 689. — WINKELMANN, R. K.: Diagnosis and treatment of lupus erythematosus, dermatomyositis, and scleroderma with emphasis on cutaneous findings. J. chron. Dis. **13**, 401 (1961).

ZELGER, J.: Ein Beitrag zur Calcinosis cutis bei Dermatomyositis. Derm. Wschr. **140**, 1289 (1959). — ZIFF, M.: Genetics, hypersensitivity and the connective tissue diseases. Amer. J. Med. **30**, 1 (1961).

Aktinische Dermatosen

Von

Hans Kuske-Bern

Mit 19 Abbildungen (davon 2 farbige)

Einleitung

Mit dem Begriff aktinische Dermatosen bezeichnet man diejenigen Hautkrankheiten, welche durch Licht hervorgerufen werden. Ihre Auslösung durch

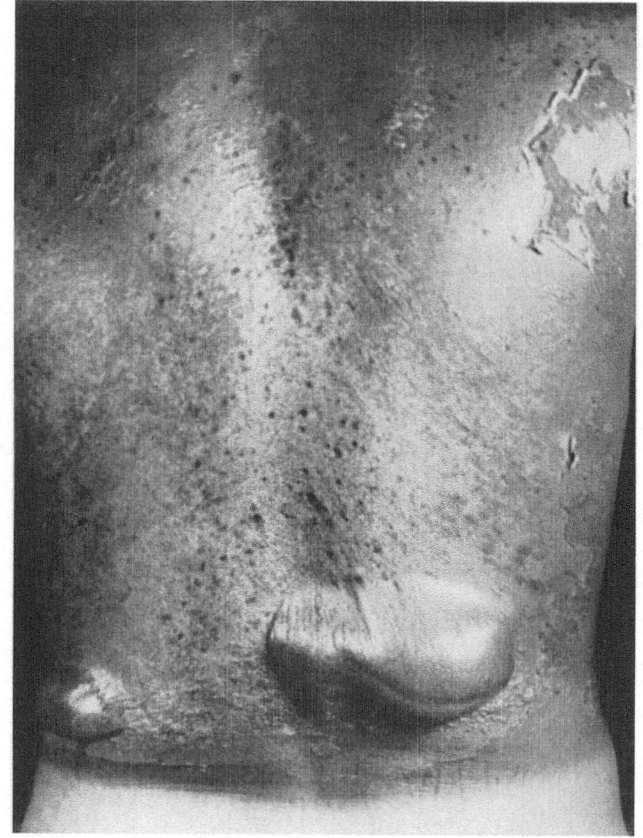

Abb. 1. *Dermatitis solaris bullosa* nach übermäßiger Besonnung. Sie ist häufig die Ursache bleibender Hyperpigmentierungen in Form von multiplen großen Naevi spili

Lichtstrahlen drückt sich in ihrer Erscheinungsform und ihrem Verlauf aus. Ist das Licht nicht alleinige Ursache der Erkrankung, wirkt es doch mindestens als wesentlicher pathogenetischer Faktor am Geschehen mit. Im Gegensatz zu der früheren Definition von Bering und Barnewitz werden hier nicht nur die ultravioletten Lichtstrahlen genannt, denn in Sonderfällen hat auch das sichtbare Spektrum für die Entstehung von Krankheitserscheinungen Bedeutung.

Die Krankheitsgruppe der aktinischen Dermatosen hat immer wieder großes Interesse gefunden und ist wiederholt zusammenfassend bearbeitet worden. Die Autoren der bedeutendsten Monographien zum Thema der Lichtkrankheiten werden im folgenden angeführt: JESIONEK (1912), SAIDMAN (1925), HAUSMANN und HAXTHAUSEN (1929), BERING und BARNEWITZ (1932), JAUSION und PAGÈS (1933), CARRIÉ (1936), VANNOTTI (1937), BLUM (1941), ELLINGER (1941), HOLLÄNDER (1956), MEYER (1956), BÉNARD, GAJDOS und GAJDOS-TÖRÖK (1958), BURCKHARDT (1959), IPPEN (1959), SCHUPPLI (1959), WULF (1959), MIESCHER (1960).

Von KIMMIG und WISKEMANN wurden im Abschnitt Lichtbiologie und Lichttherapie dieses Ergänzungswerkes bereits die physiologischen Lichtwirkungen eingehend bearbeitet (Bd. V/2). Auf ihren Beitrag sei als wichtige Grundlage für das Verständnis besonders hingewiesen. Dort wird, neben den physiologischen Wirkungen, auch die Dermatitis solaris bullosa mit ihren Nachwirkungen besprochen (Abb. 1).

Man kann das Stoffgebiet der Lichtdermatosen auf verschiedene Weise unterteilen. Weil aber noch viele Unklarheiten bestehen, wird keine Einteilung ganz befriedigen. Der folgenden Gruppierung wurde der Vorzug gegeben:

1. Eigentliche Lichtkrankheiten.
a) Xeroderma pigmentosum.
b) Porphyrinkrankheiten.
c) Eczema solare und polymorphe Lichtdermatose.
d) Frühlingslichtdermatose.
e) Cheilitis exfoliativa actinica.
f) Lichturticaria.

2. Photosensibilisierung und Photoallergie.

3. Das Licht als fakultative, zusätzliche oder provozierende Noxe.

I. Eigentliche Lichtkrankheiten

1. Xeroderma pigmentosum

Das Xeroderma pigmentosum ist ein eindrückliches Krankheitsbild. Es gehört zu den schwersten Lichtdermatosen, die wir kennen, und hat meistens eine infauste Prognose. Wir dürfen annehmen, daß die Mehrzahl der Fälle früher oder später in fachärztliche Beobachtung gelangt und meistens auch publiziert oder demonstriert wird.

Die Auffassungen über das Krankheitsbild haben sich in den vergangenen Jahrzehnten kaum verändert. Die früheren Darstellungen (KAPOSI, BERING) behalten ihre volle Gültigkeit. Nach wie vor muß eine erbliche Veranlagung angenommen werden. Der Prozentsatz der Verwandtenehen in der Aszendenz der Patienten mit Xeroderma pigmentosum ist hoch (zwischen 17—59%), die Wahrscheinlichkeit für ein recessives krankmachendes Gen darum gegeben. Weil der Prozentsatz von Befallenen den zu erwartenden Wert nicht erreicht, ist man zur Annahme einer unregelmäßig recessiven Vererbung gezwungen (SIEMENS und KOHN).

Die Krankheit zeigt sich in der Regel schon in der frühen Kindheit, in 80% der Fälle in den ersten Lebensjahren, nämlich wenn die veranlagten Kinder erstmals intensiverer Lichtbestrahlung ausgesetzt werden. Die allerersten Hautsymptome kommen selten in ärztliche Beobachtung, doch darf aus den übereinstimmenden Schilderungen der Laien gefolgert werden, daß sich fleckige, entzündliche Rötungen ausbilden, die bald nur relativ umschrieben, meist aber großflächig, erysipelartig mit akuter Hyperämie, Schwellung und Schuppung an den belichteten Stellen auftreten. Akute Exacerbationen können sich wiederholen, wobei offenbar wie bei anderen Lichtkrankheiten eine Häufung in die Frühlingsmonate fällt. Besonderheiten der Strahlung in dieser Jahreszeit spielen eine Rolle, vielleicht auch die fehlende Lichtgewöhnung. Anschließend bilden sich Pigmentanomalien aus, teils als diffuse Braunfärbung, teils als ephelidenartige Flecken und Hyperpigmentierungen, wie man sie ähnlich auch als Folge von übermäßig starker Lichtschädigung bei Normalempfindlichen auftreten sieht. Auch an den Schleimhäuten können derartige Pigmentflecken auftreten. Damit stellt sich die Frage, ob man nicht früher zu einseitig alle Krankheitserscheinungen des Xeroderma pigmentosum ausschließlich auf die schädigende Einwirkung des Sonnenlichtes zurückgeführt hat.

In späteren Stadien der Erkrankung gesellen sich atrophische Veränderungen hinzu, die Haut bekommt ein glattes oder runzeliges Aussehen, teils bilden sich scharf umschriebene Depigmentierungen mit oder ohne Konsistenzveränderung der befallenen Bezirke aus. Die Mischung von Hyperpigmentierung und Pigmentmangel und das Auftreten von Teleangiektasien führen zu einem Bilde, das an poikilodermatische Zustände oder an das Aussehen röntgenatrophischer Bezirke erinnert. Auch kommen Angiome und teils sternförmige Teleangiektasien an den Schleimhäuten, an Lippen, im Mund und an den Conjunctiven vor, so daß zur Erklärung der Genese ähnliche Überlegungen erlaubt sind, wie sie für die Pigmentflecken geäußert wurden.

Narbig atrophische Veränderungen führen schließlich besonders im Gesicht zu Verstümmelungen, zu Ektropion der Augenlider, zu Ohrmuscheldefekten und Verkleinerung der Nase. In diesem Stadium sind differentialdiagnostisch die Porphyria congenita und verschiedene Poikilodermien, ferner Röntgenatrophie und senile Degeneration der Haut zu berücksichtigen. Mit großer Regelmäßigkeit kommt es schließlich beim Xeroderma pigmentosum zur Ausbildung warziger Elemente, die den senilen Keratomen gleichgestellt werden. Eine verfrühte Vergreisung ist vielen Beobachtern aufgefallen und vereinfachend als Wesen der Erkrankung dargestellt worden. Die Ähnlichkeit mit Seemanns- oder Landmannshaut kann außerordentlich groß sein; in letzter Zeit mehren sich die Stimmen, die in den ausgesprochen chronischen, durch Licht bedingten Veränderungen dieses Krankheitsbildes abortive Formen oder formes frustes von Xeroderma pigmentosum sehen wollen (LEHMANN).

Als Xeroderma pigmentosum tardivum bezeichnet man Erkrankungsfälle, die z.B. erst im dritten Lebensjahrzehnt auftreten. Sie wären als Bindeglieder zwischen Xeroderma pigmentosum und den formes frustes der Krankheit aufzufassen (ANDERSON und BEGG). BERLIN und TAGER anerkennen milde Verlaufsformen, möchten aber mit Recht die Seemannshaut nicht dem Xeroderma pigmentosum gleichstellen.

Die warzigen Efflorescenzen sind die Vorläufer für die maligne Entartung in Spinaliome. Daneben wurden beim Xeroderma pigmentosum aber auch Basalzellencarcinome, Sarkome und maligne Melanome beschrieben, wobei die malignen Neubildungen z.T. auch aus scheinbar unveränderter Haut entstehen. Ihr relativ rasches Wachstum stellt eine ernste Bedrohung des Patienten dar. Ständige ärztliche Überwachung und frühzeitige Excision verdächtiger Efflorescenzen müssen darum gefordert werden. Zwei Drittel der Patienten sterben vor dem 15. Lebensjahr. Geistige Defekte und seelische Anomalien sollen beim Xeroderma pigmentosum vermehrt vorkommen. Beide Geschlechter werden gleich häufig befallen.

Histologie

In Frühstadien findet man nur sehr wenige charakteristische Veränderungen: Infiltrate in der unmittelbaren Umgebung der Gefäße und der Anhangsgebilde, besonders im Papillarkörper. In vereinzelten Fällen besteht Exsudation von sanguinolentem Serum, die bis zur hämorrhagischen Infarzierung reichen kann. Später fällt der große Pigmentreichtum von Epidermis und Cutis auf. Je nach den Entnahmestellen wird die Atrophie, die frühe und hochgradige Degeneration von elastischen und kollagenen Fasern besonders stark hervortreten. Eine weitere Reihe von histologischen Veränderungen, von der Acanthose und Hyperkeratose bis zur infiltrierend wachsenden Epithelwucherung reichend, ist beschrieben worden (NÖDL). Mesodermale Geschwülste hingegen kommen nur selten vor. Man darf folgern, daß nicht eine allgemeine Disposition zur Bildung maligner Geschwülste vererbt wird, sondern — wie schon immer angenommen wurde — eine Veranlagung zur vorzeitigen Degeneration der Haut und zur Hautkrebsbildung unter Lichteinfluß.

Für die auslösende Rolle des Lichtes liegen eine Menge von beweisenden klinischen Argumenten vor. Erwähnt sei nur die Lokalisation der Hautveränderungen an belichteten Körperstellen und Verschlimmerungen nach intensiveren Sonnenbestrahlungen.

Wie bei anderen Lichtkrankheiten kommt der Frage nach dem auslösenden Spektralbereich allerhöchste Bedeutung zu; wie so oft, ist aber diese Frage von den Beobachtern nicht immer mit der wünschbaren Klarheit beantwortet worden (BERLIN, BERLIN u. TAGER, MARTENSTEIN und BOBOWITSCH, ZOON). Meist wurde eine Auslösung durch den ultravioletten Anteil festgestellt. Dabei ist bemerkenswert, daß nicht einfach eine verstärkte Reaktion auftritt, sondern ein pathologischer Reaktionsablauf verfolgt werden kann, nämlich verzögerte Rückbildung und Auftreten von Teleangiektasien auf dem Höhepunkt der Entzündung. Die Empfindlichkeit soll mosaikartig auf bestimmte Hautbezirke beschränkt sein (ROTHMAN). Gegenüber Röntgen-, Radium- und Thorium-X-Bestrahlungen wurden nur vereinzelt pathologische Reaktionen beschrieben (MARTENSTEIN und BOBOWITSCH), neuerdings für Röntgen- und Grenzstrahlen (BERLIN und TAGER). Photodynamisch aktive Substanzen sind nicht nachgewiesen worden. Weil aber das Wesen der krankhaften Reaktion auf die Lichtwirkung noch keineswegs abgeklärt werden konnte, bleibt auch diese Frage noch offen. Bei neu zur Beobachtung kommenden Fällen werden Untersuchungen über den auslösenden Spektralbereich, über die Art und den Ablauf der Licht-, Röntgen-Grenzstrahlen-Reaktion und ihre Residuen von größtem Wert sein.

2. Porphyrinkrankheiten oder Porphyrien

Während wir im vorangehenden Abschnitt betonen mußten, daß sich seit den klassischen Beschreibungen des Xeroderma pigmentosum nicht viel Neues habe erarbeiten lassen, gilt für die Lichtdermatosen aus der Porphyrie-Gruppe das Gegenteil. BERING und BARNEWITZ faßten noch alles Hierhergehörige unter dem Begriff der Hydroa vacciniformis zusammen. Heute erlauben die tieferen Kenntnisse über den Porphyrinstoffwechsel eine Unterteilung in verschiedene Porphyrien. Die Umgruppierung und Änderung der Nomenklatur fördert das Verständnis und erlaubt uns eine Scheidung in Krankheitsbilder von sehr unterschiedlicher praktischer Bedeutung, die früher immer durcheinander geworfen wurden. Vereinzelt kommen allerdings auch Übergangsfälle, die nur mit Schwierigkeiten eingeordnet werden können, zur Beobachtung. In diesem Handbuch (dritter Band, erster Teil) werden die Porphyrien durch LEVER im Kapitel „Ablagerungskrankheiten körpereigener Stoffwechselprodukte“ ebenfalls abgehandelt, wobei intern-medizinische Gesichtspunkte vermehrt in den Vordergrund gestellt sind.

a) Physiologie und biologische Chemie des Porphyrinstoffwechsels. Experimentelle Porphyrinurien

Die historische Entwicklung unserer Kenntnisse über den Porphyrinstoffwechsel ist in modernen Monographien wiederholt dargestellt worden. Wir müssen auf diese Arbeiten hinweisen (VANNOTTI, WALDENSTRÖM, SHEMIN, BÉNARD, GAJDOS-TÖRÖK, R. SCHMID).

Hier soll nur kurz das zum Verständnis unbedingt Notwendige erörtert werden.

Das Porphyringerüst besteht aus vier durch Methinbrücken untereinander verbundenen Pyrrolringen. Der einfachste Vertreter, das Porphyrin, kommt nicht natürlich vor; er wurde von FISCHER synthetisiert. Uro-, Kopro- und Protoporphyrine unterscheiden sich in der Struktur durch verschiedene Anordnung der Substituenten an den vier Pyrrolringen. Von vier möglichen Isomeren der *Ätioporphyrine* kommen nur deren zwei natürlich vor, nämlich die Bautypen- bzw. Isomerenreihen I und III. Es sind verschiedene Seitenketten möglich; in der menschlichen Pathologie spielen besonders *Koproporphyrin* und *Uroporphyrin* eine wichtige Rolle.

Koproporphyrin I- und III-Ausscheidung finden wir normalerweise in jedem Harn. Die physiologisch vorkommenden Tagesmengen werden allerdings verschieden angegeben. VANNOTTI erwähnt normale Mengen bis 80 γ, SCHUPPLI anerkennt noch Ausscheidungsmengen bis 300 γ als physiologisch und normal, ebenso R. SCHMID, der 100—300 γ angibt. Sicher ist die Ausscheidung starken Schwankungen unterworfen. Immer hat man sich auf die 24stündige Ausscheidung zu beziehen. Bei wissenschaftlichen Untersuchungen ist von sorgfältig gesammelten Tagesurinmengen auszugehen. Da unter verschiedenen äußeren Bedingungen auch sehr verschiedene Mengen von Porphyrin-Vorstufen noch umgewandelt werden können, muß auf Nebenumstände wie p_H, Licht- und Lufteinwirkung und besonders auf die Anwesenheit von oxydierenden Substanzen geachtet werden. Manche Unstimmigkeiten in der Literatur dürften darauf zurückzuführen sein, daß diesen besonderen Bedingungen nicht genügend Rechnung getragen wurde.

Koproporphyrin wird nach verschiedenen Intoxikationen (Blei, Barbitursäurederivate, Sulfonal, Sedormid) vermehrt ausgeschieden. Für Porphyrinausscheidungen im Gefolge von Vergiftungen verwendet man besser den Ausdruck Porphyrinurie und nicht Porphyrie bzw. Porphyrinkrankheit.

Uroporphyrin ist immer ein pathologisches Ausscheidungsprodukt. Es entsteht, wenn man sich die Methylgruppen (CH_3 durch Carboxymethylen, CH_2COOH) ersetzt denkt, und zwar an den Stellen 1, 3, 6 und 8 am Porphyringerüst.

Bei gewissen Porphyrinkrankheiten wird Uroporphyrin als Isomer I und III ausgeschieden. Über die modernen Bestimmungsmethoden, die vereinheitlicht werden sollten, geben neuere Zusammenfassungen (SZODORAY und SÜMEGI, BÉNARD u. Mitarb. 1958) nähere Auskunft.

Weil bei der Hidroa vacciniformia-Gruppe früher oft keine pathologischen Porphyrinausscheidungen nachgewiesen werden konnten, wurde auch immer an die Bedeutung farbloser Vorstufen gedacht (SACHS). Solche Chromogene spielen heute für die Erklärung des Porphyrinaufbaus und -stoffwechsels wieder eine große Rolle. Die derzeitigen biochemischen Anschauungen über den Aufbau der

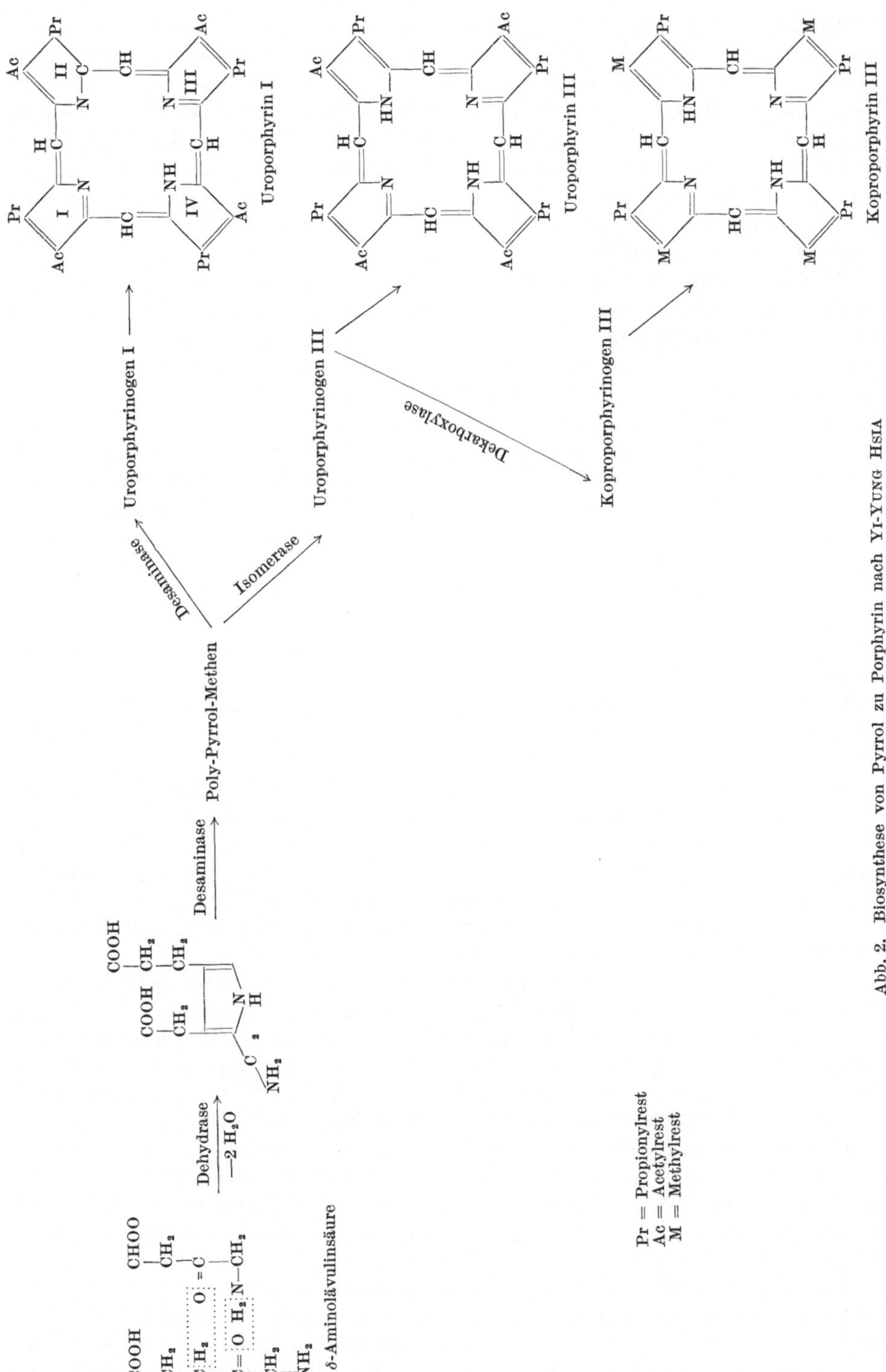

Abb. 2. Biosynthese von Pyrrol zu Porphyrin nach YI-YUNG HSIA

Porphyrine ersieht man am eindrücklichsten aus einem Schema über die Biosynthese von Pyrrol zu Porphyrin (s. Abb. 2) nach DAVID YI-YUNG HSIA.

Ausgangspunkt sind zwei Moleküle der ϑ-Deltaaminolävulinsäure, die durch eine Dehydrase unter Abspaltung von $2\,H_2O$ zu Porphobilinogen kondensiert werden. Eine Desaminase führt Porphobilinogen anaerob in Uroporphyrinogen I über, das seinerseits durch Autoxydation zu Uroporphyrin I wird. Ein zweites Enzym, eine Isomerase, verwandelt in Zusammenarbeit mit der Desaminase Porphobilinogen zu Uroporphyrinogen III, das sich zu Uroporphyrin III umwandelt. Schließlich führt ein weiteres Enzym, eine Decarboxylase, Uroporphyrinogen III in Koproporphyrinogen III über, das wiederum zu Koproporphyrin III umgewandelt wird.

Wird Deltaaminolävulinsäure einem Gesunden per os verabreicht, kann keine Porphyrinurie nachgewiesen werden. Verabfolgt man diese Verbindung hingegen Patienten mit Porphyrie, so wird es zu Porphobilinogen umgewandelt und erscheint im Urin. Beim Kaninchen kann durch die Deltaaminolävulinsäure Porphyrinurie ausgelöst werden. SCHUPPLI fand auch bei Kaninchen mit derart provozierter, sehr hoher Porphyrinausscheidung gar keine erhöhte Lädierbarkeit der Haut. Sie war gegen physikalische, chemische oder aktinische Reize nicht vermehrt empfindlich. Bei anderen Versuchstieren, Meerschweinchen und Ratten, gelang ihm die experimentelle Erzeugung von Porphyrinurie nur in ganz vereinzelten Fällen. Das Kaninchen scheint somit für diese Forschungen ein besonders günstiges biologisches Objekt zu sein. Beim Menschen wird Porphobilinogen — wie Uroporphyrin — nur unter pathologischen Bedingungen gefunden.

Neben Koproporphyrin findet man normalerweise noch Deuteroporphyrin aus der Darmfäulnis und Protoporphyrin, aus der Autolyse des Fleisches stammend (VANNOTTI).

Die normale Erythropoiese liefert nur geringe Mengen von Protoporphyrin III und Koproporphyrin I, während sie in größeren Mengen in der Leber gebildet werden.

Man kennt einen Porphyrinkreislauf zwischen Darmtrakt, Pfortaderkreislauf, Leber, Galle und zurück zum Darm, ähnlich wie er für das Urobilin bekannt ist. Über nähere Einzelheiten des enterohepatischen Porphyrinumsatzes sind aber die Spezialwerke der Physiologie (SHEMIN) und der inneren Medizin (WALDENSTRÖM) zu konsultieren. Das gleiche gilt von den Beziehungen der Porphyrine zum Auf- und Abbau des Hämoglobins und anderer häminhaltiger Pigmente und Fermente der Zellen (Cytochrom, Katalasen, Oxydasen).

Über die pharmakologischen, toxischen oder lichtsensibilisierenden Wirkungen der Porphyrine bestehen noch recht große Unklarheiten. Jedenfalls lassen sich nicht alle Symptome bei Porphyrinkrankheiten oder -stoffwechselstörungen einfach auf diese Körper direkt zurückführen. Bei der Interpretation muß vorsichtig vorgegangen werden. Vor allem besteht kein direkter Zusammenhang zwischen Porphyrinausscheidung und Lichtempfindlichkeit, wird doch etwa bei Bleiintoxikation viel Porphyrin ausgeschieden, ohne daß Lichtsensibilisierung auftritt, und das gleiche gilt für gewisse klinische Formen der Porphyrie. Mit Recht wird auch immer wieder darauf hingewiesen, daß der berühmte Selbstversuch von MEYER-BETZ mit Hämatoporphyrin (NENCKI) durchgeführt worden ist, also nicht mit einem natürlichen Porphyrin.

Auch die Photosensibilisierungsversuche an der weißen Maus (HAUSMANN) dürfen nur mit größter Vorsicht auf die Verhältnisse beim Menschen übertragen werden. Auch sie wurden mit Hämatoporphyrin durchgeführt, eine Substanz übrigens, deren direkt toxische Wirkungen von den photosensibilisierenden Eigenschaften nach GREITHER nur schwer abgegrenzt werden können. Man darf erwarten, daß die neueren Versuche von SCOTT, der nach Verabreichung von Deltaaminolävulinsäure beim Menschen eine starke Lichtsensibilisierung auftreten sah, noch mehr zum Verständnis der Porphyrinkrankheiten beitragen werden, als die älteren erwähnten und klassisch gewordenen Versuche. Diese Resultate von SCOTT stehen allerdings im Widerspruch zu anderen Arbeiten, und es ist denkbar, daß es sich um latente Porphyrien aus belasteten Familien gehandelt hat.

Andere pharmakologische Eigenschaften der Porphyrine, z.B. Beeinflussung der glatten Muskulatur des Darmes oder der Nervenfunktionen, konnten bisher auch nicht eindeutig nachgewiesen werden, was wiederum die Erklärung internistischer Symptome gewisser Porphyrieformen fast unmöglich macht.

b) Klinische Formen von Porphyrinkrankheiten

Die verschiedenen, immer wieder beobachteten Symptomenkomplexe bei den Porphyrien lassen sich am besten nach den jetzt vielerorts üblichen Einteilungen nach WATSON, WALDENSTRÖM, BRUNSTING oder SCHMID unterteilen. Sie weichen nur unwesentlich voneinander ab. Nach dem Sitz der Störung wird eine *Porphyria erythropoetica* von der Gruppe der *hepatischen Porphyrien* abgetrennt. Die letztere umfaßt den sog. *akut intermittierenden Typ* mit abdominalem und nervösem Symptomenbild, aber ohne Hautläsionen, den *Porphyria cutanea tarda-Typus* mit Bullosis mechanica et actinica und schließlich *Mischtypen*, bei denen gleichzeitig oder aber alternierend Hauterscheinungen und Darm- und Nervensymptome gesehen werden. Dieser Typ entspricht in vielen Zügen dem Bild beim sog. südafrikanischen Typus der hepatogenen Porphyrie mit dominanter Vererbung. Wenn auch diese Einteilung nicht allen Fällen gerecht wird, so erlaubt sie doch die Aufteilung in Symptom-Gruppierungen, die wirklich als abgerundete Krankheitsbilder gelten dürfen.

α) Die Porphyria erythropoetica

Die damit bezeichnete Krankheit ist identisch mit der von GÜNTHER beschriebenen kongenitalen Porphyrie, die man auch als Morbus Günther kennt. Hidroa aestivale bei Porphyrinuria congenita (HAUSMANN, HAXTHAUSEN) und Hidroa vacciniformis (BAZIN) und Porphyria mutilans sind lediglich Synonyma für das gleiche Krankheitsbild. Diese Erbkrankheit ist außerordentlich selten. Wenn nur die schwer mutilierenden Formen hinzugerechnet werden, gehört sie sogar zu den Raritäten, die man an Kongressen ab und zu einmal zu Gesicht bekommt, im eigenen Patientenmaterial aber kaum je antrifft (SCHWARTZ u. SUNDBERG). Nach einer neuesten Zusammenstellung sind in der Weltliteratur bis 1960 nur 41 sichere hierhergehörige Fälle aufzufinden (SCHMID, SCHWARTZ u. SUNDBERG).

Die Hauterscheinungen treten sehr früh, in den ersten Lebensjahren schon, auf. Nach Besonnung zeigen sich an den unbedeckten Körperstellen Rötungen und Schwellungen, die akut von Brennen begleitet auftreten. Anschließend bilden sich Bläschen und Blasen von verschiedener Größe, die rundlich sind und an Varicellen oder an Erythema exsudativum multiforme erinnern mögen. Es fehlen aber Kokarden, und es bilden sich rasch blutige Krusten aus. Nach Abheilung der Schorfe zeigen sich Narben, die zu Mutilationen führen können. Besonders dort, wo sich Blasenschübe immer wiederholen, über der Nase, an den Ohren, ausgesprochen auch an den Fingern, kommt es zur verstümmelnden Narbenbildung. Superinfektion ist an diesen Endausgängen mitbeteiligt. Die Nägel fallen ab, die Fingerendglieder werden atrophisch. Oft sieht man Hyperpigmentierung und Hypertrichosis, bzw. sehr stark ausgeprägte flaumige Lanugobehaarung. An den Schläfen, über den Jochbogen oder an den Vorderarmen ist dieses Symptom meist stark ausgeprägt zu finden. Bei milderen Formen wiederholen sich die Hautveränderungen nur in den sonnenreichen Monaten, im Herbst und Winter kommt es zur Abheilung. Die Verstümmelungen zeigen sich möglicherweise erst nach Jahren. Die Hauterscheinungen und der Verlauf sind natürlich vom Verhalten der Patienten und von den Möglichkeiten, das Licht als Noxe auszuschalten, abhängig.

Hämolytische Anämie, Milz- und auch Lebervergrößerungen sind beschrieben worden. Sie gehören zum Krankheitsbild und lassen sich zwanglos nach dem Schema von STICH erklären. Neurologische und abdominelle Symptome, wie kolikartige Darmkrämpfe und Blähungen, sollten hingegen bei dieser Form nicht vorkommen.

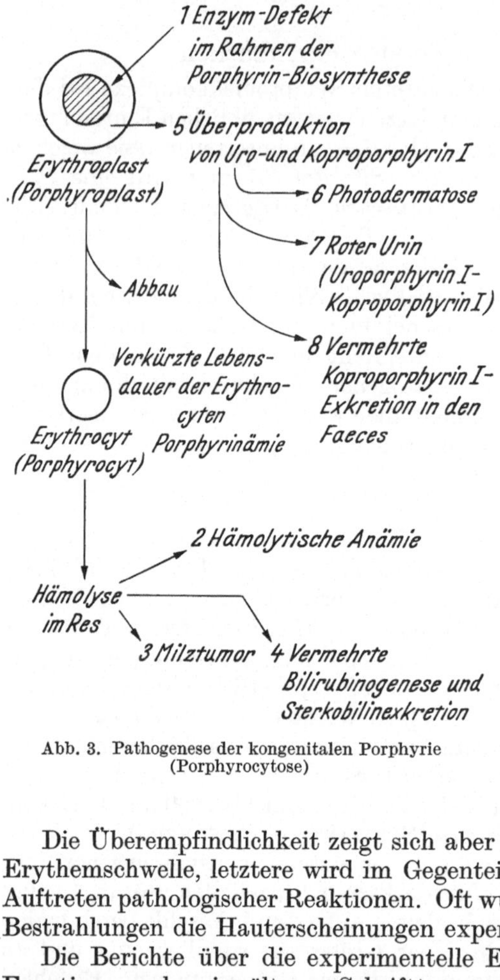

Im Urin wird Uroporphyrin I in beträchtlichen Mengen ausgeschieden. Dieser Befund ist für die Unterscheidung und Klassifizierung der Porphyriefälle ebenfalls sehr wichtig. Koproporphyrin findet man in normalen Mengen oder nur unwesentlich vermehrt. Porphobilinogen soll nicht ausgeschieden werden. Das Porphyrin verfärbt auch ab und zu die Zähne (Erythrodontie), die im Wood-Licht rot fluorescieren. Auch in den Knochen, im Knochenmarksausstrich (Nuclei der Normoblasten), in vereinzelten roten Blutkörperchen (Porphyrocyten) und in Hautschnitten sind im Fluorescenzmikroskop rot fluorescierende Granula nachgewiesen worden (WATSON, SCHMID, SCHWARTZ u. SUNDBERG).

Der auslösende Spektralbereich wird verschieden angegeben. Man darf annehmen, daß das langwellige Ultraviolett (3200—4500 Å), wie bei anderen Erkrankungen, verantwortlich ist.

Abb. 3. Pathogenese der kongenitalen Porphyrie (Porphyrocytose)

Die Überempfindlichkeit zeigt sich aber nicht einfach in einer herabgesetzten Erythemschwelle, letztere wird im Gegenteil meist normal gefunden, sondern im Auftreten pathologischer Reaktionen. Oft wurde beschrieben, daß erst wiederholte Bestrahlungen die Hauterscheinungen experimentell provozieren können.

Die Berichte über die experimentelle Erzeugung von Hidroa vacciniformia-Eruptionen gehen im älteren Schrifttum weit auseinander. Von experimentellen Untersuchungen mit Porphyrininjektionen und nachfolgenden Bestrahlungen sind die Resultate von JEAN MEYER bemerkenswert. Er fand ab und zu photoallergische Reaktionen, nicht Veränderungen der Empfindlichkeitsschwelle, wohl aber pathologische Reaktionsabläufe.

Differentialdiagnostisch kommen bei der Porphyria congenita das Xeroderma pigmentosum, die Epidermolysis bullosa dystrophicans und natürlich die anderen Porphyrinkrankheiten in Betracht.

Alle Symptome finden eine befriedigende Erklärung als Folge einer angeborenen Porphyrinstoffwechselstörung im erythropoetischen System, die mit krankhafter Reaktion auf Lichtstrahlen einhergeht. (Die Krankheit wird daher neuerdings auch als erythropathische, hämolytische Anämie oder als Porphyrocytose beschrieben [STICH 1958]) (Abb. 3).

Die Behandlung hat wenig Aussichten auf Erfolg. Immerhin soll nach WATSON die Lichtempfindlichkeit nach Splenektomie verschwinden. GRAY u. NEUBERGER beobachteten ein Absinken der Uroporphyrinausscheidung im Urin nach Splenektomie. Im übrigen wird man alles Augenmerk auf die Fernhaltung der bekannten Noxe richten. Werden Lichtschutzmittel angewandt, so müssen sie so ausgewählt werden, daß auch das langwellige UV abgehalten wird. Im allgemeinen erwiesen sich solche Maßnahmen als nur wenig wirksam.

β) Porphyria hepatica-Gruppe

Als Porphyria *hepatica* werden vier Formen zu einer Gruppe vereinigt. Davon ist die eine ein internistisches Leiden ohne Hautsymptome. Diese Form, der *akute intermittierende Typ* — auch oft als *akute Porphyrie*, als *akute idiopathische Porphyrie*, als *akute toxische Porphyrie* oder als *abdominell-nervöse Porphyrie* bezeichnet —, wurde früher sicher viel verkannt. Sie führte unter dem Bilde des akuten Abdomens zu unnötigen chirurgischen Eingriffen oder wurde wegen hysteriformer oder halluzinatorischer Symptome auch in psychiatrische Kliniken eingewiesen. Die Urinuntersuchung sollte aber die Situation rasch abklären. Es wird entweder ein portweinfarbener oder ein normal aussehender, dann aber rasch nachdunkelnder Harn ausgeschieden. Allerdings wechseln die Befunde oft rasch, so daß sie, wenn nicht speziell daran gedacht wird, übersehen werden könnten. Ausgeschieden werden Uroporphyrin III und I und Porphobilinogen. Es wurde auch Deltaaminolävulinsäure im Urin nachgewiesen.

Die verschiedenen Symptome: Erbrechen, Obstipation, sehr schmerzhafte Krampfzustände in verschiedenen Darmabschnitten mit gleichzeitiger Erschlaffung und Meteorismus anderer Abschnitte ergeben ein charakteristisches klinisches Bild. Der Dermatologe muß es auch kennen, weil er diese Symptomatologie bei den sog. Mischformen — aus Cutanea tarda-Typus und akutem intermittierendem Typ - wieder antreffen kann. Das gleiche gilt für neuritische Symptome wie Paraesthesien, Hyperaesthesien und Analgesien, für Augenmuskellähmungen, für Muskelatrophien und die psychischen Veränderungen unter dem Bilde von Depressionen, Halluzinationen oder Hysterie, die aber als Intoxikationspsychosen zu erklären wären.

Nach den Angaben von WALDENSTRÖM führt das lebensbedrohliche Krankheitsbild im hohen Prozentsatz von 60% zum Tode. Nur 50% leben noch länger als ein Jahr nach dem ersten Anfall. Die Krankheit verläuft in Schüben; Barbiturate provozieren das Leiden, und die Leber muß sorgfältig geschont werden. Es bestehen keine wirklich befriedigenden Behandlungsmöglichkeiten.

c) Porphyria cutanea tarda

Unter allen mit Störungen des Porphyrinstoffwechsels einhergehenden Krankheiten verdient die als Porphyria cutanea tarda bezeichnete Form die besondere Beachtung der Dermatologen. Es handelt sich um eine scharf und ohne Schwierigkeiten abgrenzbare Untergruppe mit sehr charakteristischen Hautsymptomen. Das Krankheitsbild ist überdies relativ häufig.

In der Regel werden Individuen des mittleren und höheren Alters befallen. Die Hauterscheinungen bleiben ganz auf die unbedeckten, dem Sonnenlicht ausgesetzten Körperpartien beschränkt. Im Gegensatz zu anderen Lichtausschlägen wird aber dem Kranken der Zusammenhang mit der Belichtung in der Regel nicht oder erst spät bewußt. Während ein Patient, der an Eczema solare oder an Lichturticaria leidet, den Arzt bei der Schilderung seiner Krankheitssymptome meistens auch auf den unmittelbaren pathogenetischen Zusammenhang mit einer Besonnung aufmerksam macht, weiß der Kranke mit Porphyria cutanea tarda oft nicht um eine solche Beziehung. Ihm ist meistens nur aufgefallen, daß sich besonders an den Händen, und zwar vorwiegend an den Streckseiten der Finger und an den Handrücken, auf geringfügige Traumen hin blasige Abhebungen der Epidermis ausbilden. Ähnlich wie bei der Epidermolysis bullosa hereditaria genügen nämlich unbedeutende mechanische Insulte wie Reiben, Scheuern und Anstoßen, um an diesen Hautstellen flache oder prall mit Serum gefüllte Blasen entstehen zu lassen. Sehr oft ist deren Inhalt leicht sanguinolent. Es liegt also eine *erhöhte mechanische Lädierbarkeit* vor, eine sog. *Bullosis mechanica.* Im Gegensatz zu den verschiedenen vererbten Formen der Epidermolysis bullosa findet man aber meistens keine familiäre Häufung. Wir haben ferner fast immer den sehr späten Beginn im 4. oder 5. Lebensdezennium zu verzeichnen, und außerdem handelt es sich um ein Syndrom, das auffällig wechselt, indem Remissionen und Exacerbationen miteinander alternieren. Auch bei der Epidermolysis bullosa hereditaria simplex erwähnen zwar die Patienten sehr oft, daß die traumatische Blasenentstehung besonders im Sommer sehr ausgesprochen ist, und daß durch das Schwitzen an Händen und Füßen die Lädierbarkeit zunehme. Die Abgrenzung und Trennung der beiden Krankheitsbilder kann also hin und wieder etwas schwer fallen, und es sind denn auch früher viele Fälle von Porphyria cutanea tarda verkannt und in die Gruppe der Epidermolysis bullosa tarda ohne nachweisbare Vererbung eingereiht worden. Nur die genaue Urinuntersuchung auf Porphyrine kann vor diesem diagnostischen Fehler schützen. Auch muß man berücksichtigen, daß die traumatische Blasenbildung bei Porphyria cutanea tarda auf die dem Licht exponierten Hautpartien beschränkt bleibt, daß also unter gewöhnlichen Bedingungen die Füße praktisch immer frei bleiben. Vor der Einführung der Krankheitsbezeichnung Porphyria cutanea tarda wurden denn auch die meisten hierher gehörenden Beobachtungen als *Bullosis mechanica et actinica*

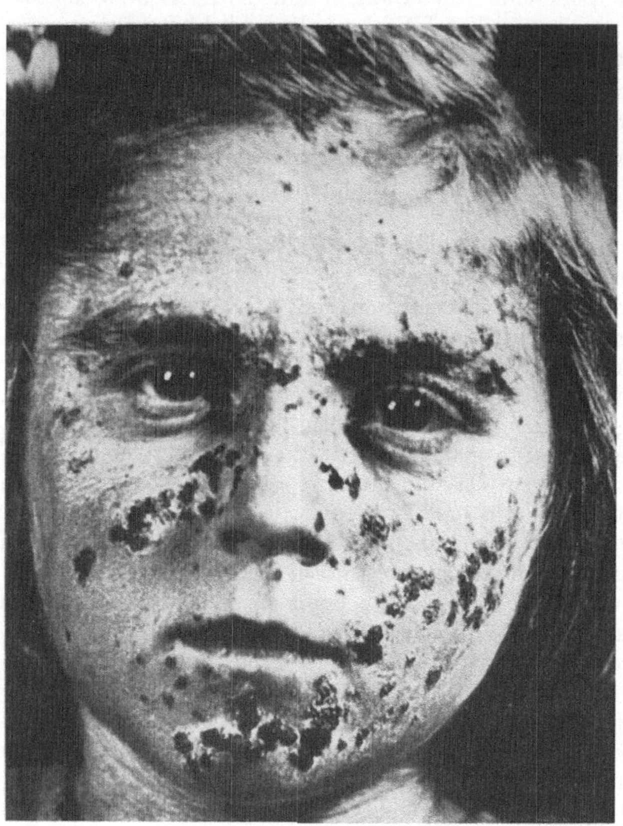

Abb. 4. *Porphyria cutanea*, relativ früh bei einem 8jährigen Mädchen auftretend. (Diese Bilder wurden seinerzeit als Hidroa aestivalis mit Porphyrinurie bezeichnet)

cum porphyrinuria (GOTTRON-ELLINGER) beschrieben. Andere Synonyma sind: Hidroa vesiculo-bullosa oder bullöse Porphyrindermatose (TAPPEINER) (Abb. 4, 5, 6).

Die richtige Erkennung des Syndroms wird oft noch dadurch erschwert, daß im Zeitpunkt der Untersuchung durch den Arzt die Blasen schon nicht mehr vorhanden sind, weil sie sich in krustöse Elemente umgewandelt haben (Abb. 4, 7, 8, 9). Diese Krusten sind meistens braunschwarz und trocken, wenn das Bild nicht durch eine Superinfektion getrübt und verwischt worden ist. Für die Diagnose recht wertvoll sind dann noch eine auffällige diffuse Pigmentierung der Haut, ferner Residuen nach Abheilung früherer Schübe in Form von Milien und gruppierten Horncystchen. Diese Epidermiscystchen sehen wir allerdings auf der

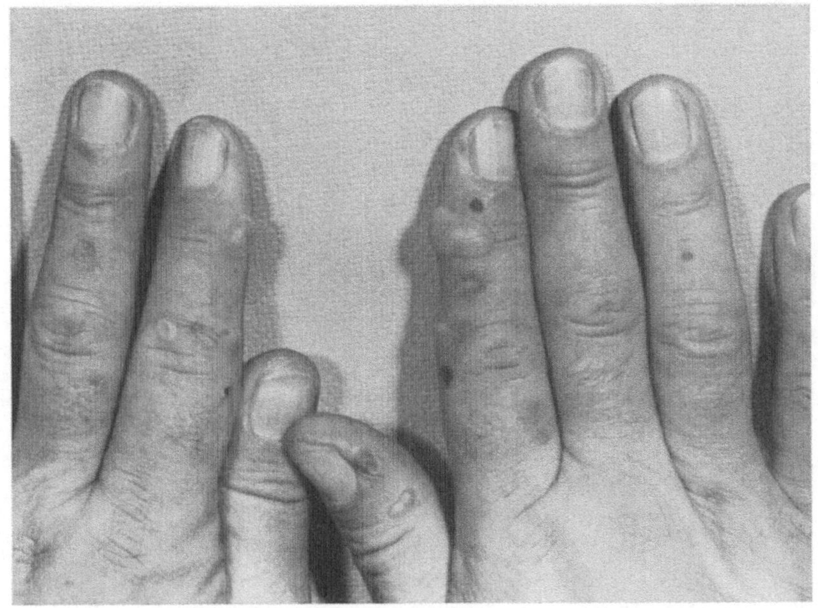

Abb. 5. *Porphyria cutanea tarda.* Blasen und Krusten an den Fingern

anderen Seite auch bei Epidermolysis bullosa, überhaupt bei vielen blasigen Affektionen, bei denen eine rasche Epithelisierung im Laufe der Ausheilung erfolgen kann. Abgeheilte Efflorescenzen hinterlassen bei der Porphyria cutanea tarda manchmal auch weißliche atrophische Flecken, seltener ausgesprochene Narben. Schließlich sei noch erwähnt, daß ab und zu neben der Hyperpigmentierung eine leichte flaumige Hypertrichose, z. B. in der Schläfengegend, die Diagnose Porphyria cutanea tarda erleichtert. Das morphologische Bild der Porphyria cutanea tarda ist somit ein eher einheitliches. Man ist immer wieder überrascht, wie genau sich die Symptomatologie wiederholt, wie sich die Beobachtungen an verschiedenen Kranken bis in alle Einzelheiten decken. Wer einmal einen Fall gesehen und richtig gedeutet hat, wird später keine Schwierigkeiten mehr haben, weitere Einzelbeobachtungen anzugliedern.

Wenn nun aus den beobachteten Hauterscheinungen — vor allem wegen der Bullosis mechanica et actinica — der Verdacht auf eine blasige Porphyrindermatose geschöpft wird, so hat die genaue Urinuntersuchung abzuklären, ob tatsächlich eine Porphyrinurie vorliegt.

In der Regel findet man eine stark vermehrte Ausscheidung von Uroporphyrin III und I. Beim Nachweis der Porphyrinurie in dieser Untergruppe der

Porphyrinkrankheiten ist es nicht unwichtig, immer daran zu denken, daß gerade hier die Ausscheidung pathologischer Porphyrine durch den Harn mengenmäßig

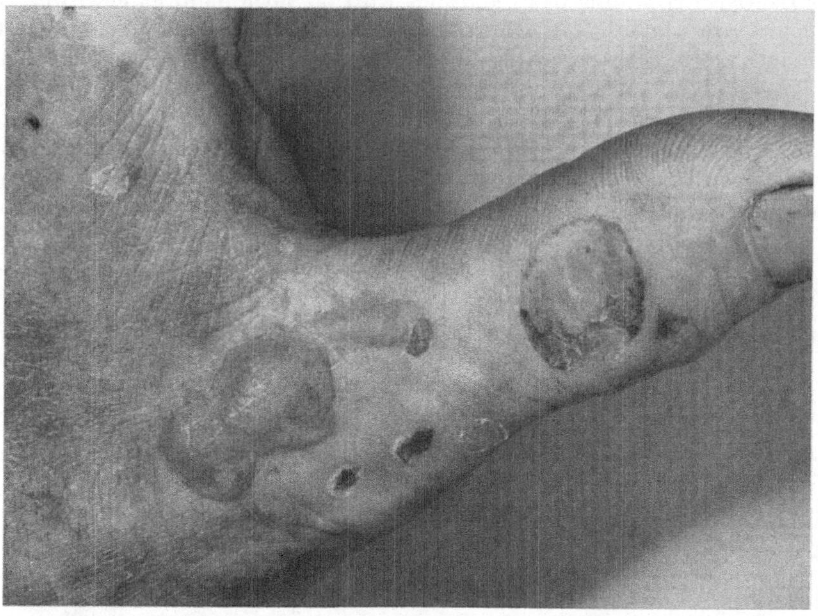

Abb. 6. *Porphyria cutanea tarda.* Detailaufnahme, Blasen in verschiedenen Stadien und Krusten an abheilenden Stellen. Bild der sog. Bullosis actinica et mechanica

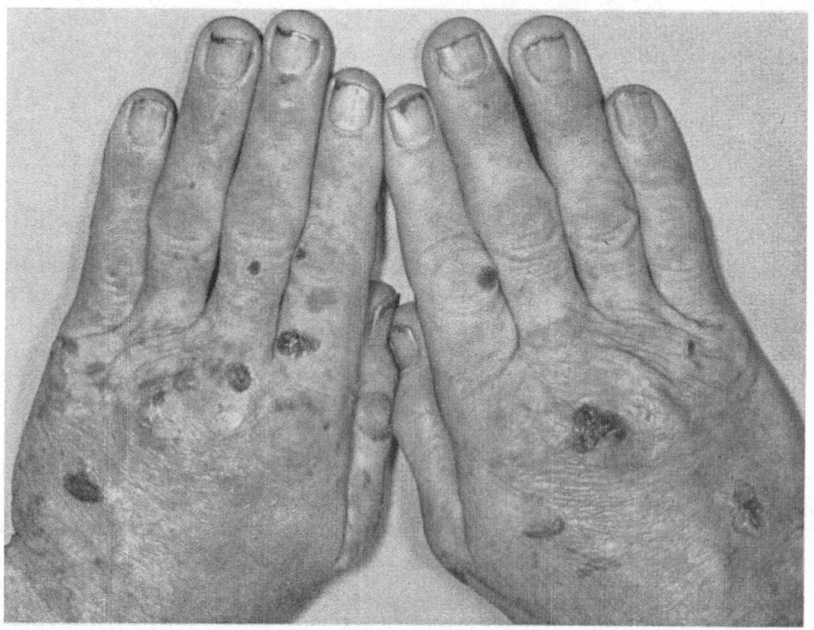

Abb. 7. *Porphyria cutanea tarda,* typischer Befall der Hände

sehr stark und periodisch wechseln kann. Wir müssen deshalb oft mehrmals untersuchen, weil sonst die zugrunde liegende Störung nicht erfaßt werden könnte.

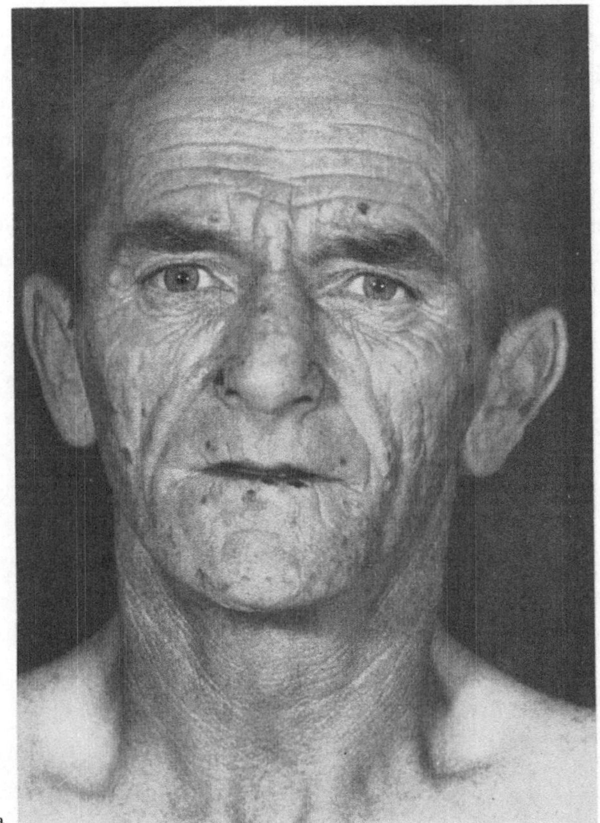

a

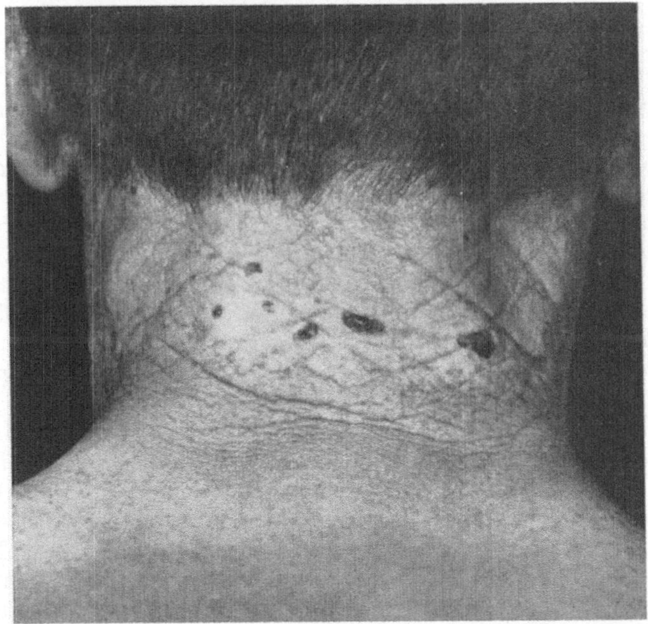

b

Abb. 8a u. b. *Porphyria cutanea tarda.* Abheilende Elemente im Gesicht und am Nacken

Bei der Porphyria cutanea tarda weist die abnorme Porphyrinausscheidung im Urin auf einen Leberschaden hin. Es ist dabei von besonderer klinischer Bedeutung, daß Hauterscheinungen und Porphyrinurie hier offenbar recht häufig die allerersten faßbaren Symptome des Leberleidens sind. In der übergroßen Mehrzahl der bisher beobachteten Fälle handelte es sich um eine chronische Schädigung durch Alkoholabusus. Die Porphyria cutanea tarda wird denn auch in 80—90% bei Männern und nur in 10—20% bei Frauen beobachtet. Neben dem Alkoholismus spielen, besonders bei Frauen, auch andere leberschädigende Faktoren eine Rolle; man hat das Syndrom im Anschluß an Hepatitis, nach Occlusionsikterus, bei chronischem Schlafmittelabusus usw. beobachtet. Immer aber müssen wir an eine — evtl. noch weitgehend latent gebliebene — Leberschädigung denken, und

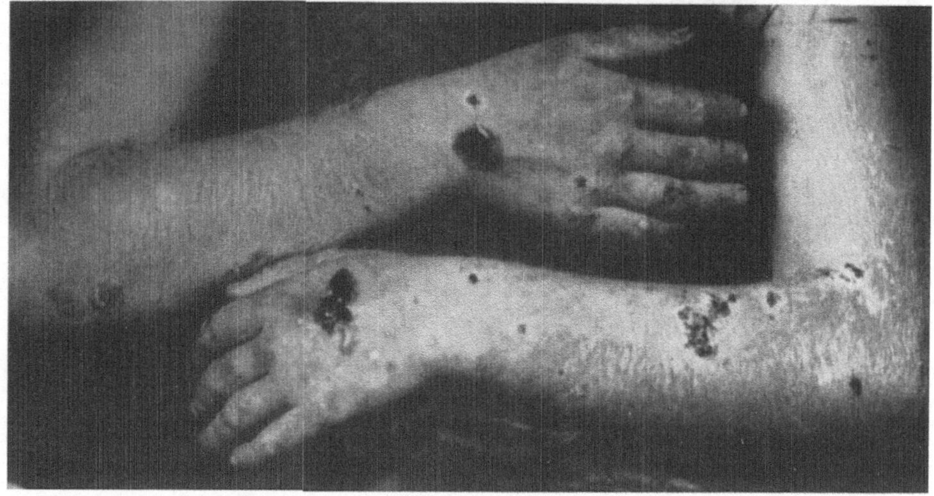

Abb. 9. *Bullös-krustöse Porphyria cutanea* bei einem 8jährigen Mädchen. Starke Hypertrichose

gerade darin haben wir den großen diagnostischen Wert der geschilderten Hautveränderungen zu erblicken.

Werden nun aber auch andere Untersuchungen angestellt, die uns über den Grad der Leberschädigung Auskunft geben könnten, ist man recht oft eher enttäuscht, d.h. außer einer meist positiven Kephalin-Probe sind kaum weitere pathologische Reaktionen zu erwarten. Takata, Galaktose-Belastung usw. ergeben in der Regel noch durchaus normale Werte. Belastungsproben mit Bromsulphalein und Testacid werden noch am ehesten pathologisch ausfallen (IPPEN).

Ich habe mehrmals beobachtet, daß bei einsichtigen Patienten die Hauterscheinungen nach rigoroser Einschränkung des Alkoholkonsums dauernd verschwanden und der Leberschaden keine weiteren Fortschritte mehr machte. In anderen Fällen allerdings geht der Prozeß weiter und endet mit dem gewöhnlichen Bild der schweren alkoholischen Lebercirrhose.

Den Dermatologen interessiert bei dieser bullösen Hautaffektion der histologische Aufbau der Primärefflorescenz (Abb. 10). Das Bild ist bemerkenswert einheitlich. Immer handelt es sich um eine subepitheliale Hohlraumbildung; die Trennung erfolgt stets an der Cutis-Epidermisgrenze unter der Basalmembran. Dabei ragen die nackten Papillen als Fransen in den Spaltraum vor, im Blaseninhalt fehlen zellige Elemente fast vollständig, und auch sonst sind kaum begleitende Entzündungsvorgänge erkennbar (BOLGERT, CANIVET, LE SOURD). Man hat wiederholt versucht, mit speziellen Färbungen die Ursache der erhöhten mechanischen

Lädierbarkeit zu klären. Bisher ist es aber noch nicht gelungen, histochemische Veränderungen an der Epidermis-Cutisgrenze festzustellen, welche uns die spezifische Lockerung der Verbindung und die Neigung zur Spaltbildung erklären könnten. Abgesehen von einigen fluorescenzmikroskopischen Untersuchungen mit gelungenem Nachweis von Porphyrinen auch im Blaseninhalt, sind die histologischen und histochemischen Untersuchungen in bezug auf die Erklärung der Bullosis mechanica resultatlos verlaufen.

Bei Bestrahlungsexperimenten haben unter anderem WISKEMANN und WULF für die Porphyria cutanea tarda nachgewiesen, daß mit langwelligem UV bei niedriger Schwelle kräftige erythematöse Reaktionen auftreten, dies in einem

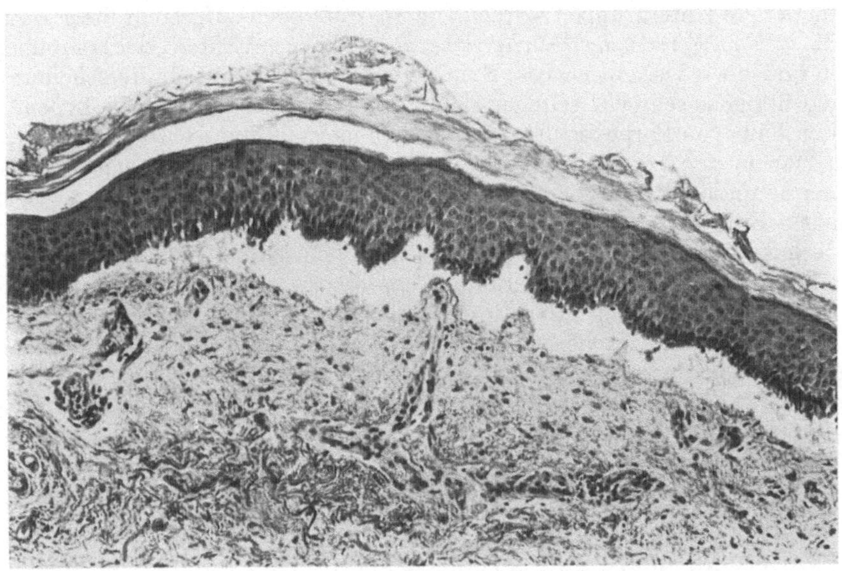

Abb. 10. *Porphyria cutanea tarda*, subepitheliale Blasenbildung

Strahlenbereich, welcher der Absorptionszone der ausgeschiedenen Porphyrine entspricht. Auch bei wiederholter Bestrahlung am gleichen Ort entstanden keine Blasen.

MAGNUS, PORTER und RIMINGTON gelang es, mit einem sehr lichtstarken Monochromator im Wellenlängenbereich 400—600 μ Erytheme und Schwellungen, unter 400 μ bei genügender Bestrahlungsdosis sogar hämorrhagische Blasen hervorzurufen.

Dem Syndrom der Bullosis mechanica et actinica kommt eine große praktisch-diagnostische Bedeutung bei der Erkennung von Leberschäden zu. Genauso, wie uns oft eine chronische Balanitis oder eine Intertrigo der Genitocruralfalten auf das Vorliegen eines Diabetes oder aber das Adenoma sebaceum Pringle auf eine tuberöse Hirnsklerose aufmerksam macht, führt uns hier der bullöse Ausschlag an den Händen auf die Diagnose des latenten, bzw. noch nicht erkannten Leberschadens. Es handelt sich, wie der bekannte Berner Internist SCHÜPBACH humorvoll zu sagen pflegte, um eine internistische Diagnostik über die Hintertreppe der dermatologischen Untersuchung.

Über die Therapie der Porphyria cutanea tarda kann man sich kurz fassen, weil — wie schon erwähnt — in der übergroßen Mehrzahl der beobachteten Fälle ein offensichtlicher Zusammenhang mit chronischem Alkoholabusus besteht.

Wenn es gelingt, den Patienten von der Notwendigkeit der rigorosen Einschränkung des Alkoholgenusses zu überzeugen, und wenn er die dahingehenden Weisungen des Arztes befolgt, so darf mit einer prompten Besserung gerechnet werden. In den Ausnahmefällen, in denen andere Ursachen für den Leberschaden ermittelt werden können, muß man das Grundleiden internistisch behandeln, wobei die allgemein gültigen Regeln der Schondiät, Zufuhr von Vitaminen des B-Komplexes, von Litrison usw. zu befolgen sind. Resochin- oder Nivaquine-Behandlung in der Absicht, die Empfindlichkeitsschwelle für Licht zu erhöhen, kann nicht empfohlen werden, da TAPPEINER, ARESU u. LOSTIA nach solchen Versuchen Exacerbationen beobachtet haben. Von anderer Seite wurde hingegen diese Behandlung mehrfach angegeben.

Als weitere Untergruppen wurden von WATSON noch aufgestellt die *gemischten* und die *latenten Formen der Porphyria hepatica*. Bei gemischten oder kombinierten Fällen finden wir visceral-nervöse Symptome kombiniert mit Hauterscheinungen; sie sind übrigens sehr viel seltener als die beiden vorher umrissenen Typen. Die latenten Fälle von Porphyria hepatica werden meistens dann entdeckt und erfaßt, wenn man in der Verwandtschaft von Kranken mit Porphyria hepatica acuta, weniger häufig bei Patienten mit Porphyria cutanea tarda, nach weiteren Trägern ähnlicher Stoffwechselabweichungen forscht. Es sei nicht verschwiegen, daß gerade mit der Aufstellung der Gruppen der gemischten und latenten Formen viele Schwierigkeiten früherer Einteilungsversuche einfach umgangen worden sind. Die klare Trennung in erythropoetische und hepatische Porphyrien bleibt aber das wesentliche Verdienst der neuen Einteilung von WATSON und wird ihr sicher zu allgemeiner Anerkennung verhelfen. Ebenso wichtig scheint mir die Erkenntnis zu sein, daß die beiden Formen der Porphyria acuta und der Porphyria cutanea tarda relativ häufig zur Beobachtung kommen, während alle anderen Porphyrien zu den ganz seltenen Erkrankungen gehören. Der Besprechung der Porphyria cutanea tarda mußte darum hier etwas mehr Platz eingeräumt werden.

3. Eczema solare und chronisch polymorphe Lichtdermatose

Man ist berechtigt, die Krankheitserscheinungen, die teils als *Eczema solare* (VEIEL), teils als *chronisch polymorpher Lichtausschlag* (HAXTHAUSEN) beschrieben werden, in einem einzigen Kapitel zusammenzufassen. Eine scharfe Trennung dieser Krankheitsbilder ist mit großen Schwierigkeiten verbunden und nicht immer mit der wünschbaren Klarheit möglich. In einigen Dermatologen-Schulen werden als Eczema solare mehr die akuten, stark an Kontaktekzem gemahnenden Bilder zusammengefaßt, als chronisch polymorphe Lichtdermatose hingegen die über längere Zeit ständig rezidivierenden, prurigoartigen Verläufe verstanden, die viel mehr an endogenes oder konstitutionelles Ekzem erinnern. Allerdings muß eine ganz eindeutige Abhängigkeit von der Belichtung und von der Jahreszeit den Beweis liefern, daß nicht banale Krankheiten aus dem Formenkreis des Ekzems vorliegen. Es werden auch andere Einteilungen verwendet. So unterscheidet WULF den ekzematösen, den erythematoiden und den erythematösen Typ innerhalb der Gruppe der chronisch polymorphen Lichtausschläge.

In unseren Breiten sehen wir Fälle von *Eczema solare* vor allem im Frühling und Frühsommer an den belichteten Körperstellen, also besonders im Gesicht, am Hals und Halsausschnitt und an den Armen und Händen auftreten. Bei diesen Patienten — meistens Mädchen oder Frauen — tritt die Lichtgewöhnung relativ rasch ein. Nach einigen Wochen kann die Empfindlichkeit schon ganz verschwunden sein, und erst im nächsten Frühjahr zeigen sich nach den ersten und folgenden Besonnungen erneut Hauterscheinungen. Es ist noch zu wenig abgeklärt, ob die besondere jahreszeitliche Strahlung oder zusätzlich auch die rasche Lichtgewöhnung durch Hornhautverdickung (MIESCHER) für das Zusammendrängen der Krankheitserscheinungen in diese Jahreszeit — der wir ja auch bei anderen Lichtdermatosen begegnen — verantwortlich zu machen ist. In eigenen Beobachtungen ist mir aufgefallen, daß Patientinnen im Februar in den Skiferien im Gebirge nicht erkrankten, wohl aber regelmäßig im April—Mai und Juni im Tiefland, und zwar über mehr als ein Jahrzehnt.

Die chronisch polymorphen Lichtausschläge können sich über viele Monate hinziehen. Hin und wieder sieht man gleichzeitig Lichtüberempfindlichkeit der Conjunctiven (Abb. 11).

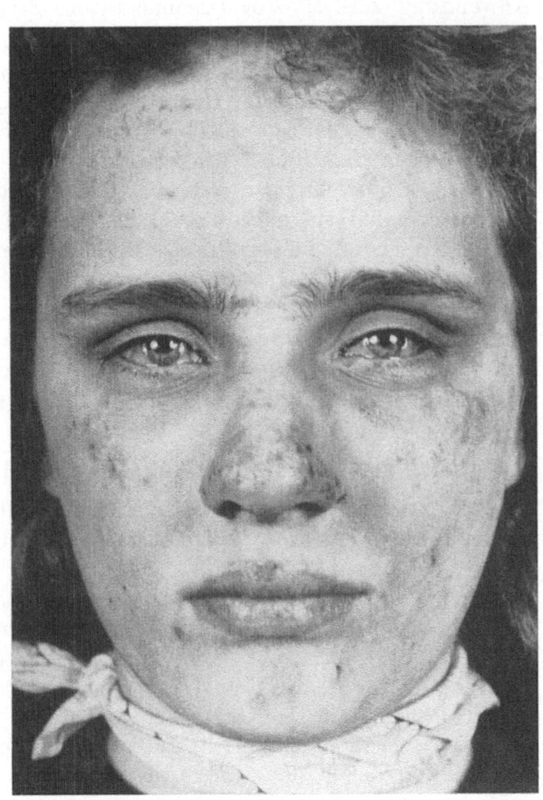

Abb. 11. *Polymorpher Lichtausschlag.* Jahrelang im Frühling und Sommer rezidivierend, später Spontanheilung, evtl. gefördert durch länger dauernde Resochintherapie

Die Differentialdiagnose gegenüber Neurodermitis und Prurigo aestivalis — letztere wahrscheinlich eine Unterform des konstitutionellen Ekzems — kann oft sehr schwierig sein. Vor allem vermissen wir Labormethoden, die unsere Diagnose eindeutig stützen könnten. Porphyrine werden in der Regel nicht vermehrt ausgeschieden. Hingegen hat KIMMIG 1946 im Harn solcher Patienten sog. „Lichtbandstoffe“ mit einer starken Absorption zwischen 480—520 μ nachgewiesen. Es wurde sehr große Mühe auf deren chemische Abklärung verwandt, ohne daß bisher ganz eindeutige Resultate vorliegen. Eiweißspaltprodukte aus dem Tryptophanstoffwechsel scheinen eine besondere Rolle zu spielen. Als ein wichtiger Bestandteil im Harn solcher Patienten wurde N-[β-(Indolyl-(3))-acryloyl]-glycin gefunden (KIMMIG, STICHERLING, TSCHESCHE und URBACH).

Über die Ursache und Pathogenese der Lichtempfindlichkeit in dieser Gruppe bestehen z.T. nur Vermutungen. BARBER und HOWITT fanden oft Achylia gastrica, in deren Gefolge Dysbakterie im Darmtrakt mit Indicanurie, ähnlich LANGHOF und SPRÖSSIG.

Als auslösender Spektralbereich wurden schon immer das UV und Anteile des sichtbaren Lichtes angegeben. Die Untersuchungen von WISKEMANN und WULF ergaben für die Mehrzahl der Untersuchten ein Maximum von pathogener Strahlenwirkung im langwelligen Ultraviolett zwischen 320—400 μ. Auch sichtbares Licht wirkte in einigen Fällen provozierend. Die Erythemschwelle für die Strahlung der Quecksilberdampflampe war nur bei einem Teil der Untersuchten unter die Norm herabgesetzt. Interessant ist ferner, daß ein großer Teil dieser Patienten im Gegensatz zu gesunden Kontrollpersonen im Spektralbereich 300—350 μ nicht direkt pigmentieren kann (WISKEMANN und WULF).

Zur Behandlung wird man je nach den vorliegenden Laborbefunden in erster Linie auf die Darmflora einzuwirken versuchen. Achylie und Anacidität wären mit Säure- und Fermentpräparaten zu bekämpfen, und damit wird sich oft automatisch wieder eine normale Darmflora einstellen. Wie bei anderen Lichtdermatosen sind vor allem Vitamine des B-Komplexes immer wieder versucht worden. Symptomatischen Wert besitzen die Corticosteroide, vor allem auch in lokaler Anwendung, z.B. Hydrocortisonacetat 1—2‰ in einer weichen Kühlpaste.

Resochin kann versucht werden, um die Lichtempfindlichkeit herabzusetzen.

Die gewöhnlichen äußerlichen Lichtschutzmittel sind ungenügend, weil sie im langwelligen UV in der Regel nicht oder nur zu wenig absorbieren. Zinkoxyd- oder titandioxydhaltige Deckpasten oder Schüttelpinselungen, wie sie zum Schutz gegen die Hochgebirgsstrahlung verwendet werden müssen, eignen sich am ehesten auch als Prophylaxe für den polymorphen Lichtausschlag. Kosmetisch können sie allerdings nicht befriedigen und werden darum von den Kranken meist nicht regelmäßig und andauernd verwendet. Als befriedigende Lösung des Problems wird von Ippen die Anwendung der Contralum-Salbe empfohlen.

Die pathologische Lichtempfindlichkeit verschwindet oft scheinbar spontan, jedenfalls ohne ersichtlichen Grund. In anderen Erkrankungsfällen wieder erlebt man oft über eine Periode von vielen Jahren regelmäßig Rezidive.

4. Frühjahrslichtdermatose (Dermatitis vernalis aurium)

Burckhardt hat 1942 „Über eine im Frühling besonders an den Ohren auftretende Lichtdermatose" berichtet; das gleiche Krankheitsbild wurde 1940 von Keining als Frühlingsperniosis beschrieben. Merkwürdigerweise fehlte ein entsprechender Abschnitt sowohl in unseren früheren Handbüchern als auch in den Spezialwerken über das Licht und die lichtbedingten Krankheiten. Eine Arbeit von Julius Heller aus dem Jahre 1907 ist offenbar völlig in Vergessenheit geraten. Unter dem Titel: Über das gehäufte Vorkommen einer eigenartigen Affektion der Haut der Ohrmuscheln bei den Schülern einer Schule (Dermatitis pustularis vernalis aurium) hatte er nämlich damals schon auf diese eigenartige Erkrankung der Kinder hingewiesen. Seine Beschreibung deckt sich mit den späteren Beobachtungen von Burckhardt und Keining und mit den Erfahrungen, die jeder Dermatologe fast alljährlich bei einigen jungen Patienten sammeln kann. Es kann kein Zweifel bestehen, daß es sich um die gleiche harmlose, aber oft in ganzen Gruppen auftretende Lichtaffektion handelt. Die Bezeichnung von Heller scheint mir gut gewählt, nur würde man gerne das Adjectivum „pustularis" durch „papulo-vesiculosa" oder „vesicularis" ersetzen, handelt es sich doch primär um rein papulöse Elemente, die sich z.T. in flache Bläschen weiterentwickeln und nur ausnahmsweise eigentlich pustulös werden. In einem Aufsatz, den ich 1959 über das Krankheitsbild veröffentlichte, habe ich das Beiwort absichtlich aus dem Titel weggelassen.

Die Affektion wird vorwiegend im Kindesalter beobachtet. Neben Einzelfällen findet man sie recht oft bei ganzen Gruppen von Schülern; den Schulärzten dürfte diese Häufung oft begegnen. Wahrscheinlich werden Knaben sehr viel häufiger befallen als Mädchen. Erwachsene und Mädchen bleiben aber nicht immer verschont. Bei Gruppenerkrankungen spielt sicher die gleiche, starke Exposition eine Rolle. Bei denjenigen Fällen, bei welchen sich Jahr für Jahr die Hauterscheinungen im Frühling wieder zeigen, wird man eher an eine besondere Disposition, an einen individuellen Faktor erinnert, wie er ja auch sicher beim echten Eczema solare eine Rolle spielt. Die Knaben erkranken häufiger, weil bei kurzgeschnittenem Haar die Exposition viel kräftiger erfolgt. Oft wird uns von den Eltern der Kinder mitgeteilt, die gleichen Veränderungen seien schon vor einem Jahr oder vor 2 Jahren zur gleichen Saison beobachtet worden. Auch die Laien vermuten meist richtig, daß das Sonnenlicht der auslösende Faktor sei. Bei Erwachsenen konnten wir die Affektion nur sehr selten feststellen. Hin und wieder wurde dann von den Patienten darauf hingewiesen, daß sich die Erkrankung bis in die Schulzeit zurückverfolgen lasse. Sie sei mehr oder weniger regelmäßig alljährlich nach intensiver Frühlingsbesonnung aufgetreten. Meistens befällt die Entzündung beide Ohrmuscheln, wobei der freie Rand in der Regel besonders stark betroffen wird. Interessant sind Beobachtungen von einseitigem Auftreten bei ganzen Schülergruppen, bei welchen dann nur die den Fenstern bzw. dem direkten Sonnenlicht zugewandte Seite erkrankt war (Abb. 12).

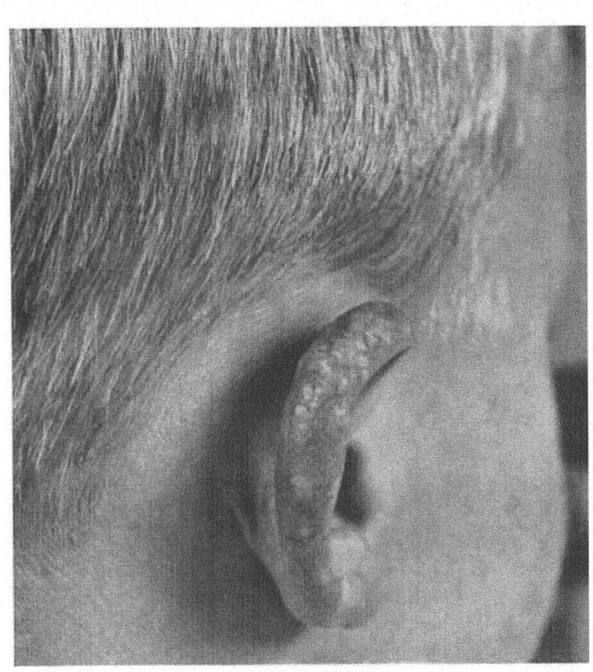

Abb. 12. *Frühlingslichtdermatose*, BURCKHARDT 1942. Dermatitis vernalis aurium, HELLER 1907. Frühlingsperniosis, KEINING 1940

Unter intensivem Brennen oder Jucken entwickeln sich die Hauterscheinungen am Ohrrand in relativ kurzer Zeit. Die Betroffenen fühlen sich im übrigen nicht krank, sondern sind wohlauf. Oft wird die Affektion auch gar nicht weiter beachtet, und weil sie relativ rasch spontan heilt, ist die Beiziehung eines Arztes auch gar nicht nötig. Sieht man die Kranken frühzeitig, so kann man eine vorübergehende diffuse entzündliche Rötung der befallenen Ohrpartie erkennen. Nachher bleiben einzelne Papeln von Stecknadelkopf- bis Linsengröße bestehen. Diese entwickeln sich ganz oder doch zentral zu Bläschen weiter. Letztere trocknen nach kurzem Bestand ein, und unter Abschuppung erfolgt in durchschnittlich 8—10 Tagen die Abheilung. Für einige Zeit sind vielleicht Residuen der durchgemachten Entzündung, rotbraune Verfärbung, Schuppung, Reste von Bläschensäumen noch erkennbar. Im Frühling sehen wir bei Knaben schon abgeheilte Fälle oft noch als Nebenbefund bei Konsultation wegen anderer Hautkrankheiten, was darauf hinweist, daß die Affektion viel häufiger vorkommen muß, als man etwa nach der Diagnosenstatistik einer Poliklinik annehmen könnte.

Eine Behandlung ist in den allermeisten Fällen unnötig, denn die Dermatitis heilt ohne Komplikationen spontan wieder ab. Bei Fällen, die Jahr für Jahr wieder rezidivieren, stellt sich hingegen die Frage einer vorbeugenden Therapie. Sowohl die lokale Anwendung von Lichtschutzmitteln als die interne Verabreichung von Nivaquine und Resochin müßten sich erwartungsgemäß günstig auswirken.

Differentialdiagnostisch ergeben sich meistens keine Schwierigkeiten. Eine gewisse Ähnlichkeit mit dem Erythema exsudativum multiforme ist hervorzuheben, besonders da von BURCKHARDT festgestellt wurde, daß auch histologisch ein ähnliches Bild mit subepithelialer Blasenbildung vorliegt. Besonders zu erwähnen ist die Hidroa vacciniformis, haben wir doch hier Analogien sowohl in der Morphologie (auch die Hidroa vacciniformis befällt mit Vorliebe die Ohren, daneben aber auch Nasenspitze und Wangen, evtl. die Hände) als in der Pathogenese. Man wird besonders bei Erwachsenen die Ausscheidung von Porphyrin untersuchen, um nicht eine Porphyria cutanea tarda zu übersehen. In der Arbeit von HELLER werden die Hydroa puerorum Unna und die Dermatitis recurrens aestivalis Ratcliffe Cocker als in der Differentialdiagnose zu berücksichtigende Affektionen genannt. Für die heutigen Dermatologen ist es allerdings schwer, sich unter diesen Bezeichnungen Krankheitsbilder vorzustellen, die noch Bestand haben.

Weil die Dermatitis vernalis aurium hin und wieder ganze Gruppen von Schülern erfaßt, ist natürlich auch der Gedanke an ein epidemieartiges infektiöses Geschehen aufgetaucht. Schon KEINING vermutete, daß die von KOCH und KÖHLER in den Monaten April und Mai beobachteten Epidemien von infektiösem Erythema exsudativum multiforme wahrscheinlich eher seiner Frühjahrsperniosis oder also HELLERs Dermatitis vernalis aurium zuzurechnen seien. In der Tat findet man kaum je Infektionsketten von Erythema exsudativum multiforme, was ich hier nicht als Argument gegen seine infektiöse Natur anführen möchte, denn auch bei Zoster und bei Herpes simplex fallen solche Infektionsketten selten auf. Ihre infektiöse Natur bleibt aber durch experimentelle Übertragungen trotzdem bewiesen. Die pathogenetische Erklärung, die KEINING für die „Frühlingsperniosis" anführt, sei kurz erwähnt und besprochen. Er weist auf die besonderen Witterungsbedingungen in der Zeit zwischen Mitte April bis Mitte Mai hin, auf die Kombination von Morgenfrösten und starker Insolation in den Nachmittagsstunden. Er glaubt, daß Vasoconstriction unter dem Kältereiz und sehr rasche Wiedererwärmung unter dem Einfluß der Sonnenstrahlung eine wichtige Rolle spielen und erklärt die Krankheit so als kombinierten Kälte-Strahlenschaden. Bei einem Großteil der eigenen Beobachtungen kann allerdings diese Erklärung nicht zutreffen, weil wir die Erscheinungen sehr oft zu einer Jahreszeit auftreten sehen, in welcher die Kälte keine Rolle mehr spielen konnte. Auch sahen wir die Veränderungen ausschließlich an den Ohren, hingegen nicht die Kombination an Ohren und Hand- und Fingerrücken, wie sie von KEINING als Frühjahrsperniosis beschrieben wird. Bei derartigen Kombinationen ist differentialdiagnostisch auch an atypischen Erythematodes disseminatus zu denken, an ein Krankheitsbild, bei dem Lichtprovokation und Lichtlokalisation immer wieder vorkommen.

5. Cheilitis exfoliativa actinica (S. AYRES jr.), Sommercheilitis (MARCHIONINI)

Die lichtbedingte Entzündung der Unterlippe wurde 1923 zuerst von S. AYRES jr. beschrieben. Später wurde das Leiden auch in Europa und im vorderen Orient beobachtet (GOUGEROT, KATZENELLENBOGEN, GRIN, DOJMI). Eine eingehende Bearbeitung stammt von MARCHIONINI und TOR, welche diese besondere Cheilitisform bei ständig im Freien arbeitenden Personen im Hochland gehäuft feststellen konnten.

Die klinischen Erscheinungen der Cheilitis actinica wechseln in der Intensität je nach Jahreszeit mit der Sonnenstrahlung und vielleicht auch im Zusammenhang mit anderen Klimafaktoren. In akuten Stadien sieht man eine entzündliche Schwellung der Unterlippe mit lividroter Verfärbung, und der Patient klagt über schmerzhaftes Spannungsgefühl. Es treten Bläschen auf, die in dieser Lokalisation rasch aufplatzen und so Erosionen und Krusten entstehen lassen. Es können auch etwas tieferreichende Ulcerationen auftreten, und durch Sekundärinfektion sind verschiedene morphologische Abweichungen zu erklären.

Die Erkrankung kann sich über Monate hinziehen, wobei sie meist wochenlang noch ein desquamatives Stadium durchläuft. Im Herbst und Winter erfolgt dann Abheilung, und zwar meistens ohne Residuen; nach geschwürigen Stadien bleiben allerdings Narben zurück. In den folgenden Jahren kann die Erkrankung rezidivieren, wobei oft ein von Jahr zu Jahr verschlimmertes Bild beobachtet wurde. Bei derartigen chronisch-rezidivierenden Verlaufsformen geht die Cheilitis möglicherweise in eine Präcancerose über, und als weitere Folgekrankheit schließt sich ein Stachelzellcarcinom an. Ob dabei das Licht als eigentlich cancerogener Faktor wirkt, oder ob der chronisch entzündliche Prozeß aus anderen Gründen zur Präcancerose wird — wie auch bei chronischen Verlaufsformen der Cheilitis glandularis —, steht vorderhand noch nicht fest. Der genauere Mechanismus der krebserzeugenden Lichtwirkung bedarf auch sonst noch der näheren biochemischen Abklärung. Die Kombination von Cheilitis actinica mit Heterotopie der Schleimspeicheldrüsen der Unterlippen wurde von MICHALOWSKI hervorgehoben.

Als Ursache der Cheilitis actinica betrachtet man allgemein den kurzwelligen Anteil des Sonnenspektrums. Photosensibilisierende Substanzen scheinen dabei nicht beteiligt zu sein. Geringe Luftfeuchtigkeit wird aber durch Austrocknung den Prozeß fördern. Individuen mit einer vollen, vorgewölbten Unterlippe scheinen mehr als andere an Cheilitis actinica zu erkranken, was sich wohl am einfachsten mit den die Absorption besonders begünstigenden Lichteinfallswinkeln erklären läßt.

Über Prophylaxe und Therapie ist bisher relativ wenig bekannt. Der Schutz der Lippen vor zu starker Ultraviolettbestrahlung ist auch im Hochgebirge ein schwieriges Problem. Die gewöhnlichen Lichtschutzmittel werden von vielen Personen durch ticartiges, ständiges Befeuchten der Unterlippe oft ganz rasch wieder entfernt, so daß sie gar nicht wirken können. In solchen Fällen versprechen nur dicke Deckpasten, die sich schwer wegwischen lassen, oder aber das Verbinden von Tüchern und das Tragen breitrandiger Sommerhüte Erfolg.

6. Lichturticaria (Urticaria solaris)

Die Lichturticaria kann in einem System der Hautkrankheiten an verschiedenen Stellen eingeordnet werden. Man würde sie in einem Lehrbuch mit Recht bei den cutan-vasculären Allergien vom Typus des Nesselfiebers abhandeln und sie einfach den anderen bekannten sog. *physikalischen Allergien* — der Kälte- oder Wärme-Urticaria und der Urticaria factitia — beiordnen. Es soll ihr aber hier ein kurzer Abschnitt gewidmet sein, weil doch einige Besonderheiten hervorgehoben werden müssen und weil die z.T. neueren Ergebnisse über den auslösenden Strahlungsbereich uns zum Vergleich mit den Befunden bei anderen Lichtdermatosen anregen können.

Die Lichturticaria wird sehr viel seltener beobachtet als das Kälte- und Wärmenesselfieber oder gar die Urticaria factitia. Wenige Minuten nach der Besonnung entstehen auf der Haut Rötungen, Schwellungen und Quaddeln, die von starkem Jucken begleitet sind. Vor allem sind es Körperpartien, die normalerweise nicht belichtet werden, welche stark reagieren können. Die Hauterscheinungen respektieren die Grenzen zwischen belichteten und bedeckten Gebieten ziemlich streng. Vor allem sind, im Gegensatz zu den Verhältnissen bei Urticaria factitia und Urticaria e frigore, Fernquaddeln an nicht belichteter Haut kaum je beobachtet worden. Hingegen hat WUCHERPFENNIG darauf hingewiesen, daß bei experimenteller Auslösung das Ödem die bestrahlte Zone nur einige Millimeter überschreitet, so daß man auf eine diffundierende Mittlersubstanz schließen darf.

Eine Sonderstellung muß der familiären, protoporphyrinämischen Lichturticaria (LANGHOF, MÜLLER u. RIETSCHEL) eingeräumt werden. Bei dieser Untergruppe werden nach intensiver Bestrahlung auch Quaddeln in der Umgebung der Bestrahlungsfelder beobachtet, es kommt weiter zu pellagraartigen Hyperkeratosen an den Handrücken, ferner zu Degenerationen, die an Kolloidmilium erinnern. Es scheint sich um eine kongenitale protoporphyrinämische Lichtdermatose zu handeln, die mit Aminacidurie, Sideropenie und Störungen der Blutgerinnung gekoppelt ist. Die Diagnose ist schwierig, denn das im Überschuß vorhandene Protoporphyrin erscheint nicht im Urin. Hingegen ist es für die Rotfluorescenz der Erythroblasten und Erythrocyten im UV-Licht verantwortlich, ferner für eine rot-braune Fluorescenz der Epidermis im Gefrierschnitt, welche aber nach etwa 30 sec Belichtung im Fluorescenzmikroskop erlöscht.

Die Lichturticaria tritt plötzlich ohne ersichtlichen Grund meist bei Menschen im mittleren Alter auf. Wie bei der Kälteurticaria verschwindet sie evtl. später wieder, ohne daß auch hierfür eine stichhaltige Begründung gefunden werden könnte.

Die Reproduktion der Krankheitserscheinungen im Bestrahlungsversuch gelingt ohne Schwierigkeit, sofern man eine normalerweise wenig belichtete Hautstelle für diesen Test auswählt.

Sehr auffällig ist nun, daß, je nach dem auslösenden Strahlenbereich, offenbar verschiedene Typen von Lichturticaria aufgefunden worden sind (BLUM, BAER und SULZBERGER, BURCKHARDT, WISKEMANN und WULF), wobei sich überdies noch Unterschiede in der passiven Übertragbarkeit der Allergie nach PRAUSNITZ-KÜSTNER ergaben. Es ist recht bezeichnend für die heutige Situation in der modernen Dermatologie, daß ein scheinbar so einfaches Symptomenbild, wie die Lichturticaria, bei genauer Analyse noch in Unterformen aufgeteilt werden muß, die sich immerhin durch einen wesentlichen Punkt — eben die passive Übertragbarkeit — voneinander unterscheiden.

Was löst beim Patienten mit Lichturticaria die allergische Reaktion an den cutanen Gefäßen aus? Man wird in erster Linie an eine Mittlersubstanz denken, an einen körpereigenen chemischen Stoff, der normalerweise bei allen Bestrahlten entsteht, auf den nun aber der Patient *überempfindlich ist bzw. geworden ist* (BURCKHARDT). Auch FINDELSBERGER und LINDENMAYR nehmen ein „Sekundärallergen“ an, um die Quaddelbildung durch das Licht erklären zu können.

Als Behandlung kommen desensibilisierende Bestrahlungen in Betracht, die offenbar eine Gewöhnung erzwingen können. Über den Wert der Antihistaminica wird sehr unterschiedlich geurteilt. BURCKHARDT hatte jedenfalls bei seiner Beobachtung guten Erfolg mit Antergan.

Will man zur Prophylaxe lokal lichtschützende Substanzen anwenden, muß bei ihrer Wahl der auslösende Strahlenbereich berücksichtigt werden.

II. Photosensibilisierung und Photoallergie

Von der physiologischen Lichtwirkung und den Lichtschädigungen, welche nach Überschreitung der tolerierten Dosis unweigerlich auftreten, wollen wir eine besondere Gruppe von Reaktionen abtrennen, bei der *Vermittlersubstanzen*, sog. Sensibilisatoren, eine Rolle spielen. Man kennt diese Erscheinungen schon lange unter dem Begriff der photodynamischen Reaktion (RAAB, JODLBAUER und TAPPEINER). Die ersten, grundlegenden Erkenntnisse wurden in pharmakologischen Versuchen an Paramaecien erarbeitet. Während im Dunkeln gehaltene Infusorien den Zusatz fluorescierender Substanzen (Acridin, Eosin usw.) zum Medium bis zu einer gewissen Konzentration anstandslos ertragen, gehen die gleichen Tiere unter sonst identischen Bedingungen bei zusätzlicher Belichtung rasch ein, wobei meistens ein Exzitationsstadium vorausgeht. Ähnliche Versuche mit weitgehend übereinstimmenden Resultaten wurden auch an Warmblütern, an weißen Mäusen und an Kaninchen gemacht. Ferner lassen sich eine ganze Reihe von Erkrankungen der Weidetiere nur erklären, wenn man als pathogenes Prinzip photodynamische Erscheinungen annimmt.

Die Versuche von HAUSMANN und HAXTHAUSEN müssen als Grundlagen für unsere Vorstellungen über die photodynamischen Erscheinungen gewertet werden. Auch der bekannte Selbstversuch von MEYER-BETZ, bei dem nach intravenöser Hämatoporphyrin-Injektion schwere akute Photosensibilisierungserscheinungen und auch mildere Zeichen von Lichtüberempfindlichkeit, ausgelöst durch glasgefiltertes Sonnenlicht, auftraten, gehört zu den fundamentalen Kenntnissen. GREITHER hat einen Teil der Hausmannschen Versuche wieder aufgenommen und an den bisherigen Erklärungen Kritik geübt. Bei künftigen experimentellen Untersuchungen wären auch seine Ergebnisse zu berücksichtigen. Solche pharmakologischen Analysen können auf breiter Basis notwendig werden, spielen doch in neuerer Zeit bei Einführung von Pharmaka teils Photosensibilisierung, teils Lichtallergie als Ursache für Nebenerscheinungen eine große Rolle.

Die meisten photosensibilisierenden Substanzen fluorescieren. Es besteht aber kein direkter Zusammenhang zwischen photodynamischen Erscheinungen und Ausstrahlung von Fluorescenzlicht; die Fluorescenz ist lediglich ein Anzeichen dafür, daß wir es mit einem Molekül zu tun haben, welches strahlende Energie in Form von Lichtquanten aufnimmt, sich anregen läßt und dann unter anderem evtl. Fluorescenzlicht ausstrahlt. Wichtiger als die Ausstrahlung von Fluorescenzlicht durch das angeregte Molekül ist die Übertragung von Energie auf Nachbarmoleküle, der photochemische Zerfall und die Auslösung von Kettenreaktionen in der Umgebung des Sensibilisators. Wenn auch gewisse Einzelheiten noch als unbewiesene Hypothesen zu beurteilen sind, so darf doch angenommen werden, daß wir es primär mit einem physikochemischen Vorgang zu tun haben und daß wir auch alle unsere Kenntnisse aus der Photochemie mit Sensibilisatoren (KUHN) auf diese Erscheinungen bei Mensch und Tier anwenden dürfen. Es sei an dieser Stelle nur an die in letzter Zeit etwas in Vergessenheit geratenen Versuche von KITCHEVATZ erinnert, der mit pflanzlichen Photosensibilisatoren die Rückenhaut behandelte und dann durch ein photographisches Negativ hindurch bestrahlte, worauf die Haut mit Entzündungserscheinungen reagierte, welche die Landschaft auf dem Negativ als Positiv erkennen ließen. Der Sensibilisator macht die menschliche Haut für einen Strahlenbereich, das langwellige UV, empfindlich, der ohne Einschaltung einer Vermittlersubstanz normalerweise kaum Entzündungserscheinungen auslösen kann, wohl aber in einem Teil der Fälle die Sofortpigmentierung herbeiführt (HENSCHKE, SCHULZE; MIESCHER und MINDER).

Bei der Photosensibilisierung spielt die individuelle Empfindlichkeit keine oder doch nur eine ganz untergeordnete Rolle. Bei richtiger Versuchsanordnung läßt sich, immer wieder reproduzierbar, das gleiche Resultat erreichen. Wir sprechen darum am besten von *obligater Photosensibilisierung* und hätten nur noch weiter zu unterscheiden, ob der Sensibilisator von außen percutan oder von außen peroral bzw. parenteral (intramuskulär oder intravenös) zugeführt wird. BURCKHARDT nennt in einem anerkennenswerten Einteilungsversuch der Lichtdermatosen diese Wirkungen die phototoxischen photodynamischen Erscheinungen, denen die photoallergischen Erscheinungen gegenübergestellt werden.

Unter allergischen Photosensibilisierungserscheinungen (ST. EPSTEIN) haben wir diejenigen Befunde zusammenzufassen, bei denen wir zwar auch eine von außen einwirkende Vermittlersubstanz kennen, bei denen wir ferner das Licht als auslösenden Faktor brauchen, aber außerdem noch auf irgendeine Weise ein persönlicher Überempfindlichkeitsfaktor mit im Spiele ist. Paradigmata für diese Gruppe von Lichtdermatosen sind gewisse Arzneimittelexantheme nach Sulfonamiden und nach Phenothiazinderivaten (s. unten, Kapitel Photoallergie).

Photodynamische Erscheinungen spielen auch bei einem Teil der eigentlichen oder idiopathischen Lichtkrankheiten eine Rolle. Das Prinzip ist bei gewissen Porphyrien wirksam, vermutlich auch bei den sog. polymorphen Lichtausschlägen, die aber in Anlehnung an früher übliche Einteilungen des Stoffes schon im vorangehenden Abschnitt besprochen worden sind.

1. Hautveränderungen, ausgelöst durch obligate Photosensibilisierung

Unsere Kenntnisse von den obligaten, meist percutanen Photosensibilisierungen beruhen vorwiegend auf den alten Erfahrungen, die im Laufe von Jahrzehnten mit *Teer und Teerprodukten*, mit *Acridinfarbstoffen* und mit *verschiedenen Pflanzen* gemacht worden sind (Phytophotodermatosen).

Am geläufigsten sind dem Hautarzt die durch *Steinkohlenteer* verursachten *Photosensibilisierungen.* Während oder unmittelbar nach der Teerbehandlung von Ekzemen treten starke Entzündungserscheinungen auf, wenn sich die Patienten ungeschützt der Sonne aussetzen. Zu dieser Sensibilisierung kommt es vor allem dann, wenn der Teer ziemlich gut, aber doch unvollständig entfernt worden ist. Bleiben größere Reste von Teerpasten oder ein Teerfirnis zurück, so verhindern sie möglicherweise durch Absorption der Strahlung eine photodynamische Reaktion (Filterwirkung). Meistens merkt der Patient selbst, daß seine Haut nach einer Teerbehandlung für die Besonnung überempfindlich geworden ist. Er spürt schon nach kurzer Expositionszeit ein Brennen in der Haut und unterbricht darum oft die Besonnung, oder er sucht sich zu schützen. Vielleicht sieht man aus diesem Grunde nur selten hochgradige Reaktionen. Meist bleibt es bei Rötungen und Schwellungen mit nachfolgender besonders kräftiger Pigmentierung.

Auch als Berufskrankheit wird Teer-Photosensibilisierung beobachtet, z.B. in Korksteinfabriken, in Kabelwerken (LEWIN), beim Arbeiten mit Karbolineum (HERXHEIMER u. NATHAN), wahrscheinlich auch beim Straßenbau, wenn nämlich Gasteer oder Asphalt verwendet wird und gleichzeitig kräftige Sonnenbestrahlung einwirkt (FOERSTER u. SCHWARTZ, ROSS).

Experimentell wurden diese Teer-Photosensibilisierungen durch FLEISCHHAUER, BAYER und BURCKHARDT u.a. abgeklärt. Vor allem eignet sich der belichtete Epicutantest; es kann aber auch einfach eine dünne Teerlösung oder eine Lösung der wirksamen Teerfraktion auf die Haut aufgepinselt werden, die dann mit natürlichem Sonnenlicht oder mit gefiltertem Licht der Quecksilberdampflampe oder eines Kohlenbogens bestrahlt wird. Die folgenden Teerbestandteile erwiesen sich als stark sensibilisierend: Anthracen, B-Methyl-Anthracen, Pyren, Fluoranthren, Benzpyren. Nach Untersuchungen von BURCKHARDT sind hingegen Stilben, Fluoren, Reten, Acenaphthen, Naphthalin, Phenanthren, Carbazol, Krysen und Methylcholanthren nicht photodynamisch aktiv.

Zu den häufig beobachteten percutanen Photosensibilisierungen gehören die Phytophotodermatosen, die, soweit man das heute übersehen kann, fast ausschließlich durch Furocumarine (KUSKE) ausgelöst werden.

Die Dermatitis bullosa striata pratensis (OPPENHEIM 1917) bildete die eine Grundlage für alle weiteren Forschungen; die *Berlock-* oder *Kölnischwasser-Dermatitis* (FREUND 1916) war die andere Basis, von der aus die Abklärung weiter vorangetrieben werden konnte. Einzelheiten über den Gang der Abklärung der Photosensibilisierung durch pflanzliche Wirkstoffe können in den Arbeiten von KUSKE und von IPPEN, der den Ausdruck Photodermatitis pigmentata für alle hierhergehörenden Beobachtungen vorschlägt, nachgelesen werden.

Das 1940 von mir mehr oder weniger abschließend bearbeitete Kapitel hat seit den Mitteilungen von ägyptischen Autoren (EL MOFTY) einen neuen Aspekt bekommen. Die Angaben über erfolgreiche Behandlungen von Vitiligo mit Präparaten aus Ammi majus, einer ägyptischen Umbellifere, wurden mit höchstem Interesse aufgenommen und überall nachgeprüft. Die anfänglichen Hoffnungen wurden allerdings weitgehend enttäuscht. Bald stellte sich heraus, daß unter bisher ungebräuchlichen Namen (Ammoidin, Majudin, Ammidin) die altbekannten Furocumarine (Xanthtoxin = 8-Methoxypsoralen, Bergapthen = Methoxypsoralen und Imoeratoxin = 8-Isoamylenoxypsoralen) neu beschrieben wurden. Diese vom Chemiker SPÄTH rein dargestellten Furocumarine hatten KUSKE mit weiteren Vertretern aus der Stoffklasse schon 1939 für seine Experimente zur Verfügung gestanden.

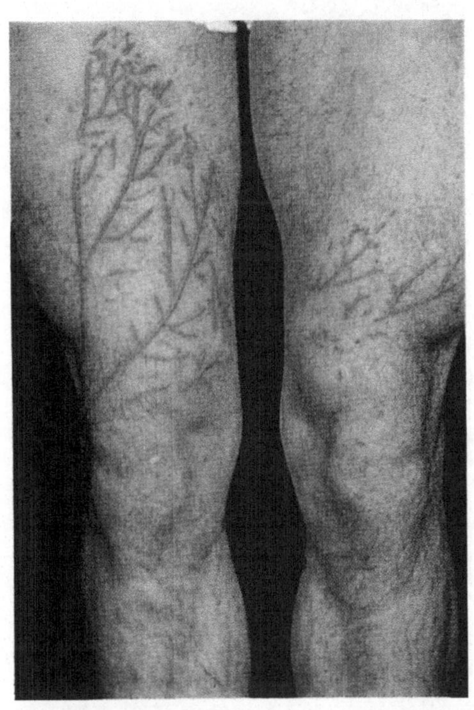

Abb. 13. Phyto-Photodermatose durch Heracleum mantegazzianum

Neu und aufsehenerregend war vorerst die perorale Verabreichung der Sensibilisatoren. Sie hat sich bis zu einem gewissen Grade bewährt. In Nachprüfungen haben auch wir durch alleinige perorale Gaben von Meladinin und Sonnenlichtbestrahlungen in Einzelfällen sehr schöne Repigmentierungen erzielen können. Leider lohnt sich die aufgewendete Mühe kaum, weil nach Absetzen der Therapie das neugebildete Pigment rasch wieder verlorengeht. Auch ist eine einheitliche kosmetisch wirklich befriedigende Repigmentierung kaum je zu erreichen. Von der percutanen Sensibilisierung ist eher abzuraten, weil Überdosierungen schwer zu vermeiden sind. Hochgradige bullöse Dermatitis mit bleibenden Pigmentverschiebungen werden beobachtet.

Von der Einnahme von Furocumarinen lediglich zur Verstärkung der Bräunung bei *Sonnen*bädern muß man ebenfalls abraten. Die zuverlässigsten Angaben über Erfolge und Mißerfolge mit photosensibilisierender Behandlung finden sich bei JARRET u. SZABÓ, die auch eine Einteilung der Vitiligo in verschiedene Schweregrade als Grundlage für alle kritischen Beurteilungen der therapeutischen Methode vorschlagen.

Phytophotodermatosen werden in Europa besonders häufig durch den wild wachsenden Pastinak (Pastinaca sativa) und durch die kultivierte, aber leicht verwildernde Riesenbärenklau (Heracleum Mantegazzianum) ausgelöst (Abb. 13, 14, 15). Je nach der geographischen Lage spielen auch die Feige (Ficus carica) oder andere furocumarinhaltige Pflanzen die auslösende Rolle (Peucedanum Ostruthium, Angelica officinalis, Ruta graveolens, Citrus Bergamiae, Ammi majus, Dictamnus alba).

Bei der kurzen Besprechung der Meladininbehandlung der Vitiligo haben wir das Kapitel der percutanen Photosensibilisierung z. T. schon verlassen und über Sensibilisierung nach peroraler Einnahme des Sensibilisators gesprochen.

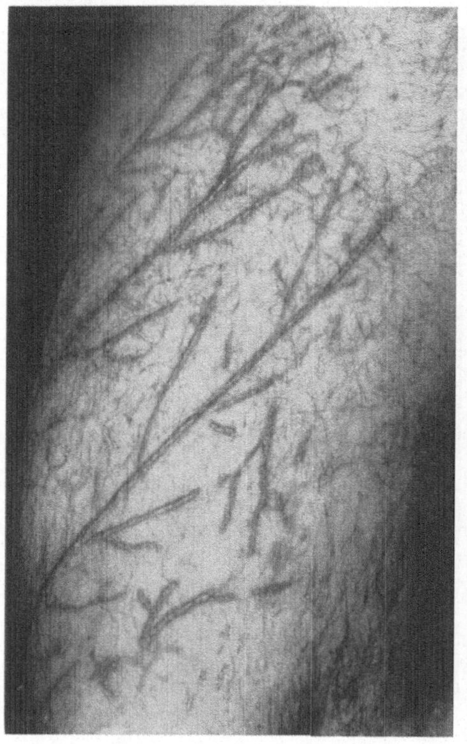

Abb. 14

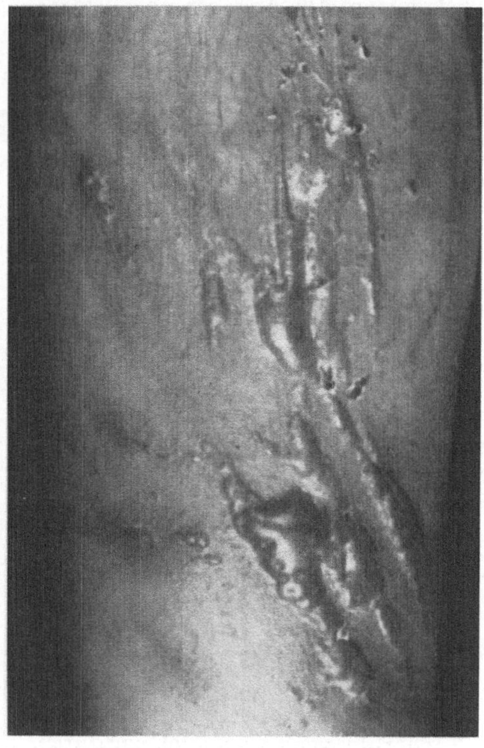

Abb. 15

Abb. 14 u. 15. *Phyto-Photodermatitis* (Dermatitis bullosa striata pratensis) nach Kontakt mit Blättern des „Riesenbärenklau" (Heracleum Mantegazzianum). Häufiger entstehen diese Badeausschläge nach Kontakt mit der wild wachsenden Pastinaca sativa. Hier entstand der Ausschlag, weil sich Badende auf Blätter der verwildert wachsenden Riesen-Umbellifere gelegt hatten und sich anschließend der Sonnenbestrahlung aussetzten. Beim unter gleichen Bedingungen badenden Kinde sind die Blattabdrücke weniger gut erkennbar (Abb. 15). Es sind größere streifenförmige Blasen entstanden

Derartige Photosensibilisierungen wurden früher nach Eosinbehandlungen, die seither obsolet geworden sind, und nach Einnahme von Acridinfarbstoffen (Coups de lumière acridinique JAUSION) beobachtet. Sie leiten über zum Kapitel der Photoallergien, denn es ist denkbar, daß die Gonacrinfälle nicht durch obligate Photosensibilisierung ausgelöst wurden, sondern daß ein allergisches Phänomen auch für jene Fälle von Arzneimittelausschlägen postuliert werden muß (BURCKHARDT).

Im Anschluß an die Besprechung der obligaten percutanen und oralen Photosensibilisierung muß hier aber noch auf das interessante Kapitel der *Lichtdermatosen beim Tier* verwiesen werden. Raummangel erlaubt nicht, darauf genauer einzutreten. Neuere Zusammenfassungen mit Literaturhinweisen finden sich vor allem bei KRÁL und NOVAK und bei WULF. Meist handelt es sich dabei um Fütterungskrankheiten mit obligater Photosensibilisierung durch pflanzliche

Sensibilisatoren. Beim sog. Geeldikop (Geil-der-Kopf = Dickkopf), einer Schafkrankheit Südafrikas, verursacht durch Tribulus terrestris, soll aber eine toxische Leberschädigung vorausgehen, die dann im Darm zu einer Entstehung von Phylloerythrin aus Chlorophyll führt. Auch die kongenitale Porphyrie der Rinder und Ferkel wäre aus dieser Gruppe herauszunehmen, da sie der Porphyria erythropoetica gleichgesetzt werden muß.

2. Photoallergie oder allergische Photosensibilisierung

Der Begriff *Photoallergie* wurde von Epstein eingeführt. Beobachtungen von Sulfonamidexanthemen, bei denen offensichtlich eine Lichtbeteiligung zur Erklärung der Standorte angenommen werden mußte, bildeten den Ausgangspunkt. Die Lokalisation an belichteten Hautpartien berechtigt uns noch nicht, einen photoallergischen Prozeß anzunehmen. Im Kapitel über das Licht als fakultative, zusätzliche oder provokatorische Noxe wird unter anderem auch von solchen Beobachtungen die Rede sein.

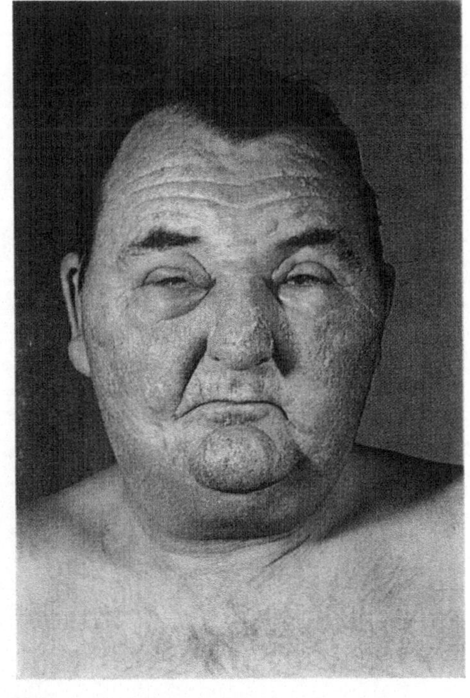

Abb. 16. Photoallergisches Exanthem durch Sulfocillin

Bei den echten photoallergischen Erscheinungen nach Epstein und Burckhardt fallen nicht nur die stärker ausgeprägten Hautveränderungen an den Lichtlokalisationen auf, auch die Anamnese ergibt meist, daß das Licht einen foudroyanten Ausbruch provoziert hat. Wenn dann eine Testprobe, die ohne Belichtung negativ ausfällt, nach teilweiser Belichtung nur im bestrahlten Anteil positiv reagiert, so darf das als Beweis für die photoallergische Natur der Erkrankung gelten.

In dieser Weise reagieren nur sehr wenige Individuen, die unter Sulfonamidwirkung stehen, und diesem Umstand muß auch bei der genaueren Erklärung der Pathogenese unbedingt Rechnung getragen werden. Um die Abklärung haben sich vor allem Burckhardt, dann Schwarz und Speck besonders bemüht. Burckhardt gelang es, vorerst durch eine intracutane Einspritzung von 1%iger Sulfanilamidlösung und nachfolgender Bestrahlung mit Sonne oder mit dem langwelligen Anteil der Quarzlampe, eine Reaktion in Form einer roten Papel zu erzielen. Nichtbestrahlte Quaddeln ergaben keine Reaktion, und die durch Sulfonamid + Licht ausgelösten Reaktionen heilten wieder ab.

Bei einigen Versuchspersonen aber traten nach einer Latenz von 8—10 Tagen an den Hautstellen, die auf die Kombination positiv reagiert hatten, merkwürdige Aufflammphänomene in Erscheinung: Rötungen, Schwellungen und Bläschenbildung. Es hatte somit eine Präparierung, Allergisierung oder Sensibilisierung stattgefunden. In der Folge reagierten sie jedenfalls bei Wiederholung der Versuche rascher und intensiver, ferner mit eindeutig ekzematiformen Erscheinungen.

Auch genügten schon minimale Mengen, um in Kombination mit Bestrahlung das Phänomen auszulösen. Die Experimente von SCHWARZ und SPECK an Meer-

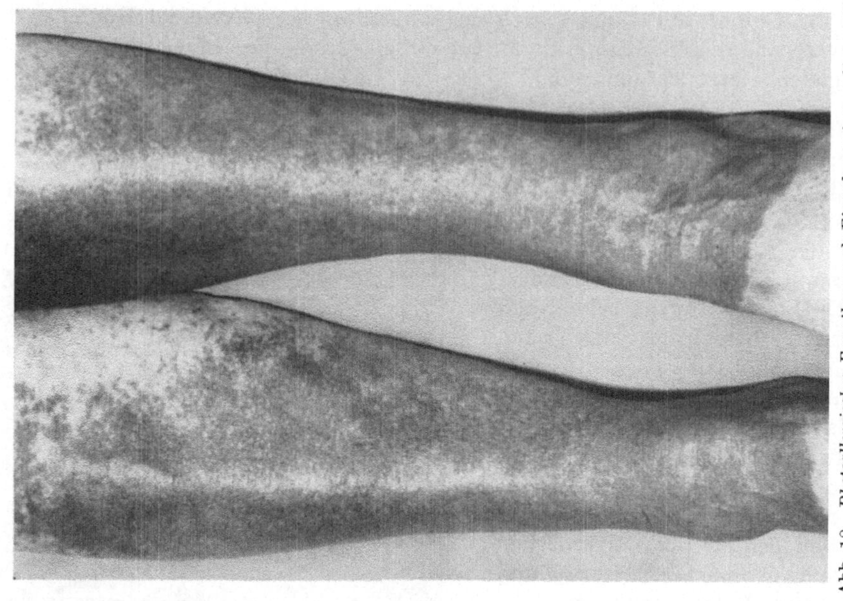

Abb. 18. *Photoallergisches Exanthem* nach Einnahme eines sulfonamidhaltigen Medikamentes. Die Lichtlokalisation wird deutlich erkennbar an der Begrenzung über den Fußrücken (2. Schub)

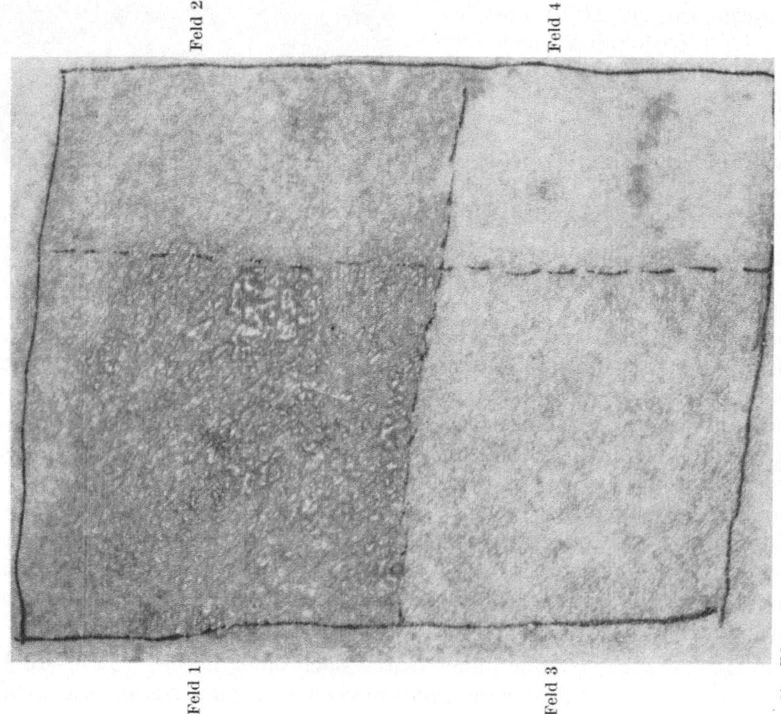

Abb. 17. *Photoallergisches Arzneimittelexanthem.* Bestrahlte Läppchenprobe. Feld 1 und 3 wurden für 24 Std mit einem Sulfocillin-Salbenlappen vorbehandelt; Feld 1 und 2 wurden anschließend bestrahlt, 3 und 4 blieben während der Besonnung bedeckt. Kräftige vesiculöse Reaktion im Sinne eines photoallergischen Ekzems nur auf Feld 1, Feld 2 zeigt eine leichte normale Strahlenreaktion als Kontrollbezirk

schweinchen zielen auf den Nachweis des eigentlichen Allergens, das sie in einem Oxydationsprodukt des Sulfonamids vermuten. Im klinischen Krankengut trifft man ab und zu auf Fälle, die sich als derartige photoallergische Sulfonamidexantheme herausstellen und durch entsprechende Testung abklären lassen. Bei Ekzemen mit scharfen Übergängen von bedeckten zu unbedeckten Hautstellen und anderen Anzeichen für Lichtlokalisation ist vor allem auch an diese Pathogenese zu denken (Abb. 16, 18). Da auch die *oralen Antidiabetica* als Sulfonamidderivate schon derartige photoallergische Exantheme ausgelöst haben (BURCKHARDT und SCHWARZ, SCHREUS und IPPEN), muß in Zukunft vermehrt mit diesem besonderen Typus der Arzneimittelnebenwirkung gerechnet werden (Abb. 16, 17, 18).

IPPEN sah auch nach Anwendung des Antimykoticums Jadit photoallergische Erscheinungen auftreten.

Phenothiazinderivate

Vertreter dieser Stoffgruppe fanden vorerst als Histaminantagonisten (Phenergan) Eingang in den Heilmittelschatz. Nachdem dann darüber hinaus zentraldämpfende, aber auch beinahe spezifische Wirkungen bei gewissen Psychosen entdeckt wurden, nahmen diese Medikamente einen ungeahnten Aufschwung und wurden in der ganzen Welt in vielen Varianten als Psychopharmaka verwendet. Neben den gewöhnlichen allergischen Nebenwirkungen an der Haut, wie Urticaria, Ekzem usw., wurden auch eindeutige photoallergische Erscheinungen nachgewiesen. Der Verdacht ergab sich schon aus der klinischen Beobachtung an Anstaltspatienten und an ambulant Weiterbehandelten. Sehr bemerkenswert war nun die Tatsache, daß besonders das Pflegepersonal psychiatrischer Kliniken und auch die Ärzte in einem relativ hohen Prozentsatz an photoallergischen Berufsdermatosen erkrankten. Merkwürdigerweise genügte schon der Umgang mit Tabletten und Ampullenlösungen vollauf, um die Sensibilisierung zu erwirken. Seit die Industrie die Phenothiazine nur noch mit Überzügen als Dragées in den Handel bringt, ist die Exanthemhäufigkeit stark zurückgegangen. Experimentelle Grundlagen zur Phenothiazin-Photosensibilisierung — und zwar zur gewöhnlichen obligaten — lieferten SCHULZ, WISKEMANN und WULF, SCHÖN und WULF. Sowohl im Paramaecienlichttest als im Belichtungsversuch an weißen Mäusen wurden photodynamische Wirkungen der Phenothiazine nachgewiesen. Wie bei den entsprechenden Sulfonamidausschlägen wird man auch hier die Technik bestrahlter Epicutantestproben heranziehen müssen, um Verdachtsfälle gründlich abzuklären.

Eine weitere Stoffgruppe, die photoallergische Erscheinungen auslösen kann, sei noch erwähnt, die sog. „*Weißmacher*" oder *Blancophore.* Es handelt sich um fluorescierende Stoffe, die fast allen modernen Waschmitteln zugesetzt werden. Sie fluorescieren im Ultraviolett und verwandeln diese absorbierte Energie in langwelliges sichtbares Licht; damit kann dann die so behandelte Wäsche „weißer als weiß" erscheinen. BURCKHARDT hat 1955 als erster über das Auftreten photoallergischer Ekzeme durch die optischen Aufheller in den modernen Waschmitteln berichtet. Seither sind auch noch weitere Beobachtungen gemeldet worden.

Große praktische Bedeutung haben die Krankheitserscheinungen, ausgelöst durch diese chemische Gruppe, aber noch nicht erlangt. Sie ist übrigens strukturchemisch völlig uneinheitlich zusammengesetzt.

III. Das Licht als zusätzliche, fakultative Noxe

Schon bei der Besprechung der eigentlichen idiopathischen Lichtkrankheiten mußte auffallen, daß das Licht nicht immer die alleinige auslösende Ursache sein kann, sondern daß z.B. eine vererbte Disposition im Sinne hochgradiger Lichtempfindlichkeit beim Xeroderma pigmentosum oder eine vererbte Anomalie im

Porphyrinstoffwechsel bei der Porphyria erythropoetica den Krankheitsbildern zugrunde liegt. Das Licht ist aber doch der wichtige, die Hauterscheinungen auslösende oder realisierende Faktor. Immer mehr müssen wir in der Medizin vom rein kausalen zum konditionalen Denken übergehen. Zum Verständnis pathologisch-physiologischer Vorgänge brauchen wir meist nicht nur eine Ursache und eine Wirkung, sondern eine Reihe von Bedingungen müssen erfüllt sein, um diese oder jene Abweichung zu begründen. Wir haben uns daran gewöhnt, unter Umständen recht komplizierte ätiologisch-pathogenetische Konstellationen anzunehmen.

Im Kapitel der Lichtkrankheiten finden wir vielleicht besonders viele und sprechende Beispiele für ein derartiges Zusammenwirken verschiedenster Faktoren oder Noxen. Bei der Porphyria cutanea tarda — um ein Beispiel zu nennen — haben wir erkannt, daß meist Alkoholabusus einen Leberschaden setzt. Es treten pathologische Porphyrine auf, welche die Haut gegen Licht sensibilisieren. Gleichzeitig entsteht offenbar eine erhöhte mechanische Lädierbarkeit. Die typischen Blasen an den belichteten Hautpartien bilden sich erst dann aus, wenn mechanische Mikrotraumen die Epidermisdecke abschieben.

In einem kurzen Abschnitt soll nun noch von Hautkrankheiten die Rede sein, bei denen das Licht nur fakultativ als Noxe in Betracht kommt. Die Strahlung kann eine untergeordnete Rolle als Teilfaktor in der Pathogenese spielen, in anderen Fällen wirkt sie *provozierend* oder auch nur *lokalisierend*. Über derartige Zusammenhänge haben ROST und KELLER im alten Handbuchbeitrag: „Die Wirkungen des Lichtes auf die Haut" schon berichtet. Ihren Ausführungen kann eigentlich nicht viel Neues beigefügt werden. Eine knappe Darstellung ist auch darum gerechtfertigt, weil bei der Besprechung derartiger Krankheitsbilder an anderen Stellen dieses Handbuches auf Lichtprovokation und Lichtlokalisation speziell eingegangen wird.

Bei der *Pellagra* sind frühere Erklärungen als Lichtkrankheit und die Suche nach photosensibilisierenden Substanzen in der Nahrung überholt. Die Pellagra kann heute als komplexe Mangelkrankheit befriedigend erklärt werden, deren Symptome auch ohne Mitwirkung von Licht auftreten. In Einzelfällen dürfte aber eine erhöhte Lichtempfindlichkeit vorhanden sein. Oft sind es nicht die klassischen Nicotinsäureamid-Avitaminosen, die zu dieser Deutung Anlaß geben, wohl aber pellagraähnliche Ausschläge, die sog. Pellagroide. Wahrscheinlich ist diese ganze Gruppe nicht einheitlich. Neben Fällen, die als unvollständig ausgebildete Pellagra aufgefaßt werden müssen (GOUGEROT, J. MEYER, OFERLÉ und UHRY), werden darin Erkrankungsfälle untergebracht, die nicht genau abgeklärt werden konnten, bei denen aber sehr oft eine eindeutige Lichtlokalisation, eine Phototopie, erkennbar war.

Beim *Erythematodes* sind Provokation und Exacerbation durch starke Besonnung seit langem bekannt und immer wieder diskutiert worden. Die moderne Behandlung mit Atebrinderivaten erhöht zwar die Lichttoleranz, ihre therapeutische Wirksamkeit beim Erythematodes ist aber damit nicht zu begründen. Auch beim Erythematodes acutus und vor allem bei der Dermatomyositis kann ab und zu Lichtempfindlichkeit und Phototopie beobachtet werden. Wieweit bei diesen Fällen auch vermehrt Porphyrine oder Lichtbandstoffe ausgeschieden werden, ist noch unklar.

Sowohl Erythematodes wie Erythema exsudativum multiforme sieht man oft in früher durch Licht geschädigten Bezirken sich ansiedeln. Sehr deutlich kann das immer wieder im Sterno-Clavicular-Dreieck nachgewiesen werden (KUSKE). Die Hautveränderungen, die als Folge wiederholter intensiver Bestrahlungen aufgetreten sind, bilden einen locus minoris resistentiae. Auch das allergische Kontaktekzem und die Psoriasis bevorzugen manchmal solche Gebiete.

Hin und wieder geht eine Sonnendermatitis in psoriatische Veränderungen über; das Licht wirkt als isomorpher Reiz. Verschlimmerungen unter Belichtung beobachtet man besonders bei exsudativen und vesiculo-bullösen Affektionen. Seit den Arbeiten von FINSEN wird das besonders für Variola-Exantheme angenommen. Ob die Pocken aber einer „negativen Phototherapie im Rotzimmer" zugänglich sind, wird heute eher angezweifelt.

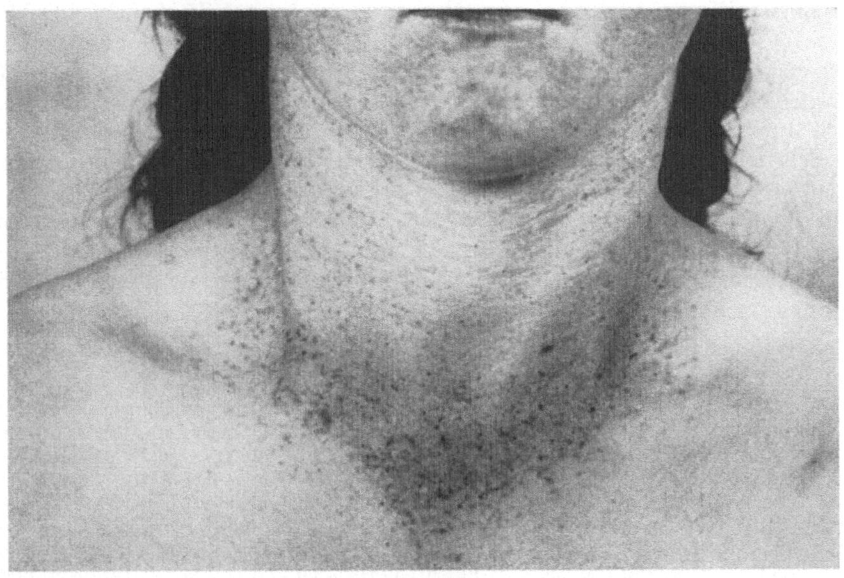

Abb. 19. Isomorpher Reizeffekt bei Morbus Darier. Aussaat von Efflorescenzen im belichteten Gebiet des Halsausschnittes

Klinisch und experimentell wurden Lichtlokalisationen beim *Morbus Darier* beobachtet. In einem von PREISSMANN mitgeteilten Fall ließen sich durch Höhensonnenerytheme die Dyskeratosen der Darierschen Erkrankung ganz eindeutig provozieren (Abb. 19). Ähnliche Beobachtungen macht man ab und zu mit Röntgentherapie oder mit mechanischen Reizen, die die Haut treffen. In einer eigenen Beobachtung waren die Veränderungen der Darierschen Krankheit unter einem Stützkorsett besonders stark ausgebildet. Wenn man beim Darier UV- und Röntgenstrahlen, mechanische Reibung oder Druck als auslösende Faktoren anerkennen muß, wird eben auch die Erklärung solcher Beobachtungen als isomorpher Reizeffekt bzw. Köbner-Phänomen nahegelegt.

Es ist wohl kein Zufall, daß diejenigen Krankheiten, bei denen häufig isomorphe Reizeffekte vorkommen (Lichen ruber, Psoriasis, Erythema exsudativum multiforme und Erythematodes disseminatus), auch jene Dermatosen sind, bei denen ab und zu Lichtlokalisation oder -provokation gesehen werden können.

Auch der *Herpes simplex* ist — allerdings in etwas anderer Weise — durch Licht provozierbar. Besonders die Hochgebirgssonne löst bei Alpinisten oft einen Herpes labialis aus. Es muß aber kein eigentliches Phototrauma vorausgehen, denn selbst die milden ersten Bestrahlungen mit Frühlingssonne im Tiefland können beim Herpetiker die genau gleiche Wirkung haben. Solche Beobachtungen würden mehr unter den Begriff des Biotropismus von MILIAN fallen.

Untersucht man übrigens die Streuphänomene im Verlauf des Ekzems genauer, so wird man immer wieder feststellen können, daß in der Großzahl der Fälle lichtexponierte Stellen besonders stark mitreagieren, was zu einem charakteristischen Verteilungsschema von Streuherden führen kann (W. LINDEMAYR).

IV. Lichtexantheme bei Lymphogranuloma inguinale

Im Verlaufe von Infektionen mit dem Virus des Lymphogranuloma inguinale kommen Lichtexantheme zur Beobachtung, die offenbar eine Sonderstellung einnehmen. Die Ausschläge sind nach SONCK streng auf die belichteten Hautgebiete beschränkt und treten schon einige Stunden nach Besonnung auf. Sie setzen sich aus mikropapulösen Efflorescenzen zusammen oder aus größeren, teils urticariellen, teils papulösen Morphen. Bläschen sollen nur selten vorkommen. Neben Juckreiz sind Allgemeinerscheinungen wie Kopfschmerzen, Schüttelfrost und Schwindel beschrieben worden. Falls weitere Provokationen vermieden werden können, heilt die Erkrankung rasch spontan ab.

Die Beobachtungen sind nicht einfach zu erklären und schwer richtig einzuordnen. Um photoallergische, medikamentöse Exantheme soll es sich nicht handeln. Eher käme ein cutanes Mikrobid in Betracht, das als Auswirkung eines Photobiotropismus gedeutet werden müßte.

Literatur

D'AGOSTINO, M., P. A. VIGLIOGLIA y M. GRINSTEIN: Porfiria mutilante. Rev. argent. Dermatosif. **41**, 31 (1957). — ANDERSON, T. E., and M. BEGG: Xeroderma pigmentosum of mild type. Brit. J. Derm. **62**, 402 (1950). — ARESU, G., e A. LOSTIA: Crisi porfirica acuta in un paziente affetto da porfiria cutanea tarda sintomatica sottoposto a trattamento clorochinico. Dermatologia (Napoli) **11**, 17 (1960). Ref. Zbl. Haut- u. Geschl.-Kr. **107**, 54 (1960). — ARRIGHI, F., P. GROUES et TOLEDANS: Porphyrie cutanée tardive (forme mixte). Bull. Soc. franç. Derm. Syph. **65**, 230 (1958). — ASBECK, F.: Photoaktivierung und Vitiligo. Hautarzt **7**, 118 (1956). — AURICCHIO, G., e A. RIBUFFO: Porfiria cutanea tarda con rare complicanze oculari. Dermatologia (Napoli) **9**, 257 (1958). Ref. Zbl. Haut- u. Geschl.-Kr. **106**, 136 (1960). — AYRES jr., S.: Chronic actinic cheilitis. J. Amer. med. Ass. **81**, 1183 (1923).

BAER, R. L., and H. J. COHEN: Polymorphus light eruption (plaque type). (Response to treatment with chorionic gonadotropin.) Arch. Derm. **81**, 129 (1960). Ref. Zbl. Haut- u. Geschl.-Kr. **107**, 47 (1960). — BARBER u. HOWITT: Zit. nach WULF (1954). — BARNES, H. D., u. J. MARSHALL: Porphyrie in Südafrika. Ann. Derm. Syph. (Paris) **79**, 521 (1952). Ref. Zbl. Haut- u. Geschl.-Kr. **85**, 177 (1953). — BAYER, E.: Die Lichtsensibilisierung der Haut durch Teerderivate. Arch. Derm. Syph. (Berl.) **183**, 142 (1942). — BAZIN, A. E. P.: Leçons théoriques et pratiques sur les affections géniriques de la peau. Paris 1862. — BECKER jr., S. W.: Use and abuse of psoralens. J. Amer. med. Ass. **173**, 1483 (1960). — BÉNARD, H., A. GADJOS et M. GADJOS-TÖRÖK: Porphyries. Etudes cliniques et biologiques. Paris: Baillière 1958. — BÉNARD, H., A. GADJOS, M. GADJOS-TÖRÖK et G. PÉQUIGNOT: Porphyrie aiguë avec atteinte hépatique et quelques particularités des troubles porphyriniques. Sem. Hôp. Paris **1953**, 2817—2819. Ref. Zbl. Haut- u. Geschl.-Kr. 88, 274 (1954). — BENSON, A., W. D. FOSTER and F. T. G. PRUNTY: Porphyrin excretion in a patient with delayed light-sensitive porphyria. Brit. med. J. **1954 I**, No 4868, 965. Ref. Zbl. Haut- u. Geschl.-Kr. **90**, 119 (1954/55). — BERGLUND, H., and K. G. PAUL: Two cases of Porphyria cutanea tarda, treated with Vit. B_{12}. Acta med. scand. **147**, Suppl. 287, 91—92 (1953). Ref. Zbl. Haut- u. Geschl.-Kr. **89**, 163 (1954). — BERGWEIN, K.: Sonnenschutz-Schaum-Aerosole, unsichtbar fettend. Seifen-Öle-Fette-Wachse **85**, 253 (1959). — BERING, F., u. U. v. BARNEWITZ: JADASSOHNs Handbuch der Haut- und Geschlechtskrankheiten, Bd. IV, Aktinische Dermatosen, S. 128. Berlin: Springer 1932. — BERLIN, CH.: Xeroderma pigmentosum (Recherches sur la sensibilité de la peau à l'égard de divers rayons). Rev. franç. Derm. Vénér. **14**, 213 (1938). Ref. Zbl. Haut- u. Geschl.-Kr. **61**, 61 (1939). — BERLIN, CH., and A. TAGER: Xeroderma pigmentosum. Report of eight cases of mild to moderate type and course; a study of response to various irradiations. Dermatologica (Basel) **116**, 27 (1958). — BERMAN, J., A. BRAUN and V. VOLEK: Liver biopsy and its clinical evaluation in porphyria cutanea tarda. Acta univ. carol. Med. Nr. 8, 589—595 mit engl. Zus.fass. (1959) [Tschechisch]. Ref. Zbl. Haut- u. Geschl.-Kr. **107**, 154 (1960). — BERNSTEIN, F.: Beiträge zu den physikalischen Idiosynkrasien der Haut. IV. Mitt. Spezifische

Sensibilisierung als Ursache idiosynkrasischer Lichtdermatosen. Arch. Derm. Syph. (Berl.) **168**, 177 (1933). — BETTLEY, F. R., u. F. PAGE: Wirkung des Mepacrin auf die Photosensibilität beim Lupus erythematodes. Bull. Soc. franç. Derm. Syph. **61**, 198 (1954). — Ref. Derm. Wschr. **133**, 227 (1956). — BLAICH, W., u. U. GERLACH: Zum Wirkungsmechanismus des Resochin beim Erythematodes. Hautarzt **6**, 267 (1955). — BLUM, H. F.: Photodynamic action and diseases caused by light. Amer. Chemical Society Monograph Series No 85. New York: Reinhold Publ. Corporation 1941. — The physiological effects of sunlight on man. Physiol. Rev. **25**, 483 (1945). — Carcinogenesis by ultraviolet light. Princeton, N.J.: Princeton University Press 1959. — Photobiological research with particular reference to skin. Report to the Committee. J. Amer. med. Ass. **173**, 1353 (1960). — BLUM, H. F., R. L. BAER and M. B. SULZBERGER: Studies in hypersensitivity to light. II. Urticaria solare. J. invest Derm. **7**, 99 (1946). — BODE, O.: Eine einfache Methode zur Bestimmung des Gesamtporphyrins im Harn und ihre klinische Anwendung. Ärztl. Forsch. **4**, (I) 617—(I) 628 (1950). — BOLGERT, M., et J. CANIVET: La porphyrie cutanée de l'adulte. Bull. Soc. franç. Derm. Syph. **61**, 219 (1954). — Brit. J. Derm. **66**, 312 (1954). — Derm. Wschr. **133**, 228 (1956). — BOLGERT, M., J. CANIVET et J. LÉPINE: A propos de l'identité de l'hydroa vacciniforme de Bazin et de la porphyrie cutanée. Ann. Derm. Syph. (Paris) **83**, 18 (1956). — BOLGERT, M., J. CANIVET et M. LE SOURD: Trois nouveaux cas de Porphyrie cutanée de l'adulte à début tardif. Bull. Soc. franç. Derm. Syph. **59**, 270 (1952). Ref. Zbl. Haut- u. Geschl.-Kr. **85**, 177 (1953). — La porphyrie cutanée de l'adulte. Etude de neuf cas et description. Sem. Hôp. Paris **1953**, 1587—1608. Ref. Zbl. Haut- u. Geschl.-Kr. **87**, 241 (1954). — BOLGERT, M., M. LE SOURD et J. CANIVET: Porphyrie congénitale à révélation tardive (P. cong. Tarda). Bull. Soc. franç. Derm. Syph. **58**, 516 (1951). — BOM, FR.: Porphyria cutanea tarda mit neuropsychiatrischen Komplikationen (verursacht durch Antabusbehandlung). Nord. Med. **47**, 83—85 [Dänisch]. Ref. Zbl. Haut- u. Geschl.-Kr. **81**, 146 (1952). — BONNET, J., A. DAVIN et L. COULIER: Sensibilisation au largactil avec éruption bulleuse sur les régions ensoleillées. Bull. Soc. franç. Derm. Syph. **66**, 145 (1959). Ref. Zbl. Haut- u. Geschl.-Kr. **105**, 25 (1959/60). — BOUCAUD, DE, P. LE COULANT, L. TEXIER et FOURNIAL: Accidents de photosensibilisation chez des malades mentaux, traités par hautes doses de largactil. Bull. Soc. franç. Derm. Syph. **62**, 245 (1955). Ref. Zbl. Haut- u. Geschl.-Kr. **93**, 287 (1956). — BRAUN, A., and J. BERMAN: Pathological anatomy in porphyria cutanea tarda. Acta Univ. Carol. Med. (Praha) Nr. 8, 597 (1959) [Tschechisch]. Ref. Zbl. Haut- u. Geschl.-Kr. **107**, 153 (1960). — BRESLER, R. R.: Cutaneous burns due to fluorescent light. J. Amer. med. Ass. **140**, 1334 (1949). — BRETT, R.: Beitrag zur internen Therapie der Lichtdermatosen und lichtbeeinflußbaren Krankheiten. Dtsch. med. Wschr. **1950**, 800. — Ref. Derm. Wschr. **123**, 504 (1951). — BROCKMANN, H., E. H. v. FALKENHAUSEN, R. NEEFF, A. DORLARS u. G. BUDDE: Die Konstitution des Hypericins. Chem. Ber. **84**, 865 (1951). — BROCKMANN, H., ERHARD WEBER u. GOTTFRIED PAMPUS: Protofagopyrin und Fagopyrin, die photodynamisch wirksamen Farbstoffe des Buchweizens. Justus Liebigs Ann. Chem. **575/576**, 53 (1952). — BROCQ, L.: De l'Hydroa vacciniforme. Ann. Derm. Syph. (Paris) **5**, 1133—1147 (1894). — BRODTHAGEN, H., and J. V. CHRISTIANSEN: Polymorphic light eruptions: Relation to ultraviolet light intensity and hours of sunshine. Brit. J. Derm. **68**, 261 (1956). Ref. Zbl. Haut- u. Geschl.-Kr. **97**, 42 (1957). — BRUGSCH jr., J.: Zum Begriff der toxischen Porphyrie. Verh. dtsch. Ges. inn. Med. **58**, 761 (1952). Ref. Zbl. Haut- u. Geschl.-Kr. **84**, 371 (1953). — Zum Problem der cutanen Porphyrien. Vortrag geh. i. d. Derm. Ges. b. d. Univ. Berlin. 15. Sitzg am 4. 12. 1954. Ref. Zbl. Haut- u. Geschl.-Kr. **94**, 127 (1956). — Hämochromatose und Melanodermieporphyrie als verschiedene Formen der Hämsynthesestörung bei Pigmentzirrhose und Bronzediabetes. Z. ges. inn. Med. **13**, 411 (1958). Ref. Zbl. Haut- u. Geschl.-Kr. **102**, 289 (1958/59). Klinische Erkennung und Bedeutung der Porphyrien. Z. ges. inn. Med. **13**, 781 (1958). Ref. Zbl. Haut- u. Geschl.-Kr. **103**, 55 (1959). — Zur Bedeutung des Hämoglobinaufbaus als klinisch-ärztliches Problem. Ther. Rdsch. **19**, 53 (1962). — BRUGSCH, J., u. D. GRÜMER: Die Stellung der Leber im Porphyrinstoffwechsel. (60. Kongr. München, 25.—29. 4. 1954.) Verh. dtsch. Ges. inn. Med. **1954**, 520 Ref. Zbl. Haut- u. Geschl.-Kr. **92**, 74 (1955). — BRUGSCH, J., D. KLAUS u. A. BIENENGRÄBER: Ein weiterer Fall von Melanodermie-Porphyrie mit Leberzirrhose. Z. ges. inn. Med. **12**, 877 (1957). Ref. Zbl. Haut- u. Geschl.-Kr. **100**, 229 (1958). — BRUGSCH, J. TH.: Zum qualitativen Porphyrinnachweis im Harn (Porphyrinschnellprobe). Münch. med. Wschr. **1934**, 1546. — Untersuchungen des quantitativen Porphyrinstoffwechsels beim gesunden und kranken Menschen. Z. ges. exp. Med. **95**, 471 (1935). — Fluorometrisches Mikroverfahren zur Erkennung und Differenzierung von Kopro- und Hämatoporphyrin im Gemisch. Untersuchung der Eigenschaften des Hämoporphyrins. Über ein neues Hämatoporphyrinderivat von Tetramethyl-Mono-Vinyl-Mono-alpha-Oxyaethyl-Porphin-Dipropionsäure-Typ. XII. Mitt. Z. ges. inn. Med. **2**, 645 (1947). Ref. Zbl. Haut- u. Geschl.-Kr. **74**, 290 (1950). — Porphyrine-Leipzig: Johann Ambrosius Barth 1952. — BRUNSTING, L. A.: Die chronische Porphyrie des Erwachsenen und ihre Hauterscheinungen. Hautarzt **4**, 536 (1953). — Observations on porphyria cutanea tarda. Arch. Derm. **70**, 551 (1954). — BRUNSTING, L. A., I. T. BRUGSCH and

P. A. O'LEARY: Quantitative investigation of porphyrin metabolism in diseases of the skin. Arch. Derm. Syph. (Chic.) **39**, 294 (1939). — BRUNSTING, L. A., and J. H. EPSTEIN: Solar urticaria. Dermatologica (Basel) **115**, 171 (1957). — BRUNSTING, L. A., and H. L. MASON: Porphyria with cutaneous manifestations. Arch. Derm. **60**, 66 (1949). — BRUNSTING, L. A., H. L. MASON u. R. A. ALDRICH: Chronische Porphyrie mit Hautveränderungen beim Erwachsenen. Bericht über 17 einschlägige Fälle. J. Amer. med. Ass. **146**, 1207 (1951). Ref. Zbl. Haut- u. Geschl.-Kr. **80**, 368 (1952). — BUCK, H. W., I. A. MAGNUS and A. C. PORTER: The action spectrum of 8-Methoxypsoralen for erythema in human skin. Brit. J. Derm. **72**, 249 (1960). — BURCKHARDT, W.: Zur Frage der photosensibilisierenden Wirkung des Teers. Schweiz. med. Wschr. **1939**, 83. — Untersuchungen über die Photoaktivität einiger Sulfonamide. Dermatologica (Basel) **83**, 63 (1941). — Über eine im Frühling, bes. an den Ohren, auftretende Lichtdermatose. Dermatologica (Basel) **86**, 85 (1942). — Ein Fall von Lichturticaria. Dermatologica (Basel) **94**, 202 (1947). — Photoallergisches Ekzem durch optisches Aufhellungsmittel als Bestandteil eines Waschmittels. Dermatologica (Basel) **111**, 229 (1955). — Photoallergische Ekzeme durch Blankophore (optische Aufheller). Hautarzt **8**, 486 (1957). — Versuch zur Einteilung der Lichtdermatosen nach ihrer Pathogenese. Dermatologica (Basel) **116**, 223 (1958a). — Versuch einer pathogenetischen Einteilung der Lichtdermatosen. Schweiz. med. Wschr. **1958b**, 1319. — Licht-Allergie. Akt. Probl. Derm. **1**, 301 (1959). — BURCKHARDT, W., u. K. SCHWARZ: Photobiologie der Haut. Hautarzt **5**, 377 (1954). — BURCKHARDT, W., K. u. M. SCHWARZ-SPECK: Photoallergische Ekzeme durch Nadisan. Schweiz. med. Wschr. **1957**, 954.

CAHN, M. M., and E. I. LEVY: Ultraviolet light factor in chlorpromazine dermatitis. Arch. Derm. **75**, 40 (1957). — CAHN, M. M., J. LEVY and B. SHAFFER: Polymorphous light eruption. The effect of chloroquine phosphate in modifying reactions to ultraviolet light. J. invest. Derm. **26**, 201 (1956). Ref. Zbl. Haut- u. Geschl.-Kr. **96**, 125 (1956). — CAHN, M. M., E. J. LEVY, B. SHAFFER and H. BEERMAN: Lupus erythematosus and polymorphous light eruptions. J. invest. Derm. **21**, 375 (1953). — CAHN, M. M., E. J. LEVY, J. M. VANDENBELT and B. SHAFFER: Spectrophotometric and electrophoretic patterns of sera of patients with polymorphous light eruption. J. invest. Derm. **31**, 93 (1958). — CALNAN, C. D.: Drug photosensitivity with chlorpromazine. Proc. 11. internat. Congr. Dermat. Stockholm 1957, **3**, 485—489 (1960). Ref. Zbl. Haut- u. Geschl.-Kr. **108**, 54 (1960/61). — Studies in contact dermatitis. V. Photosensitivity from chlorpromazine. Symposium. Trans. St. John's Hosp. derm. Soc. (Lond.) **1958**, Nr 41, 26. Ref. Zbl. Haut- u. Geschl.-Kr. **106**, 47 (1960). — CALVERT, R. J., and C. RIMINGTON: Porphyria cut. tarda in relapse, a case report. Brit. med. J. **1953**, No 4846, 1131—1134. Ref. Zbl. Haut- u. Geschl.-Kr. **91**, 74 (1955). — CANIVET, J.: Troubles de la pigmentation cutanée au cours de porphyries. Rev. Prat. (Paris) **1957**, 3099—3102. Ref. Zbl. Haut- u. Geschl.-Kr. **100**, 228 (1958). — CANIVET, J., u. P. FALLOT: Die Porphyrien, Beobachtungen an 43 Fällen. Dtsch. med. Wschr. **84**, 63 (1959). — CARN, V. L., et J. LÉPINE: Un cas de porphyrie cutanée de l'adulte d'origine bretonne. Bull. Soc. franç. Derm. Syph. **61**, 330 (1954). Ref. Zbl. Haut- u. Geschl.-Kr. **91**, 388 (1955). — CARRIÉ, CURT: Die Porphyrine. Ihr Nachweis, ihre Physiologie und Klinik. Leipzig: Georg Thieme 1936. — Die Ursache der Porphyrin-Fluoreszenz in der Mundhöhle und auf der Haut. Derm. Z. **70**, 189 (1943). Ref. Zbl. Haut- u. Geschl.-Kr. **51**, 177 (1935). — CERUTTI, P.: Sindrome porfirica con manifestazioni cutanee. Atti Soc. med.-chir. Padova **11**, 882 (1934). Ref. Zbl. Haut- u. Geschl.-Kr. **48**, 560 (1934). — Manifestazioni cutanee e ipersensibilità alla luce nella porfiria. Arch. ital. Derm. **11**, 3 (1935). Ref. Zbl. Haut- u. Geschl.-Kr. **50**, 584 (1935). — CHAUDHURI, AMALA, J. NAG. CHAUDHURI and K. C. CHAUDHURI: Congenital porphyria in siblings. (With a brief review of congenital and hereditary porphyrias.) Indian J. Pediat. **25**, 157 (1958). Ref. Zbl. Haut- u. Geschl.-Kr. **104**, 248 (1959). — CHRISTIANSEN, J. V., and H. BRODTHAGEN: The treatment of polymorphic light eruptions with chloroquine. Brit. J. Derm. **68**, 204 (1956). — Therapeutic problems in chronic polymorphous light-sensitivity eruptions. Proc. 11. internat. Congr. Dermat. Stockholm 1957, **3**, 535—537 (1960). — *Ciba Foundation Symposium* on Porphyrin biosynthesis and metabolism. 70 fig. 8°. VII, 308 p. London 1955. Editors for the Ciba Foundation, Churchill Ltd. Ref. Schweiz. med. Wschr. **1956**, 1036. — CLAESSON, S., L. JUHLIN and G. WETTERMARK: The action of ultraviolet light on skin with and without horny layer. The effect of 48/80 and methotrimeprazine. Acta derm.-venereol. (Stockh.) **39**, 3 (1959). — COLOMB, D.: Trois cas de porphyrie cutanée tardive de l'adulte et deux cas de lucite ayant bien réagi à un traitement par la nivaquine. Bull. Soc. franç. Derm. Syph. **64**, 420 (1957). Ref. Zbl. Haut- u. Geschl.-Kr. **101**, 118 (1958). — COLOMB, D., et J. FAYOLLE: A propos d'un cas de porphyrie de l'adulte. Bull. Soc. franç. Derm. Syph. **62**, 176 (1955). Ref. Zbl. Haut- u. Geschl.-Kr. **93**, 300 (1956). — COMFORT, A., H. MOORE and M. WEATHERALL: Normal human urinary porphyrins. Biochem. J. **58**, 177 (1954). Ref. Zbl. Haut- u. Geschl.-Kr. **92**, 7 (1955). — COOKSON, G. H., and C. RIMINGTON: Porphobilinogen: chemical constitution. Nature (Lond.) **171**, 875 (1953). — CORNBLEET, TH.: Cutaneous appearance of porphyria by ultraviolet light. Arch. Derm. **73**, 34 (1956). — COSTA, O. G.: Porfiria ampollar y erosiva asociada con hidroa vacciniforme. Consideraciones sobre la lamada epidermolisis ampollar porfirica. Arch.

argent. Derm. **4**, 363 (1954). Ref. Zbl. Haut- u. Geschl.-Kr. **94**, 78 (1956). — CURWEN, W. L., and O. F. JILLSON: Light hypersensitivity a simplified office procedure for diagnosis of contact photodermatitis. J. invest. Derm. **34**, 207 (1960).

DANIELS, F., and L. BERGERON: Vasomotor studies in ultraviolet erythema. J. invest. Derm. **35**, 329 (1960). — DANNENBERG, H., u. H. REINWEIN: Zur Klinik der Porphyria cutanea tarda (Haematoporphyria chronica Günther). Dtsch. Arch. klin. Med. **202**, 214 (1955). Ref. Zbl. Haut- u. Geschl.-Kr. **93**, 202 (1955/56). — DAVIS, M. J., and D. E. VANDER PLOEG: Akute porphyria and coproporphyrinuria following chloroquine therapy. Arch. Derm. **75**, 796 (1957). — DEAN, G., and H. D. BARNES: The inheritance of porphyria. Brit. med. J. **1955 II**, No 4931, 89—94. Ref. Zbl. Haut- u. Geschl.-Kr. **93**, 300 (1956). — Porphyria. A South African screening experiment. Brit. med. J. **1958 I**, No 5066, 298—301. — DÉROT, M., et J. CANIVET: Nouveau cas de porphyrie cutanée de l'adulte. Presse méd. **1955**, 97. Ref. Zbl. Haut- u. Geschl.-Kr. **92**, 76 (1955). — DILLAHA, C. J., u. W. HICKLIN: Versuchsweise Behandlung der chronischen Porphyrie mit Vitamin B_{12}. J. invest. Derm. **19**, 489 (1952). Ref. Zbl. Haut- u. Geschl.-Kr. **85**, 313 (1953). — DISCOMBE, G., and C. S. TREIP: Cutaneous manifestation of Porphyria. Brit. med. J. **1953 II**, No 4846, 1134—1136. Ref. Zbl. Haut- u. Geschl.-Kr. **91**, 74 (1955). — DOJMI, L.: Ist Cheilitis aestivalis eine Avitaminose? Zus.fass. in Zbl. Haut- u. Geschl.-Kr. **61**, 401 (1939). — DURET, R. L.: Biochimie des porphyrines. Arch. belges Derm. **12**, 148 (1956). Ref. Zbl. Haut- u. Geschl.-Kr. **97**, 340 (1957). — DURST, J. B., and M. A. KREMBS: Porphyria and pregnancy. J. Amer. med. Ass. **160**, 165 (1956).

ELIOZISVILI, K. M.: Akutes Frühlingsödem. Klin. Med. **27**, 31 Medgis-Moskau, 1949. Derm. Wschr. **123**, 504 (1951). — ELLINGER, F.: The biologic fundamentals of radiation therapy. New York 1941. — ELSCHNER, H., u. R. ANDRADE: Beitrag zur Ätiologie der aktinisch-traumatisch-bullösen Porphyrin-Dermatose. Derm. Wschr. **137**, 114 (1958). — EPSTEIN, J. H., and L. A. BRUNSTING: Topical application of chloropromazine; its effect on the erythema response to ultraviolet light. J. invest. Derm. **30**, 91 (1958). — EPSTEIN, J. H., L. A. BRUNSTING, M. C. PETERSEN and E. E. SCHWARZ: A study of photosensitivity occurring with chloropromazine therapy. J. invest. Derm. **28**, 329 (1957). — EPSTEIN, S., and R. J. ROWE: Photoallergy and photocross-sensitivity to phenergan. J. invest. Derm. **29**, 319 (1957). — EPSTEIN, ST.: Experimentelle Eruption bei Hydroa vacciniformis durch Thorium X. Arch. Derm. Syph. (Berl.) **168**, 67 (1933). — Allergische Lichtdermatosen. Dermatologica (Basel) **80**, 291 (1939a). — Photoallergy and primary photosensitivity to sulfanilamide. J. invest. Derm. **2**, 43 (1939b). — Allergic photocontact dermatitis from promethazine (Phenergen). Arch. Derm. **81**, 175 (1960).

FALK, M. S.: Light sensitivity due to demethylchlortetracycline. Report of four cases. J. Amer. med. Ass. **172**, 1156 (1960). — FASSOTTE, CH.: Les porphyrinuries congénitales et acquises. Arch. belges Derm. **9**, 259 (1953). Ref. Zbl. Haut- u. Geschl.-Kr. **88**, 278 (1954). — FELDAKER, M., H. MONTGOMERY and L. A. BRUNSTING: Histopathology of Porphyria cutanea tarda. J. invest. Derm. **24**, 131 (1955). — FERRARI, A. V.: Pseudo milio colloide e porfiria. Minerva derm. **29**, 104 (1954). Ref. Zbl. Haut- u. Geschl.-Kr. **90**, 32 (1954/55). — FINDELSBERGER, G., u. W. LINDENMAYR: Zit. nach WULF. — FINDLAY, G. H.: Light eruptions and the ATP mechanism. Brit. J. Derm. **70**, 242 (1958). — FINSEN, N. R.: Neue Untersuchungen über die Einwirkung des Lichtes auf die Haut. Mitt. Finsens Lysinst. **1**, 8 (1900). — FISCHER, H.: Über die Giftigkeit, die sensibilisierende Wirkung, das spektroskopische Verhalten der natürlichen Porphyrine. Hoppe-Seylers Z. physiol. Chem. **97**, 109 (1916). — Über Porphyrinurie und natürliche Porphyrine. Münch. med. Wschr. **1923**, 1143. — Über Porphyrine und ihre Synthesen. Ber. dtsch. chem. Ges. **60**, 2611 (1927). — FISCHER, H., u. G. W. KORTING: Über Eisenmangel bei chronisch-polymorphem Lichtausschlag. Arch. klin. exp. Derm. **209**, 111 (1959). Ref. Zbl. Haut- u. Geschl.-Kr. **105**, 220 (1959/60). — FISCHER, H., u. W. ZERWECK: Über den Harnfarbstoff bei normalen und pathologischen Verhältnissen und seine lichtschützende Wirkung. Zugleich einige Beiträge zur Kenntnis der Porphyrinurie. Hoppe-Seylers Z. physiol. Chem. **137**, 176 (1924). — FLECK, F.: Zur Entstehung und Behandlung von Dyschromien im seitlichen Halsbereich. Derm. Wschr. **138**, 1133 (1958). — FLEISCHHAUER, L.: Über die sensibilisierende Wirkung des Teerpräparates Liantral. Strahlentherapie **36**, 144 (1930). — FOERSTER, H. R., and L. SCHWARTZ: Industrial dermatitis and melanosis due to photosensitization. Arch. Derm. **39**, 55 (1939). — FRANK, L.: Photodynamischer Effekt von Rohsteinkohlenteer auf der Haut. Arch. Derm. **60**, 597 (1949). — Ref. Derm. Wschr. **123**, 211 (1951). — FRANK, O., u. V. LACHNIT: Zum Porphyrinnachweis bei Bleiarbeitern. Wien. Z. inn. Med. **32**, 413 (1951). Ref. Zbl. Haut- u. Geschl.-Kr. **81**, 57 (1952). — FRENCK, G.: Photosensibilisation chez le lapin par injection intradermique de porphyrines naturelles purifiées. Arch. belges Derm. **15**, 27 (1959). Ref. Zbl. Haut- u. Geschl.-Kr. **104**, 217 (1959). — FREUND, E.: Über bisher noch nicht beschriebene künstliche Hautverfärbungen. Derm. Wschr. **63**, 931 (1916). — FREUND, L.: Physiologische und therapeutische Studien über Lichtwirkungen auf die Haut. Wien. klin. Wschr. **1912**, 191. — FRIEDERICH, H. C., H. HÖRING u. G. W. KORTING: Berlockdermatitis, bisheriges Wissen und Problematik. Z. Haut- u. Geschl.-Kr. **27**, 255 (1959).

Galambos, J. T.: Porphyria cutanea tarda without skin lesions in an American Negro. Amer. J. Med. 25, 315 (1958). Ref. Zbl. Haut- u. Geschl.-Kr. 102, 289 (1958/59). — Garcin, R., A. Escalier, A. Gajdos, Gajdos-Török, S. Godlewski et J. Lapresle: Porphyrie aiguë avec présence dans les urines à côté de l'uroporphyrine III de porphyrines à 3,5 et 7 carboxyles. Etude clinique et bio-chimique. Presse méd. 1953, 959. Ref. Zbl. Haut- u. Geschl.-Kr. 90, 119 (1954/55). — Garrod, A.: A bypath of medicine (congenital porphyrinuria). Glasg. med. J. 98, 135 (1922). — Gheorghiu, Gh., P. P. Danila u. Al. Coltoiu: Bemerkungen zur Ätiologie der kutanen Porphyrie. Derm.-Vener. (Buc.) 4, 219 (1959). Ref. Zbl. Haut- u. Geschl.-Kr. 106, 56 (1960). — Giese, J.: Über eine kolorimetrische Vergleichsbestimmung von 2 „Nichtporphyrinfarbstofftypen" im menschlichen Harn bei kutaner Porphyrie. Z. ges. inn. Med. 7, 1007 (1952). — Gilbert, J. A. L., H. M. Toupin u. R. E. Bell: Akute Porphyrie. Canad. med. Ass. J. 65, 585 (1951). Ref. Zbl. Haut- u. Geschl.-Kr. 81, 316 (1952). — Gillesberger, W.: Bemerkungen zum Lichtschutz der Haut und ein Bericht über die Erprobung eines Lichtschutzmittels in alkoholischer Lösung an Hautkranken und Gesunden. Med. Kosmet. 8, 60 (1959). Ref. Zbl. Haut- u. Geschl.-Kr. 106, 219 (1960). — Glaubersohn, S. A., u. M. M. Goldenberg: Zur Lehre über die Photodermatosen. Derm. Wschr. 91, 1625 (1930). — Göggel, K. H.: Neue Behandlungsmöglichkeit der akuten Porphyrie. Vorl. Mitt. Ärztl. Wschr. 14, 145 (1959). Ref. Zbl. Haut- u. Geschl.-Kr. 103, 55 (1959). — Gold, S.: Congenital Porphyria. Proc. 10th internat. Congr. of Dermat. London 1952, p. 420—421 (1953). Ref. Zbl. Haut- u. Geschl.-Kr. 89, 304 (1954). — Goldberg, A., A. C. Macdonald and C. Rimington: Acute porphyria. Experimental treatment with ACTH. Brit. med. J. 1952 II, No 4795, 1174. Ref. Zbl. Haut- u. Geschl.-Kr. 84, 376 (1953). — Goldsmith, W. N.: Porphyria cutanea tarda in siblings. Proc. 10th internat. Congr. of Dermat. London 1952, p. 419—420 (1953). Ref. Zbl. Haut- u. Geschl.-Kr. 89, 304 (1954). — Gottron, H. A.: Druckurticaria bei Porphyrie. Schles. Dermat. Ges. Sitzg v. 11. 12. 1937. Ref. Zbl. Haut- u. Geschl.-Kr. 59, 7 (1938). — Gottron, H., u. F. Ellinger: Beitrag zur Klinik der Porphyrie. Arch. Derm. Syph. (Berl.) 164, 11 (1931). — Klinische und experimentelle Befunde bezüglich der Reaktion des Gefäßbindegewebsapparates der Haut bei der Porphyrie. Arch. Derm. Syph. (Berl.) 167, 325 (1933). — Gougerot, L.: Les dyschromies par photo-sensibilisation. (Porphyries et pellagre exclues.) Rev. Prat. (Paris) 1957, 3091. Ref. Zbl. Haut- u. Geschl.-Kr. 100, 228 (1958). — Gougerot, H.: Chéilites solaires. Lucites solaires labiales et causes sensibilisantes. Bull. Soc. franç. Derm. Syph. 43, 1592 (1936). — Gougerot, H., J. Meyer, Oferlé et P. Uhry: Pellagre et erythème pellagroide. Formes de transition. La pellagroide est une pellagre incomplète et atténuée. Bull. Soc. franç. Derm. Syph. 36, 1018 (1929). — Graciansky, P. de, et S. Boulle: Forme ulcéreuse de la porphyrie chronique, discussion nosologique. Arch. belges Derm. 13, 329 (1957). Ref. Zbl. Haut- u. Geschl.-Kr. 101, 118 (1958). — Grafe, G.: Porphyrinurie nach Urethan bzw. Colchicinbehandlung. Dtsch. Gesundh.-Wes. 3, 50 (1948). Ref. Zbl. Haut- u. Geschl.-Kr. 73, 361 (1949). — Granick, S., and H. G. Schrieck: Porphobilinogen and delta amino-laevulinic acid in acute porphyria. Proc. Soc. exp. Biol. (N.Y.) 88, 270 (1955). — Gray, C. H., and A. Neuberger: Effect of splenectomy in a case of congenital Porphyria. Lancet 1952 I, 851. — Greither, A.: Über das Wesen des sogenannten akuten Lichtausschlages auf Grund seiner Beeinflussung durch Antihistamine und Rutin. Klin. Wschr. 30, 175 (1952). — Experimentelle Haematoporphyrinvergiftung und akute Lichtkrankheit. Proc. 10th internat. Congr. of Dermat. London 1952, p. 391—392 (1953). — Griffin, A. C., R. E. Hakim and J. Knox: The wave length effect upon erythemal and carcinogenic response in psoralen treated mice. J. invest. Derm. 31, 289 (1958). — Grin: Zit. nach Wulf (1954). — Grogg, E.: Zur medikamentösen Beeinflussung der experimentellen Porphyrie des Kaninchens. Bull. schweiz. Akad. med. Wiss. 16, 309 (1960). — Gross, P.: Berlock Dermatitis (Due to Juice of Persian Limes). Arch. Derm. 63, 272 (1951). — Das Köbner-Phänomen in seiner Beziehung zur Photosensibilität. Arch. Derm. 74, 43 (1956). — Derm. Wschr. 135, 202 (1957). — Grossfeld, E.: Acute porphyria with unusual features. Brit. med. J. 1951 I, No 4717, 1240—1241. Ref. Zbl. Haut- u. Geschl.-Kr. 87, 355 (1954). — Grupper, Ch.: Die Behandlung der Lichtdermatosen mit Nivaquin. Vorl. Mitt. Bull. Soc. franç. Derm. Syph. 61, 325 (1954). — Derm. Wschr. 133, 251 (1956). — Günther, H.: Die klinischen Symptome der Lichtüberempfindlichkeit. Derm. Wschr. 68, 177, 203, 213, 230, 243 (1919). — Die Hämatoporphyrie. Dtsch. Arch. klin. Med. 105, 89 (1911). — Gutniak, O.: Identification of porphyrins in urine of a patient suffering from porphyria cutanea tarda. Przegl. derm. 47, 93 (1960). Ref. Zbl. Haut- u. Geschl.-Kr. 108, 62 (1960).

Hakim, R. E., A. C. Griffin and J. M. Knox: Erythema and tumor formation in methoxsalen-treated mice exposed to fluorescent light. Arch. Derm. 82, 572 (1960). — Haranghy, L.: Durch enterales Porphyrin hervorgerufene tödliche Überempfindlichkeit gegen Sonnenlicht. Zbl. allg. Path. path. Anat. 54, 161 (1932). Ref. Zbl. Haut- u. Geschl.-Kr. 42, 215 (1932). — Harber, L. C., A. M. Lashinsky, and R. L. Baer: Skin manifestations of photosensitivity due to chlorothiazide and hydrochlorothiazide. Preliminary and short report. J.

invest. Derm. **33**, 83 (1959). — HARBER, L. C., A. M. LASHINSKY and R. L. BAER: Photosensitivity due to chlorothiazide and hydrochlorothiazide. New Engl. J. Med. **261**, 1378 (1959). Ref. Zbl. Haut- u. Geschl.-Kr. **106**, 226 (1960). — HARL, J.: Les Porphyrinuries. France méd. **15**, 21 (1952). Ref. Zbl. Haut- u. Geschl.-Kr. **83**, 378 (1953). — HARMEL-TOURNEUR, L., et G. DROPSY: Porphyrie cutanée tardive traitée par le B.A.L. Bull. Soc. franç. Derm. Syph. **66**, 543 (1959). — HAUSMANN, W.: Über die giftige Wirkung des Hämatoporphyrins auf Warmblüter durch Belichtung. Wien. klin. Wschr. **52** (1910a). — Die sensibilisierende Wirkung des Haematoporphyrins. Biochem. Z. **30**, 276 (1910b). — HAUSMANN, W., u. H. HAXTHAUSEN: Sonderbände zur Strahlentherapie. Bd. XI: Die Lichterkrankungen der Haut. Berlin: Urban & Schwarzenberg 1929. — HAUSMANN, W., u. O. KRUMPEL: Über die Absorption der Porphyrine im Ultraviolett. Biochem. Z. **186**, 203 (1927). Ref. Zbl. Haut- u. Geschl.-Kr. **25**, 194 (1928). — HAXTHAUSEN, H.: Ein Fall von Hydroa aestivale ähnelndem Lichtausschlag bei einem Patienten mit Hämatoporphyrinurie, hervorgerufen durch Luminal. Derm. Wschr. **84**, 827 (1927). — HELLER, J.: Über das gehäufte Vorkommen einer eigenartigen Affektion der Haut der Ohrmuscheln bei Schülern einer Schule. Dermatitis pustularis vernalis aurium. Med. Klin. **3**, 1131 (1907). — HENSCHKE, U., u. R. SCHULZE: Methodik von Ekzem und Pigmentversuchen. Strahlentherapie **63**, 236 (1938). — Über Pigmentierung durch langwelliges UV. Strahlentherapie **64**, 14 (1939). — HERXHEIMER, K., u. E. NATHAN: Über Sensibilisierung der Haut durch Carboneol gegenüber Sonnenlicht und eine dadurch bedingte Dermatitis solaris. Derm. Z. **24**, 385 (1917). — HIJMANS VAN DEN BERGH, A. A.: On porphyrin in the mouth. Lancet **1928 I**, 281. Ref. Zbl. Haut- u. Geschl.-Kr. **27**, 759 (1928). — HIJMANS V. D. BERGH, A. A., P. MULLER and A. HIJMANS: On porphyrin-modalities. Afd. Natuurk. **38**, 15 (1929). Ref. Zbl. Haut- u. Geschl.-Kr. **31**, 613 (1929). — HJORTH, N.: Polymorphous photogenic eruption. Ichthyosis. Acta derm.-venereol. (Stockh.) **39**, 171 (1959). Ref. Zbl. Haut- u. Geschl.-Kr. **105**, 208 (1960). — HOEDE, K.: Erblichkeit der Lichtkrankheiten. Strahlentherapie **61**, 633 (1938). — Erbpathologie der menschlichen Haut. In: Handbuch der Erbbiologie des Menschen, Bd. III/1, S. 441. Berlin: Springer 1940. — HOERBURGER, W., u. W. SCHULZE: Klinische und chemische Befunde bei einem Fall von Porphyrie. Arch. Derm. Syph. (Berl.) **175**, 671 (1937). — HOESCH, K.: Über die akute Porphyrie. Zbl. inn. Med. **1942**, 321—333, 363—372. Ref. Zbl. Haut- u. Geschl.-Kr. **69**, 671 (1942/43). — HOFMANN, E.: Über die Vererbung der Hydroa vacciniforme. Derm. Z. **53**, 301 (1928). — HOLLAENDER, A.: Radiation biology. Vol. II: Ultraviolet and related radiations. 1955. Vol. III: Visible and near visible light. 1956. New York: McGraw-Hill Book Co. — HOLTI, G., C. RIMINGTON, B. C. TATE and G. THOMAS: An investigation of porphyria cutanea tarda. Quart. J. Med., N.S. **27**, 1 (1958). Ref. Zbl. Haut- u. Geschl.-Kr. **101**, 279 (1958). — HOWELL, J. B.: The sunlight factor in aging and skin cancer. Arch. Derm. **82**, 865 (1960). — HÜBNER, K.: Porphyrinuntersuchungen bei einer Gruppe von Dermatosen. Arch. Derm. Syph. (Berl.) **180**, 289 (1940).

IMBRIE, J. D., L. L. BERGERON and TH. B. FITZPATRICK: Further studies demonstrating an increased erythemal threshold following oral methoxsalen. J. invest. Derm. **35**, 69 (1960). — IPPEN, H.: Photodermatitis phytogenica. Münch. med. Wschr. **1958**, 109. — Neuere Ergebnisse der Lichtforschung. Med. Kosmet. **7**, 345 (1958). Ref. Zbl. Haut- u. Geschl.-Kr. **103**, 43 (1959). — Porphyria cutanea tarda. I. Allgemeines und Klinik. Arch. klin. exp. Derm. **208**, 223 (1959a). — Porphyria cutanea tarda. II. Das Urinsyndrom, Untersuchungsmethoden, Befunde, experimentelle Studien. Arch. klin. exp. Derm. **209**, 466 (1959b). — Zur Diagnostik der kutanen Porphyrien. Verslg Ver. Rhein.-Westf. Derm. 4. 5. 1958, Essen. Derm. Wschr. **139**, 60 (1959c). — Lichtdermatosen und Porphyrin-Photosensibilisierung. Arch. klin. exp. Derm. **210**, 496 (1960a). — Porphyria cutanea tarda. III. Porphyrinvorkommen in Organen, Körperflüssigkeiten und -ausscheidungen (außer Urin). Arch. klin. exp. Derm. **210**, 252 (1960b). — Porphyria cutanea tarda und Beruf. Berufsdermatosen **7**, 256 (1959). Ref. Zbl. Haut- u. Geschl.-Kr. **106**, 56 (1960c). — Entstehung und Behandlung der Porphyria cutanea tarda (chron. hepatische Porphyrie). Vorl. Mitt. Klin. Wschr. **1960** d, 89. — Zur Spezifität der Photoallergie. Verh. Dtsch. Derm. Ges. 1958. Arch. klin. exp. Derm. **211**, 261 (1960e). — Photoallergische Ekzeme durch das Antimykotikum 4-Chlor-2-hydroxybenzoesäure-N-n-butylamid (Jadit). Z. Haut- u. Geschl.-Kr. **31**, 185 (1961a). — Zur Pathogenese der Porphyria cutanea tarda. Arch. klin. exp. Derm. **212**, 467 (1961b). — IPPEN, H., u. H. RUHRMANN: Photodermatitis pigmentaria Freund („Berloque-Dermatitis") durch Kölnisch Wasser-Stift. Z. Haut- u. Geschl.-Kr. **23**, 230 (1957). Ref. Zbl. Haut- u. Geschl.-Kr. **100**, 114 (1958).

JAEGER, H., u. A. VANNOTTI: Porphyria cutanea tarda. 36. Kongr. Schw. Ges. f. Dermat., Lausanne 1954. Dermatologica (Basel) **110**, 389 (1955). — JAFFE, L., and J. G. SHADE: Porphyria (congenital? mixed?). Arch. Derm. **78**, 129 (1958). Ref. Zbl. Haut- u. Geschl.-Kr. **102**, 288 (1958/59). — JAMES, A. P. R.: Sensitivity of the skin to fluorescent light. Arch. Derm. **44**, 256 (1941). — JANOFF, A., J. J. POUTAS and D. YOUNG: Acute intermittent porphyria. Prompt response to therapy with corticotropin. Arch. intern. Med. **91**, 389. Ref.

Zbl. Haut- u. Geschl.-Kr. **87**, 241 (1954). — JARRET, A., and G. SZABÓ: The pathological varieties of vitiligo and their response to treatment with meladinine. Brit. J. Derm. **68**, 313 (1956). — JAUSION, H., P. COURET et B. EL KOHEN: Les dérivés métalloporphyriniques principes, et possibles applications thérapeutiques. (Com. prélimin Marseille.) Soc. franç. Dermat. **1951**, 323. Ref. Zbl. Haut- u. Geschl.-Kr. **80**, 18 (1952). — JAUSION, H.: Les dermatoses causées par le soleil. Arch. belges Derm. **12**, 341 (1957). Ref. Zbl. Haut- u. Geschl.-Kr. **98**, 273 (1957). — JAUSION, H., et F. PAGÈS: Les maladies de lumière et leur traitement. Paris: Masson & Cie. 1933. — JAUSION, M. H.: Les variations de la photo-pathologie en fonction des climats et des saisons. Bull. Soc. franç. Derm. Syph. **1938**, 1692. — JESIONEK, A.: Lichtbiologie und Lichtpathologie. Wiesbaden: J. F. Bergmann 1912. — JIRÁSEK, L., and R. SCHWANK: Photodermatitis after chlortetracycline. Čs. Derm. **34**, 379 (1959). Ref. Zbl. Haut- u. Geschl.-Kr. **107**, 13 (1960). — JODLBAUER, A.: Die Sensibilisierung der fluoreszierenden Stoffe (photodynamische Erscheinung). Strahlentherapie **2**, 71 (1913). — JODLBAUER, A., u. H. v. TAPPEINER: Dtsch. Arch. klin. Med. **82**, 520 (1905). Zit. nach HOLLAENDER: Photodynamic Action. — Die Beziehung zwischen der photodynamischen Wirkung der fluoreszierenden Stoffe und ihrer Fluoreszenz. Strahlentherapie **2**, 84 (1913). — JONQUIÈRES, E. D. L., M. ANGEL MAZZINI y H. J. SÁNCHEZ CABALLEROS: Actinodermatitis papulofigurada eritematoide recidivante. Arch. argent. Derm. **8**, 105 (1958). Ref. Zbl. Haut- u. Geschl.-Kr. **103**, 246 (1959). — JOULIA, P., DULONG, DE RESNAY, L. TEXIER u. DULUC: Ein vierter Fall von Hautporphyrie. Bull. Soc. franç. Derm. Syph.) **61**, 281 (1954).

KÄMMERER, H.: Über die klinische Bedeutung der Porphyrine. Klin. Wschr. **1930 II**, 1658. — Ausgewähltes über Porphyrin, Hämatin, Hämverbindungen. Dtsch. Arch. klin. Med. **195**, 388 (1949). Ref. Zbl. Haut- u. Geschl.-Kr. **80**, 129 (1952). — KÄMMERER, H., u. H. WEISBECKER: Über die sensibilisierende Wirkung der Porphyrine, besonders des Fäulnisporphyrins, gegenüber Licht- und Röntgenstrahlen. Naunyn-Schmiedeberg's Arch. exp. Path. Pharmak. **111**, 263 (1926). — KANOF, N. B.: Hautschutz gegen Sonnenlichtschädigung. Örtliche oder allgemeine Maßnahmen. Arch. Derm. **74**, 46 (1956). — KANSKY, A.: Porphyrinausscheidung im Harn bei Erythematodes discoides chronicus. Hautarzt **12**, 231 (1961). — KAPOSI, H.: Verhandlungsberichte über Xeroderma pigmentosum in Wien. med. Jb. **1882**, 619. — KATZENELLENBOGEN, I.: Cheilitis exfoliativa actinica. Acta derm.-venereol. (Stockh.) **18**, 319 (1937). — KEHL, R.: Ein quantitatives und qualitatives Verfahren zur Bestimmung der Porphyrinisomeren mittels Papierchromatographie. Verh. dtsch. Ges. inn. Med. **1954**, 517. Ref. Zbl. Haut- u. Geschl.-Kr. **92**, 10 (1955). — KEHOE, E. L., ST. NEWMAN and BRUCE CHANDLER: Acute porphyria. A problem in medical diagnosis. U.S. Armed Forces med. J. **4**, 1119 (1953). Ref. Zbl. Haut- u. Geschl.-Kr. **87**, 355 (1954). — KEINING, E.: Die Frühlingsperniosis zum Unterschied von der Herbstperniosis. Derm. Wschr. **110**, 26 (1940). — KENCH, J. E., F. R. FERGUSON and G. S. GRAVESON: Observation on three cases of acute Porphyria. Lancet **1953 I**, 1072. Ref. Zbl. Haut- u. Geschl.-Kr. **87**, 134 (1954). — KENNARD, J.: Nature (Lond.) **171**, 876 (1953). Zit. bei W. SIEDEL, Der Stoffwechsel der Porphyrine. In: FLASCHENTRÄGER und LEHNARTZ, Physiologische Chemie, Bd. II/1 b, S. 996 ff. Berlin-Göttingen-Heidelberg: Springer 1954. — KESTEN, BEATRICE MAHER: Photosensitivity in various dermatoses ecc. (Symp. on Photosensit. in Dermat. Bronx Dermat. Soc. Bronx 15. 12. 1955). Arch. Derm. **74**, 40 (1956). — KESTEN, B. M., and M. SLATKIN: Diseases related to light sensitivity. Arch. Derm. **67**, 284 (1953). — KIMMIG, J.: Ursache und Behandlung der Lichtdermatosen. In: Fortschritte der praktischen Dermatologie und Venerologie. Berlin-Göttingen-Heidelberg: Springer 1952. — Biochemische Erkenntnisse zu den polymorphen Lichtdermatosen. Proc. 11. internat. Congr. Dermat. Stockh. 1957, **3**, 515 (1960). Ref. Zbl. Haut- u. Geschl.-Kr. **108**, 44 (1960). — KIMMIG, J., W. STICHERLING, R. TSCHESCHE u. H. G. URBACH: N-(beta[Indolyl-(3)]-acryloyl)-glycin Isolierung aus Harn und Synthese. Hoppe-Seylers Z. physiol. Chem. **311**, 234 (1958). — KIMMIG, J., u. A. WISKEMANN: Lichtbiologie und Lichttherapie. In: Handbuch der Haut- und Geschlechtskrankheiten, Ergänzungswerk, Bd. V/2, S. 1021. Berlin-Göttingen-Heidelberg: Springer 1959. — KITAGAWA, KIYOSHI: Über Hämatoporphyria congenita. III. Mitt. Experimentelle Untersuchungen über die Porphyrinphotosensibilisation beim Kaninchen. Jap. J. Derm. **28**, 851 u. dtsch. Zus.fass. 61 (1928). Ref. Zbl. Haut- u. Geschl.-Kr. **30**, 197 (1929). — KITCHEVATZ, M.: Etiologie et pathogenèse de la dermatose striée. Photodermite actino-calorique chlorophyllienne. Ann. Derm. Syph. (Paris) **1934**, 3. — Nouvelles recherches sur la photosensibilisation de la peau. Bull. Soc. franç. Derm. Syph. **1936**, 581. — KNOX, J. M., A. C. GRIFFIN and R. E. HAKIM: Effect of chloroquine on erythematous and carcinogenic response to ultraviolet light. Arch. Derm. **81**, 570 (1960). — Protection from ultraviolet carcinogenesis. J. invest. Derm. **34**, 51 (1960). — KOCH u. H. KÖHLER: Zit. nach KEINING. — KÖHLER, H.: Epidemisches Auftreten von Erythema exsudativum multiforme. Med. Welt **1938**, 1631. — KÖNIGSDÖRFFER, H.: Zur Kenntnis der Porphyrie. Strahlentherapie **28**, 132 (1928). Ref. Zbl. Haut- u. Geschl.-Kr. **29**, 54 (1929). — KOSAKI, T.: Über die Pathogenese der Porphyrie, insbesondere der toxischen, nach Gaben von Sulfonalderivaten. J. Biochem. (Tokyo) **38**, 317 (1951). Ref. Zbl. Haut- u. Geschl.-Kr. **82**,

341 (1953). — KOSENOW: Zur Diagnostik der Porphyrindermatosen. Dtsch. Derm. Ges., 22. Tgg Frankfurt a. Main, 16. 9. 1953. Ref. Zbl. Haut- u. Geschl.-Kr. 88, 4 (1954). — Arch. Derm. Syph. (Berl.) **200**, 89 (1955). — KRÁL, F., and B. J. NOVAK: Veterinary dermatology. Philadelphia: J. B. Lippincott Company 1953. — KRAUSKOPF, J., J. MAREK and R. KRUCH: Two cases of photosensitization after aureomycin. Čs. Derm. **34**, 383 (1959). Ref. Zbl. Haut- u. Geschl.-Kr. **106**, 191 (1960). — KREIBICH, C.: Sklerodermieartige Lichtdermatosen. Arch. Derm. Syph. (Berl.) **144**, 454 (1923). — KREN u. HAITINGER: Porphyria congenita (Leichenmaterial). Österr. Derm. Ges., Wien, 20. 5. 1937. Ref. Zbl. Haut- u. Geschl.-Kr. **57**, 651 (1938). — KUHN, W.: Physikalisch-chemische Grundlagen biologischer Vorgänge. In: B. FLASCHENTRÄGER u. E. LEHNARTZ, Physiologische Chemie, Bd. I, S. 8. Berlin-Göttingen-Heidelberg: Springer 1951. — KUSKE, H.: Experimentelle Untersuchungen zur Photosensibilisierung der Haut durch pflanzliche Wirkstoffe. I. Mitt. Lichtsensibilisierung durch Furokumarine als Ursache verschiedener phytogener Dermatosen. Arch. Derm. Syph. (Berl.) **178**, 112 (1938). — Über die Lokalisation verschiedenartiger Hautausschläge im Sternoclaviculardreieck. Gleichzeitig ein Beitrag zur Resistenzverminderung des Integumentes durch Lichteinflüsse. Dermatologica (Basel) **80**, 6 (1939). — Perkutane Photosensibilisierung durch pflanzliche Wirkstoffe. Dermatologica (Basel) **82**, 273 (1940). — Zum Problem der Hautveränderungen bei Porphyrie. Dermatologica (Basel) **92**, 149 (1946). — Dermatitis vernalis aurium. Minerva derm. **34**, 248 (1959a). — Phytophotodermatitis vom Typus der Dermatitis bullosa striata pratensis (Oppenheim). Dermatologica (Basel) **118**, 349 (1959b).

LAMB, J. H.: The effects of sunlight on the skin. N.Y. St. J. Med. **59**, 59 (1959). Ref. Zbl. Haut- u. Geschl.-Kr. **103**, 305 (1959). — LAMB, J. H., P. E. JONES and T. B. MAXWELL: Solar dermatitis. Arch. Derm. **75**, 171 (1957). — LAMB, J. H., P. E. JONES, G. REBELL and H. D. ALSTON: Sensitivity to fluorescent (blue-green) light. Arch. Derm. **77**, 519 (1958). — LANG, R., and J. WALKER: Cutaneous manifestations of porphyria. South African cases. Brit. J. Derm. **65**, 352 (1953). Ref. Zbl. Haut- u. Geschl.-Kr. 88, 115 (1954). — LANGEN, C. D. DE: Einige Probleme aus dem Porphyrinstoffwechsel. Ned. Geneesk **1947**, 3761. Ref. Zbl. Haut- u. Geschl.-Kr. **72**, 387 (1949). — LANGEN, C. D. DE, u. J. A. G. TEN BERG: Porphyrin im Urin als erstes Symptom der Bleivergiftung. Acta med. scand. **130**, 37 (1948). Ref. Zbl. Haut- u. Geschl.-Kr. **72**, 267 (1949). — LANGHOF, H.: Zur Therapie der cutanen Porphyrie. (Sitzg.ber. d. Derm. Ges. Berlin, 13. 12. 1958. Ref. Zbl. Haut- u. Geschl.-Kr. **105**, 87 (1959a). — Untersuchungs- und Behandlungsergebnisse bei cutaner Porphyrie. Dtsch. Gesundh.-Wes. **140**, 1267 (1959b). — Familiäre Lichturticaria. Z. Haut- u. Geschl.-Kr. **28**, 353 (1960). — LANGHOF, H., u. G. GASSEN-BATKE: Hauterkrankungen durch Lichtsensibilisation. Derm. Wschr. **1960**, 972. — LANGHOF, H., u. G. MIDSCHLAG: Aktinisch-traumatisch-bullöse Porphyrindermatose, kombiniert mit beginnender Hämochromatose. Arch. Derm. Syph. (Berl.) **199**, 21 (1955). — LANGHOF, H., H. MÜLLER u. L. RIETSCHEL: Untersuchungen zur familiären, protoporphyrinämischen Lichturticaria. Arch. klin. exp. Derm. **212**, 506 (1961). — Dermatitis solaris subita recidivans. Med. Bild **5**, H. 4, 97 (1962). — LANGHOF, H., u. M. SPRÖSSIG: Zur Pathogenese und Therapie des Lichtekzems. Arch. Derm. Syph. (Berl.) **197**, 303 (1954). — LANGHOF, H., u. G. SCHNEIDER: Beitrag zur Ätiologie von Lichtdermatosen. Arch. klin. exp. Derm. **208**, 181 (1959). — LANGLO, L.: Der Erfolg lokaler Anwendung von Chloroquine und Mepacrine bei der Verhütung des Effektes der UV-Strahlen an der menschlichen Haut. Acta derm.-venereol. (Stockh.) **37**, 85 (1957 I). — Ref. Derm. Wschr. **137**, 162 (1958). — LANGLO, L., u. P. H. NEXMAND: Erfolglose Lokalbehandlung mit Hydrocortison zur Vermeidung des Effektes der UV-Strahlen an der menschlichen Haut. Acta derm.-venereol. (Stockh.) **37**, 82 (1957). — LATOTZKI, H.: Zum Vorkommen von Porphyrie bei Diabetes mellitus. Z. ges. inn. Med. **14**, 785 (1959). Ref. Zbl. Haut- u. Geschl.-Kr. **105**, 217 (1959/60). — LAZZARI, G.: Su un caso di porfiria. Atti Accad. med.-chir. Perugia **5**, 35 (1954). Ref. Zbl. Haut- u. Geschl.-Kr. **92**, 248 (1955). — LE COULANT, P., DULONG, DE ROSNAY et LAVIELLE: Un cas de Porphyrie cutanée. Bull. Soc. franç. Derm. Syph. **61**, 184 (1954). Ref. Zbl. Haut- u. Geschl.-Kr. **90**, 230 (1954/55). — LEHMANN: Xeroderma pigmentosum, Plattenepithelcarcinom. Sitzg Südwestdtsch. Derm. Ver. Ref. Zbl. Haut- u. Geschl.-Kr. **104**, 7 (1959a). — Bullöse Lichtdermatose. Sitzg Südwestdtsch. Derm. Ver. Ref. Zbl. Haut- u. Geschl.-Kr. **104**, 6 (1959b). — LEIDER, M.: Skin changes with Porphyria. Arch. Derm. **67**, 104 (1953). Ref. Zbl. Haut- u. Geschl.-Kr. 88, 152 (1954). — LEONHARDI, G., u. M. BAIER: Die cutane Form der hepatitischen Porphyrie und die Porphyrinausscheidung im Harn. Arch. klin. exp. Derm. **207**, 554 (1958). — LEVAL, M.: The treatment of vitiligo with psoralen derivates. Arch. Derm. **78**, 597 (1958). — LEVY, E. J., M. M. CAHN, J. G. REINHOLD and B. SHAFFER: Delta-amino levulinic acid determinations in patients with polymorphous light eruptions. J. invest. Derm. **31**, 305 (1958). — LEWIN, L.: Über photodynamische Wirkungen von Inhaltsstoffen des Steinkohlenteerpechs am Menschen. Münch. med. Wschr. **1913**, 1529. — LIECHTI, A., E. FEISTMANN u. L. GUGGENHEIM: Über die biologische Wirkung von Sensibilisatoren im langwelligen sichtbaren Licht. Strahlentherapie **64**, 353 (1939). — LIGNAC, G. O. E.: Über die Beeinflussung der Porphyrinwirkung im tierischen

Organismus durch Calciumsalze. Krankheitsforsch. **1**, 177 (1925). Ref. Zbl. Haut- u. Geschl.-Kr. **17**, 321 (1925). — LINDEMAYR, W.: Bullöse Porphyrindermatose der Erwachsenen bei Enteritis. S.-B. Österr. Derm. Ges. 28. 10. 1954. Ref. Zbl. Haut- u. Geschl.-Kr. **90**, 168 (1954/55). — Lichtpurpura. Hautarzt **12**, 174 (1961). — LIPSON, R. L., and E. J. BALDES: The photodynamic properties of a particular hematoporphyrin derivate. Arch. Derm. **82**, 508 (1960a). — Photosensitivity and heat. Arch. Derm. **82**, 517 (1960b). — LONDON, J. D.: Porphyria cutanea tarda. Arch. Derm. **75**, 801 (1957). — LÓPEZ GONZÁLES, G., S. ZIZZIAS, O. COSTA, C. PUGA y C. SUÁREZ: Porfirias. (Aguda intermitente, cutánea tarda.) Arch. argent. Derm. **8**, 301 (1958). Ref. Zbl. Haut- u. Geschl.-Kr. **105**, 31 (1959). — LORINCZ, A. L.: Physiological and pathological changes in skin from sunburn and suntan. J. Amer. med. Ass. **173**, 1227 (1960). — LOWRY, P. T., V. HAWKINSON u. C. J. WATSON: Isotopenversuch am Porphyrin vom Typ III und am Hämoglobinstoffwechsel bei einem gewöhnlichen Fall von „gemischter" Porphyrie. Metabolism **1**, 149 (1952). Ref. Zbl. Haut- u. Geschl.-Kr. **84**, 327 (1953). — LYNCH, F. R.: Porphyria (mixed type), hepativ form. Arch. Derm. **65**, 627 (1952). Ref. Zbl. Haut- u. Geschl.-Kr. **83**, 125 (1953).

MACGREGOR, A. G., R. E. H. NICHOLAS u. C. RIMINGTON: Porphyria cutanea tarda. Untersuchung eines Falles, einschließlich Isolation von einigen bisher nicht beschriebenen Porphyrinen. Arch. intern. Med. **90**, 483 (1952). Ref. Zbl. Haut- u. Geschl.-Kr. **84**, 326 (1953). — MACKEY, L., and A. E. GARROD: On congenital porphyrinuria, associated with hydroa aestivale and pink teeth. Quart. J. Med. **15**, 319 (1922). Ref. Zbl. Haut- u. Geschl.-Kr. **7**, 97 (1923). — MAGNUS, I. A.: Testing patients for photosensitivity. In: Progress in the biological sciences in relation to dermatology, p. 405ff. Cambridge: University Press 1960. — MAGNUS, I. A., and A. D. PORTER: The investigation of skin diseases due to light. Trans. St. John's Hosp. derm. Soc. (Lond.) **1958**, 58. Ref. Zbl. Haut- u. Geschl.-Kr. **106**, 38 (1960). — A case of urticaria solaris studied with a monochromator. Brit. J. Derm. **71**, 51 (1959). — MAGNUS, I. A., A. D. PORTER, K. J. MCCREE, J. D. MORELAND and W. D. WRIGHT: A monochromator. An apparatus for the investigation of the responses of the skin to ultraviolet, visible and near infra-red radiation. Brit. J. Derm. **71**, 261 (1959). — MAGNUS, I. A., A. D. PORTER and C. RIMINGTON: The action spectrum for skin lesions in porphyria cutanea tarda. Lancet **1959 I**, 912. Ref. Zbl. Haut- u. Geschl.-Kr. **105**, 31 (1959). — MALKINSON, F. D.: Porphyria cutanea tarda type. Arch. Derm. **72**, 83 (1955). Ref. Zbl. Haut- u. Geschl.-Kr. **93**, 300 (1956). — MARCHIONINI, A., u. S. TOR: Zur Klimatophysiologie und -pathologie der Haut. I. Mitt. Die Sommercheilitis in Zentralanatolien. Arch. Derm. Syph. (Berl.) **179**, 421 (1939). — MARQUARDT: Porphyrinbestimmung im Urin und ihre Bedeutung bei Hauterkrankungen. Ver. Rhein.-Westf. Derm., Sitzg in Köln, 30. 11.—1. 12. 1935. — MARSDEN, C. W.: Porphyria during chloroquine therapy. Brit. J. Derm. **71**, 219 (1959). — MARTENSTEIN, H.: Experimentelle Untersuchungen bei Hydroa vacciniforme. Arch. Derm. Syph. (Berl.) **140**, 300 (1923a). — Hydroa aestivale. Strahlentherapie **14**, 734 (1922). Ref. Zbl. Haut- u. Geschl.-Kr. **8**, 134 (1923b). — MARTENSTEIN, H., u. A. BOBOWITSCH: Über Strahlenempfindlichkeit bei Xeroderma pigmentosum. Arch. Derm. Syph. (Berl.) **150**, 165 (1926). — MARTIN, P., et J. CANIVET: Porphyrie cutanée tardive de l'adulte. Episode aigu, fébrile, douloureux et digestif avec décharge porphyrinurique massive. Bull. Soc. franç. Derm. Syph. **64**, 714 (1957). Ref. Zbl. Haut- u. Geschl.-Kr. **101**, 342 (1958). — MEJORANA, P. F., J. BLANCO DIEZ u. J. OTERO DE LA GANDERA: Bestimmung der Porphyrine im Urin, Reinigung der Extrakte. Arch. Med. exp. (Madr.) **15**, 327 (1952). Ref. Zbl. Haut- u. Geschl.-Kr. **85**, 6 (1953). — MEJORANA, F. P., J. O. DE LA GANDARA u. J. G. ALVAREZ: Eine neue Methode zur Bestimmung des Porphyrins in den Erythrocyten. Arch. Med. exp. (Madr.) **15**, 319 (1952). Ref. Zbl. Haut- u. Geschl.-Kr. **85**, 5 (1953). — MELLINGER, G. W., and C. C. PEARSON: Acute porphyria. Ann. intern. Med. **38**, 862 (1953). Ref. Zbl. Haut- u. Geschl.-Kr. **87**, 134 (1954). — MERTENS, E.: Über das Vorkommen von Koproporphyrin III bei chronischer genitaler Porphyrie. Vorl. Mitt. Hoppe-Seylers Z. physiol. Chem. **258**, I—II (1939). Ref. Zbl. Haut- u. Geschl.-Kr. **63**, 486 (1939). — MEYER, A. E. H., u. E. O. SEITZ: Ultraviolette Strahlen. Ihre Erzeugung, Messung und Anwendung in Medizin, Biologie und Technik. Berlin: W. de Gruyter & Co. 1949. — MEYER, J.: Lucites allergiques à la porphyrine irradiée. IX. Congr. des Derm. de langue franç. (Ed. Médecine et Hygiène, Genève, 1956). — La protoporphyrie aux porphyrines irradiées. Atti del 2 congr. di fotobiologia Torino 1957(a). Ed. Minerva medica, p. 233. — La sensitometrie actinique en dermatologie. Ann. Derm. Syph. (Paris) **84**, 45 (1957b). — La photoallergie aux porphyrines irradiées. Proc. 11. internat. Congr. Dermat. Stockholm, 1957, **3**, 490 (1960). — MEYER, J., et C. KELLERSHOHN: Les ultraviolets en Médecine. Paris: Doin & Cie. 1956. — MICHALOWSKI R.: La cheilite actinique et l'hétérotopie labiale de glandules salivaires — Un syndrome inédit. Dermatologica (Basel) **114**, 373 (1957). — MICHELI, F., u. G. DOMINICI: Über zwei Fälle von familiärer Porphyrie mit letalem Ausgang. Dtsch. Arch. klin. Med. **171**, 154 (1931). Ref. Zbl. Haut- u. Geschl.-Kr. **40**, 88 (1932). — MICHELSON, H. E.: Hydroa aestivale and porphyrin dermatoses. Arch. Derm. **71**, 628 (1955). Ref. Zbl. Haut- u. Geschl.-Kr. **93**, 33 (1955/56). — MIDANA, A.: Sul comportamento delle porfirine ematiche ed urinarie in alcuni casi di idroa vacciniforme ed estivale, dermatiti solari ed epidermolisi. Boll. Sez. region. Soc. ital. Derm. **3**, 245 (1936). Ref. Zbl. Haut- u. Geschl.-Kr. **56**, 188 (1937). — MIESCHER, G.: Das Problem des Lichtschutzes und der Lichtgewöhnung. Strahlentherapie **35**, 403 (1930). — Untersuchungen über die Bedeutung des Pigments für den UV-Lichtschutz der Haut. Strahlentherapie **45**, 201 (1932). — Zur Histologie der lichtbedingten Reaktionen. Dermatologica (Basel) **115**, 345 (1957). — Biologie und Pathologie des sichtbaren Lichtes des Ultravioletts und des Infrarots. Handbuch der allgemeinen Pathologie, Bd. 10/I, S. 289. 1960. — MIESCHER, G., u. H. MINDER: Untersuchungen über die durch langwelliges UV hervorgerufene Pigmentdunkelung. Strahlentherapie **66**, 6 (1939). — MIKULOWSKI, W.: A fatal case of diarrhea with melanodermia and porphyrinuria in an eight months' old child. Urol. cutan. Rev. **34**, 759 (1930). Ref. Zbl. Haut- u. Geschl.-Kr. **36**, 791 (1931). — MILIAN, G.: Le biotropisme. Paris: Baillière 1929. — MOBITZ: Kongenitale Porphyrinurie. Münch. Derm. Ges., Sitzg v. 25. 6. 1923. Ref. Zbl. Haut- u. Geschl.-Kr. **9**, 439 (1923). — MÖLLER, M.: Der Einfluß des Lichtes auf die Haut. Bibl. med. Abt. D II. Dermatologie und Syphilidologie, H. 8, 13 (1900). — EL MOFTY, A., A. M. EL MOFTY, H. ABDELAL and M. F. S. EL HAWARY: Studies on the mode of action of psoralen derivatives. I. Their effect on copper and glutathione levels in blood and liver. J. invest. Derm. **32**, 645 (1959). — EL MOFTY, A. M.: Observations on the use of Amni majus Linn. in Vitiligo. Brit. J. Derm. **64**, 431 (1952). — MORIAMÉ, G.: Etude clinique de quelques cas de porphyrie cutanée. Arch. belges Derm. **12**, 142 (1956). Ref. Zbl. Haut- u. Geschl.-Kr. **97**, 340 (1957). — MORONI, P.: Ulteriori ricerche sull'effetto Kimmig. (Kimmigsches Lichtband.) Arch. ital. Derm. **29**, 277 (1959). Ref. Zbl. Haut- u. Geschl.-Kr. **105**, 219 (1959/60). — MORRIS, W. E.: Photosensitivity due to tetracycline derivative. J. Amer. med. Ass. **172**, 1155 (1960). — MÜLLER, A. H.: Beitrag zur Kenntnis der Porphyria congenita Günther. Z. klin. Med. **127**, 460 (1934). Ref. Zbl. Haut- u. Geschl.-Kr. **50**, 584 (1935). — MÜLLER, I. L.: The pathogenesis of so-called chronic polymorphic light eruption. Derm. Wschr. **132**, 737 (1955). — Brit. J. Derm. **68**, 36 (1956).

NEFF, L.: Bericht über eine Massenverätzung einer Schulklasse durch ein schierlingähnliches Doldengewächs. Münch. med. Wschr. **1957**, 1680. — NENCKI, M., u. N. SIEBER: Über das Haematoporphyrin. Naunyn-Schmiedeberg's Arch. exp. Path. Pharmak. **24**, 430 (1888). — NÖDL, F.: Über mesenchymale und epitheliale Neubildungen bei Xeroderma pigmentosum. Arch. Derm. Syph. (Berl.) **199**, 287 (1955). — NOEHRING, M.: Der qualitative Porphyrinnachweis. Porphyrinschnellprobe nach Brugsch. Zbl. inn. Med. **4**, 182 (1949). Ref. Zbl. Haut- u. Geschl.-Kr. **74**, 357 (1950). — NORINS, A. L.: Chlorothiazide drug eruption involving photosensitization. Arch. Derm. **79**, 592 (1959). Ref. Zbl. Haut- u. Geschl.-Kr. **105**, 30 (1959/60).

OBERSTE-LEHN, H., u. K. H. SCHROEDER: Die Porphyria cutanea tarda als Wehrdienstbeschädigung. Kasuistische Mitt. Berufsdermatosen **7**, 179 (1959). Ref. Zbl. Haut- u. Geschl.-Kr. **105**, 218 (1959/60). — O'LEARY, P. A., H. MONTGOMERY, L. A. BRUNSTING, R. R. KIERLAND and H. PERRY: Porphyria cutanea tarda (probably mixed type). Arch. Derm. **71**, 277 (1955a). — Porphyria cutanea tarda, chronic discoid lupus erythematosus. Arch. Derm. **71**, 278 (1955b). — OPPENHEIM, M., u. FESSLER: Über eine streifenförmige bullöse Dermatitis (Freibad- und Wiesenpflanzendermatitis). Derm. Wschr. **86**, 183 (1928). — OPSAHL, R.: Porphyrin- bzw. Porphyrinogenausscheidung im Urin bei akuter idiopathischer Porphyrie. Fehlerquellen bei Harnanalysen; eine neue Methode zum klinischen Gebrauch. Norsk Mag. Laegevidensk. **96**, 66 u. dtsch. Zus.fass. 78 (1935). Ref. Zbl. Haut- u. Geschl.-Kr. **51**, 470 (1935). — ORBANEJA, J. G., u. H. C. MENDOZA: Dermatosen und Porphyrie. Dermatologica (Basel) **94**, 327 (1947). — OTTO, H.: Die Bedeutung der toxischen Porphyrinurie in der Gewerbemedizin unter besonderer Berücksichtigung von Untersuchungen an Tetrachlorkohlenstoff- und Phosphorarbeitern. Z. ges. inn. Med. **8**, 1114 (1953). Ref. Zbl. Haut- u. Geschl.-Kr. **89**, 282 (1954). — OTTOLENGHI-LODIGIANI, F.: Le porfirie primitive e secondarie. Rass. Derm. Sif. **6**, 79 (1953). Ref. Zbl. Haut- u. Geschl.-Kr. **91**, 314 (1955). — Studi sulla porfiria congenita. Nota III. Il metabolismo del ferro nelle porfiria congenita. G. ital. Derm. **95**, 450 (1954). Ref. Zbl. Haut- u. Geschl.-Kr. **92**, 17 (1955). — OTTOLENGHI-LODIGIANI, F., u. G. SERCHI: Die Porphyrine und ihr Stoffwechsel bei der kongenitalen Porphyrie. I. Mitt. Untersuchungen der Porphyrinverbindungen im Urin. G. ital. Derm. **92**, 77, (1951). Ref. Zbl. Haut- und Geschl.-Kr. **82**, 293 (1953).

PANCONESI, E., G. MANTELLASSI and B. GIANOTTI: First observations on behaviour of porphyrins in electrophoresi. Ital. gen. Rev. Derm. **1**, 26 (1959). Ref. Zbl. Haut- u. Geschl.-Kr. **105**, 260 (1959/60). — PARISER, H.: Critical evaluation of the psoralens. J. Amer. med. Ass. **170**, 19 (1959). — PATHAK, M. A., and T. B. FITZPATRICK: Bioassay of natural and synthetic furocoumarins (psoralens). J. invest. Derm. **32**, 509 (1959). — PAUL, K. G.: The photooxidation of porphyrins. Proc. 11. internat. Congr. Dermat. Stockholm 1957, **3**, 512 (1960). Ref. Zbl. Haut- u. Geschl.-Kr. **108**, 61 (1960). — PAUL, K. G., and H. THYRESSON: The effect of BAL on a case of cutaneous porphyria. Acta derm.-venereol. (Stockh.) **34**, 403 (1954). — PERRY, H. O., and L. A. BRUNSTING: Porphyria cutanea tarda simulating dermatitis factitia.

Report of a case. Arch. Derm. **74**, 198 (1956). Ref. Zbl. Haut- u. Geschl.-Kr. **97**, 339 (1957). — PETERS, H. A.: BAL therapy of acute porphyria. Neurology (Minneap.) **4**, 477 (1954). Ref. Zbl. Haut- u. Geschl.-Kr. **90**, 182 (1954/55). — PETTIT, J. H. S., and F. G. ANDERSON: Chronic familial Porphyria, with associated changes in long bones. Brit. J. Derm. **65**, 356 (1953). Ref. Zbl. Haut- u. Geschl.-Kr. **88**, 153 (1954). — PEVZNER, E. S., et G. N. PLÉNINA: Porphyrinurie au moment de quelques maladies cutanées. Zit. Zbl. Haut- u. Geschl.-Kr. **107**, 317 (1960). — PIERINI, L. E., u. J. M. BORDA: Die Porphyrienatur des kolloiden Pseudomilium. Ses. Dermatol. en Homenaje al Prof. Luis E. Pierini, **1950**, 419. Ref. Zbl. Haut- u. Geschl.-Kr. **79**, 274 (1952). — PIMENTA DE MELLO, R.: Die kombinierte Wirkung von Rose Bengale und UV-Licht auf die Porphyrinausscheidung beim Kaninchen. Proc. Soc. exp. Biol. (N.Y.) **72**, 292 (1949). Ref. Zbl. Haut- u. Geschl.-Kr. **76**, 323 (1951). — PREISSMANN, M.: Sur l'action provocatrice de la lumière dans la maladie de Darier. Dermatologica (Basel) **91**, 28 (1945). — PRUNTY, F. T. G.: Natrium- und Chloridhaushalt bei akuter Porphyrie und Beziehung zur Nebennierenfunktion. J. clin. Invest. **28**, 690 (1949). Ref. Zbl. Haut- u. Geschl.-Kr. **76**, 41 (1951).

RAAB, O.: Über die Wirkung fluoreszierender Stoffe auf Infusorien. Z. Biol. **39**, 524 (1900). — RAAB, O., A. JODLBAUER u. H. v. TAPPEINER: Die sensibilisierende Wirkung fluoreszierender Substanzen. Leipzig 1907. — RAJAM, R. V., N. VERGHESE and P. N. RANGIAH: Porphyria with a case report of the chronic mixed type. Indian J. med. Sci. **13**, 293 (1959). Ref. Zbl. Haut- u. Geschl.-Kr. **106**, 56 (1960). — RAJKA, G.: Berufliche Photoallergosen. Berufsdermatosen **4**, 261 (1956). — RANDAK: Porphyrin bei Lupus erythematodes disseminatus acutus. Wien. Derm. Ges., Sitzg 23. 10. 1924. Ref. Zbl. Haut- u. Geschl.-Kr. **16**, 382 (1925). — RATCLIFFE COCKER: Zit. nach HELLER. — REDEKER, A. G., R. E. STERLING and B. ARCHER: Porphyria cutanea tarda. Report of a case effectively treated with dimer caprol (BAL). Arch. intern. Med. **104**, 779 (1959). Ref. Zbl. Haut- u. Geschl.-Kr. **106**, 56 (1960). — ROEDERER, J., et J. ZIMMER: Un cas de porphyrie cutanée chez un adulte. Bull. Soc. franç. Derm. Syph. **62**, 188 (1955). Ref. Zbl. Haut- u. Geschl.-Kr. **93**, 300 (1956). — ROLLIER, R., et G. DELEUZE: La porphyrie cutanée tardive. Maroc méd. **36**, 798 (1957). Ref. Zbl. Haut- u. Geschl.-Kr. **100**, 228 (1958). — ROSENTHAL, I. M., E. L. LIPTON and G. ASTROW: Effect of splenectomy on porphyria erythropoietica. Pediatrics **15**, 663 (1955). — ROSS, P.: Occupational skin lesions due to pitch and tar. Brit. med. J. **1948 II**,, No 4572 369. — ROST, A. G., u. PH. KELLER: JADASSOHNs Handbuch der Haut- und Geschlechts krankheiten, Bd. V/2, Die Wirkung des Lichtes auf die gesunde und kranke Haut, S. 1. Berlin: Springer 1929. — ROTH, I., L. GORECZKY, J. MOLNAR u. I. SÜMEGI: Neuere Untersuchungen auf dem Gebiete der Porphyrinopathien. Z. ges. inn. Med. **12**, 707 (1957). Ref. Zbl. Haut- u. Geschl.-Kr. **100**, 227 (1958). — ROTHMAN, S.: Research on Xeroderma pigmentosum. Arch. Derm. Syph. (Berl.) **144**, 440 (1923). — ROTTIER, P. B., and J. C. VAN DER LEUN: Hyperaemia of the deeper cutaneous vessels after irradiation of human skin with large doses of ultraviolet and visible light. Brit. J. Derm. **72**, 256 (1960).

SACHS, P.: Ein Fall von akuter Porphyrie mit hochgradiger Muskelatrophie. Klin. Wschr. **1931**, 1123. — SAIDMAN, J.: Les rayons ultraviolets. Paris 1925. — Les rayons ultraviolets et associés en thérapeutique. Paris: Doin 1928a. — La sensitométrie de la peau. Bull. Soc. franç. Derm. Syph. **35**, 296 (1928b). — SAINT, E. C., D. CURNOW, R. PATON and I. B. STOKES: Diagnosis of acute Porphyria. Brit. med. J. **1954 I**, No 4872, 1182. — SAMS, W. M.: Kontaktphotodermatitis. Arch. Derm. **73**, 142 (1956). — Ref. Derm. Wschr. **134**, 1215 (1956). — Photosensitizing therapeutic agents. J. Amer. med. Ass. **174**, 2043 (1960a). — Contact photodermatitis from sun screen agents. Proc. internat. Congr. Dermat. (Stockholm) 1957, **3**, 496 (1960b). — SANNINO, M.: Sul trattamento dell'orticaria solare. (Considerazioni patogenetiche a proposito di un caso clinico.) Dermatologia (Napoli) **9**, 4 (1958). Ref. Zbl. Haut- u. Geschl.-Kr. **101**, 197 (1958). — SCHENCK, R. R.: Controlled trial of methoxsalen in solar dermatitis of chippewa indians. J. Amer. med. Ass. **172**, 1134 (1960). — SCHIFF, M., and O. F. JILLSON: Photoskin tests in Hydroa vacciniforme. Arch. Derm. **82**, 812 (1960). — SCHMID, R.: Klinische und experimentelle Porphyrie. Schweiz. med. Wschr. **1952**, 1121. — Symposium der Ciba Foundation über Biosynthese und Stoffwechsel der Porphyrine. Schweiz. med. Wschr. **1955**, 565. — SCHMID, R., S. SCHWARTZ and D. SUNDBERG: Erythropoietic (congenital) porphyria: a rare abnormality of the normoblasts. Blood **10**, 416 (1955). — SCHMID, R., S. SCHWARTZ u. C. J. WATSON: Neuere Ergebnisse auf dem Gebiete der Porphyrien. Acta haemat. (Basel) **10**, 150 (1953). Ref. Zbl. Haut- u. Geschl.-Kr. **89**, 163 (1954). — SCHMID, R.: The porphyrias. In: J. B. STANBURY, J. B. WYNGAARDEN and D. S. FREDRICKSON, The metabolic basis of inherited disease, p. 939ff. New York-Toronto-London: McGraw-Hill Book Co. 1960. — SCHMIDT, P. R.: Neurologische und psychische Störungen bei den P.-Krankheiten. Fortschr. Neurol. Psychiat. **20**, 422 (1952). Ref. Zbl. Haut- u. Geschl.-Kr. **88**, 274 (1954). — SCHMITZ, R., u. W. WAGNER: Lichturtikaria bei Porphyrinurie. Derm. Wschr. **134**, 765 (1956). — SCHNEIDER, W.: Prophylaxe und Rezidivverhütung von Dermatosen einschließlich Lichtdermatosen mit besonderer Berücksichtigung der dermatologischen Praxis. Verslg Südwestdtsch. Derm.-Verein. 26./27. 10. 1957, Frankfurt a. M. Derm. Wschr.

138, 1183 (1958). — SCHÖLMERICH P.: Zur Symptomatologie der akuten Porphyrie. Ärztl. Wschr. **1955**, 618. — SCHREUS, H. TH..: Kongenitale Porphyrinurie. Herbsttagg d. Ver. Rhein.-Westfäl. Derm. Düsseldorf, Sitzg v. 8. 11. 1931. Ref. Zbl. Haut- u. Geschl.-Kr. **40**, 582 (1932). — SCHREUS, H. TH.: Ergebnisse und Probleme der Porphyrinforschung. Klin. Wschr. **1934**, 121. — Porphyrie und Krankheitssymptome durch Porphyrine (Porphyrinopathien). Strahlentherapie **61**, 649 (1938). — SCHREUS, H. TH., u. C. CARRIÉ: Über die Einwirkung von Leber auf Kopro- und Uroporphyrin. Strahlentherapie **40**, 340 (1931 a). — Beitrag zur Methodik des Porphyrinnachweises im Harn. Klin. Wschr. **1931 I** b, 1017. — Beobachtungen bei einem Fall von kongenitaler Porphyrie. Derm. Z. **62**, 347 (1931 c). — Zur Physiologie und Pathophysiologie der Porphyrin-Ausscheidung. Klin. Wschr. **1933**, 745. — SCHREUS, H. TH., u. H. IPPEN: Photoallergie, hervorgerufen durch ein orales Antidiabetikum. Dtsch. med. Wschr. **1958**, 98, 108. — SCHULZ, K. H., A. WISKEMANN u. K. WULF: Klinische und experimentelle Untersuchungen über die photodynamische Wirksamkeit von Phenothiazin-Derivaten, insbesondere Megafen. Arch. klin. exp. Derm. **202**, 285 (1956). — SCHUMM, O.: Über die natürlichen Porphyrine. Hoppe-Seylers Z. physiol. Chem. **126**, 169 (1923). Ref. Zbl. Haut- u. Geschl.-Kr. **11**, 45 (1924). — SCHUMM, O., F. BECKERMANN u. G. KNOP: Über den Porphyringehalt des Blutes bei Krankheiten und nach Zufuhr von Hämatoporphyrin Nencki oder Protoporphyrin. Naunyn-Schmiedeberg's Arch. exp. Path. Pharmak. **205**, 98 (1948). Ref. Zbl. Haut- u. Geschl.-Kr. **73**, 80 (1949). — SCHUPPLI, R.: Klinische und experimentelle Untersuchungen über den Porphyrinstoffwechsel. Dermatologica (Basel) **116**, 289 (1958). — Weitere Untersuchungen über den Porphyrinstoffwechsel. Dermatologica (Basel) **118**, 248 (1959 a). — Porphyrin und Porphyrinkrankheiten. Akt. Probl. Derm. **1**, 411 (1959 b). — Experimentelle Untersuchungen über Porphyrinstoffwechsel und Lichtdermatosen. Proc. 11. internat. Congr. Dermat. Stockholm 1957, **3**, 501 (1960). — SCHWARZ, G. A., and J. A. L. MOULTON: Porphyria. A clinical and neuropathologic report. Dep. of Neurol. Univ. of Pennsylv., Philadelphia. Arch. intern. Med. **94**, 221 (1954). Ref. Zbl. Haut- u. Geschl.-Kr. **92**, 248 (1955). — SCHWARZ, K., and M. SCHWARZ-SPECK: Experimentally induced photoallergy to sulfonamide. Acta allerg. (Kbh.) Suppl. **7**, 224 (1960). — SCHWARZ, K., u. M. SPECK: Experimentelle Untersuchungen zur Frage der Photoallergie der Sulfonamide. Dermatologica (Basel) **114**, 232 (1957). — SCOLARI, E. G.: Porfiriogenesi e porfirie. Minerva derm. **24**, 189 (1954). — SCOTT, J. J.: The metabolism of delta-aminolaevulinic acid. In: Porphyrin biosynthesis and metabolism. London: Ciba Foundation 1955. — SCOTT, F. P., and S. M. C. MOLHUYSEN-V. D. WALLE: Light dermatoses. Dermatologica (Basel) **116**, 96 (1958). — SELLEI, J.: Purpura papulosa aestivalis. Arch. Derm. Syph. (Berl.) **161**, 29 (1930). — SERRA, J. B.: A proposito del „paaj" y otras fitodermatosis. (Estudio de un caso.) Rev. argent. Dermatosif. **41**, 113 (1957). Ref. Zbl. Haut- u. Geschl.-Kr. **102**, 185 (1958/59). — SERTOLI, P.: Konstitutionelles Syndrom der „Bullosis traumatica" und Lichtsensibilisierung bei einem Albino auf wahrscheinlicher Grundlage einer Porphyrinurie. Derm. Wschr. **123**, 191 (1951). — SHEMIN, D.: The biosynthesis of porphyrins. In: O. KRAYER, E. LEHNARTZ, A. v. MURALT, H. H. WEBER, Ergebnisse der Physiologie, biologischen Chemie und experimentellen Pharmakologie. Berlin-Göttingen-Heidelberg: Springer 1957. — SHIBUYA, HISAO: Über die sensibilisierende Wirkung der Porphyrine. Strahlentherapie **17**, 412 (1924 a). — Über die Sensibilisation von Warmblütern durch Serum-Porphyringemenge. Zur Kenntnis des Hydroaharnes. Strahlentherapie **18**, 710 (1924 b). — SHIMODA, CH., and R. HASEGAWA: Urticaria solare. Jap. J. Derm. **68**, 1046 u. Abstr. 190 (1958). Ref. Zbl. Haut- u. Geschl.-Kr. **104**, 175 (1959). — SIDI, E., et M. HINCKY: Traitement des dermites par photosensibilisation. Thérapeutique **35**, 512 (1959). Ref. Zbl. Haut- u. Geschl.-Kr. **105**, 24 (1959/60). — SIEDEL, W.: Der Stoffwechsel der Porphyrine. In: FLASCHENTRÄGER u. LEHNARTZ, Physiologische Chemie, Bd. II/1 b, S. 996 ff. Berlin-Göttingen-Heidelberg: Springer 1954. — SIEMENS, H. W.: Studien über Vererbung von Hautkrankheiten. Arch. Derm. Syph. (Berl.) **140**, 314 (1922). — SIEMENS, H. W., u. E. KOHN: Studien über Vererbung von Hautkrankheiten. IX. Xeroderma pigmentosum (mit Mitt. von fünf neuen Fällen). Z. indukt. Abstamm.- u. Vererb.-L. **38**, 1 (1925). — SLEPYAN, A. H.: Polymorphous light eruption. Arch. Derm. **80**, 109 (1959). Ref. Zbl. Haut- u. Geschl.-Kr. **105**, 207 (1959/60). — SNAPPER, J.: Porphyrinurie mit und ohne Koliken. Dtsch. med. Wschr. **1922**, 619. Ref. Zbl. Haut- u. Geschl.-Kr. **6**, 221 (1923). — SONCK, C. E.: Über die Photosensibilität bei Lymphogranuloma inguinale. Acta derm.-venereol. (Stockh.), Suppl. VI, Helsingfors 1941. — SOYSAL, S. S., M. BILGER et O. NEYZI: A propos de deux cas de porphyrie du type „cutanea tarda". Arch. franç. Pédiat. **16**, 1084 (1959). Ref. Zbl. Haut- u. Geschl.-Kr. **106**, 136 (1960). — SPÄTH, E.: Die natürlichen Cumarine und ihre Wirkung auf Fische. Mh. Chem. **69**, 75 (1936). — STEGMAIER, O. C.: Chronic porphyria. Arch. Derm. **71**, 415 (1955). Ref. Zbl. Haut- u. Geschl.-Kr. **92**, 323 (1955). — Methoxsalen and sun-tanning. Arch. Derm. **79**, 148 (1959). Ref. Zbl. Haut- u. Geschl.-Kr. **103**, 43 (1959). — STEINIGER, F.: Erbbiologie und Erbpathologie des Hautorgans der Säugetiere. IV. Keratose, unvollständige Hautbildung, Ödeme, Lichtüberempfindlichkeit, Ekzeme, Tumoren. In: Handbuch der Erbbiologie des Menschen, Bd. III/1, S. 375. Berlin: Springer 1940. — STEVANOVIC, D. V.: Polymorphic light eruption. Brit. J. Derm. **72**, 261 (1960). — Sun screening substances. Their physical evaluation and clinical application. Brit. J. Derm. **72**, 271 (1960). — Stich, W.: Die Vitamintherapie der Porphyrinkrankheiten. Dtsch. med. Wschr. **1951**, 967. — Über einen neuen biochemischen Unterschied zwischen humaner akuter Porphyrie und experimenteller Porphyrie. Klin. Wschr. **1958** a, 386. — Die kongenitale Porphyrie, eine erythropathische hämolytische Anämie (Porphyrocytose). Schweiz. med. Wschr. **1958** b, 1042. — Humane und experimentelle Porphyrinkrankheiten. Münch. med. Wschr. **1959** a, 455, 514. — Klinik und Biochemie der Porphyrinkrankheiten. Münch. med. Wschr. **1959** b, 1718. — Neue Ergebnisse über Porphyrinstoffwechsel und Porphyrinkrankheiten. Klin. Wschr. **1959** c, 681. — Sümegi, St.: Über die kongenitale tierische Porphyrie. Dermatologica (Basel) **90**, 242 (1944). — Sümegi, St., u. L. Szodoray: Ein einfaches Verfahren zur Bestimmung der Porphyrine im Harn und im biologischen Material. Dermatologica (Basel) **90**, 233 (1944). — Sulzberger, M. B., and R. L. Baer: Studies in hypersensitivity to light. I. Preliminary report. J. invest. Derm. **6**, 345 (1945). — Sulzberger, M. B., and A. B. Lerner: Suntanning, potentiation with oral medication. J. Amer. med. Ass. **167**, 2077 (1958). — Svendsen, I. B.: Urticaria solaris. Acta derm.-venereol. (Stockh.) **39**, 170 (1959). Ref. Zbl. Haut- u. Geschl.-Kr. **105**, 207 (1959/60). — Szodoray, L., u. St. Sümegi: Über die Nosologie der chronischen kutanen Porphyrie. Dermatologica (Basel) **90**, 224 (1944).

Tappeiner, S.: Die bullöse Porphyrindermatose beim Erwachsenen (Zeligman-Baum). Abstracts of short papers. In: The tenth internat. congr. of Dermatology, London, 1952. Proceedings, p. 407. — Wien. klin. Wschr. **1953**, 143. — 3 Fälle von bullöser Porphyrindermatose. Österr. Derm. Ges., Sitzg v. 29. 10. 1953. Ref. Zbl. Haut- u. Geschl.-Kr. **88**, 353 (1954). — Porphyria cutanea tarda. Derm. Wschr. **133**, 305 (1956). — Tappeiner, S., u. H. Tirschek: Das Syndrom der aktinisch-traumatischen bullösen Porphyrindermatose. Arch. Derm. Syph. (Berl.) **196**, 65 (1953). — Tataru, C., A. Opris, I. Capusan u. A. Marinescu: Phyto-Photodermatitis in Verbindung mit einer Massenerkrankung. Derm. Wschr. **137**, 106 (1958). — Templeton, H. J., and C. J. Lunsford: Eczema solare and Porphyria. Arch. Derm. **25**, 691 (1932). Ref. Zbl. Haut- u. Geschl.-Kr. **42**, 215 (1932). — Teodorescu, St., Al. Badaniou u. Gh. Gheorghiu: Über einen eigenartigen Zwischenfall im Verlaufe der Behandlung der kutanen Porphyrie des Erwachsenen mit synthetischen weißen Antipaludika. Derm. Wschr. **139**, 445 (1959). — Thiers, H.: Das Syndrom von Ekchymosen nach Anstrengung ohne Urticaria: Porphyrinurie, Besserung nach Verabreichung starker Dosen von Nikotinsäureamid. Bull. Soc. franç. Derm. Syph. **59**, 177 (1952). — Thiers, H., D. Colomb, J. Fayolle, B. Taine et G. Moulin: Porphyrie cutanée tardive de l'adulte avec décharges porphyrinuriques aigues fébriles. Bull. Soc. franç. Derm. Syph. **64**, 302 (1957). — Thiers, H., D. Colomb et J. Thévénon: Nouveau cas de porphyrie cutanée tardive de l'adulte. Bull. Soc. franç. Derm. Syph. **64**, 44 (1957). — Thiers, H., u. I. Thivolet: Chronische Porphyrie mit Pigmentation der Haut und der Schleimhäute. Bull. Soc. franç. Derm. Syph. **59**, 176 (1952). — Tio, Tiong Hoo, and B. Leijnse: Porphyria cutanea tarda. Arch. Derm. **77**, 568 (1958). — Todd, C. M.: Die Laboratoriumsdiagnostik der Porphyrie mit Bemerkungen über einen akuten Fall. N. Z. med. J. **51**, 37 (1952). Ref. Zbl. Haut- u. Geschl.-Kr. **83**, 124 (1953). — Toleff, J.: Pellagra acuta oder Atriplizismus? Derm. Wschr. **139**, 258 (1959). — Torre, D.: Porphyria cutanea tarda. Arch. Derm. **78**, 120 (1958). — Totter, J. R., E. S. Amos u. C. K. Keith: Der Einfluß der Pteroylglutaminsäure (PGS) auf Glycin und auf den Porphyrinstoffwechsel. J. biol. Chem. **178**, 847 (1949). Ref. Zbl. Haut- u. Geschl.-Kr. **75**, 203 (1950/51). — Toyama, J.: The further course of the congenital porphyrinurie anemia previously reported. Jap. J. Derm. Urol. **23**, 440 (1923). Ref. Zbl. Haut- u. Geschl.-Kr. **11**, 44 (1924). — Trainito, R., u. V. Prato: Klinischer Beitrag zur Frage der Porphyrie mit Polyglobulie. Minerva med. **1953 I**, 72. — Tropp, C., u. L. Penew (Sofia): Quantitative klinische Harnporphyrinuntersuchungen. II. Mitt. Lebercirrhosen, Hepatopathien (außer Cirrhosen), Tuberkulose und andere Krankheiten. (Zugleich ein Beitrag zur Verbesserung und Vereinfachung der Bestimmungsmethode.) Dtsch. Arch. klin. Med. **180**, 411 (1937). — Turner, W. J., and M. E. Obermayer: Studies on porphyria. Arch. Derm. Syph. (Chic.) **37**, 549 (1938).

Unna, G. P.: Histopathologie der Hautkrankheiten. Berlin 1894. — Unna, G. P.: Zit. nach Heller. — Urbach, E.: Lichtdermatosen und Eiklar- und Eigelb-Überempfindlichkeit. Ref. Zbl. Haut- u. Geschl.-Kr. **55**, 181 (1937). — Urbach, W., u. J. Konrad: Über eine durch den langwelligen Anteil des Sonnenspektrums erzeugte Lichtdermatose vom Typus der Prurigo aestivalis Hutchinson. Die lichtschützende Wirkung des Resorcins. Strahlentherapie **32**, 193 (1929).

Vankos, J., u. A. Gerö: Photodermatose, hervorgerufen durch Sulfanilylbutylharnstoff. Medizinische **1959**, 1115. Ref. Zbl. Haut- u. Geschl.-Kr. **105**, 23 (1959). — Vannotti, A.: Klinik und Pathogenese der Porphyrien. Ergebn. inn. Med. Kinderheilk. **49**, 337 (1935). — Porphyrine und Porphyrinkrankheiten. Berlin: Springer 1937. — Les porphyrines en biologie et en clinique. Helv. med. Acta **6**, 658 (1939). Ref. Zbl. Haut- u. Geschl.-Kr. **66**, 636 (1941). — Porphyrinurie und Porphyrinkrankheiten. In: Handbuch der inneren Medizin (begr. von

MOHR u. STAEHLLIN, 4. Aufl. Herausgeg. von BERGMANN, FREY, SCHWIEGK), Bd. 7: Innersekretorische und Stoffwechselkrankheiten, Teil 2: Stoffwechselkrankheiten, bearbeitet von GRAFE, KOLLER, KÜHNAU, LÖFFLER, SCHETTLER, SCHREIER u. VANNOTTI. Berlin-Göttingen-Heidelberg: Springer 1955. — VEIEL: Über einen Fall von Eczema solare. Vjz. Derm. **19**, 1113 (1887). — VIGLIOGLIA, P., R. O. LINARES, J. VIGLIOGLIA y J. VIDIELLA: Porfiria mutilante. Una nueva observación. Pren. méd. argent. **45**, 3671 (1958). Ref. Zbl. Haut- u. Geschl.-Kr. **105**, 31 (1959/60). — VILANOVA, X., u. P. AGUADE: Beitrag zum Studium der chronischen Porphyrien. Act. dermo-sifiliogr. (Madr.) **43**, 497, 585 (1952). — VILANOVA, X., J. PINOL u. J. REIG: Ein Fall von chronischer Porphyrie. Act. dermo-sifiliogr. (Madr.) **42**, 17 (1950). Ref. Zbl. Haut- u. Geschl.-Kr. **80**, 368 (1952).

WALDENSTRÖM, J.: Untersuchungen über Harnfarbstoffe, hauptsächlich Porphyrine, mittels der chromatographischen Analyse. Dtsch. Arch. klin. Med. **178**, 38 (1935). — Studien über Porphyrie. Acta med. scand., Suppl. **82**, 1 (1937). — The porphyrias as inborn errors of metabolism. Amer. J. Med. **22**, 758 (1957). — WATSON, C. J.: Porphyria advances in international medicine. Year Book Publ. **6**, 235 (1954). — Porphyrin metabolism. In: G. G. DUNCAN, Diseases of metabolism: Detailed methods of diagnosis and treatment, ed. 3, p. 1079—1103. Philadelphia: W. B. Saunders Company 1952. — WATSON, C. J.: Porphyria: Clinical manifestations in relation to chemical findings. Minneapolis, Minn., University of Minnesota Staff Meeting Bulletin **22**, No 7, Nov. 7 (1950). — WAWERSIG, R.: Beitrag zum Krankheitsbild der Porphyria cutanea tarda. Z. Haut- u. Geschl.-Kr. **23**, 154 (1957). Ref. Zbl. Haut- u. Geschl.-Kr. **100**, 42 (1958). — WEIDNER, H., u. G. A. HUNOLD: Porphyrinbestimmung im Urin von Bleiarbeitern. Zbl. Arbeitsmed. **2**, 187 (1952). Ref. Zbl. Haut- u. Geschl.-Kr. **87**, 350 (1954). — WELLS, G. C., and C. RIMINGTON: Studies on a case of Porphyria cutanea tarda. Brit. J. Derm. **65**, 337 (1953). Ref. Zbl. Haut- u. Geschl.-Kr. 88, 153 (1954). — WEYERS, H., u. H. BICKEL: Photodermatose mit Aminoacidurie, Indolaceturie und cerebralen Manifestationen (Hartnup-Syndrom). Klin. Wschr. **1958**, 893. — WIGGINS, C. A.: Tödlicher Fall von akuter Porphyrie bei einem Neger. Brit. med. J. **1950 II**, No 4684, 866. — WILEY, M. SAMS: Contact photodermatitis. Arch. Derm. **73**, 142 (1955). — WINKELMANN, R. K., E. J. BALDES and P. E. ZOLLMAN: Squamous cell tumors induced in hairless mice with ultraviolet light. J. invest. Derm. **34**, 131 (1960). — WISKEMANN, A.: Zur Diagnose des chronisch polymorphen Lichtexanthems. Hautarzt **7**, 162 (1956). — WISKEMANN, A., u. K. WULF: Zur Kenntnis der Lichturticaria mit besonderer Berücksichtigung der auslösenden Spektralbereiche. Arch. klin. exp. Derm. **203**, 394 (1956). — Untersuchungen über den auslösenden Spektralbereich und die direkte Lichtpigmentierung bei chronischen und akuten Lichtausschlägen. Arch. klin. exp. Derm. **209**, 443 (1959a). — Zur Lichtprovokation der Porphyrin-Dermatosen. Arch. klin. exp. Derm. **209**, 454 (1959b). — WITH, T. K.: Porphyrins and porphyria with particular reference to photogenic eruption. Acta derm.-venereol. (Stockh.) **39**, 168 (1959). — WRIGHT, E. T., and L. H. WINER: Histopathology of allergic solar dermatitis. J. invest. Derm. **34**, 103 (1960). — WUCHERPFENNIG, V.: Pathologische Lichtüberempfindlichkeit in qualitativer und quantitativer Hinsicht, nebst Untersuchungen zur Lichtquaddel. Arch. Derm. Syph. (Berl.) **156**, 520 (1928). — WULF, K.: Beitrag zur Ätiologie der Lichtdermatosen. Mit experimentellem Nachweis endogen gebildeter photodynamisch wirksamer Urinsubstanzen unter besonderer Berücksichtigung der chronischen polymorphen Lichtausschläge. Arch. Derm. Syph. (Berl.) **197**, 209 (1954). — Zur derzeitigen Kenntnis der Ätiologie und Pathogenese der chronisch polymorphen Lichtausschläge. Atti del 2 congr. internat. di fotobiologia, Torino 1957. Minerva med. **1957** a, 229. — Untersuchungen zur photodynamischen Wirksamkeit einiger praktisch bedeutsamer Phenothiazin-Derivate. Derm. Wschr. **135**, 475 (1957b). — Lichtdermatosen. In: GOTTRON u. SCHÖNFELD, Dermatologie und Venerologie, Bd. III/1, S. 107. Stuttgart: Georg Thieme 1959. — Experimentelle Untersuchungen über die photodynamische Wirksamkeit einiger Phenothiazinderivate. Proc. 11. internat. Congr. Dermat. Stockholm 1957, **3**, 505 (1960). — WULF, K., A. WISKEMANN u. K. ULLERICH: Zur Ätiologie und derzeitigen Therapie der Keratokonjunktivitis photoallergica. Derm. Wschr. **140**, 1236 (1959).

YI YUNG HSIA, DAVID: Inborn errors of metabolism. Chicago: Year Book Publ. Co. 1960. — YU KUANG-YUAN: Observations on dermatitis solaris in China. Proc. 11. internat. Congr. Dermat. Stockholm 1957, **3**, 538 (1960).

ZELIGMAN, I.: Porphyrins, porphyrinuria and porphyria. Arch. Derm. **74**, 33 (1956). — ZIMMER, J.: Etude de l'élimination des porphyrines dans un cas d'épidermolyse bulleuse dystrophique. Bull. Soc. franç. Derm. Syph. **60**, 324 (1953). Ref. Zbl. Haut- u. Geschl.-Kr. 88, 158 (1954). — ZIMMERMANN, M.: Chronic porphyria (Porphyria hepatica, mixed or „cutanea tarda" type) bullosis actinica et mechanica, hydroa vacciniforme. Arch. Derm. **69**, 504 (1954). — Porphyria with pseudoskleroderma. Arch. Derm. **71**, 546 (1955). — Ultraviolet light therapy. Utilization of tubular fluorescent lamps in a cabinet for generalized simultaneous irradiation. Arch. Derm. **78**, 646 (1958). — ZOON, J.: Untersuchungen über die Empfindlichkeit der Haut für ultraviolette Strahlen bei zwei Patienten mit Xeroderma pigmentosum. Strahlentherapie **61**, 486 (1938).

Epidermolysis bullosa

Von

Walter F. Lever-Boston (Mass., USA)

Mit 1 Abbildung

Einleitung

In seiner 1931 veröffentlichten Darstellung im Jadassohnschen Handbuch teilte RIECKE die Epidermolysis bullosa in zwei Formen ein, und zwar in die vorwiegend dominant vererbte Epidermolysis bullosa simplex und die vorwiegend recessiv vererbte Epidermolysis bullosa dystrophica. Nach RIECKE besitzen diese die folgenden Hauptmerkmale:

Epidermolysis bullosa simplex. Gewöhnlich beginnt diese Krankheit bei der Geburt oder im frühen Säuglingsalter, gelegentlich aber erst im 2. oder 3. Lebensjahr oder selbst erst im Schulalter. Die Blasen treten vor allem an den Händen und Füßen und in der Nähe der großen Gelenke auf. Hyperhidrosis der Handflächen und Fußsohlen findet sich häufig, und zugleich mit gesteigerter Schweißabsonderung nimmt im Sommer die Blasenbildung oft erheblich zu. Die Blasen heilen ohne die Bildung von Narben oder Milien ab. Die Schleimhäute sind nur sehr selten befallen, in nur etwa 2% der Fälle. Auch fehlen gewöhnlich Veränderungen an den Nägeln. Der Allgemeinzustand und die Entwicklung des Patienten sind normal. Oft bessert sich der Hautzustand zur Zeit der Pubertät.

Epidermolysis bullosa dystrophica. Das Alter bei Beginn der Krankheit ist ungefähr das gleiche wie bei der Simplex-Form. Die Hände, Füße, Ellbogen und Knie sind ebenfalls Prädilektionsorte, aber auch der Kopf, der Stamm und die Extremitäten sind oft befallen. An den Schleimhäuten treten Blasen häufig auf, besonders im Munde, gelegentlich aber auch im Pharynx, im Oesophagus, im Respirationstractus und an den Conjunctiven. Charakteristisch für die dystrophische Form sind Hautatrophien, die oft schwer sind und dann zu Mutilationen und zu einem Zusammenwachsen von Fingern führen können. Oft bilden sich Milia beim Abheilen der Blasen. Nageldefekte können schon bei der Geburt vorliegen; gewöhnlich treten aber Nagelanomalien erst später auf. In seltenen Fällen kommt es auch zu Atrophie an der Mundschleimhaut, im Kehlkopf, im Oesophagus und an den Conjunctiven sowie zu Trübungen der Hornhaut. Das Allgemeinbefinden und die Entwicklung des Patienten sind oft beeinträchtigt.

Bereits 2 Jahre nach dem Erscheinen von RIECKES Beitrag, d.h. im Jahre 1933, stellte COCKAYNE eine dritte Form der Epidermolysis bullosa auf, nämlich die dominant-dystrophische Epidermolysis bullosa, da er erkannte, daß die dominant vererbten dystrophischen Fälle sich in wesentlichen Zügen von den recessiv vererbten Fällen unterschieden. Eine vermeintlich vierte Form, die Epidermolysis bullosa letalis, wurde 1937 von HERLITZ beschrieben. Es hat sich aber in den letzten Jahren ergeben, daß diese lediglich eine schwere und daher mit dem Tode endende Verlaufsart der recessiv-dystrophischen Epidermolysis bullosa darstellt. Als Sonderformen der Epidermolysis bullosa sind heute anerkannt: die von COCKAYNE im Jahre 1938 beschriebene Epidermolysis bullosa der Hände und Füße als eine Sonderform der Epidermolysis bullosa simplex, die Epidermolysis bullosa albo-papuloidea als eine Sonderform der dominant-dystrophischen Epidermolysis bullosa und die Epidermolysis bullosa ulcero-vegetans als eine Sonderform der recessiv-dystrophischen Epidermolysis bullosa. Von Interesse ist auch, daß Oesophagusstenosen sowie Carcinombildung in den Krankheitsherden bei der recessiv-dystrophischen Epidermolysis bullosa, obwohl bereits von RIECKE kurz erwähnt, letzthin mehrere Male beschrieben worden sind.

Die Einteilung der Epidermolysis bullosa ist, dem heutigen Stande der Literatur entsprechend, die folgende:

1. Epidermolysis bullosa simplex (dominant). Sonderform: Epidermolysis bullosa simplex der Füße und Hände.

2. Dominant-dystrophische Epidermolysis bullosa. Sonderform: Epidermolysis bullosa albo-papuloidea.

3. Recessiv-dystrophische Epidermolysis bullosa. Sonderformen: Epidermolysis bullosa ulcero-vegetans, Epidermolysis bullosa letalis.

1. Klinische Beschreibung

a) Epidermolysis bullosa simplex der Füße und Hände

COCKAYNE (1938, 1947) stellte diese Form als ein genetisch von den anderen Formen der Epidermolysis bullosa unabhängiges Krankheitsbild auf und behielt daher die erstmalig von F. PARKES WEBER (1926) benutzte Bezeichnung bei: „Recurrent bullous eruption of the feet." Mehrere Autoren sind heute jedoch der Ansicht, daß es sich hier nur um eine Sonderform der Epidermolysis bullosa simplex handelt (s. unten).

Blasen bilden sich dabei gewöhnlich nur an den Füßen, manchmal aber sowohl an den Händen als auch an den Füßen im Anschluß an ein oft nur geringfügiges Trauma. Vielfach bilden sich Blasen nur bei warmem Wetter, und bei vielen Patienten besteht Hyperhidrose an den Handflächen und Fußsohlen. Die Blasen heilen stets ohne Narbenbildung. Die Krankheit kann solitär, d.h. ohne Familienanamnese, auftreten, wie schon in dem von PARKES WEBER beschriebenen Falle. Vielfach besteht jedoch ausgesprochene dominante Vererbung, so daß zahlreiche Familienmitglieder über mehrere Generationen hin befallen sind (COCKAYNE 1938; LEIDER und BAER; FRANKS und DAVIS). Bei weitem das größte Familienvorkommen beobachteten JOHNSON und TEST, die einen Familienstammbaum veröffentlichten, in dem unter 356 Personen in acht Generationen 125 befallen waren. Gewöhnlich treten die Blasen schon kurz nach der Geburt auf; aber tardive Fälle kommen vor. So haben FRANKS und DAVIS das Auftreten im Alter von 18 Jahren, WAISMAN im Alter von 20 Jahren und WINER und ORMAN im Alter von 31 Jahren mitgeteilt. Bei all diesen Patienten trat die Blasenbildung erstmalig während des Heeresdienstes in Erscheinung, wahrscheinlich weil während diesem die Füße mehr als sonst strapaziert werden. ROBINSON jedoch berichtete das Auftreten von Blasen ohne jeglichen äußeren Grund bei sowohl Vater als auch Sohn erst im Alter von 43 Jahren. Besonders bei solitär auftretenden oder tardiven Fällen ist die Diagnose vielfach verfehlt worden und die Blasen wurden dann als Dermatomykose oder Kontaktdermatitis diagnostiziert (FRANKS und DAVIS).

Es besteht keine Übereinstimmung darüber, ob die Epidermolysis bullosa simplex der Füße und Hände lediglich eine abgeschwächte Form der Epidermolysis bullosa simplex darstellt oder ob die beiden Krankheiten Phaene verschiedener dominanter Genloci darstellen. Der Grund dafür, daß z.B. COCKAYNE (1938, 1947), HALDANE und POOLE, JOHNSON und TEST sowie ANNING die Krankheit als eine selbständige Einheit angesehen haben, liegt darin, daß die klinischen Anzeichen gerade bei Familien mit vielen Befallenen auffallend gleichartig sind und Blasen nicht anderswo als an den Füßen und Händen und in manchen Familien nur an den Füßen auftreten. Fälle von intrafamiliärem Alterieren mit der Epidermolysis bullosa simplex, wie sie z.B. GREENBERG, FRANK sowie ROBINSON berichtet haben, würden nach der der Ansicht dieser Autoren der Epidermolysis bullosa simplex zugeteilt werden, die sich ja auch gelegentlich bei leichteren Fällen auf die Füße und Hände beschränken kann. Andere Autoren, wie z.B. WAISMAN und auch SCHNYDER, JUNG und SALAMON, sehen in solchen Fällen den Beweis dafür, daß die beiden Formen formalgenetisch zusammengehören. In der Tat sprechen Fälle, wie sie Greenberg, Frank sowie Robinson berichtet haben, sehr für diese Ansicht. Greenbergs Patient hatte, wie seine Mutter und seine zwei Schwestern, immer nur Blasen an den Füßen und Händen mit einer einzigen Ausnahme: Als er einmal ritt, brachen an seinen Oberschenkeln große Blasen aus, so daß er mehrere Wochen im Bett verbringen mußte. In der von Frank mitgeteilten Familie hatte unter 19 Merkmalsträgern einer einmal eine Blase außerhalb der Hände und Füße, nämlich am Halse nach dem Tragen eines steifen Kragens. In der von Robinson beobachteten Familie hatte der Urgroßvater Blasen nur an den Füßen und Händen, während unter 17 Merkmalsträgern in den drei folgenden Generationen fünf Blasen nur an den Füßen und Händen hatten, während sechs gelegentlich Blasen auch an anderen Hautstellen hatten.

b) Dominant-dystrophische Epidermolysis bullosa

Diese zeigt in ihrem klinischen Bild große Ähnlichkeit mit leichten Fällen von recessiv-dystrophischer Epidermolysis bullosa (Schnyder und Eichhoff). Das Leiden tritt bei Geburt oder bald nachher auf. Tardive Fälle sind bis jetzt noch nicht beobachtet worden. Die Blasen kommen vor allem im Bereich der Hände und Füße sowie an den Ellbogen und Knien vor. Mundschleimhautblasen werden in ungefähr 20% der Fälle vorgefunden (Touraine). Abheilung erfolgt teils mit und teils ohne Narbenbildung. Die Narben sind vorwiegend vom atrophischen Typ; gelegentlich aber kommen hypertrophische Narben und Hyperkeratosen vor. Milien bilden sich recht oft im Bereich der Narben. Nagelstörungen sind häufig und bestehen oft aus klauenartigen Nagelverdickungen. Hyperhidrose der Handflächen und Fußsohlen besteht in vielen Fällen. Der Allgemein- und Ernährungszustand sind gut und die Intelligenz ist normal.

Bei Mitgliedern zweier Familien, über die Sakaguchi bzw. Hensler berichtet haben, wurde eine schwere dystrophische Epidermolysis bullosa in zwei aufeinanderfolgenden Generationen festgestellt und diese daher als dominant vererbt betrachtet. Wie aber Schnyder und Eichhoff nachweisen konnten, handelte es sich hier um Familien mit Verwandtschaftsehen, so daß in Wirklichkeit bei allen Merkmalsträgern recessive Vererbung vorlag. Dagegen bestand bei einer Familie, in der der Vater und zwei Kinder schwere dystrophische Veränderungen aufwiesen und ein drittes Kind im Alter von 4 Monaten an Epidermolysis bullosa verstorben war, nach den Angaben von Fuchs keine Verwandtschaftsehe; aber eine eingehende Untersuchung des Stammbaums war nicht durchgeführt worden.

c) Epidermolysis bullosa albo-papuloidea

Bei dieser zuerst von Pasini beschriebenen dominant-dystrophischen Form von Epidermolysis bullosa findet man Blasenbildung hauptsächlich an den Extremitäten, während die albo-papuloiden Veränderungen vorwiegend am Stamm auftreten. Aber auch die Extremitäten und gelegentlich die Mundschleimhaut, besonders im Bereich des harten Gaumens, können albo-papuloideEfflorescenzen zeigen (Gasser und Walther). Die albo-papuloiden Veränderungen treten meist erst im 2. Lebensjahrzehnt in Erscheinung, während die Bereitschaft zur Blasenbildung schon in früher Kindheit auftritt. Es handelt sich bei den albo-papuloiden Veränderungen um primär auftretende Herde und nicht um eine Folgeerscheinung der Blasenbildung. Die albo-papuloiden Herde bestehen aus weißlichen oder elfenbeinfarbenen, runden oder ovalären, etwas über das Hautniveau erhabenen, flachen Knötchen oder Plaques, die keine entzündliche Reaktion aufweisen (Götz und Meinicke). Die Zahl der albo-papuloiden Herde ist gewöhnlich recht groß und kann mehrere Hundert betragen (Gasser und Walther). In seltenen Fällen findet man im Bereich der albo-papuloiden Veränderungen sekundär Blasenbildung.

Die Frage, ob die Epidermolysis bullosa albo-papuloidea und die dominant-dystrophische Epidermolysis bullosa formalgenetisch zusammengehören, kann auf Grund der verhältnismäßig wenigen Fälle von Epidermolysis bullosa albo-papuloidea nicht mit Sicherheit entschieden werden. Es scheint aber, daß in Familien mit Epidermolysis bullosa albo-papuloidea alle Merkmalsträger, wenn auch erst später im Leben, albo-papuloide Veränderungen aufweisen. SCHNYDER und EICHHOFF betrachten daher die Epidermolysis bullosa albo-papuloidea als eine möglicherweise genetisch selbständige Form der Epidermolysis bullosa.

d) Epidermolysis bullosa ulcero-vegetans

Die erste Mitteilung über diese Sonderform der recessiv-dystrophischen Epidermolysis bullosa, die 1913 von NICOLAS, MOUTOT und CHARLET veröffentlicht worden war, wird von RIECKE erwähnt. Seitdem haben MIESCHER, MARCHIONINI, BRAIN, VILANOVA und PIÑOL, KEINING und WOHNLICH sowie LEINBROCK weitere Fälle mitgeteilt. Bei dieser Sonderform findet man außer Blasen, Epitheldefekten und atrophischen Herden vegetierendes, schwammiges Granulationsgewebe und sich daraus sekundär durch Zerfall bildende Ulcerationen. Gelegentlich bestehen Narbenbildungen an der Hornhaut (MARCHIONINI; BRAIN; KEINING und WOHNLICH) und im Kehlkopf, besonders an den Stimmbändern (NICOLAS et al.; MARCHIONINI). Im Fall VILANOVA bestand eine starke Hypertrophie des Zahnfleisches. Die Patienten zeigen oft allgemeine Unterentwicklung. In dem von BRAIN berichteten Patienten starb ein Zwilling an dieser Krankheit im Alter von $1^1/_2$ Jahren. Bei den zwei Patienten, über die MIESCHER bzw. MARCHIONINI berichteten, bestand eine sekundäre Amyloidose, und MIESCHERs Patient starb daran.

In vier der sieben Mitteilungen bestand ein erbliches Vorkommen der Krankheit bei Geschwistern und einmal auch bei Vettern (NICOLAS; MARCHIONINI; BRAIN; KEINING). In all diesen Fällen hatten die befallenen Verwandten ebenfalls die ulcero-vegetative Form der Epidermolysis bullosa, so daß die Möglichkeit besteht, daß diese Form genetisch selbständig ist.

e) Epidermolysis bullosa letalis

Im Jahre 1935 beschrieb HERLITZ an Hand von acht eigenen Fällen, die er in drei Familien beobachtet hatte, und von 14 Fällen, die er aus der Literatur gesammelt hatte, die Epidermolysis bullosa letalis, die gewöhnlich schon in den ersten Lebensmonaten tödlich endet. Er betrachtete sie als eine selbständige Form der Epidermolysis bullosa. Ein tödlicher Ausgang der Epidermolysis bullosa galt zu RIECKEs Zeiten noch als höchst ungewöhnlich, und RIECKE führte insgesamt nur drei Mitteilungen auf, die 13 Todesfälle in vier Familien betrafen und die überdies alle erst seit 1927 veröffentlicht worden waren. Nach dem Erscheinen der Herlitzschen Arbeit wurden aber recht viele letale Fälle von Epidermolysis bullosa veröffentlicht, so daß jetzt fest steht, daß ein tödlicher Ausgang bei der Epidermolysis bullosa keineswegs selten ist. Es erscheint aber, im Gegensatz zu der von HERLITZ gehaltenen Ansicht, nicht als wahrscheinlich, daß die Epidermolysis bullosa letalis eine besondere Form der Epidermolysis bullosa darstellt. Vielmehr schließt sie besonders schwere Fälle der recessiv-dystrophischen Epidermolysis bullosa ein, bei denen es wegen des raschen tödlichen Verlaufs gewöhnlich nicht zur Bildung von Narben kommt (s. unten).

Die Epidermolysis bullosa letalis, die stets recessiv vererbt ist, zeichnet sich dadurch aus, daß große Blasen und Epitheldefekte entweder schon bei der Geburt vorhanden sind oder spätestens binnen weniger Tage nach der Geburt auftreten (Abb. 1). Die Zahl und Größe der Blasen nimmt allmählich zu. Wegen der schlechten Heilungstendenz dehnen sich die Epitheldefekte immer weiter aus. Wenn sie aber heilen, so vollzieht sich dies ohne Narbenbildung. Schon auf geringe Berührung hin bilden sich Blasen und das Nikolski-Zeichen ist gewöhnlich positiv. Mundschleimhautveränderungen sind regelmäßig vorhanden. Die Nägel können schon bei Geburt dystrophisch sein und lösen sich später oft ab (LAMB und HALPERT).

Meistens tritt der Tod binnen weniger Tage oder Monate ein, gelegentlich aber erst später, wie bei dem von KAGEN et al. berichteten Fall, bei dem der Tod erst im Alter von 16 Monaten eintrat. In mehreren Berichten waren die befallenen Kinder zur Zeit des Berichtes noch am Leben. In WALTHERs Bericht war das lebende Kind 22 Monate alt, in KLUNKERs Bericht $2^1/_4$ Jahre alt, in ROSSETs Bericht $2^1/_3$ Jahre alt und in EBERHARTINGERs Bericht $2^1/_2$ Jahre alt. Dabei entwickelten sich bei dem von KLUNKER beobachteten Kind Atrophie der Haut an den Fingern und Zehen und ein Zusammenwachsen mehrerer Zehen, und bei dem von EBERHARTINGER beschriebenen Kinde bestand Atrophie an den Endphalangen

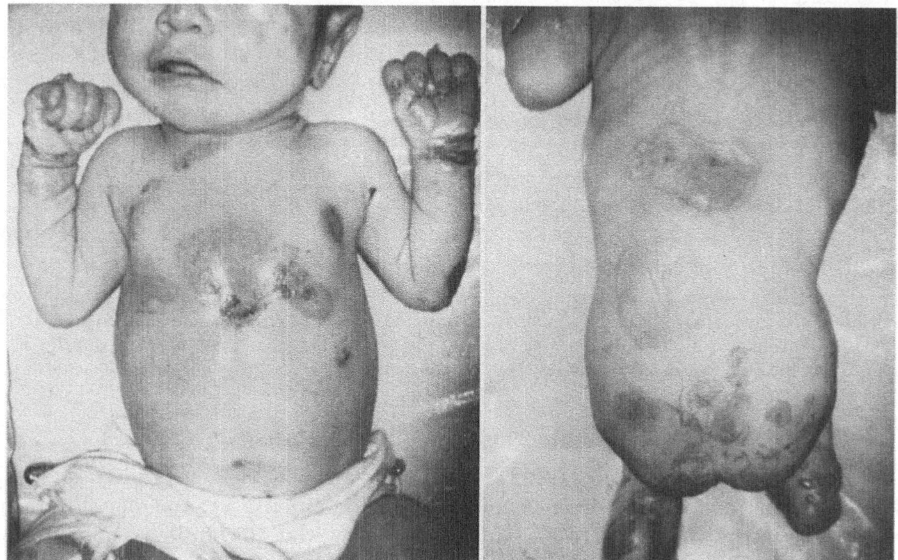

Abb. 1. *Epidermolysis bullosa letalis.* 2 Monate alter Säugling. Der Tod trat 2 Wochen später ein. Auf dem Rücken befinden sich zwei sehr große Blasen

der Finger. Besonders eindrucksvoll ist der Verlauf der Krankheit bei dem erst von SILVER und später von M. L. JOHNSON beobachteten Kinde. Dieses Kind, das schwere Blasenbildungen seit Geburt aufwies und von dem ein Bruder im Alter von 18 Monaten an Epidermolysis bullosa starb, war im Frühjahr 1964 bereits 9 Jahre alt. Es besaß durchschnittliche Intelligenz, war aber körperlich behindert infolge einer Ankylose der Sprunggelenke und hatte nie zu gehen gelernt. Es bestanden Verwachsungen zwischen den Fingern sowie Narbenbildungen an der Haut in der Nähe der Knie- und Sprunggelenke.

Auf Grund seiner Beobachtungen kam EBERHARTINGER zu dem Schluß, daß es Übergangsformen zwischen der Epidermolysis bullosa letalis und der recessiv-dystrophischen Epidermolysis bullosa gäbe; und KLUNKER betrachtete die Epidermolysis bullosa letalis lediglich als die letale Variante der recessiv-dystrophischen Epidermolysis bullosa. Er wies darauf hin, daß bereits TOURAINE im Jahre 1942 diese Meinung vertreten habe. Ferner sah KLUNKER eine beträchtliche Unterstützung seines Standpunktes in den in der Literatur mitgeteilten Geschwisterschaften mit recessiv-dystrophischer Epidermolysis bullosa, die in bezug auf Letalität diskordant waren. So haben unter anderen TILBURY FOX, PETRINI-GALATZ, P. LINSER, HENSLER, BAUMANN und KRAUSE sowie RUSSELL und RIDLEY Geschwisterschaften beschrieben, bei denen ein Geschwister in den ersten Lebenstagen oder Monaten mit Blasen verstarb, während ein anderes Geschwister mit recessiv-dystrophischer Epidermolysis bullosa aufwuchs.

Am bemerkenswertesten in dieser Beziehung ist die große schweizer Sippschaft, über die MUGGLER im Jahre 1963 kurz nach dem Erscheinen von KLUNKERs Arbeit berichtete und die nach MUGGLERs Ansicht den Beweis für die Wesenseinheit der Epidermolysis bullosa letalis und der recessiv-dystrophischen Epidermolysis bullosa erbringt. In dieser Sippschaft mit mehrfach vorkommender Verwandtenheirat befanden sich im Verlauf von über 200 Jahren (festgestellt teilweise auf Grund von Einträgen in das Sterberegister) 30 Fälle von recessiv-dystrophischer Epidermolysis bullosa (von denen sieben Fälle bereits von HENSLER mitgeteilt worden waren; s. S. 598). Unter diesen 30 Fällen befanden sich einige, die bereits im Säuglingsalter am „Blasenausschlag" verstorben waren, während die meisten Befallenen aufwuchsen und dann schwere Hautatrophien und teilweise auch Verstümmelungen an den Händen und Füßen aufwiesen.

f) Oesophagusstenosen bei der recessiv-dystrophischen Epidermolysis

Während RIECKE nur zwei Fälle von Oesophagusstenose erwähnt, finden sich in der 1963 erschienenen Übersicht von BERGENHOLTZ et al. 18 Fälle von Oesophagusstenose. Bei sechs dieser Patienten hatte die durch die Oesophagusstenose hervorgerufene Dysphagie ihren Anfang in frühester Kindheit, während bei der Mehrzahl der Patienten die Beschwerden erstmalig im 3. oder 4. Dezennium auftraten. Die Lokalisation der Oesophagusveränderungen war nicht einheitlich, da sie bei sieben Patienten im oberen Drittel des Oesophagus gelegen waren, bei fünf Patienten im unteren Drittel und bei vier Patienten sich über den ganzen Oesophagus erstreckten.

g) Carcinomentwicklung bei der recessiv-dystrophischen Epidermolysis bullosa

RIECKE referierte einen Fall von Zungencarcinom, 1913 von KLAUSNER berichtet. Seitdem hat SCHILLER das Vorkommen eines Zungencarcinoms und RÖCKL das Vorkommen eines Carcinoms an der Unterlippe mitgeteilt. Da bei beiden Patienten schwere, durch die Epidermolysis bullosa hervorgerufene Veränderungen an der Mundschleimhaut bestanden, sahen beide Autoren die Carcinombildung als eine Folgeerscheinung der Epidermolysis bullosa an.

Ferner ist die Entwicklung eines spinocellulären Carcinoms auf dem Boden ulcerierter Hautherde an den Beinen mehrmals beschrieben worden. Erstmalig wurde darüber 1947 von HALPERN berichtet. Ferner haben CALNAN und PORTER sowie LEINBROCK je einen Fall und RASPONI drei Fälle von Carcinombildung beschrieben. Bei dem von CALNAN beschriebenen Fall und bei einem der drei Fälle von RASPONI (1950) bestanden Carcinombildungen sogar an beiden Beinen. In dem letzteren Falle kam es zur Bildung von Metastasen in den regionären Lymphknoten.

2. Histologie und Elektronenmikroskopie

a) Histologie

RIECKE stellte fest, daß in der Regel die Blase bei der Epidermolysis bullosa simplex subcorneal gelegen sei, bei der Epidermolysis bullosa dystrophica aber subepidermal. Er wies jedoch darauf hin, daß Ausnahmen vorkämen und daß daher die Histologie für die Differentialdiagnose nicht verläßlich sei. Derselbe Standpunkt wurde 1942 von TOURAINE und 1953 von DUPERRAT vertreten, mit dem Zusatz, daß bei der dominant-dystrophischen Form die Blasen entweder subcorneal oder subepidermal gelegen seien. Auf Grund neuerer Untersuchungen, bei denen entweder ganz frische oder experimentell hervorgerufene Blasen (siehe unten) untersucht wurden, steht wohl nun fest, daß sich die Blasen bei allen Formen der Epidermolysis bullosa nahe der dermo-epidermalen Grenze bilden; aber bei der Epidermolysis bullosa simplex und der dominant-dystrophischen Epidermolysis bullosa regeneriert wegen der guten Heilungstendenz die Epidermis am Blasenboden rasch, so daß man Blasen, die älter als 2 Tage sind, oft subcorneal gelegen auffindet.

Wenn der Rand ganz frischer Blasen histologisch untersucht wird, kann man gewöhnlich Unterschiede in der Art der Blasenbildung zwischen der Epidermolysis bullosa simplex und der recessiv-dystrophischen Form feststellen (s. unten); da aber die voll entwickelten Blasen bei beiden Formen subepidermal liegen, ist eine histologische Differenzierung der beiden Formen nicht verläßlich.

b) Histogenese

Bei der Epidermolysis bullosa simplex scheinen sich die Blasen infolge einer Degeneration innerhalb der Basalzellen zu bilden, wie Schnyder, Jung und Salamon an frischen Blasen und Pearson und Spargo an experimentell erzeugten Blasen feststellen konnten. Die degenerierten Basalzellen heben sich entweder mit der Blasendecke ab (Pearson und Spargo) oder bleiben vollständig oder teilweise am Blasenboden zurück (Schnyder, Jung und Salamon), wo sie dann aber mit Ausnahme einiger zurückbleibender Epithelinseln bald zerfallen. Der PAS-positive Grenzstreifen erscheint normal. Die Dermis weist keine stärkeren Veränderungen auf.

Bei der recessiv-dystrophischen Epidermolysis bullosa scheint sich die Blase nicht innerhalb, sondern unterhalb der Basalzellen zu bilden. Die abgehobene Epidermis erscheint daher zu Beginn verhältnismäßig normal. Der PAS-positive Grenzstreifen ist meistens schlecht färbbar (Pearson) und gelegentlich erscheint er dissoziiert, d.h. ein Teil lagert sich der Blasendecke an, während der andere Teil der Dermis anliegt (Schnyder, Jung und Salamon). In der obersten Dermis, besonders in den Papillarkörpern, erscheinen die Kollagenfasern und die Elastica fragmentiert (Pearson). van der Meiren et al. haben auf das Verschwinden der vertikal verlaufenden Retikulinfasern in der obersten Lage der Dermis hingewiesen.

Bei der Epidermolysis bullosa letalis beginnt anscheinend die Blasenbildung, ähnlich wie bei der Simplex-Form, mit Vacuolisierung der Basalzellen, wie zuerst von Roberts et al. festgestellt wurde und von Pearson sowie von Klunker und von Lapière et al. bestätigt wurde. Die Epidermis löst sich aber stets, im Gegensatz zur Simplex-Form, vollständig ab. Der PAS-positive Grenzstreifen und die Dermis weisen keinen Schaden auf (Roberts et al., Klunker).

Über die Blasenbildung bei der dominant-dystrophischen Epidermolysis bullosa liegen bisher Mitteilungen von Touraine, von Duperrat sowie von Schnyder und Eichhoff vor. Demnach findet man sowohl subepidermale als auch (infolge Regeneration?) subcorneale Blasen.

Die Möglichkeit, daß der Epidermolysis bullosa eine Unterentwicklung oder selbst ein Fehlen des elastischen Gewebes in den obersten Schichten der Dermis zugrunde liegt, ist, seit dies von Engman und Mook im Jahre 1905 zuerst erwähnt wurde, recht oft erwogen worden. Letzthin haben Leoni sowie Ritzenfeld sich dafür eingesetzt. Nach der Ansicht beider Autoren fehlen bei der Epidermolysis bullosa die feinen elastischen Fasern, die angeblich normalerweise in die „Basalmembran“ eindringen. Das Fehlen der elastischen Fasern in den obersten Dermisschichten ist aber wohl eine Folgeerscheinung, die auch bei anderen blasenbildenden Krankheiten, z.B. beim Erythema exsudativum multiforme, vorkommt (van der Meiren et al.). Elektronenmikroskopische Untersuchungen haben keinen Anhalt dafür ergeben, daß elastische Fasern zu dem Anhaften der Basalzellen an die elektronenoptische Basalmembran beitragen.

c) Elektronenmikroskopie

Bei der Epidermolysis bullosa simplex fanden Pearson und Spargo in experimentell erzeugten Blasen Degenerationserscheinungen im Cytoplasma der Basalzellen, insbesondere ein Verschwinden der Tonofilamente sowie Formveränderungen der Mitochondria. An einigen Stellen zeigten auch die Stachelzellen Anzeichen von Degeneration. Die Verbindung der Basalzellen mit der Basalmembran war dagegen erhalten. Die Autoren zogen den Schluß, daß bei der Epidermolysis bullosa simplex der primäre Schaden die Basalzellen betreffe.

Bei der recessiv-dystrophischen Form fand Pearson, daß sich die Blasen auf Grund eines in der obersten Dermis stattfindenden Zerfalls von Kollagenfasern bildeten. Nekrotische Kollagenfasern wurden dabei von Makrophagen phagocytiert. Die Basalmembran, die keinen größeren Schaden aufwies, löste sich bei der Blasenbildung mit der Epidermis ab.

Bei der Epidermolysis bullosa letalis beobachtete PEARSON, daß bei Bildung von Blasen die Trennung zwischen der Basalmembran und den Basalzellen stattfand. LAPIÈRE et al. fanden dagegen in ihrem Fall von Epidermolysis bullosa letalis den Primärschaden innerhalb der Basalzellen. Diese zeigten schwere Degenerationserscheinungen, insbesondere Schwund der Tonofilamente und der Desmosomen, einschließlich der Halbdesmosomen, die die Basalzellen mit der Basalmembran verbinden. Bei der Blasenbildung, die größtenteils unterhalb der Basalzellen stattfand, blieben manchmal Bruchstücke von degenerierten Basalzellen an der Basalmembran haften.

3. Ätiologie und Pathogenese

Obwohl über die Ätiologie der Epidermolysis bullosa nichts bekannt ist, kann doch bezugs der Pathogenese das folgende festgestellt werden: Während die Epidermolysis bullosa simplex eine rein ektodermale Strukturkrankheit ist, trägt bei der recessiv-dystrophischen Form der Epidermolysis bullosa die Dermis wesentlich zu dem Kohäsionsverlust zwischen Epidermis und Dermis bei.

Es erscheint recht unwahrscheinlich, daß die gelegentlich beobachteten Störungen in der Blutgerinnung eine ätiologische Bedeutung besitzen. Mehrere Autoren haben eine Verkürzung der Blutgerinnungszeit festgestellt (LANGHOF; BAUMANN und KRAUSE; LEINBROCK; TIO et al.). BAUMANN und KRAUSE fanden außerdem bei der Antithrombinbestimmung eine Erniedrigung der Heparinansprechbarkeit; und TIO et al. fanden bei fast allen ihren Patienten, die neun verschiedenen Familien entstammten, nicht nur, wie BAUMANN und KRAUSE, eine verkürzte Gerinnungszeit und ein abgeschwächtes Ansprechen auf intravenös verabreichtes Heparin, sondern auch paradoxerweise ein verstärktes Ansprechen auf Heparin in vitro. Andere Autoren dagegen, wie FINZI und auch SCHNYDER, JUNG und SALAMON, konnten keine Störung des Gerinnungsmechanismus nachweisen. Die negativen Resultate, die allgemein bei Behandlung mit Heparin erzielt wurden, sprechen ebenfalls gegen einen kausalen Zusammenhang zwischen der Epidermolysis bullosa und der gelegentlich beobachteten Gerinnungsbeschleunigung.

Mechanismus der Blasenbildung

Früher waren manche Autoren der Ansicht, daß zwar bei der Epidermolysis bullosa simplex die Blasen sich nur auf Trauma hin bildeten, dagegen bei der Epidermolysis bullosa dystrophica auch „spontan" auftreten könnten (TOURAINE). Es ist jedoch wahrscheinlich, daß bei allen Formen der Epidermolysis bullosa ein Trauma die auslösende Rolle bei der Blasenbildung spielt; nur bedarf es eines intensiveren Traumas bei der Simplex-Form als bei der recessiv-dystrophischen oder der Letalis-Form. So fand SIMON bei drei Patienten mit recessiv-dystrophischer Epidermolysis bullosa, daß es keiner Reibung bedurfte, um Blasen hervorzurufen. Mehrfaches Beklopfen einer Hautstelle mit einem Reflexhammer rief erst ein Erythem hervor und weiteres Beklopfen dann Ablösung der Epidermis. Auch kann ein verlängertes Intervall zwischen dem Trauma und der Blasenbildung den Eindruck spontaner Blasenbildung erwecken. HÖCKER beobachtete z.B. bei einer Patientin mit Epidermolysis bullosa dystrophica, daß sich erst am 5. Tage nach mechanischem Reiben der Haut an der Stelle des Insultes Blasen bildeten.

4. Differentialdiagnose

Zwei Krankheiten zeigen gelegentlich genügend Übereinstimmung mit der Epidermolysis bullosa, so daß sie mit ihr verwechselt worden sind. Diese sind die Rittersche Krankheit und die Porphyrien.

α) Die **Rittersche Krankheit**, die eine schwere Impetigo bullosa der Neugeborenen darstellt und früher auch Pemphigus neonatorum genannt wurde, weist, wie die Epidermolysis bullosa letalis, große Blasen und ausgedehnte Epitheldefekte auf (LEE et al.). Die folgenden Unterschiede bestehen zwischen den beiden Krankheiten: *Beginn:* Bei der Epidermolysis bullosa letalis bilden sich Blasen schon bei der Geburt oder jedenfalls kurz nach der Geburt; bei der Ritterschen Krankheit treten sie gewöhnlich erst einige Tage nach der Geburt auf. *Mundschleimhaut:* Bei der Epidermolysis bullosa letalis ist diese regelmäßig befallen; bei der Ritterschen Krankheit nur gelegentlich. *Nägel:* Bei der Epidermolysis bullosa letalis sind diese oft dystrophisch oder fehlen; bei der Ritterschen Krankheit sind sie nur sekundär befallen. *Verlauf:* Bei der Epidermolysis bullosa letalis ist der Verlauf gewöhnlich langsam mit allmählicher Verschlimmerung und Eintritt des Todes meistens nicht vor dem Ende des ersten Monats; bei der Ritterschen Krankheit ist der Verlauf akut und endet entweder mit dem Tode binnen weniger Tage oder mit Erholung. *Familienanamnese:* Bei der Epidermolysis bullosa letalis können wegen der recessiven Vererbung früher geborene Geschwister befallen gewesen sein; bei der Ritterschen Krankheit können wegen der Ansteckungsmöglichkeit gleichzeitig andere Familienmitglieder mit Impetigo befallen sein. *Behandlung:* Bei der Epidermolysis bullosa letalis tritt keine Besserung auf Behandlung mit Antibiotica ein; bei der Ritterschen Krankheit folgt gewöhnlich rasche Besserung. Daher sollen in Zweifelsfällen Antibiotica stets verabreicht werden.

β) Die **Porphyrien** haben mit der Epidermolysis bullosa gemeinsam das Auftreten von Blasen nach Traumen und das Abheilen mit Atrophie und Milien. Es gibt vier Formen von Porphyrie mit Hauterscheinungen, nämlich die kongenitale erythropoetische Porphyrie, die erythropoetische Protoporphyrie, die Porphyria cutanea tarda und die kombinierte Porphyrie (Protokoproporphyrie) (s. Band III, Teil 1, S. 197ff.). Bei diesen vier Formen der Porphyrie ist jedoch im Gegensatz zur Epidermolysis bullosa eine Einwirkung von Sonnenlicht erforderlich, in dessen Folge erst ein Trauma Blasen hervorbringt. So kommt es bei den vier Arten von Porphyrien nur an den lichtexponierten Hautpartien zur Blasenbildung und nicht z.B. an den Füßen und Knien, die bei der Epidermolysis bullosa fast stets befallen sind. Auch sind bei den Porphyrien die Handflächen verschont, während die Handrücken bei beiden Krankheiten befallen sein können (TIO). Außerdem finden sich als Unterscheidungsmerkmale von der Epidermolysis bullosa bei der kongenitalen erythropoetischen Porphyrie Erythrodontie und hämolytische Anämie, bei der erythropoetischen Protoporphyrie Lichturticaria (LANGHOF et al.), bei der Porphyria cutanea tarda Ansetzen im späteren Leben sowie Hyperpigmentierung und Hypertrichose, und bei der kombinierten Porphyrie Koliken und oft auch nervale und psychische Symptome. Der Nachweis von Porphyrinen ist gewöhnlich leicht; denn bei der kongenitalen erythropoetischen Porphyrie und der Porphyria cutanea tarda fluoresciert der Urin bei Bestrahlung mit der Woodschen Lampe, bei der kombinierten Porphyrie fluoresciert entweder der Urin oder der Stuhl und bei der erythropoetischen Protoporphyrie fluorescieren die Erythrocyten. Außerdem kann natürlich auch das Vorhandensein von Porphyrinen mit Hilfe von chemischen Reaktionen nachgewiesen werden (s. Bd. III/1, S. 195).

Behandlung

Eine befriedigende Behandlung der Epidermolysis bullosa besteht nicht. Corticotropin und die Corticosteroide sind meistens ohne Nutzen, wie bereits 1951 CANNON u. Mitarb. in einem Bericht darlegten, der zwei Patienten mit dystrophischer Epidermolysis bullosa betraf, denen sie recht hohe Dosen von Cortison verabreicht hatten. Negative Ergebnisse sind bei der recessiv-dystrophischen Form unter anderen von BERGENHOLTZ und bei der Epidermolysis bullosa letalis von LEVER, von EBERHARTINGER und NIEBAUER, von LELAND und HIRSCHL und von WALTHER mitgeteilt worden. Einige Autoren haben jedoch bei Behandlung mit Corticosteroiden ein temporäres Sistieren der Blasenbildung festgestellt, z.B. PLENERT in einem Fall von Epidermolysis bullosa simplex, HAUSTEIN in einem Fall von Epidermolysis bullosa albo-papuloidea, COSTE et al., VERNIER und PRINGUET sowie HARNACK in Fällen von recessiv-dystrophischer Epidermolysis bullosa und ROSSET in einem Fall von Epidermolysis bullosa letalis. In dem letzteren Falle schrieb ROSSET das Überleben auf ein Alter von über 2 Jahren (s. S. 600) dieser Behandlung zu. Ferner erzielte MOYNAHAN bei einem Patienten mit einer Pharynxstenose, die durch eine recessiv-dystrophische Epidermolysis bullosa verursacht war, mittels Verabreichung von Corticosteroiden eine Lumenerweiterung von 2 auf 7 mm. Jedoch handelte es sich bei dieser Besserung nicht um eine Unterdrückung von Blasen, sondern um die Verringerung eines Ödems. Bei den anderen berichteten Fällen, bei denen eine Unterdrückung von Blasenbildung beobachtet wurde, kann man die Frage stellen, ob die Besserung nicht durch die schonende Krankenhauspflege hervorgebracht worden war.

Auch der Wert von Chloroquin ist sehr fraglich. T. BAER berichtete 1961 über gute Resultate bei zwei Patienten mit Epidermolysis bullosa und SCHNYDER, JUNG und SALAMON beobachteten partielle Unterdrückung der Blasenbildung bei sechs Kindern mit Epidermolysis bullosa simplex. Andere Beobachter (R. L. BAER und WITTEN; eigene Ergebnisse) konnten jedoch keine Besserung feststellen.

Literatur

ANNING, S. T.: Recurrent bullous eruption of the feet. Brit. J. Derm. **63**, 104 (1951).

BAER, R. L., and V. H. WITTEN: Comment in The Year Book of Dermatology, 1961—1962 Year Book Series, p. 65. Chicago: Year Book Medical Publ. 1962. — BAER, T.: Epidermolysis bullosa hereditaria treated with antimalarials. Arch. Derm. **84**, 503 (1961). — BAUMANN, R., u. S. KRAUSE: Kasuistischer Beitrag zur Epidermolysis bullosa hereditaria dystrophica. Derm. Wschr. **130**, 1003 (1954). — BERGENHOLTZ, A., O. OLSSON, T. ARWILL u. N. R. LUNDSTRÖM: Die Epidermolysis bullosa hereditaria dystrophica mit Oesophagusveränderungen. Arch. klin. exp. Derm. **217**, 518 (1963). — BRAIN, R. T.: Epidermolysis bullosa dystrophica vegetans. Acta derm.-venereol. (Stockh.) **32** (Suppl. 29), 56 (1952).

CALNAN, C. D., and A. D. PORTER: Recessive epidermolysis bullosa with unusual features. Trans. St. John's Hosp. derm. Soc. (Lond.) **33**, 62 (1954). — CANNON, A. B., J. G. HOPKINS, G. C. ANDREWS, H. F. COLFER, P. GROSS, C. T. NELSON, and C. M. HOWELL jr.: Pituitary adrenocorticotropic hormone (ACTH) and cortisone in diseases of the skin. I. Pemphigus vulgaris and other bullous dermatoses. J. Amer. med. Ass. **145**, 201 (1951). — COCKAYNE, E. A.: Inherited abnormalities of the skin and its appendages, p. 118. New York: Oxford University Press 1933. — Recurrent bullous eruption of the feet. Brit. J. Derm. **50**, 358 (1938). — Recurrent bullous eruption of the feet. Brit. J. Derm. **59**, 109 (1947). — COSTE, F., B. PIGUET et J. CIVATTE: Un cas d'épidermolyse bulleuse polydysplasique ameliorée par l'A.C.T.H. Bull. Soc. franç. Derm. Syph. **59**, 89 (1952).

DUPERRAT, B.: Les épidermolyses bulleuses congénitales. Gaz. méd. Fr. **60**, 1077 (1953).

EBERHARTINGER, C., u. G. NIEBAUER: Zur Herlitzschen Sonderform von Epidermolysis bullosa. Z. Kinderheilk. **82**, 227 (1959). — ENGMAN, M. F., and W. H. MOOK: A study of some cases of epidermolysis bullosa with remarks upon the congenital absence of elastic tissue. J. cutan. Dis. **24**, 55 (1905).

FINZI, A. F.: Osservazioni su due casi di epidermolisi bullosa distrofica con riferimento a recenti vedute patogenetiche. Rass. Derm. Sif. **12**, 239 (1959). — FOX, T.: Notes on unusual or rare forms of skin disease. IV. Congenital ulceration of skin (two cases) with pemphigus eruption and arrest of development generally. Lancet **1879 I**, 766. — FRANK, S. B.: An unusual variant of epidermolysis bullosa. Recurrent bullous eruption of the feet. Arch. Derm. Syph. (Chic.) **47**, 327 (1943). — FRANKS, A. G., and M. I. J. DAVIS: Epidermolysis bullosa. Arch. Derm. Syph. (Chic.) **47**, 647 (1943). — FUCHS, F.: Epidermolysis bullosa hereditaria dystrophica. Derm. Wschr. **125**, 303 (1952).

Gasser, I., u. H. Walther: Zur Kenntnis der Epidermolysis bullosa et albopapuloidea Pasinii. Derm. Wschr. **120**, 417 (1949). — Götz, H., u. K. Meinicke: Zur Klinik und Therapie der Epidermolysis bullosa et albo-papuloidea Pasini. Derm. Wschr. **131**, 481 (1955). — Greenberg, S. I.: Epidermolysis bullosa. Arch. Derm. Syph. (Chic.) **49**, 333 (1944).

Haldane, J. B. S., and R. Poole: A new pedigree of recurrent bullous eruption of the feet. J. Hered. **33**, 17 (1942). — Halpern, L. K.: Development of squamous cell epithelioma in epidermolysis bullosa. Arch. Derm. Syph. (Chic.) **56**, 517 (1947). — Harnack, K.: Epidermolysis bullosa dystrophica et polydysplastica (Touraine). Derm. Wschr. **145**, 369 (1962). — Haustein, U. F.: Klinisch-therapeutische Anmerkung zur Epidermolysis bullosa dystrophica albo-papuloidea (Pasini). Derm. Wschr. **148**, 689 (1963). — Hensler, K.: Epidermolysis bullosa dystrophica mit dominantem Erbgang und großen Manifestationsschwankungen. Dermatologica (Basel) **93**, 155 (1946). — Herlitz, G.: Kongenitaler, nicht syphilitischer Pemphigus. Acta paediat. (Uppsala) **17**, 315 (1935). — Höcker, H.: Untersuchungen über die Epidermolysis bullosa hereditaria. Arch. Derm. Syph. (Berl.) **193**, 406 (1951).

Johnson, M. L.: Persönliche Mitteilung am 9. April 1964. — Johnson, S. A. M., and A. R. Test: Epidermolysis bullosa simplex of the hands and feet. Arch. Derm. Syph. (Chic.) **53**, 610 (1946).

Kagen, M. S., L. Williams, W. Griffin, and R. Wiley: Epidermolysis bullosa hereditaria in a newborn. Wis. med. J. **51**, 766 (1952). — Keining, E., u. H. Wohnlich: Epidermolysis bullosa hereditaria hyperplastica. Derm. Wschr. **127**, 418 (1953). — Klausner, E.: Zungenkrebs als Folgezustand bei einem Falle von Epidermolysis bullosa (dystrophische Form). Arch. Derm. Syph. (Berl.) **116**, 71 (1913). — Klunker, W.: Zur nosologischen Stellung der Epidermolysis bullosa hereditaria letalis Herlitz (mit Kasuistik). Arch. klin. exp. Derm. **216**, 74 (1963).

Lamb, J. H., and B. Halpert: Epidermolysis bullosa of the newborn. Arch. Derm. Syph. (Chic.) **55**, 369 (1947). — Langhof, H.: Zur Epidermolysis bullosa. Derm. Wschr. **126**, 764 (1952). — Langhof, H., H. Muller u. L. Rietschel: Untersuchungen zur familiären protoporphyrinämischen Lichturticaria. Arch. klin. exp. Derm. **212**, 506 (1961). — Lapière, L., S. Castermans-Elias u. H. Firket: Elektronenmikroskopische Untersuchungen über die Ultrastruktur der Epidermolysis bullosa letalis bei einem Säugling mit familiärer Belastung. Hautarzt **15**, 30 (1964). — Lee, H. F., R. B. Wilson, C. E. Brown, and T. P. Reed: Impetigo and acute infectious exfoliative dermatitis of the newborn infant (Ritter's disease). J. Pediat. **41**, 159 (1952). — Leider, M., and R. L. Baer: Epidermolysis bullosa hereditaria. Arch. Derm. Syph. (Chic.) **46**, 419 (1942). — Leinbrock, A.: Epidermolysis bullosa dystrophica et albo-papuloidea (Pasini) et ulcero-vegetans (cum Carcinoma) mit diffuser Hämangiomatose bei Schilddrüsen-Dysfunktion. Hautarzt **7**, 395 (1956). — Leland, L. S., and D. Hirschl: Epidermolysis bullosa hereditaria letalis in newborn twins: Report of two cases with failure to respond favorably to cortisone. Amer. J. Dis. Child. **87**, 321 (1954). — Leoni, A.: Recherches sur le mécanisme de formation des bulles dans l'épidermolyse bulleuse simple. Ann. Derm. Syph. (Paris) VIII, **10**, 501 (1950). — Lever, W. F.: In der Diskussion zu I. Zeligman u. H. M. Robinson jr., Epidermolysis bullosa hereditaria. Arch. Derm. Syph. (Chic.) **63**, 669 (1951). — Linser, P.: Über die Epidermolysis bullosa hereditaria und ihren Zusammenhang mit der Raynaudschen Krankheit. Arch. Derm. Syph. (Berl.) **84**, 369 (1907).

Marchionini, A.: Über Epidermolysis bullosa dystrophica vegetans. Arch. Derm. Syph. (Berl.) **176**, 347 (1938). — Meiren, L. van der, G. Achten et M. Ledoux-Corbusier: A propos d'un cas d'épidermolyse bulleuse. La jonction dermo-épidermique des maladies bulleuses. Arch. belges Derm. **15**, 169 (1959). — Miescher, G.: Epidermolysis bullosa vegetans mit Amyloid. Derm. Z. **76**, 1 (1937). — Moynahan, E. J.: Epidermolysis bullosa dystrophica with severe deformity of hands and pharyngeal stenosis, relieved by cortisone. Proc. roy. Soc. Med. **54**, 693 (1961). — Muggler, F.: Häufung von Epidermolysis bullosa hereditaria dystrophica recessiva in einer großen Aargauer Sippe. Helv. paediat. Acta **18**, 323 (1963).

Nicolas, J., H. Moutot et L. Charlet: Dermatose congénitale et familiale à lésions trophiques progressives et chroniques ulcéro-végétantes, à début pemphigoide, avec dystrophies ungéales, variété nouvelle de pemphigus congénital de forme dystrophique. Ann. Derm. Syph. (Paris) V, **4**, 385 (1913).

Pasini, A.: Dystrophie cutanée bulleuse atrophiante et albopapuloide. Ann. Derm. Syph. (Paris) VI, **9**, 1044 (1928). — Pearson, R. W.: Studies on the pathogenesis of epidermolysis bullosa. J. invest. Derm. **39**, 551 (1962). — Pearson, R. W., and B. Spargo: Electron microscope studies of dermal-epidermal separation in human skin. J. invest. Derm. **36**, 213 (1961). — Petrini - Galatz: Contribution à l'étude clinique et histopathologique de l'épidermolyse bulleuse dystrophique et congénitale. Ann. Derm. Syph. (Paris) **7**, 766 (1906). — Plenert, W.: Studie zur Blasenbildung bei der Epidermolysis bullosa. Z. Kinderheilk. **78**, 329 (1956).

Rasponi, L.: Il cancro sull'epidermolisi bollosa distrofica. Arch. ital. Derm. **23**, 19 (1950). — Epiteliomatosi multipla delle gambe su epidermolisi bollosa distrofica in leutico con note distrofiche dello scheletro degli arti inferiori. Arch. ital. Derm. **24**, 353 (1951). —

RIECKE, E.: Epidermolysis bullosa. In: Handbuch der Haut- und Geschlechtskrankheiten, hrsg. von J. JADASSOHN, Bd. VII, Teil 2, S. 222. Berlin: Springer 1931. — RITZENFELD, P.: Histologische Untersuchungen zur Pathogenese der Epidermolysis bullosa hereditaria. Arch. klin. exp. Derm. **215**, 369 (1962). — ROBERTS, M. H., D. R. S. HOWELL, J. L. BRAMHALL, and B. REUBNER: Epidermolysis bullosa letalis. Pediatrics **25**, 283 (1960). — ROBINSON, M. M.: Epidermolysis bullosa hereditaria. Urol. cutan. Rev. **50**, 545 (1946). — RÖCKL, H.: Carcinom bei Epidermolysis bullosa dystrophica. Hautarzt **7**, 463 (1956). — ROSSET, M.: Epidermolysis bullosa of the newborn. Canad. med. Ass. J. **75**, 507 (1956). — RUSSELL, B., and C. M. RIDLEY: Epidermolysis bullosa (with unusual features). Brit. J. Derm. **75**, 125 (1963).

SAKAGUCHI, Y.: Über die Epidermolysis bullosa hereditaria Köbner. Arch. Derm. Syph. (Berl.) **121**, 379 (1915/16). — SCHILLER, F.: Zungencarcinom bei Epidermolysis bullosa dystrophica. Arch. klin. exp. Derm. **209**, 643 (1960). — SCHNYDER, U. W., u. D. EICHHOFF: Zur Klinik und Genetik der dominant-dystrophischen Epidermolysis bullosa hereditaria. Arch. klin. exp. Derm. **218**, 62 (1963). — SCHNYDER, U. W., E. G. JUNG u. T. SALAMON: Zur Klassifizierung, Histogenetik, Gerinnungsphysiologie und Therapie der hereditären Epidermolysen. Arch. klin. exp. Derm. **220**, 38 (1964). — SILVER, H. K.: Epidermolysis bullosa hereditaria „letalis": Report of a case surviving for two and a half years. Arch. Dis. Childh. **32**, 216 (1957). — SIMON, C. R.: The effect of certain types of trauma in epidermolysis bullosa. J. Pediat. **47**, 750 (1955).

TIO, T. H.: The differential diagnosis between epidermolysis bullosa hereditaria and porphyria cutanea tarda. Dermatologica (Basel) **115**, 112 (1957). — TIO, T. H., P. J. WAARDENBURG, and H. J. VERMEULEN: Blood coagulation in epidermolysis bullosa hereditaria. Arch. Derm. 88, 24 (1963). — TOURAINE, A.: Classification des epidermolyses bulleuses. Ann. Derm. Syph. (Paris) VIII, **2**, 309 (1942).

VERNIER, P., et G. PRINGUET: Un cas de guérison complète d'épidermolyse bulleuse dystrophique congénitale par d'A.C.T.H. Bull. Soc. franç. Derm. Syph. **60**, 58 (1953). — VILANOVA, X., u. J. PIÑOL AGUADÉ: Beitrag zur Kenntnis der Epidermolysis bullosa dystrophica ulcero-vegetans. Hautarzt **3**, 514 (1952).

WAISMAN, M.: Recurrent bullous eruption of the feet and hands (Weber-Cockayne). J. Amer. med. Ass. **124**, 1247 (1944). — WALTHER, T.: Epidermolysis bullosa hereditaria letalis. A review and report of two own cases. Ann. paediat. (Basel) **180**, 382 (1953). — WEBER, F. P.: Recurrent bullous eruption on the feet of a child. Proc. roy. Soc. Med. **19**, 72 (1926). — WINER, M. N., and J. M. ORMAN: Epidermolysis bullosa. A suggestion as to possible causation. Arch. Derm. Syph. (Chic.) **52**, 317 (1945).

Pemphigus. Pemphigoid. Pemphigus familiaris benignus

Von

Walter F. Lever-Boston (Mass., USA)

Mit 61 Abbildungen (davon 2 farbige)

A. Pemphigus

Seit RIECKEs Darstellung des Pemphigus sind auf Grund histologischer, cytologischer und elektronenmikroskopischer Untersuchungen beträchtliche Fortschritte in der Diagnose und Klassifizierung der verschiedenen Arten von Pemphigus gemacht worden. Die Erkennung der Acantholyse als das entscheidende diagnostische Merkmal des Pemphigus durch CIVATTE im Jahre 1943 hat eine Herausnahme von zwei chronischen blasenbildenden Krankheiten aus der Pemphigusgruppe zur Folge gehabt, die dann die Bezeichnung Pemphigoid erhielten. Diese zwei Krankheiten sind das bullöse Pemphigoid und das gutartige Schleimhautpemphigoid. Ein bedeutender Fortschritt ist auch die Einführung der Corticosteroide in die Behandlung des Pemphigus. In vielen Fällen wirkt diese Behandlung lebensrettend.

I. Die Einteilung des Pemphigus

Vier Krankheiten, die alle das charakteristische histologische Bild der Acantholyse aufweisen, gehören zur Pemphigusgruppe, nämlich:

Pemphigus vulgaris,
Pemphigus vegetans,
Pemphigus foliaceus,
Pemphigus erythematosus.

Die Einteilung des Pemphigus kann noch weiter vereinfacht werden, denn der Pemphigus vegetans stellt eigentlich nur eine Sonderform des Pemphigus vulgaris dar, „ein Reaktionsstadium des Patienten mit Pemphigus vulgaris in Richtung eines erhöhten Widerstandes gegen die Krankheit“ (DIRECTOR 1952b), und der Pemphigus erythematosus stellt entweder ein Frühstadium oder eine gemilderte Form des Pemphigus foliaceus dar (obwohl einige Autoren der Meinung sind, daß der Pemphigus erythematosus in manchen Fällen ein Frühstadium oder eine gemilderte Form des Pemphigus vulgaris darstellt; s. S. 636). So gibt es also, genau wie zu HEBRAs Zeiten, nur zwei Formen von Pemphigus, nämlich den Pemphigus vulgaris und den Pemphigus foliaceus.

1. Pemphigus vulgaris

Eine Unterscheidung zwischen dem Pemphigus vulgaris und dem bullösen Pemphigoid ist gewöhnlich nicht nur auf Grund des histologischen Bildes, sondern auch auf Grund des klinischen Aussehens möglich (LEVER 1953). Die Unterschiede im klinischen Aussehen werden bei der Beschreibung der beiden Krankheiten betont werden. Eine klinische Beschreibung erscheint angebracht, da RIECKE in seiner Beschreibung des Pemphigus vulgaris die beiden Krankheitsbilder nicht voneinander trennte; denn zu jener Zeit war ja das charakteristische histologische Bild des Pemphigus vulgaris noch nicht bekannt. Es muß allerdings darauf hingewiesen werden, daß nicht alle Autoren solcher strengen Scheidung zustimmen (s. S. 661).

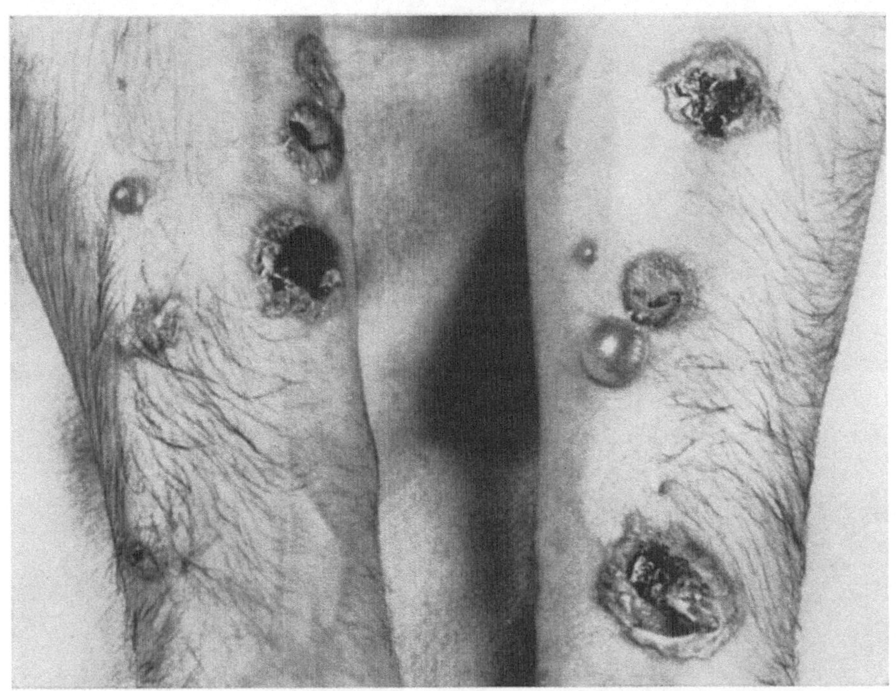

a

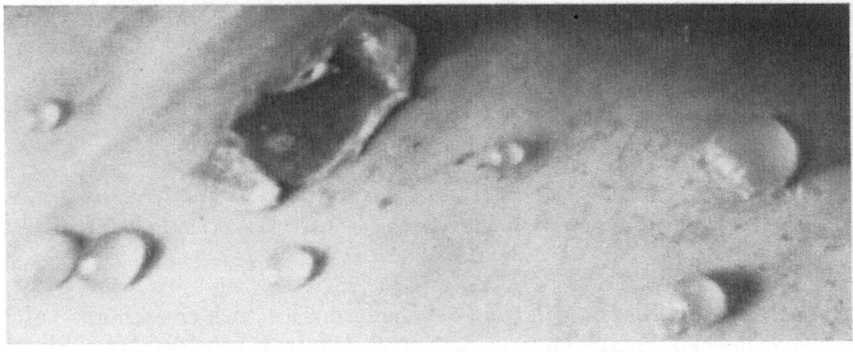

b

Abb. 1a u. b. Pemphigus vulgaris. Die Blasen brechen leicht und hinterlassen Epitheldefekte, die sich fortschreitend vergrößern

a) Hauterscheinungen

Beim Pemphigus vulgaris sind die Blasen auf der Haut oft von Anfang an schlaff. Sie mögen prall sein, wenn sie zuerst auftreten; sie werden aber schlaff, sobald sie an Größe zunehmen (Abb. 1). Die Blasen brechen leicht (wegen der in der Epidermis stattfindenden Degeneration) und erreichen daher nur selten eine beträchtliche Größe. Die Epitheldefekte, die entstehen, wenn die Blasen brechen, vergrößern sich durch fortschreitende Ablösung der Epidermis an ihrer Peripherie. Häufig zeigen die Epitheldefekte daher an ihrer Peripherie einen „Kragen" von abgelöster Epidermis (Abb. 2). Im fortgeschrittenen Stadium der Krankheit

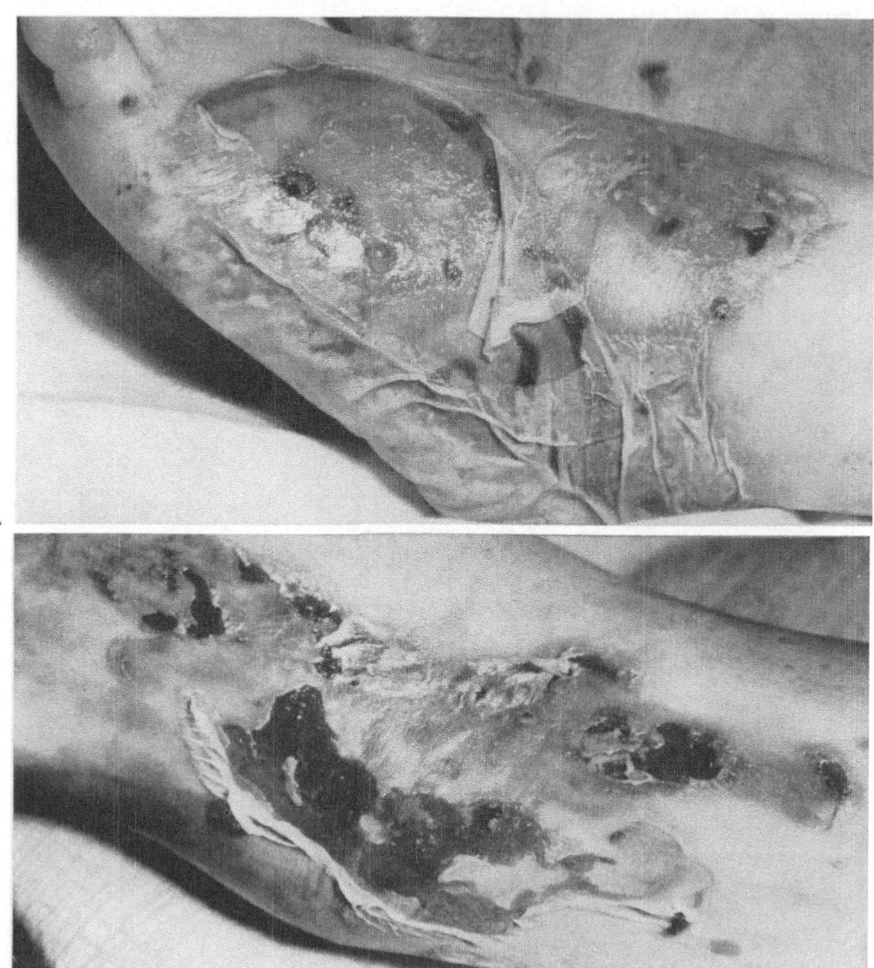

Abb. 2a u. b. Pemphigus vulgaris. Die Epitheldefekte zeigen an ihrer Peripherie einen „Kragen" abgelöster Epidermis

bilden sich oft keine Blasen mehr und die Epidermis löst sich einfach ab. Infolgedessen stellen beim Pemphigus vulgaris ausgedehnte Epitheldefekte und nicht, wie beim bullösen Pemphigoid, Blasen das hervorstechendste klinische Merkmal dar (Abb. 3). Die Epitheldefekte zeigen gewöhnlich nur eine geringe Heilungstendenz. Ältere Epitheldefekte sind häufig mit hämorrhagischen Krusten bedeckt. Wenn sie abheilen, tritt dabei gewöhnlich keine atrophische Vernarbung, wohl aber Pigmentierung auf (Abb. 4). Jucken fehlt entweder oder ist gering. Jedoch sind die ausgedehnten Epitheldefekte sehr schmerzempfindlich und verursachen daher dem Patienten viel Qual.

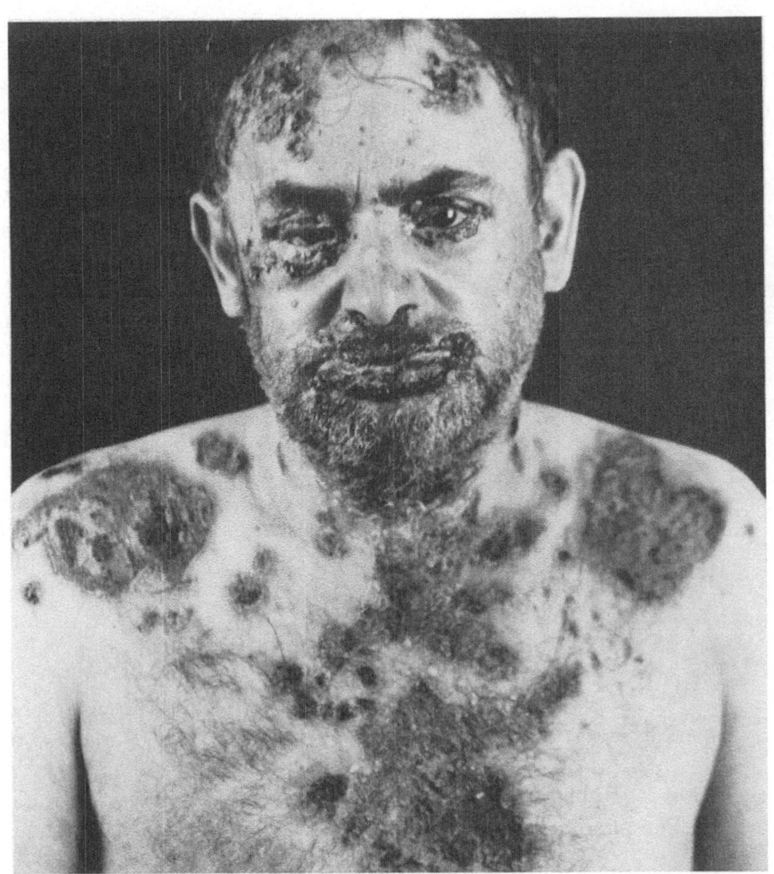

Abb. 3. Pemphigus vulgaris. Ausgedehnte Epitheldefekte und nicht Blasen kennzeichnen das klinische Bild bei fortgeschrittenen Fällen

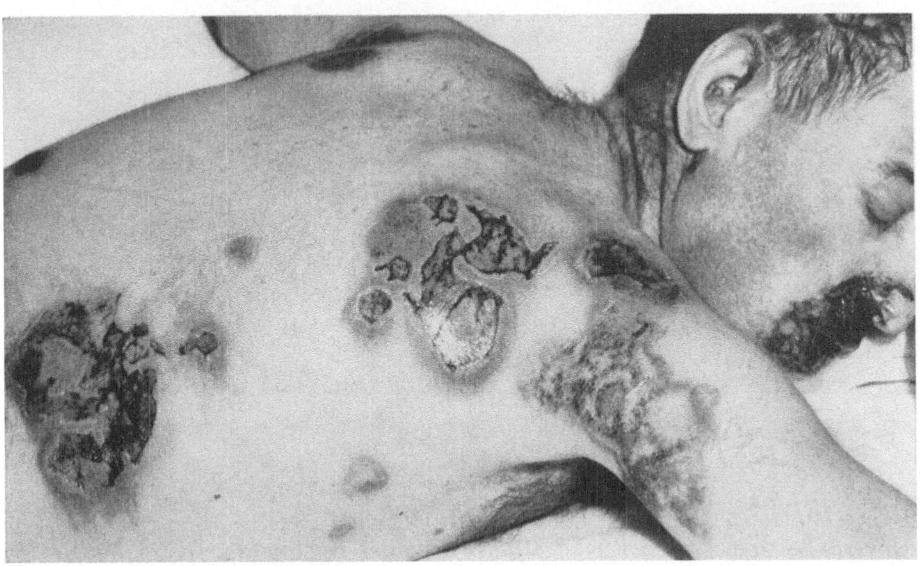

Abb. 4. Pemphigus vulgaris. Der Patient befindet sich in teilweiser spontaner Abheilung. Die abgeheilten Stellen zeigen beträchtliche Pigmentierung

Die Verteilung der Hautherde folgt keiner Regel; da aber Druck zu Epithelablösungen führt, sind oft Hautgebiete, die Druck und Reibung ausgesetzt sind, wie der Rücken, das Gesäß und die Füße, schwer befallen. Verhältnismäßig häufig findet man Efflorescenzen auch in der Umgebung des Mundes und an den Augenlidern. Gelegentlich sind die Nagelfalten befallen. Die damit verbundene Gewebsschwellung ruft das Bild einer akuten Paronychie hervor. Recht oft zeigen einige Krankheitsherde, besonders solche, die in intertriginösen Regionen, wie die Achselhöhlen und Leistenbeugen, gelegen sind, Granulationen und heilen mit verruköser Hypertrophie ab (Abbildung 5). Solche Herde haben dann dasselbe Aussehen, wie man es beim Pemphigus vegetans findet. Somit kann man keine scharfe Trennungslinie zwischen dem Pemphigus vulgaris und dem Pemphigus vegetans ziehen.

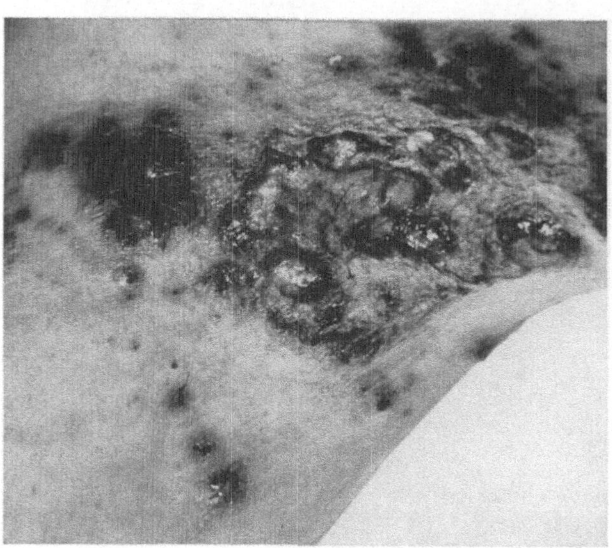

Abb. 5. Pemphigus vulgaris. Ein Epitheldefekt in der Axilla zeigt Heilung mit Bildung von Granulationen und nimmt so das Aussehen von Pemphigus vegetans an

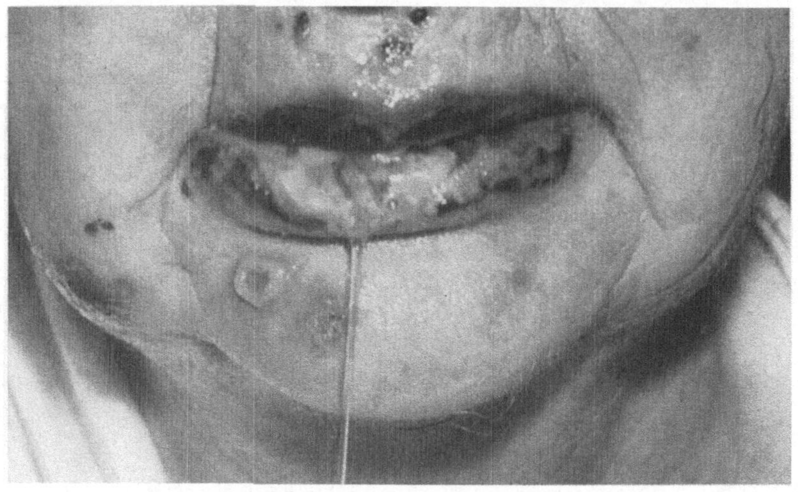

Abb. 6. Pemphigus vulgaris. Das Lippenrot ist schwer befallen

b) Schleimhauterscheinungen

Die Mundschleimhaut ist bei fast allen Patienten befallen, und zwar meistens schwer. Bei mehr als der Hälfte der Patienten beginnt die Krankheit an der Mundschleimhaut (s. Tabelle 1, S. 613). Das Aussehen der Mundschleimhauterscheinungen ist dem der Hauterscheinungen ähnlich. Unversehrte Blasen findet man

Tabelle 1. *Sterblichkeit bei den persönlich beobachteten Patienten mit Pemphigus oder Pemphigoid vor der Erhältlichkeit der Corticosteroide (1936—1949)*

	Gesamtzahl der Patienten	Zahl der jüdischen Patienten	Zahl der Patienten mit Mundschleimhauterscheinungen	Zahl der Patienten mit Beginn im Munde	Sterblichkeit in bezug auf das Alter des Patienten bei Beginn der Krankheit							
					Alle Patienten		Alter bis 49 Jahre		Alter, 50 bis 65 Jahre		Alter über 65 Jahre	
					Zahl	Tod	Zahl	Tod	Zahl	Tod	Zahl	Tod
Pemphigus vulgaris . . .	33	22	33	19	33	31	9	8	18	17	6	6
Pemphigus vegetans . .	3	1	3	3	3	1						
Pemphigus foliaceus . .	30	7	2	0	30	18	14	2	7	7	9	9
Pemphigus erythematosus	2	1	0	0	2	0						
Bullöses Pemphigoid . . .	33	2	11	3	33	8	5	0	14	0	14	8
Benignes Schleimhautpemphigoid .	29	1	26	7	29	1	6	0	10	0	13	1

nur selten, da sie bald nach ihrem Auftreten brechen. Genau wie auf der Haut, bilden sich oft gar keine Blasen, sondern das Schleimhautepithelium löst sich einfach ab. Die Epitheldefekte vergrößern sich durch periphere Ausbreitung, so daß weite Flächen des Mundes befallen sein können. Von besonderer Bedeutung bei der Diagnose ist die Ausdehnung des Krankheitsprozesses auf das Lippenrot (Abb. 6) und oft auch auf die daran angrenzende Haut. Der Rachen und Kehlkopf können befallen sein, was dann Heiserkeit zur Folge hat. Andere Schleimhäute, wie die Nasenschleimhaut, die Bindehaut, die Vulva und der After können auch Epitheldefekte zeigen, die wie die auf der Haut gelegenen nur wenig spontane Heilungstendenz zeigen; wenn sie aber abheilen, geschieht dieses ohne Narbenbildung.

c) Verlauf

Der häufige Beginn des Pemphigus vulgaris in einem umschriebenen Bezirk ist oft betont worden (Oppenheim und Cohen). Am häufigsten befinden sich die Initialefflorescenzen im Munde; sie können aber auch anderswo auftreten, besonders an der Kopfhaut, im Gesicht, in den Achselhöhlen und um die Nägel herum. Während dieses Initialstadiums, das sich über mehrere Wochen oder Monate erstrecken kann, ist die Diagnose oft schwer zu stellen. Immerhin ist das Auftreten von Blasen und Epitheldefekten im Mund verdächtig entweder für den Pemphigus vulgaris oder für das benigne Schleimhautpemphigoid. Eine histologische Untersuchung ist dabei von großem Werte.

Die Prognose war beim Pemphigus vulgaris sehr ernst, bevor die Corticosteroide erhältlich waren, denn fast alle Patienten starben. Gelegentlich schritt die Krankheit rasch fort und der Tod trat bereits nach einigen Wochen ein. Gewöhnlich dauerte es aber, selbst vor Erhältlichkeit der Corticosteroide, mehrere Monate und gelegentlich mehrere Jahre, bevor der Patient seiner Krankheit erlag. Nur selten überlebte ein Patient die Krankheit. (Von 33 Patienten mit Pemphigus vulgaris, die von mir am Massachusetts General Hospital beobachtet wurden, bevor ACTH und die Corticosteroide erhältlich waren, starben 31 und nur 2 überlebten die Krankheit; s. Tabelle 1.)

d) Alter, Geschlecht, Herkunft

Die meisten Patienten mit Pemphigus vulgaris stehen im mittleren Alter. Bei Kindern kommt er kaum jemals vor. Nur STEIGLEDER hat über einen histologisch fundierten Fall bei einem 12jährigen Mädchen berichtet. Auch bei Personen über 70 Jahren tritt die Krankheit nur selten auf, und fast niemals in einem Alter über 75 Jahre. (Unter 65 persönlich beobachteten Patienten war keiner unter 20 Jahre oder über 75 Jahre alt bei Beginn der Krankheit, und nur 4 standen im Alter zwischen 71 und 75; LEVER 1953, LEVER und WHITE.) Beide Geschlechter werden gleich betroffen. Ein großer Prozentsatz der Patienten ist jüdischer Herkunft. In vier verschiedenen Berichten von New York (GELLIS und GLASS; COMBES und CANIZARES; ELLER und KEST; COSTELLO et al.), die 399 Patienten mit Pemphigus vulgaris oder foliaceus betrafen, waren 238 oder 60% jüdisch. SHEKLAKOV berichtete 1961 aus Moskau, daß 65 seiner 162 Patienten mit Pemphigus vulgaris, d.h. 40%, jüdisch waren. Unter meinen eigenen Patienten waren von 33 Patienten mit Pemphigus vulgaris, die am Massachusetts General Hospital beobachtet wurden, bevor die Corticosteroide erhältlich waren, 22, d.h. 66%, jüdisch (Tabelle 1), obwohl weniger als 10% der Patienten in diesem Krankenhaus jüdisch sind. In einer darauf folgenden Serie von mit Corticosteroiden behandelten Patienten waren von 32 Patienten mit Pemphigus vulgaris 17, d.h. 53%, jüdisch (LEVER und WHITE). Auch scheint die Krankheit im Durchschnitt bei jüdischen Patienten fulminanter zu verlaufen als bei nicht-jüdischen (s. unter Behandlung).

e) Histologie

Es ist das große Verdienst von CIVATTE, das typische histologische Aussehen der Pemphigusblase zuerst erkannt zu haben. In seiner 1943 erschienenen Arbeit stellte er fest, daß die grundlegende Veränderung innerhalb der Epidermis stattfindet und aus dem Verschwinden der Intercellularbrücken besteht, was zu einem Verlust des Zusammenhaltes zwischen den Epidermiszellen führt. Diesen Vorgang, den er als Acantholyse bezeichnete, fand CIVATTE nicht nur beim Pemphigus vulgaris, sondern auch beim Pemphigus vegetans und Pemphigus foliaceus. Dies betrachtete er als Beweis, daß diese drei Krankheiten miteinander verwandt seien. Dagegen fand er in den Blasen der Dermatitis herpetiformis niemals Acantholyse, sondern stets subepidermale Blasenbildung.

Die Befunde von CIVATTE haben weitgehend Bestätigung gefunden und die Mehrzahl der Dermatologen nimmt heute den Standpunkt ein, daß der Nachweis der Acantholyse eine Vorbedingung für die Diagnose des Pemphigus ist. Unter diesen befinden sich z.B. in Argentinien CORDERO, in Belgien DUPONT und PIÉRARD, in Deutschland HAENSCH (1955 [I]) sowie KEINING und BRAUN-FALCO, in Frankreich DEGOS, in Großbritannien HABER wie auch PERCIVAL (1957) und ROOK und WHIMSTER, in Israel KATZENELLENBOGEN und SANDBANK sowie SAGHER, in Italien TOSTI und NAZZARO, in Japan NIKI, in Österreich EBERHARTINGER und EBNER sowie TAPPEINER und PFLEGER, in Polen JABLONSKA et al., in der Sowjetunion SHEKLAKOV und in den Vereinigten Staaten BRENNAN und MONTGOMERY, DIRECTOR (1952), LEVER (1951) und SANDERS, BRODY und NELSON. Einige Autoren bezweifeln jedoch, daß der Pemphigus vulgaris Acantholyse zeigen muß und glauben, daß selbst beim Bestehen von nicht-acantholytischen, subepidermalen Blasen ein Pemphigus vulgaris vorliegen kann. Zu diesen gehören HERZBERG (1955, 1958) und STEIGLEDER in Deutschland, HELLIER in Großbritannien, FÖLDVÁRI in Ungarn und CHARGIN et al. in den Vereinigten Staaten. (Eine Besprechung dieser Ansicht findet sich unter Bullöses Pemphigoid, S. 661.)

Die frühzeitigste histologische Veränderung, die beim Pemphigus vulgaris stattfindet, bevor klinisch sichtbare Änderungen auf der Haut vorhanden sind, besteht aus einem intercellulärem Ödem in den unteren Schichten der Epidermis, besonders zwischen der Basalzellenschicht und der direkt darüber gelegenen Zellschicht (Abb. 7). Innerhalb solcher Gebiete zeigen die Epidermiszellen entweder

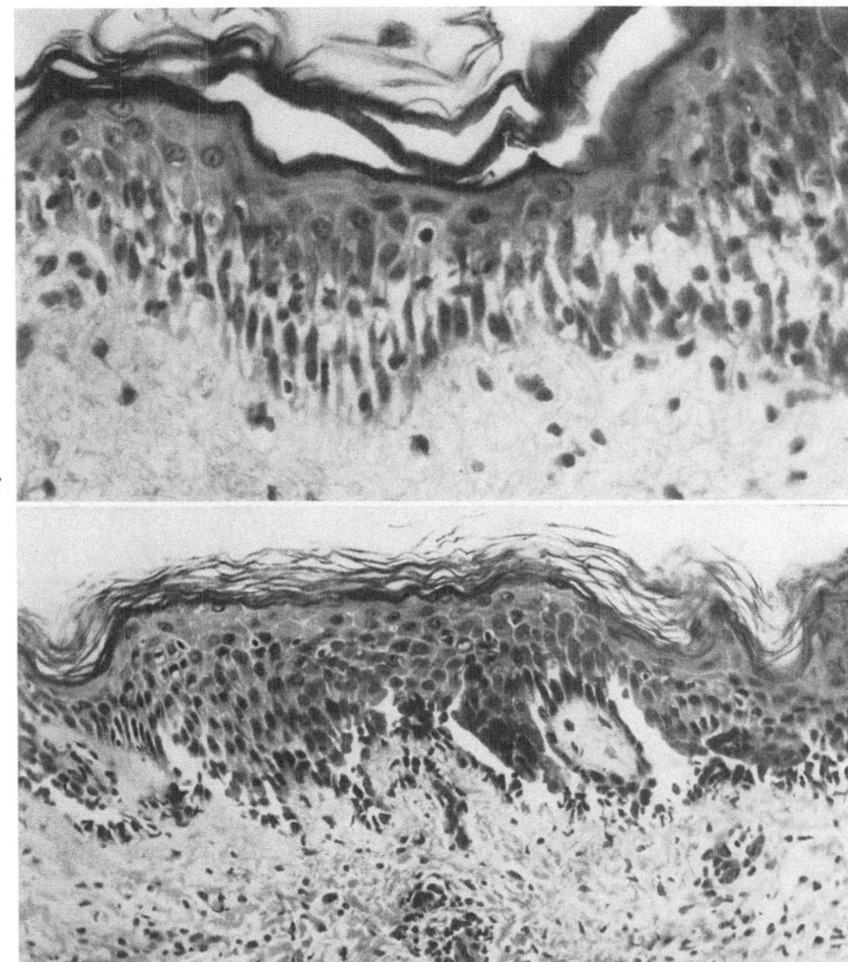

Abb. 7

Abb. 8

Abb. 7. Pemphigus vulgaris. Die frühzeitigste histologische Änderung besteht aus intercellulärem Ödem innerhalb und über der Basalzellenschicht. Die Zellen in der unteren Epidermis haben ihre Intercellularbrücken verloren (400mal)

Abb. 8. Pemphigus vulgaris. Ein Spalt hat sich direkt über derBasalzellenschicht gebildet (200mal)

keine Intercellularbrücken mehr oder nur noch Reste davon. Die Basalzellen sind in die Länge gezogen und können somit eine spindelige Gestalt aufweisen.

Wo das intercelluläre Ödem am ausgesprochensten ist, entwickeln sich Spalten innerhalb der Epidermis (Abb. 8). Fast immer befinden sich diese direkt über der Basalzellenschicht. Wenn sich einmal der Spalt gebildet hat, sind die Basalzellen nicht mehr in die Länge gezogen, sondern nehmen wieder ihre kubische oder zylindrische Gestalt an. Da die Intercellularbrücken zwischen den Basalzellen größtenteils verloren gegangen sind, liegen die Basalzellen durch kleine Zwischenräume voneinander getrennt. Dies gibt der Basalzellenschicht das Aussehen einer „Reihe von Grabsteinen“ (DIRECTOR 1952a). (Eine Erklärung, warum die Basal-

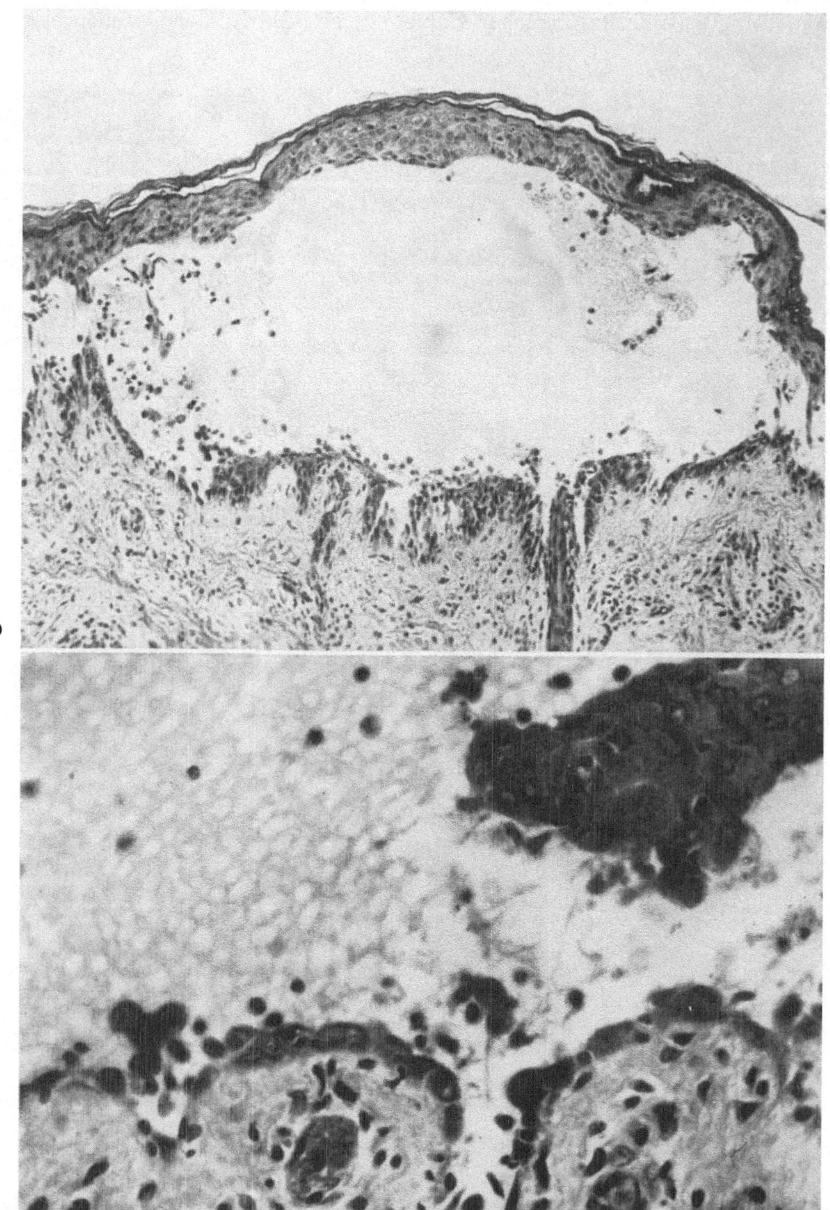

Abb. 9

Abb. 10

Abb. 9. Pemphigus vulgaris. Die Blase liegt vorwiegend suprabasal und läuft an der Peripherie in suprabasale Spalten aus (100mal)

Abb. 10. Pemphigus vulgaris. Der Blasenboden zeigt die Basalzellenschicht an die Dermis anhaftend. Die Blasenhöhle zeigt einzelne wie auch Gruppen abgelöster, degenerierter Epidermiszellen (400mal)

zellen an der Dermis haften bleiben, geben die elektronenmikroskopischen Befunde; s. S. 622.)

Das nächste Stadium ist die Bildung einer Blase. Frisch entstandene Blasen liegen manchmal in ihrer ganzen Ausdehnung zwischen der Basalzellenschicht

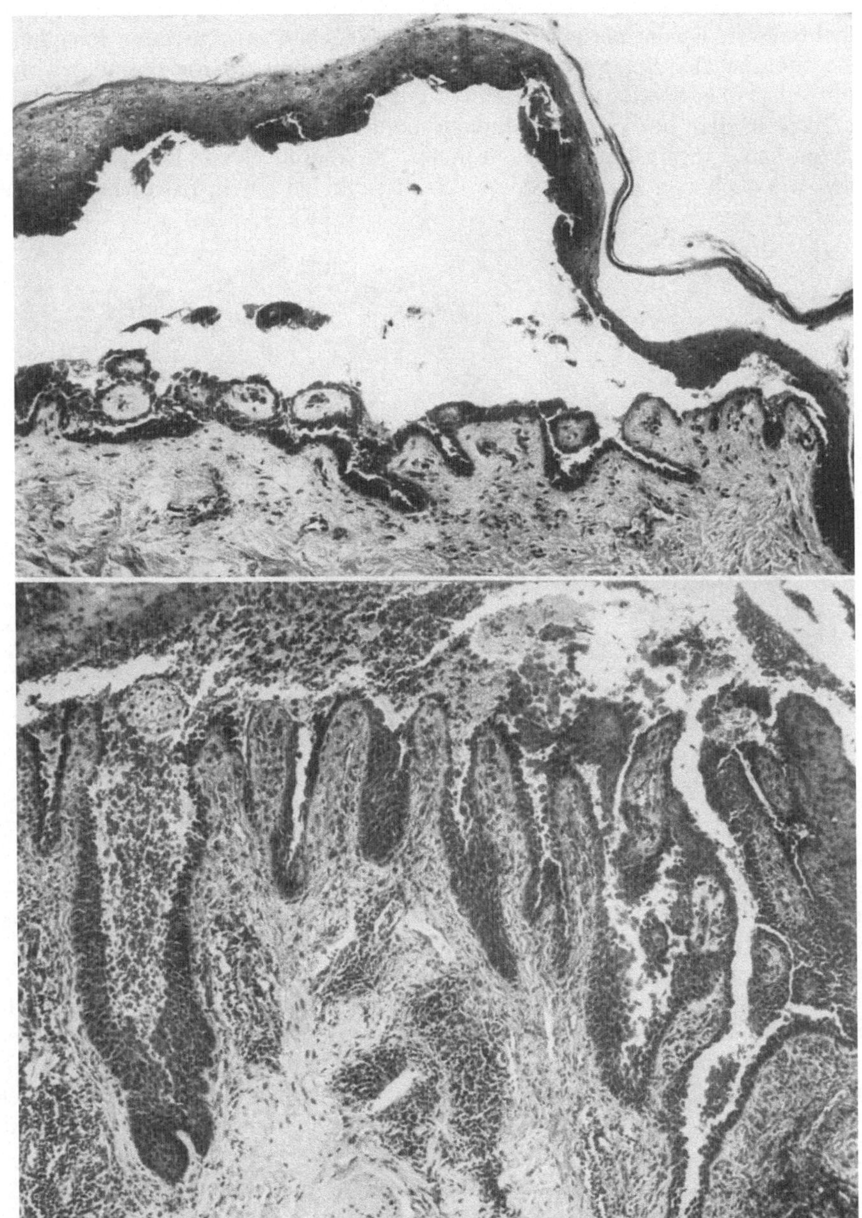

Abb. 11

Abb. 12

Abb. 11. Pemphigus vulgaris. Der Blasengrund zeigt hinaufwuchernde Papillarkörper, die mit einer einzelnen Lage von Epidermiszellen überzogen sind (100mal)

Abb. 12. Pemphigus vulgaris. Ein Vegetationen aufweisender Hautherd zeigt ausgesprochenes Hinaufwuchern von Papillarkörpern und Hinunterwuchern von Epidermissträngen (100mal)

und der übrigen Epidermis (Abb. 9). In vielen Blasen besteht aber der Boden, besonders in der Mitte der Blase, aus mehr als einer Schicht von Epidermiszellen;

und in seltenen Fällen ist die Blase vollständig in der Mittelschicht der Epidermis gelegen. Es ist wahrscheinlich, daß in solchen Fällen die verhältnismäßig hohe Lage der Blase durch eine Regeneration von Epidermiszellen am Blasenboden hervorgerufen ist. Subepidermal oder subcorneal gelegene Blasen kommen jedenfalls nicht vor. Auch die Tatsache, daß viele Blasen, die in der Mitte mehrere Schichten von Epidermiszellen am Blasenboden besitzen, an ihrer Peripherie in einen suprabasalen Spalt übergehen, weist darauf hin, daß die Blasen gewöhnlich unmittelbar über der Basalzellenschicht entstehen. Viele der Epidermiszellen, die am Blasenboden und am Blasendach nahe der Blasenhöhlung gelegen sind, besitzen keine Intercellularbrücken mehr. So kommt es zur Loslösung einzelner Zellen wie auch von Zellgruppen in die Blasenhöhle hinein (Acantholyse). Viele

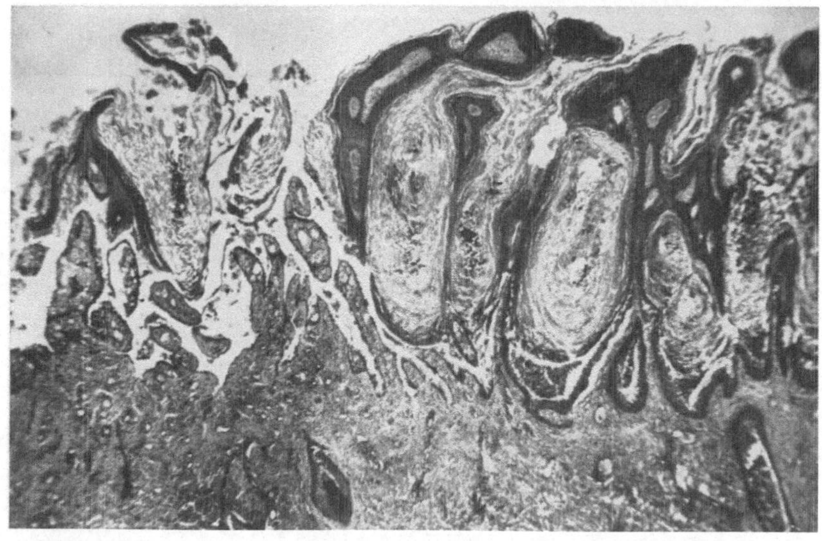

Abb. 13. Pemphigus vulgaris. Ein in Heilung begriffener Hautherd zeigt beträchtliche Papillomatose, Acanthose und Hyperkeratose (50mal)

der in der Blasenhöhlung gelegenen Epidermiszellen zeigen degenerative Veränderungen (Abb. 10). Ihre Kerne sind hyperchromatisch und das Cytoplasma erscheint an der Zellperipherie verdichtet. Manche Zellen haben an Größe zugenommen, so daß sie den Ballonzellen des Zoster ähnlich sehen. Der Grad von Acantholyse ist unterschiedlich: Der abgehobene Anteil der Epidermis sieht an manchen Stellen fast normal aus, während an anderen Stellen zahlreiche Zellen ihren Zusammenhang miteinander verloren haben und infolgedessen in der Blasenhöhle gelegen sind. Im allgemeinen ist jedoch der Verlust der Intercellularbrücken und die dadurch hervorgerufene Akantholyse beim Pemphigus vulgaris weniger ausgesprochen als beim Pemphigus familiaris benignus (s. S. 687).

Der Blasenboden zeigt in frischen Blasen oft nur etwas Wellung, normalen Papillarkörpern entsprechend. Häufig findet man jedoch, besonders in älteren Blasen, unregelmäßig aufwärts gewachsene Papillarkörper, die mit nur einer Lage von Epidermiszellen überzogen sind, sowie Stränge von Epidermiszellen, die zwischen Papillarkörpern in die Dermis hineingewuchert sind (Abb. 11).

Frisch entstandene Epitheldefekte zeigen gewöhnlich noch eine der Dermis aufliegende Schicht von Basalzellen. Ältere Epitheldefekte besitzen manchmal keine Epidermiszellen mehr auf ihrer Oberfläche.

Krankheitsherde, die klinisch Granulationen aufweisen, zeigen ein sehr ausgesprochenes Hinaufwachsen von Papillarkörpern und Hinunterwachsen von Epithelsträngen (Abb. 12). Das histologische Bild ähnelt dann dem des Pemphigus vegetans sehr. Intraepidermale eosinophile Abscesse fehlen zwar, aber diese sind ja selbst beim Pemphigus vegetans nicht regelmäßig vorhanden. Wenn solche Granulationen heilen, bildet sich außer der Papillomatose oft auch beträchtliche Acanthose und Hyperkeratose aus (Abb. 13).

Die Acantholyse kann auch das Epithelium der Haarfollikel, der Talgdrüsen und der Schweißdrüsenausführungsgänge ergreifen. Wie bei der Oberflächenepidermis entstehen auch hier die Spalten bevorzugt unmittelbar über der Basalzellen- oder äußeren Zellschicht.

An der Mundschleimhaut ist der histologische Befund dem an der Haut analog. Man findet vorwiegend suprabasale Acantholyse. Oft findet man recht ausgesprochene Papillomatose.

Es ist ratsam, die Probeexcision an einer recht frischen Blase vorzunehmen und vorzugsweise an einer kleinen Blase, die in ihrer Gesamtheit, möglichst mit etwas umgebender Haut, excidiert werden kann; denn dann fehlen sekundäre Veränderungen, die durch Zellregeneration oder durch Sekundärinfektion hervorgerufen werden können und die die Diagnose recht erschweren können.

Ein histologisches Bild, das dem einer frischen Blase des Pemphigus vulgaris ähnelt, findet sich nur bei zwei anderen Krankheiten, nämlich beim Frühstadium des Pemphigus vegetans und beim Pemphigus familiaris benignus. Beim Pemphigus vegetans ist die Ähnlichkeit leicht zu verstehen, da ja der Pemphigus vegetans lediglich eine Variante des Pemphigus vulgaris darstellt. Dagegen ist die histologische Ähnlichkeit zwischen dem Pemphigus vulgaris und dem Pemphigus familiaris benignus merkwürdig, da zwischen den beiden Krankheiten nur wenig klinische Ähnlichkeit besteht. Diese histologische Differentialdiagnose ist auf S. 687 besprochen. Betreffs histologischer Unterscheidung des Pemphigus vulgaris vom Pemphigus foliaceus s. S. 632; und vom bullösen Pemphigoid s. S. 672.

f) Cytologische Untersuchung

Tzanck beschrieb 1948 einen recht einfachen Test, nämlich die Untersuchung des Blasengrundausstriches, für den schnellen Nachweis von acantholytischen Zellen in den Blasen des Pemphigus vulgaris. Dieser Test stellt eine wertvolle Hilfe in der Diagnose des Pemphigus dar (Rook und Whimster; Blank und Burgoon; Haensch 1955 [I]; Steigleder). Er sollte aber nur als eine vorläufige Untersuchung gewertet werden und nicht die histologische Untersuchung ersetzen.

Zur Ausführung des Testes öffnet man die Blasendecke einer möglichst frischen Blase mit einem kleinen Skalpell und legt den Blasenboden frei. Mit einem Mulltupfer wird die Blasenflüssigkeit seitlich abgesaugt. Sodann schabt man den Blasenboden vorsichtig mit dem Skalpell, ohne eine Blutung hervorzurufen. Das abgeschabte Material wird dann auf einem Objektträger dünn ausgestrichen. Sobald der Ausstrich an der Luft getrocknet hat, wird er in Methylalkohol fixiert und dann mit Giemsa-Lösung gefärbt.

Das auffallendste Merkmal, durch welches sich diese Ausstriche von denen anderer Blasen unterscheiden, ist das Vorhandensein zahlreicher Epithelzellen. Dies kann man schon mit schwacher Vergrößerung feststellen. Infolge des Verlustes ihrer Intercellularbrücken (Acantholyse) liegen die Epithelzellen voneinander getrennt und sind abgerundet. Sie zeigen ferner Anzeichen von Degeneration: Das Cytoplasma erscheint als ein heller Hof um den Zellkern (wegen der dort vorhandenen Zusammenballung von Tonofilamenten, wie man bei der elektronenmikroskopischen Untersuchung erkennen kann) und ist an der Peripherie verdichtet (Abb. 14).

Im Gegensatz dazu zeigen Ausstriche von Blasen des bullösen Pemphigoids und der Dermatitis herpetiformis viele entzündliche Zellen und nur wenige Epithelzellen. Die letzteren besitzen entweder noch ihre Intercellularbrücken oder sie sind völlig nekrotisch.

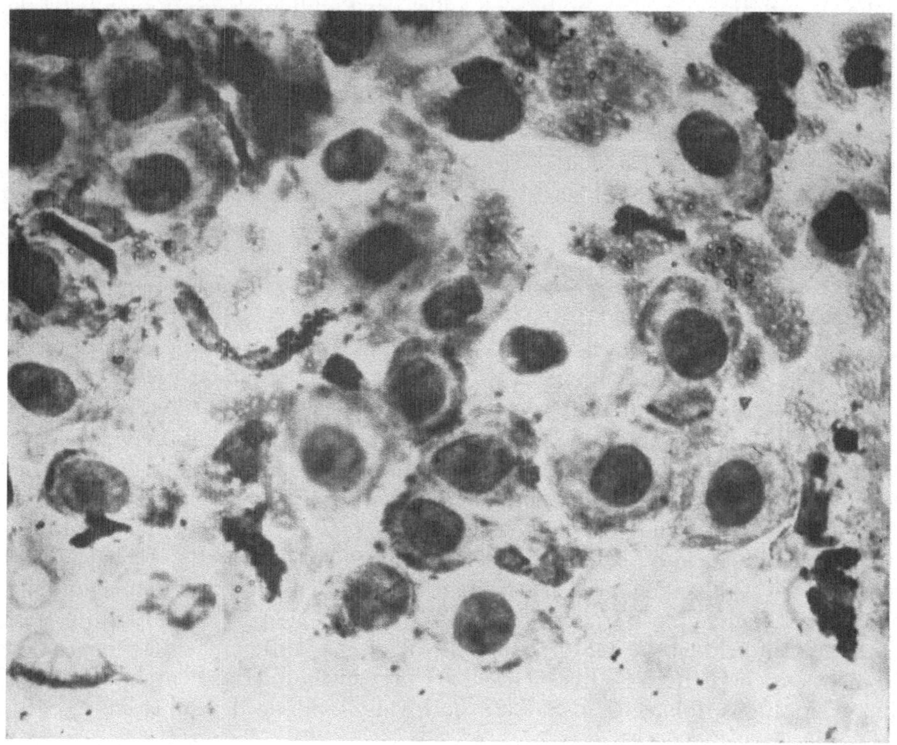

Abb. 14. Pemphigus vulgaris. Blasengrundausstrich. Die Epithelzellen liegen infolge Acantholyse voneinander getrennt. Sie zeigen Verdichtung des Cytoplasmas an der Peripherie. Giemsa-Färbung (600mal)

g) Histochemie

Bei Anwendung der Hotchkiss-McManus-Färbung ist der PAS-positive Grenzstreifen in den Blasen des Pemphigus vulgaris gut erhalten, während er in subepidermal entstehenden Blasen oft Schaden aufweist oder gar fehlt (BRAUN-FALCO 1960).

h) Polarisationsmikroskopie

NELEMANS et al. sowie NIEUWMEIJER untersuchten den Zustand der Tonofibrillen bei verschiedenen Arten von Blasen mittels des Polarisationsmikroskops, da unter diesem die Tonofibrillen doppeltbrechend sind. Beide Untersuchungen ergaben, daß, während bei spongiotischen Blasen und bei sich subepidermal bildenden Blasen die Tonofibrillen erhalten blieben, sie bei acantholytischen Blasen weitgehend degeneriert und selbst verschwunden waren.

i) Elektronenmikroskopie

Nach den von WILGRAM, CAULFIELD und LEVER (1961, 1963) durchgeführten Untersuchungen besteht beim Pemphigus vulgaris die früheste Veränderung in den Epidermiszellen aus einer Ablösung der Tonofilamente von ihren Desmosomen

(Intercellularbrücken). Infolgedessen kommt es zu einer Retraktion und Zusammenballung der Tonofilamente in der perinucleären Zone (Abb. 15). Im Anschluß an die Ablösung der Tonofilamente gehen die meisten Desmosomen

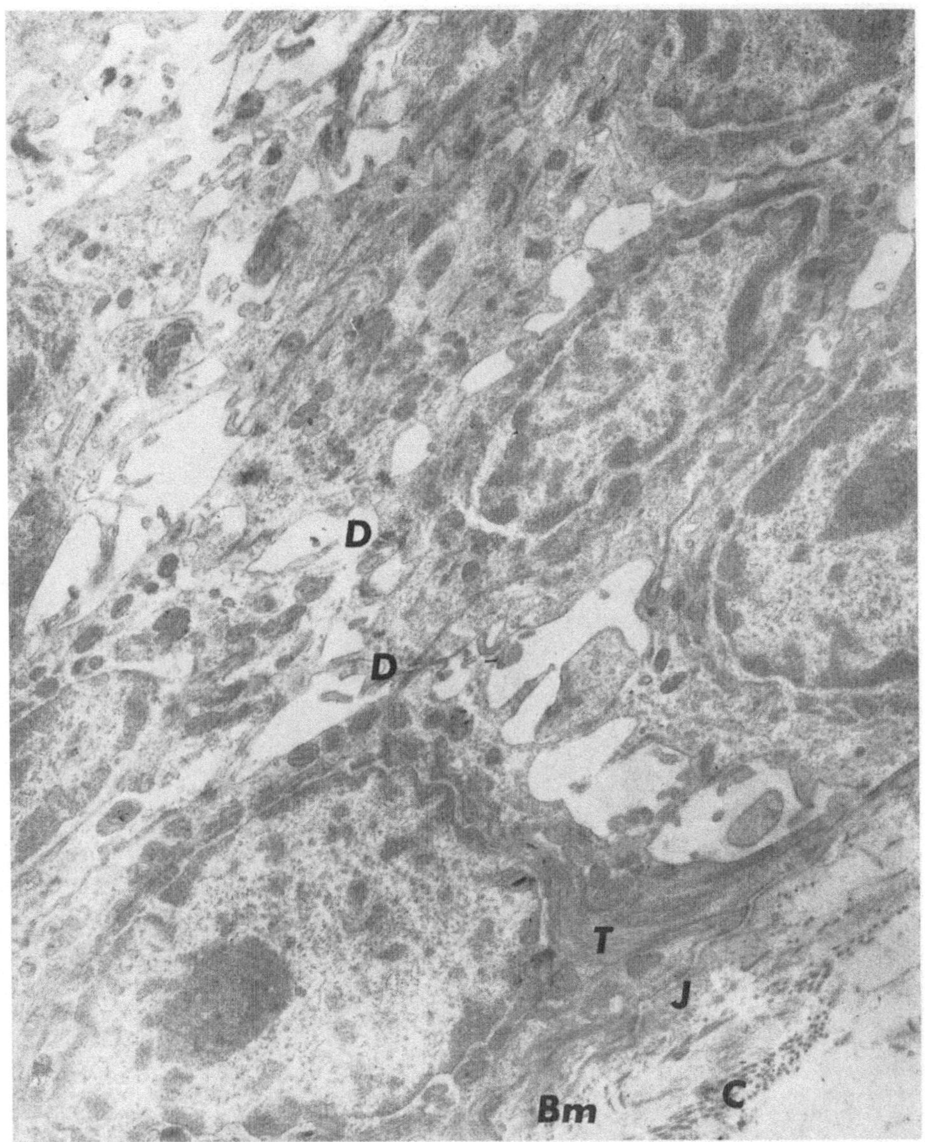

Abb. 15. Pemphigus vulgaris. Frühes Stadium der Blasenbildung. Nur wenige Desmosomen (*D*) (Intercellularbrücken) sind noch vorhanden. Selbst zwischen den beiden Basalzellen sind die Desmosomen verschwunden. Da aber die Basalmembran (*Bm*) und die Halbdesmosomen (*J*) ziemlich gut erhalten bleiben, haften die beiden Basalzellen der Basalmembran an. Während in den Basalzellen die Tonofilamente (*T*) noch mit den Halbdesmosomen verbunden sind, haben sie sich in den oberen Zellagen retrahiert und liegen perinucleär. *C* Kollagen (20000mal)

zugrunde. Infolge des Verschwindens der Desmosomen verlieren die Epidermiszellen ihren Zusammenhang miteinander. Dieser Verlust des Zusammenhaltes betrifft vor allem die Basalzellen und die an sie angrenzenden Stachelzellen; aber trotz des Verlustes ihres lateralen Zusammenhanges bleiben die Basalzellen an der Basalmembran haften, da die Basalmembran wie auch die Halbdesmosomen, die die Basalzellen mit der Basalmembran verbinden, erhalten bleiben (Abb. 16).

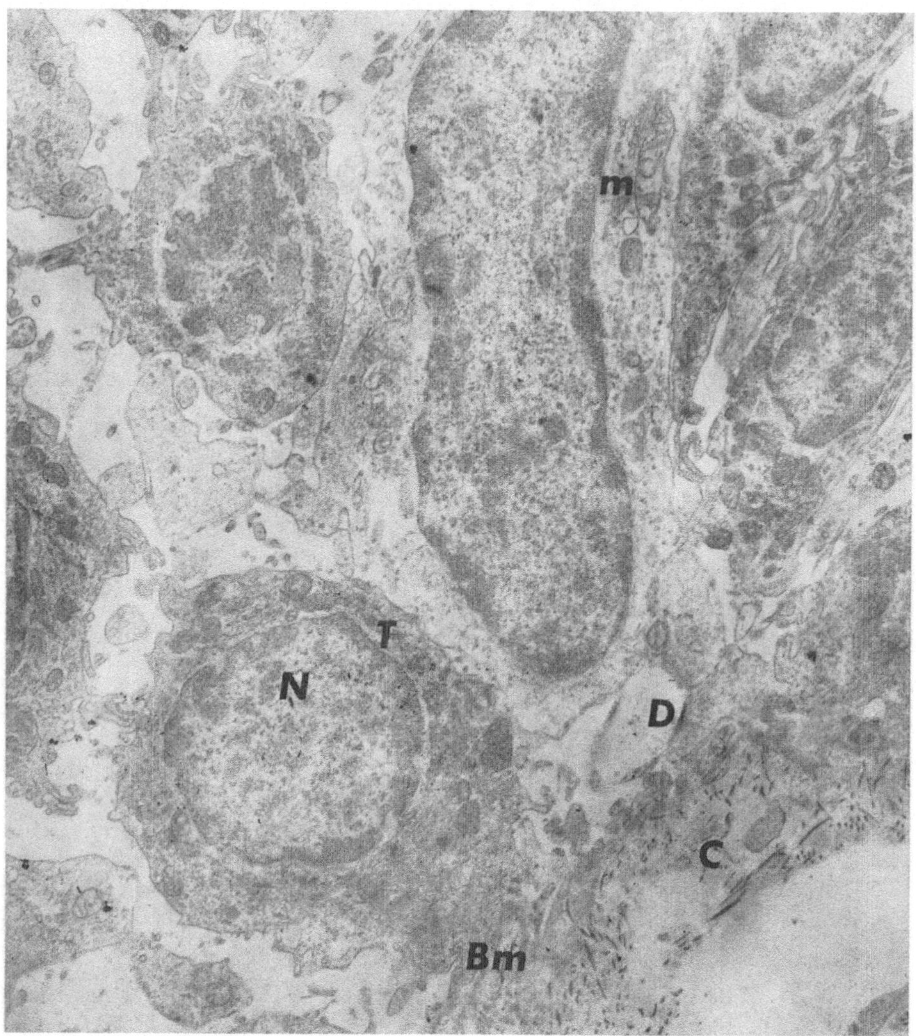

Abb. 16. Pemphigus vulgaris. Etwas weiter fortgeschrittenes Stadium. Obwohl die Basalmembran (*Bm*) verwaschen aussieht, haften ihr die Basalzellen doch an. Nur sehr wenige Desmosomen (*D*) sind noch vorhanden. In den oberen Zellagen zeigen Cytoplasma und Tonofilamente (*T*) degenerative Veränderungen. *C* Kollagen; *N* Zellkern; *m* Mitochondrien (14000mal)

Im Anschluß an das Verschwinden der Desmosomen verlieren die zusammengeballten Tonofilamente wie auch das Zellcytoplasma ihre strukturellen Einzelheiten (Abb. 17). Das Cytoplasma der acantholytischen Zellen nimmt ein granuläres Aussehen an. Die Mitochondrien degenerieren und die Zellkerne zeigen unregelmäßige Zackenbildung. Schließlich kommt es zu einer völligen Degeneration der acantholytischen Zellen, die jede Keratinisierung, selbst die Bildung von dyskeratotischem Material, verhindert.

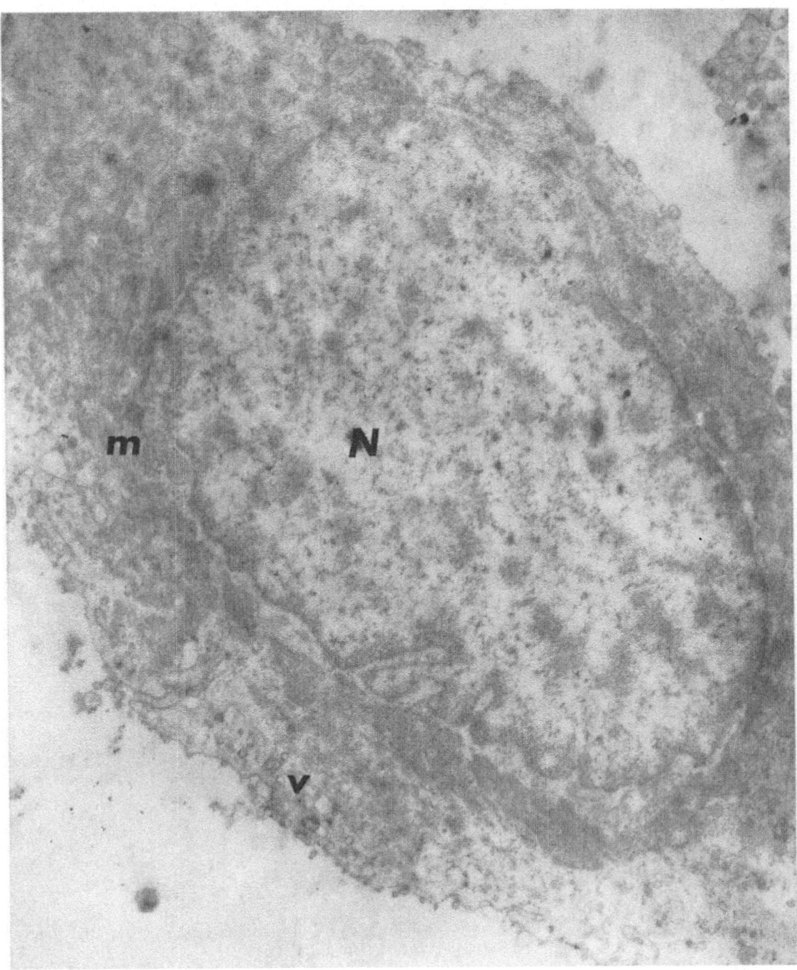

Abb. 17. Pemphigus vulgaris. Eine vereinzelt gelegene Epidermiszelle besitzt keine Desmosomen mehr. Pinocytotische Bläschen (*v*) sind am Zellrand wie auch innerhalb des Cytoplasma gelegen. Trotz der Degeneration im Cytoplasma sind noch einige Mitochondrien (*m*) vorhanden. Die Tonofilamente, die um den Zellkern (*N*) herum liegen, haben infolge Degeneration teilweise ihre fibrilläre Struktur verloren und zeigen ein granuläres Aussehen (24000mal)

2. Pemphigus vegetans

Der Pemphigus vegetans stellt eine Variante des Pemphigus vulgaris dar. Er tritt in einer malignen Form auf, dem sog. Neumann-Typ, und einer gutartigen Form, dem sog. Hallopeau-Typ (Pyodermite végétante), der allerdings in die maligne Form übergehen kann.

a) Die maligne Form des Pemphigus vegetans

Die maligne Form des Pemphigus vegetans, zuerst von NEUMANN beschrieben, beginnt und endet meistens als Pemphigus vulgaris, wie schon von RIECKE festgestellt wurde. Der maligne Pemphigus vegetans unterscheidet sich in klinischer Hinsicht vom Pemphigus vulgaris nur dadurch, daß viele Epitheldefekte mit papillomatösen Wucherungen, den sog. Vegetationen, heilen (Abb. 18). Frische

Vegetationen sind feucht und oft mit kleinen Pusteln besetzt, während ältere Vegetationen ein trockenes, verruköses und hyperkeratotisches Aussehen haben. Die Krankheit beginnt, wie der Pemphigus vulgaris, häufig im Munde. Späterhin ist die Mundschleimhaut wohl immer befallen. Entsprechend der Auffassung Directors (1952b), daß der Pemphigus vegetans ein Reaktionsstadium des Patienten mit Pemphigus vulgaris in Richtung eines erhöhten Widerstandes gegen die

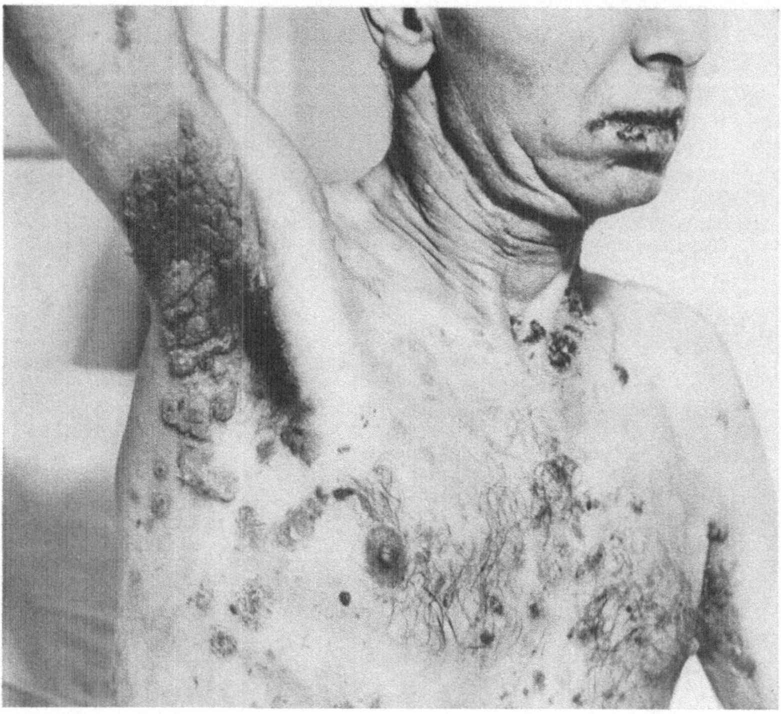

Abb. 18. Pemphigus vegetans, maligne Form. Die Abheilung der Epitheldefekte ist mit der Bildung verruköser Vegetationen vor sich gegangen

Krankheit darstellt, ist der Verlauf gewöhnlich mehr protrahiert als beim Pemphigus vulgaris, und längere Spontanremissionen, die beim Pemphigus vulgaris sehr selten sind, können vorkommen. Jedoch endete die Krankheit, bevor die Corticosteroide erhältlich waren, meistens mit dem Tode. Doch kommen Ausnahmen vor, wie schon Frühwald in seiner 1915 erschienenen Monographie über den Pemphigus vegetans auf Grund von zwei Patienten nachweisen konnte. Weitere Beispiele eines gutartigen Verlaufs beim Pemphigus vegetans vom Neumann-Typ sind erst vor kurzem von Director (1952b) und von Wentholt und Jansen mitgeteilt worden. Gewöhnlich treten bei einem gutartigen Verlauf allmählich mehr und mehr Vesico-Pusteln und Pusteln auf, so daß dann das klinische Bild von einem Pemphigus vegetans vom Hallopeau-Typ ununterscheidbar ist.

Histologie. Die Blasen haben dasselbe histologische Aussehen wie beim Pemphigus vulgaris. In den meisten, aber doch nicht in allen Blasen findet man in größerem Ausmaß als beim Pemphigus vulgaris ein unregelmäßiges Aufwärtswuchern der Papillarkörper und ein Hinunterwuchern von Epithelsträngen in die Dermis hinein.

Die mit Pusteln besetzten Vegetationen zeigen histologisch Papillomatose, Hyperkeratose und Eindringen von dicken Strängen von Epidermiszellen tief in die Dermis hinein. Acantholyse und Spaltenbildung in der Epidermis sind gewöhnlich vorhanden. Auffallend und von hohem diagnostischen Wert ist das Vorhandensein von intraepidermalen Abscessen, die fast ausschließlich aus Eosinophilen bestehen. Diese Abscesse stellen das histologische Substrat der

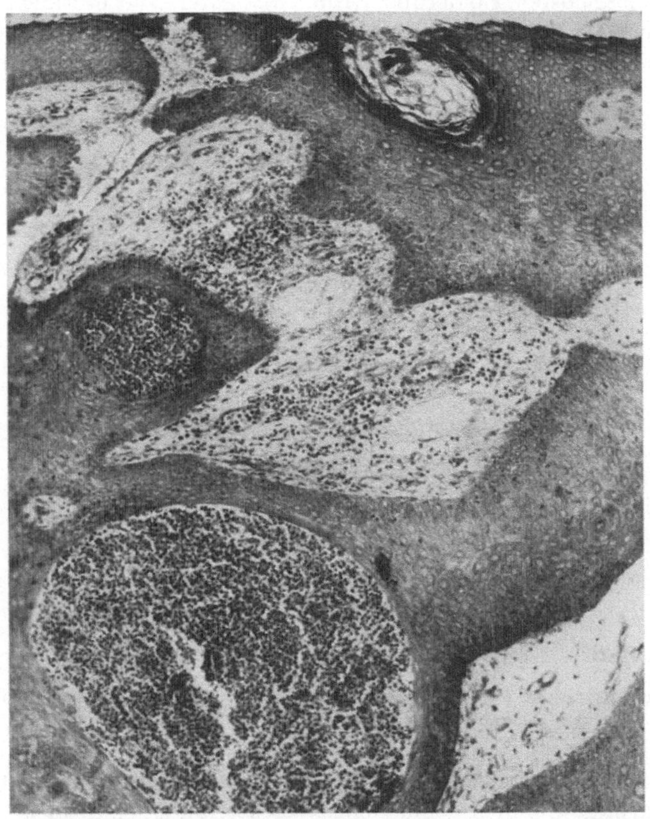

Abb. 19. Pemphigus vegetans, maligne Form. Ein älterer Krankheitsherd zeigt tief in die Dermis eingedrungene Epidermisstränge. Zwei intraepidermale Abscesse, die fast gänzlich aus Eosinophilen bestehen, sind vorhanden (100mal)

klinisch sichtbaren Pusteln dar. Man findet sie nicht nur in der Oberflächenepidermis, sondern auch innerhalb der dicken Epidermisstränge, die tief in die Dermis eingedrungen sind (Abb. 19). Gewöhnlich sind die intraepidermalen Abscesse von mehreren Schichten von Epidermiszellen umgeben und somit nicht suprabasal gelegen. Die schnelle Proliferation der Epidermis um die Abscesse herum ist wahrscheinlich die Erklärung dafür, daß man sie selten in suprabasaler Lage vorfindet. Die Dermis enthält gewöhnlich viele entzündliche Zellen, von denen ein großer Teil Eosinophile sind.

Ältere Vegetationen, die klinisch keine Pusteln mehr zeigen, weisen auch keine eosinophile Abscesse mehr auf. Man findet lediglich beträchtliche Papillomatose und Hyperkeratose. Ihr histologisches Aussehen ist somit nicht diagnostisch.

b) Pyodermite végétante

Diese Form von Pemphigus vegetans, die zuerst von HALLOPEAU (1896) beschrieben wurde, der aber RIECKE keine Sonderstellung einräumte, verdient Beachtung wegen des relativ gutartigen Verlaufs. Hierbei stellen Pusteln und nicht Blasen die Primärefflorescenz dar. Den Pusteln folgen recht bald verruköse Vegetationen, die mit Pusteln besetzt sind. Diese Vegetationen breiten sich peripher aus. Solange sie sich ausbreiten, findet man an ihrem Rande einen „Kragen“ losgelöster Epidermis (Abb. 20). Ältere Vegetationen zeigen keine Pusteln mehr. Die intertriginösen Hautgebiete sind hauptsächlich befallen. Durch peripheres Ausbreiten und Zusammenfließen benachbarter Krankheitsherde

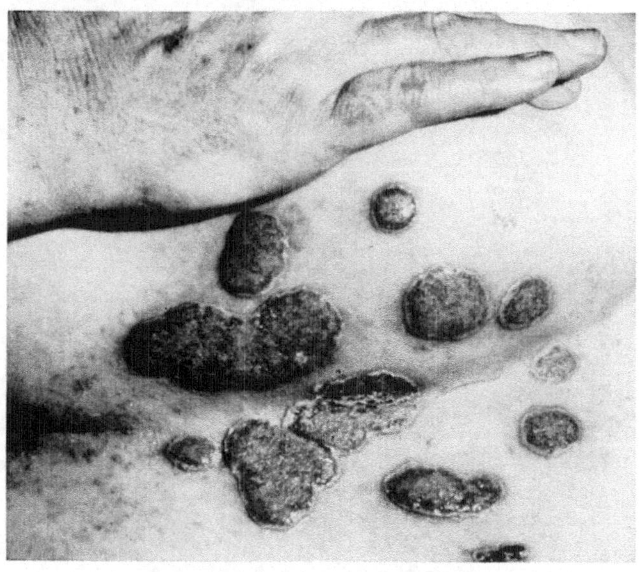

Abb. 20. Pemphigus vegetans, Pyodermite végétante. Peripher sich ausdehnende Vegetationen zeigen an ihrem Rande einen „Kragen“ von losgelöster Epidermis

können recht große Hautflächen befallen werden (Abb. 21). Im Gegensatz zur Haut, wo man gewöhnlich keine Epitheldefekte findet, sind solche an der Mundschleimhaut vorhanden. In manchen Fällen von Pyodermite végétante bilden sich nie Blasen, sondern ausschließlich Pusteln, und die Krankheit nimmt einen chronischen, gutartigen Verlauf. Spontane Remissionen kommen vor und anscheinend auch Heilung (WALLHAUSER; TSCHOPP; POSTMA; GOLDSMITH; SANTORI; LEVER und WHITE). Bei einigen Patienten entwickeln sich aber schließlich, wie schon HALLOPEAU (1898) feststellte, schlaffe Blasen und Epitheldefekte auf der Haut, so daß dann die Krankheit im Aussehen wie auch im Verlauf mit dem malignen Pemphigus vegetans von NEUMANN identisch ist.

Histologie. Die Pusteln, die hier die Primärefflorescenzen bilden, zeigen oft eine suprabasale Lage und beträchtliche Acantholyse. Sie enthalten außer degenerierten Epidermiszellen zahlreiche Eosinophile. Ein entzündliches Infiltrat, das fast ausschließlich aus Neutrophilen und Eosinophilen besteht, durchsetzt die Epidermis wie auch die obere Dermis.

Die mit Pusteln besetzten Vegetationen zeigen beträchtliche Hyperplasie der Epidermis und viele intraepidermale Eosinophil-Abscesse (Abb. 22). Ältere Krankheitsherde zeigen ausgesprochene Papillomatose und Hyperkeratose ohne

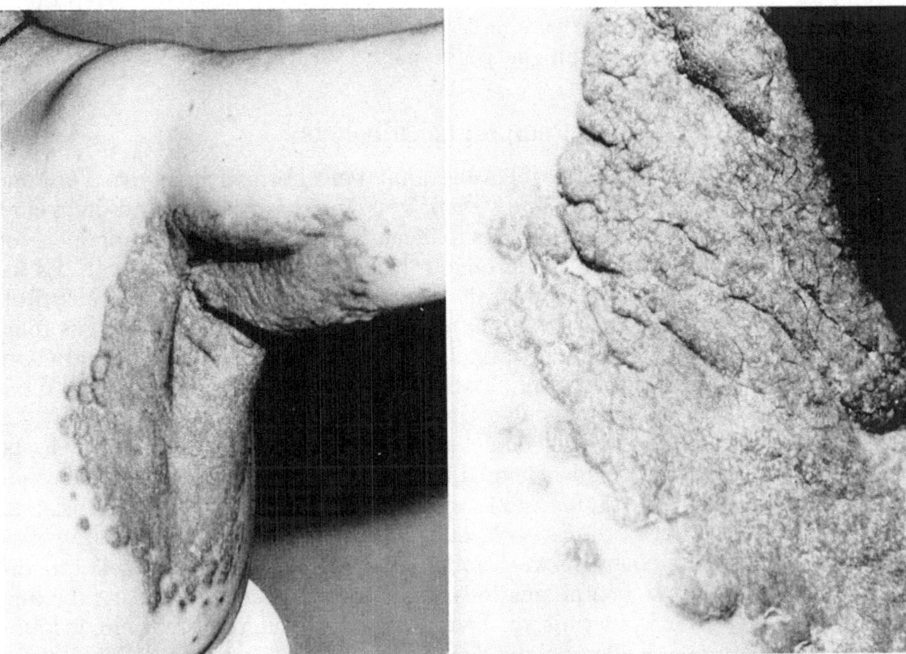

Abb. 21. Pemphigus vegetans, Pyodermite végétante. Ein großer Herd von Vegetationen ist in der Axilla vorhanden (links). Nahaufnahme desselben Herdes (rechts)

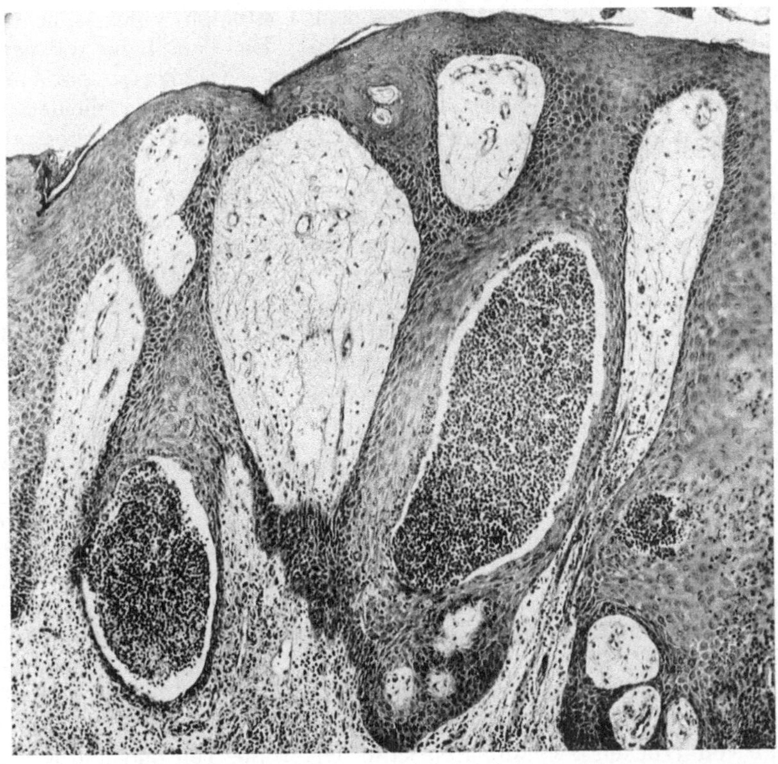

Abb. 22. Pemphigus vegetans, Pyodermite végétante. Es findet sich beträchtliche nach unten gerichtete Proliferation der Epidermis mit Bildung von intraepidermalen Eosinophil-Abscessen (50mal)

Eosinophil-Abscesse. Das histologische Bild der Pusteln wie auch der Vegetationen bei der Pyodermite végétante ist somit dasselbe, wie das der Pusteln und Vegetationen beim malignen Pemphigus vegetans.

3. Pemphigus foliaceus

Riecke sieht im Pemphigus foliaceus „nur eine Formvarietät des Verlaufes eines gewöhnlichen Pemphigus“ und spricht von einer häufigen Abwandlung eines Pemphigus vulgaris in einen Pemphigus foliaceus und das häufige Vorkommen von schweren Mundschleimhautveränderungen beim Pemphigus foliaceus. Es ist meine Ansicht, in Übereinstimmung mit Percival (1949), Vilanova und Piñol, Watrin und Merand, Herzberg (1958) sowie Perry, daß der Pemphigus foliaceus eine wesenseigene Krankheit darstellt. Im Gegensatz zu Combes und Canizares, Chargin et al., Michelson, Fisher (1962) sowie Tappeiner und Wodniansky wurde von mir niemals eine Umwandlung eines Pemphigus vulgaris in einen Pemphigus foliaceus oder umgekehrt, beobachtet. Ferner habe ich, im Gegensatz zu Riecke, Mundschleimhautveränderungen nur sehr selten beim Pemphigus foliaceus angetroffen, und zwar nur zweimal unter 41 Fällen (Lever 1953; Lever und White). Es ist wohl anzunehmen, daß Beobachtungen, wie sie Riecke erwähnt, auf einer Verwechslung zwischen den Krankheitsbildern des Pemphigus vulgaris und Pemphigus foliaceus beruhen. Anscheinend ist die ausgedehnte Ablösung der Epidermis, die beim Pemphigus vulgaris vorkommen kann, von einigen Autoren als Pemphigus foliaceus angesehen worden. Die Art der Ablösung oder Exfoliation ist aber bei den beiden Krankheiten verschieden. Beim Pemphigus foliaceus findet man nur eine oberflächliche Exfoliation der Epidermis, ohne die Bildung von Epitheldefekten wie beim Pemphigus vulgaris, bei dem sich die Epidermis fast in ihrer ganzen Dicke ablöst. Der Pemphigus foliaceus stellt somit ein eigenes Krankheitsbild dar, das sich vom Pemphigus vulgaris nicht nur im klinischen Aussehen, im Verlauf und in der Prognose unterscheidet, sondern auch im histologischen Bilde, obwohl Acantholyse bei beiden vorkommt.

a) Hauterscheinungen

Im Frühstadium des Pemphigus foliaceus sind Blasen gewöhnlich vorhanden. Manchmal fehlen sie aber. Die Blasen sind klein und schlaff. Sie brechen leicht und wegen ihrer oberflächlichen Lage führen sie nicht zu Epitheldefekten, sondern nur zu einer Exfoliation der oberen Epidermisschichten. Man sieht von Anfang an nicht nur Blasen, sondern auch erythematöse Flächen mit Schuppen, serösem Exsudat und Krusten.

Die ersten Erscheinungen finden sich oft in der Gesichtsmitte, wo sie eine „Schmetterlingsform“ annehmen können (Abb. 23). Auch auf der Kopfhaut, der Brust und dem oberen Rücken können sich die ersten Herde befinden. Wenn, wie es im Frühstadium der Krankheit oft der Fall ist, die Kopfhaut, das Gesicht, die Brust und der obere Rücken allein befallen sind, dann sind die Verteilung wie auch das Aussehen der Krankheitsherde die gleichen wie beim Pemphigus erythematosus (s. S. 637). Obwohl manchmal die Krankheit auf diese Hautgegenden beschränkt bleibt, findet doch in der Mehrzahl der Fälle eine allmähliche Ausbreitung statt. Solange sich die erythematösen Flächen durch periphere Ausbreitung vergrößern, haben sie einen scharf begrenzten, oft serpiginösen Rand, an dem sich die oberflächlichen Epidermisschichten ablösen (Abb. 24). Allmählich im Laufe von Wochen oder Monaten kann der größte Teil und häufig sogar die ganze Hautoberfläche befallen werden (Abb. 25).

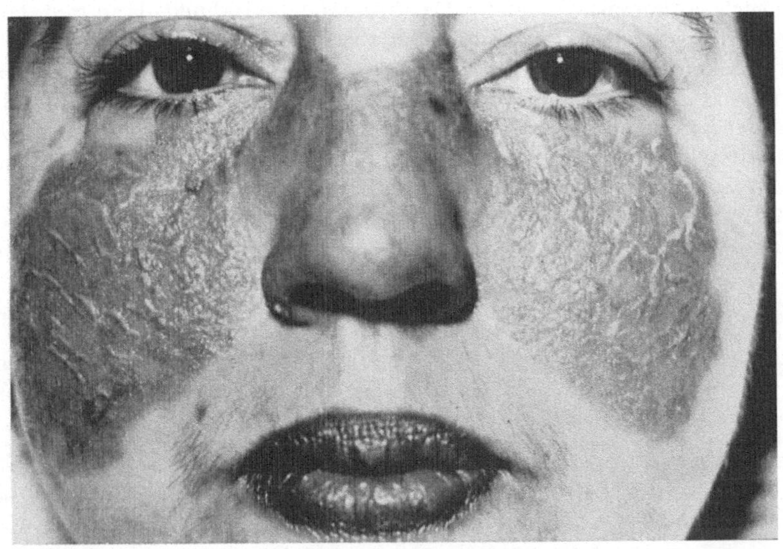

Abb. 23. Pemphigus foliaceus. Im Frühstadium können die Krankheitsherde am Gesicht „Schmetterlingsform" zeigen

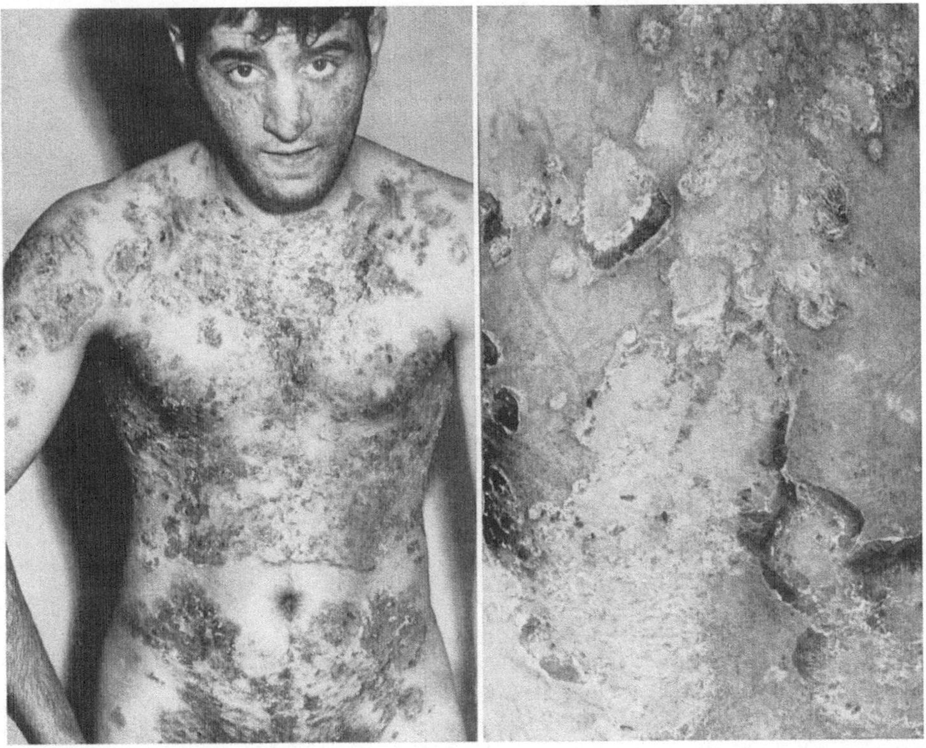

Abb. 24. Pemphigus foliaceus. Die Krankheitsherde haben während ihrer peripheren Ausbreitung oft einen serpiginösen Rand

Im vorgerückten Stadium der universalen Exfoliierung finden sich wenige oder gar keine Blasen, mit Ausnahme der Handflächen und Fußsohlen, wo sie noch gelegentlich vorkommen können. Das klinische Bild ähnelt dann dem einer exfoliierenden Erythrodermie, von der sich aber der Pemphigus foliaceus durch sein positives Nikolski-Zeichen unterscheidet. Ohne Behandlung hält das Stadium der universalen Exfoliierung gewöhnlich für viele Jahre an, vorausgesetzt, daß der Patient der Krankheit nicht erliegt. Manchmal bilden sich, besonders am Gesicht, fest anhaftende, dicke, hyperkeratotische Schuppen, die, wenn entfernt, auf ihrer Unterseite, wie beim Lupus erythematodes, dornenartige Fortsätze zeigen, die in die Haarfollikel hineinpassen (Abb. 26). In Fällen von langer Dauer findet man oft solch hyperkeratotische Schuppen über weite Hautgebiete verteilt (Abb. 27).

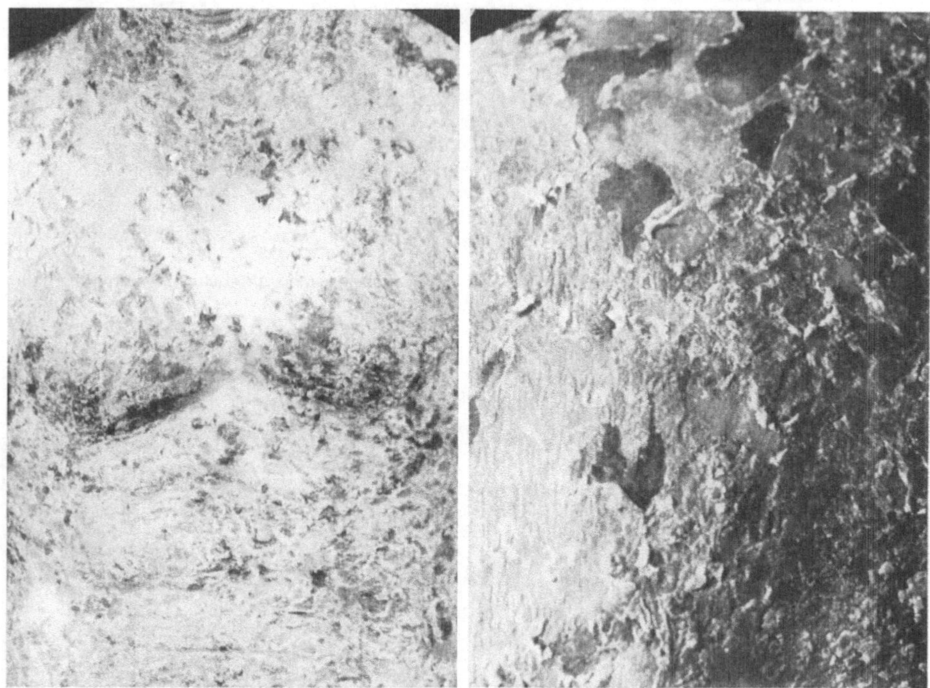

Abb. 25. Pemphigus foliaceus. Die ganze Hautfläche ist befallen und zeigt Rötung, Schuppung und Krustenbildung. Man sieht oberflächliche Exfoliation der Epidermis, aber keine Epithledefekte

Gelegentlich sieht der Pemphigus foliaceus im Frühstadium wegen einer gruppierten Anordnung der Bläschen einer Dermatitis herpetiformis ähnlich. Eine vermeintliche „Umwandlung“ einer Dermatitis herpetiformis in einen Pemphigus foliaceus ist mehrere Male beschrieben worden, z.B. von Low und Senear. Letzthin haben Floden und Gentele (1955), Doepfmer sowie Winkelmann und Roth über insgesamt vier Patienten berichtet, bei denen das klinische Bild einer Dermatitis herpetiformis ähnelte, die histologische Untersuchung aber die Diagnose Pemphigus foliaceus ergab. Die Hauterscheinungen bestanden bei diesen Patienten aus symmetrisch angeordneten rötlichen Flächen mit gruppierten Papeln und Bläschen.

b) Schleimhauterscheinungen

In der großen Mehrzahl der Patienten ist die Mundschleimhaut nicht befallen. In den seltenen Fällen, in denen Mundschleimhauterscheinungen vorhanden sind, bestehen sie aus kleinen, oberflächlich erodierten Herden. Nur bei Patienten, bei denen die Krankheit einen raschen und schweren Verlauf nimmt, kann ausnahmsweise diffuse Rötung mit oberflächlicher Exfoliierung des Mundschleimhautepithels vorhanden sein. Wenn die Augenlider befallen sind, ist die tarsale Bindehaut häufig gerötet und geschwollen mit profuser, sero-purulenter Sekretbildung; jedoch kommen Blasen und Exfoliierung dort nicht vor.

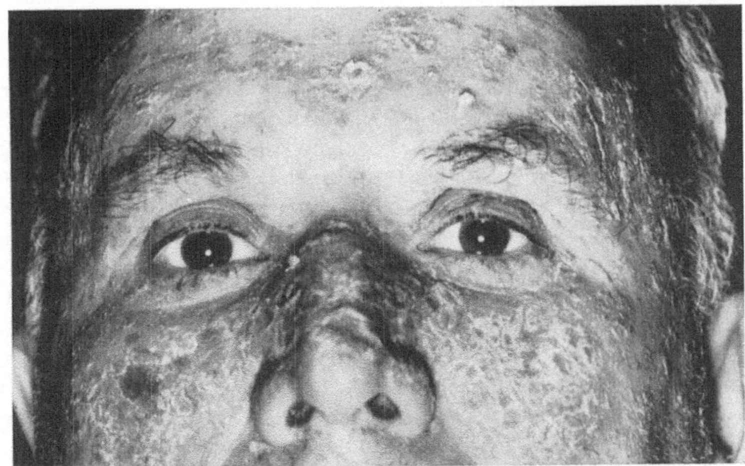

Abb. 26a u. b. Pemphigus foliaceus. Dicke, fest anhaftende, hyperkeratotische Schuppen befinden sich am Gesicht. Die Nahaufnahme (b) einer solchen Schuppe zeigt an ihrer Unterfläche dornenartige Fortsätze, die in die Haarfollikel hineinpassen

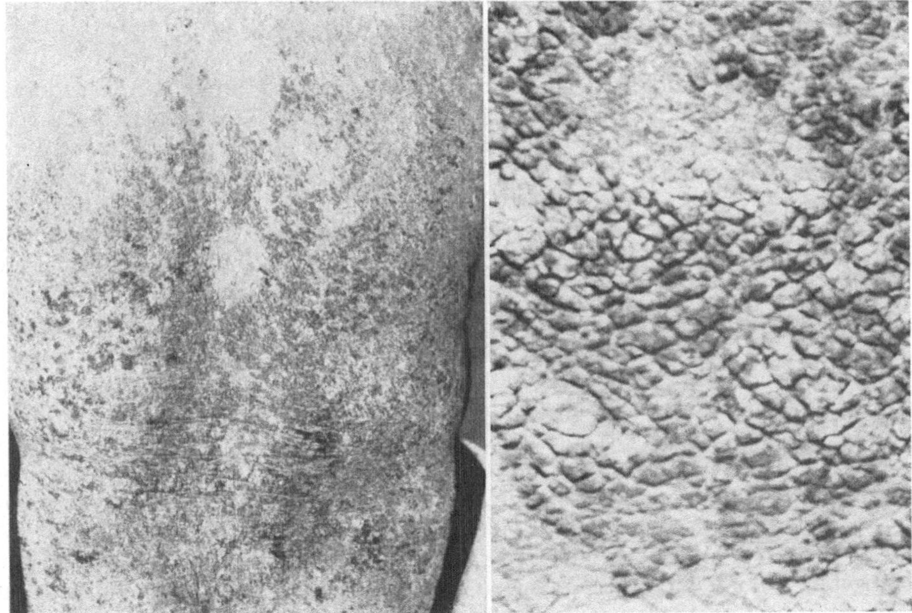

Abb. 27. Pemphigus foliaceus. Bei diesem Patienten, dessen Krankheit schon seit 15 Jahren besteht, ist der Rücken mit dicken, hyperkeratotischen Schuppen bedeckt

c) Verlauf

Gelegentlich breitet sich der Pemphigus foliaceus recht schnell aus und führt binnen weniger Wochen zu universeller Exfoliierung. Bei den meisten Patienten nimmt die Krankheit jedoch einen chronischen Verlauf, der sich über viele Jahre erstreckt (Perry). Bevor die Corticosteroide erhältlich waren, hing die Prognose hauptsächlich davon ab, ob die Krankheit einen schnellen oder langsamen Verlauf nahm und wie alt der Patient war. Bei Patienten, bei denen die Krankheit sich schnell ausbreitete, endete sie oft tödlich. Gleichfalls bei Patienten, die bei Beginn der Krankheit über 50 Jahre alt waren, endete der Pemphigus foliaceus selbst bei sehr langsamem Verlauf oft tödlich, da die Krankheit den Patienten schwächte und oft Komplikationen, wie Bronchopneumonie oder pyogene Infektionen, eintraten. So starben unter den von mir vor der Einführung der Corticosteroide beobachteten Patienten nur zwei unter den 14 Patienten, bei denen die Krankheit vor dem Alter von 50 Jahren begonnen hatte; während alle 16 Patienten starben, bei denen sie in späterem Alter aufgetreten war (Lever 1953). Bei den jüngeren Patienten bildete sich die Krankheit allmählich spontan zurück, nachdem sie für eine Zeitspanne von 2—30 Jahren in einem aktiven Stadium gewesen war. Während dieser Zeit war der allgemeine Gesundheitszustand der jüngeren Kranken oft nicht sehr beeinträchtigt, obwohl der Zustand ihrer Haut ihnen das Leben recht beschwerlich machte. Der Grund, daß bei Patienten mit Pemphigus foliaceus der Allgemeinzustand weniger als beim Pemphigus vulgaris beeinträchtigt ist, liegt wohl darin, daß beim Pemphigus foliaceus die Epidermis nur in ihren oberen Schichten exfoliiert. So ist der Grad der Zerstörung der Epidermis eher mit dem zu vergleichen, der bei einer exfoliierenden Erythrodermie vorliegt, als mit dem, der beim Pemphigus vulgaris vorkommt.

Der Pemphigus foliaceus beginnt häufiger als der Pemphigus vulgaris bei jungen Erwachsenen und kommt gelegentlich bei Kindern vor (Perry). Es besteht eine leichte Bevorzugung für Juden, aber dies ist keineswegs so ausgesprochen wie beim Pemphigus vulgaris. Unter den 41 persönlich beobachteten Patienten waren neun, d.h. 22%, jüdisch (Lever 1953; Lever und White).

d) Histologie

Die früheste Veränderung beim Pemphigus foliaceus besteht aus Acantholyse in den oberen Epidermisschichten, gewöhnlich in der Körnerzellenschicht oder direkt darunter. Dies führt zur Bildung von Spalten in oberflächlicher, oft subcornealer Lage (Abb. 28).

Wenn sich der Spalt vergrößert, bildet sich gelegentlich eine Blase in oberflächlicher, oft subcornealer Lage, in der man Acantholyse sowohl am Boden wie auch in der Blasendecke findet (Abb. 29). Häufiger jedoch führt die Vergrößerung der Spalte zu einer Ablösung der obersten Epidermisschichten ohne Blasenbildung (Abb. 30). Der sich ablösende Epidermisanteil besteht manchmal nur aus der Hornzellenschicht, in anderen Fällen aber aus der Horn- und Körnerzellenschicht oder aus diesen beiden Schichten zusammen mit den obersten Stachelzellschichten. Die übrige Epidermis bleibt in Zusammenhang mit der Dermis. Viele der Epidermiszellen, die an solche Spalten angrenzen, besitzen keine Intercellularbrücken mehr, so daß sie sich ablösen und in die Spalten hineintreiben. Häufig entwickeln sich sekundäre Spalten, die tiefer in die Epidermis hineinführen und zu Ablösungen in den Mittelschichten der Epidermis führen. Eine Ablösung der Epidermis direkt über der Basalzellenschicht wie beim Pemphigus vulgaris kommt aber nur sehr selten vor und dann nur an einigen Stellen. Außerdem findet man an solchen Stellen, im Gegensatz zum Pemphigus vulgaris, keinen Verlust der Intercellularbrücken zwischen den Basalzellen.

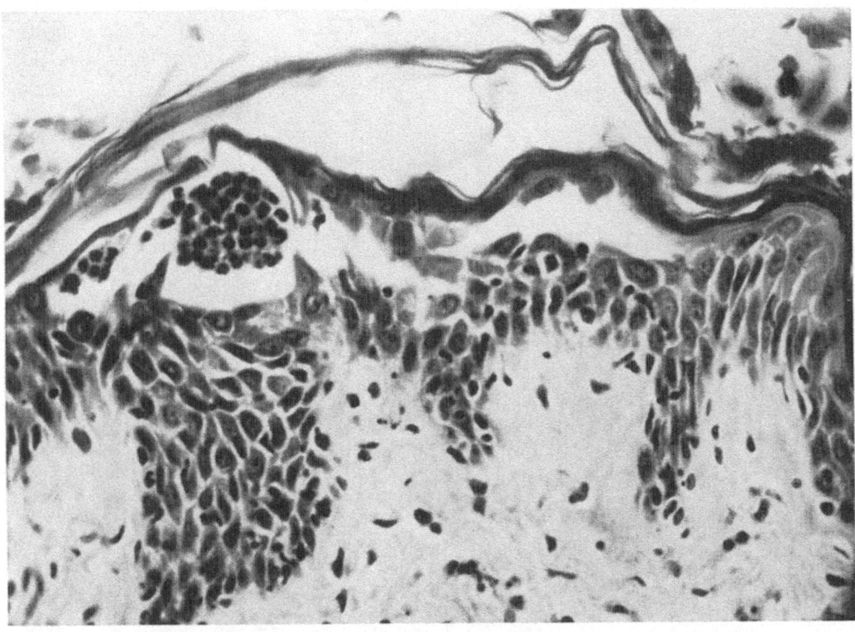

Abb. 28. Pemphigus foliaceus. Die früheste Veränderung besteht in der Bildung einer kleinen, oberflächlichen teilweise subcornealen Blase. Die Epidermiszellen unterhalb der Blase zeigen Degeneration mit Verlust der Intercellularbrücken (400mal)

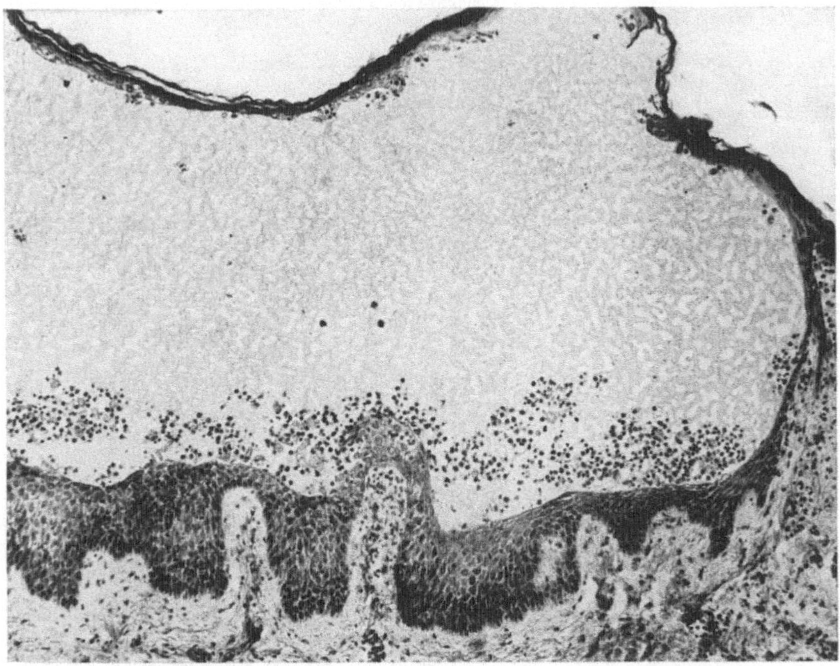

Abb. 29. Pemphigus foliaceus. Eine Blase befindet sich in oberflächlicher, teilweise subcornealer Lage (100mal)

Ältere Krankheitsherde zeigen Acanthose, etwas Papillomatose und außerdem Hyperkeratose, Parakeratose und oft auch Dyskeratose. Die parakeratotischen

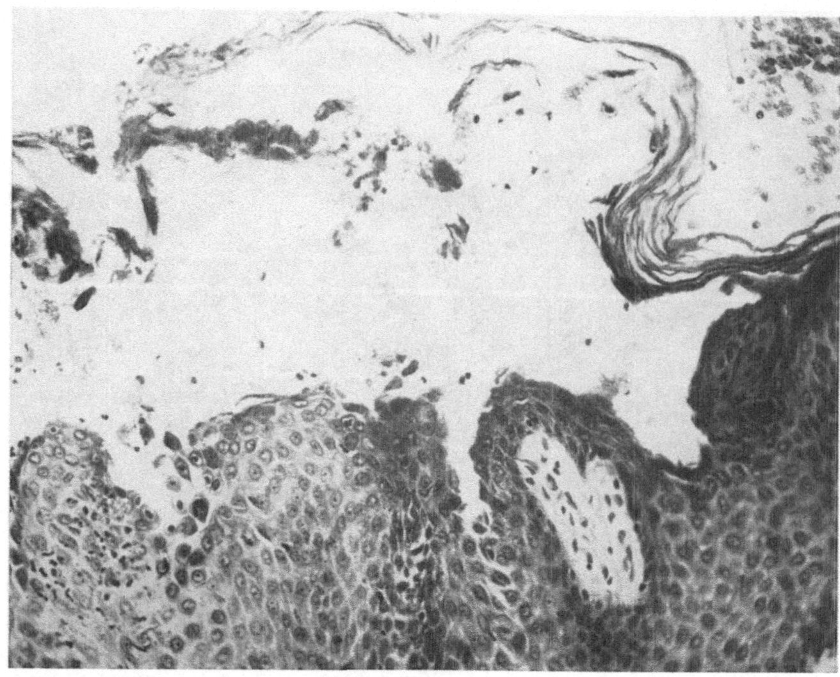

Abb. 30. Pemphigus foliaceus. Ein frisch entwickelter Krankheitsherd zeigt Ablösung der Horn- und Körnerzellenschicht ohne Blasenbildung. Die Epidermiszellen unmittelbar unter dem Spalt zeigen Verlust ihrer Intercellularbrücken (200mal)

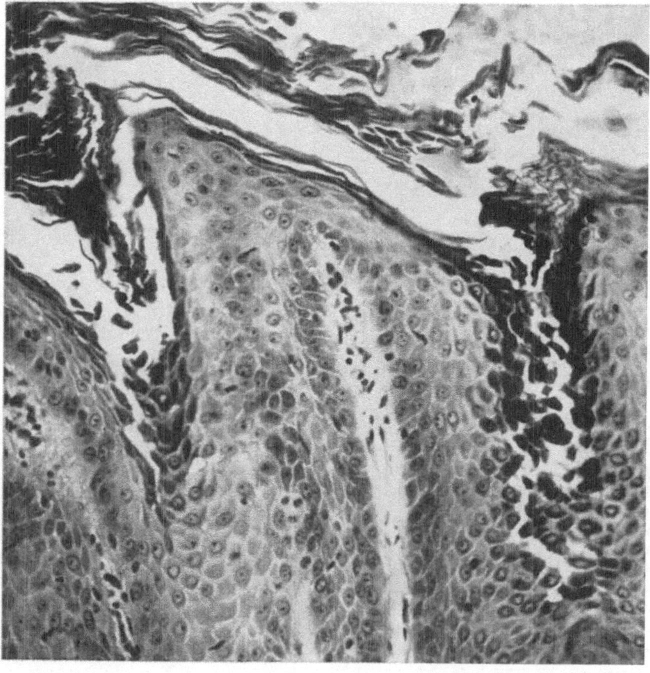

Abb. 31. Pemphigus foliaceus. Ein seit langem bestehender Krankheitsherd zeigt beträchtliche Acanthose und Hyperkeratose mit Spaltbildung in der Horn- und Körnerzellenschicht. Die Körnerzellen erscheinen degeneriert; sie sehen den Grains des Morbus Darier sehr ähnlich (200mal)

Zellen sind oft mit Neutrophilen und Lymphocyten und mit eingetrocknetem Plasma vermischt. In Krankheitsherden von langer Dauer kann beträchtliche Hyperkeratose bestehen, die auch in die Haarfollikel hinabreicht. Es können mehrere acantholytische Spalten vorhanden sein. Sie sind dann übereinander gelagert und durchsetzen die verdickte Hornzellenschicht wie auch die Körnerzellenschicht und die oberen Stachelzellenschichten. Ein auffallendes Zeichen, das recht häufig in älteren Herden beobachtet wird und für den Pemphigus foliaceus kennzeichnend ist, da es beim Pemphigus vulgaris nicht vorkommt, ist eine besondere Art von Degeneration der Körnerzellen. Die betroffenen Körnerzellen liegen infolge Acantholyse voneinander getrennt. Die in ihnen enthaltenden Körner sind vermehrt, größer als normal und zusammengeballt, so daß man den Zellkern oft nicht mehr erkennen kann. Solche Zellen erscheinen dann tief basophil und besitzen große Ähnlichkeit mit den „Grains", die man beim Morbus Darier sieht (Abb. 31). Diese dyskeratotischen Veränderungen der Körnerzellen sind oft am ausgesprochensten innerhalb der hyperkeratotischen Haarfollikel.

e) Elektronenmikroskopie

Die Veränderungen in der Epidermis sind, wie WILGRAM und CAULFIELD festgestellt haben, beim Pemphigus foliaceus denen ähnlich, die beim Pemphigus vulgaris vorkommen; doch sind sie weniger ausgesprochen. Obwohl man auch beim Pemphigus foliaceus bereits in der Basalzellenschicht die Ablösung einiger Tonofilamente von ihren Desmosomen feststellen kann, kommt es doch erst in den oberen Epidermislagen, besonders in der Körnerzellschicht, zu einem nahezu vollkommenen Schwinden der Desmosomen und damit zur Acantholyse (Abb. 32). Ferner, während beim Pemphigus vulgaris die Epidermiszellen unter Zerfall der

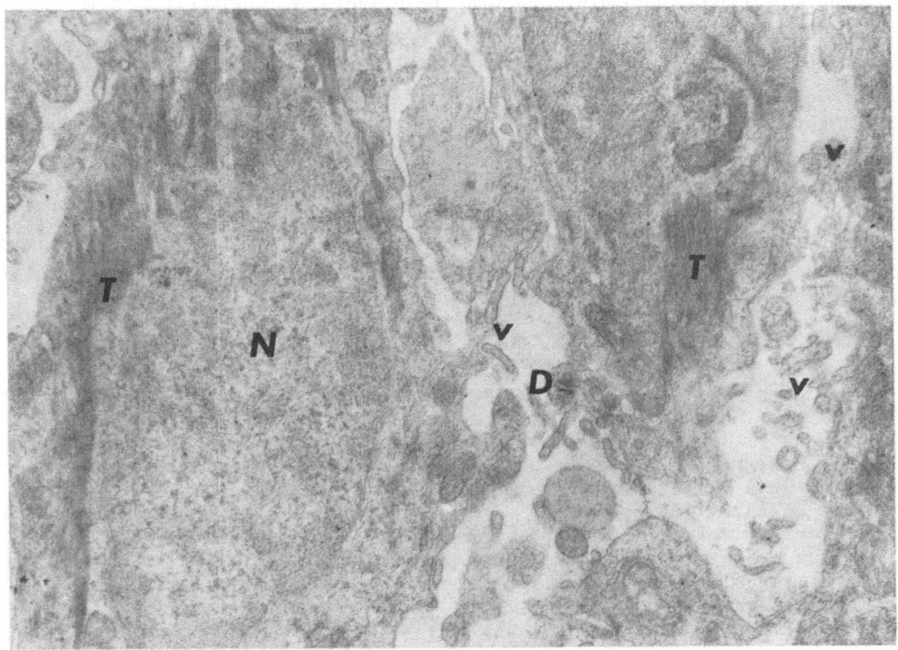

Abb. 32. Pemphigus foliaceus. In den oberen Zellagen der Epidermis befinden sich acantholytische Zellen, die den acantholytischen Zellen des Pemphigus vulgaris ähnlich sehen (s. Abb. 16). Nur wenige Desmosomen (*D*) sind übriggeblieben; aber zahlreiche Mikrovilli (*v*) sind als Überreste der Intercellularbrücken vorhanden. *N* Zellkern; *T* Tonofilamente (22000mal)

Tonofilamente nekrotisch werden, behalten sie beim Pemphigus foliaceus eine gewisse Lebensfähigkeit, so daß sie Verhornung zeigen, die allerdings unvollständig und abnorm ist. Die Verhornung besteht nämlich darin, daß sich die Tonofilamente, nachdem sie den Zusammenhalt mit ihren Desmosomen verloren haben, sich perinuclear in dichten Massen von dyskeratotischem Material zusammenballen.

4. Pemphigus erythematosus (Senear-Usher-Syndrom)

Der Pemphigus erythematosus, im Jahre 1926 von SENEAR und USHER zuerst beschrieben, wird von RIECKE nicht erwähnt. Er ist jedoch letzthin viel in der Literatur diskutiert worden. SENEAR und USHER berichteten ursprünglich über elf Patienten, die klinische Züge sowohl von Pemphigus als auch von Lupus erythematodes aufwiesen. In einer späteren Arbeit, die im Jahre 1949 erschien, definierten SENEAR und KINGERY den Pemphigus erythematosus als ein chronisches Hautleiden von begrenzter Ausdehnung, bei dem die Hauterscheinungen Ähnlichkeit mit dem Pemphigus, der seborrhoischen Dermatitis und dem Lupus erythemadodes zeigen, und das in seiner Ausdehnung begrenzt bleiben kann und dann gutartig verläuft oder sich in einen Pemphigus vulgaris oder Pemphigus foliaceus weiterentwickeln kann und dann dieselbe Prognose hat wie diese Pemphigusarten.

Eine Durchsicht der veröffentlichten Fälle von Pemphigus erythematosus einschließlich der 122 Fälle, die RICHTER (1950 [I]) in seiner Arbeit vom Jahre 1950 zusammengefaßt hat, ergibt ein recht unterschiedliches klinisches Bild bei den veröffentlichten Fällen. Im allgemeinen zeigten die Patienten jedoch gerötete, schuppende, hyperkeratotische oder krustöse Herde an der Nase und den Wangen. Ähnliche Herde, mit oder ohne Blasen, waren gewöhnlich auch auf der Kopfhaut und am Körper, besonders am oberen Teil des Rückens und in der Sternalgegend, vorhanden. Manche Patienten zeigten Mundschleimhautherde und andere zeigten keine. Obwohl die Krankheit bei einigen Patienten in ihrer Ausdehnung beschränkt blieb, schritt sie doch bei den meisten Patienten, die lange gnug unter Beobachtung standen, zu einem Pemphigus vulgaris oder Pemphigus foliaceus fort.

a) Nosologie

Die *nosologische Stellung des Pemphigus erythematosus* ist bis jetzt noch nicht völlig geklärt. Während zuerst Fälle von Lupus erythematodes mit Blasen in das Krankheitsbild einbezogen wurden, stimmen jetzt fast alle Autoren darin überein, daß der Pemphigus erythematosus eine Variante des Pemphigus ist. Nur RICHTER (1955) hält eine abweichende Ansicht, indem er die Meinung vertritt, daß es sich beim Pemphigus erythematosus „um ein autonomes Krankheitsbild handelt, das sowohl vom Pemphigus vulgaris und foliaceus, als auch vom Erythematodes disseminatus acutus abzutrennen ist“. Man kann wohl mit TOURAINEs Feststellung (1951) übereinstimmen, daß die zwei Fälle, die RICHTER im Jahre 1950 unter der Diagnose Pemphigus erythematosus veröffentlichte, Fälle von Lupus erythematodes acutus waren.

Es besteht allerdings keine Einigung darüber, wie der Pemphigus erythematosus in die Pemphigusgruppe eingeordnet werden soll. Einige sehen ihn als eine selbständige Variante des Pemphigus an; andere erkennen dem Pemphigus erythematosus zwar Selbständigkeit zu, weisen aber darauf hin, daß eine Fortentwicklung zu einem Pemphigus vulgaris oder Pemphigus foliaceus stattfinden kann; wiederum andere sehen ihn als ein Frühstadium des Pemphigus vulgaris an; und eine weitere Gruppe betrachtet ihn als einen örtlich begrenzten Pemphigus foliaceus.

Unter denjenigen, die die Ansicht vertreten, daß der Pemphigus erythematosus eine selbständige Variante des Pemphigus sei, mögen TOURAINE und LORTAT-JACOB sowie WORINGER und FLODEN und GENTELE (1953) genannt werden. TOURAINE und LORTAT-JACOB stellten 1941 fest, daß keine der anderen drei Formen des Pemphigus, nämlich vulgaris, vegetans und foliaceus, die Trias zeigt, die den Pemphigus erythematosus auszeichnet, nämlich Herde vom Aussehen des Lupus erythematodes, solche vom Aussehen der seborrhoischen Dermatitis wie auch pemphigusartige Blasen. Wegen der seborrhoischen Komponente schlugen sie die Bezeichnung „pemphigoide séborrhéique“ vor. Im Jahre 1954 änderte TOURAINE (1954, 1955) jedoch seine Ansicht über die Selbständigkeit der Krankheit, da es sich herausgestellt hatte, daß die von ihm beobachteten Fälle fast alle entweder in einen Pemphigus vulgaris oder einen Pemphigus foliaceus übergegangen waren. Er schlug die Bezeichnung „pemphigus séborrhéique" an Stelle von „pemphigoide séborrhéique" vor. WORINGER wie auch FLODEN und GENTELE (1953) haben die Autonomie des Pemphigus erythematosus innerhalb der Pemphigusgruppe betont; aber die von ihnen veröffentlichten histologischen Abbildungen sind recht typisch für den Pemphigus foliaceus.

Die Ansicht, daß sich der Pemphigus erythematosus entweder in einen Pemphigus vulgaris oder in einen Pemphigus foliaceus fortentwickeln kann, wird nicht nur von SENEAR und von TOURAINE (1954, 1955) vertreten, sondern auch von TAPPEINER und WODNIANSKY, CHARGIN et al. und FISHER (1962). Diese Autoren betrachten übrigens den Pemphigus vulgaris und den Pemphigus foliaceus lediglich als Varianten derselben Krankheit, die ineinander überwechseln können.

Ein ausgesprochener Repräsentant der Ansicht, daß der Pemphigus erythematosus ein Frühstadium des Pemphigus vulgaris darstelle, war WISE (1942, 1946). Dieselbe Meinung wurde auch von DOUCAS und KAPETANAKIS sowie von COSTELLO (1961) ausgesprochen.

Der erste Autor, der dafür eintrat, daß der Pemphigus erythematosus eine lokalisierte Form des Pemphigus foliaceus darstelle und nicht mit dem Pemphigus vulgaris in Beziehung stehe, war GRAY im Jahre 1938. Im folgenden Jahr berichtete GRAY (1939), daß der Patient, bei dem er einen Pemphigus erythematosus diagnostiziert hatte, nun einen universellen Pemphigus foliaceus habe. PERCIVAL stellte 1949 fest, daß klinisch und histologisch der Pemphigus foliaceus und der Pemphigus erythematosus identisch seien. „Beide stellen dieselbe Krankheit dar, deren Schwere über einen großen Spielraum variieren kann." Die gleiche Ansicht ist von WATRIN und MERAND, KEINING, VILANOVA und PIÑOL sowie PERRY ausgesprochen worden. PERRY kam zu dieser Meinung, da im Grunde genommen bei den 39 Patienten, deren Krankheit an der Mayo Clinic als Pemphigus foliaceus angesehen wurde, und bei den 16 Patienten, bei denen daselbst die Diagnose Pemphigus erythematosus gestellt worden war, die klinischen Erscheinungen und die histologischen Befunde die gleichen waren.

Der Widerspruch der Meinungen über das Wesen des Pemphigus erythematosus kann nur dadurch gelöst werden, daß man dem Begriff des Pemphigus eryththematosus nicht nur eine klinische, sondern auch eine histologische Definition gibt. Auf Grund histologischer Merkmale gibt es nur zwei Arten von Pemphigus: Pemphigus vulgaris und Pemphigus foliaceus. Beide können sich für eine beträchtliche Zeitspanne auf nur einige Stellen beschränken (s. S. 613 und 628). Beim Pemphigus vulgaris breitet sich die Krankheit früher oder später aus und nimmt fast stets einen tödlichen Verlauf, wenn der Patient nicht mit Corticosteroiden behandelt wird. Beim Pemphigus foliaceus dagegen breitet sich die Krankheit nicht immer aus, sondern kann für viele Jahre lokalisiert bleiben und dann schließlich spontan abheilen. Es unterliegt keinem Zweifel, daß einige Autoren das Initialstadium des Pemphigus vulgaris, andere das Initialstadium des Pemphigus foliaceus, und wiederum andere das Initialstadium beider Krankheiten als Pemphigus erythematosus bezeichnet haben.

Da nun aber der Pemphigus vulgaris und der Pemphigus foliaceus zwei verschiedene Krankheiten sind, zwischen denen es kein Überwechseln gibt, erscheint es nicht logisch, ein Krankheitsstadium anzuerkennen, das in zwei verschiedene Krankheiten auslaufen kann. Ferner scheint es unnötig, dem Initialstadium des Pemphigus vulgaris eine besondere Bezeichnung zu geben, da dieses Stadium stets von beschränkter Dauer ist und, falls nicht mit massiven Dosen von Corticosteroiden behandelt wird, der Tod infolge generalisierten Pemphigus vulgaris eintreten wird.

Andererseits besteht eine gewisse Berechtigung, dem Initialstadium des Pemphigus foliaceus eine Sonderstellung einzuräumen, weil ein Fortschreiten in einen generalisierten Pemphigus foliaceus nicht immer eintritt und die Krankheit einen gutartigen Verlauf nehmen kann, der nicht einmal die interne Verabreichung von Corticosteroiden erfordert. Dies ist der Grund, warum ich es bevorzuge, wie zuerst von GRAY vorgeschlagen, den Pemphigus erythematosus als ein Frühstadium des Pemphigus foliaceus zu definieren, das lokalisiert bleiben kann oder in einen generalisierten Pemphigus foliaceus fortschreiten kann.

b) Hauterscheinungen

Die Hauterscheinungen des Pemphigus erythematosus befinden sich, wie beim Frühstadium des Pemphigus foliaceus, vor allem im Gesicht, an der Kopfhaut, auf der Brust und auf dem oberen Teil des Rückens. Im Gesicht können die Herde eine schmetterlingsartige Ausbreitung zeigen (Abb. 23). Die Hauterscheinungen bestehen aus geröteten Arealen, die Schuppung, Nässen und leichte Krustenbildung zeigen. Nach Entfernung der Schuppen und Krusten sieht man oberflächliche Erosionen. Schlaffe Bläschen finden sich zwar nur sehr selten im Gesicht, ziemlich häufig aber auf der Brust und dem Rücken.

Eine gewisse Ähnlichkeit hat der Pemphigus erythematosus mit dem Lupus erythematodes und der seborrhoischen Dermatitis sowohl in der Lokalisation als auch im Aussehen. So kann z.B. beträchtliche follikuläre Hyperkeratose wie beim Lupus erythematodes bestehen, besonders im Gesicht. Atrophie findet man dagegen nicht. Der Pemphigus vulgaris zeigt im Frühstadium häufig Bildung dicker Krusten, nach deren Ablösung entweder Epitheldefekte oder Vegetationen zutage treten. Weder dicke Krusten noch Epitheldefekte oder Vegetationen findet man beim Pemphigus erythematosus. Auch sind beim Pemphigus vulgaris Mundschleimhauterscheinungen häufig schon im Frühstadium vorhanden, während sie beim Pemphigus erythematosus stets fehlen.

c) Verlauf

Der Pemphigus erythematosus kann wohl während des ersten Jahres seines Bestehens in einen Pemphigus foliaceus übergehen. Danach ist es nicht mehr wahrscheinlich. Statt dessen bleibt er dann gewöhnlich über viele Jahre hin unverändert bestehen, bis er allmählich spontan heilt (Lever und White).

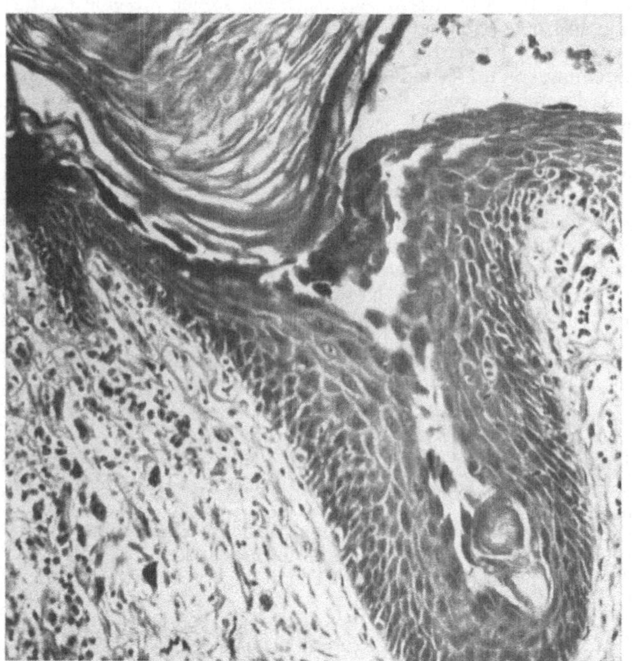

Abb. 33. Pemphigus erythematosus. Ein Spalt hat sich unterhalb der Körnerzellenschicht gebildet. Die Körnerzellen zeigen Degeneration (200mal)

d) Histologie

Die histologischen Befunde sind beim Pemphigus erythematosus dieselben wie beim Pemphigus foliaceus. Oft besteht beim Pemphigus erythematosus ausgesprochene follikuläre Hyperkeratose wie beim Pemphigus foliaceus. Acantholyse und Dyskeratose der Körnerzellen innerhalb der hyperkeratotischen Haarfollikel treten oft recht ausgesprochen zu tage (Abb. 33).

Die histologische Abgrenzung des Pemphigus erythematosus vom Lupus erythematodes ist gewöhnlich ohne große Schwierigkeit möglich; denn, obwohl beide Krankheiten follikuläre Hyperkeratose zeigen, kommt es nur beim Pemphigus erythematosus zu Acantholyse und Dyskeratose der Körnerzellen. Hydropische Degeneration der Basalzellen findet sich dagegen nur beim Lupus erythematodes. Wenn Blasen vorhanden sind, befinden sie sich in den obersten Epidermislagen beim Pemphigus erythematosus, während sie beim Lupus erythematodes subepidermal gelegen sind, wo sie sich sekundär zu der hydropischen Degeneration der Basalzellen bilden.

II. Differentialdiagnose

1. Pemphigus acutus

In seiner eingehenden Abhandlung über den Pemphigus acutus kommt RIECKE zu dem Schluß, daß dieser in drei Krankheitsbilder aufgeteilt werden kann: Erstens akute Verlaufsformen des Pemphigus vulgaris, zweitens Pemphigus acutus non contagiosus, der eigentliche Repräsentant des Krankheitsbegriffes, von dem er glaubt, daß er wahrscheinlich kein auf die Dauer haltbarer Typ ist, und drittens Pemphigus acutus infectiosus sive contagiosus, der kein Pemphigus sensu strictiore sei, sondern verdiene, als Septicaemia bullosa aus der Pemphigusgruppe ausgeschieden zu werden.

Seit RIECKEs Darstellung ist über den Begriff des Pemphigus acutus keine einheitliche Anschauung zustande gekommen. Manche Autoren haben Zweifel an dem Bestehen eines Pemphigus acutus ausgedrückt. So betrachten PILLSBURY et al. den Ausdruck Pemphigus acutus als überholt. Sie nehmen an, daß schwere Pyodermien und verschiedene Arten von Erythema exsudativum multiforme damit bezeichnet wurden. Andere Autoren halten an dem Begriff des Pemphigus acutus fest. MICHELSON erkennt, neben einem akuten Verlauf des Pemphigus vulgaris, einen echten Pemphigus acutus an, der eine Sepsis darstelle und binnen 1–3 Wochen tödlich ende. Auch LAUSECKER hat den Pemphigus acutus als einen septischen Prozeß mit Hervortreten von Hauterscheinungen definiert. PROPPE sowie RICHTER (1950[II]) glauben, daß der Pemphigus acutus der Ausdruck eines Sanarelli-Shwartzman-Phänomens sei. Sie nehmen an, daß „Staphylokokken, Streptokokken, Pneumokokken, Colibacillen u. a., auch Viren, einen Entzündungsherd schaffen, der als vorbereitendes Moment wirkt, und daß dann andere Erreger oder eine unbelebte organische Substanz das auslösende Moment darstellen" (RICHTER 1950 [II]).

Eine eingehende Durchsicht der in der Literatur als Pemphigus acutus bezeichneten Fälle erweckt den Eindruck, daß diese entweder als Fälle von Pemphigus vulgaris mit akutem Verlauf oder als Fälle von schwerem Erythema exsudativum multiforme angesehen werden können. Daß das Erythema exsudativum multiforme eine schwere und selbst tödliche Krankheit sein kann, ist eine recht neue Auffassung. Anscheinend wurden bis in die zwanziger Jahre hinein Fälle mit schweren, akuten Blasenausschlägen größtenteils unter der Diagnose Pemphigus acutus veröffentlicht. Dann stellten drei Autoren in drei verschiedenen Ländern kurz hintereinander solche Fälle als eine neue Krankheitseinheit auf. FIESSINGER und RENDU beschrieben im Jahre 1916 Fälle mit akuten Blasenausschlägen und schweren Schleimhauterscheinungen unter der Bezeichnung „ectodermose érosive pluriorificielle". STEVENS und JOHNSON führten im Jahre 1922 die Bezeichnung „eruptive fever with ophthalmia" ein und BAADER prägte im Jahre 1925 die Bezeichnung „Dermatostomatitis". Seither hat sich die Auffassung allgemein durchgesetzt, daß die von diesen drei Autoren beschriebenen Krankheitsbilder eine schwere Form der Erythema exsudativum multiforme darstellen (LEVER 1944; KLAUDER; COSTELLO 1947; BOHNSTEDT; FRIEDMANN und PATHÉ); und viele solche Fälle sind beschrieben worden. Andererseits sind seit Einführung des Begriffes einer schweren und möglicherweise tödlichen Form von Erythema exsudativum multiforme Fälle von Pemphigus acutus nur sehr selten in der Literatur berichtet worden.

Ausschlaggebend gegen die Zuteilung von Fällen mit akuten, febrilen Blasenausschlägen zum echten Pemphigus ist die Tatsache, daß solche Fälle subepidermale Blasenbildung zeigen, wie schon CIVATTE in seiner grundlegenden Veröffentlichung aus dem Jahre 1943 feststellte. Dieses konnten wir an Hand von drei Fällen bestätigen (LEVER 1953).

2. Brasilianischer Pemphigus (Fogo selvagem)

Diese Krankheit, von RIECKE nicht erwähnt, ist in einigen Gegenden von Brasilien endemisch. Nach Schätzungen von VIEIRA, FONZARI und GOLDMAN gab es im Jahre 1954 ungefähr 3000 Fälle in der endemischen Zone. Der brasilianische Pemphigus sieht dem Pemphigus foliaceus klinisch wie auch histologisch in einem solchen Ausmaß ähnlich, daß eine Unterscheidung unmöglich ist. Wie beim Pemphigus foliaceus beginnt die Krankheit gewöhnlich mit Blasen und geröteten, schuppenden Herden am Gesicht, der Brust und dem oberen Teil des Rückens (VIEIRA, FONZANI und GOLDMAN). Dem frühen Blasenstadium folgt das chronische exfoliierende Stadium. Das Nikolski-Zeichen ist positiv. Mundschleimhauterscheinungen bestehen nicht. Meistens verläuft die Krankheit sehr chronisch; sie kann aber gelegentlich recht akut verlaufen, so daß der Patient schon im Blasenstadium stirbt. Außerdem gibt es Abortivformen, die nach der Ansicht von VIEIRA (1948) und von VILANOVA und PIÑOL dem Pemphigus erythematosus sehr ähnlich sehen. Nach BROWN sterben ungefähr 40% der Patienten innerhalb der ersten 2 Jahre. Die anderen 60% leben für 10—30 Jahre mit nur geringem Fluktuieren im Krankheitsbild. Nur bei 25% der Patienten heilt die Krankheit völlig ab. Die Ursache ist unbekannt.

Mehrere brasilianische Autoren, wie z.B. VIEIRA (1940, 1948) und COSTA, nehmen an, daß der brasilianische Pemphigus eine Infektionskrankheit sei, weil er in umschriebenen Gebieten vorkommt und gelegentlich mehrere Familienmitglieder davon befallen sind. Aber kein infektiöses Agens ist bisher gefunden worden.

Es ist zur Zeit unmöglich, die Beziehungen zwischen dem brasilianischen Pemphigus und dem Pemphigus foliaceus festzulegen. Die Ähnlichkeit, wenn nicht Gleichheit im klinischen und histologischen Bilde wie auch im Verlauf deuten auf eine nahe Verwandtschaft der beiden Krankheiten hin. So betrachten die meisten brasilianischen Autoren, wie VIEIRA (1948), ZILBERBERG, FURTADO und ferner ANGULO und FERRAZ-MAZZONI, die beiden Krankheiten als identisch. Aber, wie schon SENEAR und KINGERY festgestellt haben, auf Grund seines endemischen Auftretens sollte doch der brasilianische Pemphigus vom Pemphigus foliaceus getrennt werden, bis eine gemeinsame Ursache für beide Krankheiten gefunden worden ist.

Hinsichtlich der Differentialdiagnose zwischen dem Pemphigus vulgaris und dem *bullösen Pemphigoid* s. S. 672; und zwischen dem Pemphigus vulgaris und dem *Pemphigus familiaris benignus* s. S. 687.

III. Pathologie der inneren Organe

RIECKE hat die beim Pemphigus vulgaris, Pemphigus foliaceus und Pemphigus vegetans erhobenen Sektionsbefunde eingehend besprochen und dabei den am Zentralnervensystem beobachteten Veränderungen besondere Beachtung geschenkt. Veränderungen an den Nebennieren werden dagegen von ihm nicht erwähnt. RIECKE stellte fest, daß eine Fülle verschiedenartigster Organveränderungen gefunden worden sind. Er betrachtete all diese Befunde als unspezifisch. Viele neue Sektionsbefunde sind seitdem mitgeteilt worden. Sie besitzen aber auch keine spezifische Bedeutung. Besonders erwähnt wurden letzthin diffuse Gefäßveränderungen und Veränderungen an den Spinalganglien und Nebennieren.

Diffuse Gefäßveränderungen wurden von CHARPY, FRAMIER und STAHL beschrieben. Sie fanden Hyalinisierung der Gefäßwände von Arteriolen und Venülen zusammen mit Wandverdickung, Endothelproliferation und Thrombosierung. Diese Veränderungen hielten sie für die von ihnen festgestellten weitverbreiteten Änderungen an den parenchymatösen Organen und den Spinalganglien verantwortlich. Obwohl sie zugeben, daß die Gefäßveränderungen für den Pemphigus nicht spezifisch sind, betrachten sie diese trotzdem nicht als sekundär.

BALÓ und FÖLDVÁRI fanden bei der Sektion von 54 Patienten mit Pemphigus schwere Veränderungen in den Spinalganglien, nämlich Degeneration von Ganglienzellen, Schwellung und Verdickung der um die Ganglienzellen gelegenen Kapseln und Bildung von großen, schon makroskopisch sichtbaren Cysten. In einem Fall von Pemphigus vulgaris mit Munderscheinungen fanden FÖLDVÁRI und BALÓ die gleichen Veränderungen im Ganglion Gasseri. Sie schlossen daraus, daß die Pemphiguserscheinungen auf der Haut und im Munde durch eine Degeneration von Ganglien hervorgerufen seien. GAWALOWSKI et al. konnten diese Befunde nicht bestätigen. Ferner haben SULZBERGER und BAER darauf hingewiesen, daß das Fehlen jeglicher segmentaler Anordnung der Hautherde und das gute Ansprechen der Krankheit auf die Behandlung mit Corticosteroiden es unwahrscheinlich mache, daß die Hauterscheinungen durch eine irreversible Degeneration von Spinalganglien verursacht seien.

Veränderungen in den Nebennieren sind beim Pemphigus vulgaris mehrfach beschrieben worden. TALBOTT, LEVER und CONSOLAZIO berichteten im Jahre 1940 über eine schwere hämorrhagische Nekrose der Nebennieren bei zwei Fällen und leichtere Veränderungen bei zwei weiteren Fällen. Im Jahre 1945 sammelte GOLDZIEHER 13 Fälle von Pemphigus vulgaris aus der Literatur und berichtete über sechs eigene Fälle, bei denen die Nebennieren akute Degeneration und Entzündung mit nachfolgender Vernarbung und Regeneration zeigten. KUHN und IVERSON fanden ähnliche, doch weniger ausgesprochene Veränderungen in den Nebennieren. Man kann wohl annehmen, wie es KUHN und IVERSON tun, daß die Nebennierenveränderungen beim Pemphigus vulgaris sekundär entstehen und denen gleichen, die man in der Folge von vielen anderen schweren Krankheiten findet. Wenn die Veränderungen so ausgesprochen sind, wie bei den von TALBOTT et al. und GOLDZIEHER beschriebenen Fällen, kann es wohl zu Funktionsstörungen der Nebennieren kommen. (Siehe betreffs Serumelektrolyte auf S. 644 und betreffs Nebennierenfunktionsprüfungen auf S. 645.)

IV. Biochemische Veränderungen in Blut, Urin und Blasenflüssigkeit

Der Pemphigus vulgaris verursacht beträchtliche Veränderungen in den Werten für die Proteine, Enzyme und Elektrolyte im Blutserum sowie Veränderungen im Plasmavolumen und im interstitiellen Flüssigkeitsvolumen und im Blutbild. Häufig besteht auch eine reduzierte Ausscheidung von 17-Ketosteroiden und 17-Hydroxysteroiden im Urin. Bei den anderen Formen von Pemphigus und beim bullösen Pemphigoid finden sich ähnliche, aber viel mildere Veränderungen. Sie sind die Folge und keineswegs die Ursache der Krankheit und sind daher unspezifisch. Die Anwendung der Corticosteroide verhindert die Entwicklung dieser biochemischen Veränderungen und normalisiert die Veränderungen bei Patienten, bei denen sie sich schon entwickelt haben.

1. Veränderungen im Blut

a) Gesamtprotein im Blutserum

Im Frühstadium des Pemphigus vulgaris ist der Wert für das Gesamtprotein im Blutserum entweder normal oder etwas verringert. Mit dem Fortschreiten der Krankheit sinkt der Wert allmählich ab und, falls keine Corticosteroide verabreicht werden, kann er fast auf die Hälfte des Normalwertes absinken (BRØCHNER-MORTENSEN; MULVEHILL; STARCK). Bei 14 Patienten, die untersucht wurden, bevor die Corticosteroide erhältlich waren, fand LEVER (1953) als niedrigste Werte im Durchschnitt 4,9 g/100 cm³ (Normalwert 6,5—7,5 g/100 cm³).

b) Elektrophoretische Untersuchungen der Serumproteine

Elektrophoretische Bestimmungen der Serumproteine wurden mittels freier (Tiselius) Elektrophorese von ROBERT, LEVER (1950 [I]) und LEINBROCK durchgeführt, während RÖCKL und JAROSCHKA, HAENSCH (1954), FELDAKER et al. und

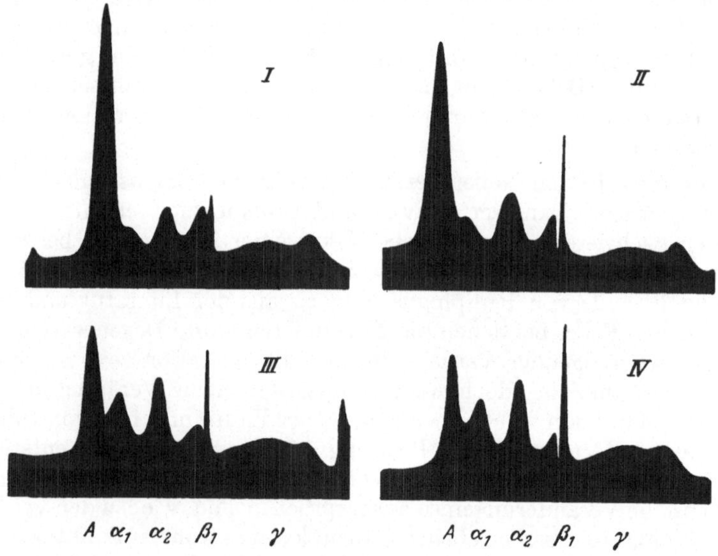

Abb. 34. Elektrophoretische Analyse der Serumproteine mittels freier (Tiselius) Elektrophorese bei einem Patienten mit Pemphigus vulgaris während des allmählichen Fortschreitens der Krankheit. Das Albumin fiel von 55 auf 23% der Gesamtproteine, während die α_1- und α_2-Globuline anstiegen, das α_1-Globulin von 6 auf 18% und das α_2-Globulin von 12 auf 21%

MATRAS und STÖBERL Papierelektrophorese anwandten. Die Befunde stimmen gut überein. Im Frühstadium des Pemphigus vulgaris ist das elektrophoretische Proteinspektrum fast normal. Mit dem Fortschreiten der Krankheit fällt der Wert für Albumin allmählich ab, während die Werte für die α_1- und α_2-Globuline ansteigen (Abb. 34). Im vorgeschrittenen Stadium sind die Relativwerte des Albumins stark reduziert, oft auf Werte niedriger als ein Drittel des Normalwertes. Dagegen sind die Werte für die α_1- und α_2-Globuline stark vermehrt, oft zu Relativwerten, die zwei- bis dreimal so hoch sind wie normal. Die Relativwerte für die β_1- und β_2-Globuline sind gewöhnlich normal. Das γ-Globulin steigt mit der Dauer der Krankheit an, aber viel langsamer als die α-Globuline, so daß eine wesentliche Erhöhung erst nach einigen Monaten konstatiert wird. Bei Patienten, die seit vielen Monaten erkrankt sind, kann der Relativwert für das γ-Globulin auf das Dreifache erhöht sein. [Die durchschnittlichen Normalwerte betragen bei freier (Tiselius) Elektrophorese: Albumin 55% des Gesamtproteins; α_1-Globulin 5%; α_2-Globulin 10%; β_1-Globulin 15%; β_2-Globulin 4%; γ-Globulin 11%.]

Umrechnung der elektrophoretischen Relativwerte auf absolute Werte mit Hilfe der quantitativen Bestimmung des Gesamtproteins zeigt den Abfall der Albuminwerte bei Patienten mit fortgeschrittenem Pemphigus vulgaris noch viel deutlicher. Normalerweise beträgt der Albuminwert bei Bestimmung mittels freier (Tiselius) Elektrophorese ungefähr 3,7 gm/100 cm³. Bei sieben Patienten mit fortgeschrittenem Pemphigus vulgaris lagen die niedrigsten Werte zwischen 1,5 und 0,76 gm/100 cm³, mit einem Durchschnittswert von 1,17 gm/100 cm³ (LEVER 1950 [I]).

Es mag darauf hingewiesen werden, daß mit der für die Bestimmung des Albumins und der Globuline oft gebrauchten Aussalzungsmethode der Globuline nach HOWE die starke Verminderung der Albumine nicht voll in Erscheinung tritt, denn bei dieser Methode wird ein großer Teil der α-Globuline, die beim Pemphigus vulgaris ja erhöht sind, nicht ausgefällt, sondern bleibt mit dem Albumin in Lösung und wird als Albumin gewertet. Die Verminderung des Albumins wird somit durch den Anstieg der α-Globuline verschleiert (LEVER 1950 [I]).

Bedeutung der Albuminverminderung. Eine solch bedeutende Erniedrigung des Albumins im Blutserum, wie beim Pemphigus vulgaris, kommt sonst nur bei der Nephrose vor. Worin liegt nun die Ursache für die starke Albuminverminderung beim Pemphigus vulgaris? Es ist wohl bekannt, daß bei allen fieberhaften und schweren Krankheiten das Albumin im Blutserum vermindert ist; aber die Verminderung ist nicht so ausgesprochen wie beim Pemphigus vulgaris. Bei diesem besteht der zusätzliche Faktor des Verlustes großer Mengen von Proteinen durch die ausgedehnten Epitheldefekte. Dieser Verlust ist vergleichbar mit dem renalen Proteinverlust bei der Nephrose. Wie durch die Niere bei der Nephrose, wird aber durch die Epitheldefekte beim Pemphigus vulgaris nicht ausschließlich Albumin verloren. Elektrophoretische Analyse von Blasenflüssigkeit (s. S. 646) hat ergeben, daß alle Proteinfraktionen durch die Haut verlorengehen. So liegt die Ursache für die Hypalbuminämie anscheinend darin, daß Albumin, im Gegensatz zu den Globulinen, in nicht zureichenden Mengen regeneriert wird. Albumin wird in der Leber gebildet. Da nun aber Leberfunktionsprüfungen beim Pemphigus vulgaris im allgemeinen normal ausfallen, ist die einzig mögliche Erklärung für die ungenügende Regeneration von Albumin, daß die Menge von Albumin, die selbst in einer normalen Leber gebildet werden kann, kleiner ist als die Menge, die beim Pemphigus vulgaris durch die Epitheldefekte verlorengeht. In der Tat haben Untersuchungen an Hunden nach Plasmapherese ergeben, daß selbst bei normaler Leberfunktion Albumin bedeutend langsamer regeneriert wird als die Globuline (ZELDIS und ALLING).

Da Albumin für die Regelung des kolloid-osmotischen Druckes der Serumproteine von großer Wichtigkeit ist, stellt die Entwicklung einer ausgesprochenen Erniedrigung des Serumalbumins beim Pemphigus vulgaris eine ernste Komplikation dar. Seit der Einführung der Corticosteroide in die Behandlung des Pemphigus ist die Entwicklung einer schweren Hypalbuminämie allerdings kaum mehr zu befürchten; und selbst bei Patienten, bei denen sich bereits vor der Behandlung mit Corticosteroiden eine ausgesprochene Hypalbuminämie entwickelt hat, steigt der Albuminspiegel unter der Behandlung mit Corticosteroiden an, sobald die Haut zu heilen beginnt (LEVER, HURLEY und BLANEY).

c) Bestimmung der Glykoproteine und Lipoproteine im Serum

Chemische Fraktionierung und Analyse der Serumproteine mittels der Mikromodifizierung der Cohnschen Methode 10 (LEVER, GURD et al.) ergab bei vier Patienten mit Pemphigus vulgaris, daß die Menge der α_1- und α_2-Glykoproteine im Durchschnitt auf das Dreifache angestiegen ist (LEVER, HURLEY und BLANEY). Man kann daraus schließen, daß die erhebliche Vermehrung der α_1- und α_2-Globuline, die man bei der elektrophoretischen Analyse findet, größtenteils durch einen Anstieg der in den beiden α-Globulinen enthaltenen Glykoprotein-Anteile hervorgerufen ist. Die Werte für die α_1-und β_1-Lipoproteine waren stets normal.

Diese Befunde sind durch die Untersuchungen von WEBER, BRAUN-FALCO und THAESLER sowie von BURBACH (1955) und von MATRAS und STÖBERL bestätigt worden. So fanden WEBER et al. im Serum eines Patienten mit Pemphigus vulgaris eine Erhöhung der proteingebundenen Polysaccharide (Hexosen und Glucosamin); BURBACH beobachtete bei drei Patienten mit Pemphigus vulgaris eine beträchtliche Erhöhung der Serum-Mucoproteine, welche zur α_1-Globulinfraktion in Beziehung stehen; und MATRAS und STÖBERL stellten mittels Papierelektrophorese eine Erhöhung der Glykoproteine in den α_1- und α_2-Globulinfraktionen fest, während die Menge der Lipoproteine in den verschiedenen Proteinfraktionen normal war.

d) Bestimmung des Fibrinogens im Blutplasma

Wie bei den meisten entzündlichen Krankheiten ist beim Pemphigus vulgaris die Menge des Fibrinogens im Plasma erhöht, gelegentlich auf das Doppelte des normalen Wertes, der 29 mg/100 cm^3 beträgt (LEVER, HURLEY und BLANEY).

e) Blutsenkungsreaktion

Eine Erhöhung der Senkungsgeschwindigkeit der Erythrocyten findet sich stets, wenn Hypalbuminämie mit einer Erhöhung der Globuline, besonders der α-Globuline und des Fibrinogens, verbunden ist. Da beim Pemphigus vulgaris diese Proteinveränderungen bestehen, ist die Senkungsgeschwindigkeit erhöht, und zwar oft beträchtlich (LEVER, HURLEY und BLANEY). Zu einem gewissen Maße spiegelt die Senkungsgeschwindigkeit den Aktivitätsgrad und die Schwere der Krankheit wider.

f) Enzymaktivität im Blutserum

Die glykolytischen Enzyme Aldolase und Milchsäure-Dehydrogenase können im Blutserum von Patienten mit Pemphigus vulgaris eine etwas erhöhte Konzentration aufweisen, während die beiden Transaminasen, die Glutaminsäure-Oxalessigsäure-Transaminase und die Glutaminsäure-Brenztraubensäure-Transaminase, nicht erhöht sind (WEBER 1958 [I], 1958 [II]; WÜST). Wie WÜST hervorhebt, ist es überraschend, daß die Aktivität dieser vier Enzyme im Blutserum nicht oder nur geringfügig vermehrt ist, da doch diese Enzyme in recht hoher Konzentration in der Epidermis und auch in der Blasenflüssigkeit (s. S. 647) vorhanden sind.

Die Aktivität der Leucin-Aminopeptidase ist zwar im Blutserum von Patienten mit Pemphigus erhöht; jedoch ist eine solche Erhöhung unspezifisch, da sie auch im Serum von Patienten mit weit ausgedehnter Dermatitis gefunden wird (BRAUN-FALCO und SALFELD).

g) Elektrolyte im Blutserum

Die Werte für Natrium, Chloride und Calcium im Blutserum sind beim Pemphigus vulgaris oft beträchtlich erniedrigt, während der Wert für Kalium erhöht sein kann (TALBOTT, LEVER und CONSOLAZIO; LEVER und TALBOTT 1944). Wie beim Albumin hängt der Grad der Erniedrigung von der Schwere des Krankheitsbildes ab. Im Frühstadium, wenn nur wenige Krankheitsherde vorhanden sind, sind die Werte gewöhnlich noch normal. Bei Patienten mit fortgeschrittenem Pemphigus vulgaris können die Werte für Natrium auf 120 Millieq./L. erniedrigt sein (Normalwert 140 Millieq./L.) und die Werte für die Chloride auf 90 Millieq./L. (Normalwert 102 Millieq./L.). Eine Erhöhung des Kaliumspiegels findet sich nicht so regelmäßig wie die Erniedrigung der Natrium-, Chlorid- und Calciumwerte.

Die Veränderungen in den Elektrolytwerten sind sekundär. Der Hauptgrund für die Erniedrigung der Werte für Natrium, Chloride und Calcium liegt ohne Zweifel, wie beim Protein, in ihrem Verlust in dem Exsudat, das durch die Epitheldefekte ausgeschieden wird. Es liegen beim Pemphigus vulgaris in dieser Beziehung ähnliche Verhältnisse vor wie bei ausgedehnten Verbrennungen, bei denen MOORE et al. einen beträchtlichen Verlust von Natrium und Chloriden durch die Brandwunden feststellten und gleichzeitig erniedrigte Werte für Natrium und Chloride im Serum fanden.

Bei Patienten mit erblich erniedrigten Natriumwerten glaubten TALBOTT, LEVER und CONSOLAZIO, daß Nebenniereninsuffizienz einen weiteren Grund für die Erniedrigung darstellte, zumal sie außerdem gelegentlich hohe Serumwerte für Kalium fanden und Untersuchung der Nebennieren während der Sektion bei vier ihrer Fälle Nekroseherde ergab. Sie nahmen an, daß beim Pemphigus vulgaris, genau wie bei schweren Infektionskrankheiten, wegen Erschöpfung der Nebennieren die Menge von Nebennierenrindenhormon vermindert sei. Aus diesem Grunde behandelten sie Patienten mit Pemphigus vulgaris mit hohen Dosen von Nebennierenrindenextrakt und hatten damit, wie sie 1940 und 1944 berichteten, wenigstens temporäre Erfolge (TALBOTT, LEVER und CONSOLAZIO; LEVER und TALBOTT 1944). Es ist wahrscheinlich, daß die hohen Dosen von Nebennierenrindenhormon, die sie anwandten (bis 20 cm^3 pro Tag), genügend Cortison enthielten, um ähnlich wie die Verabreichung von Cortison zu wirken.

h) Plasma- und interstitielles Flüssigkeitsvolumen

Im fortgeschrittenen Stadium des Pemphigus vulgaris sind das Plasmavolumen und das interstitielle Flüssigkeitsvolumen stark vermehrt. So fanden TALBOTT, LEVER und CONSOLAZIO sowie LEVER und MACLEAN bei sieben Patienten eine durchschnittliche Vermehrung des Plasmavolumens um 60% und einen Anstieg des interstitiellen Flüssigkeitsvolumen um 7—10 kg über den Normalwert. Der Grad für den Anstieg des Plasma- und interstitiellen Flüssigkeitsvolumen ist unbekannt, aber Hypoproteinämie und entzündliches Ödem der befallenen Haut tragen zweifellos zu dem Anstieg des interstitiellen Flüssigkeitsvolumen wesentlich bei.

i) Erythrocytenzahl und Hämoglobin

Die Zahl der Erythrocyten und somit der Hämatokrit und die Konzentration des Hämoglobins vermindern sich bei Patienten mit Pemphigus vulgaris allmählich mit dem Fortschreiten der Krankheit (HÖCKER). Bei Patienten, die sich kurz vor ihrem Tode befinden, kann die Anämie bedeutend sein.

j) Eosinophile Zellen im Blut

Bei vielen Patienten mit Pemphigus vulgaris ist der prozentuale Anteil der Eosinophilen unter den weißen Blutzellen mäßig erhöht. Jedoch kann solch eine Vermehrung fehlen. Bei schwerkranken und moribunden Patienten wurde oft ein Verschwinden der eosinophilen Zellen festgestellt, selbst wenn deren Zahl vorher erhöht war (GRACE). Bei Patienten mit Pemphigus vegetans wird fast stets und bei solchen mit Pemphigus foliaceus wird häufig eine Eosinophilie des Blutes gefunden (LEVER 1953).

2. Steroidausscheidung im Urin

Bei Patienten mit Pemphigus vulgaris, besonders in schweren Fällen, ist die Ausscheidung der 17-Ketosteroide und der 17-Hydroxysteroide im Urin häufig reduziert.

Im Jahre 1953 berichtete LEVER über die 17-Ketosteroidausscheidung bei zehn Patienten mit Pemphigus vulgaris. Bei den meisten Patienten bestand eine verringerte Ausscheidung; denn während die normale Ausscheidung mittels der angewandten Methode (TALBOT et al.) pro 24 Std bei Frauen 5—10 mg und bei Männern 8—15 mg beträgt, betrug die Ausscheidung im Durchschnitt bei sieben weiblichen Patienten 2,3 mg und bei drei männlichen Patienten 3,8 mg. Ebenfalls im Jahre 1953 berichteten CACCIALANZA et al. eine reduzierte Ausscheidung der 17-Ketosteroide und 17-Hydroxysteroide bei acht Patienten mit Pemphigus vulgaris, wobei die niedrigsten Werte bei den Patienten mit der längsten Krankheitsdauer gefunden wurden. Eine Injektion von 20 Einheiten von Corticotropin ergab entweder einen geringen oder keinen Anstieg der Werte. In gleicher Weise fanden Quiroga und Corti bei acht Patienten mit Pemphigus vulgaris stets eine niedrige Ausscheidung der 17-Ketosteroide, nämlich zwischen 2,02 und 3,45 mg in 24 Std. Nach einer Injektion von Corticotropin konnten sie keinen Anstieg dieser Werte feststellen. Nazzaro und Valenti fanden die niedrigsten Werte für die 17-Ketosteroidausscheidung und zugleich das geringste Ansprechen auf eine Injektion von Corticotropin bei Patienten, die sich in einem fortgeschrittenen Krankheitsstadium befanden, während zu Beginn der Krankheit keine signifikanten Abweichungen von der Norm bestanden.

Im Gegensatz zu diesen Beobachtern fanden Dostrovsky und Sulman sowie Cohen, Ullmann und Dostrovsky wie auch Csóka und Vadász beträchtliche Variationen. So bemerkten z.B. Dostrovsky und Sulman, daß nicht alle Patienten mit Pemphigus vulgaris eine erniedrigte Ausscheidung von 17-Ketosteroiden aufwiesen und daß die Patienten mit erniedrigter Ausscheidung nicht immer diejenigen waren, die ihre Krankheit am längsten hatten. Ferner bestand nicht immer ein paralleles Verhalten zwischen dem Grad, in dem die Ausscheidung der 17-Ketosteroide erniedrigt war, und dem Ansprechen auf eine Test-Injektion von Corticotropin, so daß einige Patienten mit einer reduzierten Ausscheidung auf Corticotropin gut ansprachen, während andere, die eine gute Ausscheidung der 17-Ketosteroide aufwiesen, auf Corticotropin nicht ansprachen. Nichtsdestoweniger fanden Dostrovsky und Sulman, daß unter ihren 15 Patienten mit Pemphigus vulgaris elf auf eine Test-Injektion von Corticotropin schlecht oder gar nicht ansprachen.

Aus den dargelegten Daten kann man wohl schließen, daß beim Pemphigus vulgaris keine primäre Unterfunktion der Nebennieren vorliegt. Jedoch besteht beim Pemphigus vulgaris, wie bei anderen schweren chronischen Krankheiten, ein erhöhtes Bedürfnis des Organismus für adrenocorticales Hormon. Der Patient, dessen Nebennieren nicht in der Lage sind, dieses erhöhte Bedürfnis zu befriedigen, wird Anzeichen einer relativen Nebenniereninsuffizierung zeigen (Furtado et al.). Bei solchen Patienten würde dann, bevor die Corticosteroide erhältlich waren, die Sektion möglicherweise auch degenerative Veränderungen an der Nebennierenrinde ergeben haben (s. S. 641).

3. Blasenflüssigkeit

a) Gesamtprotein

Die Konzentration von Protein in der Blasenflüssigkeit ist fast immer niedriger als im entsprechenden Blutserum (Lever und Talbott 1942; Lever 1950 [II]; Leinbrock; Haensch 1955 [II]; Matras und Stöberl). Im Durchschnitt beträgt das Verhältnis der Proteinkonzentration in der Blasenflüssigkeit zu der Konzentration im entsprechenden Blutserum 0,75 (Lever 1950 [II]). Es besteht jedoch eine beträchtliche Variationsbreite in diesem Verhältnis; denn Blasen in tiefliegenden Hautgebieten, wie an den Unterschenkeln oder Unterarmen, weisen gewöhnlich eine niedrige Proteinkonzentration auf, da sie oft einen beträchtlichen Anteil von eiweißarmer Ödemflüssigkeit enthalten.

b) Elektrophoretische Untersuchungen

Freie (Tiselius) Elektrophorese der Proteine in der Blasenflüssigkeit, von Lever (1950 [II]) und Leinbrock durchgeführt, ergab in allen Fällen eine große Ähnlichkeit zwischen dem elektrophoretischen Proteinspektrum der Blasenflüssigkeit und dem Spektrum des entsprechenden Blutserums. Jede bedeutende Abweichung vom Normalen, die im elektrophoretischen Diagramm des Blutserums vorhanden war, fand sich auch im Diagramm der Blasenflüssigkeit (Abb. 35). Trotz dieser auffallenden Übereinstimmung fanden Lever wie auch Leinbrock, daß der relative Albnminanteil in der Blasenflüssigkeit stets etwas höher war als im zugehörigen Serum. Außerdem fand Lever, daß die Relativwerte für β_1-Globulin etwas niedriger und jene für β_2-Globulin etwas höher in der Blasenflüssigkeit als im Serum waren. Vielfach erschien das β_2-Globulin im

Diagramm der Blasenflüssigkeit als ein kleiner Gipfel, während es im Diagramm des zugehörigen Serums nur teilweise das Tal zwischen den β_1- und γ-Gipfeln füllte. HAENSCH (1955 [II]) sowie MATRAS und STÖBERL, die ihre Untersuchungen mittels Papierelektrophorese ausführten, konnten dagegen keine Unterschiede zwischen Serum und Blasenflüssigkeit aufdecken. Der Grund dafür liegt wohl darin, daß die papierelektrophoretische Methode quantitativ weniger genau ist als die freie Elektrophorese.

Die Beobachtung, daß der Gesamtproteinwert in der Blasenflüssigkeit fast immer niedriger ist als im entsprechenden Blutserum, während die Relativwerte für die einzelnen Eiweißfraktionen fast gleich sind, deutet darauf hin, daß die Blasenflüssigkeit im wesentlichen aus Blutserum besteht, das mit Gewebsflüssigkeit verdünnt ist. Gewebsflüssigkeit enthält ja nur verhältnismäßig geringe Mengen von Protein. Daß der Relativwert für Albumin in der Blasenflüssigkeit etwas höher ist als im entsprechenden Serum, mag wohl daran liegen, daß das Albumin mit seinem verhältnismäßig niedrigem Molekulargewicht von 69000 (COHN et al.) leichter die Capillarwände durchtritt als die Globuline. Die Tatsache, daß die Blasenflüssigkeit relativ mehr β_2-Globulin enthält als das entsprechende Blutserum, kann damit erklärt werden, daß in der Blasenflüssigkeit im Gegensatz zum Blutserum selbst nach vollständiger Koagulation noch etwas Fibrinogen vorhanden ist, wie HERRMANN mit SCHULZ mittels Immunoelektrophorese nachweisen konnten.

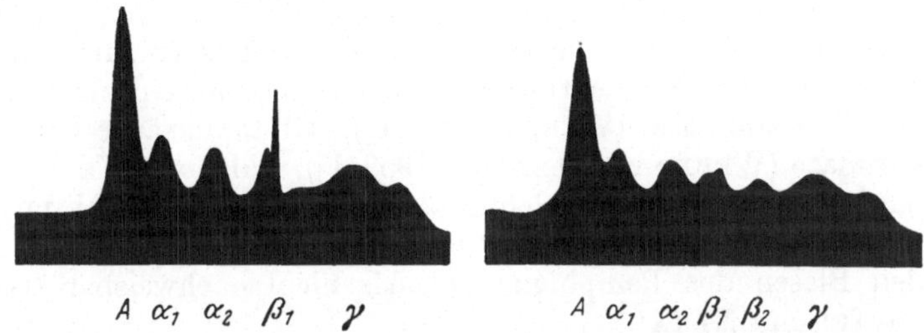

Abb. 35. Elektrophoretische Analyse mittels freier (Tiselius) Elektrophorese des Blutserums (links) und der Blasenflüssigkeit (rechts) bei einem Patienten mit Pemphigus vulgaris. In beiden Diagrammen ist das Albumin erniedrigt, während die α_1-, α_2- und γ-Globuline erhöht sind. Obwohl sich die beiden Diagramme recht ähnlich sehen, erscheint doch das β_2-Globulin im Diagramm der Blasenflüssigkeit (im Gegensatz zu dem des Blutserums) als ein kleiner Gipfel

c) Immunoelektrophoretische Untersuchungen

Die immunoelektrophoretischen Untersuchungen von HERRMANN und SCHULZ ergaben, daß alle 18 Proteinfraktionen, die im Blutplasma vorhanden sind, auch in der Blasenflüssigkeit gefunden werden. Bei der Analyse von Blasenflüssigkeit verschiedener Krankheiten, einschließlich des Pemphigus vulgaris, beobachteten sie drei Unterschiede zwischen Blasenflüssigkeit und Blutplasma. Erstens enthielt die Blasenflüssigkeit selbst nach vollständiger Koagulation noch etwas Fibrinogen; zweitens besaßen alle drei vorhandene Lipoproteine, nämlich die α_1-, α_2- und β_1-Lipoproteine, eine größere Wanderungsgeschwindigkeit in der Blasenflüssigkeit als im Blutplasma, wahrscheinlich infolge des Vorhandenseins einer Lipase; und drittens besaßen in mehreren der untersuchten Blasen die α- und β-Glykoproteine eine verminderte Wanderungsgeschwindigkeit, wahrscheinlich infolge des Vorhandenseins von Neuraminidase.

d) Enzymaktivität

Daß die Blasenflüssigkeit Enzymaktivität besitzt, wiesen erstmalig ZAMECNIK, STEPHENSON und COPE im Jahre 1945 nach, als sie in zellfreier Blasenflüssigkeit, die sie von Brandblasen der menschlichen Haut gewonnen hatten, eine Peptidase nachweisen konnten. Seitdem hat es sich ergeben, daß Hautblasenflüssigkeit, unabhängig ihrer Genese, beträchtliche Enzymaktivität besitzt. Fast alle Enzyme finden sich in der Blasenflüssigkeit in höherer Konzentration als im entsprechenden Blutserum. Dieser Unterschied wird noch deutlicher, wenn man die Enzymaktivitäten, wie WEBER (1960) vorgeschlagen hat, nicht auf das Flüssigkeitsvolumen, sondern auf den Stickstoffgehalt der jeweiligen Untersuchungsflüssigkeit bezieht. Es besteht jedoch keine Berechtigung, die hohe Enzymaktivität der Blasenflüssigkeit als Beweis dafür anzusehen, daß die Hautblasen gewisser Krankheiten durch Enzyme verursacht sind. Wahrscheinlich diffundieren, wie WEBER und THEISEN (1959 [II]) annehmen, die Enzyme aus beschädigten Epidermiszellen in die Blasenflüssigkeit, da Epidermiszellen Enzyme in hoher Konzentration enthalten.

In der Blasenflüssigkeit von Patienten mit Pemphigus vulgaris sind die folgenden Enzyme in hoher Konzentration nachgewiesen worden: Glutaminsäure-Oxalessigsäure-Transaminase (WEBER 1958 [I]), Glutaminsäure-Brenztraubensäure-Transaminase (WEBER und THEISEN 1959 [I]), Aldolase (WEBER 1958 [II], STÜTTGEN und WÜST), Milchsäuredehydrogenase (WEBER und WILDNER) und Leucin-Aminopeptidase (BRAUN-FALCO und SALFELD). Andererseits ist Hyaluronidase in den Blasen des Pemphigus vulgaris nicht nachweisbar (GRAIS und GLICK; FÖLDVÁRI und NÉKÁM).

Der Nachweis proteolytischer Aktivität in der Blasenflüssigkeit verschiedener Krankheiten, einschließlich des Pemphigus vulgaris und des bullösen Pemphigoids, ist durch HERZBERG und ROHDE auf die folgende Weise erbracht worden: Einer Hühnerembryo-Fibroblastenkultur setzten sie zellfreie, sterile Blasenflüssigkeit hinzu. Dies führte zu Cytolyse, die gewöhnlich nach 19 Std einsetzte und nach 125 Std in völliger Auflösung der Kultur endete. Inkubation für 30 min bei 56° hob die proteolytische Aktivität der Blasenflüssigkeit auf. Im Gegensatz zur Blasenflüssigkeit wies keines der untersuchten Blutsera proteolytische Aktivität auf.

e) Elektrolyte

Die Konzentration von Natrium, Chloriden, Kalium und Calcium in der Blasenflüssigkeit von Patienten mit Pemphigus vulgaris war stets der Konzentration im entsprechenden Blutserum sehr ähnlich (LEVER und TALBOTT 1942; FISHER 1952). Wenn abnormale Konzentrationen im Blutserum bestanden, fanden sich diese auch in der Blasenflüssigkeit.

V. Ätiologie

Die Ursache des Pemphigus ist unbekannt und nicht einmal eine plausible Theorie gibt es zur Zeit für seine Entstehung. Unter den verschiedenen Theorien sind letzthin vor allem die Möglichkeit einer Virusinfektion oder einer Enzymstörung erörtert worden.

1. Theorie der Kochsalzretention

RIECKE bespricht eingehend die vielfach gemachte Beobachtung, daß beim Pemphigus vulgaris eine stark verminderte Ausscheidung von Kochsalz im Urin besteht und deutet dieses, wie alle Autoren vor ihm, als eine Kochsalzretention. Er erblickt darin eine Schutzreaktion des kranken Organismus zum Zwecke einer Eiweißeinsparung. Doch weist RIECKE, wie schon vor ihm URBACH, darauf hin, daß solch eine Kochsalzretention nicht nur beim Pemphigus, sondern auch bei anderen stark konsumierenden Leiden zur Beobachtung kommt. Die ersten

Zweifel daran, daß beim Pemphigus die verminderte Kochsalzausscheidung im Urin durch Kochsalzretention verursacht war, äußerte PRAKKEN (1935). Er bestimmte bei einem Patienten mit Pemphigus vulgaris den Verlust von Kochsalz in dem durch die Hautherde ausgeschiedenen Exsudat und errechnete einen recht hohen Verlust von Kochsalz, nämlich 2,4 g pro Tag. Da Unterdrückung des Schwitzens mittels Atropins keine Erhöhung der Kochsalzausscheidung im Urin verursachte, nahm er an, daß der Kochsalzverlust durch erhöhtes Schwitzen keine wesentliche Rolle spielte. Er folgerte, daß der Verlust von Natriumchlorid durch die Epitheldefekte und nicht eine Kochsalzretention für die geringe Ausscheidung von Natriumchlorid im Urin verantwortlich war (PRAKKEN 1936).

Der Kochsalzstoffwechsel von Patienten mit schweren Verbrennungen ähnelt dem von Pemphiguspatienten. Eine Verminderung des Serumchloridspiegels bei Patienten mit Verbrennungen wurden zuerst von DAVIDSON im Jahre 1926 festgestellt. MOORE und seine Mitarbeiter fanden in eingehenden Stoffwechseluntersuchungen, daß bei Patienten mit schweren Verbrennungen das Exsudat von Brandwunden bis zu 95% des gesamten vom Körper ausgeschiedenen Natriums enthielt, so daß die Ausscheidung von Natrium im Urin sehr gering war. Diese Autoren fanden gleichzeitig erniedrigte Natriumwerte im Serum und schlossen daraus, wie es schon DAVIDSON getan hatte, daß die niedrige Ausscheidung von Natrium im Urin darauf beruhe, daß die Nieren Natrium einzusparen versuchen. Wenn die großen Natriumverluste durch die Brandwunden in die Stoffwechselbilanz eingeschlossen wurden, fand sich eine wirkliche Natriumretention nur während der ersten Tage nach der Verbrennung, hauptsächlich auf Grund einer Ansammlung von natriumreicher Ödemflüssigkeit in den Brandwunden und ihrer Umgebung. Das Verhalten der Chloride war dem des Natriums ähnlich.

Heute steht es fest, daß die Verminderung der Natrium- und Chloridausscheidung im Urin bei Patienten mit Pemphigus nur eine Sekundärerscheinung ist. Eine gewisse Menge von Natrium und Chloriden wird wahrscheinlich auf Grund der beträchtlichen Vermehrung des interstitiellen Flüssigkeitsvolumens (s. S. 645) im Körper zurückgehalten; aber eine große Menge von Natrium und Chloriden geht mittels des durch die Epitheldefekte ausgeschiedenen Exsudats verloren. Keine aktive Retention von Natrium oder Chloriden findet im Blute oder in den Organen von Patienten mit Pemphigus statt. Im Gegenteil, Patienten mit Pemphigus befinden sich oft wegen des beträchtlichen Verlustes von Natrium und Chloriden durch die Haut in einem Zustand der Natrium- und Chloridverarmung; und die Verminderung der Natrium- und Chloridausscheidung im Urin stellt eine Kompensationsmaßnahme dar. Ein Beweis für die Natrium- und Chloridverarmung sind die niedrigen Werte für Natrium und Chloride im Blutserum von Pemphiguspatienten (s. S. 644). Bestimmungen des Natrium- und Chloridgehaltes der Haut und inneren Organe bei Patienten mit Pemphigus hat auch keine Vermehrung gezeigt.

KARTAMISCHEW fand bei einem Patienten mit Pemphigus vulgaris die Konzentration von Natriumchlorid in der Haut sowie in allen inneren Organen mit Ausnahme der Muskeln und des Fettes vermindert. URBACH fand die Menge von Natriumchlorid in der Haut bei drei Patienten erhöht und bei zwei Patienten normal. Bei einem Patienten wurde auch der Gehalt an Natriumchlorid in Muskelgewebe, Leber und Milz bestimmt und an der unteren Grenze der Norm gefunden. Bestimmungen, die LEVER (1953) an Patienten mit Pemphigus durchführte, ergaben etwas verminderte Werte für Natrium in der normalen Haut, normale Werte in Muskelgewebe, Herz und Leber und eine leichte, aber wahrscheinlich nicht bedeutsame Erhöhung in Niere und Gehirn. In den von Pemphigus befallenen Hautbezirken war der Natriumgehalt etwas erhöht. Diese Erhöhung war jedoch nicht spezifisch für den Pemphigus, denn eine gleichartige Erhöhung des Gehaltes an Natrium wurde auch in der befallenen Haut von Patienten mit universeller Dermatitis festgestellt. FELSHER fand normale Werte für Chloride sowohl in der normalen wie in der befallenen Haut von Patienten mit Pemphigus.

2. Theorie der Virus-Infektion

Mehrere Untersucher haben den Anspruch erhoben, ein für den Pemphigus spezifisches Virus isoliert zu haben. Da aber die Untersucher recht verschiedenartige Viren fanden und ihre Befunde von Nachuntersuchern nicht bestätigt worden sind, können die Resultate nicht als gültig angesehen werden.

Es würde zu weit führen, im einzelnen alle erhobenen Befunde zu schildern. Sie sind von LEVER (1953) sowie von MARCHIONINI und NASEMANN (1955, 1957) zusammengefaßt worden. Es seien daher nur einige Experimente, insbesondere aus den letzten Jahren, aufgeführt.

a) Tierinoculationen

URBACH und seine Mitarbeiter REISS und WOLFRAM (1931, 1934, 1936) führten zwischen 1931 und 1936 viele Versuche an Kaninchen durch, bei denen sie unter anderem Ultrafiltrate der Blasenflüssigkeit und des Blutserums von Patienten mit Pemphigus intracysternal injizierten. Dies rief Lähmungserscheinungen infolge Encephalo-myelo-meningitis hervor. DOSTROVSKY et al. (1938) bestätigten diese Befunde, aber BERNHARDT sowie CAROL et al., FLECK und GOLDSCHLAG, NELEMANS und VERLINDE und MARCHIONINI und NASEMANN erhielten im wesentlichen negative Resultate. Die gegen URBACHs Befunde erhobenen Einwendungen sind: 1. Selbst normales Serum, wenn intracysternal injiziert, kann Gehirnschäden mit Lähmungen hervorrufen (FLECK und GOLDSCHLAG); 2. solche Injektionen können eine bei Kaninchen häufige, latente Infektion des Zentralnervensystems mit dem Protozoon *Encephalitozoon cuniculi* aktivieren (MARKHAM und ENGMAN); und 3. intracerebrale Injektionen von Material, das Detritus von eosinophilen Zellen enthält, kann bei Kaninchen spastisch-paralytische Symptome hervorrufen (BEHÇET et al.).

Von GRACE und SUSKIND, die ihre Versuche an mit Röntgenstrahlen vorbehandelten Mäusen durchführten, wurde ein Virus beschrieben, das nach ihren eigenen Feststellungen von dem Urbachschen Virus unterschiedlich war. Die von ihnen mittels Inoculierung von Pemphigus-Blutserum, -Blasenflüssigkeit und -Spinalflüssigkeit im Maushirn hervorgerufenen Krankheitsherde enthielten Ansammlungen von neutrophilen Zellen. MARKHAM und ENGMAN wandten dieselbe Technik an, hatten aber negative Resultate. Sie deuteten darauf hin, daß GRACE und SUSKIND pyogene Herde im Gehirn der Mäuse erzeugten, während beim Menschen jedenfalls der Pemphigus keine pyogene Krankheit wäre.

WERTH (1938, 1943) beschrieb bei Kaninchen eine schwere Panophthalmie nach Beimpfung der vorderen Augenkammer mit einem Ultrafiltrat von Pemphigusblasenflüssigkeit. Auch glaubte er, daß die Infektion Immunität verleihe, da bei Inoculation des anderen Auges nur eine sehr leichte Entzündung eintrat. Sowohl NELEMANS und VERLINDE als auch MARCHIONINI und NASEMANN wiederholten diese Experimente, erhielten aber negative Resultate.

b) Inoculation der Chorionallantois

WERTH berichtete 1938 die Entwicklung von Viruskulturen auf der Chorionalllantoismembran nach deren Inoculation entweder mit Pemphigusblasenflüssigkeit oder mit Material, das der vorderen Augenkammer inoculierter Kaninchen entnommen worden war. Positive Resultate durch Inoculation der Chorionallantoismembran haben auch MELCZER sowie MEIROWSKY mitgeteilt. Es erscheint aber durchaus möglich, daß die Paraplegien, die sie bei Hühnerembryonen hervorriefen, traumatischen Ursprunges waren. Negative Resultate mittels Inoculation der Chorionallantois erhielten unter anderen MARKHAM und ENGMAN, MEZZADRA und RABITO, NELEMANS und VERLINDE, NAZZARO und KRUSE-SPICCA sowie MARCHIONINI und NASEMANN.

c) Gewebszüchtung

GAWALOWSKI et al. berichteten 1957, daß sie ein filtrierbares und übertragbares Agens feststellen konnten, wenn sie Affennieren-Gewebskulturen entweder mit der Blasenflüssigkeit oder mit einem Homogenat der paravertebralen Ganglien von Pemphiguspatienten inoculierten; aber bisher ist keine weitere Mitteilung darüber von diesen Autoren erschienen.

BELLONE und LEONE beobachteten, daß, wenn Serum von Pemphiguspatienten Gewebskulturen menschlicher Haut zugefügt wurde, dieses in der Epidermis Acantholyse hervorbrachte. CROSTI et al. beobachteten, daß Blutserum und Blasenflüssigkeit von Pemphiguspatienten in Kulturen menschlicher Haut übertragbare Zellschädigungen in der Epidermis erzeugten. Jedoch läßt die Tatsache, daß die Autoren die gleiche Beobachtung bei Erythema exsudativum multiforme und bei Impetigo bullosa neonatorum machten, ihre Resultate fraglich erschienen.

d) Elektronenmikroskopie

Bei der Untersuchung der Blasenflüssigkeit mittels des Elektronenmikroskops fanden MELCZER sowie MEIROWSKY virusähnliche Partikel, während EVERALL und REED sowie MARCHIONINI und NASEMANN negative Resultate verzeichneten. CROSTI et al. beobachteten virusähnliche Partikel in der Nährflüssigkeit von Gewebskulturen menschlicher Haut, nachdem sie der Nährflüssigkeit entweder den Inhalt von Hautblasen oder Blutserum von Patienten mit Pemphigus beigefügt hatten.

e) Antikörpernachweis

Bereits im Jahre 1936 hatten URBACH, WOLFRAM und BRANDT im Blutserum von Pemphiguspatienten Komplement bindende Antikörper gefunden, wenn sie als Antigen ein Gehirnhomogenat von Kaninchen benutzten, die intracerebral mit Material von Pemphiguspatienten inoculiert worden waren. Jedoch betrachteten sowohl FLECK und GOLDSCHLAG wie auch PREININGER diese Komplementbindungsreaktion als unspezifisch und nicht als einen Beweis für das Vorhandensein eines Virus. So konnte z.B. PREININGER nachweisen, daß Organextrakte von Patienten, die an Pemphigus vulgaris verstorben waren, eine positive Komplementbindungsreaktion auch mit dem Blutserum von Patienten mit Syphilis ergaben.

Was den Nachweis von Autoantikörpern betrifft, teilte KOPEL 1954 mit, daß er bei drei Pemphiguspatienten mit Hilfe von serologischen Reaktionen weder im Blutserum noch in der Blasenflüssigkeit, noch in den Erythrocyten Antoantikörper nachweisen konnte. WAGNER et al. fanden dagegen, wie sie 1956 mitteilten, mit Hilfe der Collodiumagglutination nicht nur beim Pemphigus vulgaris, sondern auch bei mehreren anderen Krankheiten im Blutserum Autoantikörper gegen Extrakte, die sie aus menschlichen Organen gewonnen hatten. Beim Pemphigus vulgaris konnten diese Antikörper auch im Blaseninhalt nachgewiesen werden. Die Autoren kamen zu dem Schluß, daß die Autoantikörper unspezifisch waren und nicht als die Ursache, sondern als eine Folge der Krankheit auftraten. Andererseits demonstrierten MELCZER und VÁSÁRHELYI im Blutserum von Patienten mit Pemphigus vulgaris oder Dermatitis herpetiformis spezifische Hämagglutinine gegen im Blaseninhalt und im Spinalliquor vorhandene Antigene. Da Verbrennungsblasen keine solche Antigene enthielten, nahmen sie an, daß die im Blutserum enthaltenen Antikörper spezifischer Natur waren. Sollten diese Untersuchungen Bestätigung finden, würden sie wohl kaum dafür sprechen, wie MELCZER und VÁSÁRHELYI glauben, daß der Pemphigus vulgaris eine Viruskrankheit ist, aber sie würden ein Anzeichen dafür sein, daß er eine Krankheit des Immunmechanismus ist und vielleicht zur Gruppe der Autoimmunkrankheiten gehört.

3. Theorie einer Enzymstörung

Obwohl es jetzt feststeht, daß Enzyme als Vermittler bei der Blasenbildung mitwirken, besteht bis jetzt kein Beweis dafür, daß eine Enzymstörung in der Haut möglicherweise die Ursache des Pemphigus darstellt.

a) Blasenbildung infolge Inhibition eines Enzyms

Daß sich Blasen gleichzeitig mit der Inhibition eines Enzyms bilden können, bewiesen im Jahre 1946 PETERS, SINCLAIR und THOMPSON bei Versuchen mit Gelbkreuzgas, das auf der Haut Blasen hervorruft. Sie wiesen nach, daß sich das Arsen des Gelbkreuzgases in der Haut mit Sulfhydrylgruppen gewisser Enzyme verbindet, die dadurch inaktiv werden. So war infolge der Inaktivierung ihrer Sulfhydrylgruppen die Brenztraubensäure-Dehydrogenase unfähig, Brenztraubensäure zu oxydieren, und der oxydative Abbau von Kohlenhydraten war dadurch erheblich gestört.

Sodann fanden DIXON und NEEDHAM, daß auch ein anderes Enzym, das für den Kohlenhydratabbau wichtig ist, von den blasenbildenden Arsenpräparaten inaktiviert wurde, nämlich Hexokinase, welches Glucose-6-Phosphat phosphorylisiert. Ferner beobachteten sie, daß außer den arsenhaltigen Blasenbildnern auch andere blasenerzeugende Chemikalien, wie z.B. Methylbromid, die Hexokinase unterdrückten.

Auf Grund seiner eigenen und der von DIXON und NEEDHAM durchgeführten Experimente folgerten PETERS und THOMPSON, daß Gelbkreuzgas und andere blasenerzeugende Chemikalien durch Inaktivierung von Enzymen, die für die normale Stoffwechselfunktion der Haut notwendig sind, eine Reihenfolge von Störungen in Bewegung setzen, die schließlich zur Entwicklung von Blasen führe. Sie sprachen sogar die Vermutung aus, daß selbst nicht mit chemischen Mitteln hervorgerufene Blasen durch Inaktivierung oder Schädigung von Enzymen verursacht sein könnten. Es erscheint aber doch wahrscheinlicher, daß, mit Ausnahme der chemisch hervorgerufenen Blasen, eher Aktivierung proteolytischer Enzyme als Inhibition von Enzymen eine Rolle spielt bei der Bildung von Blasen bei verschiedenen Krankheiten.

b) Blasenbildung infolge Aktivierung von Enzymen

Da verschiedene proteolytische Enzyme in der Epidermis vorhanden sind und da Blasen sowohl in vivo als auch in vitro durch proteolytische Enzyme erzeugt werden können, erscheint es möglich, daß in Krankheiten, bei denen Blasen vorkommen, proteolytische Enzyme bei der Bildung von Blasen eine Rolle spielen. Es bestehen zwei Möglichkeiten für eine Aktivierung der proteolytischen Enzyme in der Epidermis nach der Einwirkung einer Noxe: Die eine Möglichkeit ist, daß die Protease innerhalb der Zelle in einem inhibierten Zustand vorhanden ist und nach Einwirkung der Noxe von ihrer normalen Lokalisation, z.B. innerhalb eines Mitochondrium, freigelassen wird und hierdurch aktiviert wird. Die andere Möglichkeit besteht darin, daß innerhalb der Zelle ein Inhibitor entweder zerstört oder inaktiviert wird, wonach die normalerweise inhibierte Protease ihre Wirkung frei entfalten kann (ROTHMAN).

Drei proteolytische Enzyme sind bisher in der Haut gefunden, die Proteasen oder Endopeptidasen darstellen. Die erste Protease wurde 1945 von BELOFF und PETERS (1945) nachgewiesen und als alkalische Dermoprotease bezeichnet, da sie zwischen pH 7,0 und 8,0 aktiv war. Diese Protease war gegen Hitze recht widerstandsfähig und war nur zu 25% inaktiviert, wenn sie 5 min lang einer Temperatur von 70⁰ ausgesetzt wurde, ein Hitzegrad, der schon binnen 1 min der Haut beträchtlichen Schaden zufügt. BELOFF und PETERS (1945) konnten nachweisen, daß sich bei Ratten, die hohen Temperaturen ausgesetzt wurden, der Gehalt dieser Protease in der Haut verminderte, da sie aus den Zellen der Haut in die Blutbahn abwanderte. BELOFF und PETERS (1945) schlossen daraus, daß bei Verbrennungen diese Protease aus ihrer physiologischen Position innerhalb von Zellen gelöst wird und dann auf die Epidermiszellen derart wirkt, daß sie ihren Zusammenhalt mit der Dermis verlieren. Diese Theorie wurde dadurch bestärkt, daß WELLS und BABCOCK nachweisen konnten, daß ein beträchtlicher Teil der Protease, die BELOFF und PETERS (1945) in Gesamthautstücken nachgewiesen hatten, normalerweise in der Epidermis gelegen ist.

Eine zweite Protease wurde von STÜTTGEN, HOFMANN und SIMMICH beschrieben. Sie wurde in der Epidermis wie auch in der Dermis gefunden, hatte ein pH-Optimum von 5,6 und wurde durch Inkubation bei 56⁰ für 15 min inaktiviert. STÜTTGEN und seine Mitarbeiter konnten, in ähnlicher Weise wie BELOFF und PETERS bei Verbrennungen, feststellen, daß beim Pemphigus, bei akuter Dermatitis und bei Urticaria die veränderte Haut im Vergleich zu normaler Haut eine deutliche Verringerung in der Aktivität dieser Protease zeigte, wahrscheinlich infolge Abwanderung des freigesetzten Enzyms in die Lymph- und Blutbahn.

Eine dritte Protease ist von KLASCHKA beschrieben worden, ein Kathepsin mit einem recht weitgestrecktem pH-Optimum, zwischen 3,0 und 4,5. Diese Protease war in der Epidermis und der Dermis in ungefähr gleichen Mengen nachweisbar.

Exopeptidasen, welche kleinere Polypeptidmoleküle in Aminosäuren spalten, sind ebenfalls in der Haut vorgefunden worden. Die erste in der Haut vorhandene Exopeptidase wurde 1945 durch ZAMECNIK, STEPHENSON und COPE beschrieben. Sie fanden diese sowohl in der Haut von Hunden, wie auch in der Blasenflüssigkeit, die sie von Brandwunden der menschlichen Haut gewonnen hatten. Beim Kalb und bei der Ratte fanden sie regelmäßig nach Verbrennungen einen Anstieg der Peptidasenaktivität im Serum. BELOFF und PETERS (1946) konnten das Vorkommen dieser Peptidase in Hautextrakten bestätigen. Daß noch weitere Exopeptidasen in der Haut vorhanden sind, kann daraus geschlossen werden, daß PASCHOUD et al. in der menschlichen Haut insgesamt drei Dipeptidasen und eine Tripeptidase nachweisen konnten.

c) Hervorrufen der Acantholyse in vitro

Wenn excidierte Stücke von menschlicher Haut proteolytischen Enzymen ausgesetzt werden, tritt in der Epidermis Acantholyse ein. HAMBRICK und BLANK wiesen 1954 nach, daß, wenn sie Hautstücke in einer 0,5%igen Trypsinlösung inkubierten, sowohl Ablösung der Epidermis von der Dermis als auch Acantholyse innerhalb der Epidermis eintrat. SCOTT setzte Hautstücke verschiedenen Konzentrationen von Chymotrypsin für 75 min aus. Bei einer Konzentration von 0,05% trat suprabasale Acantholyse auf, während bei höheren Konzentrationen eine Ablösung der Epidermis von der Dermis eintrat. BURBACH (1959), der eine 1%ige Trypsinlösung in excidierte Hautstücke injizierte, fand, daß das Ausmaß der Acantholyse mit der Dauer der Trypsineinwirkung zunahm, so daß nach 6 Std alle Epidermiszellen den Zusammenhang miteinander verloren hatten. STOUGHTON und BAGATELL injizierten verschiedene Enzyme in excidierte Hautstücke. Sie stellten dabei fest, daß die Injektion von Papain und von Elastase Acantholyse hervorrief, während Injektionen von mucolytischen Enzymen oder von Nucleasen, Lipasen, Carboxypeptidase oder Hyaluronidase keine Acantholyse zur Folge hatte.

Daß das Aussetzen von Hautstücken zu mäßigen Hitzegraden Acantholyse hervorruft und daß diese Acantholyse enzymatischen Ursprungs ist, haben die Untersuchungen von STOUGHTON und NOVAK gezeigt. Acantholyse war nachweisbar, wenn Hautstücke erst für eine 1 min 55° Hitze ausgesetzt und danach für 24 Std bei 37° inkubiert wurden. Da diese Acantholyse verhindert werden konnte, wenn die Hautstücke entweder vor der Hitzeeinwirkung sulfhydrylbindenden Lösungen, wie Kupfer-, Quecksilber- oder Silberlösungen, ausgesetzt wurden oder statt bei 37° bei 4° inkubiert wurden, kamen STOUGHTON und NOVAK zu dem Schluß, daß durch die Hitzeeinwirkung ein Enzymsystem stimuliert wurde, das normalerweise in der Epidermis in inaktiver Form vorhanden ist und das die Fähigkeit besitzt, die Disulfidbindungen im fibrillären Protein der Epidermiszellen zu brechen. STOUGHTON und NOVAK erwogen die Möglichkeit, daß Kathepsine die enzymatische Acantholyse hervorriefen, da Kathepsine auf Disulfidbindungen einwirken können; aber sie wiesen darauf hin, daß bisher keine Disulfidbindungen brechende Enzyme in der Haut nachgewiesen worden sind.

Die Acantholyse, die durch Cantharidin verursacht wird, wurde von STOUGHTON und BAGATELL ebenfalls als eine enzymatische Reaktion erkannt. Diese Untersucher trugen Cantharidinpulver auf excidierte Hautstücke auf, und wenn sie dann die Hautstücke bei 37° inkubierten, beobachteten sie, daß Acantholyse binnen 30 min einsetzte und gewöhnlich nach 2—4 Std zu einer vollständigen Auflösung der Epidermis geführt hatte. Die Acantholyse konnte verhindert werden, wenn vor der Auftragung des Cantharidins die Hautstücke entweder gefroren oder in die Dermis dieser Stücke niedrige Konzentrationen von Kupfersulfat, Quecksilberchlorid, Arsentrioxyd oder Jodessigsäure injiziert wurden. STOUGHTON und BAGATELL hielten es für wahrscheinlich, daß der die Acantholyse hervorrufende enzymatische Faktor, der durch Cantharidin in der Haut freigesetzt wurde, dem Faktor ähnlich oder gleich war, der in der Haut nach milden Hitzestimuli auftrat; denn das histologische Aussehen der Acantholyse war in beiden Fällen dasselbe. Später wies dann BURBACH (1961) nach, daß Cantharidin nur in der Gegenwart von Sauerstoff Acantholyse hervorrief; und WEAKLEY und EINBINDER (1962 [I]) stellten fest, daß das Hinzusetzen von Glucose oder von Malonsäure zu den Inkubationsmedien die durch Cantharidin induzierte Acantholyse verhinderte. Da Malonsäure die Umwandlung der Succinylsäure zu Fumarsäure durch Inhibition der Succinyl-Dehydrogenase verhindert, kamen WEAKLEY und EINBINDER (1962 [I]) zu dem Schluß, daß ein wahrscheinlicher Angriffspunkt des Cantharidins das Cytochromsystem sei, welches nach der Umwandlung von Succinylsäure zu Fumarsäure in Aktion tritt. Durch seine Einwirkung auf das Cytochromsystem würde Cantharidin die Bildung von Adenosintriphosphat aus Adenosindiphosphat und inorganischem Phosphor während der oxydativen Phase des Kohlenhydratstoffwechsels verhindern. Wegen der Ähnlichkeit der Cantharidin-Acantholyse mit der beim Pemphigus bestehenden Acantholyse haben WEAKLEY und EINBINDER (1962 [I]) die Möglichkeit erwogen, daß auch beim Pemphigus die Acantholyse durch eine Störung im oxydativen Kohlenhydratstoffwechsel, insbesondere durch eine Verhinderung der Bildung von Adenosintriphosphat, hervorgerufen sei. Sie geben zu, daß ihre Hypothese der biochemischen Ähnlichkeit der beiden Arten von Acantholyse geschwächt ist durch die von RAJKA gemachte und von ihnen bestätigte Beobachtung, daß eine Vorbehandlung der Versuchstiere mit Corticosteroiden keineswegs die Cantharidin-Acantholyse in vitro verhinderte; andererseits glauben sie aber nicht, daß diese Beobachtung ihre Hypothese völlig widerlegt.

d) Hervorrufen der Acantholyse in vivo

Wie EPSTEIN und KLIGMAN erstmalig mitteilten, führt beim Menschen die Auftragung einer 0,7%igen Lösung von Cantharidin in gleichen Anteilen von Aceton und Collodion, gefolgt von dem Auflegen eines Heftpflasters, zu Blasenbildung auf Grund von Acantholyse. Ferner verursachten MILLER und STOUGHTON bei Versuchspersonen mittels intradermaler Injektionen von kristallisiertem Papain, einem proteolytischen Enzym, bei ansteigender Konzentration des Papains erst Spongiose, dann Trennung zwischen Epidermis und Dermis und schließlich Acantholyse. MILLER und STOUGHTON erblickten in ihren Befunden eine Unterstützung ihrer Hypothese, daß enzymatische Vorgänge bei der Bildung aller Blasenarten eine Rolle spielen, unabhängig davon, ob die Blase in ihrer Genese spongiotisch, subepidermal oder acantholytisch ist. Sie glauben allerdings, daß proteolytische Enzyme den pathologischen Vorgang eher vermitteln als verursachen.

Diese von MILLER und STOUGHTON ausgesprochene Ansicht kann bei dem heutigen Stand unserer Kenntnisse auch auf den Pemphigus vulgaris angewandt werden: Proteolytische Enzyme spielen bei der Blasenbildung des Pemphigus zwar eine Rolle, aber sie verursachen die Blasenbildung nicht.

VI. Behandlung

Bevor Corticotropin (ACTH) und die Corticosteroide erhältlich waren, gab es keine befriedigende Behandlung für den Pemphigus. Wenn trotzdem gelegentlich gute Resultate mit einzelnen Behandlungsmethoden berichtet wurden (RIECKE widmete der Behandlung des Pemphigus 24 Seiten!), so liegt das vor allem daran, daß eine Trennung des Pemphigus vulgaris von dem bullösen Pemphigoid noch nicht bestand. Viele Fälle, bei denen gute therapeutische Resultate berichtet worden sind, waren wahrscheinlich keine Fälle von Pemphigus vulgaris, sondern waren Fälle von bullösem Pemphigoid, das ja oft schon nach einigen Monaten spontan heilt und außer bei alten, geschwächten Patienten selten zum Tode führt. Erst die vor wenigen Jahren erkannten histologischen Unterschiede ermöglichen eine objektive Trennung zwischen dem durch Acantholyse gekennzeichneten Pemphigus vulgaris und dem ohne Acantholyse einhergehenden bullösen Pemphigoid.

Die Einführung des Corticotropins (ACTH) und des Cortisons im Jahre 1949 und des Prednisons im Jahre 1954 hat die Prognose für Patienten mit Pemphigus sehr verbessert. Alle Formen von Pemphigus und Pemphigoid sprechen auf die Corticosteroide zu allen Zeiten an, vorausgesetzt, daß hinreichend hohe Dosen verabreicht werden.

1. Literaturübersicht über die Behandlung des Pemphigus

Mehrere Serien von Patienten, die über längere Zeit hin mit Corticosteroiden behandelt wurden, sind in der Literatur mitgeteilt worden. In der folgenden Übersicht können nur einige dieser Berichte erwähnt werden. In allen hier mitgeteilten Berichten war Acantholyse die Grundlage für die Diagnose Pemphigus. Wie von SANDERS et al. betont worden ist, würde das Einbeziehen von Patienten mit bullösem Pemphigoid ein zu optimistisches Bild der Resultate zur Folge haben.

COSTELLO, JAIMOVICH und DANNENBERG berichteten 1957 von New York über die Behandlung von 52 Patienten mit Pemphigus mittels Corticotropin oder Corticosteroiden. Unter diesen Patienten hatten 42 Pemphigus vulgaris, von denen 20 starben. Die Sterblichkeit war bei den jüdischen Patienten größer als bei den nicht-jüdischen Patienten. Einige Patienten waren bereits ein, zwei oder mehrere Jahre lang ohne Behandlung beschwerdefrei; aber Einzelheiten darüber fehlen in dem Bericht. Die Autoren betonen, daß hohe Anfangsdosen in schweren Fällen notwendig seien und daß die Prognose um so günstiger sei, je früher die Behandlung einsetze.

SANDERS et al. berichteten 1960 von New York über 50 Patienten mit Pemphigus. Von diesen waren 22, d.h. 44%, entweder an ihrer Krankheit oder an Behandlungskomplikationen und drei, d.h. 6%, an anderen Ursachen gestorben. Von den 37 Patienten, die Pemphigus vulgaris hatten, waren 17, d.h. 46%, an ihrer Krankheit gestorben und drei, d.h. 8%, an anderen Ursachen. Die Autoren bemerkten, daß die Prognose für solche Patienten günstig war, die die ersten drei Jahre ihrer Krankheit überlebt hatten und für solche, bei denen der Pemphigus vor dem Alter von vierzig Jahren seinen Anfang hatte. Von den überlebenden 25 Patienten waren 23 in der Lage, ihrer Beschäftigung nachzugehen, und 21 hatten keine Hauterscheinungen. Jedoch mußten alle 25 Patienten Erhaltungsdosen von Corticosteroiden einnehmen: 21 von ihnen brauchten 75 mg von Cortison-Äquivalenten pro Tag und 4 brauchten höhere Dosen. Keiner der Patienten blieb mehr als einige Wochen erscheinungsfrei, wenn die Corticosteroide abgesetzt wurden.

STEVENSON berichtete 1960 über die Resultate, die in der Behandlung des Pemphigus an einer Reihe von Londoner Krankenhäusern erzielt worden waren. Unter 61 Patienten waren 21, d.h. 34%, gestorben; 39 von den 61 Patienten hatten Pemphigus vulgaris, von denen 15 starben, d.h. 38%. Der bei 21 Patienten eingetretene Tod wurde in 8 Fällen ungenügender Dosierung der Corticosteroide zugeschrieben, in 7 Fällen Behandlungskomplikationen und in 8 Fällen anderen Krankheiten. Von den 24 Patienten mit Pemphigus vulgaris, die am Leben waren, waren 4 bereits längere Zeit ohne Behandlung erscheinungsfrei, und zwar zwei seit drei Jahren, einer seit zwei Jahren und einer seit einem Jahr.

WITTELS berichtete 1960 aus Wien über 25 Patienten mit Pemphigus, von denen 11 Pemphigus vulgaris hatten. Keiner von ihnen war jüdisch. Mit der Ausnahme eines Patienten, dessen Maximaldosis 800 mg Cortison-Äquivalente pro Tag war, erhielten alle Patienten als Maximaldosis 500 oder 600 mg pro Tag. Von den 25 Patienten waren 16 ohne Behandlung erscheinungsfrei, 5 erhielten noch Erhaltungsdosen, 3 waren nicht auffindbar und einer war an Pemphigus verstorben. Von ihren 11 Patienten mit Pemphigus vulgaris waren 9 ohne Behandlung erscheinungsfrei, 3 darunter seit über vier Jahren.

PERRY berichtete 1961 von der Mayo Clinic über 22 Patienten mit Pemphigus foliaceus und 8 mit Pemphigus erythematosus, die mit Corticotropin oder Corticosteroiden behandelt worden waren. Zwei Patienten mit Pemphigus foliaceus und ein Patient mit Pemphigus erythematosus zeigten Abheilung aller Hauterscheinungen unter Behandlung mit Corticosteroiden und waren seit $7^1/_2$, $3^1/_2$ bzw. $3^1/_2$ Jahren ohne weitere Behandlung erscheinungsfrei.

Im Jahre 1962 berichteten PER und MASHKILLEISON aus Moskau über ihre Resultate in der Behandlung von 40 Patienten mit Pemphigus. Von diesen hatten 34 Pemphigus vulgaris, 5 Pemphigus foliaceus und einer Pemphigus erythematosus. Zu Anfang der Behandlung wie auch bei Exacerbationen gaben die Autoren 300—400 mg Cortison-Äquivalente. Wenn binnen weniger Tage keine Besserung einsetzte, wurde die Dosis auf 500—900 mg pro Tag heraufgesetzt. Von ihren 40 Patienten waren 32 am Leben, und 6 von diesen waren nicht nur erscheinungsfrei, sondern hatten bereits von sechs Monaten bis zu drei Jahren keine Behandlung mehr erfordert. Die anderen 26 Patienten nahmen noch Erhaltungsdosen ein, die bei 24 Patienten eine volle oder fast volle Remission aufrechterhielten und die Patienten in die Lage versetzten, ihrer gewohnten Beschäftigung nachzugehen. Acht Patienten waren gestorben, und zwar 4 an ihrer Krankheit und 4 an Komplikationen, die sich aus der Behandlung ergeben hatten.

2. Eigene Ergebnisse bei der Behandlung des Pemphigus

Die eigenen Behandlungsergebnisse (LEVER und WHITE), die 1963 veröffentlicht wurden, betreffen 45 Patienten, von denen jeder mindestens 2 Jahre unter Behandlung gewesen war.

a) Pemphigus vulgaris

Von 32 Patienten mit Pemphigus vulgaris waren 21 am Leben. Fünf von ihnen waren, ohne Behandlung zu erhalten, erscheinungsfrei; 5 waren zwar erscheinungsfrei, brauchten aber noch Erhaltungsdosen; und 11 hatten einige Hauterscheinungen und standen noch unter Behandlung. Elf Patienten waren verstorben. Bei 6 von ihnen trat der Tod infolge Behandlungskomplikationen ein, während 5 an anderen Krankheiten gestorben waren.

Die Resultate ergaben, daß, je früher mit der Behandlung begonnen wurde, desto leichter war es, die Krankheitserscheinungen zum Abheilen zu bringen und desto seltener kam es zu Rückfällen. So bedurfte es bei allen 5 Patienten, die im Frühstadium behandelt wurden, verhältnismäßig kurzer Zeit, eine andauernde Remission herbeizuführen. Von diesen 5 Patienten waren 3 zur Zeit des Berichtes gesund, während 2 an anderen Krankheiten verstorben waren und zur Zeit ihres Todes erscheinungsfrei gewesen waren. Im Gegensatz dazu war von 17 Patienten, die ausgedehnte Erscheinungen hatten, als die Behandlung begann, nur einer ohne Behandlung erscheinungsfrei.

Der Pemphigus vulgaris nahm im Durchschnitt bei den jüdischen Patienten einen schwereren Verlauf als bei den anderen. Dies ist daraus ersichtlich, daß unter 17 jüdischen Patienten 10 verstorben waren, und zwar 5 an Behandlungskomplikationen und 5 an anderen Krankheiten. Dagegen war von den 15 nicht-jüdischen Patienten nur einer verstorben, und zwar an einer Behandlungskomplikation.

b) Pemphigus vegetans

Ein Patient mit der Hallopeau-Form, Pyodermite végétante, war seit ungefähr 5 Jahren erscheinungsfrei, ohne der Behandlung mehr zu bedürfen.

c) Pemphigus foliaceus

Von zehn Patienten mit Pemphigus foliaceus waren alle sechs, die am Leben waren, ohne Behandlung erscheinungsfrei. Die anderen vier waren an anderen Krankheiten verstorben und waren zur Zeit ihres Todes erscheinungsfrei gewesen. Bei den Patienten mit ausgedehntem Pemphigus foliaceus waren, wie bei den Patienten mit fortgeschrittenem Pemphigus vulgaris, hohe Dosen von Corticosteroiden über eine lange Zeit hin erforderlich; aber, im Gegensatz zu den fortgeschrittenen Fällen von Pemphigus vulgaris, neigten selbst die generalisierten Fälle von Pemphigus foliaceus dazu, infolge der Behandlung völlig und dauernd abzuheilen. So waren von vier Patienten mit generalisiertem Pemphigus zwei bereits seit 7 und einer seit 9 Jahren ohne Behandlung erscheinungsfrei, und nur bei einem Patienten waren stets Erhaltungsdosen nötig, bis er nach fast 6 Jahren an einer anderen Krankheit verstarb.

d) Pemphigus erythematosus

Zwei Patienten hatten Pemphigus erythematosus. Sie waren nie ernstlich krank. Nur einer von ihnen wurde für eine kurze Zeit mit Corticosteroiden behandelt. Dieser Patient hatte noch einige Hauterscheinungen zur Zeit des Berichtes. Bei dem anderen Patienten waren 16 Jahre nach Beginn der Krankheit alle Hauterscheinungen spontan geheilt und er war seit 6 Jahren erscheinungsfrei.

e) Behandlungskomplikationen

Bei sechs Patienten verursachten Behandlungskomplikationen den Tod: Eine Patientin starb an Diabetes, der zwar schon vor Krankheitsbeginn bestanden hatte, sich aber unter der Behandlung mit Corticosteroiden verschlimmerte; zwei Patienten starben an Infektionen, und zwar ein Patient an einer Pyelitis und der andere an einer Staphylokokkensepsis. Weitere Todesursachen, die mit der Corticosteroid-Behandlung in Beziehung standen, waren die folgenden: Einmal ein perforiertes Magengeschwür, einmal eine Beinvenenthrombose, gefolgt von Lungenembolie, und einmal multiple innere Blutungen.

3. Behandlungsplan beim Pemphigus vulgaris

Es ist äußerst wichtig, daß beim Pemphigus vulgaris die Behandlung mit Corticosteroiden so bald wie möglich begonnen wird. Bei schweren Fällen sollte mit Behandlung begonnen werden, sobald die Probeexcisionen durchgeführt worden sind, ohne daß man den histologischen Bericht abwartet. Je früher im Krankheitsverlauf die Behandlung begonnen wird, desto schneller kann man die Krankheitserscheinungen zum Abheilen bringen und desto leichter kann man Rückfälle vermeiden. Diese Ansicht des frühen und intensiven Behandelns beim Pemphigus vulgaris wird nicht nur durch die eigenen Ergebnisse unterstützt, sondern auch durch die von Costello et al. (1957) und von Sanders et al. gemachten Erfahrungen. Sanders et al. haben festgestellt, daß „intensive Behandlung mit vollständiger Unterdrückung aller Krankheitsherde beim Beginn der Behandlung verringert die Häufigkeit und Schwere der Rückfälle beim Pemphigus vulgaris“.

a) Wahl des Medikamentes

Corticotropin (ACTH) und Cortison werden bei der Behandlung des Pemphigus nicht mehr angewandt, weil sie eine Retention von Natrium und einen Verlust von Kalium verursachen. Es besteht kein Anlaß anzunehmen, daß irgendeines der Corticosteroide, die nach dem Prednison synthetisiert worden sind, wie z.B. Methylprednison, Triamcinolon, Dexamethason oder Betamethason, einen Vorteil über das Prednison besitzen: Wenn äquivalente Dosen verabreicht werden, sind sowohl die Wirksamkeit als auch die Nebenwirkungen die gleichen. Ungefähr äquivalent mit einer Tablette Cortison (25 mg) sind eine Tablette Prednison (5 mg), eine Tablette Methylprednison (4 mg), eine Tablette Triamcinolon (4 mg) und eine halbe Tablette Betamethasone (0,3 mg).

b) Anfängliche Behandlung

Die Dosierung der Corticosteroide soll zu Beginn der Behandlung hoch genug sein, um die Krankheitserscheinungen so bald wie möglich zur Abheilung zu bringen. Der Pemphigus vulgaris spricht auf die Behandlung mit Corticosteroiden stets an, vorausgesetzt, daß genügend hohe Dosen verabreicht werden. Es ist besser, mit einer zu hohen täglichen Dosis anzufangen, als mit einer zu niedrigen. Bei Patienten mit nur einigen Krankheitsherden ist es ratsam, mit einer täglichen Verabreichung von 24 Tabletten Prednison (120 mg) zu beginnen oder mit einer äquivalenten Dosis eines anderen Corticosteroid. Bei Patienten, die schon weiter ausgebreitete Krankheitserscheinungen haben, sollten zu Beginn 36 Tabletten Prednison (180 mg) pro Tag gegeben werden. Da beim Pemphigus vulgaris unter Behandlung mit genügend hohen Dosen eine Besserung binnen weniger Tage einsetzt, sollte man, falls nach fünf Tagen noch neue Krankheitsherde auftreten, die Zahl der Tabletten entweder von 24 auf 36 oder von 36 auf 48 pro Tag erhöhen. Selbst wenn keine neuen Herde mehr auftreten, sollte man mit der hohen Dosierung (24 oder mehr Tabletten pro Tag) fortfahren, mindestens so lange, bis alle

Epitheldefekte geheilt sind und möglicherweise darüber hinaus. Es erscheint ratsam, die Behandlung mit hohen Dosen für mindestens acht Wochen durchzuführen, da auf diese Weise Rückfälle gelegentlich verhindert werden und, falls sie eintreten, sie gewöhnlich leicht sind. Die vorgeschlagene lange Intensivbehandlung wird in der Regel von Patienten, die erstmalig mit Corticosteroiden behandelt werden, ohne ernste Nebenwirkungen vertragen. Die Gefahr ernster Behandlungskomplikationen steigert sich beträchtlich bei späteren Intensivkursen.

Nach dem völligen Abheilen aller Epitheldefekte wird die täglich verabreichte Menge von Prednison herabgesetzt, und zwar auf „logarithmische Weise", d.h. erst schnell, aber dann mit dem Absinken der Dosis immer langsamer. Obwohl die Behandlung des Pemphigus vulgaris mit Corticosteroiden individuell gehandhabt werden soll, stellt das folgende Schema ein Beispiel dar für die anfängliche Behandlung eines „Durchschnittspatienten" mit einem mäßig schweren Pemphigus vulgaris. Der Patient würde zu Beginn 36 Tabletten Prednison (180 mg) pro Tag für acht Wochen einnehmen. Dann, falls alle Krankheitserscheinungen abgeheilt sind, wird die Zahl der Tabletten pro Tag erst schnell und dann immer langsamer hinuntergesetzt, z.B.: 24 Tabletten für eine Woche; 12 Tabletten für eine Woche; 8 Tabletten für eine Woche; 7 Tabletten für eine Woche; 6 Tabletten für zwei Wochen; 5 Tabletten für vier Wochen; 4 Tabletten für sechs Wochen; 3 Tabletten für acht Wochen; und danach 2 Tabletten. Man kann nicht bei jedem Patienten die Dosierung auf 2 oder 3 Tabletten pro Tag reduzieren, und so muß die Behandlung, besonders bei Verabreichung niedriger Dosen, individuell reguliert werden. Selbst wenn zuerst die Erhaltungsdosis etwas hoch sein muß, ist es doch ratsam, nach einigen Monaten eine vorsichtige Herabsetzung der täglichen Dosis zu versuchen, vielleicht um eine halbe Tablette.

Es ist unnötig, daß man, wie von einigen Autoren vorgeschlagen worden ist, Corticotropin verabreicht, bevor man die Corticosteroide absetzt; denn eine irreversible Atrophie der Nebennierenrinde kommt selbst bei sehr lange durchgeführter Behandlung mit Corticosteroiden nicht vor (Larzelere et al.). Es ist allerdings nötig, im Bereich niedriger Dosen die täglich zu verabreichende Menge von Corticosteroiden ganz vorsichtig herabzusetzen, um der Nebennierenrinde Zeit zum Regenerieren zu geben. So soll man, nachdem der Patient 2 Tabletten Prednison (10 mg) täglich über acht Wochen hin erhalten hat, die tägliche Dosis nicht schneller als um eine halbe Tablette Prednison (2,5 mg) alle vier Wochen herabsetzen.

Es wirkt sich sogar zum Nachteil aus, wenn Corticotropin während der Herabsetzung der täglichen Dosis von Corticosteroiden verabreicht wird; denn die Behandlung mit Corticosteroiden über eine lange Zeit hin verursacht nicht nur eine Atrophie der Nebennierenrinde, sondern auch eine verringerte Synthese von Corticotropin in der Hypophyse (Farrell und Laqueur). Somit würde die Verabreichung von Corticotropin lediglich eine fortgesetzte Unterdrückung der Synthese von Corticotropin in der Hypophyse zur Folge haben (Holub et al.; Paris).

c) Behandlung von Rückfällen

Das Auftreten einiger neuer Pemphigusherde mag keinen oder nur einen kleinen Anstieg in der täglichen Dosis erforderlich machen. Jedoch, wenn der Verdacht besteht, daß ein Rückfall bevorsteht, sollte die Dosis ohne Zeitverlust auf mindestens 24 Tabletten pro Tag heraufgesetzt werden; und wie bei der anfänglichen Behandlung soll, falls eine Besserung nicht binnen fünf Tagen eintritt, eine höhere Dosis verabreicht werden (36 Tabletten pro Tag und dann 48 Tabletten pro Tag). Wird eine solche Intensivbehandlung rechtzeitig eingesetzt, dann kann der Rückfall gewöhnlich binnen zwei bis drei Wochen zur Abheilung gebracht werden. Danach kann die Dosis wieder auf „logarithmische Weise" herabgesetzt werden.

d) Verhinderung von Nebenwirkungen

Der Pemphigus vulgaris selbst stellt zwar nicht mehr eine Lebensbedrohung dar; jedoch kann die lang ausgedehnte Behandlung mit solch hohen Dosen von Corticosteroiden, wie sie zur Behandlung notwendig sind, Nebenwirkungen hervorrufen, die gelegentlich tödlich verlaufen. Vorbeugende Maßnahmen, die von einigem Wert sind, können gegen das Eintreten von Wirbelbrüchen und gegen das Eintreten von Magengeschwüren oder von Magenblutungen getroffen werden. Diese Maßnahmen sollten eingesetzt werden, sobald der Patient beginnt, hohe Dosen von Corticosteroiden einzunehmen. Andererseits ist es nicht mehr nötig, Kaliumchlorid zu verabreichen und die Menge von Salz in der Nahrung zu beschränken, wie es nötig war, als Corticotropin und Cortison für die Behandlung benutzt wurden.

Als Vorbeugung gegen *Wirbelbrüche* ist die Verabreichung von Testosteron, Oestrogen und Calciumgluconat ratsam. Für die Hormone ist die folgende tägliche Dosierung empfohlen: Für Männer 10 mg Methyltestosteron (als Linguette) und 0,5 mg Diäthylstilboestrol, und für Frauen 10 mg Methyltestosteron und 1,0 mg Diäthylstilboestrol. Männliche wie weibliche Patienten erhalten 2—5 mg Calciumgluconat pro Tag. In unserer Erfahrung haben sich diese Maßnahmen bewährt, seit sie 1953 eingeführt wurden: denn Wirbelbrüche wurden vor 1953 bei 10 von 23 Patienten mit Pemphigus beobachtet, nach 1953 aber nur bei 2 von 21 Patienten.

Als Vorbeugung gegen *Magengeschwüre* oder *Magenblutungen* sollen Säure neutralisierende Tabletten, die z. B. Magnesiumtrisilicat und Aluminiumhydroxyd enthalten, verordnet werden. Sie werden zwei- oder dreimal täglich zusammen mit den Corticosteroidtabletten eingenommen, und außerdem abends vor dem Einschlafen. Es ist ferner empfohlen, daß die Corticosteroidtabletten stets nach einer Mahlzeit eingenommen werden.

Eine routinemäßige Verabreichung von *Antibiotica* als eine Vorbeugung gegen Infektionen ist nicht ratsam. Der Grund dafür ist, daß, falls eine Infektion während der Verabreichung von Antibiotica stattfindet, diese dann durch Bakterien verursacht ist, die gewöhnlich nicht nur gegen das angewandte Antibioticum, sondern auch gegen viele andere Antibiotica resistent sind. Falls aber eine durch Bakterien verursachte Infektion eintritt, sollte diese baldigst und intensiv behandelt werden.

e) Behandlung von Nebenwirkungen

Außer Infektionen, die, wie gerade festgestellt, bei ihrem Auftreten intensiver Behandlung bedürfen, stellt der Diabetes eine Nebenwirkung dar, die möglicherweise behandelt werden muß. Bei Patienten, die bereits Diabetes haben, erhöht die Verabreichung von Corticosteroiden die für die Behandlung des Diabetes notwendige Menge von Insulin oft erheblich. Bei Patienten ohne vorhergehenden Diabetes hängt die Entwicklung eines „Corticosteroid-Diabetes" von der Fähigkeit des Patienten ab, seine Insulinerzeugung zu erhöhen. Solch ein „Corticosteroid-Diabetes" ist meistens leicht und unterscheidet sich von einem „idiopathischen" Diabetes durch die folgenden Kennzeichen: 1. ist er Insulin-resistent; 2. führt er sehr selten zu Acidosis; 3. ist er mit erhöhter Speicherung von Glykogen in der Leber verbunden; und 4. ist er reversibel (Frawley et al.). Gewöhnlich bedarf ein „Corticosteroid-Diabetes" keiner Behandlung. Die Anwendung von Insulin und einer strikten Diät ist nur in solchen Fällen indiziert, bei denen sich eine Acidosis entwickelt.

f) Zusätzliche Behandlungsmaßnahmen

Patienten im Anfangsstadium des Pemphigus vulgaris können ambulant behandelt werden. Andererseits ist bei Patienten im fortgeschrittenen Stadium der Krankheit gute Pflege im Krankenhaus nötig. Da Patienten, die für längere Zeit mit hohen Dosen von Corticosteroiden behandelt worden sind, einen verringerten Widerstand gegen Infektionen besitzen, ist es ratsam, einige Isolierungsmaßnahmen zu treffen, um das Einschleppen von Infektionen durch das Krankenhauspersonal und durch Besucher möglichst zu verhindern. Wenn ausgedehnte Schleimhautherde bestehen, kann ein Lokalanaestheticum zum Mundspülen 15 min vor dem Essen verwendet werden.

g) Laboratoriumsuntersuchungen

Die einzige notwendige Laboratoriumsuntersuchung vor dem Einleiten der Behandlung ist eine Blutzuckerbestimmung und eine Zuckerbelastungsprobe, um das Bestehen eines Diabetes oder die dazu bestehende Neigung festzustellen. Bei älteren Leuten ist außerdem eine röntgenologische Untersuchung der Wirbelsäule ratsam, um Auskunft über den schon bestehenden Grad von Osteoporose zu erhalten. Bei schweren Fällen sollte man außerdem Untersuchungen darüber anstellen, wieweit der Pemphigus den Hämatokrit, die Serumproteine und Serumelektrolyte beeinflußt hat.

Während der Behandlung sollen gelegentliche Urinzuckeruntersuchungen und, wenn diese positiv sind, Blutzuckerbestimmungen durchgeführt werden. Eine Bestimmung der Bluteosinophilen hat kaum einen praktischen Wert, da mit den vorgeschlagenen hohen Dosen von Corticosteroiden die Zahl der Eosinophilen schnell auf Null oder fast Null abfällt. Vielleicht sollte man bei Patienten, bei denen die verabreichte Menge von Corticosteroiden nicht genügend Besserung hervorruft, die Zahl der Bluteosinophilen bestimmen.

4. Behandlungsplan bei den anderen Pemphigusarten

a) Pemphigus vegetans

Die Neumann-Form des Pemphigus vegetans, die ja lediglich eine Variante des Pemphigus vulgaris darstellt und gewöhnlich in einen Pemphigus vulgaris ausläuft, soll genau so intensiv wie der Pemphigus vulgaris behandelt werden. Andererseits ist es unnötig, die recht gutartig verlaufende Hallopeau-Form des Pemphigus vegetans (Pyodermite végétante) für längere Zeit intensiv mit Corticosteroiden zu behandeln. In dem einen persönlich behandelten Patienten konnte recht gute Besserung dadurch erreicht werden, daß verschiedene Male kurze Kurse von Corticosteroiden in mäßiger Dosierung verabreicht wurden, nämlich 500 mg von Cortison-Äquivalenten pro Tag für 9—16 Tage (LEVER und WHITE). Antibiotica waren von einigem Wert in der Unterdrückung von leichteren Pustelschüben.

b) Pemphigus foliaceus

Eine Remission beim Pemphigus foliaceus herbeizuführen, erfordert gewöhnlich ebenso hohe Dosen wie beim Pemphigus vulgaris. Auch müssen diese hohen Dosen, genau wie beim Pemphigus foliaceus, über viele Wochen hin verabreicht werden. Trotzdem ist diese Intensivbehandlung bei fast allen Patienten mit Pemphigus foliaceus indiziert, ob alt oder jung. Denn bei älteren Patienten, nämlich solchen mit Krankheitsbeginn im Alter über 50 Jahre, ist diese Behandlung angebracht trotz der möglichen Nebenerscheinungen wegen der hohen Mortalität in dieser Altersgruppe (100% in unserer Serie unbehandelter Patienten; s. S. 613). Bei jüngeren Patienten hat der Pemphigus foliaceus zwar eine relativ niedrige Sterblichkeit, aber die sehr lange Dauer der Krankheit, bevor gewöhnlich eine Spontanheilung eintritt, rechtfertigt die intensive Behandlung bei jüngeren Patienten, die ja diese viel besser vertragen als ältere Patienten. Wie unsere eigenen Beobachtungen (s. S. 632) und die von PERRY (s. S. 632) zeigen, hat der Pemphigus foliaceus weniger Neigung zu Rückfällen als der Pemphigus vulgaris, wenn er einmal zum Abheilen gebracht worden ist.

c) Pemphigus erythematosus

Beim Pemphigus erythematosus, der eine lokalisierte Form des Pemphigus foliaceus darstellt, ist eine interne Corticosteroidbehandlung oft nicht nötig, da die Krankheit nicht unbedingt fortschreitet und in einen Pemphigus foliaceus übergeht. Falls ein solches Fortschreiten stattfindet, sollte derselbe Behandlungsplan wie beim Pemphigus foliaceus angewandt werden; aber gewöhnlich kann man mit niedrigerer Dosierung als beim Pemphigus foliaceus behandeln.

Die Lokalapplikation von Corticosteroidsalben ist bei der Behandlung des Pemphigus erythematosus zweifellos von Wert, wie auch bei übrigbleibenden Einzelherden von Pemphigus foliaceus (COLOMB und ABGRALL; COLOMB und JEANNEROD). Die Wirkungskraft von Corticosteroidsalben wird durch einen nach Auftragung der Salbe angelegten Okklusionsverband, der aus einem feuchten Tuch und einer plastischen Hülle besteht, bedeutend erhöht. Solch ein Okklusionsverband soll mindestens für 8 Std, am besten über Nacht, angelegt bleiben. Am

Gesicht, wo ein Okklusionsverband nicht gut möglich ist, können, um eine Hydrierung der Hornschicht herbeizuführen, heiße, feuchte Kompressen benutzt werden. Diese werden drei- oder viermal am Tage 5—10 min lang aufgelegt und danach wird die Corticosteroidsalbe gut in die Haut eingerieben (TYE, BLUMENTAL und LEVER).

B. Pemphigoid

Zwei Krankheiten, die früher allgemein, auch von RIECKE, zur Pemphigusgruppe gezählt wurden, sind 1953 von LEVER als Pemphigoid von der Pemphigusgruppe abgetrennt worden, da sie keine Acantholyse aufweisen. Diese sind das bullöse Pemphigoid und das benigne Schleimhautpemphigoid.

I. Bullöses Pemphigoid

Dieses Krankheitsbild ist letzthin mehrfach diskutiert worden. Auch sind andere Namen dafür vorgeschlagen worden, nämlich Pemphigoid (ROOK und WADDINGTON), Parapemphigus (PRAKKEN und WOERDEMAN) und, wegen des häufigen Vorkommens bei alten Leuten, Alterspemphigus (STEIGLEDER). Zwar ist das Krankheitsbild von vielen anerkannt worden (BRENNAN und MONTGOMERY; SNEDDON und CHURCH; PIÉRARD und WHIMSTER; SANDERS et al.; KIM und WINKELMANN; TAPPEINER und PFLEGER; RUPEC et al.); aber andere wollen das bullöse Pemphigoid doch dem Pemphigus vulgaris eingliedern (HERZBERG 1955, 1958; STEIGLEDER; CHARGIN et al.; FÖLDVÁRI 1959), und die meisten französischen Dermatologen (DEGOS; RIMBAUD und GUIBERT) sowie mehrere andere Autoren (LAPIÈRE; FASSOTTE; PERCIVAL) betrachten das bullöse Pemphigoid als eine bullöse Form der Dermatitis herpetiformis. Mehr wird über die nosologische Stellung des bullösen Pemphigoids nach der Beschreibung des klinischen und histologischen Bildes gesagt werden.

a) Hauterscheinungen

Das bullöse Pemphigoid stellt eine chronische, relativ gutartige und in seiner Dauer oft begrenzte Erkrankung dar. Das Hauptmerkmal des bullösen Pemphigoids, nämlich das Vorhandensein von zahlreichen großen, prallen Blasen, ist in dem Beiwort bullös zum Ausdruck gebracht.

Die Blasen beim bullösen Pemphigoid können recht groß werden und haben oft eine unregelmäßige Gestalt (Abb. 36). Sie sind prall, wenn sie entstehen, und nur nachdem ein Teil der Blasenflüssigkeit abgeflossen ist oder absorbiert worden ist, werden sie schlaff. Die Blasen brechen nicht so leicht wie beim Pemphigus vulgaris (da die Zellen der Epidermis, im Gegensatz zum Pemphigus vulgaris, keine acantholytische Degeneration aufweisen). Wenn die Blasen brechen, vergrößern sich die auf diese Weise entstandenen Epitheldefekte gewöhnlich nicht, sondern zeigen eine gute Heilungstendenz (Abb. 37). Daher beherrschen Blasen während des ganzen Krankheitsverlaufes das klinische Bild, und die Epitheldefekte sind im Gegensatz zum Pemphigus vulgaris selten ausgedehnt. Gelegentlich sind einige Blasen hämorrhagisch. Obwohl die Blasen wahllos über die ganze Hautoberfläche verstreut sein können, zeigen doch die Leistenbeugen, die Achselhöhlen und die Beugefläche der Unterarme (Abb. 38) oft die größte Anzahl von Blasen. Gewöhnlich bilden sich die Blasen auf normal aussehender Haut, nicht selten aber auch auf erythematösen Flächen, die sich bei den meisten Fällen zusätzlich zu den Blasen finden. Diese erythematösen Flächen zeigen oft etwas Ödem und können einen serpiginösen Umriß haben mit infiltriertem Rand und Abblassen in der

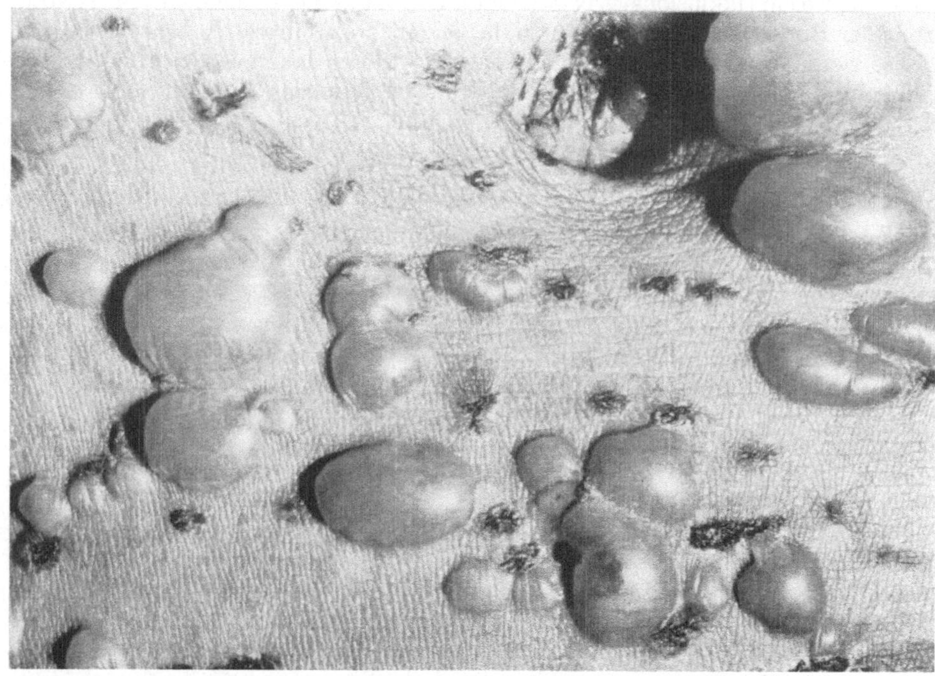

Abb. 36. Bullöses Pemphigoid. Die Blasen sind groß, prall und haben eine unregelmäßige Gestalt

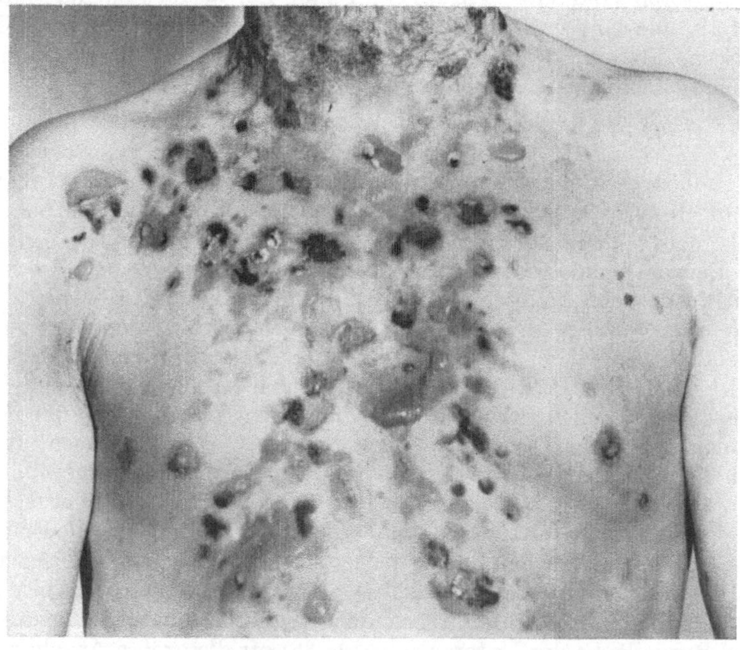

Abb. 37. Bullöses Pemphigoid. Die an der Stelle von gebrochenen Blasen gelegenen Epitheldefekte vergrößern sich nicht wesentlich und zeigen eine gute Heilungstendenz

Mitte (Abb. 39). Diese geröteten Flächen sehen denen, die man beim Erythema exsudativum multiforme sieht, sehr ähnlich, so daß diese Diagnose oft ernstlich

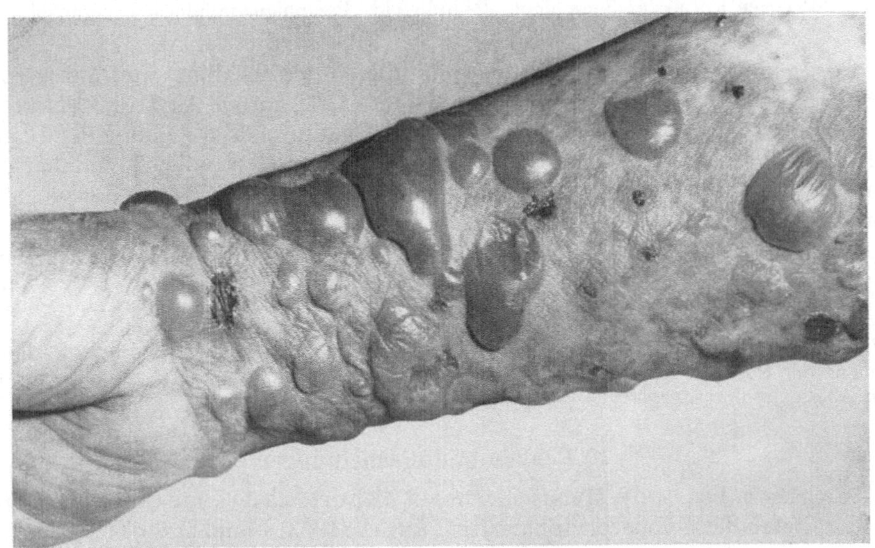

Abb. 38. Bullöses Pemphigoid. Die Beugefläche der Unterarme ist sehr häufig befallen

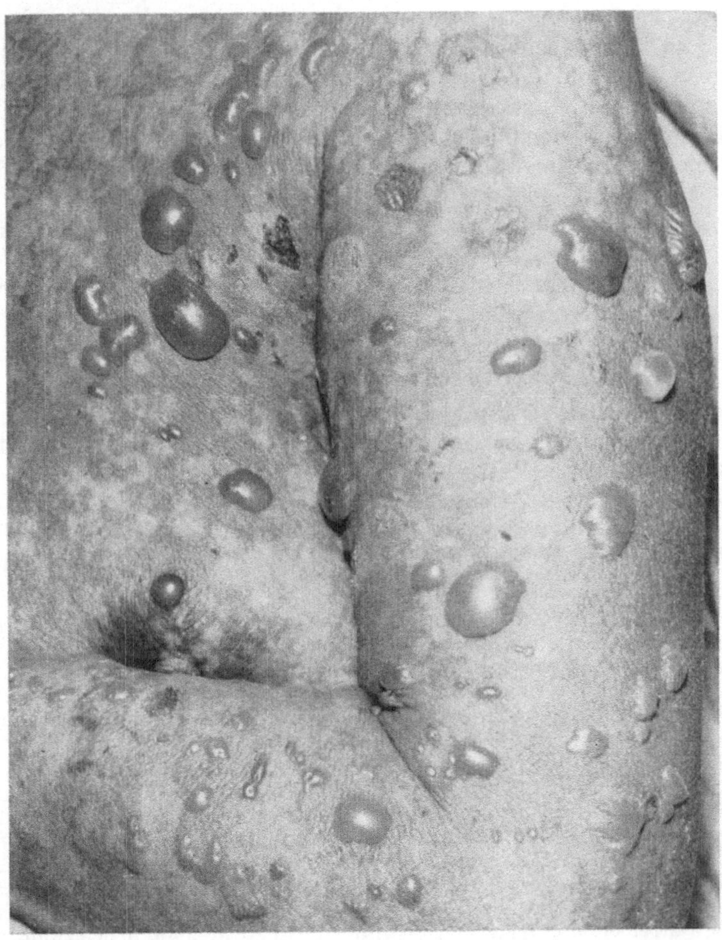

Abb. 39. Bullöses Pemphigoid. Außer Blasen sind auch unregelmäßig begrenzte erythematöse Flächen vorhanden

in Erwägung gezogen werden muß und die Unterscheidung nur auf Grund der Krankheitsdauer gemacht werden kann. Gelegentlich sind die Blasen in Gruppen angeordnet wie bei der Dermatitis herpetiformis. Abheilung der Blasen geht stets ohne Atrophie vonstatten. Jucken ist zu unterschiedlichen Graden vorhanden. Es kann fehlen; aber bei den meisten Patienten besteht Jucken, und manchmal ist es recht stark.

In seltenen Fällen bleibt der Blasenausschlag beim bullösen Pemphigoid auf ein Hautgebiet oder auf zwei, gewöhnlich symmetrisch angeordnete Gebiete beschränkt. Die häufigste Lokalisation für solch ein *lokalisiertes bullöses Pemphigoid* sind die Unterschenkel, besonders die Schienbeine (EBERHARTINGER und NIEBAUER). Am häufigsten sind ältere Personen davon befallen. Der Verlauf ist äußerst chronisch (FÖLDVÁRI 1958). Wegen der schlechten Heilungstendenz der Epitheldefekte an den Schienbeinen kommt es dort gelegentlich zu Ulceration und Abheilung mit Atrophie.

b) Schleimhauterscheinungen

In vielen Fällen ist die Mundschleimhaut nicht befallen. Unter ihren Patienten stellten Befall der Mundschleimhaut fest: LEVER (1953) 15mal unter 44 Patienten; WADDINGTON fünfmal unter 38 Patienten und KIM und WINKELMANN zweimal unter 18 Patienten. Nur selten ist die Mundschleimhaut schon zu Beginn der Krankheit befallen. Die Blasen und Epitheldefekte an der Mundschleimhaut sind gewöhnlich klein, und meistens sind sie in nur geringer Anzahl vorhanden. Sie befinden sich hauptsächlich an der Wangenschleimhaut und im Gegensatz zum Pemphigus vulgaris kommen sie kaum jemals am Lippenrot vor. Verhältnismäßig häufig kann man im Munde intakte Blasen finden, da sie nicht so leicht brechen wie die Blasen beim Pemphigus vulgaris. Auch vergrößern sich im Munde die den Blasen folgenden Epitheldefekte gewöhnlich nicht, sondern zeigen wie die auf der Haut gelegenen Epitheldefekte eine gute Heilungstendenz. So ist der Mund bei diesen Patienten nur mäßig wund, so daß Kauen und Schlucken leicht möglich sind.

Blasen können im Rachen und im Kehlkopf vorkommen. In seltenen Fällen sind auch die Bindehaut, die Vulva und die Afterschleimhaut leicht befallen.

c) Geschlecht, Herkunft, Alter

Beide Geschlechter sind in gleichem Maße betroffen. Auch findet man nicht, wie beim Pemphigus vulgaris, ein bevorzugtes Auftreten bei jüdischen Patienten. (Unter 33 persönlich am Massachusetts General Hospital beobachteten Patienten mit bullösem Pemphigoid waren nur zwei jüdisch, d.h. 6%, während unter den Patienten mit Pemphigus vulgaris 67% jüdisch waren; s. Tabelle 2.) Es besteht eine auffallende Altersverteilung, indem vor allem Kinder und alte Leute befallen werden (Abb. 40).

Unter den von LEVER (1953) berichteten 44 Patienten (33 vor und 11 nach Erhältlichkeit der Corticosteroide) waren vier Kinder, die beim Einsetzen der Krankheit $1^1/_2$, 3, $3^1/_2$ bzw. 8 Jahre alt waren. PRAKKEN und WOERDEMAN berichteten über drei Kinder, die 2, 3 bzw. 4 Jahre alt waren. Unter den 18 von KIM und WINKELMANN beobachteten Kindern waren sieben 2 Jahre alt oder jünger beim Beginn der Krankheit, vier waren zwischen 3 und 6 Jahre alt und sieben zwischen 7 und 14 Jahre alt.

Daß die meisten Patienten mit bullösem Pemphigoid alt sind, ergibt sich aus dem Folgenden: Unter den 40 erwachsenen Patienten, über die LEVER (1953) berichtete, war das Durchschnittsalter bei Krankheitsbeginn 66, und elf davon waren über 75 Jahre alt. Von den insgesamt 107 Patienten, über die ROOK und WADDINGTON, BRENNAN und MONTGOMERY, SNEDDON und CHURCH, STEIGLEDER sowie HERZBERG berichten, waren beim Beginn der Krankheit 87, d.h. 81%, über 60 Jahre alt. Gelegentlich kann aber das bullöse Pemphigoid bei jüngeren Erwachsenen auftreten: Einer unter den von LEVER (1953) berichteten Patienten war 26 Jahre alt, einer unter ROOK und WADDINGTONs Patienten war in den zwanziger Jahren, und unter BRENNAN und MONTGOMERYs Patienten waren drei unter 40 Jahre alt.

Tabelle 2. *Differentialdiagnose zwischen Pemphigus vulgaris und bullösem Pemphigoid*

	Pemphigus vulgaris	Bullöses Pemphigoid
Art der Blase	schlaff, gewöhnlich klein	prall, oft groß
Epitheldefekte	ausgedehnt, wegen peripherer Ausdehnung	klein, keine periphere Ausdehnung
Heilen der Epitheldefekte	schlecht	gut
Beginn im Munde	58%	10%
Häufigkeit von Mundschleimhauterscheinungen	100%	33%
Schwere der Mundschleimhauterscheinungen	schwer	leicht
Einbeziehung des Lippenrots	häufig	sehr selten
Jüdische Rasse	67%	6%
Durchschnittsalter beim Beginn	54 Jahre	65 Jahre (bei Erwachsenen)
Vorkommen im Kindesalter	nein	ja (9%)
Sterblichkeit vor ACTH und Corticosteroiden	alle Altersgruppen: 94% bis zu 65 Jahren: 93% über 65 Jahren: 100%	alle Altersgruppen: 24% bis zu 65 Jahren: 0% über 65 Jahren: 57%
Histologie	Acantholyse; Blasen bilden sich intraepidermal, gewöhnlich suprabasal	keine Acantholyse; Blasen bilden sich subepidermal
Serumchemie		
Albumin	stark vermindert	etwas vermindert
Natrium	stark vermindert	normal oder etwas vermindert
Chloride	stark vermindert	normal oder etwas vermindert

Die in Prozent angegebenen Zahlen beziehen sich auf die in Tabelle 1 (S. 613) angeführten Patienten.

d) Verlauf

Das bullöse Pemphigoid ist eine chronische Krankheit, die aber in ihrer Dauer begrenzt ist. Die Dauer kann sich von einigen Monaten bis zu mehreren Jahren erstrecken. Die längste Dauer, die von Lever (1953) berichtet wurde, war 8 Jahre, zu welcher Zeit der Patient an einer anderen Krankheit verstarb. Gewöhnlich beginnt das bullöse Pemphigoid allmählich; und manchmal bleibt es vor der Disseminierung für mehrere Monate auf einige Stellen lokalisiert (Rook und Waddington; Prakken und Woerdeman). Während des Stadiums des generalisierten Befalls der Haut kann es zu Verbesserungen und Verschlimmerungen kommen; und gelegentlich kann, nachdem die Krankheit monatelang oder selbst jahrelang in einer Remission war, ein Rückfall einsetzen. Meistens ist jedoch solch ein Rückfall nicht so schwer wie der erste Anfall. Die allgemeine Gesundheit ist gewöhnlich nicht besonders angegriffen, außer bei alten Patienten und in besonders schweren Fällen.

Die *Prognose* beim bullösen Pemphigoid war bereits vor der Erhältlichkeit der Corticosteroide bei Kindern und bei jungen Erwachsenen gut. Dagegen war die Sterblichkeit bei alten Patienten ziemlich hoch, und selbst bei Behandlung mit den Corticosteroiden kann gelegentlich der Tod eintreten. Jedoch ist mit wenigen Ausnahmen das bullöse Pemphigoid an sich keine tödliche Krankheit (Prakken und Woerdeman). Die häufigsten Todesursachen bei alten Patienten sind Allgemeinschwächung und Komplikationen, wie z.B. Bronchopneumonie.

Die Sterblichkeit unter den vor Erhältlichkeit der Corticosteroide gesehenen Patienten war wie folgend: Lever (1953) berichtete, daß unter 30 erwachsenen Patienten acht, d.h. 27%, starben, während sie im aktiven Stadium ihrer Krankheit waren, und daß elf, d.h. 37%, an anderen Ursachen starben. Brennan und Montgomery stellten fest, daß keiner ihrer 20 Patienten an den Folgen des bullösen Pemphigoids starb, wohl aber fünf an anderen Ursachen.

ROOK und WADDINGTON berichteten eine Sterblichkeit von 32%, da zwölf ihrer 38 Patienten verstarben; und unter den elf von SNEDDON und CHURCH beobachteten Patienten starben sieben, d.h. 64%. (Betreffs Sterblichkeit bei den mit Corticosteroiden behandelten Patienten s. unter Behandlung, S. 674.)

Daß das bullöse Pemphigoid gewöhnlich eine Krankheit von begrenzter Dauer ist, geht daraus hervor, daß bei vielen überlebenden Patienten die Hauterscheinungen abheilen und

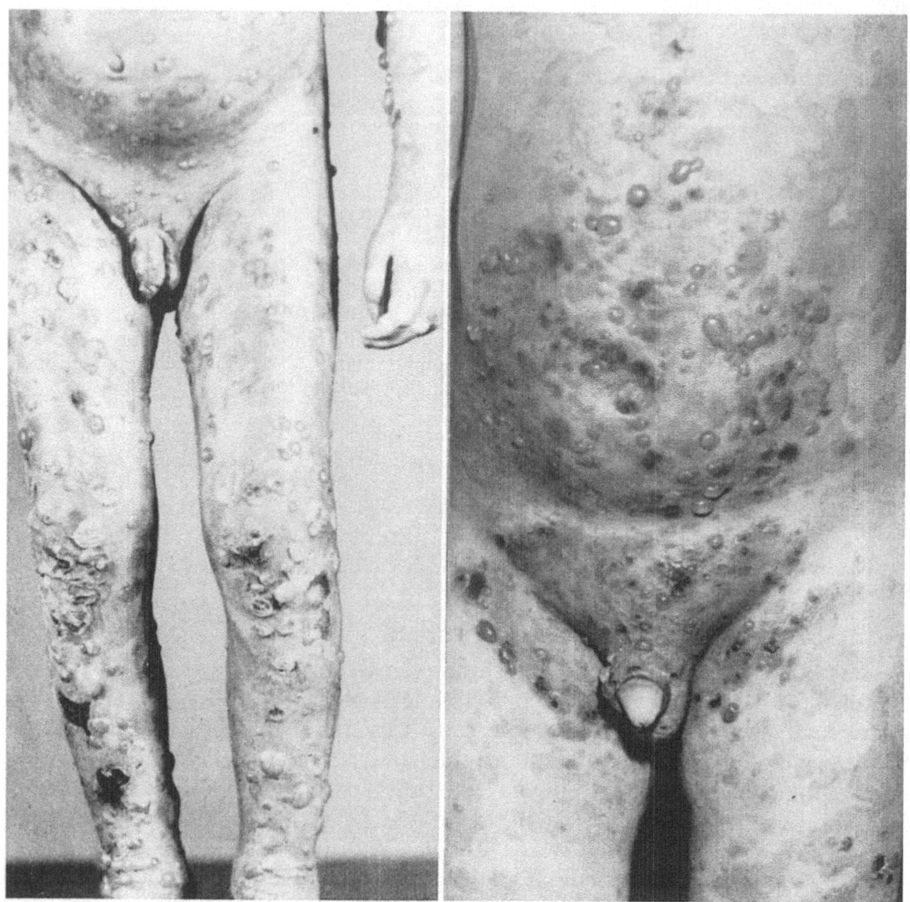

Abb. 40. Bullöses Pemphigoid. Zwei Kinder. Der Junge auf der rechten Seite zeigt nicht nur Blasen, sondern auch erythematöse Flächen mit zentraler Aufhellung

auch nicht wiederkehren. LEVER (1953) berichtete, daß von 33 vor Erhältlichkeit der Corticosteroide beobachteten Patienten 14 am Leben waren und unter diesen elf keine Krankheitserscheinungen mehr aufwiesen. Die Krankheit hatte bei diesen elf Patienten von 3—38 Monate gedauert, im Durchschnitt 15 Monate. BRENNAN und MONTGOMERY stellten fest, daß unter ihren 20 Patienten 15 noch am Leben waren und diese 15 Patienten bereits von 8 Monaten bis zu 30 Jahren keine Hauterscheinungen mehr gehabt hatten. Unter den 38 von ROOK und WADDINGTON beobachteten Patienten waren acht von einem bis zu 5 Jahren erscheinungsfrei; unter den elf Patienten, über die SNEDDON und CHURCH berichteten, waren vier Patienten bereits von 8 Monaten bis zu 2 Jahren erscheinungsfrei; und unter den 15 Kindern, die KIM und WINKELMANN unter Beobachtung hatten, wurden zehn erscheinungsfrei.

e) Histologie

Wie schon während der histologischen Beschreibung des Pemphigus betont wurde, ist es bei der histologischen Untersuchung aller Blasen äußerst wichtig, daß eine frische Blase gewählt wird, die nicht älter als 24 Std ist und die klein genug ist, so daß sie in ihrer Gesamtheit, möglichst mit etwas umgebender Haut, excidiert werden kann.

Die frühesten Veränderungen beim bullösen Pemphigoid bestehen gewöhnlich aus der Bildung zahlreicher subepidermaler Mikrovacuolen (Abb. 41) (RITZENFELD). Solche Mikrovacuolen kann man oft auch in der an die Blasen angrenzende Haut finden. In ihrem frühesten Stadium sind diese Mikrovacuolen kleiner als die Grundfläche einer Basalzelle und liegen zwischen den cytoplasmischen Fortsätzen der Basalzellen. Durch Zusammenfließen der Mikrovacuolen bilden sich große Vacuolen in subepidermaler Lage (Abb. 42), und aus diesen subepidermale Blasen.

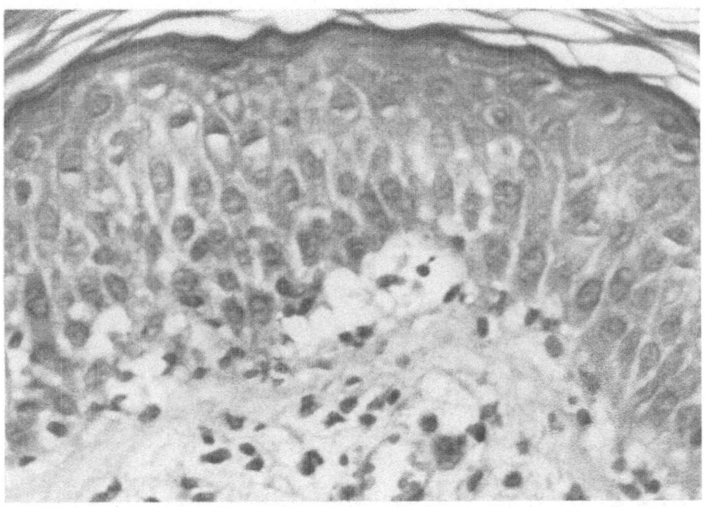

Abb. 41. Bullöses Pemphigoid. Als früheste Veränderung bilden sich zahlreiche subepidermale Mikrovacuolen (400mal)

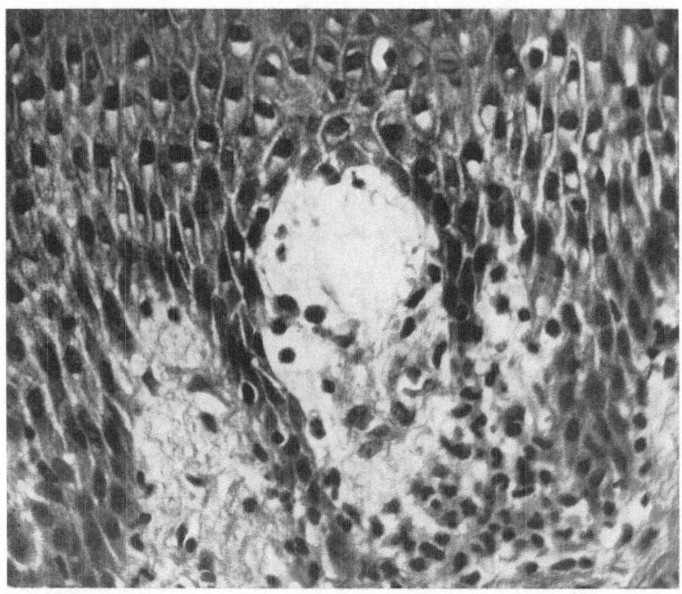

Abb. 42. Bullöses Pemphigoid. Durch Zusammenfließen von Mikrovacuolen bilden sich große Vacuolen in subepidermaler Lage (400mal)

Frische Blasen liegen vollständig subepidermal (Abb. 43), mit der Ausnahme, daß sich gelegentlich Stümpfe von Haarfollikeln oder Schweißdrüsen am Blasenboden befinden. Jedoch schon bei Blasen, die 2 Tage alt sind, kann man Anzeichen

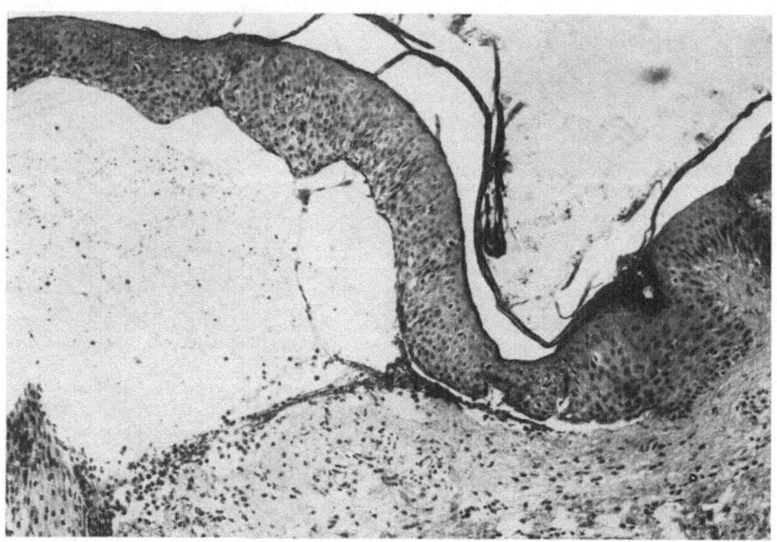

Abb. 43. Bullöses Pemphigoid. Teil einer vollständig subepidermal gelegenen Blase, die in eine subepidermale Spalte ausläuft (100mal)

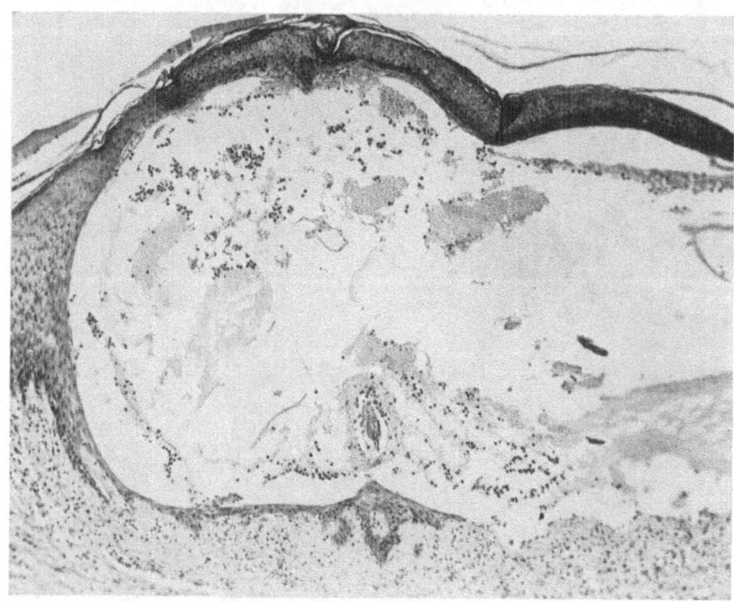

Abb. 44. Bullöses Pemphigoid. Die Blase ist in der Mitte subepidermal, an der Peripherie aber intraepidermal gelegen. Mehrere Zellagen liegen dort der Dermis auf und es besteht keine Acantholyse (100mal)

einer Regeneration der Epidermis am Blasenboden finden, besonders an der Peripherie der Blase, aber auch ausgehend von den Adnexstümpfen. Während dieses Regenerationsvorganges können die Blasen an der Peripherie intraepidermal, in der Mitte aber subepidermal gelegen sein (Abb. 44). Wenn die Regeneration am Blasenboden vollendet ist, befindet sich die Blase vollständig in intraepidermaler Lage, obwohl sie sich subepidermal gebildet hat. Es ist daher sehr wichtig, nicht die Lage einer Blase mit dem Ort der Blasenbildung gleichzusetzen. Eine Unterscheidung solcher intraepidermal gelegener Blasen von den Blasen des Pemphigus vulgaris ist gewöhnlich leicht, da sich meistens mehr als eine Zellage am Blasenboden befindet und die Basalzellen, wie in normaler Epidermis, miteinander durch Intercellularbrücken verbunden sind.

Die abgelöste Epidermis erscheint in frischen, intakten Blasen gewöhnlich normal, mit Ausnahme von etwas intercellulärem Ödem. In älteren Blasen zeigen allerdings die Zellen der abgelösten Epidermis oft beträchtliche Nekrose (Abb. 45).

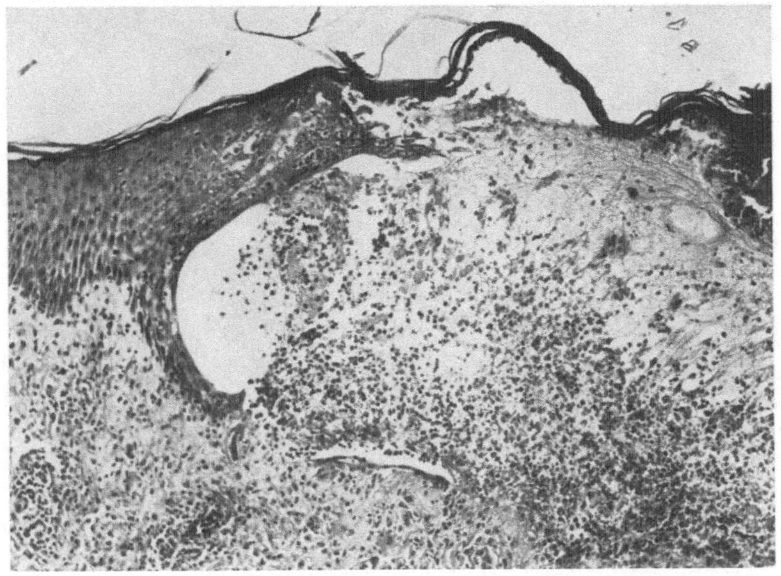

Abb. 45. Bullöses Pemphigoid. Teil einer subepidermal gelegenen Blase. Die abgehobene Epidermis hat bis auf die Hornzellenschicht Nekrose erlitten (100mal)

Während diese Nekrose vor sich geht, können einzelne Zellen sich ablösen und können dann als acantholytische Zellen in der Blasenhöhlung vorgefunden werden; aber diese Zellen zeigen ausgesprochenere Nekrose als die acantholytischen Zellen in den Blasen des Pemphigus vulgaris. (Dies stellt eine sekundäre Acantholyse dar, bei der die Acantholyse eine Folge der Blasenbildung und nicht die Ursache der Blasenbildung ist.)

Der Inhalt der Blasen besteht, abgesehen von vereinzelten nekrotischen Epidermiszellen, aus einem Fibrinnetzwerk und einer unterschiedlichen Anzahl von Zellen, hauptsächlich Eosinophile, aber auch Neutrophile und Lymphocyten. Die in der Dermis vorgefunden Änderungen hängen davon ab, ob die Probeexcision an einer Blase durchgeführt wurde, die auf normal aussehender Haut gelegen war, oder an einer, die sich auf einer erythematösen Fläche befand. Im ersteren Falle findet man in der Dermis lediglich ein geringes perivasculäres Zellinfiltrat, das aus Lymphocytes und Eosinophilen besteht. Andererseits, bei Probeexcisionen von erythematösen Flächen, finden sich oft beträchtliche Veränderungen in der Dermis. Die oberflächlichen Gefäße können dann Anzeichen einer Vasculitis zeigen, nämlich Anschwellen und Zerfall von Endothelzellen, und ein beträchtliches, perivasculär angeordnetes Zellinfiltrat, das aus Neutrophilen, Eosinophilen und

Lymphocyten besteht und in dem infolge des Zerfalls von Neutrophilen verstreute Kernfragmente zu finden sind. Das Infiltrat kann sich auch in die obersten Lagen der Dermis zur Blasenhöhle hin sowie in die Umgebung der Blase ausdehnen. Gelegentlich findet man dann, ähnlich wie bei der Dermatitis herpetiformis, Ansammlungen von Neutrophilen und Eosinophilen innerhalb von Papillen (Abb. 46) (s. unter Differentialdiagnose, S. 673, und unter Dermatitis herpetiformis, S. 703).

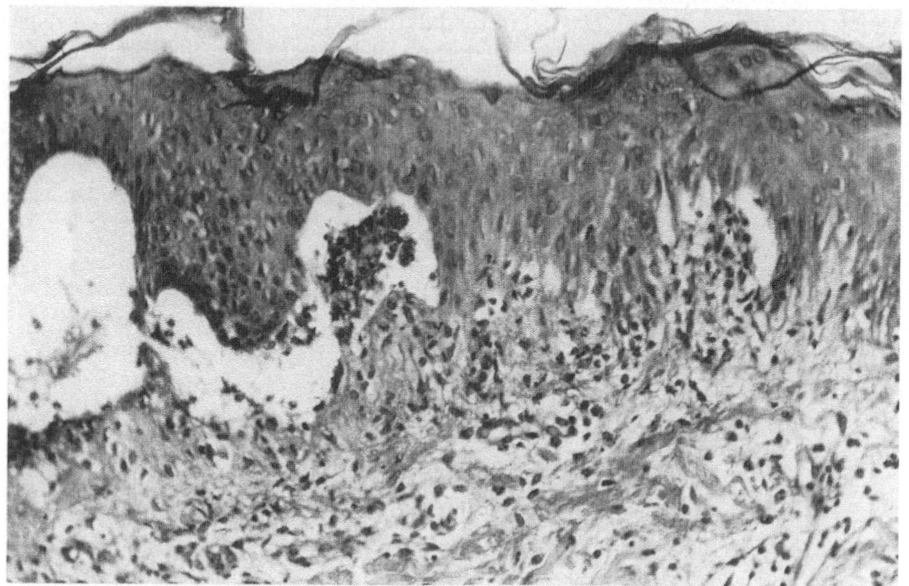

Abb. 46. Bullöses Pemphigoid. Am Rande einer Blase befinden sich subepidermale Vacuolen sowie Papillen, die Ansammlungen von Neutrophilen und Eosinophilen enthalten (200mal)

f) Histochemie

Der PAS-positive Grenzstreifen zeigt Veränderungen während der Zeit der Blasenbildung. Im frühesten Stadium, wenn Mikrovacuolen zugegen sind, ist der Grenzstreifen oft aufgesplittert, so daß die Mikrovacuolen teils unterhalb und teils oberhalb des Grenzstreifens liegen (Ritzenfeld; Rupec et al.). Im Stadium der Blasenbildung kann der Grenzstreifen verdünnt sein, besonders wenn Ödem vorliegt, und bei Vorhandensein eines Zellfiltrates kann er sogar fehlen (Achten und Corbusier-Ledoux). Wenn sich die Blase dann vergrößert, bildet sich der Grenzstreifen neu und in Blasen, die groß genug sind, um klinisch sichtbar zu sein, findet man ihn am Blasenboden der Dermis anliegend (Piérard, Dupont und Fontaine; Piérard und Whimster).

g) Polarisationsmikroskopie

Wie schon bei der Beschreibung des Pemphigus vulgaris festgestellt wurde, fanden sowohl Nelemans et al. als auch Nieuwmeijer bei ihren Untersuchungen mittels des Polarisationsmikroskops, daß beim bullösen Pemphigoid, im Gegensatz zum Pemphigus vulgaris, die Tonofibrillen in den Epidermiszellen gut erhalten waren. In der Nähe von Blasen erschienen sie in die Länge gezogen und stärker doppelbrechend als normalerweise.

h) Elektronenmikroskopie

Im Gegensatz zum Pemphigus vulgaris befinden sich nach den Untersuchungen von Charles und von Caulfied und Wilgram die frühesten Veränderungen nicht in der Epidermis, sondern in der Dermis (Abb. 47). Dort sieht man außer

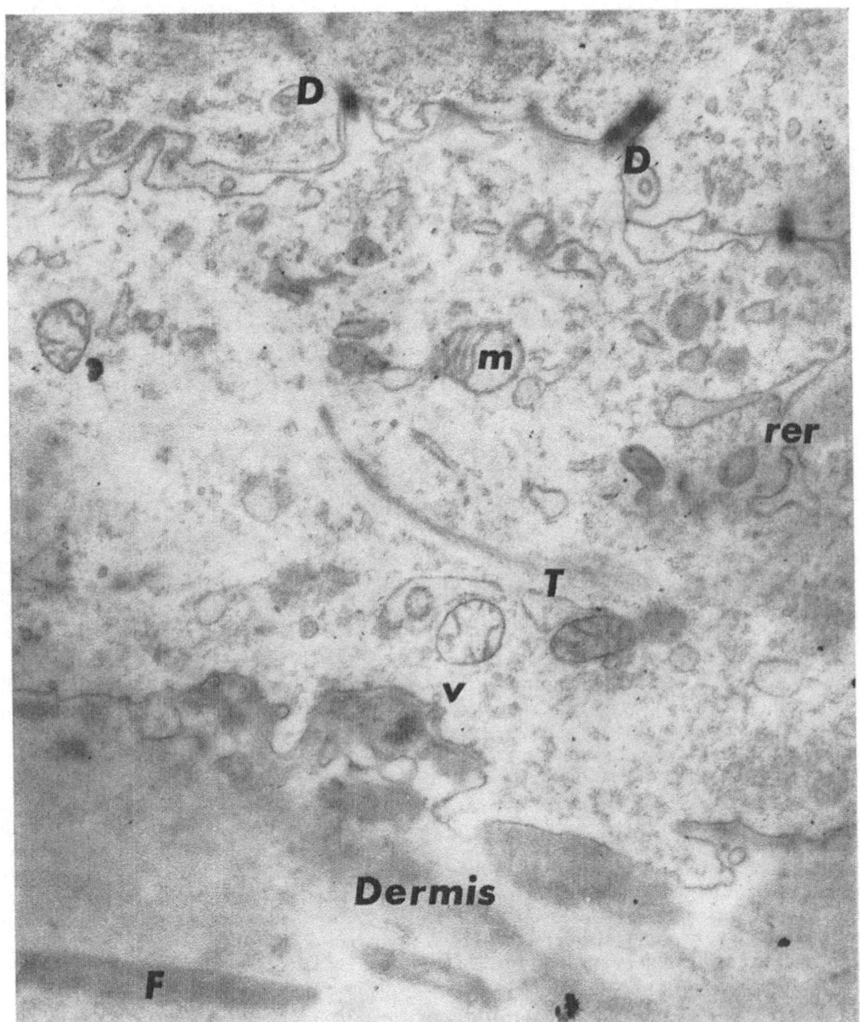

Abb. 47. Bullöses Pemphigoid. In einem Gebiet, das nahe einer subepidermalen Blase gelegen ist, zeigt die Dermis beträchtliches Ödem und enthält eine fibrinoide Substanz, die teils diffus und teils in Aggregaten (*F*) vorhanden ist. Die Basalmembran und die Halbdesmosomen sind verschwunden. Der basale Rand der hier gezeigten Basalzelle weist einige pinocytotische Bläschen (*v*) auf. Sonst sieht die Basalzelle normal aus mit unbeschädigten Zellbestandteilen, wie Desmosomen (*D*), Mitochondrien (*m*), Tonofilamenten (*T*) und endoplasmischem Reticulum (*rer*) (23000mal)

Ödem und einem Zellinfiltrat zwischen den Kollagenfibrillen und Kollagenbündeln Proteinpräcipitate. Diese Präcipitate zeigen, wenn längs geschnitten, eine Periodizität von 220 Å und stellen somit Fibrin dar. Auf die Veränderungen in der Dermis folgen solche in der Basalmembran und in den Basalzellen.

Die Veränderungen an der Basalmembran stellen wohl den auffälligsten Befund beim bullösen Pemphigoid dar. Die Basalmembran kann verdickt oder verwaschen erscheinen und kann sogar Unterbrechungen aufweisen oder an einigen Stellen fehlen. Bereits bevor sich eine Blase gebildet hat, können im Cytoplasma der Basalzellen degenerative Änderungen vorhanden sein, besonders eine Schwellung der Mitochondria und ein Schwinden der Tonofilamente, der Desmosomen wie auch der Halbdesmosomen, die die Basalzellen mit der Basalmembran verbinden. Wo sich eine Blase gebildet hat, bleibt die Basalmembran auf der Dermis liegen und bildet somit den Blasenboden. Obwohl sich bei Bildung der Blase die Basalzellen gewöhnlich vollständig von der Basalmembran ablösen, bleibt doch gelegentlich der untere Teil der Zellmembran und etwas Cytoplasma der Basalzellen an der Basalmembran hängen. Während der Reepithelisierung des Blasenbodens erscheint die Basalmembran oft aus mehreren Schichten zusammengesetzt.

i) Nosologische Stellung des bullösen Pemphigoids

Das bullöse Pemphigoid zeigt im klinischen Bilde gewisse Ähnlichkeiten mit dem Pemphigus vulgaris, der Dermatitis herpetiformis und dem Erythema exsudativum multiforme. Bevor es als eine selbständige Krankheit aufgestellt wurde, war es im allgemeinen von den anglo-sächsischen und deutschen Dermatologen mit dem Pemphigus vulgaris identifiziert, von den französischen Dermatologen aber mit der Dermatitis herpetiformis.

Gegen einen Zusammenhang zwischen dem *Pemphigus vulgaris* und dem bullösen Pemphigoid spricht vor allem die Spezifität der Acantholyse. Besonders elektronenmikroskopische Untersuchungen machen es schwer vorstellbar, daß zwei so grundverschiedene Vorgänge, wie die intraepidermal-acantholytische Blasenbildung und die subepidermale Blasenbildung, dieselbe oder ineinander übergehende Krankheiten hervorbringen könnten. So gibt es dann auch in der Literatur keinen gesicherten Fall, bei dem die beiden Arten von Blasen nebeneinander bestanden.

Nur zwei Autoren haben über Patienten mit beiden Arten von Blasen berichtet, nämlich Fisher und Hellier. Was Fisher betrifft, berichtete er 1956 das gleichzeitige Vorkommen von acantholytischen und nicht-acantholytischen Blasen bei sechs Patienten und lehnte daraufhin den Begriff des bullösen Pemphigoids ab. Jedoch erwähnte er in einer Besprechung des Pemphigus 6 Jahre später diese Befunde nicht mehr, sondern betrachtete Acantholyse als das Kennzeichen des Pemphigus vulgaris. Möglicherweise hatte Fisher denselben Vorgang beobachtet, über den Haber 1957 berichtete. Haber hatte bei drei Patienten mit Pemphigus vulgaris je einmal intraepidermal gelegene Blasen ohne Acantholyse angetroffen, während andere Probeexcisionen typische Acantholyse gezeigt hatten. Das Fehlen von Acantholyse in solchen Fällen kommt wahrscheinlich daher, daß die Blasen sich im Stadium der Regeneration befanden. Durch Probeexcisionen frischer Blasen kann solch eine Verwirrung stiftende Situation vermieden werden. In dem von Hellier berichteten Falle hatte der Patient nacheinander zwei verschiedene Krankheiten. Erst hatte der Patient mehrere akute Ausbrüche von Erythema exsudativum multiforme, und später entstand ein Pemphigus foliaceus.

Eine Erörterung des Zusammenhanges zwischen *Dermatitis herpetiformis* und bullösem Pemphigoid erfordert zunächst eine Definierung der Dermatitis herpetiformis, da ja manche Dermatologen, besonders in Frankreich, den Begriff der Dermatitis herpetiformis weiter stecken als die meisten anglo-sächsischen und deutschen Dermatologen. Zu der Dermatitis herpetiformis im weiteren Sinne rechnen die französischen Dermatologen das bullöse Pemphigoid, das die bullöse Form der Dermatitis herpetiformis darstellen soll. Jedoch erscheint mir das Einbeziehen des bullösen Pemphigoids in die Dermatitis herpetiformis nicht gerechtfertigt, da zu viele Unterschiede zwischen der Dermatitis herpetiformis im engeren Sinne und dem bullösen Pemphigoid bestehen. (Für eine klinische Beschreibung der Dermatitis herpetiformis im engeren Sinne s. S. 701.)

Das bullöse Pemphigoid unterscheidet sich von der Dermatitis herpetiformis durch die folgenden klinischen Merkmale: 1. Überwiegen von großen Blasen, die gelegentlich hämorrhagisch aussehen; 2. Prädilektion der Blasen für Beugeflächen wie die Axillae, Leistenbeugen und Handgelenke; 3. wenig oder keine Gruppierung außer in stark befallenen Hautgebieten; 4. Mundschleimhauterscheinungen bei ungefähr einem Drittel der Fälle; 5. bevorzugtes Vorkommen bei alten Leuten und Kindern; und 6. wenig oder kein Ansprechen auf Sulfapyridin oder auf die Sulfone. Auch ist in der Mehrzahl der Fälle das bullöse Pemphigoid von begrenzter Dauer und heilt spontan nach einigen Jahren ab, während die Dermatitis herpetiformis äußerst langdauernd ist und in vielen Fällen nie abheilt. Gelegentlich sind bei einem Patienten mit bullösem Pemphigoid, bei dem zuerst eine generalisierte Aussaat von Blasen bestand, im späteren Stadium nur noch vereinzelte Bläschen vorhanden, die einer Dermatitis herpetiformis ähnlich sehen; aber solche Patienten sprechen auf die Sulfone nicht an. (Für einen therapeutischen Test sind, besonders bei alten Leuten, die Sulfone vorzuziehen, da das Sulfapyridin eine schon bestehende Niereninsuffizienz oft verschlimmert; s. S. 709.)

Eine histologische Unterscheidung zwischen der Dermatitis herpetiformis und dem bullösen Pemphigoid ist nicht immer möglich. Wenn aber frische Blasen zusammen mit etwas an die Blase angrenzender Haut excidiert werden und in zweifelhaften Fällen mehrere solche Excisionen vorgenommen werden, kann eine Unterscheidung meistens getroffen werden; denn die für die Dermatitis herpetiformis typischen intrapapillären Mikroabscesse (s. S. 703) werden beim bullösen Pemphigoid nur selten angetroffen. Manche Autoren, wie PIÉRARD et al., RUPEC et al. und MACVICAR et al., haben sie nie beim bullösen Pemphigoid beobachtet, während JABLONSKA und CHORZELSKI sie bei vier Patienten mit bullösem Pemphigoid auffanden. Meine Erfahrung geht dahin, daß beim bullösen Pemphigoid die Untersuchung von Blasen, die auf erythematösen Flächen gelegen sind, gelegentlich intrapapilläre Ansammlungen von Neutrophilen und Eosinophilen ergeben kann.

In bezug auf einen Zusammenhang zwischen dem *Erythema exsudativum multiforme* und dem bullösen Pemphigoid ist darauf hinzuweisen, daß der Unterschied weniger in der Morphologie als im Verlauf liegt; denn das Erythema exsudativum multiforme ist im Gegensatz zum bullösen Pemphigoid eine akut verlaufende Krankheit, die plötzlich beginnt und binnen weniger Wochen entweder mit dem Tode oder mit Heilung endet. Was die Morphologie betrifft, gibt es kein klinisches oder histologisches Merkmal beim bullösen Pemphigoid, das nicht auch beim Erythema exsudativum multiforme vorkommt; denn auch das Erythema exsudativum multiforme weist oft außer großen, klaren Blasen flächenhafte Erytheme und nicht selten hämorrhagisch aussehende Blasen auf.

Auch ist eine histologische Unterscheidung des Erythema exsudativum multiforme vom bullösen Pemphigoid gewöhnlich nicht möglich (PIÉRARD, DUPONT und FONTAINE; PIÉRARD und WHIMSTER). Wenn Unterschiede bestehen, sind sie lediglich graduell und kommen bei solchen Fällen von Erythema exsudativum multiforme vor, die mit ausgesprocheneren Entzündungserscheinungen verlaufen, als sie beim bullösen Pemphigoid vorkommen. Solche Fälle von Erythema exsudativum multiforme zeigen im Vergleich zum bullösen Pemphigoid: 1. eine schwerere Vasculitis mit Extravasaten von Erythrocyten; 2. mehr Lymphocyten als Eosinophile; 3. in Hautgebieten ohne Blasen Einwandern von Lymphocyten in die Epidermis mit Spongiose und intraepidermalen spongiotischen Blasen und 4. in Hautgebieten mit Blasen Nekrose der Epidermis, schon bevor sich die Epidermis von der Dermis abgelöst hat.

Da sich also das Erythema exsudativum multiforme vom bullösen Pemphigoid eigentlich nur durch seine Dauer unterscheidet, ist es möglich, daß das bullöse Pemphigoid die chronische Form derjenigen Krankheit darstellt, die bei akutem

Verlauf Erythema exsudativum multiforme genannt wird (LEVER 1957). Das Erythema exsudativum multiforme gehört, wie OSLER bereits 1904 feststellte, zu der sog. Erythema-Gruppe von Krankheiten, zusammen mit Urticaria, Erythema nodosum und anaphylaktoider Purpura. Die letzteren drei Krankheiten können akut oder chronisch verlaufen. Es erscheint daher möglich, daß es eine chronische Form des Erythema exsudativum multiforme gibt, das unter dem Bilde des bullösen Pemphigoids verläuft. Da allerdings zur Zeit kein Lehrbuch der Dermatologie eine chronische Form des Erythema exsudativum multiforme anerkennt, scheint es am besten, das bullöse Pemphigoid nicht mit einer anderen Krankheit zu identifizieren, sondern es als eine wesenseigene Erkrankung anzusehen.

j) Laboratoriumsbefunde

Die chemischen Veränderungen im Blutserum sind beim bullösen Pemphigoid zwar denen, die beim Pemphigus vulgaris vorkommen, ähnlich, doch sind sie bedeutend geringer im Ausmaß und waren auch schon damals geringer, als die Corticosteroide noch nicht erhältlich waren (LEVER 1950; LEVER, HURLEY und BLANEY). Insbesondere entwickelte sich nie eine so ausgesprochene Hypalbuminämie wie beim Pemphigus vulgaris, da ausgedehnte Epitheldefekte beim bullösen Pemphigoid nicht vorkommen. Während bei sieben Patienten mit Pemphigus vulgaris die niedrigsten elektrophoretischen Albuminwerte im Durchschnitt nur 1,17 gm/100 cm^3 Serum betrugen (verglichen mit einem Normalwert von 3,74 gm), belief sich bei sieben Patienten mit bullösem Pemphigoid der Durchschnitt der niedrigsten Albuminwerte auf 2,80 gm/100 cm^3 Serum (LEVER 1953). Ebenfalls war die Erniedrigung des Natriums im Serum nicht erheblich. Während bei neun von elf Patienten mit Pemphigus vulgaris die Werte unter 131 mEq./L. Serum lagen (verglichen mit einem Normalwert von 140 mEq./L.), hatte keiner der Patienten mit bullösem Pemphigoid einen Wert unter 131 mEq./L. (TALBOTT, LEVER und CONSOLAZIO; LEVER 1953).

Die Zahl der Eosinophilen ist beim bullösen Pemphigoid recht unterschiedlich. Bei manchen Patienten findet man recht hohe Werte, während andere eine mäßige oder auch keine Erhöhung zeigen. Eine ausgesprochene Eosinophilie, d.h. über 20% Eosinophile unter den weißen Blutkörperchen, findet sich beim bullösen Pemphigoid viel häufiger als beim Pemphigus vulgaris. So wurden bei zehn von 41 am bullösen Pemphigoid Erkrankten im Blute über 20% Eosinophile gefunden, beim Pemphigus vulgaris dagegen bei nur einem von 35 Patienten (LEVER 1953).

Die Gesamteiweißkonzentration ist beim bullösen Pemphigoid wie beim Pemphigus vulgaris niedriger in der Blasenflüssigkeit als im entsprechenden Blutserum (LEVER und TALBOTT; LEVER 1950; BURBACH). Bei elektrophoretischer Bestimmung der einzelnen in der Blasenflüssigkeit vorhandenen Proteinfraktionen ergibt sich, daß beim bullösen Pemphigoid wie beim Pemphigus vulgaris die relative Konzentration der einzelnen Proteinfraktionen in der Blasenflüssigkeit der relativen Konzentration im entsprechenden Blutserum sehr ähnlich ist; aber wie beim Pemphigus vulgaris ist gewöhnlich die relative Konzentration des Albumins und des β_2-Globulins in der Blasenflüssigkeit etwas höher als im entsprechenden Blutserum (LEVER 1950 [II]).

k) Behandlung

Das bullöse Pemphigoid spricht auf die Behandlung mit Corticosteroiden gut an.

Die erste Serie von elf behandelten Patienten teilte LEVER 1953 mit. Von diesen waren drei bereits seit 8, 10 bzw. 12 Monaten ohne Behandlung erscheinungsfrei, drei hatten zwar einige Krankheitsherde, bedurften aber keiner Behandlung, vier waren noch unter Behandlung und ein Patient war an einer anderen Krankheit verstorben.

PRAKKEN und WOERDEMAN behandelten 19 Patienten. Von diesen starben drei, die alle in hohem Alter waren, während die anderen auf die Behandlung gut ansprachen.

STEVENSON berichtete 1960 über die Behandlung von 68 Patienten mit bullösem Pemphigoid. Auf Grund der Behandlungsergebnisse teilte er seine Patienten in drei Gruppen. In der ersten Gruppe, zu der 30 Patienten gehörten, konnte die Behandlung wegen Eintretens einer Remission abgesetzt werden. Bei 23 dieser Patienten betrug die Behandlungsdauer weniger als ein Jahr, bei 4 Patienten ungefähr zwei Jahre und bei 3 Patienten über drei Jahre. Die eingetretene Remission war vollständig bei 25 Patienten, während 5 Patienten gelegentlich einige Hauterscheinungen aufwiesen. Vier dieser 30 Patienten waren an anderen Krankheiten verstorben. In der zweiten Gruppe, die 32 der 68 Patienten umfaßte, konnte die Behandlung mit Corticosteroiden nicht abgesetzt werden. Sieben von diesen Patienten standen bereits länger als vier Jahre unter Behandlung, 11 länger als zwei Jahre und 14 weniger als zwei Jahre. Alle sprachen auf die Behandlung an; jedoch waren 10 der 32 Patienten gestorben, 2 davon an Behandlungskomplikationen und 8 an anderen Krankheiten. Eine dritte Gruppe von 6 Patienten sprach auf die Behandlung mit Corticosteroiden in den verabreichten Dosen nicht besonders an, aber 4 von ihnen zeigten spontane Abheilung.

CHURCH teilte 1960 seine an 37 Patienten erhaltenen Behandlungsergebnisse mit. Von diesen waren 4 kurz nach ihrer Aufnahme in das Krankenhaus gestorben, bevor eine wesentliche Besserung eingetreten war, 12 waren an anderen Krankheiten gestorben, während sie keine oder nur wenige Hauterscheinungen hatten, 18 waren erscheinungsfrei, bedurften aber noch Erhaltungsdosen (die bereits bis zu sieben Jahren gegeben worden waren), und 3 Patienten waren ohne Behandlung erscheinungsfrei. Von diesen 3 Patienten war einer bereits vier Jahre lang erscheinungsfrei, nachdem er für sechs Monate behandelt worden war, und 2 waren seit zwei Jahren erscheinungsfrei, nachdem sie für drei Jahre, bzw. zehn Monate, behandelt worden waren. CHURCH kam zu dem Schluß, daß die Behandlung mit Corticosteroiden den Verlauf des bullösen Pemphigoids derart geändert hat, daß es nicht mehr eine chronische, qualvolle und oft tödliche Krankheit darstellt, sondern eine, bei der die Hauterscheinungen binnen weniger Wochen unter Kontrolle gebracht werden können und die, wenn sie im Anfangsstadium behandelt wird, nicht einmal eine Krankenhausaufnahme mehr erforderlich macht. CHURCH schlug vor, zu Beginn der Behandlung ziemlich hohe Dosen zu verabreichen, z.B. 60 mg Prednison pro Tag.

Behandlungsplan. Die Behandlung mit Corticosteroiden ist bei fast jedem Patienten mit bullösem Pemphigoid indiziert. Bei alten Patienten ist, wenn keine wichtigen Kontraindikationen bestehen, die Behandlung trotz des mit der Behandlung verbundenen Risikos ratsam, da bei alten Leuten die Sterblichkeit infolge von Komplikationen des bullösen Pemphigoids ziemlich hoch ist. Bei jüngeren Patienten ist die Behandlung mit Corticosteroiden wegen der schnell damit verbundenen Besserung ratsam. Im allgemeinen ist es nicht nötig, die Corticosteroide in so hohen Dosen und für eine so lange Zeit zu verabreichen wie beim Pemphigus vulgaris oder Pemphigus foliaceus. Bei Patienten mit nicht zu ausgedehntem Befall kann man mit einer Tagesdosis von 16 Tabletten Prednison (80 mg) beginnen oder mit einer äquivalenten Dosis eines der anderen Corticosteroide (s. S. 657). Bei Patienten mit schweren Hauterscheinungen sollten 24 oder selbst 36 Tabletten pro Tag eingenommen werden, bis keine neuen Blasen mehr auftreten. Danach kann dann die Tagesdosis auf 16 Tabletten Prednison herabgesetzt werden. Im Gegensatz zum Pemphigus vulgaris, bei dem hohe Dosen für mindestens 8 Wochen gegeben werden sollten, um Rückfälle zu vermeiden, kann man beim bullösen Pemphigoid die Tagesdosis reduzieren, sobald gutes Abheilen eingesetzt hat; denn eine lang ausgedehnte Behandlung mit hohen Dosen stellt beim bullösen Pemphigoid ein größeres Risiko dar als die Krankheit selbst. Die Herabsetzung der Tagesdosis unter 16 Tabletten Prednison pro Tag sollte in „logarithmischer Weise" geschehen, d.h. erst schnell und dann um so langsamer, je kleiner die Tagesdosis wird (s. auch S. 658). Auf diese Weise wird die Erhaltungsdosis ausfindig gemacht. Bei der Herabsetzung der Tagesdosis kann man z.B. folgendermaßen vorgehen: 8 Tabletten für eine Woche, dann 6 Tabletten für zwei Wochen, 5 Tabletten für drei Wochen, 4 Tabletten für vier Wochen; 3 Tabletten für acht Wochen und hiernach 2 Tabletten. Zwar kann die Tagesdosis nicht bei jedem Patienten auf 3 oder gar 2 Tabletten erniedrigt werden;

aber selbst wenn die Erhaltungsdosis anfangs etwas höher liegen muß, sollte man alle zwei oder drei Monate versuchen, die Tagesdosis vielleicht um eine halbe Tablette herabzusetzen; denn das bullöse Pemphigoid ist ja eine in seiner Dauer begrenzte Krankheit. Zwecks Verhinderung von Nebenerscheinungen ist es ratsam, Methyltestosteron, Diäthylstilboestrol, Calciumgluconat und Tabletten, die die Magensäure neutralisieren, genau so wie beim Pemphigus vulgaris, zu geben (s. S. 659).

Was die Dosierung der Corticosteroide bei Kindern betrifft, sollte man bis zum Alter von 4 Jahren die Hälfte der für Erwachsene gültigen Dosis verabreichen; zwischen 5 und 8 Jahren zwei Drittel dieser Dosis und für ältere Kinder die volle Dosis.

In der Regel sind die Sulfone und das Sulfapyridin bei der Behandlung des bullösen Pemphigoids von wenig oder keinem Wert (Sneddon und Church; Kim und Winkelmann). Nur in Ausnahmefällen spricht das bullöse Pemphigoid auf sie an, wie Rook und Waddington berichtet haben. Darum lohnt sich ein Behandlungsversuch mit ihnen nicht, mit Ausnahme von solchen Fällen, die schwer von der Dermatitis herpetiformis abzutrennen sind. Im allgemeinen sind wegen der besseren Verträglichkeit die Sulfone dem Sulfapyridin für einen therapeutischen Test vorzuziehen (s. S. 673 und S. 708).

II. Benignes Schleimhautpemphigoid

Das benigne Schleimhautpemphigoid, das früher als Pemphigus conjunctivae bezeichnet wurde und jetzt gelegentlich auch vernarbendes Schleimhautpemphigoid genannt wird, stellt ein wesenseigenes Krankheitsbild dar, wie letzthin viele Autoren dargelegt haben (Lever 1942, 1944, 1953; Klauder und Cowan; Church und Sneddon; Jablonska et al. 1957; Lodin und Gentele; Degos, Lortat-Jacob und Hardy; Lortat-Jacob; McCarthy und Shklar).

Die auffallendsten Merkmale des benignen Schleimhautpemphigoids sind: 1. Bevorzugtes Auftreten an den Schleimhäuten, besonders der Bindehaut und Mundschleimhaut, 2. Neigung zu Narbenbildung und 3. ein chronischer und gewöhnlich gutartiger Verlauf. Die Schleimhäute sind fast immer befallen und in ungefähr einem Drittel der Fälle finden sich auch Hauterscheinungen. (Unter 30 persönlich beobachteten Patienten wiesen 13 Hauterscheinungen auf.) Narbenbildung findet sich stets, wenn die Bindehaut befallen ist. Vernarbung findet sich häufig auch an anderen Schleimhäuten und gelegentlich auf der Haut. Obwohl die Krankheit, wenn einmal entstanden, oft das ganze Leben hindurch andauert, kann sie doch nach vieljähriger Dauer zum Stillstand kommen.

a) Schleimhautveränderungen

Jede der hautnahen Schleimhäute kann erkranken. Dies schließt die Bindehaut und die Schleimhäute des Mundes, des Rachens, des Kehlkopfes, der Speiseröhre, der Nase, des Penis, der Vulva und des Afters ein. Die Erscheinungen an den Augen, im Munde, im Rachen und im Kehlkopf sind von Riecke beschrieben worden. Auch das Vorkommen von Speiseröhrenstrikturen ist kurz erwähnt. Nicht erwähnt dagegen sind die narbigen Veränderungen, die an den Genitalien und am After auftreten können.

Augenerscheinungen sind sehr häufig, aber doch nicht immer vorhanden; und gelegentlich sind nur die Augen befallen. Die Bindehautentzündung setzt langsam ein und schreitet nur allmählich fort. Im Anfang gleicht das klinische Bild dem einer einfachen Conjunctivitis; aber selbst in diesem Frühstadium kann man kleine fibröse Adhäsionen („Synechien“) zwischen der Bindehaut des Lides und der des Auges oder auch zwischen der Bindehaut des oberen Lides und der des unteren Lides feststellen (Abb. 48). Bläschen sieht man dabei nur sehr selten. Im Laufe der Zeit findet beträchtliche Vernarbung und Schrumpfung der Augenbindehaut statt, so daß die Conjunctivalsäcke schließlich völlig obliteriert werden (SCHRECK). Oft entwickelt sich allmählich ein Entropium, das zu einem Reiben

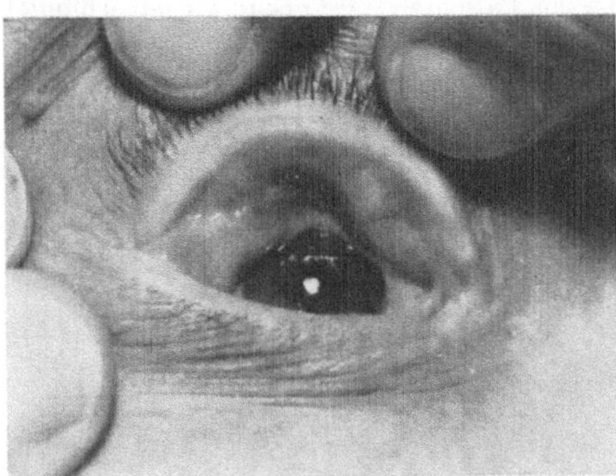

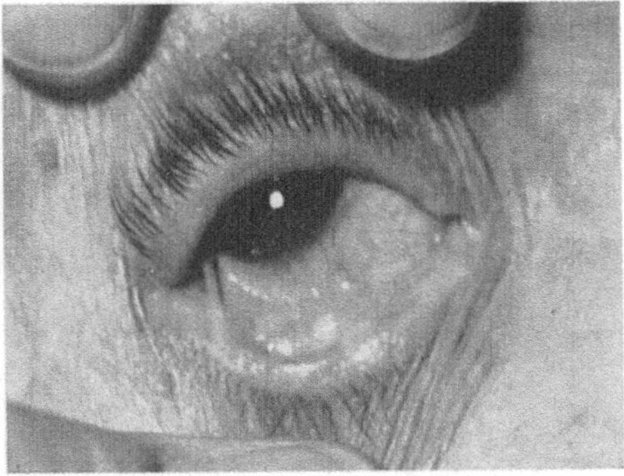

Abb. 48. Benignes Schleimhautpemphigoid. Frühstadium der Bindehauterkrankung. Die Bindehaut des oberen Lides zeigt diffuse Entzündung (links). Ein fribröses Band (Synechie) streckt sich von der Bindehaut des oberen Lides zur Bindehaut des unteren Lides

der Wimpern gegen die Hornhaut und somit zu Hornhautverletzungen führt. Mit der Zunahme der Adhäsionen zwischen der Bindehaut des Lides und der des Auges wachsen die Lider fest an das Auge an („Symblepharon“). Auch wachsen dann oft die Ecken der Lider zusammen, was eine Verengung der Lidspalten zur Folge hat („Ankyloblepharon“).

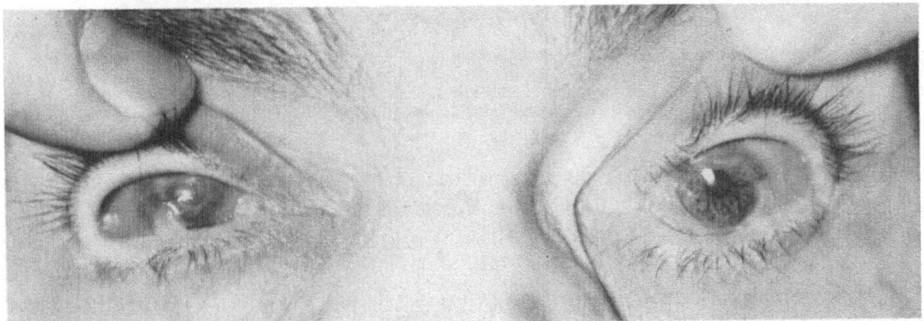

Abb. 49. Benignes Schleimhautpemphigoid. Fortschreitendes Stadium der Bindehauterkrankung. Ein Pannus erstreckt sich über die Cornea

Die Hornhaut kann auf vier verschiedene Weisen Schaden erleiden. Erstens kann die die Hornhaut umgebende Bindehautentzündung zu einer Gefäßeinwanderung in die Hornhaut und somit zu einer Trübung der Hornhaut führen; zweitens kann ein Pannus von der Bindehaut her über die Cornea wachsen (Abb. 49); drittens kann das Reiben von Wimpern gegen die Hornhaut dort Geschwürbildung und Trübungen hervorrufen; und viertens kann das Fehlen von Tränensekretion, hervorgerufen durch eine entzündliche Zerstörung der Tränendrüsen bzw. durch Obliterierung ihrer Ausführungsgänge, zu Xerosis und Degeneration der Hornhaut führen. Im Endstadium überzieht eine hornige Membran die Hornhaut (sog. Statuenauge) (Abb. 50). Allerdings kommen nicht selten die Augenerscheinungen zum Stillstand, bevor die Sehkraft völlig zerstört ist.

Unter den 30 persönlich beobachteten Patienten hatten sechs keine Augenerscheinungen (LEVER 1953). Es ist aber möglich, daß bei einigen dieser Patienten die Augen später noch erkrankten; denn häufig treten Bindehautveränderungen erst mehrere Jahre nach dem Beginn der Krankheit auf. So wurden die Augen bei zwei der 30 persönlich beobachteten Patienten erst 9 bzw. 10 Jahre nach Beginn der Krankheit befallen; und in einem von KLAUDER (1938) mitgeteilten Fall kam es erst nach 19jähriger Krankheitsdauer zu einem Befall der Bindehaut. Unter den 24 persönlich beobachteten Patienten, die Augenerscheinungen hatten, befanden sich vier Patienten, die zwar Vernarbung der Bindehaut, aber keine Entzündung mehr zeigten und deren Sehkraft noch gut erhalten war. Bei sechs Patienten waren beide Augen erblindet und bei drei weiteren Patienten war ein Auge erblindet.

Mundschleimhauterscheinungen finden sich sehr häufig. Sie sind oft das erste und für lange Zeit einzige Symptom, und gelegentlich können sie das einzige

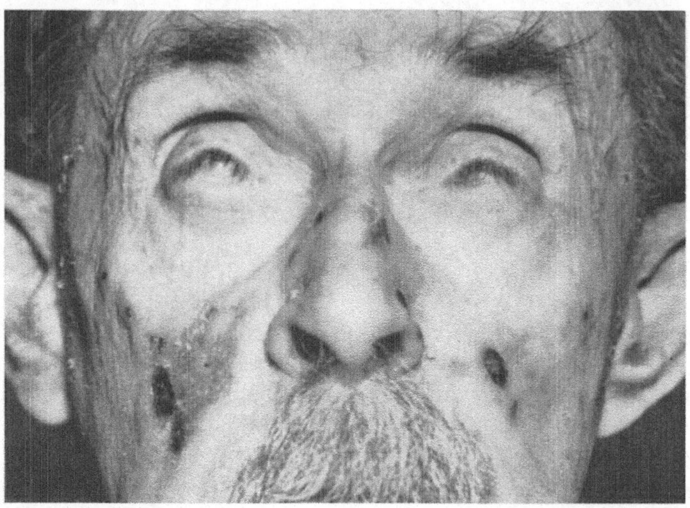

Abb. 50. Benignes Schleimhautpemphigoid. Endstadium der Bindehauterkrankung mit Erblindung. Hier finden sich Symblepharon (Verwachsung zwischen Conjunctiva bulbi und Conjunctiva tarsi) und Ankyloblepharon (partielle Verwachsung der Ränder des oberen und unteren Lides). Eine hornige Membran überzieht die Cornea. Dieser Patient zeigt außerdem Epitheldefekte und atrophische Narben an Nase und Wangen

Symptom bleiben (LEVER 1953; PACHKOV und CHEKLATOV). Im Gegensatz zur Bindehaut, wo die Entzündung stets Vernarbung hervorruft, kann Vernarbung an der Mundschleimhaut fehlen. Blasen bilden die ersten Krankheitserscheinungen. Die darauf folgenden Epitheldefekte heilen nur sehr langsam. Wegen des Auftretens von aufeinanderfolgenden Ausbrüchen von Blasen können ausgedehnte Epitheldefekte vorhanden sein. Diese Epitheldefekte unterscheiden sich von denen, die beim Pemphigus vulgaris vorkommen, in mehreren Punkten. Da sie durch Zusammenfluß benachbarter Blasen und nicht durch periphere Ausbreitung von einzelnen Blasen entstehen, zeigen sie gewöhnlich keinen Rand von abgehobenem Epithel an ihrer Peripherie. Sie bluten nicht so leicht und sind nicht so schmerzhaft wie beim Pemphigus vulgaris. Auch findet man nur geringes Ödem; und das Lippenrot, das beim Pemphigus vulgaris häufig befallen ist, ist gewöhnlich frei von Krankheitserscheinungen. Diese Unterschiede sind allerdings nicht immer verläßlich, und histologische Untersuchung stellt die einzige sichere Unterscheidung dar. Vernarbung findet sich am häufigsten am weichen Gaumen und an der Uvula. Es kann zum Schwund der Uvula und zu narbigen Verwachsungen der Gaumenbögen mit der hinteren Rachenwand kommen. Verwachsungen der oberen und unteren Lippen an den Mundecken können zu einer beträchtlichen Verkleinerung der Mundöffnung führen (Abb. 51).

Befall des Larynx verursacht Schmerzen und Heiserkeit. Bei der Untersuchung sieht man Blasen, Epitheldefekte und oft auch narbige Verwachsungen. Gelegentlich besteht dabei reichliche Schleimabsonderung. Dies kann eine Bronchopneumonie hervorrufen und so zum Tode führen, wie es bei einem unserer Patienten geschah (LEVER 1953).

Die Entwicklung von Speiseröhrenstrikturen ist ein seltenes Ereignis. Seit dem ersten von ADAM im Jahre 1910 beschriebenen Fall sind ungefähr ein Dutzend Fälle beschrieben worden, darunter vier Fälle von BENEDICT und LEVER und je ein Fall von GREITHER, SCHMITZ, HERZBERG (1959) und AUBERTIN et al. Bei Patienten mit Speiseröhrenstrikturen bleibt festes Essen, nachdem es geschluckt worden ist, oft in der Speiseröhre stecken. Röntgen-Untersuchungen des Oesophagus nach einem Bariumschluck zeigen eine oder mehrere Stellen, an denen die Speiseröhre ständig verengt ist (Abb. 52). Mit dem Oesophagoskop sieht man eine diffuse Entzündung der Schleimhaut und entweder eine oder mehrere spinnengewebeartige Membranen. Diese Membranen können das Lumen des Oesophagus durchqueren und es so in zwei Lumina aufteilen (THOST; BENEDICT und LEVER). Zu Beginn sind die Membranen weich und dehnbar und können ohne Schwierigkeiten mit dem Oesophagoskop zertrennt werden. Später aber werden sie fibrös und sind dann nicht mehr zertrennbar. Blasen sind im Oesophagus nie gesehen worden. In dem von ADAM berichteten Falle trat völliger Verschluß des Oesophagus ein und der Patient starb an den Folgen einer Perforation, die eintrat, wenn der Versuch gemacht wurde, den Oesophagus zu sondieren. Einer der persönlich beobachteten Patienten (Case Records of the Massachusetts General Hospital, Case 40111) litt von Speiseröhrenstrikturen seit 3 Jahren. Zuletzt entwickelte sich recht plötzlich eine völlige Unfähigkeit, selbst Flüssigkeiten durch die Speiseröhre gleiten zu lassen und der Patient erlag einer Aspirationspneumonie. Wichtig ist die von SCHMITZ mitgeteilte Beobachtung, daß bei seinem Patienten die Oesophagusstenose mittels Corticosteroidbehandlung fast völlig behoben werden konnte. SCHMITZ folgerte daraus, daß in diesem Falle vor allem Ödem und Spasmen für die Passagebehinderung verantwortlich waren und der narbige Anteil der Verengung gering war.

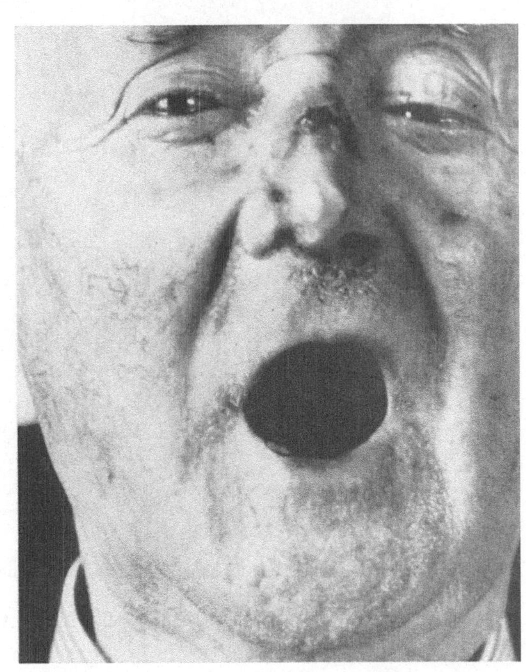

Abb. 51. Benignes Schleimhautpemphigoid. Zusammenwachsen der oberen und unteren Lippen an den Mundecken hat zu einer beträchtlichen Verkleinerung der Mundöffnung geführt. Dieser Patient zeigt außerdem Epitheldefekte und atrophische Vernarbung an der Nase

Zwischen der Glans penis und der Vorhaut können narbige Verklebungen vorkommen, die eine Phimose verursachen (KANEE). An der Vulva und in der Vagina kann sich Schleimhautatrophie entwickeln. Verwachsungen zwischen den Labia minora können zu einer Verengung der Vaginalöffnung führen. Die Afterschleimhaut kann atrophieren, aber die Verengung scheint niemals so ausgesprochen zu werden, daß es zu Schwierigkeiten während des Stuhlganges kommt.

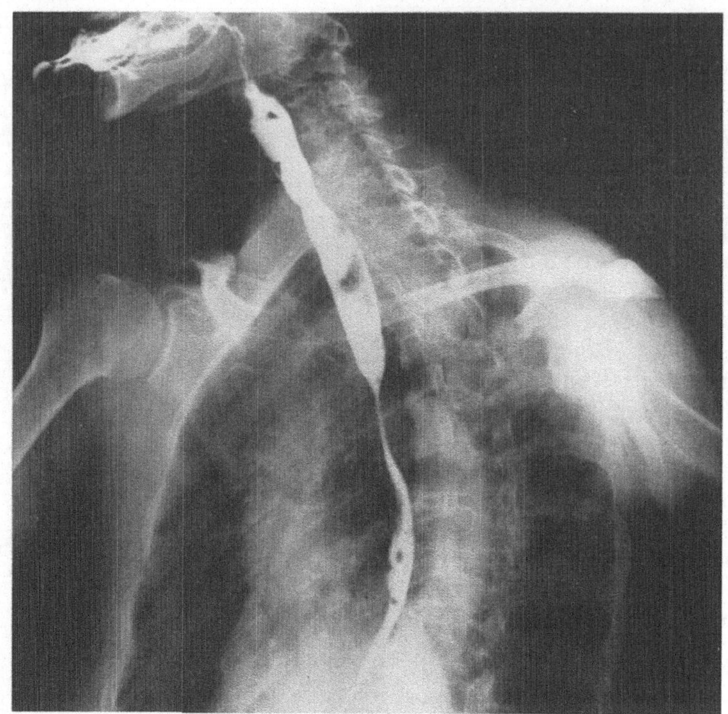

Abb. 52. Benignes Schleimhautpemphigoid. Die Röntgenaufnahme zeigt eine Striktur der Speiseröhre

b) Hauterscheinungen

Zwei Arten von Hauterscheinungen kommen beim benignen Schleimhautpemphigoid vor. Die eine Art besteht aus intermittierenden Ausbrüchen von Blasen, die ohne Vernarbung heilen. Diese Blasenausbrüche können weit ausgebreitet sein oder sich auf einige Hautgebiete beschränken. Am häufigsten findet man Blasen in der Genitalgegend und an den unteren Extremitäten. Die andere Art von Hauterscheinungen besteht aus geröteten Krankheitsherden, die gewöhnlich nur in geringer Zahl vorhanden sind, und zwar hauptsächlich im Gesicht (Abb. 53) und auf der Kopfhaut (Abb. 54) (LEVER 1942, 1944, 1953; DEGOS et al. 1957). Innerhalb dieser Herde bilden sich in unregelmäßigen Abständen schlaffe Blasen, die Epitheldefekte hinterlassen. Nach einer langen Zeit heilen diese Herde mit Atrophie ab.

Die Frage, ob das benigne Schleimhautpemphigoid gelegentlich auch ohne Schleimhauterscheinungen auftreten kann, gekennzeichnet nur durch vernarbende Hauterscheinungen, ist von BRUNSTING und PERRY aufgeworfen worden. Sie berichteten über sieben Patienten mit chronischen, rezidivierenden, auf Kopf und Hals beschränkten Blaseneruptionen, die zu Atrophie führten. Nur einer der sieben Patienten zeigte Blasen im Munde, aber ohne Narbenbildung. Die histologische Untersuchung ergab in jedem Fall subepidermale Blasenbildung. Das Bestehen einer Porphyrie konnte ausgeschlossen werden.

c) Verlauf

Der Verlauf ist äußerst chronisch. Gewöhnlich ist der allgemeine Gesundheitszustand nicht beeinträchtigt. Nur gelegentlich führt Ansammlung von Schleim im Larynx oder Obstruktion der Speiseröhre zu Bronchopneumonie und tödlichem

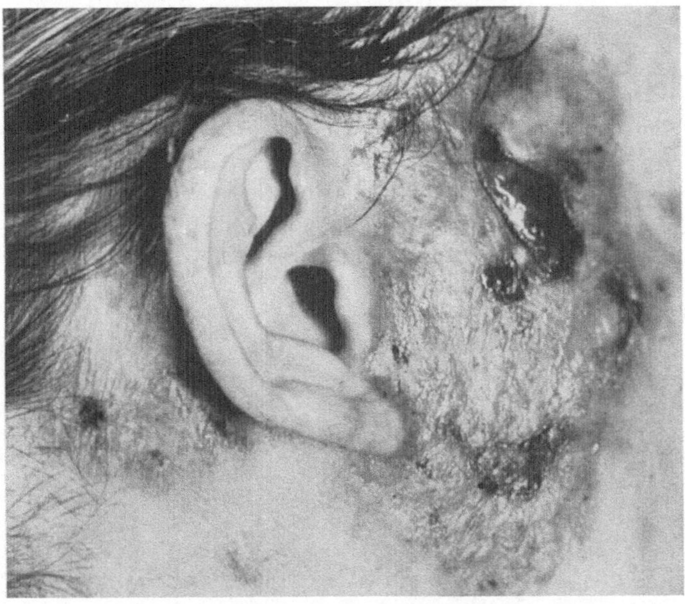

Abb. 53. Benignes Schleimhautpemphigoid. Epitheldefekte und atrophische Vernarbung finden sich vor und hinter dem Ohr

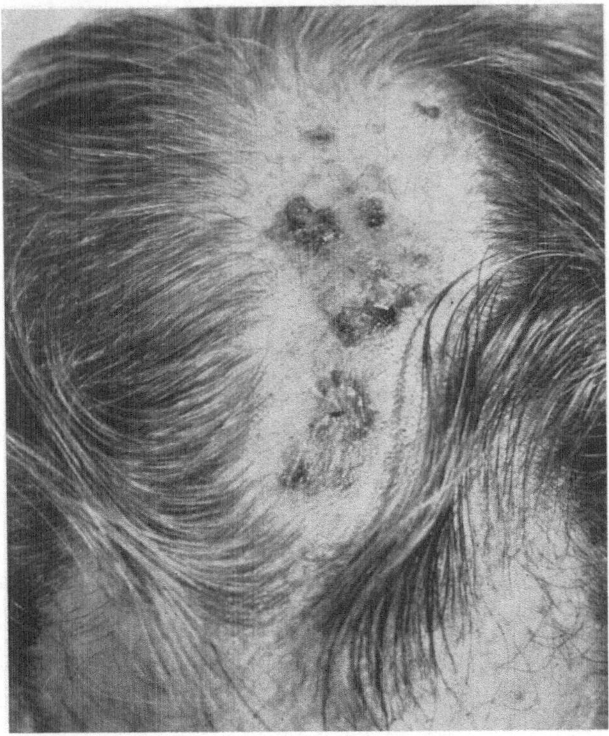

Abb. 54. Benignes Schleimhautpemphigoid. Blasen und Epitheldefekte mit beginnender atrophischer Vernarbung befinden sich auf der Kopfhaut

Ausgang. Die Mehrzahl der Patienten ist beim Beginn der Krankheit über 50 Jahre alt; doch kann die Krankheit schon bei Patienten, die zwischen 30 und 50 Jahre alt sind, beginnen. Es besteht kein bevorzugter Befall jüdischer Patienten. (Unter den 30 persönlich beobachteten Patienten waren 16 über sechzig Jahre alt beim Beginn der Krankheit. Nur einer der 30 Patienten war jüdisch.)

d) Histologie

Die Blasen der Haut und Mundschleimhaut bilden sich subepidermal und zeigen keine Acantholyse (Lever 1951; Church und Sneddon 1956; Jablonska

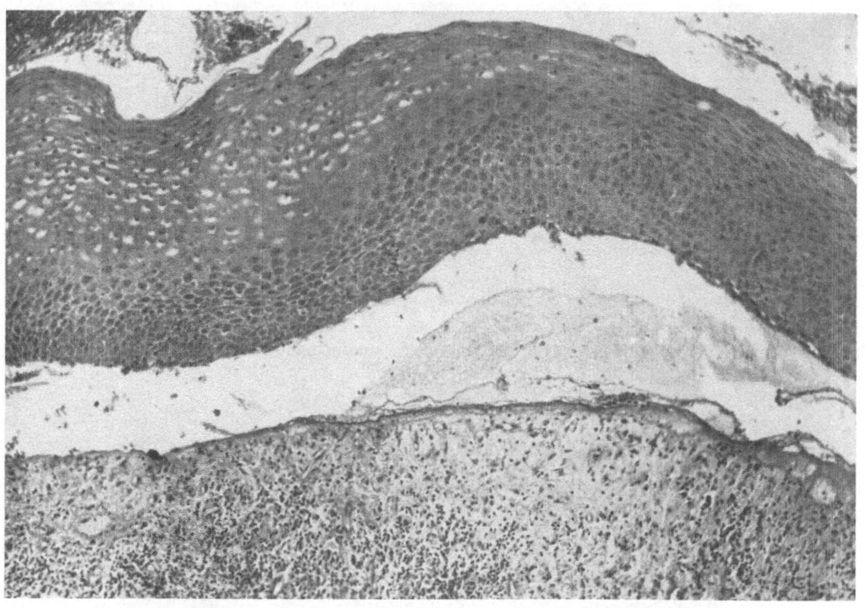

Abb. 55. Benignes Schleimhautpemphigoid. Die Blase, die von der Mundschleimhaut stammt, liegt subepidermal. In der abgehobenen Epidermis findet sich keine Degeneration (100mal)

et al. 1957) (Abb. 55). In der Dermis befindet sich ein beträchtliches entzündliches Infiltrat und späterhin auch Fibrose. Es ist wahrscheinlich, daß die Fibrose für das Auftreten von Vernarbung verantwortlich ist.

e) Behandlung

Bei der Behandlung der Krankheitserscheinungen an den Augen sind subkonjunktivale Injektionen einer Corticosteroidsuspension die Behandlung der Wahl (Lortat-Jacob). Die Häufigkeit der Injektionen muß individuell geregelt werden. Gewöhnlich werden sie zuerst alle 4—7 Tage gegeben. Als zusätzliche Behandlung können Corticosteroidtropfen in die Augen geträufelt werden; aber als alleinige Behandlung sind Einträuflungen wohl kaum von Wert. Die interne Verabreichung von Corticosteroiden ist wirkungsvoll, wenn hohe Dosen verabreicht werden (Lodin und Gentele); aber das Risiko, das eine über lange Zeit hin ausgedehnte Behandlung mit hohen Dosen von Corticosteroiden in sich trägt, ist zu groß, besonders in Hinsicht darauf, daß die meisten Patienten mit benignem Schleimhautpemphigoid im höheren Alter stehen. Jedoch kann man zu Beginn der Behandlung mit subkonjunktivalen Injektionen gleichzeitig auch intern für einige Wochen Corticosteroide verabreichen und dann auch ab und zu, wenn die subkonjunktivalen Injektionen die Bindehautentzündung nicht in Schach halten. Beim Bestehen eines Entropiums sollten die Augenwimpern mittels Elektrolyse entfernt werden, um eine Beschädigung der Hornhaut, die durch das Reiben der Wimpern gegen sie entstehen kann, zu vermeiden.

Da eine Striktur der Speiseröhre durch eine evtl. eintretende Aspirationspneumonie lebensgefährlich werden kann, ist es von Wichtigkeit, daß sie frühzeitig erkannt und behandelt wird, besonders in Hinsicht darauf, daß die Strikturen auf die Verabreichung von Corticosteroiden gut ansprechen (SCHMITZ). Nach dem anfänglichen guten Ansprechen, das von einer Verringerung des bestehenden Ödems herrührt, mag man vielleicht Sondierungen der Speiseröhre ausführen, um Adhäsionen zu beseitigen. Wiederholte interne Anwendungen von Corticosteroiden, gefolgt von Sondierung, wird wohl gewöhnlich nötig sein.

Die Mundschleimhauterscheinungen sind gewöhnlich nicht schmerzhaft genug, um die interne Anwendung von Corticosteroiden erforderlich zu machen. Oft genügt das Auftragen eines Lokalanaestheticums, wie z.B. einer $^1/_2$%igen Lösung von Tetracain, eine Viertelstunde vor dem Essen. Andererseits besteht bei Patienten in gutem Allgemeinzustand kein Grund, warum nicht gelegentlich relativ niedrige Dosen von Corticosteroiden verordnet werden können (McCARTHY und SHKLAR).

C. Pemphigus familiaris benignus

Obwohl der Pemphigus familiaris benignus nur selten klinische Ähnlichkeit mit dem Pemphigus vulgaris aufweist und gutartig verläuft, zeigt er doch eine auffallende histologische Ähnlichkeit mit dem Pemphigus vulgaris. Da Acantholyse dabei besteht, erscheint das Wort Pemphigus in der Bezeichnung dieser Krankheit berechtigt, trotz des Fehlens jeglicher Beziehungen zum Pemphigus vulgaris.

a) Geschichtlicher Überblick

Der erste Fall, auf den nachträglich die Diagnose Pemphigus familiaris benignus angewandt werden kann, wurde im März 1939 von PELS und GOODMAN unter der Bezeichnung „keratosis follicularis (Darier) with vesiculation“ veröffentlicht. Einen Monat später teilten HAILEY und HAILEY vier Krankheitsfälle bei zwei Familien mit und gaben der Krankheit die Bezeichnung „familial benign chronic pemphigus“. Im September 1939 veröffentlichten AYRES und ANDERSON einen Bericht über fünf Fälle von „recurrent herpetiform dermatitis repens“. Dieser Bericht war zwar schon vor der Veröffentlichung von HAILEY und HAILEY geschrieben worden, doch in einem Zusatz zu ihrer Arbeit erkannten AYRES und ANDERSON die Identität ihrer Fälle mit den von HAILEY und HAILEY beschriebenen an. Der erste europäische Fall wurde 1947 von CREMER und PRAKKEN veröffentlicht.

GOUGEROTS Anspruch, dieses Krankheitsbild erstmalig im Jahre 1933 beschrieben zu haben, erscheint unhaltbar. Bei dem von GOUGEROT beschriebenen Patienten waren seit Geburt Blasen vorhanden und außerdem urticarielle Herde. Da keine histologische Untersuchung durchgeführt worden war, ist es unmöglich, eine Diagnose zu stellen; aber wie PALMER und PERRY festgestellt haben: „Das Alter bei Beginn der Krankheit, der klinische Verlauf und das Bestehen von Urticaria sind nicht vereinbar mit einer Diagnose von Morbus Hailey und Hailey.“

b) Klinisches Bild

Die Primärefflorescenzen des Pemphigus familiaris benignus bestehen aus in Gruppen zusammenstehenden Bläschen, die sich entweder auf normaler oder auf geröteter Haut bilden. Zuerst ist die in ihnen enthaltene Flüssigkeit klar, aber sie trübt sich meistens bald. Die Bläschen sind schlaff und reißen leicht ein, so daß sich Epitheldefekte und feuchte Krusten bilden. Die Herde breiten sich peripher aus und zeigen dann einen circinär verlaufenden Rand, auf dem sich

Blasen und Pusteln befinden (Abb. 56). Die Herde zeigen in ihrer Mitte entweder Abheilung mit Pigmentierung oder Bildung von Vegetationen (Abb. 57). Nach einer gewissen Zeit, gewöhnlich nach Monaten, findet Abheilung unter Pigmen-

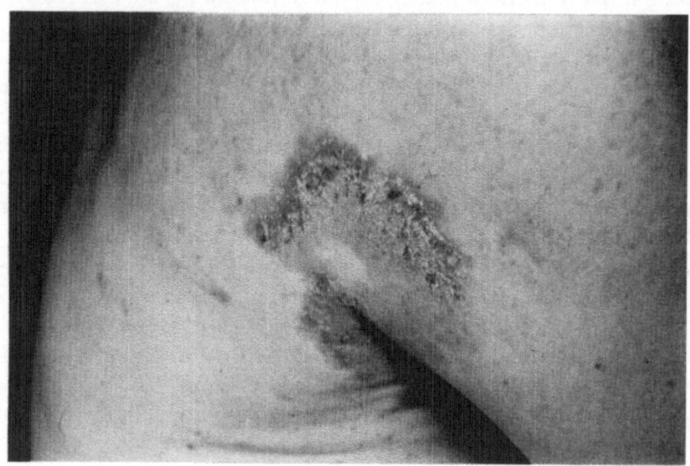

Abb. 56. Pemphigus familiaris benignus. Krankheitsherd in der linken Ellenbeuge. Man beachte den aktiven Rand mit Bläschenbildung

tierung, aber ohne Narbenbildung statt. Rezidive treten über viele Jahre hin in gleicher Lokalisierung auf.

Bei den meisten Patienten ist die Krankheit auf nur einige Körperstellen beschränkt, obwohl ausnahmsweise recht weite Ausbreitung vorkommt, wie bei

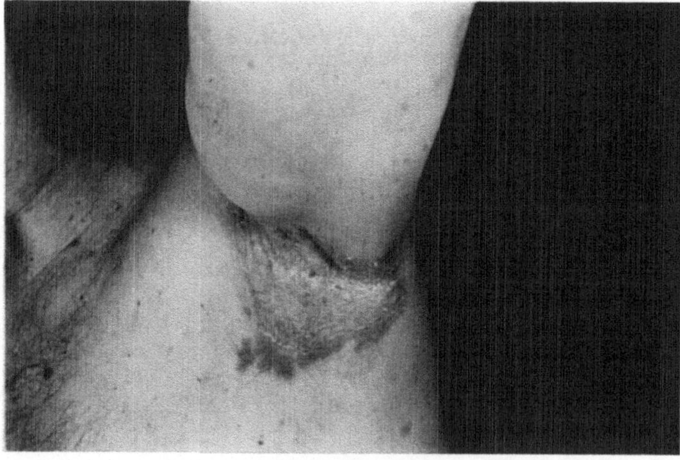

Abb. 57. Pemphigus familiaris benignus. Der Krankheitsherd, in der Axilla gelegen, zeigt in der Mitte vegetative Gewebshypertrophie

den von PELS und GOODMAN und von HERZBERG beschriebenen Fällen (Abb. 58). Die Prädilektionsstellen sind die Seiten des Halses, der Nacken und die intertriginösen Gegenden, besonders die Achselhöhlen, Leistenbeugen und Perianalgegend, gelegentlich aber auch die inframammäre Gegend und die Ellenbeugen. Weniger häufig findet man Herde am Körper oder im Bereich des Kopfes.

Das Allgemeinbefinden ist selbst bei weiter Ausbreitung kaum gestört; doch besteht oft Jucken und ein brennendes Gefühl. Zudem können Maceration und Rhagadenbildung in den intertriginösen Gegenden Schmerzen verursachen.

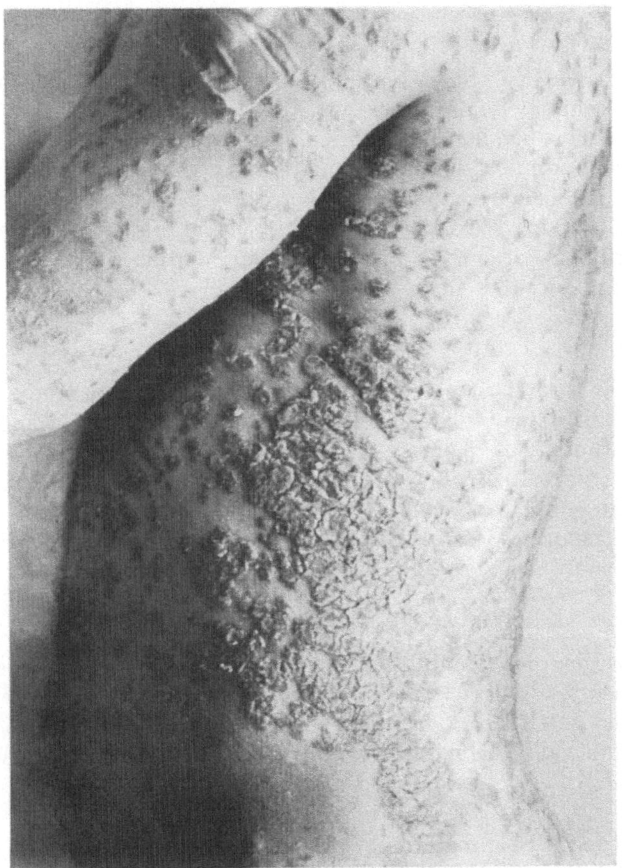

Abb. 58. Pemphigus familiaris benignus. Generalisierte Aussaat krustenbedeckter Herde. [HERZBERG, J. J.: Arch. klin. exp. Derm. **202**, 21 (1955)]

c) Schleimhautbefall

Bis vor kurzer Zeit wurde das Fehlen von Mundschleimhautherden als für den Pemphigus familiaris benignus charakteristisch angesehen. Jedoch beschrieben 1962 FISCHER und NIKOLOWSKI Mundschleimhautherde bei drei Patienten. Der erste Patient hatte lediglich einige kleine Epitheldefekte an der Wangenschleimhaut; der zweite Patient wies an der Wangenschleimhaut mit Rhagaden besetzte weißliche Herde auf, die wie Leukoplakien aussahen; und beim dritten Patienten waren im Munde Epitheldefekte und ausgedehnte Vegetationen zu sehen. Bei allen drei Patienten konnte die Diagnose histologisch verifiziert werden. In einer kurz darauf folgenden Publikation berichteten SCHNEIDER und FISCHER, daß bei dem ersten dieser drei Patienten während einer vorübergehenden Verschlimmerung das klinische wie auch das histologische Bild von einem Pemphigus vulgaris ununterscheidbar war.

d) Alter

Gewöhnlich tritt die Krankheit erstmalig im 2. oder 3. Lebensjahrzehnt auf, gelegentlich aber erst später. Beginn der Krankheit bei Personen über 50 Jahre alt ist zwar selten, ist aber z.B. von Palmer und Perry und von Wehnert beobachtet worden. Erstmaliges Auftreten bei Kindern ist höchst ungewöhnlich; jedoch haben Khandari und Singh den Beginn eines Pemphigus familiaris benignus bei einem 2jährigen indischen Kinde mitgeteilt.

e) Verlauf

Der Verlauf des Pemphigus familiaris benignus zeichnet sich durch ein Abwechseln von Remissionen und Rezidiven aus, wobei sich die Rezidive gewöhnlich auf die früher schon befallenen Hautareale beschränken. Vollständige oder partielle Remissionen können sich über Monate und selbst Jahre erstrecken. Häufig verschlimmern sich die Krankheitserscheinungen in der warmen Jahreszeit, da Schwitzen und Reibung provozierend wirken. Die Krankheit zeigt wenig Neigung, mit dem Altern des Patienten zu verschwinden; und so sind Fälle bekannt, bei denen die Krankheit über mehr als 40 Jahre hin bestanden hat (Palmer und Perry).

f) Vererbung

Bei ungefähr zwei Drittel der Patienten ergibt die Anamnese, daß andere Familienmitglieder dieselbe Krankheit haben oder hatten. Gelegentlich kann sie bei vielen Verwandten in mehreren Generationen vorkommen. So fanden z.B. Hailey und Hailey (1940) ein Vorkommen der Krankheit elfmal in vier Generationen, Becker und Obermayer 27mal unter 78 Verwandten in drei Generationen und Raaschou-Nielsen und Reymann 21mal unter 65 Verwandten in fünf Generationen. Die Vererbung ist unregelmäßig dominant.

g) Geschlecht und Rasse

Ein Überwiegen des männlichen oder weiblichen Geschlechtes oder einer bestimmten Rasse besteht nicht. Obwohl die meisten in der Literatur mitgeteilten Fälle Kaukasier betrifft, ist das Vorkommen bei Negern (Jewell und Key; Lyles et al.) und bei Mongolen (Pels und Goodman) beschrieben worden.

h) Ätiologie

Die grundliegende Störung besteht aus einer genetisch bedingten Gebrechlichkeit der Epidermis, die einen acantholytischen Zerfall der Epidermis zur Folge hat. Wie die elektronenmikroskopischen Untersuchungen von Wilgram, Caulfield und Lever (1962, 1963) gezeigt haben, besteht der zuerst erkennbare Schaden aus einer Trennung der Tonofilamente von ihren Desmosomen (s. S. 620). Diese Trennung erfolgt wahrscheinlich auf Grund einer falschen Synthese oder falschen Reifung der Tonofilamente.

Es steht jedenfalls fest, daß die Epidermis oft Reibung, wie sie durch eng anliegende Kragen oder durch Träger verursacht wird, nicht widerstehen kann. Ein weiterer wichtiger Faktor, der zur Bildung von Hauterscheinungen beim Pemphigus familiaris benignus führt, ist Infektion mit Bakterien (Loewenthal; Shelley und Pillsbury; Chorzelski). Die folgenden klinischen Beobachtungen sprechen nach Shelley und Pillsbury dafür, daß Bakterien Krankheitserscheinungen hervorrufen können: Erstens ähnelt das klinische Aussehen der Hautherde des Pemphigus familiaris benignus infolge des Vorhandenseins von schlaffen Bläschen und Krusten dem der Impetigo; zweitens wachsen oft in Kulturen von intakten Blasen Staphylokokken, und drittens spricht der Pemphigus familiaris benignus auf eine Behandlung mit Antibiotica gewöhnlich rasch an.

Daß Reizung der Haut bei Patienten mit Pemphigus familiaris benignus Krankheitsherde hervorrufen kann, hat Chorzelski nachgewiesen, der bei solchen Patienten durch eine Reihe von Reizen, wie Reiben, Vereisung mit Kohlensäureschnee, Erhitzung oder Auftragen von primär-toxischen Substanzen, typische Herde hervorrief, die auch Acantholyse aufwiesen. Die Rolle, die Bakterien bei dem Entstehen von Krankheitsherden spielen können, wurde von LOEWENTHAL in folgender Weise dargelegt: Bei drei Patienten applizierte er eine Kultur von Coagulase-positiven Staphylokokken auf ein Hautgebiet, das vorher mit Sandpapier leicht geschabt worden war. (An einer Kontrollstelle wurde die Haut wohl geschabt, aber keine Bakterien aufgetragen.) Drei Tage später zeigten Probeexcisionen bei zwei dieser drei Patienten Acantholyse auf der mit Bakterien inoculierten Stelle, aber nicht auf der Kontrollstelle.

i) Histologie

Das histologische Bild des Pemphigus familiaris benignus ähnelt dem des Pemphigus vulgaris in auffallender Weise; und gelegentlich kann in einer einzelnen

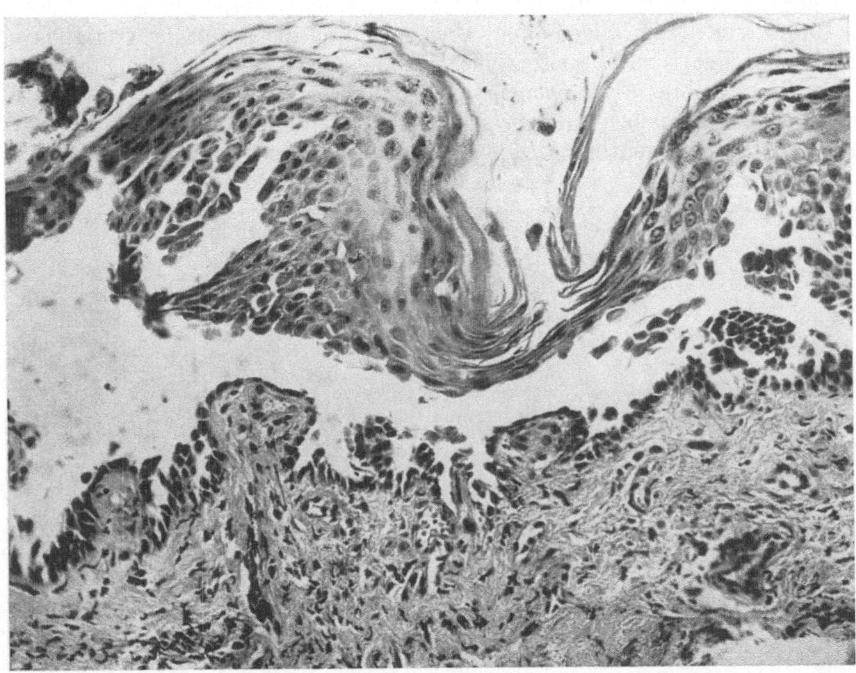

Abb. 59. Pemphigus familiaris benignus. Die Blase befindet sich in suprabasaler Lage. Man sieht einen weitgehenden Verlust der Intercellularbrücken, der zu beträchtlicher Acantholyse geführt hat. Der Blasenboden zeigt beginnende Proliferation der Papillarkörper. Das histologische Bild zeigt eine überraschende Ähnlichkeit mit dem des Pemphigus vulgaris (200mal)

Probeexcision eine Entscheidung, welche der beiden Krankheiten vorliegt, unmöglich sein; denn man findet bei beiden Krankheiten Acantholyse, die zu suprabasaler Blasenbildung führt, sowie beträchtliche Papillomatose, die mit einer Proliferation von Epidermiszellen in die Dermis hinein verbunden sein kann (Abb. 59).

Es bestehen jedoch drei Unterschiede zwischen dem histologischen Bilde des Pemphigus familiaris benignus und dem des Pemphigus vulgaris: Erstens besteht beim Pemphigus familiaris benignus eine viel ausgedehntere Acantholyse; zweitens geht die Acantholyse mit weniger Zellschaden in den acantholytischen Zellen einher (DUPONT 1951); und drittens sind an vielen Zellen trotz des weit ausgebreiteten Verlustes von Intercellularbrücken noch einige Intercellularbrücken vorhanden, so daß viele acantholytische Zellen lose miteinander verbunden sind. Dies ruft in der suprabasal abgelösten Epidermis das Aussehen einer „zerfallenden Backsteinwand" hervor (HABER und RUSSELL).

Daß die acantholytischen Zellen beim Pemphigus familiaris benignus eine gewisse Lebensfähigkeit besitzen, ist daraus ersichtlich, daß sie verhornen können.

So weisen einige acantholytische Zellen ein homogenes, leicht eosinophiles Cytoplasma auf als Anzeichen beginnender Verhornung, während andere geschrumpft erscheinen, gelegentlich zu einem solchen Grade, daß sie den „Grains" des Morbus Darier ähnlich sehen. In einigen Fällen sind in den oberen Epidermisschichten auch dyskeratotische Zellen, die den „Corps ronds" ähnlich sehen, beobachtet worden (HERZBERG, WINER und LEEB; GÖNCZÖL und SZODORAY).

j) Cytologische Untersuchung

Cytologische Abstriche von Blasen des Pemphigus familiaris benignus unterscheiden sich nicht genügend von Abstrichen, die von Blasen des Pemphigus vulgaris gewonnen wurden, um eine Unterscheidung zu ermöglichen (JABLONSKA und CHORZELSKI). Im allgemeinen aber enthalten die Abstriche von Blasen des Pemphigus vulgaris recht viele Zellen, die als Anzeichen von Degeneration eine Kondensierung ihres Cytoplasmas am Rand der Zelle zeigen, während beim Pemphigus familiaris benignus die Abstriche Zellen enthalten, die Anzeichen von Verhornung und gelegentlich Anzeichen von Dyskeratose zeigen (WINER und LEEB).

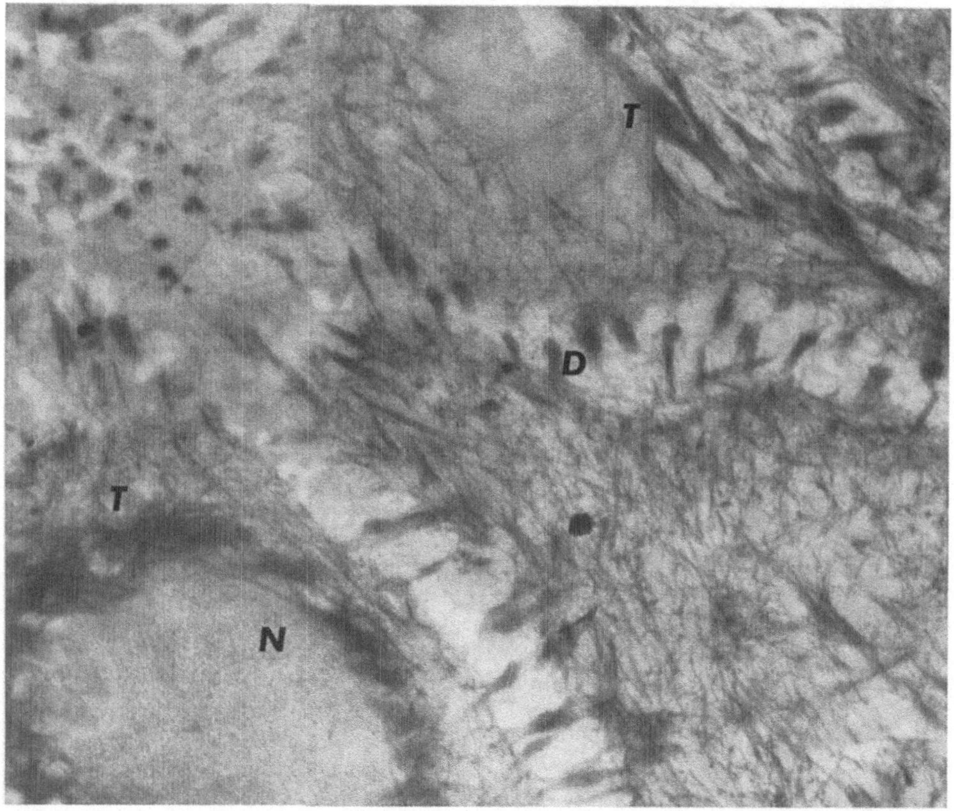

Abb. 60. Pemphigus familiaris benignus. In einem Epidermisgebiet, in dem noch keine Acantholyse eingesetzt hat, erscheinen die Desmosomen (*D*) normal. Die Tonofilamente (*T*) sind beträchtlich vermehrt und lose angeordnet. Viele Tonofilamente scheinen keine Verbindung mit Desmosomen zu haben. *N* Zellkern (20000mal)

k) Elektronenmikroskopie

Beim Pemphigus familiaris benignus bestehen anscheinend auf Grund eines Erbfehlers Veränderungen im Tonofilament-Desmosom-Komplex, während die anderen Zellbestandteile wie Kern, Mitochondrien und das endoplasmische Reticulum ziemlich intakt sind (WILGRAM, CAULFIELD und LEVER 1962, 1963).

Die elektronenmikroskopischen Befunde unterstützen die auf Grund der Histologie gewonnene Ansicht, daß beim Pemphigus familiaris benignus ein weitgehendes Schwinden der Intercellularbrücken (Desmosomen) das hervorstechendste Merkmal ist. Allerdings besteht die früheste mit dem Elektronenmikroskop erfaßbare Veränderung, wie beim Pemphigus vulgaris, darin, daß die Tonofilamente von

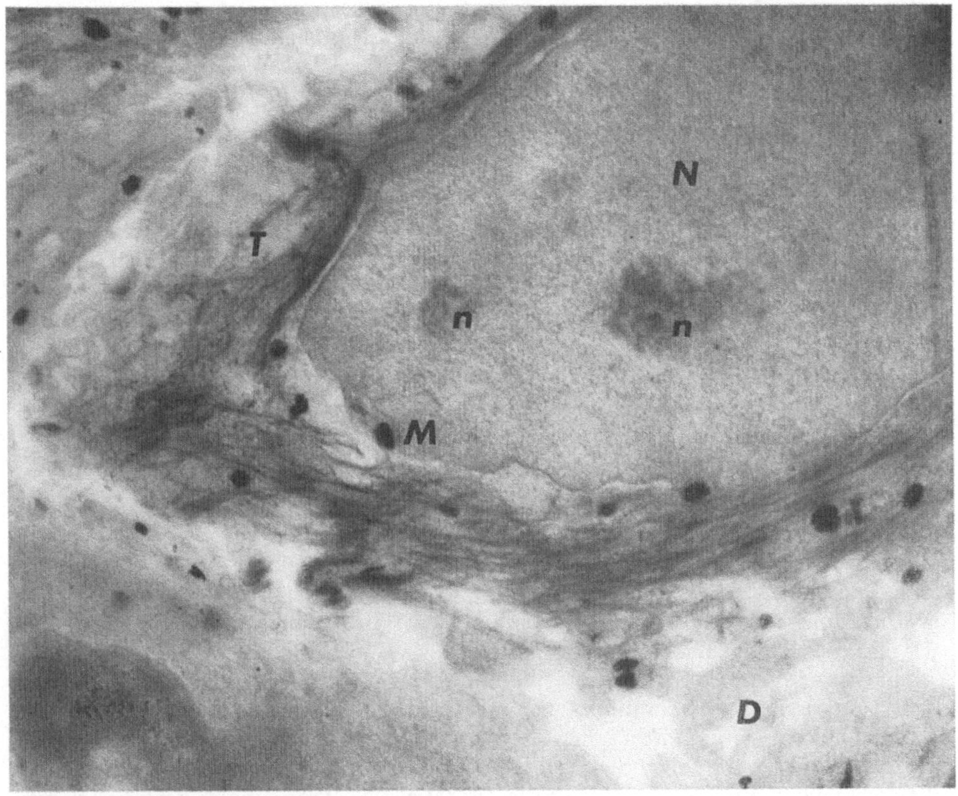

Abb. 61. Pemphigus familiaris benignus. In einer acantholytischen Zelle fehlen die Desmosomen (*D*) fast vollständig. Die Tonofilamente (*T*), die um den Zellkern (*N*) herum liegen, sind beträchtlich vermehrt, zeigen aber keine degenerative Veränderungen. Auch der Zellkern, der Nucleoli (*n*) enthält, erscheint nicht degeneriert. Viele Melaninkörner (*M*) befinden sich in dieser Zelle (24000mal)

ihren Desmosomen getrennt sind, also einem intracellulären Vorgang (Abb. 60). Es kann zur Zeit nicht entschieden werden, ob die einzelnen Tonofilamente sich von ihren Desmosomen ablösen oder sich primär während ihrer Bildung nicht mit Desmosomen verbinden. Wo die Desmosomen keine Verbindung mit Tonofilamenten besitzen, gehen die Desmosomen zugrunde. Im Gegensatz zu den Desmosomen bleiben die Halbdesmosomen und die Basalmembran intakt, so daß die Basalzellen an der Basalmembran haften bleiben.

In fortgeschrittenen Krankheitsherden zeigen viele Epidermiszellen ein Zusammenballen der in ihnen enthaltenen Tonofilamente (Abb. 61). Dieses ist am deutlichsten vorhanden in solchen Zellen, die alle ihre Desmosomen verloren haben, ist weniger vorhanden in Zellen, die noch einige Desmosomen besitzen, und ist am wenigsten vorhanden in Zellen, die noch die Mehrzahl ihrer Desmosomen aufweisen. Ein Zusammenballen der Tonofilamente findet also nicht statt, solange sie an einer

Desmosome haften. Im Gegensatz zum Pemphigus vulgaris, bei dem die Tonofilamente degenerieren, bewahren beim Pemphigus familiaris benignus die einzelnen Tonofilamente ihr normales Aussehen. Insbesondere zeigen sie dieselbe Periodizität wie die Tonofilamente in normalen Epidermiszellen. Jedoch ist die Anzahl von Tonofilamenten beträchtlich vermehrt. Keratohyalinkörner sind in den Zellen, die Aggregate von Tonofilamenten enthalten, nicht vorhanden. Diese Tatsache spricht dafür, daß es sich bei den Aggregaten von Tonofilamenten nicht nur um unreifes, sondern auch um abnormes Keratin handelt. Man ist also berechtigt, von einer Dyskeratose zu sprechen. Zellen mit besonders dichtem Zusammenballen von Tonofilamenten können eine gewisse Ähnlichkeit mit den Corps ronds des Morbus Darier zeigen; doch unterscheiden sie sich von ihnen durch das Fehlen von Keratohyalinkörnern.

l) Differentialdiagnose

Obwohl das klinische Aussehen des Pemphigus familiaris benignus gelegentlich einer Impetigo sehr ähnlich ist, kann doch eine Impetigo gewöhnlich schon durch die lange Dauer und die Lokalisation, dann aber definitiv durch den histologischen Befund ausgeschlossen werden. In Fällen, die Vegetationen aufweisen, kann ein Pemphigus vegetans vorgetäuscht werden, der ja auch gewöhnlich in intertriginösen Hautgegenden vorkommt. Zudem ist das histologische Bild der beiden Krankheiten einander recht ähnlich (s. S. 625). Eine positive Familienanamnese, das nur sehr seltene Vorkommen von Mundschleimhauterscheinungen und der chronisch-rezidivierende Verlauf beim Pemphigus familiaris benignus sind bei der Unterscheidung von Hilfe.

Von besonderem Interesse sind die Beziehungen zwischen dem *Morbus Darier* und dem Pemphigus familiaris benignus. Klinisch gesehen besteht ja recht wenig Ähnlichkeit, da der Morbus Darier eine andere Lokalisierung hat, nämlich vor allem in den seborrhoischen Hautgebieten, und ausgesprochene papillomatöse Verhornung aufweist. Bläschen kommen zwar in seltenen Fällen beim Morbus Darier vor (REISS; BOLGERT et al.; JABLONSKA und CHORZELSKI); aber sie stellen dann eine zusätzliche Krankheitserscheinung dar und nicht die Primärefflorescenz, wie beim Pemphigus familiaris benignus. Histologisch bestehen zwar gewisse Ähnlichkeiten, wie suprabasale Abtrennung der Epidermis und Papillomatose. Jedoch bestehen die folgenden drei Unterschiede, die allerdings nur graduell sind. Erstens sind beim Morbus Darier die suprabasalen Trennungen gewöhnlich von kleinerem Ausmaß als beim Pemphigus familiaris benignus und stellen daher Lakunen anstatt Bläschen dar; zweitens ist beim Morbus Darier die Acantholyse weniger ausgeprägt, und drittens findet sich beim Morbus Darier viel ausgesprochenere Dyskeratose. Obwohl man beim Pemphigus familiaris benignus, wie beim Morbus Darier, nicht selten Grains antrifft, welche geschrumpfte, teilweise verhornte Zellen darstellen, findet man ausgesprochene Dyskeratose, wie sie Corps ronds darstellen, nur sehr selten beim Pemphigus familiaris benignus und dann in geringerem Ausmaße. Andererseits sind beim Morbus Darier Corps ronds eine typische Erscheinung und sind gewöhnlich in großer Zahl vorhanden.

Seit der Zeit, daß der Pemphigus familiaris benignus im Jahre 1939 erstmalig beschrieben wurde, hat es verschiedene Meinungen darüber gegeben, ob er eine wesenseigene Krankheit ist oder eine Variante des Morbus Darier darstellt. ELLIS äußerste sich 1950 zugunsten der letzteren Ansicht und unterschied eine vesiculäre und eine trockene Form des Morbus Darier. Er kam zu dieser Ansicht, da er in neun von zehn Fällen von Pemphigus familiaris benignus Corps ronds in den histologischen Schnitten aufgefunden hatte. In demselben Jahr veröffentlichten FINNERUD und SZYMANSKI einen Fall, welcher ihrer Ansicht nach Merkmale beider Krankheiten besaß. Es ist jedoch möglich, daß dies, wie JABLONSKA und CHORZELSKI glauben, ein Fall von Morbus Darier mit Blasenbildung war.

In den letzten Jahren haben verhältnismäßig wenige Autoren die unitarische Ansicht vertreten. Unter ihnen befinden sich WINER und LEEB sowie GÖNCZÖL, die sich in ihrer Ansicht auf das Vorhandensein von Corps ronds in histologischen Schnitten stützen; und JAEGER sowie DEGOS und CIVATTE, die je einen Fall beschrieben haben, der klinisch wie auch histologisch Merkmale beider Krankheiten aufwies. Die Mehrheit der Autoren, die sich letzthin über das Problem geäußert haben, sieht die beiden Krankheiten als unterschiedlich an, unter ihnen BOLGERT et al., DUPONT (1951, 1960), HERZBERG, JABLONSKA und CHORZELSKI, PALMER und PERRY sowie WILGRAM, CAULFIELD und LEVER (1962, 1963). CAULFIELD und WILGRAM haben in ihrer elektronenmikroskopischen Untersuchung von Morbus Darier dargelegt, daß beim Morbus Darier die Verhornung der Epidermiszellen weiter fortgeschritten ist als beim Pemphigus familiaris benignus und mit dem Auftreten von Keratohyalinkörnern verbunden ist, die im allgemeinen in den vorzeitig verhornenden Zellen des Pemphigus familiaris benignus nicht vorhanden sind.

Gegen eine Identität der beiden Krankheiten sprechen auch die genetischen Studien von SVENDSEN und ALBRECTSEN und von RAASCHOU-NIELSEN und REYMANN, die darauf hindeuten, daß der Morbus Darier, bzw. der Pemphigus familiaris benignus, stets nur für sich allein bei den von der einen oder der anderen Krankheit befallenen Familien vorkommt. Gegen eine Beziehung zwischen den beiden Krankheiten spricht ferner die von CHORZELSKI gemachte Beobachtung, daß er zwar mit Hilfe verschiedener äußerer Reize bei zwei Patienten mit Pemphigus familiaris benignus Hauterscheinungen hervorrufen konnte, aber nicht bei einem Patienten mit Morbus Darier. Außerdem bestehen Unterschiede im Ansprechen der beiden Krankheiten auf therapeutische Maßnahmen: Die Hauterscheinungen des Pemphigus familiaris benignus sprechen auf die Verabreichung von Antibiotica sowie von Corticosteroiden an (s. unten), während der Morbus Darier auf diese Mittel nicht anspricht.

m) Behandlung

Da beim Pemphigus familiaris benignus eine Infektion der Haut mit Bakterien Hauterscheinungen auslösen kann (s. Ätiologie), ist es erklärlich, daß Antibiotica bei dieser Krankheit Besserungen herbeiführen. Gelegentlich sind schon lokale Applikationen von Antibiotica enthaltenden Salben von Wert (HAILEY 1953), besonders wenn das Antibioticum auf Grund von Sensibilitätstesten in Bakterienkulturen gewählt wird (LOEWENTHAL). Ein noch besseres Ansprechen kann gewöhnlich erzielt werden, wenn die Antibiotica intern verabreicht werden. Verschiedene Antibiotica haben sich dabei bewährt, unter ihnen die Sulfonamide (LYLES et al.), Penicillin (CARPENTER) und die Tetracycline (SALSBERG). Da Eruptionen nicht nur bei verschiedenen Patienten durch verschiedene Bakterienstämme hervorgerufen werden können, sondern auch aufeinanderfolgende Verschlimmerungen bei demselben Patienten, ist nicht immer dasselbe Antibioticum wirksam. SHELLEY und PILLSBURY schlagen daher vor, daß bei jeder Verschlimmerung Sensibilitätsteste in Bakterienkulturen vorgenommen werden, um das wirksamste Antibioticum für interne Verabreichung festzustellen.

Auf Grund von Berichten, wie sie WEHNERT und HERZBERG veröffentlicht haben, steht fest, daß die Hauterscheinungen des Pemphigus familiaris benignus auf die Corticosteroide ansprechen, vorausgesetzt, daß hinreichende Mengen verabreicht werden. Bei dem von WEHNERT behandelten Patienten war eine Tagesdosis von 200 mg Cortison unzulänglich, während die Verabreichung von 400 mg pro Tag rasche Besserung brachte. Bei HERZBERGs Patienten war zwar die tägliche Einnahme von 200 mg Cortison wirksam, aber bei Absetzen der Behandlung trat ein schwerer Rückfall ein, bei dem mehr Krankheitsherde als je zuvor auftraten. Es erscheint daher ratsam, bei einer so chronischen und dabei gutartigen Krankheit, wie dem Pemphigus familiaris benignus, die innere Verabreichung von Corticosteroiden möglichst zu vermeiden. Lokalbehandlung mit Corticosteroidsalben ist gewöhnlich erfolglos (SULLIVAN). Wenn jedoch das Auftragen der Corticosteroidsalbe mit einem plastischen Okklusivverband verbunden wird (s. auch S. 660), kann gewöhnlich eine temporäre Besserung erzielt werden (SAMITZ).

Literatur

A. *Pemphigus*

ANGULO, J. J., et L. E. FERRAZ-MAZZONI: Sur la fonction hypophyso-adréno-corticale dans le pemphigus foliacé. Ann. Derm. Syph. (Paris) **81**, 404 (1954).

BAADER, E.: Dermatostomatitis. Arch. Derm. Syph. (Berl.) **149**, 261 (1925). — BALÓ, J., et F. FÖLDVÁRY: L'examen des ganglions spinaux dans des cas de pemphigus. Ann. Derm. Syph. (Paris) **79**, 626 (1952). — BEHÇET, H., B. OTTENSTEIN, G. TOKSOY u. S. ESER: Tierexperimentelle Untersuchungen zur Frage der Ätiologie des Pemphigus. Dermatologica (Basel) **87**, 113 (1943). — BELLONE, A. G., e V. LEONE: Ricerche sull'influenza esercita da sieri di soggetti sani o affeti da pemfigo su pelle umana normale e pemfigosa coltivata „in vitro". G. ital. Derm. Sif. **97**, 97 (1956). — BELOFF, A., and R. A. PETERS: Observations upon thermal burns: The influence of moderate temperature burns upon a proteinase of skin. J. Physiol. (Lond.) **103**, 461 (1945). — An investigation for the presence of a skin protease inhibitory factor in burned skin. J. Physiol. (Lond.) **105**, 54 (1946). — BERNHARDT, R.: Weitere Beiträge zur Ätiologie des Pemphigus und der Duhringschen Krankheit. Arch. Derm. Syph. (Berl.) **171**, 536 (1935). — BLANK, H., and C. F. BURGOON: Abnormal cytology of epithelial cells in pemphigus vulgaris: a diagnostic acid. J. invest. Derm. **18**, 213 (1952). — BOHNSTEDT, R. M.: Das Erythema exsudativum multiforme und verwandte Krankheitsbilder. Z. Haut- u. Geschl.-Kr. **14**, 272 (1953). — BRAUN-FALCO, O.: Histochemische Befunde bei „Pemphigus mit subepidermaler Blasenbildung", gleichzeitig ein Beitrag zur Pathogenese subepidermaler Blasenbildung. Arch. klin. exp. Derm. **211**, 213 (1960). — BRAUN-FALCO, O., u. K. SALFELD: Über das Verhalten der Leucin-Aminopeptidase-Aktivität im Blutserum und Blaseninhalt. Arch. klin. exp. Derm. **205**, 103 (1957). — BRENNAN, J. G., and H. MONTGOMERY: Pemphigus and other bullous dermatoses: Correlation of clinical and pathologic findings. J. invest. Derm. **21**, 349 (1953). — BRØCHNER-MORTENSEN, K.: Hypoproteinemia in chronic pemphigus. Acta med. scand. **97**, 319 (1938). — BROWN, M. V.: Fogo selvagem (pemphigus foliaceus). Review of the Brazilian literature. Arch. Derm. Syph. (Chic.) **69**, 589 (1954). — BURBACH, J. P. E.: The serum mucoprotein level in various diseases of the skin. Dermatologica (Basel) **111**, 65 (1955). — Experiments on blister formation. I. Experiments with proteolytic enzymes and hyaluronidases. Dermatologica (Basel) **118**, 379 (1959). — Experiments on blister formation. IV. The action of cantharidin. Dermatologica (Basel) **123**, 42 (1961).

CACCIALANZA, P., F. GIANOTTI e L. LEVI: Studio della funzionalità cortico-surrenale nel pemfigo e nelle forme pemfigoidi mediante valutazione della eliminazione orinaria dei corticoidi e dei 17-chetosteroidi, prima e dopo stimulazione con ACTH. G. ital. Derm. Sif. **94**, 85 (1953). — CAROL, W. L. L., J. R. PRAKKEN, M. RUITER, E. P. SNYDERS u. D. K. WIELENGA: Untersuchungen über das Vorkommen eines filtrierbaren Virus bei Pemphigus vulgaris. Arch. Derm. Syph. (Berl.) **175**, 265 (1937). — CHARGIN, L., H. SILVER, and P. M. SACHS: Pemphigus seborrheicus. Acta derm.-venereol. (Stockh.) **38**, 137 (1958). — CHARPY, J., G. FRAMIER et A. STAHL: Les lésions viscérales du pemphigus. Arch. belg. Derm. **11**, 22 (1955) sowie Presse méd. **63**, 436 (1955). — CIVATTE, A.: Diagnostic histopathologique de la dermatite polymorphe douloureuse ou maladie du Duhring-Brocq. Ann. Derm. Syph. (Paris) **3**, 1 (1943). — COHEN, H. A., T. D. ULLMANN, and A. DOSTROVSKY: Adrenocortical dysfunction in the early stage of pemphigus vulgaris. J. invest. Derm. **30**, 207 (1958). — COHN, E. J., L. J. ONCLEY, L. E. STRONG, W. L. HUGHES jr., and S. H. ARMSTRONG jr.: The characterization of the protein fractions of human plasma. J. clin. Invest. **23**, 417 (1944). — COLOMB, D., et C. ABGRALL: Maladie de Senear-Usher; réflexions thérapeutiques. Bull. Soc. franç. Derm. Syph. **69**, 104 (1962). — COLOMB, D., et M. JEANNEROD: Nouveau cas de pemphigus séborrhéique de Senear-Usher agent bénéficié d'un traitement local d'appoint à la pomade néomycine-triamcinolone. Bull. Soc. franc. Derm. Syph. **69**, 409 (1962). — COMBES, F. C., and O. CANIZARES: Pemphigus vulgaris: a clinopathological study of 100 cases. Arch. Derm. Syph. (Chic.) **62**, 786 (1950). — CORDERO, A. A. J.: La histopatología de la dermatitis de Duhring y de los pénfigos. Rev. argent. Dermatosif. **31**, 212 (1947). — COSTA, O. G.: Brazilian pemphigus foliaceus (wild fire). Brit. J. Derm. **60**, 359 (1948). — COSTELLO, M. J.: Erythema multiforme exudativum. (Erythema bullosum malignans, pluriorificial type.) J. invest. Derm. **8**, 127 (1947). — In der Diskussion zu H. O. PERRY: Arch. Derm. **83**, 52 (1961). — COSTELLO, M. J., L. JAIMOVICH, and M. DANNENBERG: Treatment of pemphigus with corticosteroids. J. Amer. med. Ass. **165**, 1249 (1957). — CROSTI, A., F. GIANOTTI et E. HAHN: Isolement d'un singulier virus pathogène dans les malades du groupe pemphigus. Dermatologica (Basel) **121**, 121 (1960). — CSOKA, I., u. E. VADASZ: Über die Glykocorticoid-Produktionsstörungen der Neben- nierenrinde bei Pemphiguskranken. Z. Haut- u. Geschl.-Kr. **35**, 102 (1963).

DAVIDSON, E. C.: Sodium chloride metabolism in cutaneous burns and its possible significance for a rational therapy. Arch. Surg. **13**, 262 (1926). — DEGOS, R.: In der Diskussion zu „Bullous Dermatoses". Acta derm.-venereol. (Stockh.), Proc. 11th Internat. Congr.

Derm., 1957, Bd. 3, S. 301. — DIRECTOR, W.: Pemphigus vulgaris: a clinicopathological study. Arch. Derm. Syph. (Chic.) **65**, 155 (1952) (I). — Pemphigus vegetans: a clinicopathological correlation. Arch. Derm. Syph. (Chic.) **66**, 343 (1952) (II). — DIXON, M., and D. M. NEEDHAM: Biochemical research on chemical warfare agents. Nature (Lond.) **158**, 432 (1946). — DOEPFMER, R.: Über eine nosologisch ungeklärte bullöse Dermatose (Pemphigus chronicus vulgaris oder Dermatitis herpetiformis). Hautarzt **12**, 452 (1961). — DOSTROVSKY, A., L. GUREVITCH, and H. UNGAR: On the question of the aetiology of pemphigus vulgaris and dermatitis herpetiformis Duhring. Brit. J. Derm. **50**, 412 (1938). — DOSTROVSKY, A., and F. G. SULMAN: Pemphigus vulgaris under prolonged massive treatment with ACTH and cortisone. Dermatologica (Basel) **116**, 65 (1958). — DOUCAS, C., u. J. KAPETANAKIS: Über vier in Griechenland beobachtete Fälle von Senear-Usher-Syndrom. Hautarzt **4**, 336 (1953). — DUPONT, A., et J. PIÉRARD: Histologie du pemphigus chronique et de la dermatite de Duhring-Brocq. Arch. belges Derm. **5**, 275 (1949).

EBERHARTINGER, C., u. H. EBNER: Behandlungsmöglichkeiten der Dermatitis herpetiformis Duhring. Derm. Wschr. **148**, 145 (1963). — ELLER, J. J., and L. H. KEST: Pemphigus. Report of seventy-seven cases. Arch. Derm. Syph. (Chic.) **44**, 337 (1941). — EPSTEIN, W. L., and A. M. KLIGMAN: Treatment of warts with cantharidin. Arch. Derm. **77**, 508 (1958). — EVERALL, J., and R. REED: A preliminary electron microscope study of dermatitis herpetiformis and pemphigus vulgaris. Brit. J. Derm. **65**, 432 (1953).

FARRELL, G. L., and G. LAQUEUR: Reduction of pituitary content of ACTH by cortisone. Endocrinology **56**, 471 (1955). — FELDAKER, M., L. A. BRUNSTING, and B. F. MCKENZIE: Paper electrophoresis of serum proteins in selected dermatoses. J. invest. Derm. **26**, 293 (1956). — FIESSINGER, N., et R. RENDU: Sur un syndrome characterisé par l'inflammation simultanée de toutes les muqueuses externes coexistant avec une éruption vésiculeuse des quatre membres non douloureuse et non récidivante. Paris méd. **25**, 54 (1917). — FISHER, I.: Pemphigus vulgaris. A clinical and laboratory study. Arch. Derm. **66**, 49 (1952). — In der Diskussion zu Fall 12, Pemphigus foliaceus, Minnesota Derm. Soc. Arch. Derm. **85**, 678 (1962). — FLECK, L., and F. GOLDSCHLAG: Further experimental studies of pemphigus. Brit. J. Derm. **51**, 70 (1939). — FLODEN, C. H., and H. GENTELE: Two cases of „pemphigoide séborrhéique" or Senear-Usher's syndrome. Acta derm.-venereol. (Stockh.) **33**, 402 (1953). — A case of clinically typical dermatitis herpetiformis (Morbus Duhring) presenting acantholysis. Acta derm.-venereol. (Stockh.) **35**, 128 (1955). — FÖLDVÁRI, F.: Histopathologische Untersuchungen bei Pemphigus. Hautarzt **10**, 442 (1959). — FÖLDVÁRI, F., et J. BALÓ: Les altérations du ganglion de Gasser dans des cas de pemphigus de la bouche. Ann. Derm. Syph. (Paris) **81**, 507 (1954). — FÖLDVÁRI, F., u. L. NÉKÁM jr.: Die Rolle des Hyaluronsäure-Hyaluronidase-Gleichgewichtes in der Pathogenese einzelner bullöser Erkrankungen. Arch. klin. exp. Derm. **203**, 433 (1956). — FRAWLEY, T. F., H. KISTLER, and T. SHELLEY: Effects of antiinflammatory steroids on carbohydrate metabolism, with emphasis on hypoglycemic and diabetic states. Ann. N.Y. Acad. Sci. **82**, 868 (1959). — FRIEDMANN, E., et G. PATHÉ: Le syndrome de Stevens-Johnson n'est qu'une forme grave de l'érythemè polymorphe. Ann. Derm. Syph. (Paris) **80**, 132 (1953). — FRÜHWALD, R.: Pemphigus vegetans, S. 137 u. 236. Leipzig: Voss 1915. — FURTADO, T. A.: Histopathology of pemphigus foliaceus. Arch. Derm. **80**, 66 (1959). — FURTADO, T. A., O. G. MOURÃO, M. D. MORIAS, and G. BATISTA: The urinary excretion of 17-ketosteroids in pemphigus foliaceus. J. invest. Derm. **32**, 641 (1959).

GAWALOWSKI, K., J. L. BLAŽEK, E. ČERNY, J. FISCHER, V. KUBELKA et E. NEUMANN: Notions nouvelles sur le pemphigus vulgaris. Acta derm.-venereol. (Stockh.), Proc. 11th Internat. Congr. Derm. 1957, Bd. 3, S. 323. — GELLIS, S., and F. A. GLASS: Pemphigus: Survey of 170 patients admitted to Bellevue Hospital between 1911 and 1941. Arch. Derm. Syph. (Chic.) **44**, 321 (1941). — GOLDSMITH, W. N.: A case of pyodermite végétante (Hallopeau). Brit. J. Derm. **53**, 209 (1941). — GOLDZIEHER, J. W.: The adrenal glands in pemphigus vulgaris. Arch. Derm. Syph. (Chic.) **52**, 369 (1945). — GRACE, A. W.: Pemphigus vulgaris. A study of the blood picture. Arch. Derm. Syph. (Chic.) **55**, 772 (1947). — GRACE, A. W., and F. H. SUSKIND: An investigation of the etiology of pemphigus vulgaris. J. invest. Derm. **2**, 1 (1939). — GRAIS, M. L., and D. GLICK: Mucolytic enzyme systems. II. Inhibition of hyaluronidase by serum in skin diseases. J. invest. Derm. **11**, 259 (1948). — GRAY, A. M. A.: Pemphigus of the Senear-Usher type. Proc. roy. Soc. Med. **31**, 871 (1938). — In der Diskussion zu I. MUENDE, Senear-Usher syndrome. Proc. roy. Soc. Med. **32**, 420 (1939).

HABER, H.: Cytodiagnosis in dermatology. Brit. J. Derm. **66**, 79 (1954). — HAENSCH, R.: Ergebnisse der Serumelektrophorese bei schweren Dermatosen. Z. Haut- u. Geschl.-Kr. **17**, 40 (1954). — Der Tzanck-Test. Hautarzt **6**, 407 (1955) (I). — Elektrophoretische Vergleichsuntersuchungen zwischen Serum und Blasenflüssigkeit bei bullösen Dermatosen. Derm. Wschr. **132**, 1327 (1955) (II). — HALLOPEAU, H.: „Pyodermite végétante", ihre Beziehungen zur Dermatitis herpetiformis und dem Pemphigus vegetans. Arch. Derm. Syph. (Berl.) **43**, 289 (1898a). — Zweite Mittheilung über „Pyodermite végétante" (Suppurative Form der Neumann'schen Krankheit). Arch. Derm. Syph. (Berl.) **45**, 323 (1898b). — HAMBRICK jr.,

G. W., and H. BLANK: Whole mounts for the study of skin and its appendages. J. invest. Derm. 23, 437 (1954). — HEBRA, F.: Acute Exantheme und Hautkrankheiten. In: Handbuch der Speciellen Pathologie und Therapie, redigiert von RUDOLF VIRCHOW, Bd. 4, S. 572. Erlangen: Enke 1860. — HELLIER, F. F.: Anomalous findings in pemphigus. Brit. J. Derm. 66, 49 (1954). — HERRMANN, W. P., u. K. H. SCHULZ: Immunoelektrophoretische Untersuchungen an Blasenflüssigkeiten. Arch. klin. exp. Derm. 214, 493 (1962). — HERZBERG, J. J.: Kritische Betrachtungen zur histologischen Differenzierung von Pemphigus und Pemphigoiden. Arch. Derm. Syph. (Berl.) 200, 206 (1955). — Vesiculöse-bullöse Erkrankungen. In: Dermatologie und Venerologie, hrsg. von H. A. GOTTRON u. W. SCHÖNFELD, Bd. 4, Teil 1, S. 676. Stuttgart: Georg Thieme 1958. — HERZBERG, J. J., u. B. ROHDE: Über den Mechanismus der Blasenbildung. I. Nachweis der proteolytischen Aktivität des Blaseninhaltes. Dermatologica (Basel) 118, 396 (1959). — HÖCKER, H.: Die Kennzeichnung der remissionsfähigen und der malignen Verlaufsformen des Pemphigus chronicus nach dem Blutbild. Arch. Derm. Syph. (Berl.) 187, 181 (1949). — HOLUB, D. A., J. I. KITAY, and J. W. JAILER: Effects of exogenous adrenocorticotropic hormone (ACTH) upon pituitary ACTH concentration after prolonged cortisone treatment and stress. J. clin. Invest. 38, 291 (1959).

JABLONSKA, S., L. FABJANSKA, and B. MILEWSKI: The significance of cytological and histological examinations in diagnosis and differential diagnosis of bullous diseases. Acta derm.-venereol. (Stockh.), 11th Internat. Congr. Derm. 1957, Bd. 3, S. 277.

KARTAMISCHEW, A.: Zur Frühdiagnose und Wesen des Pemphigus. Arch. Derm. Syph. (Berl.) 148, 69 (1925). — KATZENELLENBOGEN, I., u. M. SANDBANK: Beitrag zum Pemphigus vulgaris der Mundschleimhaut. Hautarzt 10, 363 (1959). — KEINING, E.: In der Diskussion zu R. RICHTER, Zur nosologischen Stellung und Pathogenese des Senear-Usherschen Syndroms. Arch. Derm. Syph. (Berl.) 200, 190 (1955). — KEINING, E., u. O. BRAUN-FALCO: Dermatologie und Venerologie, S. 424. München: J. F. Lehmann 1961. — KLASCHKA, F.: Untersuchungen zur autolytischen und heterolytischen Aktivität der Proteasen normaler und pathologisch veränderter menschlicher Epidermis und Cutis. Arch. klin. exp. Derm. 215, 137 (1962). — KLAUDER, J. V.: Ectodermosis erosiva pluriorificialis. Arch. Derm. Syph. (Chic.) 36, 1067 (1937). — KOPEL, D.: Serologic reactions in pemphigus vulgaris. An attempt to detect auto-antibodies or a virus in the blood serum or blister fluid in pemphigus vulgaris. J. invest. Derm. 22, 261 (1954). — KUHN, B. H., and L. IVERSON: Pemphigus vulgaris. Arch. Derm. Syph. (Chic.) 57, 891 (1948).

LARZELERE jr., R. G., E. A. BARTHOLD, F. M. WILLETT, T. V. FEICHTMEIER, L. WILSON, and E. P. ENGLEMAN: Adrenocortical function in long-term treatment with corticoids. Arch. intern. Med. 99, 888 (1957). — LAUSECKER, H.: Zur Frage des Pemphigus acutus. Hautarzt 8, 97 (1957). — LEINBROCK, A.: Veränderungen der elektrophoretischen Proteinspektren im Serum und in der Blasenflüssigkeit und Verhalten der Serumlabilitätsteste bei verschiedenen Pemphigusformen. Arch. Derm. Syph. (Berl.) 192, 535 (1951). — LEVER, W. F.: Severe erythema multiforme. Report of two cases of the type ectodermosis erosiva pluriorificialis, with development of cicatricial conjunctivitis and keratitis in one case. Arch. Derm. Syph. (Chic.) 49, 47 (1944). — The proteins in pemphigus vulgaris. I. Electrophoretic analysis of the proteins in the blood serum of patients with pemphigus vulgaris. J. invest. Derm. 14, 205 (1950) (I). — The proteins in pemphigus vulgaris. II. Electrophoretic analysis of the proteins in the blister fluid of patients with pemphigus vulgaris. J. invest. Derm. 14, 219 (1950) (II). — Pemphigus. A histopathologic study. Arch. Derm. Syph. (Chic.) 64, 727 (1951). — Pemphigus. Medicine (Baltimore) 32, 1 (1953). — Pemphigus and Pemphigoid. Springfield (Ill.): Ch. C. Thomas 1964. — LEVER, W. F., F. R. N. GURD, E. UROMA, R. K. BROWN, B. A. BARNES, K. SCHMID, and E. L. SCHULTZ: Chemical, clinical, and immunological studies on the products of human plasma fractionation. XL. Quantitative separation and determination of the protein components in small amounts of normal human plasma. J. clin. Invest. 30, 99 (1951). — LEVER, W. F., N. A. HURLEY, and A. E. BLANEY: The proteins in pemphigus vulgaris. IV. Determination of the plasma proteins by electrophoresis and chemical fractionation in patients with pemphigus under treatment with corticotropin or cortisone. J. invest. Derm. 19, 55 (1952). — LEVER, W. F., and J. G. MACLEAN: The proteins in pemphigus vulgaris. III. The effect of infusions of human serum albumin on the proteins in the blood serum of patients with pemphigus vulgaris. J. invest. Derm. 15, 215 (1950). — LEVER, W. F., and J. H. TALBOTT: Electrolyte content of the blister fluid in pemphigus. J. invest. Derm. 5, 303 (1942). — Pemphigus. A further report on chemical studies of the blood serum and treatment with adrenocortical extracts, dihydrotachysterol or Vitamin D. New Engl. J. Med. 231, 227 (1944). — LEVER, W. F., and W. WHITE: Treatment of pemphigus with corticosteroids. Results obtained in 46 patients over a period of 11 years. Arch. Derm. 87, 12 (1963). — LOW, R. C.: Pemphigus foliaceus. Brit. J. Derm. 21, 101 (1909).

MARCHIONINI, A., and TH. NASEMANN: On the virus etiology of pemphigus and dermatitis herpetiformis Duhring. J. invest. Derm. 24, 267 (1955). — Über die Virusätiologie des Pemphigus und der Dermatitis herpetiformis Duhring. Dermatologica (Basel) 115, 320 (1957). —

MARKHAM, F. S., and M. F. ENGMAN jr.: An inquiry into the cause of pemphigus. Arch Derm. Syph. (Chic.) 41, 78 (1940). — MATRAS, A., u. R. STÖBERL: Über vergleichende elektrophoretische Untersuchungen von Serum und Blaseninhalt bei blasenbildenden Dermatosen. Derm. Wschr. 140, 828, 1213 (1959). — MEIROWSKY, E.: Experimentelle Studien zur Ätiologie des Pemphigus und der Dermatitis herpetiformis Duhring. Hautarzt 8, 389 (1957). — MELCZER, N.: Bemerkungen zu der Arbeit von E. MEIROWSKY: Experimentelle Studien zur Ätiologie des Pemphigus und der Dermatitis herpetiformis Duhring. Hautarzt 9, 328 (1958). — MELCZER, N., and P. VÁSÁRHELYI: Specific hemagglutinins in serum and spinal fluid of patients with pemphigus and dermatitis herpetiformis. Acta derm.-venereol. (Stockh.) 38, 198 (1958). — MEZZADRA, G., e C. RABITO: Tentativi di cultura su membrana corion allantoidea di embrione di pollo di un supposto virus del pemfigo e della dermatite erpetiforme. G. ital. Derm. Sif. 2, 106 (1949). — MICHELSON, H. E.: Acute forms of pemphigus. Arch. Derm. Syph. (Chic.) 65, 422 (1952). — MILLER, R. F., and R. B. STOUGHTON: Enzymatic vesication in vivo: I. Effects of papain in human skin. J. invest. Derm. 35, 141 (1960). — MOORE, F. D., J. L. LANGOHR, M. INGEBRETSEN, and O. COPE: The role of exudate losses in the protein and electrolyte imbalance of burned patients. Ann. Surg. 132, 1 (1950). — MULVEHILL, W.: Serum protein in dermatoses. Arch. Derm. Syph. (Chic.) 49, 327 (1944).

NAZZARO, P., e M. KRUSE-SPICCA: Ricerche virologiche nel pemfigo volgare. Ann. ital. Derm. Sif. 8, 377 (1953). — NAZZARO, P., e A. VALENTI: Ricerche sulla funcionalità corticosurrenale nel pemfigo. Ann. ital. Derm. Sif. 8, 290 (1953). — NELEMANS, T. G., F. J. KEUNING, T. G. RYSSEL, and M. RUITER: Histological changes in the tonofibrils in vesicular and bullous diseases of the skin. Brit. J. Derm. 64, 177 (1952). — NELEMANS, T. G., u. J. D. VERLINDE: Untersuchungen zur Frage der Virusätiologie des Pemphigus vulgaris. Dermatologica (Basel) 105, 44 (1952). — NEUMANN, I.: Pemphigus vegetans. Vjschr. Derm. Syph. 1, 382 (1896). — NIEUWMEIJER, A. H.: Tonofibrils in bullous dermatoses. A histo- and cytopathologic study. Dermatologica (Basel) 106, 379 (1953). — NIKI, F.: Comparative studies on bullous dermatoses: pemphigus, pemphigoid and dermatitis herpetiformis Duhring. Jap. J. Derm. Venereol. 66, 252 (1956).

OPPENHEIM, M., and D. COHEN: Primary lesions of pemphigus vulgaris. Arch. Derm. Syph. (Chic.) 46, 201 (1942).

PARIS, J.: Pituitary-adrenal suppression after protracted administration of adrenal cortical hormones. Proc. Mayo Clin. 36, 305 (1961). — PASCHOUD, J. M., B. SCHMIDLI u. W. KELLER: Über proteolytische Fermente der normalen menschlichen Haut. Arch. klin. exp. Derm. 201, 484 (1955). — PER, M. I., and A. L. MASCHKILLEISON: Remote results of continuous systemic corticosteroid treatment in pemphigus. Dermatologica (Basel) 124, 99 (1962). — PERCIVAL, G. H.: Diagnostic histologique du pemphigus foliacé et du syndrome de Senear-Usher. Arch. belges Derm. 5, 278 (1949). — The relationship between dermatitis herpetiformis, pemphigoid and pemphigus, on the basis of clinical and histological investigation. Acta derm.-venereol. (Stockh.), Proc. 11th Internat. Congr. Derm. 1957, Bd. 3, S. 286. — PERRY, H. O.: Pemphigus foliaceus. Arch. Derm. 83, 52 (1961). — PETERS, R. A., H. M. SINCLAIR, and R. H. S. THOMPSON: An analysis of the inhibition of pyruvate oxidation by arsenicals in relation to the enzyme theory of vesication. Biochem. J. 40, 516 (1946). — PETERS, R. A., and R. H. S. THOMPSON: The biochemistry of the skin. In: Modern trends in dermatology, hrsg. von R. M. B. MACKENNA, S. 94. New York u. London: Hoeber 1948. — PILLSBURY, D. M., W. B. SHELLEY, and A. M. KLIGMAN: Dermatology, S. 791. Philadelphia: W. B. Saunders Co. 1956. — POSTMA, C.: Ein Fall von Pemphigus vegetans. Acta derm.-venereol. (Stockh.) 12, 352 (1932). — PRAKKEN, J. R.: Zur Frage der sogenannten Kochsalzretention bei Hautkrankheiten. Acta derm.-venereol. (Stockh.) 16, 156 (1935). — Weitere Untersuchungen über die erhöhte Ausscheidung von Chlor durch die Haut bei Pemphigus. Acta derm.-venereol. (Stockh.) 17, 103 (1936). — PREININGER, T.: Beiträge zur Ätiologie des Pemphigus. Neues Antigen zur Komplementbindung bei Pemphigus. Derm. Wschr. 107, 1341 (1938). — PROPPE, A.: Pemphigus acutus febrilis gravis. Arch. Derm. Syph. (Berl.) 187, 364 (1949).

QUIROGA, M. I., y R. N. CORTI: Dosificación de los 17-cetosteroides urinários en el diagnóstico del pénfigo vulgar. Act. dermo-sifiliogr. (Madr.) 45, 233 (1954).

RAJKA jr., G.: The effect of hydrocortisone on blisters produced by threshold concentrations of cantharidin; studies on the guinea pig. Dermatologica (Basel) 117, 387 (1958). — RICHTER, R.: Das Senear-Usher Syndrom. Arch. Derm. Syph. (Berl.) 188, 724 (1950) (I). — Zur Frage der klinischen Manifestation des Sanarelli-Shwartzman-Phänomens in der Dermatologie. Arch. Derm. Syph. (Berl.) 190, 317 (1950) (II). — Zur nosologischen Stellung und Pathogenese des Senear-Usherschen Syndroms. Arch. Derm. Syph. (Berl.) 200, 190 (1955). — RIECKE, E.: Pemphigus. In: Handbuch der Haut- und Geschlechtskrankheiten, hrsg. von J. JADASSOHN, Bd. 7, Teil 2, S. 452. Berlin: Springer 1931. — ROBERT, P.: Serumuntersuchungen, insbesondere mit der Elektrophorese, bei verschiedenen Hautkrankheiten. Dermatologica (Basel) 97 (Suppl.), 89 (1948). — RÖCKL, H., and R. JAROSCHKA: Verhalten der Serumeiweißkörper bei Dermatosen. Arch. Derm. Syph. (Berl.) 196, 223 (1953). — ROOK,

A. J., and I. W. Whimster: The histologic diagnosis of pemphigus. Brit. J. Derm. **62**, 443 (1950). — Rothman, S.: Clinical implications of skin enzyme systems. Arch. Derm. **76**, 277 (1957).

Sagher, F.: Pemphigus, a disease of the ectodermal structures of skin and mucous membranes. Acta derm.-venereol. (Stockh.), 11th Internat. Congr. Derm. 1957, Bd. 3, S. 312. — Sanders, S. L., M. Brody, and C. T. Nelson: Corticosteroid treatment of pemphigus. Arch. Derm. **82**, 717 (1960). — Santori, G.: Clinica del pemfigo. Minerva derm. **30**, 350 (1955). — Scott, A.: A study of the action of chymotrypsin on the skin. J. invest. Derm. **30**, 201 (1958). — Senear, F. E.: Chronic pemphigus vulgaris. Arch. Derm. Syph. (Chic.) **65**, 429 (1952). — Senear, F. E., and L. B. Kingery: Pemphigus erythematosus. Arch. Derm. Syph. (Chic.) **60**, 238 (1949). — Senear, F. E., and B. Usher: An unusual type of pemphigus combining features of lupus erythematosus. Arch. Derm. Syph. (Chic.) **13**, 761 (1926). — Sheklakov, N. D.: Pemphigus. Moscow 1961. Ref. in Excerpta med. (Amst.), Sect. XIII **16**, 309 (1962). — Starck, V.: Changes in protein content of serum in bullous dermatoses. Acta derm.-venereol. (Stockh.) **26**, 418 (1946). — Steigleder, G. K.: Zur Differentialdiagnose des Pemphigus vulgaris aus dem Blasengrundstrich. Arch. klin. exp. Derm. **202**, 1 (1955). — Stevens, A. M., and F. C. Johnson: A new eruptive fever associated with stomatitis and ophthalmia. Amer. J. Dis. Child. **24**, 526 (1922). — Stevenson, C. J.: Treatment in bullous diseases with corticosteroid drugs and corticotrophin. Brit. J. Derm. **72**, 11 (1960). — Stoughton, R. B., and F. Bagatell: The nature of cantharidin acantholysis. J. invest. Derm. **33**, 287 (1959). — Stoughton, R. B., and N. Novak: Disruption of tonofibrils and intercellular bridges by disulfide-splitting agents. J. invest. Derm. **26**, 127 (1956). — Stüttgen, G., N. Hofmann u. W. Simmich: Die Proteolyse normaler und pathologisch veränderter Haut durch Endopeptidase. Arch. klin. exp. Derm. **205**, 381 (1957). — Stüttgen, G., u. H. Wüst: Die Blasenbildung in den Hautschichten in fermentchemischer Sicht. Arch. klin. exp. Derm. **206**, 403 (1957). — Sulzberger, M. B., and R. L. Baer: Comment. The Year Book of Dermatology and Syphilology 1953/54, S. 223. Chicago: Year Book Publ. 1954.

Talbot, N. B., A. M. Butler, E. A. MacLachlan, and R. M. Jones: Definition and elimination of certain errors in hydrolysis, extraction, and spectrochemical assay of α- and β-neutral urinary 17-ketosteroids. J. biol. Chem. **136**, 365 (1940). — Talbott, J. H., W. F. Lever, and W. V. Consolazio: Metabolic studies on patients with pemphigus. J. invest. Derm. **3**, 31 (1940). — Tappeiner, J., u. L. Pfleger: Ist der histologische Befund für die Pemphigusdiagnose entscheidend? Hautarzt **13**, 198 (1962). — Tappeiner, J., u. P. Wodniansky: Das „Senear-Usher Syndrom". Arch. klin. exp. Derm. **205**, 161 (1957). — Tosti, A., e P. Nazzaro: Istopatologia del pemfigo. Vierzigster Kongreß der Italienischen Gesellschaft für Dermatologie und Syphilographie. Minerva derm. **30** (Suppl. al No 8), 382 (1955). — Touraine, A.: La pemphigoide séborrhéique. Bull. Soc. franç. Derm. Syph. **58**, 113 (1951). — Pemphigus et pemphigoides. Ann. Derm. Syph. (Paris) **81**, 121 (1954). — Pemphigus und Pemphigoide. Arch. Derm. Syph. (Berl.) **200**, 180 (1955). — Touraine, A., et E. Lortat-Jacob: La pemphigoide séborrhéique (Syndrome de Senear-Usher). Ann. Derm. Syph. (Paris) **1**, 28 (1941). — Tschopp, W.: Zur Frage der Dermatitis herpetiformis vegetans. Acta derm.-venereol. (Stockh.) **12**, 352 (1932). — Tye, M., G. Blumental, and W. F. Lever: Pemphigus erythematosus. Favorable response to topical treatment. Arch. Derm. **90**, 307 (1964). — Tzanck, A.: Le cytodiagnostic immédiat en dermatologie. Ann. Derm. Syph. (Paris) **8**, 205 (1948).

Urbach, E.: Zur Pathochemie des Pemphigus. Arch. Derm. Syph. (Berl.) **150**, 52 (1926). — Urbach, E., u. F. Reiss: Tierexperimentelle Untersuchungen zur Frage der infektiös-toxischen Genese des Pemphigus vulgaris und der Dermatitis herpetiformis Duhring. Arch. Derm. Syph. (Berl.) **162**, 713 (1931). — Urbach, E., u. S. Wolfram: Experimentelle und histologische Studien zur Frage der Virusgenese der Pemphiguserkrankungen. Acta derm.-venereol. (Stockh.) **15**, 120 (1934). — The virus of pemphigus and dermatitis herpetiformis. Arch. Derm. Syph. (Chic.) **33**, 788 (1936). — Urbach, E., S. Wolfram u. R. Brandt: Zur Serodiagnose des Pemphigus. Klin. Wschr. **15**, 1479 (1936).

Vieira, J. P.: Pemphigus foliaceus (fogo selvagem). Arch. Derm. Syph. (Chic.) **41**, 858 (1940). — Considérations sur le pemphigus foliacé au Brasil, S. 220. São Paulo: Academia Nacional de Medicina 1948. — Vieira, J. P., M. Fonzari, and L. Goldman: Some recent studies in Brazilian pemphigus. Amer. J. trop. Med. Hyg. **3**, 868 (1954). — Vilanova, X., u. A. J. Piñol: Das Syndrom von Senear-Usher und der Pemphigus. Arch. Derm. Syph. (Berl.) **200**, 211 (1955).

Wagner, V., G. Šeba, and B. Hruščová: Demonstration of tissue antibodies in the blood serum of patients with certain skin diseases. Dermatologica (Basel) **112**, 25 (1956). — Wallhauser, H. J. F.: Dermatitis vegetans. Report of two cases of the Hallopeau type. Arch. Derm. Syph. (Chic.) **19**, 77 (1929). — Watrin, J., et A. Merand: Les aspects histologiques des maladies bulleuses. Arch. belges Derm. **8**, 168 (1952). — Weakley, D. R., and J. M. Einbinder: The mechanism of cantharidin acantholysis. J. invest. Derm. **39**, 39 (1962). —

Enzymes, acantholysis and pemphigus. Arch. Derm. **85**, 190 (1962). — WEBER, G.: Über das Verhalten der Glutaminsäure-Oxalessigsäure-Transaminase im Blutserum und der Cantharidenblasenflüssigkeit bei Dermatosen. Derm. Wschr. **137**, 257 (1958) (I). — Über das Verhalten der Aldolase-Aktivität im Blutserum und der Hautblasenflüssigkeit bei Dermatosen. Derm. Wschr. **138**, 737 (1958) (II). — Vergleichende fermentchemische Untersuchungen im Blut-, Hautblasenserum, Epidermishomogenat und in Psoriasisschuppen. Arch. klin. exp. Derm. **211**, 183 (1960). — WEBER, G., O. BRAUN-FALCO u. G. THAESLER: Zur Folge des Verhaltens proteingebundener Polysaccharide im Serum bei Dermatosen. II. Teil: Klinisch-experimentelle Ergebnisse. Arch. Derm. Syph. (Berl.) **198**, 634 (1954). — WEBER, G., u. H. THEISEN: Zur Frage des Verhaltens der Glutaminsäure-Brenztraubensäure-Transaminase im Blut- und Hautblasenserum bei Ekzem und bullösen Dermatosen. Arch. klin. exp. Derm. **208**, 93 (1959) (I). — Zum Nachweis enzymatischer Mechanismen in menschlicher Epidermis am Modell der subepidermalen Blase. Arch. klin. exp. Derm. **208**, 459 (1959) (II). — WEBER, G., u. I. WILDNER: Über die Milchsäuredehydrogenase-Aktivität im Blut und der Hautblasenflüssigkeit bei Dermatosen. Derm. Wschr. **138**, 767 (1958). — WELLS, G. C., and C. BABCOCK: Epidermal protease. J. invest. Derm. **21**, 459 (1953). — WENTHOLD, H. M. M., and E. JANSEN: Some observations on pemphigus vegetans. Dermatologica (Basel) **105**, 100 (1952). — WERTH, J.: Beitrag zur Virusätiologie des Pemphigus vulgaris. Arch. Derm. Syph. (Berl.) **176**, 382 (1938). — Neue Ergebnisse der experimentellen Pemphigusforschung. Arch. Derm. Syph. (Berl.) **183**, 483 (1943). — WILGRAM, G. F., and J. B. CAULFIELD: An electron microscopic study of acantholysis and dyskeratosis in pemphigus foliaceus with a special note on peculiar cytoplasmic bodies. J. invest. Derm. (im Druck). — WILGRAM, G. F., J. B. CAULFIELD, and W. F. LEVER: An electron microscopic study of acantholysis in pemphigus vulgaris. J. invest. Derm. **36**, 373 (1961). — Elektronenmikroskopische Untersuchungen bei Hauterkrankungen mit Acantholyse (Pemphigus vulgaris, Pemphigus familiaris benignus chronicus, Morbus Darier). Derm. Wschr. **147**, 281 (1963). — WINKELMANN, R. K., and H. L. ROTH: Dermatitis herpetiformis with acantholysis or pemphigus with response to sulfonamides. Arch. Derm. **82**, 385 (1960). — WISE, F.: In der Diskussion zu D. BLOOM, Pemphigus (Senear-Usher type). Arch. Derm. Syph. (Chic.) **45**, 781 (1942). — In der Diskussion zu M. J. COSTELLO, A case for diagnosis (Lupus erythematosus with superimposed Senear-Usher syndrome). Arch. Derm. Syph. (Chic.) **54**, 727 (1946). — WITTELS, W.: Ergebnisse der Kortikosteroidtherapie beim Pemphigus vulgaris. Derm. Wschr. **141**, 401 (1960). — WORINGER, F.: Un cas de pemphigoide séborrhéique. Acta derm.-venereol. (Stockh.) **32**, 110 (1952). — WÜST, H.: Die prognostische und diagnostische Bedeutung von Serumenzymen bei dermatologischen Erkrankungen. Arch. klin. exp. Derm. **211**, 198 (1960).

ZAMECNIK, P. C., M. L. STEPHENSON, and O. COPE: Peptidase activity of lymph and serum after burns. J. biol. Chem. **158**, 135 (1945). — ZELDIS, L. J., and E. L. ALLING: Plasma protein metabolism — electrophoretic studies. Restoration of circulating proteins following acute depletion by plasmapheresis. J. exp. Med. **81**, 515 (1945). — ZILBERBERG, B.: Pênfigo e Dermatite de Duhring-Brocq, S. 68. São Paulo: Faculdade Nacional de Medicina da Universidade do Brasil 1955.

B. Pemphigoid

ACHTEN, G., et M. CORBUSIER-LEDOUX: Contribution à l'étude histologique de la membrane basale dans les dermatoses bulleuses. Arch. belges Derm. **14**, 290 (1958). — ADAM, C.: Untersuchungen zur Pathologie des Pemphigus conjunctivae. Z. Augenheilk. **23**, 35 (1910). — AUBERTIN, LAVIGNOLLE, TEXIER, ROY et SORBE: Maladie de Duhring-Brocq à prédominance buccale avec sténose oesophagienne. Bull. Soc. franç. Derm. Syph. **67**, 58 (1960).

BENEDICT, E. B., and W. F. LEVER: Stenosis of esophagus in benign mucous membrane pemphigus. Ann. Otol. (St. Louis) **61**, 1120 (1952). — BRENNAN, J. G., and H. MONTGOMERY: Pemphigus and other bullous dermatoses: Correlation of clinical and pathologic findings. J. invest. Derm. **21**, 349 (1953). — BRUNSTING, L. A., and H. O. PERRY: Benign pemphigoid. A report of seven cases with chronic, scarring, herpetiform plaques about the head and neck. Arch. Derm. **75**, 489 (1957). — BURBACH, J. P. E.: Experiments on blister formation. II. The contents of blisters. Dermatologica (Basel) **120**, 345 (1960).

Case Records of the Massachusetts General Hospital: Case 40111. Benign mucous membrane pemphigoid. New Engl. J. Med. **250**, 478 (1954). — CAULFIELD, J. B., and G. F. WILGRAM: An electron microscopic study of blister formation in erythema multiforme. J. invest. Derm. **39**, 307 (1962). — CHARGIN, L., H. SILVER, and P. M. SACHS: Pemphigus seborrheicus. Acta derm.-venereol. (Stockh.) **38**, 137 (1958). — CHARLES, A.: Electron microscopic observations on pemphigoid. Brit. J. Derm. **72**, 439 (1960). — CHURCH, R.: Pemphigoid treated with corticosteroids. Brit. J. Derm. **72**, 434 (1960). — CHURCH, R. E., and I. B. SNEDDON: Ocular pemphigus. Brit. J. Derm. **65**, 235 (1953).

Degos, R.: In der Diskussion zu „Bullous Dermatoses". Acta derm.-venereol. (Stockh.), Proc. 11th Internat. Congr. Derm., 1957, Bd. 3, S. 301. — Degos, R., E. Lortat-Jacob et P. Hardy: La place nosologique du „pemphigus oculaire". Dermatologica (Basel) **115**, 205 (1957).

Eberhartinger, C., u. G. Niebauer: Zur Prognose und Therapie des Pemphigus vulgaris und ähnlicher Erkrankungen. Hautarzt **12**, 503 (1961).

Fassotte, C.: Les dermatites polymorphes de Duhring-Brocq d'évolution mortelles. Arch. belges Derm. **9**, 105 (1953). — Fisher, I.: Pemphigus vulgaris. A correlation of clinical and microscopic observation. Arch. Derm. **74**, 50 (1956). — Pemphigus vulgaris. Re-evaluation of management. J.-Lancet **82**, 210 (1962). — Földvári, F.: Histopathologische Untersuchungen bei Pemphigus. Hautarzt **10**, 442 (1959).

Greither, A.: Chronische Aphthose von Mundschleimhaut, Speiseröhre und Genitale mit stenosierender Atrophie und sekundärer Carcinombildung. Hautarzt **2**, 547 (1951).

Haber, H.: Some unusual histologic observations in pemphigus vulgaris. Acta derm.-venereol. (Stockh.), Proc. 11th Internat. Congr. Derm. 1957, Bd. 3, S. 322. — Hellier, F. F.: Anomalous findings in pemphigus. Brit. J. Derm. **66**, 49 (1954). — Herzberg, J. J.: Kritische Betrachtungen zur histologischen Differenzierung von Pemphigus und Pemphigoiden. Arch. Derm. Syph. (Berl.) **200**, 206 (1955). — Vesiculöse-bullöse Erkrankungen. In: Dermatologie und Venerologie, hrsg. von H. A. Gottron u. W. Schönfeld, Bd. 4, Teil 1, S. 676. Stuttgart: Georg Thieme 1958.

Jablonska, S., u. T. Chorzelski: Kann das histologische Bild die Grundlage zur Differenzierung des Morbus Duhring mit dem Pemphigoid und Erythema multiforme darstellen? Derm. Wschr. **146**, 590 (1963). — Jablonska, S., P. Segal, B. Milewski, and H. Dabrowska: Pemphigoid mucosae. The so-called pemphigus ocularis and its relation to pemphigus. Acta derm.-venereol. (Stockh.) **37**, 364 (1957).

Kanee, B.: Ocular pemphigus with scarring of the skin and mucous membranes. Arch. Derm. Syph. (Chic.) **55**, 37 (1947). — Kim, R., and R. K. Winkelmann: Dermatitis herpetiformis in children. Relationship to bullous pemphigoid. Arch. Derm. **83**, 895 (1961). — Klauder, J. V.: Argyria. Lupus erythematosus of the scalp. Essential shriveling of the conjunctiva (ocular pemphigus) with ocular, oral and vulvar lesions. Arch. Derm. Syph. (Chic.) **37**, 687 (1938). — Klauder, J. V., and A. Cowan: Ocular pemphigus and its relation to pemphigus of the skin and mucous membranes. Amer. J. Ophthal. **25**, 643 (1942).

Lapière, S.: In der Diskussion zu J. P. Clairbois, Duhring pemphigoide. Arch. belges Derm. **13**, 83 (1957). — Lever, W. F.: Pemphigus conjunctivae with scarring of the skin. Report of three cases. Arch. Derm. Syph. (Chic.) **46**, 875 (1942). — Pemphigus conjunctivae with scarring of the skin. Report of three additional cases. Arch. Derm. Syph. (Chic.) **49**, 113 (1944). — The proteins in pemphigus vulgaris. I. Electrophoretic analysis of the proteins in the blood serum of patients with pemphigus vulgaris. J. invest. Derm. **14**, 205 (1950) (I). — The proteins in pemphigus vulgaris. II. Electrophoretic analysis of the proteins in the blister fluid of patients with pemphigus vulgaris. J. invest. Derm. **14**, 219 (1950) (II). — Pemphigus. Medicine (Baltimore) **32**, 1 (1953). — Bullous dermatoses. Acta derm.-venereol. (Stockh.), Proc. 11th Internat. Congr. Derm. 1957, Bd. 3, S. 293. — Lever, W. F., N. A. Hurley, and A. E. Blaney: The proteins in pemphigus vulgaris. IV. Determination of the plasma proteins by electrophoresis and chemical fractionation in patients with pemphigus under treatment with corticotropin or cortisone. J. invest. Derm. **19**, 55 (1952). — Lever, W. F., and J. H. Talbott: Electrolyte content of the blister fluid in pemphigus. J. invest. Derm. **5**, 303 (1942). — Lodin, A., and H. Gentele: Benign mucous membrane pemphigoid (pemphigus conjunctivae). Acta derm.-venereol. (Stockh.) **37**, 357 (1957). — Lortat-Jacob, E.: Benign mucosal pemphigoid. Dermatite bulleuse muco-synéchante et atrophiante. Brit. J. Derm. **70**, 361 (1958).

MacVicar, D. N., J. H. Graham, and C. F. Burgoon jr.: Dermatitis herpetiformis, erythema multiforme and bullous pemphigoid: A comparative histopathological and histochemical study. J. invest. Derm. **41**, 289 (1963). — McCarthy, P. L., and G. Shklar: Benign mucous-membrane pemphigus. New Engl. J. Med. **258**, 726 (1958).

Nelemans, T. G., F. J. Keuning, T. G. van Ryssel, and M. Ruiter: Histological changes in the tonofibrils in vesicular and bullous diseases of the skin. Brit. J. Derm. **64**, 177 (1952). — Nieuwmeijer, A. H.: Tonofibrils in bullous dermatoses. A histo- and cytopathologic study. Dermatologica (Basel) **106**, 379 (1963).

Osler, W.: On the visceral manifestations of the erythema group of skin diseases. Amer. J. med. Sci. **127**, 1 (1904).

Pachkov, B. M., and N. D. Cheklatov: Pemphigus benignus non acantholyticus mucosae oris. Dermatologica (Basel) **123**, 288 (1961). — Percival, G. H.: The relationship between dermatitis herpetiformis, pemphigoid and pemphigus, on the basis of clinical and histological investigation. Acta derm.-venereol. (Stockh.), Proc. 11th Internat. Congr. Derm. 1957, Bd. 3, S. 286. — Piérard, J., A. Dupont et A. Fontaine: Les critères du diagnostic histopathologique de la dermatite herpétiforme de Duhring et de l'erythème polymorphe. Arch. belges Derm. **13**, 370 (1957). — PIÉRARD, J., and I. WHIMSTER: The histological diagnosis of dermatitis herpetiformis, bullous pemphigoid and erythema multiforme. Brit. J. Derm. **73**, 253 (1961). — PRAKKEN, J. R., and M. J. WOERDEMAN: „Pemphigoid" (parapemphigus): Its relationship to other bullous dermatoses. Brit. J. Derm. **67**, 92 (1955).

RIECKE, E.: Pemphigus. In: Handbuch der Haut- und Geschlechtskrankheiten, hrsg. von J. JADASSOHN, Bd. 7, Teil 2, S. 452. Berlin: Springer 1931. — RIMBAUD, P., et H. L. GUIBERT: La dermatite de Duhring-Brocq. Remarques cliniques et histologiques. Ann. Derm. Syph. (Paris) **83**, 241 (1956). — RITZENFELD, P.: Zur Histologie der Entstehung subepidermaler Blasen. Dermatitis herpetiformis und benignes Schleimhautpemphigoid. Arch. klin. exp. Derm. **216**, 521 (1963). — ROOK, A., and E. WADDINGTON: Pemphigus and pemphigoid. Brit. J. Derm. **65**, 425 (1953). — RUPEC, M., A. KINT u. O. BRAUN-FALCO: Zur Frage der Histopathologie der peribullösen Veränderungen bei Dermatitis herpetiformis Duhring und ihrer Differentialdiagnose. Z. Haut- u. Geschl.-Kr. **34**, 121 (1963).

SANDERS, S. L., M. BRODY, and C. T. NELSON: Corticosteroid treatment of pemphigus. Arch. Derm. **82**, 717 (1960). — SCHMITZ, R.: Oesophagusverengung bei Pemphigus vulgaris. Z. Haut- u. Geschl.-Kr. **24**, 36 (1958). — SCHRECK, E.: Über einander zugeordnete Erkrankungen der Haut, der Schleimhäute und der Deckschicht des Auges (cutaneo-muco-oculo-epitheliale Syndrome). Arch. Derm. Syph. (Berl.) **198**, 221 (1954). — SNEDDON, I. B., and R. CHURCH: Diagnosis and treatment of pemphigoid. Report on 22 cases. Brit. med. J. **1955 II**, 1360. — STEIGLEDER, G. K.: Zur Differentialdiagnose des Pemphigus vulgaris aus dem Blasengrundstrich. Arch. klin. exp. Derm. **202**, 1 (1955). — STEVENSON, C. J.: Treatment in bullous diseases with corticosteroid drugs and corticotrophin. Brit. J. Derm. **72**, 434 (1960).

TALBOTT, J. H., W. F. LEVER, and W. V. CONSOLAZIO: Metabolic studies on patients with pemphigus. J. invest. Derm. **3**, 31 (1940). — TAPPEINER, J., u. L. PFLEGER: Ist der histologische Befund für die Pemphigusdiagnose entscheidend? Hautarzt **13**, 198 (1962). — THOST, A.: Über Schleimhautpemphigus. Arch. Laryng. Rhin. (Berl.) **31**, 599 (1918).

C. Pemphigus familiaris benignus

AYRES jr., S., and N. P. ANDERSON: Recurrent herpetiform dermatitis repens. Arch. Derm. Syph. (Chic.) **40**, 402 (1939).

BECKER, S. W., and M. E. OBERMAYER: Bullous disease. Bullous Darier's disease (Pels and Goodman). Familial benign pemphigus (Hailey and Hailey). Herpetiform dermatitis repens (Ayers and Anderson). Arch. Derm. Syph. (Chic.) **41**, 1170 (1940). — BOLGERT, M., G. LEVY, C. MIKOL, M. KAHN et R. DELUZENNE: Lésions bulleuses des aisselles dans un cas de maladie de Darier avec études histologique et cytologique. Ann. Derm. Syph. (Paris) **81**, 33 (1954).

CARPENTER, C. C.: Treatment of familial benign chronic pemphigus. Arch. Derm. Syph. (Chic.) **58**, 80 (1948). — CAULFIELD, J. B., and G. F. WILGRAM: An electronmicroscope study of dyskeratosis and acantholysis in Darier's disease. J. invest. Derm. **41**, 57 (1963). — CHORZELSKI, T.: Experimentally induced acantholysis in Hailey's benign pemphigus. Dermatologica (Basel) **124**, 21 (1962). — CREMER, G., and J. R. PRAKKEN: Hailey's disease. Dermatologica (Basel) **94**, 207 (1947).

DEGOS, R., et J. CIVATTE: Pemphigus bénin de Hailey-Hailey et maladie de Darier bulleuse. Bull. Soc. franç. Derm. Syph. **67**, 854 (1960). — DUPONT, A.: Note sur l'histologie du pemphigus familial héréditaire bénin (maladie de Gougerot-Hailey). Ann. Derm. Syph. (Paris) **78**, 703 (1951). — Sind Dyskeratosis follicularis Darier und Pemphigus familiaris hereditarius benignus Hailey-Hailey zwei verschiedene Krankheiten? Hautarzt **11**, 75 (1960).

ELLIS, F. A.: Vesicular Darier's disease (so-called benign familial pemphigus). Arch. Derm. Syph. (Chic.) **61**, 715 (1950).

FINNERUD, C. W., and F. J. SZYMANSKI: Chronic benign familial pemphigus, a possible vesicular variant of keratosis follicularis. Arch. Derm. Syph. (Chic.) **61**, 737 (1950). — FISCHER, H., u. W. NIKOLOWSKI: Die Mundschleimhaut beim Pemphigus benignus familiaris chronicus. Arch. klin. exp. Derm. **214**, 261 (1962).

GÖNCZÖL, I., u. L. SZODORAY: Hailey-Hailey'sche Pemphigus-Fälle bei Großvater und Enkel. Dermatologica (Basel) **120**, 214 (1960). — GOUGEROT, H.: La priorité du pemphigus chronique familial héréditaire bénin. Ann. Derm. **10**, 361 (1950).

HABER, H., and B. RUSSELL: Sisters with familial benign chronic pemphigus (Gougerot, Hailey and Hailey). Brit. J. Derm. **62**, 458 (1950). — HAILEY, H.: Familial benign chronic pemphigus. Sth. med. J. (Bgham, Ala.) **46**, 763 (1953). — HAILEY, H., and H. HAILEY: Familial benign chronic pemphigus. Arch. Derm. Syph. (Chic.) **39**, 679 (1939). — Familial benign chronic pemphigus. Sth. med. J. (Bgham, Ala.) **33**, 477 (1940). — HERZBERG, J. J.: Pemphigus Gougerot/Hailey-Hailey. Arch. klin. exp. Derm. **202**, 21 (1955).

JABLONSKA, S., u. T. CHORZELSKI: Zur Klassifikation des Pemphigus Hailey-Hailey. Dermatologica (Basel) **117**, 24 (1958). — JAEGER, H., J. DELACRETAZ et H. CHAPUS: Morbus Darier (actuellement en phase vésiculo-bulleuse rapellant le Morbus Hailey-Hailey). Dermatologica (Basel) **110**, 378 (1955). — JEWELL, E. W., and M. M. KEY: Familial benign chronic pemphigus (Hailey-Hailey) in Negroes. Arch. Derm. **75**, 715 (1957).

KANDHARI, K. C., and G. SINGH: Chronic benign pemphigus of Hailey and Hailey in an Indian child. Brit. J. Derm. **75**, 212 (1963).

LOEWENTHAL, L. J. A.: Familial benign chronic pemphigus. Arch. Derm. **80**, 318 (1959).— LYLES, T. W., J. M. KNOX and J. B. RICHARDSON: Atypical features in familial benign chronic pemphigus. Arch. Derm. **78**, 446 (1958).

PALMER, D. D., and H. O. PERRY: Benign familial chronic pemphigus. Arch. Derm. **86**, 493 (1962). — PELS, I. R., and M. H. GOODMAN: Criteria for the histologic diagnosis of keratosis follicularis (Darier). Arch. Derm. Syph. (Chic.) **39**, 438 (1939).

RAASCHOU-NIELSEN, W., and F. REYMANN: Familial benign chronic pemphigus. Acta derm.-venereol. (Stockh.) **39**, 280 (1959). — REISS, F.: Generalized bullous dyskeratosis (generalized bullous Darier's disease), with special reference to the histogenesis and metabolic changes. J. invest. Derm. **9**, 17 (1947).

SALSBERG, R. H.: Treatment of familial benign chronic pemphigus (Hailey and Hailey syndrome). Arch. Derm. Syph. (Chic.) **62**, 568 (1950). — SAMITZ, M. H.: Clinical evaluation of topical fluocinolone acetonide cream. Curr. ther. Res. **4**, 589 (1963). — SCHNEIDER, W., u. H. FISCHER: Passagere Gestaltswandel eines Pemphigus benignus familiaris chronicus (Gougerot-Hailey-Hailey) unter dem Bilde des Pemphigus vulgaris. Arch. klin. exp. Derm. **217**, 1 (1963). — SHELLEY, W. B., and D. M. PILLSBURY: Specific systemic antibiotic therapy in familial benign chronic pemphigus. Arch. Derm. **80**, 554 (1959). — SULLIVAN, C. N.: Familial benign chronic pemphigus (Hailey and Hailey). Arch. Derm. **74**, 329 (1956). — SVENDSEN, I. B., and B. ALBRECTSEN: The prevalence of dyskeratosis follicularis (Darier's disease) in Denmark. Acta derm.-venereol. (Stockh.) **39**, 256 (1959).

WEHNERT, R. A.: Familial benign chronic pemphigus (Hailey and Hailey) treated with cortisone. Acta derm.-venereol. (Stockh.) **33**, 211 (1953). — WILGRAM, G. F., J. B. CAULFIELD, and W. F. LEVER: An electron microscopic study of acantholysis and dyskeratosis in Hailey and Hailey's disease. J. invest. Derm. **39**, 373 (1962). — Elektronenmikroskopische Untersuchungen bei Hauterkrankungen mit Akantholyse (Pemphigus vulgaris, Pemphigus familiaris benignus chronicus, Morbus Darier). Derm. Wschr. **147**, 281 (1963). — WINER, L. H., and A. J. LEEB: Benign familial pemphigus. Arch. Derm. Syph. (Chic.) **67**, 77 (1953).

Dermatitis herpetiformis. Herpes gestationis. Subcorneale pustulöse Dermatose

Von

Walter F. Lever-Boston (Mass., USA)

Mit 8 Abbildungen

I. Dermatitis herpetiformis

Der wesentlichste Fortschritt in bezug auf die Dermatitis herpetiformis seit RIECKEs Beschreibung liegt in ihrer Behandlung.

a) Klinische Abgrenzung des Krankheitsbegriffes

Wie bereits bei der Besprechung des bullösen Pemphigoids hervorgehoben wurde (s. S. 672), besteht keine einheitliche Auffassung bezüglich der Abgrenzung der Dermatitis herpetiformis. Eine ganze Reihe von Dermatologen ziehen die Grenzen der Dermatitis herpetiformis ziemlich weit und schließen das bullöse Pemphigoid in den Begriff der Dermatitis herpetiformis ein. Unter diesen befinden sich besonders Angehörige der französischen Schule, z.B. DEGOS und CIVATTE sowie WORINGER, aber auch mehrere andere europäische Dermatologen, z.B. PERCIVAL, JABLONSKA sowie KORTING.

Andere Dermatologen ziehen dagegen die Grenzen der Dermatitis herpetiformis recht eng. Unter ihnen befinden sich die meisten Angehörigen der anglo-sächsischen Schule, z.B. TOLMAN et al., LIVINGOOD sowie KIM und WINKELMANN, aber auch eine Reihe von europäischen Dermatologen, wie EBERHARTINGER und EBNER, KIMMIG sowie SPIER und THIES und PIÉRARD und WHIMSTER. Nach der Auffassung dieser Autoren stellt die Dermatitis herpetiformis statt eines Symptomenkomplexes ein recht einheitliches Krankheitsbild dar. Dieser Ansicht stimme ich bei, und somit auch der Beschreibung der Dermatitis herpetiformis, die PIÉRARD und WHIMSTER kürzlich gegeben haben:

„Die Dermatitis herpetiformis ist eine gutartige, aber chronische und rezidivierende Krankheit, deren Hauterscheinungen pleomorphisch und symmetrisch sind. Sie bestehen aus rötlichen Flächen, die oft ein Urticaria-artiges Ödem aufweisen und eine serpiginöse Begrenzung haben. Auf diesen Flächen entwickeln sich Papeln, Bläschen sowie kleine, pralle Blasen, entweder diffus oder gruppiert. Die Hauterscheinungen finden sich vor allem an den Streckseiten der Extremitäten, an den Schultern, in der Sacralgegend und am Gesäß (Abb. 1). Sie jucken, und ihrem Auftreten geht ein Gefühl des Brennens voraus."

Dieser Definition kann man die Merkmale zufügen, die TOLMAN et al. in einer Arbeit aufgeführt haben, der sie die Überschrift gaben: „Dermatitis herpetiformis: Specific entity or clinical complex?" Darin führen sie die folgenden Merkmale auf: Vorkommen hauptsächlich bei jungen Erwachsenen, Fehlen von Schleimhauterscheinungen und Ansprechen auf Sulfapyridin und auf die Sulfone. TOLMAN et al. schlossen ausdrücklich von der Dermatitis herpetiformis aus: vorwiegend großblasige Hauterkrankungen mit Befall der Mundschleimhaut und ohne Gruppierung in der Anordnung der Hauterscheinungen sowie großblasige Erkrankungen bei Kindern und bei alten Leuten und ferner Herpes gestationis.

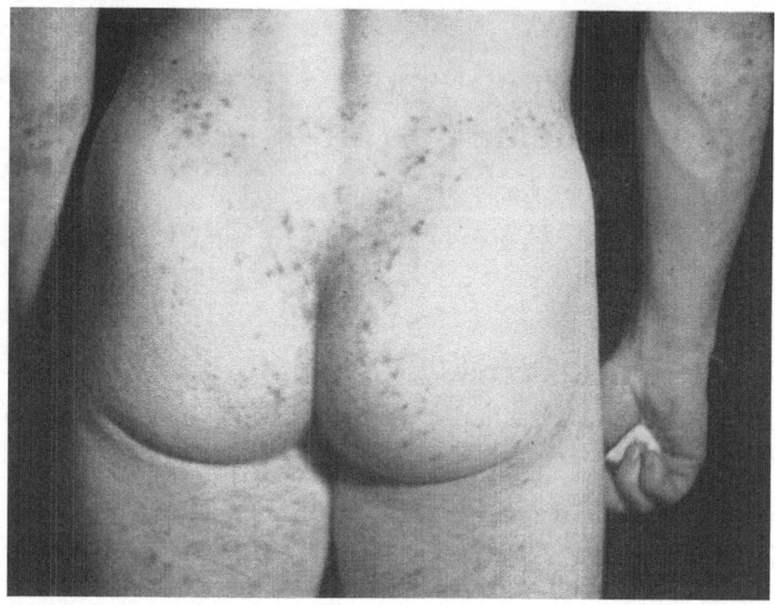

Abb. 1. Dermatitis herpetiformis. Bei einem Mann sind Papeln und Bläschen in gruppierter, symmetrischer Anordnung in der Sacralgegend und an den Ellbogen zu sehen

b) Verlauf

Der Verlauf der Dermatitis herpetiformis ist äußerst chronisch und bei recht vielen Patienten bleibt sie, wenn einmal aufgetreten, bis an das Lebensende bestehen. Doch kommt Abheilung vor, wenn auch erst gewöhnlich nach vielen Jahren. So stellten EYSTER und KIERLAND fest, daß unter 203 Patienten, die mindestens 10 Jahre lang unter ihrer Beobachtung gestanden hatten, 72, d.h. 35%, eine Abheilung ihrer Hauterscheinungen zeigten. Die kürzeste Zeit bis zur Abheilung unter diesen 72 Patienten war 2 Jahre gewesen und die längste Zeit 40 Jahre.

Obwohl die Dermatitis herpetiformis, wie TOLMAN et al. betont haben, gewöhnlich bei jungen Erwachsenen erstmalig auftritt, können in seltenen Fällen Kinder von ihr befallen werden (Abb. 2). Wie KIM und WINKELMANN betonen, besteht die Dermatitis herpetiformis auch bei Kindern aus stark juckenden papulovesiculären Efflorescenzen, die hauptsächlich an den Knien und Ellbogen vorkommen. Sie zeigt eine geringere Heilungstendenz als das bullöse Pemphigoid und dauert daher bis in das erwachsene Alter an. Männer sind häufiger befallen als Frauen. So betrug das Verhältnis unter den von EYSTER und KIERLAND beobachteten Patienten 2,7:1.

Die Beziehung zwischen Dermatitis herpetiformis und Schwangerschaft ist von besonderem Interesse wegen der immer noch von einigen Autoren vertretenen Ansicht, daß der Herpes gestationis lediglich eine während der Schwangerschaft auftretende Dermatitis herpetiformis darstelle (s. unter Herpes gestationis, S. 712). Abgesehen von Unterschieden im klinischen Bilde ist besonders hervorzuheben, daß eine bestehende Dermatitis herpetiformis sich oft während der Schwangerschaft bessert und die Besserung so lange wie die Schwangerschaft anhält. BROCQ beschrieb bereits im Jahre 1889 einen Fall von Dermatitis herpetiformis, bei dem die Hauterscheinungen für die Dauer der Schwangerschaft in voller Remission waren; und letzthin haben EYSTER und KIERLAND wie auch BJÖRNBERG und HELLGREN über je zwei Fälle mit völliger Abheilung und HANSEN und PETERKIN über je einen Fall mit Besserung der Dermatitis herpetiformis

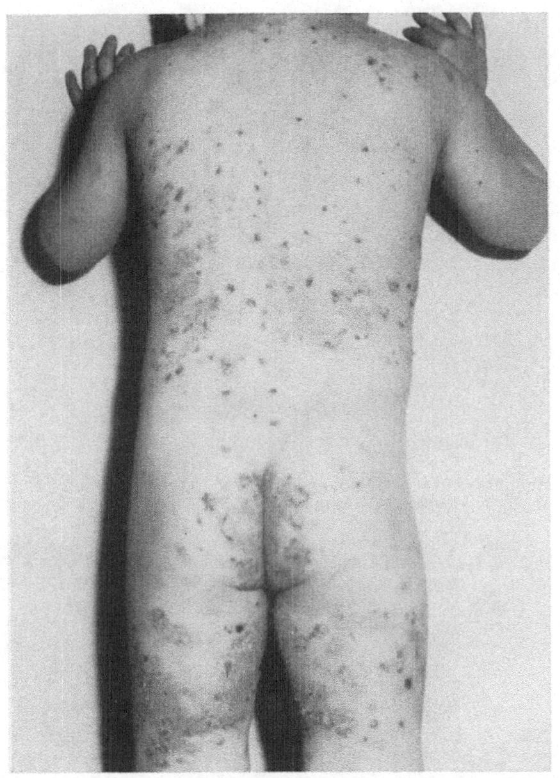

Abb. 2. Dermatitis herpetiformis. Bei einem 3jährigen Knaben bestehen rötliche Flächen, auf denen sich Papeln, Bläschen und kleine Blasen in gruppierter und teilweise in serpiginöser Anordnung befinden

während der Schwangerschaft berichtet. Daß eine Besserung während der Schwangerschaft aber nicht immer eintritt, beweist ein von RUSSELL und THORNE berichteter Fall.

c) Histologie

Die für die Dermatitis herpetiformis typischen histologischen Veränderungen findet man am besten in frischen erythematösen Herden, in denen klinisch noch keine Blasen sichtbar sind, sowie in der Umgebung frischer Bläschen. Diese Veränderungen wurden 1954 erstmalig von ALLEN kurz beschrieben, dann aber 1957 von PIÉRARD, DUPONT und FONTAINE in Einzelheiten dargestellt. Die früheste histologische Veränderung besteht bei der Dermatitis herpetiformis aus einer Ansammlung von Neutrophilen und Eosinophilen, zuerst innerhalb der Papillen und später in deren oberen Teil. Auf diese Weise bilden sich dort Mikroabscesse und gleichzeitig degeneriert das Kollagen innerhalb der Papillen und erscheint dann amorph. Diese Degeneration des Kollagens hat eine Kontinuitätstrennung zwischen den oberen Papillenenden und der Epidermis zur Folge (Abb. 3). Zuerst bleiben die interpapillären Reteleisten der Epidermis noch mit der Dermis in

Zusammenhang, so daß die Bläschen der Dermatitis herpetiformis im ersten Stadium ihrer Bildung multilocular sind (Abb. 4). Aber bereits nach 24—36 Std verlieren die Epidermisleisten, wie MACVICAR et al. nachgewiesen haben, ihren

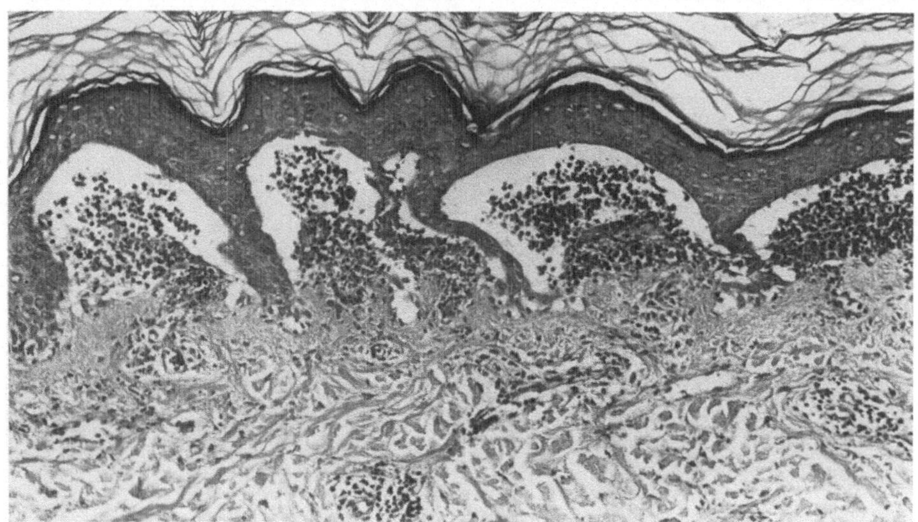

Abb. 3. Dermatitis herpetiformis. Ein in der Bildung begriffenes Bläschen ist multilocular und zeigt im oberen Teil der Papillen Mikroabscesse, die aus eosinophilen Leukocyten bestehen (200mal)

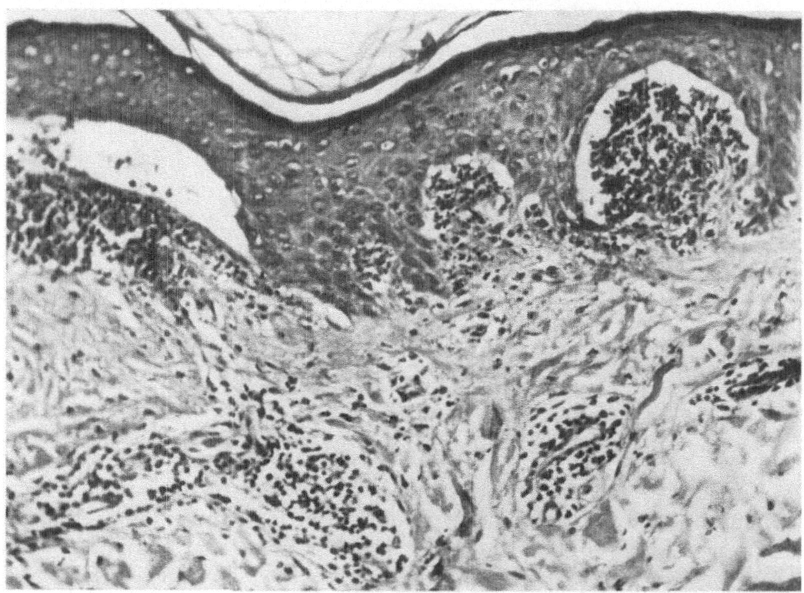

Abb. 4. Dermatitis herpetiformis. Am Rande eines Bläschens finden sich drei intrapapilläre Mikroabscesse (200mal)

Zusammenhang mit der Dermis und die Blasen sind dann unilocular (Abb. 5). Oft kann man zu diesem Zeitpunkt noch an der Peripherie solcher unilocularen Blasen die charakteristischen Mikroabscesse sehen (Abb. 4). Aus diesem Grund sollte man für die histologische Untersuchung zusammen mit einem frischen Bläschen stets etwas peribullöse Haut excidieren. PIÉRARD hat sogar darauf hingewiesen, daß oft die erythematösen Herde, auf denen noch keine Bläschen sichtbar sind, die intrapapillären Mikroabscesse am ausgesprochensten zeigen.

In den oberen Dermisschichten findet sich bei der Dermatitis herpetiformis gewöhnlich ein ziemlich ausgeprägtes celluläres Infiltrat, das oft recht viele Eosinophile enthält. Dabei kann manchmal recht ausgesprochene Leukocytoklasie bestehen, zusammen mit einer Degeneration von Endothelzellen der Gefäße, so daß das Bild einer Vasculitis vorliegt (RUPEC et al.).

Es erscheint zur Zeit noch zweifelhaft, ob das eben beschriebene histologische Bild für die Dermatitis herpetiformis absolut spezifisch ist. Anscheinend kann ein

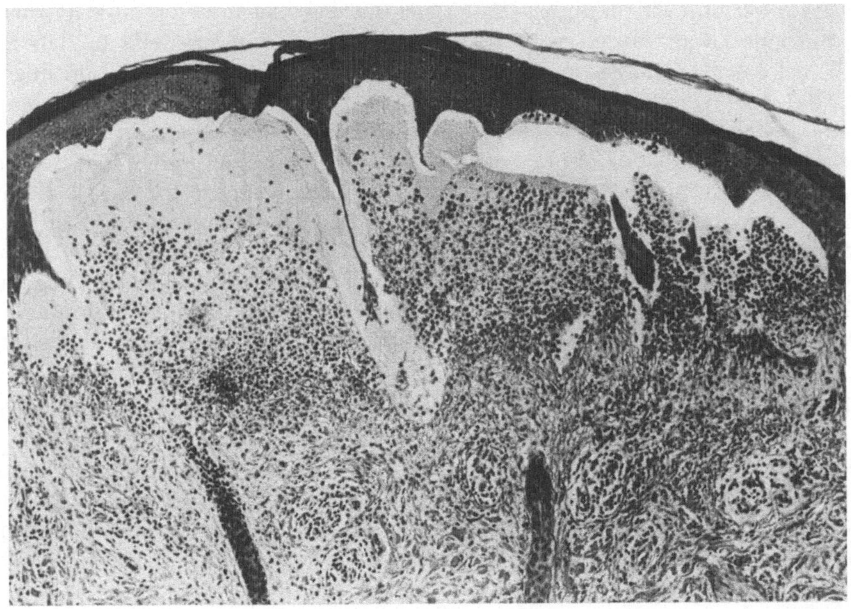

Abb. 5. Dermatitis herpetiformis. Die ältere Blase ist nicht mehr multilocular, sondern unilocular. Zahlreiche eosinophile Leukocyten befinden sich innerhalb der Blase; aber inrapapilläre Mikroabscesse sind nicht mehr erkennbar (100mal)

ähnliches histologisches Bild gelegentlich auch beim bullösen Pemphigoid gefunden werden, wenn man für die histologische Untersuchung Blasen, die auf erythematösen Flächen gelegen sind, wählt (JABLONSKA und CHORZELSKI) (s. auch S. 669).

d) Laboratoriumsbefunde

Trotz des regelmäßigen Bestehens einer Gewebseosinophilie im Gebiet der Hautherde, findet sich eine Bluteosinophilie nur gelegentlich. EYSTER und KIERLAND sowie ALEXANDER (1961) fanden eine ausgesprochene Bluteosinophilie nur bei Patienten mit sehr ausgedehnten Hauterscheinungen. Als Durchschnittswert berichtete NILES bei 37 Patienten mit Dermatitis herpetiformis 3,1% Eosinophile unter den weißen Blutkörperchen und ALEXANDER (1961) bei 33 Patienten 3,6% Eosinophile. EYSTER und KIERLAND stellten unter 116 Patienten fest, daß zwar 46 Patienten, d.h. 40%, über 4% Eosinophile hatten, aber nur 14 Patienten, d.h. 12%, über 10% Eosinophile hatten. ALEXANDER (1961) hat daher bestritten, daß die Zählung der Eosinophile bei der Stellung der Diagnose Dermatitis herpetiformis von Wert ist.

e) Halogenempfindlichkeit

EYSTER und KIERLAND stellten bei einem Krankengut von 121 Patienten mit Dermatitis herpetiformis fest, daß bei epicutanem Testen 50% der Patienten eine positive Reaktion zu Kaliumjodid und 31% zu Kaliumbromid aufwiesen. Nach interner Verabreichung kleiner Dosen von Kaliumjodid zeigten 78% der Patienten eine Verschlimmerung ihrer Hauterkrankung. Die Verfasser kamen zu dem Schluß, daß eine Jodüberempfindlichkeit nicht so regelmäßig bestehe, um diagnostischen Wert zu besitzen.

SPIER u. Mitarb. sahen dagegen die Verschlimmerung der Hauterscheinungen bei der Dermatitis herpetiformis durch kleine perorale Jodmengen als klinisch sichergestellt an. Sie glaubten, daß es sich hierbei eher um eine „Jod-Pathergie" als um eine cutan-vasculäre Jod-Allergie handelte. Andererseits fanden SPIER et al. bei epicutanem Testen mit Jodid, Rhodanid, Nitrat und Bromid ungefähr dieselbe Zahl von positiven Reaktionen bei Patienten mit Dermatitis herpetiformis wie bei solchen mit anderen Hauterkrankungen. Die Prozentsätze der positiven Reaktionen entsprachen der Hofmeister-Reihe: Rhodanid = Jodid > Nitrat = Bromid. Bei dem Aussetzen von Hautstücken zu diesen Halogen-Anionen und anschließender histologischer Untersuchung fanden SPIER et al., daß die Halogen-Anione eine Quellung der Epidermis hervorriefen. Sie werteten daher den Epicutantest mit Jodid und den anderen Halogen-Anionen als ein unspezifisches Epidermis-toxisches Anionenphänomen, das in keinem Zusammenhang stehe mit der Auslösbarkeit klinischer Symptome durch peroral zugeführtes Jodid.

FELSHER vertritt andererseits den Standpunkt, daß in Hinsicht darauf, daß Rhodanid, Jodid und Bromid in vitro eine Quellung des Kollagens hervorrufen, die bei der Dermatitis herpetiformis beobachteten Reaktionen auf extern appliziertes, wie auch auf intern verabreichtes Jodkali oder Bromid darauf beruhen, daß bei der Dermatitis herpetiformis eine Quellung des Kollagens leichter als gewöhnlich eintrete auf Grund eines veränderten physiko-chemischen Zustandes des Kollagens. Die Schwellung des Kollagens führe zu einer Trennung zwischen Dermis und Epidermis und so zur Blasenbildung.

f) Ätiologie

Die Möglichkeit, daß der Dermatitis herpetiformis eine Allergie zu Bakterien zugrunde liegt, ist von mehreren Autoren erwogen worden, die feststellten, daß bei Patienten mit Dermatitis herpetiformis intradermale Injektionen von Bakterien-Vaccinen an den Injektionsstellen Blasen hervorriefen. So beobachtete BERNHARDT Blasenbildung nach Injektionen eines Streptococcus-Vaccins oder von Trichophytin. LEONE stellte Blasenbildung auch nach Injektionen von Staphylococcus- oder Gonococcus-Vaccin fest, und CALLAWAY und STERNBERG sahen Blasenbildung nach der Injektion eines Pneumococcus-Vaccins. SWARTZ und LEVER erzeugten Blasen bei fünf von zwölf Patienten mittels eines E. coli-Vaccins, und außerdem konnten sie bei je einem dieser fünf Patienten mittels eines Staphylococcus- resp. eines Streptococcus-Vaccins Blasen hervorrufen. Ferner beobachtete EPSTEIN bei zwei Patienten Blasenbildung nach der intradermalen Injektion von Streptokokkenantigenen. Während LEONE seine Resultate lediglich als einen isomorphen Reizeffekt ansah, hielten die anderen Autoren doch eine Allergie zu Bakterien für möglich. SWARTZ betonte, daß eine bakterielle Allergie nicht unbedingt eine Allergie zu pathogenen Mikroben bedeute. Er erwog bei der Dermatitis herpetiformis die Möglichkeit einer Sensibilisierung zu normalerweise vorhandenen, nicht pathogenen Bakterien.

g) Differentialdiagnose

Das bullöse Pemphigoid und der Herpes gestationis können in ihrem klinischen Aussehen gelegentlich der Dermatitis herpetiformis ähnlich sehen. Für die Differenzierung der Dermatitis herpetiformis vom bullösen Pemphigoid s. S. 672, und von dem Herpes gestationis s. S. 712.

h) Therapie

Inorganische Arsenpräparate, die zu Rieckes Zeiten „zum eisernen Bestand der Duhringtherapie“ gehörten, werden nicht mehr angewandt, denn sie sind weniger wirksam als die neueren Behandlungsmittel und bei Verabreichung über längere Zeit besteht die Gefahr der Bildung von Arsenkeratosen und Arsencarcinomen.

Die beiden heute am meisten verwandten Mittel sind das Sulfapyridin (Eubasin) und die Sulfone. Dabei sind die Sulfone vorzuziehen, da sie seltener gefährliche Nebenwirkungen hervorbringen als das Sulfapyridin (s. unten). Zwar unterdrücken noch mehrere andere Mittel die Hauterscheinungen der Dermatitis herpetiformis; aber sie werden kaum jemals angewandt, entweder weil ihre Wirkung verhältnismäßig gering ist, wie z.B. beim Sulfanilamid, beim Sulfathiazol und bei der Nicotinsäure, oder weil ernste Nebenwirkungen häufig sind, wie z.B. beim 3-Sulfanilamido-6-methoxypyridazin (Kynex, Lederkyn) (Perry und Winkelmann) und bei den Corticosteroiden. Vor Darlegung der Behandlungspläne für die Sulfone und das Sulfapyridin mögen einige Worte über deren bisher noch nicht völlig erkannte Wirkungsweise gesagt werden.

Wirkungsweiese der Sulfonamide und Sulfone. Eine antibakterielle Wirkung der Sulfonamide wurde des öfteren erwogen, seit sie erstmalig im Jahre 1938 für die Behandlung der Dermatitis herpetiformis angewandt wurden (Lain und Lamb). Jedoch stellte Welsh fest, daß die Wirkung des Sulfapyridins bei der Dermatitis herpetiformis nicht beeinträchtigt war, wenn es zusammen mit p-Aminobenzoesäure verabreicht wurde, obwohl die p-Aminobenzoesäure bei bakteriellen Infektionen als Antagonist der Sulfonamide wirkt. Dafür, daß vielleicht der Sulfanyl-Anteil wirksam war, sprach die Tatsache, daß mehrere Sulfonamide bei der Dermatitis herpetiformis wirksam waren; aber Schulz konnte nachweisen, daß beim Sulfapyridin der Sulfanyl-Anteil für die Behandlung der Dermatitis herpetiformis nicht nötig war, da keine Verringerung der Wirkung eintrat, als er im Sulfapyridin die Sulfongruppe durch eine Carbonylgruppe ersetzte. Für eine Wirksamkeit des Pyridin-Anteils im Sulfapyridin sprach, daß auch die Nicotinsäure und das 3-Sulfanilamido-6-methoxypyridazin (Kynex) wirksam sind. Aber dies ist nicht wahrscheinlich, da das pyridinhaltige Antihistaminicum Pyribenzamin wirkungslos ist.

Die chemische Verwandtschaft zwischen dem Sulfapyridin und dem Diaminodiphenylsulfon ist nicht so groß, wie man nach der Ähnlichkeit der chemischen

$$H_2N—C_6H_4—SO_2—NH—C_5H_4N$$

Sulfapyridin

$$H_2N—C_6H_4—SO_2—C_6H_4—NH_2$$

Diaminodiphenylsulfon

Formeln denken würde; denn es besteht, wie Morgan et al. betonen, ein großer Unterschied zwischen der Bindung C—SO_2—NH und der Bindung C—SO_2—C, und die chemischen Eigenschaften des Pyridinrings im Sulfapyridin 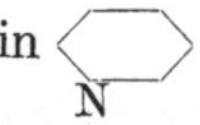 sind recht verschieden von den Eigenschaften des im Diaminodiphenylsulfon vorhandenen Ringes 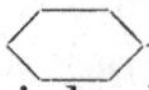 —NH_2. Wahrscheinlich hat SCHULZ recht, daß dem 2-Aminopyridid bei der Behandlung der Dermatitis herpetiformis eine Wirkung zukommt, denn sowohl Sulfapyridin als auch das von ihm substituierte Sulfapyridin besitzen einen 2-Aminopyridinrest.

Worin die Wirkung des Diaminodiphenylsulfons und des Sulfapyridins besteht, ist nicht bekannt. LORINCZ und PEARSON vermuten, daß sie sich mit im Gewebe oder in Bakterien vorhandenen Polysacchariden verbinden und auf diese Weise die Reaktivität dieser Polysaccharide ändern.

α) Sulfone. Es macht keinen Unterschied, ob das Diaminodiphenylsulfon (DDS, Dapson oder Avlosulfon) oder die substituierten Sulfonpräparate Diason oder Promacetin verabreicht werden; denn die letzteren sind erst wirksam, nachdem sie im Körper zu Diaminodiphenylsulfon hydrolysiert worden sind. Daher besteht auch kein Grund, sie statt dem DDS anzuwenden.

Die ersten Berichte über gute Erfolge mit Sulfonen bei der Dermatitis herpetiformis stammen aus dem Jahre 1951, als CORNBLETT über die Anwendung von Diason bei 13 Patienten berichtete, und aus dem Jahre 1952, als KRUIZINGA und HAMMINGA über die Anwendung des DDS bei zwölf Patienten berichteten. In rascher Folge kamen danach Mitteilungen über gute Resultate und viele Autoren haben betont, daß sie wegen der Seltenheit von ernsten Nebenwirkungen die Sulfone bei der Behandlung der Dermatitis herpetiformis als das Mittel der Wahl ansähen. Unter diesen befinden sich ALEXANDER (1955), CALNAN, GRANROTH, MORGAN et al., SKOG und WIKSTRÖM sowie SPIER und THIES. Der Erfolg ist bei richtiger Dosierung so sicher, daß, wie SPIER und THIES und auch MARCH und SAWICKY festgestellt haben, bei einem Versagen von DDS die Richtigkeit der Diagnose Dermatitis herpetiformis überprüft werden sollte.

Die Dosierung variiert etwas von Patienten zu Patienten und hängt auch von der Schwere der Hauterscheinungen ab. Als Anfangsdosis werden 200—300 mg DDS pro Tag empfohlen, und nach Abklingen der Hauterscheinungen als Erhaltungsdosis 100—200 mg pro Tag (ALEXANDER 1955; GRANROTH). Jedoch ist es bei einigen Patienten möglich, die Erhaltungsdosis auf 50 mg DDS pro Tag zu reduzieren. Die Wirkung des DDS tritt binnen weniger Tage ein, oft schon binnen eines Tages. Falls nach 3 Tagen keine Besserung eingetreten ist, sollte die Dosierung für einige Tage auf 400 mg pro Tag und dann auf 500 mg pro Tag erhöht werden. Beim Ausbleiben einer Besserung kann dann die Diagnose Dermatitis herpetiformis aufgegeben werden.

Ernste Nebenerscheinungen sind bei der Behandlung mit DDS selten. Recht häufig entwickelt sich während der ersten 2—3 Wochen vorübergehend eine normocytäre, bisweilen hypochrome Anämie, bei der die Zahl der Erythrocyten auf 2500000 per mm^3 absinken kann. Diese Anämie stellt aber keinen Grund dar, das Medikament abzusetzen; denn fast immer steigt die Zahl der Erythrocyten in der 3. oder 4. Woche wieder an und stabilisiert sich ungefähr in der 6. Woche in der Nähe von 4000000 per mm^3. Nur wenn kein Ansteigen stattfindet, muß das Absetzen des DDS erwogen werden. Das anämische Stadium ist gelegentlich mit Depression, Schwächegefühl und Kopfschmerzen verbunden. Die Erklärung für diese temporäre Anämie liegt darin, daß das DDS zu einer vermehrten Zerstörung der älteren Erythrocyten führt. Allmählich wird aber durch eine Vermehrung der jüngeren Erythrocyten ein Gleichgewicht hergestellt (DESFORGES et al.).

Ferner entwickelt sich unter der Behandlung mit dem DDS oft eine Methämoglobinämie, die mit Cyanose verbunden ist. Obwohl diese Methämoglobinämie andauern kann, solange das DDS verabreicht wird, kommt ihr keine ernste Bedeutung zu (Calnan).

Als ernste Nebenerscheinungen, die ein Absetzen des DDS erforderlich machen, gelten hämolytische Anämie, Agranulocytose und Neuropathien peripherer Nerven. Das Vorliegen einer hämolytischen Anämie ist gekennzeichnet durch eine progressive ausgesprochene Anämie, durch eine erhöhte Anzahl von Reticulocyten und durch das Vorhandensein von sog. Heinz-Körperchen in mehr als 20% der Erythrocyten (Smith und Alexander; Hutchinson et al.). (Die Heinz-Körperchen bestehen aus Körnchen, die sich mittels Methylviolett anfärben; sie stellen ein Degradierungsprodukt von Hämoglobin dar.) Schwere hämolytische Anämien erfordern die Anwendung von Corticosteroiden, die wirkungsvoll sind, da die durch DDS hervorgerufenen hämolytischen Anämien ein allergisches Phänomen darstellen. Agranulocytosen kommen zwar nur selten vor; sie können aber tödlich verlaufen (Samuel und Wiesendanger). Neuropathien heilen spontan nach Absetzen des DDS.

β) Sulfapyridin, erstmalig von Costello 1939 für die Behandlung der Dermatitis herpetiformis angewandt, wird heute bei der Dermatitis herpetiformis viel weniger angewandt als das DDS, weil ernste Nebenwirkungen dabei häufiger vorkommen als beim DDS. Es sei aber trotzdem erwähnt, da das Sulfapyridin bei Unverträglichkeit des DDS angewandt werden kann. Wie beim DDS muß die Dosierung des Sulfapyridins individuell geregelt werden. Meistens ist als Anfangsdosis 3—4 g pro Tag erforderlich und als Erhaltungsdosis 2—3 g pro Tag. Während einige Patienten mit niedrigeren Erhaltungsdosen auskommen, wie 0,5 g pro Tag, gibt es schwere Fälle, bei denen 4—6 g Sulfapyridin erforderlich sind (Granroth), und bei einem persönlich beobachteten Fall waren 6—8 g Sulfapyridin pro Tag erforderlich (Lever). Patienten, die Sulfapyridin erhalten, sollen angewiesen werden, besonders im Sommer, reichliche Flüssigkeitsmengen zu trinken und von 2—6 g Natrium bicarbonicum täglich einzunehmen, um ein Auskristallisieren des Sulfapyridins in den Nierentubuli zu vermeiden.

Unter den Nebenwirkungen überwiegen solche, die harmlos, aber recht störend sind, wie Magenerscheinungen, Kopfschmerzen, Schwäche und Schwindelgefühl. Sodann kommen Exantheme vor, die aus Erythemen, Blasen, Purpura oder einer generalisierten Erythrodermie bestehen können und tödlich verlaufen können, falls nicht rechtzeitig Corticosteroide in großen Dosen verabreicht werden (Sherlock und White; Oliver). Ferner können Leukopenie und Agranulocytose auftreten, so daß besonders im Anfang der Behandlung Zählungen der weißen Blutkörperchen regelmäßig ausgeführt werden sollten. Eine sehr ernste Komplikation stellt die Verstopfung der Nierentubuli durch auskristallisiertes Sulfapyridin dar, da dies zu Urämie und so zum Tode führen kann (Hopkins). Selbst die prophylaktische Anwendung von Natrium bicarbonicum kann diese Komplikation bei älteren Leuten mit beeinträchtigter Nierenfunktion oder bei jüngeren Leuten mit bestehender Niereninsuffizienz nicht immer vermeiden. Daher sollte das Sulfapyridin bei solchen Patienten nie angewandt werden.

II. Herpes gestationis

Das Hauptproblem beim Herpes gestationis stellt immer noch, wie zu Rieckes Zeiten, die Ursache dieser Schwangerschaftsdermatose dar. Auch besteht immer noch keine Einigkeit über die Beziehung des Herpes gestationis zur Dermatitis herpetiformis. In der Behandlung des Herpes gestationis sind jedoch Fortschritte gemacht worden, da die Krankheit auf die Corticosteroide gut anspricht.

a) Klinisches Bild

Der Herpes gestationis setzt oft mit Jucken ohne Hauterscheinungen ein. Es entwickeln sich dann papulo-vesiculöse Efflorescenzen, bevor serpiginös begrenzte, erythematöse und großblasige Hauterscheinungen auftreten (Abb. 6). Demnach besteht oft zu Beginn der Krankheit eine gewisse Ähnlichkeit mit der Dermatitis herpetiformis, während später, worauf RUSSELL und THORNE hinweisen, die Ähnlichkeit mit dem bullösen Pemphigoid oder mit dem Erythema exsudativum multiforme recht groß ist. Die Hauterscheinungen sind oft auf der Haut des

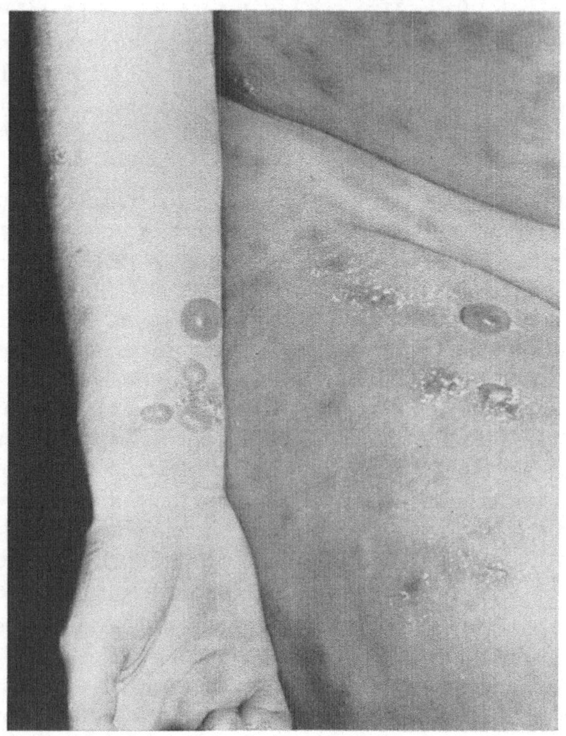

Abb. 6. Herpes gestationis. Schwangere im 8. Monat. Große pralle Blasen beherrschen das Krankheitsbild

Abdomens am zahlreichsten vorhanden. An den Extremitäten sind die Beugeseiten ebenso stark wie die Streckseiten befallen. Mundschleimhauterscheinungen kommen gelegentlich vor (RUSSELL und THORNE).

b) Häufigkeit und Verlauf

Der Herpes gestationis tritt ungefähr einmal unter 4000 Schwangeren auf (CRAWFORD und LEEPER; RUSSELL und THORNE). Den Verlauf hat RIECKE wie folgend beschrieben:

„Meistens erfolgt in der zweiten Schwangerschaftshälfte der Beginn des Leidens. Manchmal setzt das Exanthem schon früher ein oder erst im Puerperium. Bei erneuter Schwangerschaft tritt das Exanthem häufig etwas vorzeitiger auf als zuvor und bei jeder weiteren Gravidität zeigt sich zu einem immer früheren Zeitpunkt der pruriginöse Ausschlag. Häufig verschwindet das Exanthem kurz vor der Entbindung, manchmal schon 1—2 Monate zuvor, um dann 24—48 Std post partum in meist sehr starker Weise wieder auszubrechen. Meistens vergehen die Hauterscheinungen einige Wochen oder einige Monate post partum. In einzelnen Fällen jedoch hat man auch unabhängig von neuer Schwangerschaft Rezidive gesehen."

Auch nach den Erfahrungen anderer Autoren heilt der Herpes gestationis gewöhnlich binnen eines Monats, fast immer aber binnen 6 Monaten nach der Entbindung ab. Jedoch hat unter anderen Fox über eine Patientin berichtet, bei der über 2 Jahre hin mit jeder Menstruation einige Bläschen auftraten.

Todesfälle, die direkt auf einen Herpes gestationis zurückzuführen waren, sind bei Patientinnen mit Herpes gestationis nie beschrieben worden. Jedoch kommen Spontanaborte oder Todgeburten anscheinend häufiger als normalerweise vor (Russell und Thorne; Toussaint und Schoysman).

c) Ätiologie

Es ist natürlich naheliegend, eine endokrine Störung als die Ursache für den Herpes gestationis anzunehmen. Da aber der Herpes gestationis mit keiner bestimmten Periode der Schwangerschaft verbunden ist und mehrere Monate lang nach der Entbindung andauern kann, ist es schwierig, ein bestimmtes Hormon für die Hauterscheinungen verantwortlich zu halten. Trotzdem haben Keaty, Jones und Lamb eine Vermehrung des Gonadotropins im Blutserum als eine Ursache des Herpes gestationis angesehen. Sie fanden bei sieben von zehn Schwangeren mit Herpes gestationis die Konzentration des Gonadotropins im Serum während der späteren Schwangerschaftsmonate stark vermehrt, im Durchschnitt auf 3125 Ratteneinheiten pro 100 cm^3 Serum. (Die gewöhnliche Konzentration ist während dieser Periode 500—700 Ratteneinheiten.) Die Untersucher nahmen an, daß dieser Überproduktion von Gonadotropin eine Unterproduktion von Progesteron zugrunde liege; und in einigen Fällen sahen sie eine Besserung des Herpes gestationis unter Behandlung mit Progesteron. Zugunsten ihrer Theorie, daß eine Vermehrung von Gonadotropin einen Herpes gestationis hervorrufen kann, führen Keaty u. Mitarb. den von Elliott berichteten Fall an, bei dem ein Herpes gestationis im Zusammenhang mit einem Chorionepitheliom auftrat und bei dem sich die Hauterscheinungen um so mehr verschlimmerten, als der Titer von chorionischem Gonadotropin im Blute anstieg. Weitere Fälle von Herpes gestationis in Verbindung mit einem Chorionepitheliom sind von Whitfield et al. und von Tillman berichtet worden. In dem letzteren Fall brachte eine Besserung des Chorionepithelioms durch Röntgenbestrahlung eine Abheilung der Hauterscheinungen mit sich.

Wahrscheinlicher als eine hormonale Störung ist eine Sensibilisierung zu autolytischen Produkten der Placenta oder vielleicht zu tryptischen Enzymen, die von Zellen des chorionischen Gewebes herstammen. Sensibilisierung als Ursache des Herpes gestationis ist besser vereinbar mit dem Auftreten der Hauterscheinungen zu verschiedenen Zeiten der Schwangerschaft und würde fernerhin erklären, warum, wie es häufig geschieht, bei weiteren Schwangerschaften derselben Patientin der Zeitpunkt der Erkrankung sich weiter nach vorne verlagert (Fisher; Rimbaud und Guibert; Lindemann et al.; Russell und Thorne). Auch die Spätfälle im Wochenbett könnte man auf diese Weise erklären; denn nicht sofort nach der Geburt ist jedes kleinste Placentateilchen aus dem Körper eliminiert; im Gegenteil, die Grundlagen zur Aufnahme von autolytischen Produkten sind besonders günstig, da eine große Placentawundfläche besteht, durch die eine ungehinderte Resorption stattfinden kann (Hollenweger-Mayr). Das Vorkommen von Herpes gestationis beim Bestehen eines Chorionepithelioms (s. oben) könnte auf dieselbe Weise erklärt werden. Auch das gute Ansprechen des Herpes gestationis auf die Corticosteroidè weist auf einen Sensibilisierungsprozeß hin.

Cawley u. Mitarb. erwogen die Möglichkeit, daß Isosensibilisierung zum Rhesus-Faktor bei Rh-negativen Müttern, die ein Rh-positives Kind tragen, einen Herpes gestationis verursachen könnte. Es hat sich jedoch erwiesen, daß viele Mütter mit Herpes gestationis Rh-positiv sind (FISHER; RUSSELL und THORNE).

d) Beziehung zur Dermatitis herpetiformis

Autoren, die die Grenzen der Dermatitis herpetiformis recht weit ziehen, wie z.B. Angehörige der französischen Schule, schließen den Herpes gestationis (wie das bullöse Pemphigoid) in den Begriff der Dermatitis herpetiformis ein und betrachten den Herpes gestationis als eine an die Schwangerschaft gebundene Dermatitis herpetiformis (WATRIN und JEANDIDIER; RIMBAUD und GUIBERT; LAPIÈRE). Auch RIECKE sympathisierte mit dieser Möglichkeit: „Ebenso wie bei der Impetigo herpetiformis die Gestation nur eine der äußeren Bedingungen der Manifestation des Krankheitszustandes ist, so könnte die Gestation bei dem Herpes gestationis einen Teilfaktor für den Ausbruch des Exanthems bilden.“ RIECKE wies darauf hin, daß ja auch das Jod für die Dermatitis herpetiformis ein auslösendes Moment sein kann. Das gelegentliche Ansprechen des Herpes gestationis auf Sulfathiazol (LEWIS) oder Sulfapyridin (DOWNING und JILLSON) ist ebenfalls als ein Anzeichen einer engen Beziehung zur Dermatitis herpetiformis gewertet worden.

Andererseits trat in der großen Mehrzahl der Patientinnen, bei denen Sulfapyridin angewandt wurde, keine Besserung ein (TURNER und ZAKON; MUELLER und LAPP; LINDEMANN et al.; FOX; RUSSELL und THORNE; CASTERMANS-ELIAS); und auch die Sulfone haben versagt (RUSSELL und THORNE; TOUSSAINT und SCHOYSMAN). Aber der Herpes gestationis und die Dermatitis herpetiformis zeigen nicht nur unterschiedliches Ansprechen auf die Behandlung, sondern auch Unterschiede in ihrem klinischen Aussehen und in ihrem Verlauf. In bezug auf das klinische Aussehen findet man bei der Dermatitis herpetiformis im Gegensatz zum Herpes gestationis kein Vorwiegen großer Blasen und keine Mundschleimhauterscheinungen, und die Hauterscheinungen haben als Prädilektionsstellen die Ellbogen, die Knie, die Schultern und das Gesäß; und in bezug auf den Verlauf zeigt die Dermatitis herpetiformis eher Besserung als Verschlimmerung während der Schwangerschaft (s. S. 702). Wegen dieser Unterschiede erscheint es ratsam, die beiden Krankheiten nicht als miteinander identisch anzusehen, solange deren Ursache noch unbekannt ist (BÄFVERSTEDT; RUSSELL und THORNE; TOLMAN et al.).

e) Behandlung

Wegen des starken Juckens, den der Herpes gestationis verursacht, ist eine effektive Behandlung äußerst wünschenswert. Die Corticosteroide stellen die einzige verläßliche Behandlung dar, denn den vereinzelten Erfolgen mit Sulfonamiden stehen viele Mißerfolge gegenüber. Auch die von KEATY et al. angeregte Behandlung mit Progesteron hat sich nicht bewährt (FISHER; FOX; RUSSELL und THORNE). Ferner konnte die Wirksamkeit des Pyridoxins (Vitamin B_6) beim Herpes gestationis, über die FOSNAUGH et al. an Hand von vier Fällen berichtet haben, von BAER und WITTEN nicht bestätigt werden.

Die Corticosteroide verursachen schnelle Besserung und unterdrücken die Hauterscheinungen, solange sie in genügender Menge verabreicht werden. Die Dosierung hängt natürlich von der Schwere des Falles ab. Oft scheinen aber verhältnismäßig kleine Dosen zu genügen, wie z.B. bei der von LINDEMANN et al. beschriebenen Patientin, bei der 100 mg Cortison pro Tag die Hauterscheinungen fast völlig unterdrückten, nachdem sich allerdings 50 mg als ungenügend erwiesen hatten. TOUSSAINT und SCHLOYSMAN fanden ebenfalls 100 mg Cortison pro Tag als Anfangsbehandlung ausreichend, während RUSSELL und THORNE diese Dosis zwar bei einer Patientin für ausreichend befanden, nicht aber bei einer weiteren Patientin, bei der 150 mg pro Tag für die Unterdrückung der Hauterscheinungen erforderlich waren. Sowohl FISHER als auch FOX fanden, daß nach anfänglichen Dosen von erst 200 mg und dann 100 mg Cortison pro Tag, 50 mg pro Tag als Erhaltungsdosis genügten.

Es wird allgemein angenommen, daß die Corticosteroide in den empfohlenen Dosen keinen nachteiligen Einfluß auf die Entwicklung der Schwangerschaft ausüben (DE COSTA und ABELMAN). Jedoch können Neugeborene, deren Mütter für längere Zeit und bis zur Zeit der Geburt hin Corticosteroide erhalten haben, Anzeichen von Nebenniereninsuffizienz aufweisen und bedürfen daher der prophylaktischen Behandlung mit kleinen Dosen von Corticosteroiden. Nicht selten bessert sich aber der Herpes gestationis gegen das Ende der Schwangerschaft hin, so daß man dann ohne die Corticosteroide auskommen kann. Die nicht selten vorkommenden Exacerbationen nach der Geburt können dann ohne weiteres mit Corticosteroiden behandelt werden.

III. Subcorneale pustulöse Dermatose

Die subcorneale pustulöse Dermatose wurde erstmalig unter diesem Namen von SNEDDON und WILKINSON im Jahre 1956 als ein selbständiges Krankheitsbild aufgestellt. Diese Autoren beschrieben sieben eigene Fälle und fügten diesen drei Fälle hinzu, die unter verschiedenen fraglichen Diagnosen von SIMPSON (1948), CARNEY (1952) und CIPOLLARO (1954) mitgeteilt worden waren. Eigentlich war der erste unzweifelhafte Fall von subcornealer pustulöser Dermatose bereits 1932 von RUITER nebst histologischer Beschreibung berichtet worden; aber die Sonderstellung dieser Erkrankung wurde von ihm damals nicht erkannt. Auch der 1944 von HALL unter der Diagnose Impetigo herpetiformis berichtete Fall stellte eine subcorneale pustulöse Dermatose dar. Der Mitteilung von SNEDDON und WILKINSON folgten zahlreiche Veröffentlichungen solcher Fälle, so daß SCHRÖPL im Jahre 1962 bereits über 70 Fälle in der Literatur vorfand. Demnach ist die subcorneale pustulöse Dermatose keineswegs eine allzu seltene Krankheit.

a) Klinisches Bild

Die Primärefflorescenz ist entweder eine Pustel oder ein Bläschen, das sich aber rasch zu einer Pustel umwandelt. Die Pusteln zeigen gewöhnlich einen schmalen rötlichen Randsaum (Abb. 7). Meistens sind die Pusteln nur wenige Millimeter groß; gelegentlich finden sich aber recht große Eiterblasen, die schlaff sind und in denen der Eiter als ein Hypopyon zu sehen ist (BURNS und FINE). Während diese größeren, Eiter enthaltenden Blasen gewöhnlich allein stehen, sind die Pusteln oft in Gruppen angeordnet. Aus solchen Gruppen von Pusteln bilden sich allmählich auf Grund von peripherem Ausbreiten, das mit zentraler Abheilung einhergeht, circinäre, zum Teil polycyclisch begrenzte Herde. Deren aktive Randpartien weisen entweder einen Saum von Pusteln oder nach deren Eintrocknung einen Saum von gelblichen Krusten auf. Abheilung der Herde erfolgt gewöhnlich binnen einiger Wochen oder Monate unter Hinterlassung von Hyperpigmentierung.

Die Hauterscheinungen werden vor allem am Rumpf und an den proximalen Teilen der Extremitäten angetroffen. Dabei sind die intertriginösen Gegenden, wie die Axillen, die Submammärregion und die Inguinalfalten, oft bevorzugt befallen. Der Kopf bleibt wohl immer verschont. Auch die Fußsohlen und die Handteller sind nur selten befallen; jedoch wurde dies von HELLIER, von HABER und auch von REYNAERS beobachtet. Auch Mundschleimhauterscheinungen fehlen fast immer. Nur GREENBAUM und LEE stellten bei ihrer Patientin das Vorhandensein von zwei Bläschen im Munde fest.

Das Allgemeinbefinden wird durch die Hauterscheinungen nicht beeinträchtigt. Obwohl in einigen Fällen ausgesprochener Juckreiz bestand (DUPERRAT; HADIDA und SAYAG; SCHUPPENER und THAL), fehlt dieser doch meistens oder ist

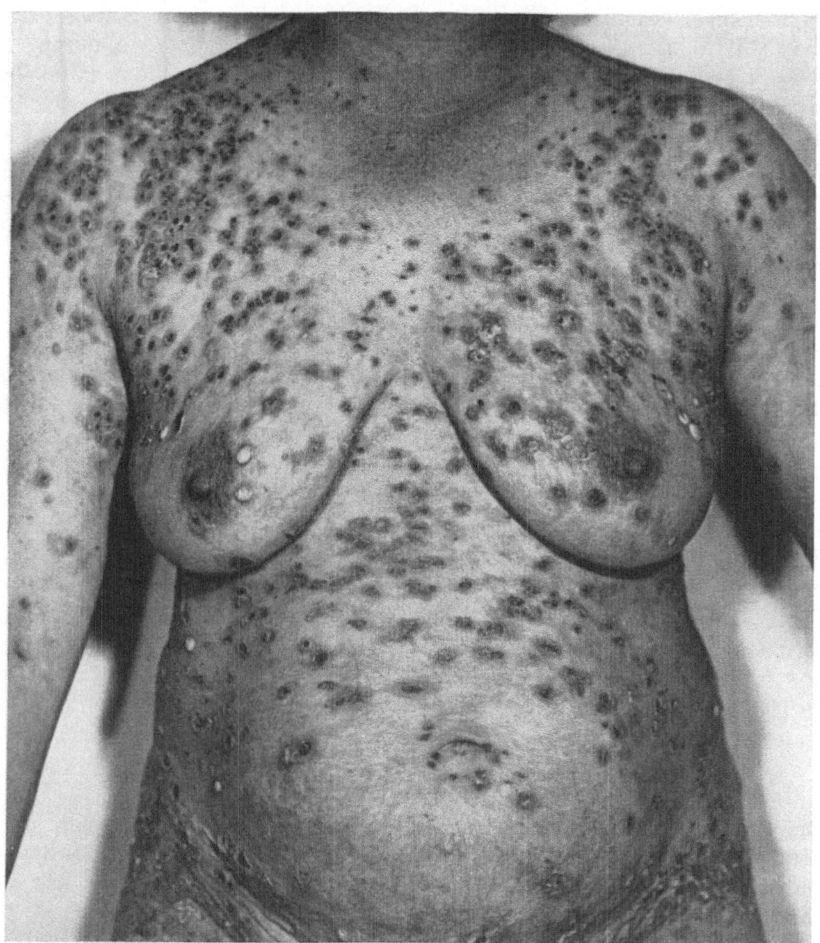

Abb. 7. Subcorneale pustulöse Dermatose. Es bestehen einzeln stehende große Eiterblasen und Gruppen kleinerer Pusteln, die teilweise eine circinäre Anordnung aufweisen. [DUPERRAT, B.: Ann. Derm. Syph. (Paris) 8, 514 (1957)]

unbedeutend, so daß dieses als ein differentialdiagnostisch wichtiges Zeichen zur Abgrenzung gegen die Dermatitis herpetiformis gewertet werden kann (SNEDDON und WILKINSON).

b) Verlauf

Die subcorneale pustulöse Dermatose zieht sich in der Regel über viele Jahre hin. Die längste bisher beobachtete Dauer, nämlich 20 Jahre, wurde von SCHOENFELD berichtet. Während des Krankheitsverlaufes kommt es häufig zu spontanen Verbesserungen und Verschlimmerungen. Dabei kann es sogar zu einer vorübergehenden völligen Abheilung kommen, die gelegentlich mehrere Monate und selbst mehrere Jahre anhält (SCHOENFELD). Bei neuen Pustelschüben werden dann gewöhnlich die vorher erkrankten Hautpartien wieder befallen.

c) Geschlecht, Alter, Herkunft

Es besteht ein deutliches Überwiegen des weiblichen Geschlechtes. So fand SCHRÖPL unter 55 Patienten mit subcornealer pustulöser Dermatose das Verhältnis weiblicher zu männlichen Patienten 2,3:1, während dieses Verhältnis bei der Dermatitis herpetiformis nach den Erhebungen von EYSTER und KIERLAND 1:2,7 beträgt.

Die meisten Patienten sind beim Erstauftreten der Hauterscheinungen zwischen 40 und 70 Jahre alt. Doch kann die Krankheit gelegentlich früher beginnen. Das früheste bisher beobachtete Auftreten fand sich bei einer Patientin, die 20 Jahre alt war (ELLIS).

In bezug auf Herkunft der Patienten läßt sich feststellen, daß unter den aus den Vereinigten Staaten berichteten Fällen recht viele Neger sind (ELLIS; SCHOENFELD; BARSKY und CORNBLEET).

d) Laboratoriumsuntersuchungen

Die Pusteln der subcornealen pustulösen Dermatose sind zwar steril, wenn sie zuerst auftreten. Wegen der leicht eintretenden Sekundärinfektion finden sich aber bei bakteriologischen Untersuchungen recht oft Staphylokokken und gelegentlich Streptokokken (RÖCKL).

e) Histologie

Die Bläschen und Pusteln bilden sich stets subcorneal (Abb. 8). Der Pustelinhalt besteht hauptsächlich aus polymorphkernigen neutrophilen Leukocyten; nur selten findet man darin auch einige eosinophile Leukocyten. Einige acantholytische Zellen sind recht häufig vorhanden: Entweder stehen diese noch teilweise mit der am unteren Rand der Pustel gelegenen Epidermis in Verbindung oder sie liegen bereits frei im Pustelinhalt (ELLIS; BARSKI und CORNBLEET; BURNS und FINE; SCHUPPENER und THAL; SCHRÖPL). Es handelt sich aber dabei um eine sekundäre Acantholyse; denn die Bläschen oder Pusteln bilden sich ja nicht auf Grund einer Acantholyse. Vielmehr tritt die Acantholyse erst im Anschluß an die Bildung der Pustel auf, wahrscheinlich infolge der im Pustelinhalt vorhandenen proteolytischen Enzyme (BURNS und FINE). Eine Bildung von spongiformen Pusteln, wie bei der Psoriasis pustulosa, der Acrodermatitis continua (s. S. 725) oder der Impetigo herpetiformis (s. S. 731), kommt bei der subcornealen pustulösen Dermatose nicht vor. Höchstens kann man gelegentlich eine angedeutete spongiforme Pustelbildung an den Rändern der Pustel finden, wie es SCHUPPENER und THAL beobachteten. (Die von SCHWANK und TRAPL sowie von LAPIÈRE und CASTERMANS-ELIAS berichteten Fälle von subcornealer pustulöser Dermatose mit spongiformer Pustelbildung sind wahrscheinlich Fälle von pustulöser Psoriasis.)

Die der Pustel unterliegende Epidermis kann geringe Acanthose und etwas Spongiose aufweisen. Vereinzelt liegen neutrophile Leukocyten zwischen den Epidermiszellen. Die obere Dermis enthält ein vorwiegend perivasculäres Infiltrat, das vor allem Lymphocyten, aber auch Histiocyten, neutrophile Leukocyten und gelegentlich einige eosinophile Leukocyten enthält (DUPERRAT; WINSTON).

f) Differentialdiagnose

Das klinische und histologische Bild der subcornealen pustulösen Dermatose ist so kennzeichnend, daß es gewöhnlich nicht schwierig ist, diese Hauterkrankung von anderen zu unterscheiden. Jedoch besteht vom klinischen Standpunkt aus gelegentlich Ähnlichkeit entweder mit der Dermatitis herpetiformis oder mit der Impetigo herpetiformis bzw. der Psoriasis pustulosa; und vom histologischen

Standpunkt aus entweder mit der Impetigo oder mit dem Pemphigus foliaceus bzw. erythematosus. Die *Dermatitis herpetiformis*, die zwar auch gewöhnlich eine

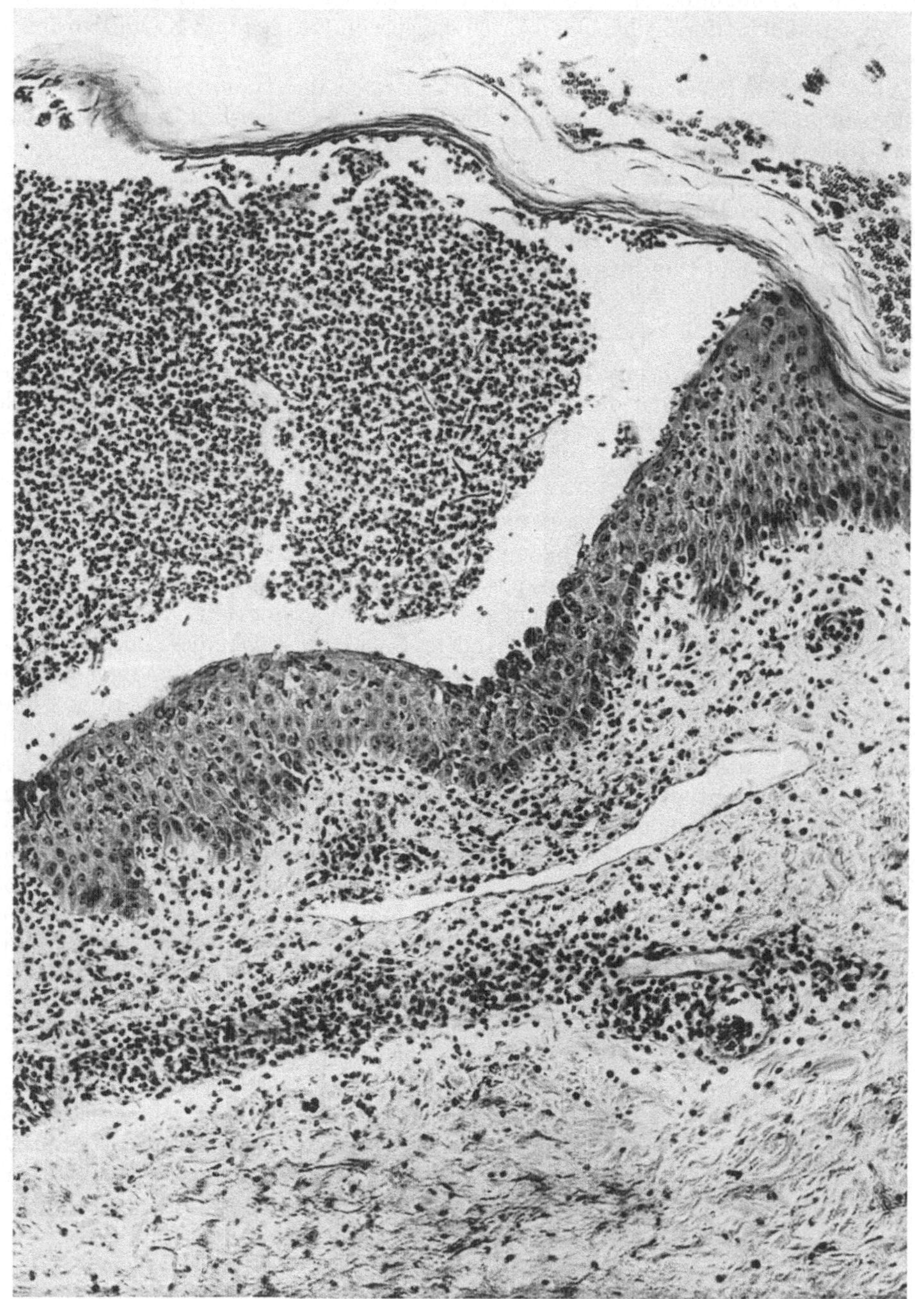

Abb. 8. Subcorneale pustulöse Dermatose. Eine subcorneale Pustel ist dargestellt (200mal). [DUPERRAT, B.: Ann. Derm. Syph. (Paris) **84**, 514 (1957)]

gruppierte Anordnung ihrer Efflorescenzen zeigt, unterscheidet sich von der subcornealen pustulösen Dermatose 1. durch die Polymorphie ihrer Primäreffloreszenzen rescenzen, 2. durch eine andere Lokalisation ihrer Hauterscheinungen und 3. durch stärkeren Juckreiz (s. S. 701). Auch überwiegt bei der Dermatitis herpetiformis das männliche Geschlecht. Bei der histologischen Untersuchung befinden sich die Blasen bei der Dermatitis herpetiformis subepidermal und enthalten viele eosinophile Leukocyten (s. S. 704). Bei der *Impetigo herpetiformis* und der *pustulösen Psoriasis* bestehen zusätzlich zu den Pusteln erythematöse und oft auch schuppende Flächen und das Allgemeinbefinden ist meistens recht beeinträchtigt. Ferner ergibt die histologische Untersuchung spongiforme Pustelbildung (s. S. 725).

Die *Impetigo* hat dasselbe histologische Aussehen wie die subcorneale pustulöse Dermatose, und als Impetigo circinata kann sie selbst in ihrem klinischen Aussehen große Ähnlichkeit mit der subcornealen pustulösen Dermatose besitzen, da auch bei der Impetigo cricinata die Pusteln eine polycyclische Anordnung haben. Da infolge Sekundärinfektion auch die Pusteln der subcornealen pustulösen Dermatose ein Wachstum von Staphylokokken aufweisen können, hängt die Unterscheidung vor allem von der Dauer der Erkrankung und der Lokalisation der Hauterscheinungen ab. Sollten Zweifel bestehen, ist ein therapeutischer Test mit Diaminodiphenylsulfon (DDS) angezeigt (s. unten). Die histologische Unterscheidung des *Pemphigus foliaceus resp. erythematosus* von der subcornealen pustulösen Dermatose kann schwierig sein (Feuerman-Pogorzelski); denn bei beiden Krankheiten kann man subcorneale Blasen mit Acantholyse vorfinden, die zwar gewöhnlich, aber nicht immer beim Pemphigus foliaceus viel ausgesprochener ist. In seinem klinischen Aussehen unterscheidet sich der Pemphigus foliaceus resp. erythematosus von der subcornealen pustulösen Dermatose dadurch, daß er 1. fast immer Krankheitsherde im Gesicht und auf dem Kopf aufweist und 2. mit erythematösen Hautflächen einhergeht, die Schuppung, Nässen und leichte Krustenbildung zeigen und ein positives Nikolski-Zeichen besitzen.

g) Behandlung

Die Behandlung der subcornealen pustulösen Dermatose ist die gleiche wie die der Dermatitis herpetiformis (s. S. 707). Die Sulfone, das Sulfapyridin und die Corticosteroide unterdrücken die Krankheitserscheinungen, vorausgesetzt, daß sie in genügend hohen Dosen verabreicht werden. Wie bei der Dermatitis herpetiformis ist das Diaminodiphenylsulfon (DDS) wegen der geringen Nebenwirkungen das Mittel der Wahl.

Was die Dosierung des DDS anbelangt, hat es den Anschein, daß bei der subcornealen pustulösen Dermatose oft kleinere Dosen als bei der Dermatosis herpetiformis wirksam sind. Gelegentlich verursachen schon 50 mg DDS pro Tag eine Remission (Sneddon und Wilkinson; Meara und Calnan). Meistens bedarf es aber 100 mg pro Tag (Schröpl) und gelegentlich mehr (Sneddon und Wilkinson). Oft können die Erhaltungsdosen niedriger gehalten werden als die Anfangsdosen, d.h. 50 mg oder sogar 25 mg pro Tag (Schröpl).

Literatur

I. Dermatitis herpetiformis

Alexander, J. O'D.: Dapsone in the treatment of dermatitis herpetiformis. Lancet **1955 II**, 1201. — Is eosinophilia of diagnostic importance in dermatitis herpetiformis? Brit. J. Derm. **73**, 267 (1961). — Allen, A.: The Skin, p. 273. St. Louis: C. V. Mosby Co. 1954.

Bernhardt, R.: Zur Ätiologie des Pemphigus und der Duhringschen Krankheit. Acta derm.-venereol. (Stockh.) **14**, 165 (1933). — Björnberg, A., and L. Hellgren: Dermatitis herpetiformis. A laboratory and clinical investigation based on a numerical study of 53 patients and matched controls. Dermatologica (Basel) **125**, 205 (1962). — Brocq, L.: Über die Dermatitis herpetiformis Duhring. IV. Polymorphe, pruriginöse, recidivierende Schwangerschafts-Dermatitis (Herpes gestationis). Mh. prakt. Derm. **9**, 69 (1889).

CALLAWAY, J., and T. H. STERNBERG: Bacterial allergy: An etiologic factor in dermatitis herpetiformis. Arch. Derm. Syph. (Chic.) **43**, 956 (1941). — CALNAN, C. D.: A note on sulphone treatment of dermatitis herpetiformis. Trans. St. John's Hosp. derm. Soc. (Lond.) **33**, 53 (1954). — CORNBLEET, T.: Sulfoxone (Diasone) sodium for dermatitis herpetiformis. Arch. Derm. Syph. (Chic.) **64**, 684 (1951). — COSTELLO, M. J.: Dermatitis herpetiformis treated with sulfapyridine. Arch. Derm. Syph. (Chic.) **41**, 134 (1940).

DEGOS, R., and J. CIVATTE: Unusual histological appearances in Duhring-Brocq's disease. Brit. J. Derm. **73**, 295 (1961). — DESFORGES, J. F., W. W. THAYER, and J. P. DAWSON: Hemolytic anemia induced by sulfone therapy, with investigations into the mechanism of its production. Amer. J. Med. **27**, 132 (1959).

EBERHARTINGER, C., u. H. EBNER: Behandlungsmöglichkeiten der Dermatitis herpetiformis Duhring. Derm. Wschr. **148**, 145 (1963). — EPSTEIN, S.: Bullous reactions to bacterial antigens in dermatitis herpetiformis. J. invest. Derm. **33**, 31 (1959). — EYSTER jr., W. H., and R. R. KIERLAND: Prognosis of dermatitis herpetiformis, treated and untreated. Arch. Derm. Syph. (Chic.) **64**, 1 (1951).

FELSHER, Z.: Skin chlorides in dermatitis herpetiformis and pemphigus. J. invest. Derm. **31**, 47 (1958).

GRANROTH, T.: Dermatitis herpetiformis treated with D.A.D.P.S. (diaminodiphenylsulfone). Acta derm.-venereol. (Stockh.) **36**, 474 (1956).

HANSEN, P.: Über die Prognose bei Dermatitis herpetiformis. Acta derm.-venereol. (Stockh.) **18**, 452 (1937). — HOPKINS, H. H.: Dermatitis herpetiformis. Treatment with sulfonamides. Bull. Johns Hopk. Hosp. **92**, 1 (1953). — HUTCHINSON, H. E., J. M. JACKSON, and P. CASSIDY: Drug-induced hemolytic anemia in dermatitis herpetiformis. The importance of Heinz bodies in its recognition. Brit. J. Derm. **75**, 161 (1963).

JABLONSKA, S.: Therapeutische Umfrage. Derm. Wschr. **145**, 57 (1962). — JABLONSKA, S., u. T. CHORZELSKI: Kann das histologische Bild die Grundlage zur Differenzierung des Morbus Duhring mit dem Pemphigoid und Erythema multiforme darstellen? Derm. Wschr. **146**, 590 (1963).

KIM, R., and R. K. WINKELMANN: Dermatitis herpetiformis in children. Relationship to bullous pemphigoid. Arch. Derm. **83**, 895 (1961). — KIMMIG, J.: Therapeutische Umfrage. Derm. Wschr. **145**, 59 (1962). — KORTING, G. W.: Therapeutische Umfrage. Derm. Wschr. **145**, 61 (1962). — KRUIZINGA, E. E., and H. HAMMINGA: Treatment of dermatitis herpetiformis with diamino-diphenyl-sulphone (D.D.S.). Dermatologica (Basel) **106**, 387 (1953).

LAIN, E. S., and J. H. LAMB: Treatment of a pemphigoid eruption with sulfanilamide. Arch. Derm. Syph. (Chic.) **37**, 840 (1938). — LEONE, R.: Dermatite erpetiforme e streptococco. G. ital. Derm. Sif. **79**, 365 (1938). — LEVER, W. F.: In der Diskussion zu A. L. LORINCZ and R. W. PEARSON: Arch. Derm. **85**, 15 (1962). — LIVINGOOD, C. S.: In der Diskussion zu M. M. TOLMAN, S. L. MOSCHELLA and R. N. SCHNEIDERMAN: J. invest. Derm. **32**, 560 (1959). — LORINCZ, A. L., and R. W. PEARSON: Sulfapyridine and sulfone type drugs in dermatology. Arch. Derm. **85**, 2 (1962).

MACVICAR, D. N., J. H. GRAHAM, and C. F. BURGOON: Dermatitis herpetiformis, erythema multiforme and bullous pemphigoid. A comparative histopathological and histochemical study. J. invest. Derm. **41**, 289 (1963). — MARCH, C., and H. H. SAWICKY: Diaminodiphenylsulfone in dermatitis herpetiformis. Arch. Derm. **85**, 751 (1962). — MORGAN, J. K., C. W. MARSDEN, J. G. COBURN, and J. M. MUNGAVIN: Dapsone in dermatitis herpetiformis. Lancet **1955 I**, 1197.

NILES, H. D.: In der Diskussion zu M. H. GOODMAN: Dermatitis herpetiformis. Arch. Derm. Syph. (Chic.) **43**, 254 (1941).

OLIVER, E. A.: In der Diskussion zu M. J. COSTELLO, Sulfapyridine in the treatment of dermatitis herpetiformis. Arch. Derm. Syph. (Chic.) **56**, 625 (1947).

PERCIVAL, G. H.: The relationship between dermatitis herpetiformis, pemphigoid and pemphigus, on the basis of clinical and histological investigation. Acta derm.-venereol. (Stockh.), Proc. 11th Internat. Congr. Derm. 1957, Bd. 3, S. 286. — PERRY, H. O., and R. K. WINKELMANN: Adverse reactions to sulfamethoxypyridazine (Kynex). Its use in the treatment of dermatitis herpetiformis. J. Amer. med. Ass. **169**, 127 (1959). — PETERKIN, G. A. GRANT: Dermatitis herpetiformis. A follow-up and survey of treatment. Brit. J. Derm. **63**, 1 (1951). — PIÉRARD, J.: De l'aspect histologique des plaques érythémateuses de la dermatite herpétiforme de Duhring. Ann. Derm. Syph. (Paris) **90**, 121 (1963). — PIÉRARD, J., A. DUPONT et A. FONTAINE: Les critères du diagnostic histopathologique de la dermatite herpétiforme de Duhring et de l'erythème polymorphe. Arch. belges Derm. **13**, 370 (1957). — PIÉRARD, J., and I. WHIMSTER: The histological diagnosis of dermatitis herpetiformis, bullous pemphigoid and erythema multiforme. Brit. J. Derm. **73**, 253 (1961).

RIECKE, E.: Dermatitis herpetiformis. In: Handbuch der Haut- und Geschlechtskrankheiten, hrsg. von J. JADASSOHN, Bd. 7, Teil 2, S. 549. Berlin: Springer 1931. — RUPEC, M., A. KINT u. O. BRAUN-FALCO: Zur Frage der Histopathologie der peribullösen Veränderungen bei Dermatitis herpetiformis Duhring und ihrer Differentialdiagnose. Z. Haut- u. Geschl.-Kr. **34**, 121 (1963). — RUSSELL, B., and N. A. THORNE: Herpes gestationis. Brit. J. Derm. **69**, 339 (1957).

SAMUEL, H. S., and P. H. WIESENDANGER: Agranulocytosis following treatment with dapsone. Brit. J. Derm. **74**, 383 (1962). — SCHULZ, K. H.: Zur Therapie der Dermatitis herpetiformis Duhring. Hautarzt **10**, 129 (1959). — SHERLOCK, S., and J. C. WHITE: Fatal purpura after sulphapyridine. Brit. med. J. **1944II**, 401. — SKOG, E., and K. WIKSTRÖM: A comparative study of the effects of different sulfa products and sulfone products in dermatitis herpetiformis. Acta derm.-venereol. (Stockh.) **39**, 372 (1959). — SMITH, R. S., and S. ALEXANDER: Heinz-body anemia due to dapsone. Brit. med. J. **1959I**, 625. — SPIER, H. W., C. G. SCHIRREN, U. DESSIN u. T. EWINGER: Zur Frage der Jodempfindlichkeit bei der Dermatitis herpetiformis Duhring. Arch. Derm. Syph. (Berl.) **195**, 105 (1952). — SPIER, H. W., u. W. THIES: Zur Sulfonbehandlung der Dermatitis herpetiformis Duhring. Hautarzt **6**, 415 (1955). — SWARTZ, J. H.: In der Diskussion zu M. J. COSTELLO, Sulfapyridine in the treatment of dermatitis herpetiformis. Arch. Derm. Syph. (Chic.) **56**, 614 (1947). — SWARTZ, J. H., and W. F. LEVER: Dermatitis herpetiformis. Immunologic and therapeutic considerations. Arch. Derm. Syph. (Chic.) **47**, 680 (1943).

TOLMAN, M. M., S. L. MOSCHELLA, and R. N. SCHNEIDERMAN: Dermatitis herpetiformis: Specific entity or clinical complex? J. invest. Derm. **32**, 557 (1959).

WELSH, A. L.: In der Diskussion zu S. ROTHMAN and J. H. MCCREARY: Dermatitis herpetiformis. Arch. Derm. Syph. (Chic.) **60**, 889 (1949). — WORINGER, F.: Therapeutische Umfrage. Derm. Wschr. **145**, 66 (1962).

II. Herpes gestationis

BÄFVERSTEDT, B.: Case of herpes gestationis treated with anterior pituitary hormone. Acta derm.-venereol. (Stockh.) **31**, 470 (1951). — BAER, R. L., u. V. H. WITTEN: Kommentar zu R. P. FOSNAUGH et al., The Year Book of Dermatology 1961/62, p. 59. Chicago: Year Book Medical Publ. 1962.

CASTERMANS-ELIAS, S.: Herpès gestationis. Arch. belges Derm. **18**, 50 (1962). — CAWLEY, E. R., C. E. WHEELER, and P. A. WILHITE: Herpes gestationis and the Rh factor. Sth. med. J. (Bgham, Ala.) **45**, 827 (1952). — COSTA, E. J. DE, and M. A. ABELMAN: Cortisone and pregnancy: An experimental and clinical study of the effects of cortisone on gestation. Amer. J. Obstet. Gynec. **64**, 746 (1952). — CRAWFORD, G. M., and A. W. LEEPER: Diseases of the skin in pregnancy. Arch. Derm. Syph. (Chic.) **61**, 753 (1950).

DOWNING, J. G., and O. F. JILLSON: Herpes gestationis. New Engl. J. Med. **241**, 906 (1949).

ELLIOTT, J. A.: Bullous dermatoses of toxic origin: Report of a case involving an association with choriocarcinoma. Arch. Derm. Syph. (Chic.) **37**, 219 (1938).

FISHER, A. A.: Herpes gestationis (Rh-positive, type 0) treated with cortisone and progesterone. Arch. Derm. Syph. (Chic.) **68**, 449 (1953). — FOSNAUGH, R. P., H. G. BRYAN, and R. L. ORDERS: Pyridoxine in the treatment of herpes gestationis. Arch. Derm. **84**, 90 (1961). — FOX, E. C.: Herpes gestationis (dermatitis herpetiformis). Arch. Derm. Syph. (Chic.) **70**, 331 (1954).

HOLLENWEGER-MAYR, B.: Herpes gestationis, entstanden nach dem Absterben einer Extrauterinfrucht. Zbl. Gynäk. **72**, 569 (1950).

KEATY, C., P. E. JONES, and J. H. LAMB: Progesterone therapy in dermatoses of pregnancy. Arch. Derm. Syph. (Chic.) **63**, 675 (1951).

LAPIÈRE, A.: In der Diskussion zu S. CASTERMANS-ELIAS. Arch. belges Derm. **18**, 51 (1962). — LEWIS, G. M.: Herpes gestationis. Successful treatment with sulfathiazole: Report of a case. Arch. Derm. Syph. (Chic.) **46**, 841 (1942). — LINDEMANN, C., W. W. ENGSTROM, and R. T. FLYNN: Herpes gestationis: Results of treatment with adrenocorticotropic hormone (ACTH) and cortisone. Amer. J. Obstet. Gynec. **63**, 167 (1952).

MUELLER, C. W., and W. A. LAPP: Herpes gestationis. With a report of two cases and a survey of the literature. Amer. J. Obstet. Gynec. **48**, 170 (1944).

RIECKE, E.: Herpes gestationis (Milton). In: Handbuch der Haut- und Geschlechtskrankheiten, hrsg. von J. JADASSOHN, Bd. 7, Teil 2, S. 637. Berlin: Springer 1931. — RIMBAUD, P., et H. L. GUIBERT: La dermatite de Duhring-Brocq. Remarques cliniques et histologiques. Ann. Derm. Syph. (Paris) **83**, 241 (1956). — RUSSELL, B., and N. A. THORNE: Herpes gestationis. Brit. J. Derm. **69**, 339 (1957).

TILLMAN, W. G.: Herpes gestationis with hydatiform mole and chorion epithelioma. Brit. J. Med. **1**, 1471 (1950). — TOLMAN, M. M., S. L. MOSCHELLA, and R. N. SCHNEIDERMAN: Dermatitis herpetiformis: Specific entity or clinical complex? J. invest. Derm. **32**, 557 (1959). — TOUSSAINT, P., et R. SCHOYSMAN: Herpès gestationis. Étude anatomocliniques des lésions foetales. Arch. belges Derm. **13**, 149 (1957). — TURNER, S. J., and S. J. ZAKON: Herpes gestationis. Amer. J. Obstet. Gynec. **41**, 527 (1941).

WATRIN, J., et P. JEANDIDIER: Sur douze cas de maladie de Duhring. Ann. Derm. Syph. (Paris) **78**, 551 (1951). — WHITFIELD, J. M., L. SMITH, and R. C. MANSON: Chorioepithelioma with herpes gestationis. Virginia med. Mth. **73**, 257 (1946).

III. Subcorneale pustulöse Dermatose

BARSKY, S., and T. CORNBLEET: Subcorneal pustular dermatosis. J. invest. Derm. **32**, 69 (1959). — BURNS, R. E., and G. FINE: Subcorneal pustular dermatosis. Arch. Derm. **80**, 72 (1959).

CARNEY, J. W.: Case for diagnosis: Duhring's disease (dermatitis herpetiformis)? Impetigo herpetiformis? Moniliids? Arch. Derm. Syph. (Chic.) **66**, 421 (1952). — CIPOLLARO, A. C.: A case for diagnosis (dermatitis herpetiformis; impetigo herpetiformis?). Arch. Derm. Syph. (Chic.) **70**, 390 (1954).

DUPERRAT, B.: Pustulose thoracique amicrobienne récidivante: maladie de Duhring? maladie de Sneddon-Wilkinson? Ann. Derm. Syph. (Paris) **84**, 514 (1957).

ELLIS, F. A.: Subcorneal pustular dermatosis. Arch. Derm. **78**, 580 (1958). — EYSTER jr., W. H., and R. R. KIERLAND: Prognosis of dermatitis herpetiformis, treated and untreated. Arch. Derm. Syph. (Chic.) **64**, 1 (1951).

FEUERMAN-POGORZELSKI, E. J.: Subcorneal pustular dermatosis Sneddon-Wilkinson with face lesions. Acta derm.-venereol. (Stockh.) **41**, 240 (1961).

GREENBAUM, C. H., and J. B. LEE: Subcorneal pustular dermatosis. Arch. Derm. **77**, 512 (1958).

HABER, H., and G. C. WELLS: Subcorneal pustular dermatosis of the soles. Brit. J. Derm. **71**, 253 (1959). — HADIDA, E., et J. SAYAG: Syndrome de Sneddon-Wilkinson (Dermatose pustuleuse sous-cornée). Ann. Derm. Syph. (Paris) **89**, 301 (1962). — HALL, A. F.: Impetigo herpetiformis in the male. Report of one case with response to sulfapyridine. Arch. Derm. Syph. (Chic.) **50**, 107 (1944). — HELLIER, F. F.: Generalized pustular bacterid. Its relationship to the pustular dermatosis of Sneddon and Wilkinson. Brit. J. Derm. **68**, 395 (1956).

LAPIÈRE, S., et S. CASTERMANS-ELIAS: Étude clinique et histologique de plusieurs cas de pustulose sous-cornée multiloculaire du type Sneddon-Wilkinson. Arch. belges Derm. **18**, 22 (1962).

MEARA, R. H., and C. D. CALNAN: Sub-corneal pustular dermatosis. Trans. St John's Hosp. derm. Soc. **37**, 23 (1956).

REYNAERS, H.: Pustulose sous-cornée récidivante bénigne, maladie de Sneddon et Wilkinson, ou variété pustuleuse de la dermatite herpetiforme de Duhring? Arch. belges Derm. **14**, 337 (1958). — RÖCKL, H.: Subcorneale pustulöse Dermatose (Dermatitis pustulosa subcornealis). Fortschr. prakt. Derm. Venereol. **3**, 79 (1960). — RUITER, M.: Zum Bilde der Pyodermia chronica papillaris et exulcerans (Horncystenbildung) und über ihr Auftreten bei Dermatitis herpetiformis Duhring. Arch. Derm. Syph. (Berl.) **166**, 184 (1932).

SCHOENFELD, R. J.: Subcorneal pustular dermatosis. Arch. Derm. **78**, 589 (1958). — SCHRÖPL, F.: Zur nosologischen Stellung der subcornealen pustulösen Dermatose. Hautarzt **13**, 107 (1962). — SCHUPPENER, H. J., u. M. THAL: Die subcorneale Pustulose. Hautarzt **10**, 312 (1959). — SCHWANK, R., and J. TRAPL: Dermatosis subcornealis pustulosa (Sneddon-Wilkinson). Derm. Wschr. **142**, 846 (1960). — SIMPSON, J. R.: Pustular eruption: for diagnosis. Brit. J. Derm. **60**, 418 (1948). — SNEDDON, J. B., and D. S. WILKINSON: Subcorneal pustular dermatosis. Brit. J. Derm. **68**, 385 (1956).

WINSTON, M.: Subcorneal pustular dermatosis. Arch. Derm. **87**, 489 (1963).

Acrodermatitis continua. Impetigo herpetiformis

Von

Walter F. Lever-Boston (Mass., USA)

Mit 6 Abbildungen (davon 2 farbige)

I. Acrodermatitis continua

Zu dem klinischen Bilde der Acrodermatitis continua (Hallopeau) ist seit RIECKEs Veröffentlichung nichts Wesentliches hinzugefügt worden. Die Beziehungen der Acrodermatitis continua zur Psoriasis pustulosa haben sich jedoch etwas geklärt. Auch hat sich herausgestellt, daß die Acrodermatitis continua ein charakteristisches, wenn auch nicht pathognomonisches histologisches Bild besitzt. In bezug auf die Behandlung ist durch die Corticosteroide, besonders durch deren Lokalanwendung, ein Fortschritt erzielt worden.

a) Klinisches Bild nach RIECKE

Bereits RIECKE beschrieb eine lokalisierte und eine generalisierte Form.

Bei der *lokalisierten Form* treten die ersten Erscheinungen meistens an den Endgliedern der Phalangen, insbesondere perionychial auf. Der den Nagel umsäumende Pustelkranz schreitet peripher weiter, sowohl zu den Fingerkuppen als auch zu den zweiten und ersten Phalangen. Es bilden sich Erythemflächen, in die die Pusteln flach und breit eingelagert sind. Später weisen die Endglieder der Finger und Zehen Atrophie der Haut und Schrumpfung der unterliegenden Weichteile auf, so daß sich die Gestaltung von Trommelschlegelfingern ergibt, die distal zugespitzt sind. Auch zu Knochenatrophien und Flexionskontrakturen kann es kommen. Im abklingenden Stadium kann Desquamation vorherrschen, und bei der geröteten Basis dann durchaus das Bild der Psoriasis imitiert werden. Üblicherweise bilden die Hand- bzw. Fußgelenke die Grenze für die proximale Ausdehnung der Hautveränderungen. Bei diesen lokalisierten Krankheitsbildern pflegt das Allgemeinbefinden kaum verändert zu sein.

Bei der *disseminierten Form* finden sich die ersten Krankheitserscheinungen bisweilen an proximalen Hautstellen statt an den Händen oder Füßen. Es kommen auch Krankheitsbilder zur Beobachtung, die lange Zeit auf Hände und Füße beschränkte Erscheinungen der Acrodermatitis continua darbieten und dann plötzlich weitere Partien der Körperdecke befallen. Dabei entstehen auf der Basis von Erythemen Pusteleruptionen. Das Gesamtbefinden ist gestört und Schüttelfröste und Fieber stellen sich ein. Erscheinungen an der Schleimhaut, insbesondere der Mundschleimhaut, aber auch der Vulva, können auftreten. Todesfälle sind nach RIECKE sehr selten, da er nur fünf tödlich verlaufende Fälle in der Literatur auffand.

b) Beziehungen zur Psoriasis pustulosa

Eine im Jahre 1936 von der Dermatologischen Wochenschrift durchgeführte Umfrage ergab, daß alle Befragten, nämlich FRÜHWALD, MATRAS, RAMEL und RIECKE, die Acrodermatitis continua (Hallopeau) und die Psoriasis pustulosa (Zumbusch) als unterschiedliche Krankheiten betrachteten, obwohl zugegeben wurde, daß die Abgrenzung manchmal recht schwierig sei. Dieser Standpunkt wurde auch vor kurzem von FRÜHWALD (1953) und von KEINING und JUNG-GRIMM vertreten. FRÜHWALD führte einen über 26 Jahre hin beobachteten Fall von disseminierter Acrodermatitis continua an, bei dem er niemals einen für die Psoriasis typischen Herd gesehen hatte. KEINING und JUNG-GRIMM wiesen darauf hin, daß die Acrodermatitis continua (Abb. 1—3), im Gegensatz zur Psoriasis pustulosa, zu atrophischen und sklerotischen Hautveränderungen und Knochenatrophien an den Endphalangen führe und Mundschleimhauterscheinungen zeige. Nach KEINING und JUNG-GRIMM stellt die Psoriasis pustulosa den stärksten „Eruptionsdruck" dar, zu dem eine Psoriasis fähig sei, und trete daher als ein akutes, große Flächen des Körpers einnehmendes Exanthem auf.

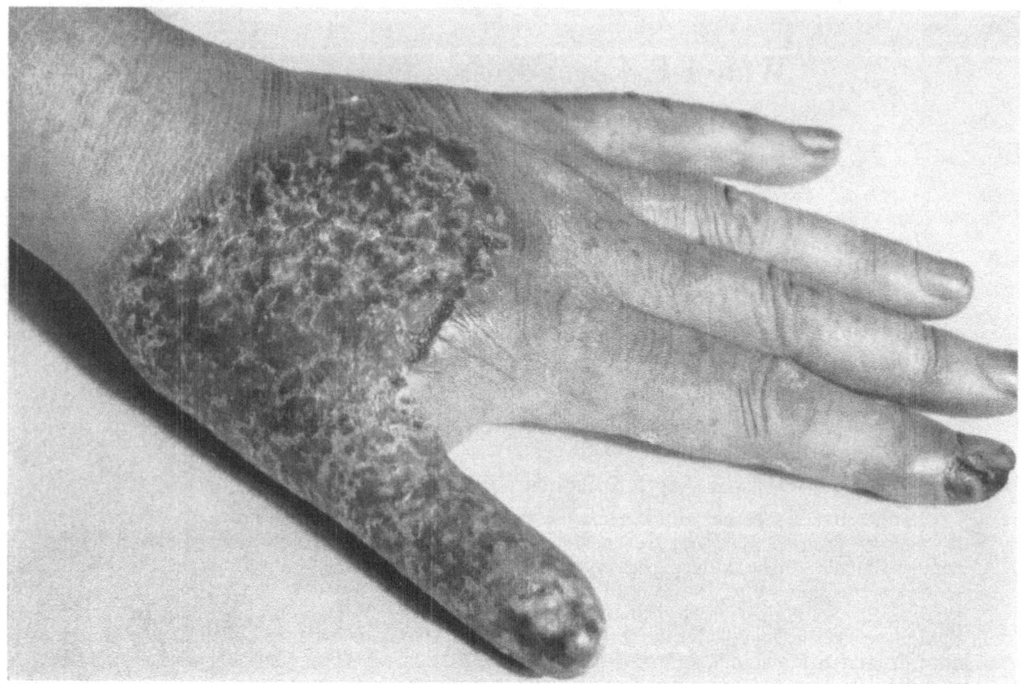

Abb. 1. *Lokalisierte Acrodermatitis continua.* Die Krankheitsherde bestehen seit 11 Jahren. Am Daumen findet sich Atrophie

Dem gegenüber sind in den letzten Jahren zahlreiche Berichte erschienen, in denen die Acrodermatitis continua als eine Variante der Psoriasis pustulosa betrachtet worden ist. Als starkes Argument für diese Ansicht wird das Vorkommen von gewöhnlichen Psoriasisherden bei Patienten mit Acrodermatitis continua hervorgehoben. So berichteten z.B. LANGHOF u. Mitarb. bei einem Patienten über das gleichzeitige Auftreten einer Acrodermatitis continua und einer Psoriasis vulgaris; LAPIÈRE et al., BRÜCK, SKOG, SOLTERMANN, LANGHOF et al. sowie KOGOJ (1962) beobachteten das spätere Auftreten von Psoriasisherden bei Patienten mit Acrodermatitis continua; und BERNHARDT, CARRIÉ sowie SOLTERMANN sahen eine Acrodermatitis continua bei bereits bestehender Psoriasis auftreten.

Insofern als die Acrodermatitis continua nicht immer zuerst an den Fingern und Zehen auftritt (CARRIÉ; SOLTERMANN; EPSTEIN et al.) und auch die Psoriasis pustulosa dort auftreten kann (MÖSLEIN) und die disseminierte Acrodermatitis continua wie die Psoriasis pustulosa akute, fieberhafte Schübe zeigen kann, scheinen die einzigen wesentlichen Unterschiede zwischen den beiden Krankheiten darin zu liegen, daß bei der Acrodermatitis continua, im Gegensatz zur Psoriasis pustulosa, Atrophie und Osteoporose an den Fingern sowie Krankheitsherde an der Mundschleimhaut vorkommen können. Jedoch hängt wahrscheinlich die Entwicklung von Atrophie und Osteoporose an den Fingern lediglich von der Dauer und Intensität der Krankheit in dieser Lokalisation ab (BERNHARDT).

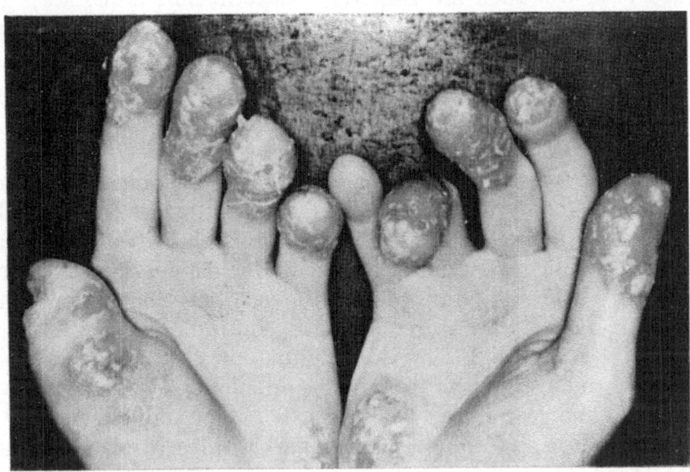

Abb. 2. *Disseminierte Acrodermatitis continua.* Neun Finger zeigen Pusteln, Zerstörung ihrer Nägel und Atrophie der Haut

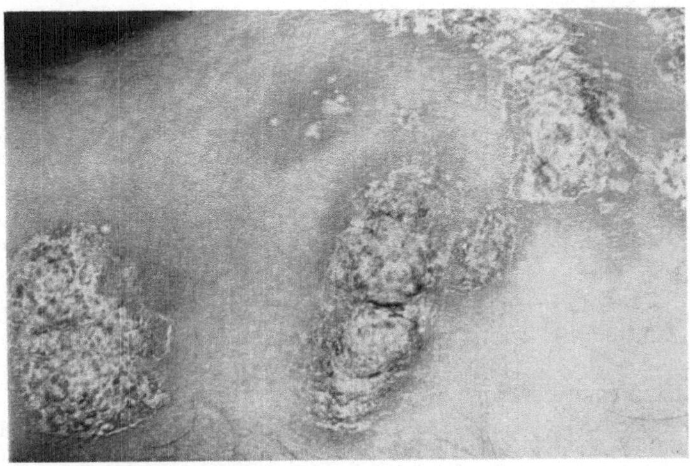

Abb. 3. *Disseminierte Acrodermatitis continua.* Derselbe Patient wie auf Abb. 2. Die Innenseite des rechten Knies ist dargestellt. In der Mitte des Bildes sieht man einen neuen Herd, der Pusteln auf erythematösem Grund zeigt. Die älteren Herde sind mit dicken Krusten bedeckt

Zudem ist einerseits die anscheinend bestehende Atrophie rückbildungsfähig (LAUSECKER) und andererseits können auch bei typischer Psoriasis pustulosa gelegentlich sekundäre Hautatrophien entstehen (SCHUPPENER 1958). Der bereits von RIECKE hervorgehobene Differenzierungspunkt, daß bei der Acrodermatitis continua häufig Mundschleimhautherde aufträten, nicht aber bei der Psoriasis pustulosa, kann nicht länger aufrechterhalten werden, da Mundschleimhauterscheinungen auch bei als Psoriasis pustulosa beschriebenen Fällen des öfteren beobachtet worden sind (DANBOLT; SCHUPPENER 1959, 1960).

Zu der klinischen Ähnlichkeit zwischen der Acrodermatitis continua und der Psoriasis pustulosa kommt auch noch die völlige Übereinstimmung im histologischen Bilde (s. unten). Somit unterliegt es keinem Zweifel mehr, daß diese beiden Krankheiten eng verwandt sind. Die Acrodermatitis continua und die Psoriasis pustulosa, wie auch die Impetigo herpetiformis (s. S. 728), gravitieren, wie BERNHARDT es ausgedrückt hat, nach einem gemeinsamen Brennpunkt, der atypischen Psoriasis. LANGHOF u. Mitarb. haben sogar vorgeschlagen, die Acrodermatitis continua als Psoriasis pustulosa Typ Hallopeau zu bezeichnen.

c) Beziehungen zur Dermatitis repens (Crocker)

Während RIECKE, wie schon HALLOPEAU, das Bestehen einer vesiculösen, abortiven Form der Acrodermatitis continua anerkannte, die er mit der Dermatitis repens von CROCKER in Beziehung setzte, ist man sich heute wohl darüber einig, daß die Pustel die obligate Primärefflorescenz der Acrodermatitis continua darstellt. Somit fällt jede Beziehung der Acrodermatitis continua zur Dermatitis repens fort; denn während die Acrodermatitis continua eine pustulöse, trockene, chronische und destruktive Erkrankung darstellt, ist die Dermatitis repens vesiculös, feucht, in ihrer Dauer begrenzt und nicht destruktiv (LEVER 1944). Histologisch weist die Dermatitis repens auch keine Ähnlichkeit mit der Acrodermatitis continua auf, da die Bläschen innerhalb des Stratum Malpighi liegen wie bei einer Dermatitis, und nicht spongiform sind wie bei der Acrodermatitis continua (s. unten).

d) Beziehungen zur Pustulosis palmaris et plantaris

Der Name Pustulosis palmaris et plantaris (LEVER 1961) bezeichnet eine Dermatose, die auch unter mehreren anderen Namen bekannt ist. DORE beschrieb sie zuerst im Jahre 1928 als „Acrodermatitis perstans". Sodann schlug BARBER als Bezeichnung „pustular psoriasis of the palms and soles" vor, ANDREWS und MACHACEK „pustular bacterids of the hands and feet" und SACHS, MACKEE und ROTHSTEIN „Acrodermatitis pustulosa perstans". Es handelt sich bei der Pustulosis palmaris et plantaris um eine chronische, fast symptomenfreie Erkrankung, die sich gewöhnlich auf die Handflächen und Sohlen beschränkt und durch das schubweise Auftreten von Pusteln innerhalb von scharf begrenzten, geröteten und schuppenden Herden gekennzeichnet ist. Obgleich die Pustulosis palmaris et plantaris zu der Acrodermatitis continua (Hallopeau) wie auch zu der Psoriasis pustulosa (Zumbusch) wohl keine Beziehungen hat, sind doch Beziehungen zwischen der Pustulosis palmaris et plantaris und diesen beiden Krankheiten mehrfach angenommen worden.

Wie bereits BARBER nahm auch EVERALL an, daß die Pustulosis palmaris et plantaris mit der Psoriasis in Beziehung stünde und durch eine „Kombinierung von Psoriasis mit gewöhnlicher Ekzematisierung" zustande käme. Er wies darauf hin, daß unter den 70 von ihm beobachteten Patienten mit Pustulosis palmaris et plantaris 13, d.h. 19%, Herde von Psoriasis an anderen Körperstellen aufwiesen. SCHUPPENER und KOBER stellten die Pustulosis palmaris et plantaris als Psoriasis pustulosa Typ Barber der Psoriasis pustulosa Typ Zumbusch gegenüber und behaupteten, daß eine Abgrenzung des Typ Barber gegen den Typ Zumbusch nicht immer exakt möglich wäre, denn es gäbe zahlreiche Zwischenformen, und auch beim Typ Barber wäre eine Generalisierung möglich. INGRAM vereinigte zu einer Gruppe Acrodermatitis continua, Psoriasis pustulosa und „pustular bacterid", da sie lediglich Varianten einer klinischen Einheit wären. Im Gegensatz zu diesen Autoren haben ANDREWS und MACHACEK sowie SACHS und SCANNONE ihre Überzeugung ausgesprochen, daß die Pustulosis palmaris et plantaris eine wesenseigene Krankheit sei.

Gegen eine Beziehung der Pustulosis palmaris et plantaris zur Acrodermatitis continua sprechen die folgenden Tatsachen: Bei der Pustulosis palmaris et plantaris sind erstens die Finger- und Zehenspitzen nur sehr selten befallen; zweitens entwickelt sich bei ihr keine Atrophie; drittens kommt bei ihr (im Gegensatz zur Auffassung von SCHUPPENER und KOBER) keine Generalisierung vor; und viertens zeigt ihr histologisches Bild keine Anklänge an die Acrodermatitis continua oder an die Psoriasis, denn es finden sich bei der Pustulosis palmaris et plantaris tief in der Epidermis gelegene, einkämmerige Pusteln.

e) Histologie

Es ist das Verdienst von KOGOJ (1927, 1937), als erster darauf hingewiesen zu haben, daß die Acrodermatitis continua auf Grund der sog. spongiformen Pustel ein charakteristisches histologisches Aussehen besitzt. Das Bestehen der spongiformen Pustel bei der Acrodermatitis continua ist seitdem vielerseits bestätigt worden (LAPIÈRE et al.; LAUSECKER; KEINING und JUNG-GRIMM). Allerdings kommt die spongiforme Pustel nicht nur bei der Acrodermatitis continua vor, sondern auch bei der Psoriasis pustulosa Zumbusch (SCHUPPENER 1960), der Impetigo herpetiformis (KOGOJ 1938; LEONHARDI und MICHEL), dem Morbus REITER (WEINBERGER; BOHNSTEDT) und, in allerdings nur angedeuteter Weise, in frischen Efflorescenzen der Psoriasis vulgaris (STREITMANN; KEINING und JUNG - GRIMM; LEVER 1961).

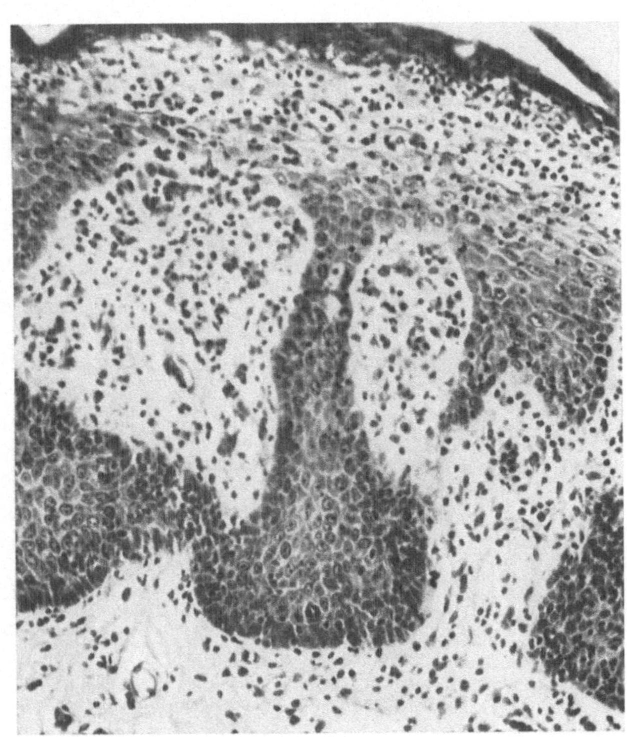

Abb. 4. *Acrodermatitis continua*. Eine sich eben bildende Pustel ist dargestellt. Die obere Epidermis enthält eine spongiforme Pustel: Die Zellwände geschwollener Epidermiszellen bilden ein schwammartiges Netzwerk, in dessen Maschen neutrophile Leukocyten liegen (200mal)

Die spongiforme Pustel bildet sich in den obersten Lagen des Stratum Malpighi infolge des Einwanderns von neutrophilen Leukocyten in ödematös geschwollene Stachelzellen. Mit diesem Einwandern geht eine Auflösung des Cytoplasma und ein Zerfall des Zellkern einher. Die Zellwände bleiben aber zunächst bestehen und bilden so ein schwammartiges Netzwerk, in dessen Zwischenräumen sich neutrophile Leukocyten weiterhin ansammeln (Abb. 4). Mit Größerwerden der Pustel zerfallen in der Mitte der Pustel die Zellwände allmählich, so daß sich dort eine größere Blasenhöhlung bildet (Abb. 5). An der Peripherie solch einer großen Pustel erhält sich jedoch das Netzwerk viel länger (Abb. 6). Wenn nun die Pustel eintrocknet und in das Stratum corneum hinaufrückt, nimmt sie das Aussehen eines Munroschen Mikroabscesses an (STREIMANN; KEINING und JUNG-GRIMM; LEVER 1961). Somit scheinen die spongiforme Pustel und der Munrosche Mikroabsceß miteinander in Beziehung zu stehen. Der Munrosche Mikroabsceß stellt entweder eine eingetrocknete spongiforme Pustel oder eine Abortivform derselben dar.

Außerhalb der spongiformen Pustel sehen die Veränderungen in der Epidermis denen ähnlich, die bei der Psoriasis vorkommen; denn man findet oft Parakeratose und eine Verlängerung der Reteleisten. Ein Infiltrat von Lymphocyten und Neutrophilen befindet sich in den oberen Schichten der Dermis. Oft sieht man ein Einwandern vieler Leukocyten in die Epidermis.

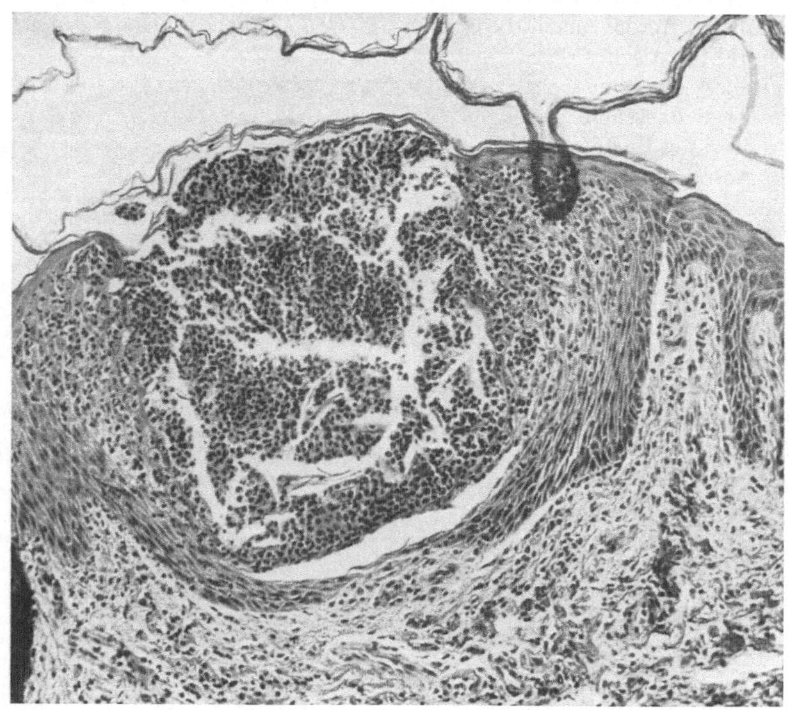

Abb. 5. *Acrodermatitis continua.* Große, ältere Pustel. Es besteht eine ziemlich große Blasenhöhle. An den Seiten der Pustel sieht man aber noch ein spongiformes Netzwerk (50mal)

Auf Grund der Tatsache, daß die spongiforme Pustel bei mehreren Krankheiten gefunden wird, sprach ihr KOGOJ (1951) keine ätiologische Bedeutung zu. Trotzdem ist es wohl kein Zufall, daß die spongiforme Pustel als charakteristisches Merkmal in einer Gruppe von Krankheiten vorkommt, die alle in ihrem klinischen Aussehen Ähnlichkeit mit der Psoriasis besitzen und möglicherweise ätiologisch mit der Psoriasis in Beziehung stehen.

f) Behandlung

Bevor die Corticosteroide aufkamen, gab es für die Acrodermatitis continua keine wirksame innere Behandlung. In zwei von SULZBERGER und von LEVER (1944) mitgeteilten Fällen war zwar Sulfapyridin wirksam, solange es verabreicht wurde, aber seitdem sind keine weiteren Erfolge mit Sulfapyridin mitgeteilt worden.

Die Corticosteroide sind äußerst wirkungsvoll, wenn sie in genügend hohen Dosen verabreicht werden, wie die von MILFORT, von CARRIÉ sowie von KEINING und JUNG-GRIMM berichteten Fälle darlegen, bei denen die Anfangsdosen 150 bis

200 mg Cortison betrugen. Die interne Anwendung der Corticosteroide ist jedoch nur bei äußerst akuten und lebensbedrohenden Fällen angezeigt, da das Absetzen der Corticosteroide, in ähnlicher Weise wie bei der Psoriasis, zu einer bedeutenden Exacerbation führen kann. So kam es bei dem von CALKINS et al. beobachteten Patienten mit lokalisierter Acrodermatitis continua bei Reduzierung der Dosis zu einer schweren Dissemination.

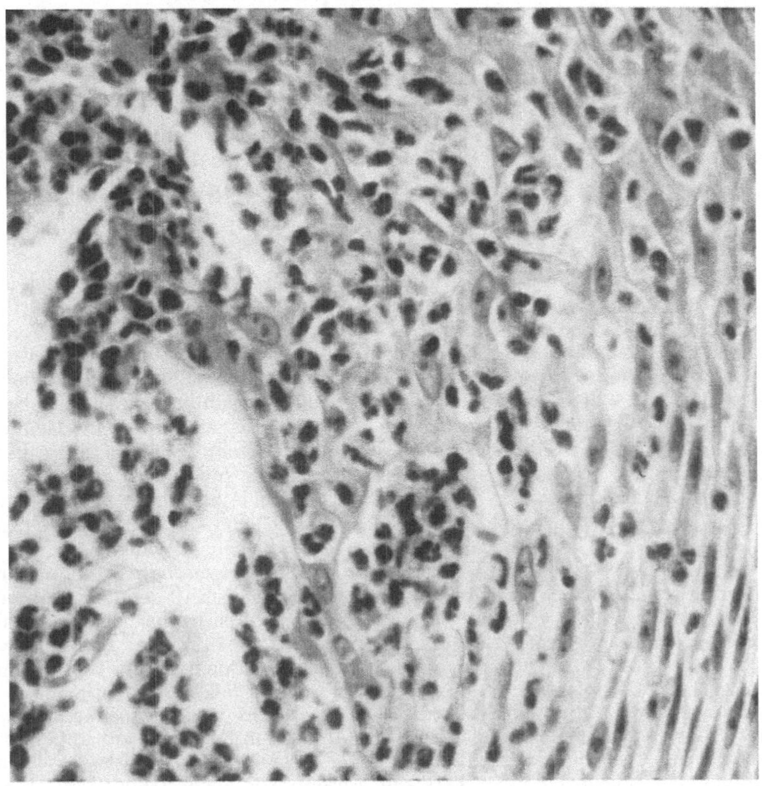

Abb. 6. *Acrodermatitis continua.* Vergrößerung der rechten Pustelwand aus der vorhergehenden Abbildung. Man sieht deutlich das spongiforme Netzwerk (400mal)

Bei dem von CALKINS et al. behandelten Patienten war die Acrodermatitis continua über 39 Jahre auf die Hände beschränkt gewesen. Hohe Dosen, nämlich 150 mg Prednisolon pro Tag (750 mg Cortison entsprechend), waren für die Abheilung erforderlich. Nach völliger Abheilung wurde die Dosis allmählich herabgesetzt. Als nur noch 5 mg Prednisolon gegeben wurden, entwickelten sich plötzlich zahlreiche, weitverbreitete, mit Pusteln besetzte Erythemherde, so daß das klinische Bild einer disseminierten Acrodermatitis continua bestand. Hohe Dosen von Prednisolon waren nötig, um diesen Ausbruch zur Abheilung zu bringen. Die Dosis wurde dann sehr vorsichtig reduziert; und nach Ablauf von 6 Monaten betrug die Erhaltungsdosis 12 mg Prednisolon (60 mg Cortison entsprechend).

Die Lokalbehandlung mit Corticosteroidsalben ist meistens nur dann wirksam, wenn ein Okklusionsverband nach Auftragen der Salbe angelegt wird. Bei auf die Hände beschränkter Acrodermatitis continua werden als Okklusionsverband angefeuchtete dünne Baumwollhandschuhe und darüber plastische Handschuhe für einen Zeitraum von 8—16 Std getragen. Außerhalb der Hände befindliche Herde bedeckt man, wie es von TYE et al. für die Behandlung der Psoriasis vorgeschlagen worden ist, nach Einreiben der Corticosteroidsalbe erst mit einem angefeuchteten dünnen Baumwolltuch (z.B. mit einem Teil eines alten Bettlakens) und dann mit einer plastischen Folie. Die Folie wird mittels eng anliegender Kleidungsstücke, elastischer Bandagen oder plastischen Heftpflasters an die Haut fixiert und von 8—16 Std am Orte belassen. Zu Beginn der Behandlung sollte, falls möglich, ein Okklusionsverband jeden Abend angelegt werden, und später dann jeden zweiten oder dritten Abend.

II. Impetigo herpetiformis

Ein recht bedeutungsvoller Fortschritt seit dem Erscheinen von Rieckes Abhandlung über die Impetigo herpetiformis stellt die Behandlung dieser Krankheit mit AT 10 oder Vitamin D dar. Ferner hat sich ergeben, daß die Hauterscheinungen der Impetigo herpetiformis auf die Corticosteroide gut ansprechen. Auch sind das histologische Bild der Impetigo herpetiformis und die Beziehungen der Impetigo herpetiformis zur Psoriasis pustulosa weithin geklärt worden.

a) Klinisches Bild nach Riecke

Bei der Impetigo herpetiformis entwickeln sich Pustelgruppen auf entzündlich geschwollener Basis. Da randständig neue Pusteln entstehen, findet sich oft eine ringförmige oder serpiginöse Anordnung der Pusteln. In der Regel bricht die Pustulosis plötzlich und heftig hervor, um zunächst einmal als solche für lange Zeit unter fortgesetzten Exacerbationen und Remissionen zu bestehen. Diesem sog. „Stadium der Pustelbildung" kann ein exfoliatives erythrodermatisches sog. „Stadium der Exfoliation" folgen. Während diesem erfolgen oft an einzelnen Stellen noch eine Zeitlang typische Pustelausbrüche. Obwohl die Genito-Crural-Region und die Mammae Prädilektionsstellen darstellen, besteht doch eine rechte Inkonstanz der Lokalisation. Auch an den Nägeln und ihrer Umgebung spielen sich gelegentlich bei der Impetigo herpetiformis krankhafte Vorgänge ab. Die Mundschleimhaut und die Vulva sind recht oft befallen. In der Mehrzahl der Fälle zeigt sich eine starke Beeinträchtigung des Allgemeinbefindens. Das Leiden nimmt häufig einen tödlichen Ausgang.

Was die Ätiologie betrifft, prädisponiert zwar die Schwangerschaft zum Ausbruch einer Impetigo herpetiformis; jedoch ist diese kein an die Schwangerschaft gebundener Krankheitsprozeß. Eine unverkennbare Beziehung besteht zwischen Impetigo herpetiformis und Funktionsausfall der Glandulae parathyreoideae, wie durch die zwei 1921 von Schardorn berichteten Fälle erwiesen wurde, bei denen nach einer Kropfoperation erst eine Tetanie und später eine Impetigo herpetiformis auftrat. Autoptisch wurde bei beiden Patientinnen ein Fehlen der Epithelkörperchen festgestellt. Nach Rieckes Ansicht steht jedoch nicht allein die durch Epithelkörperchenschädigung bedingte Dysfunktion in Beziehung zur Impetigo herpetiformis, sondern eine Reihe anderer inkretorischer Organe kann höchstwahrscheinlich im gleichen Sinne bei Störungen ihrer Tätigkeit wirken, vor allem Hypophyse, Thyreoidea, Thymus und Genitaldrüsen.

Eine Abgrenzung bzw. Differenzierung der Psoriasis pustulosa von der Impetigo herpetiformis erscheint nach Riecke oft schwierig; andererseits glaubt er, daß die v. Zumbuschsche Vermutung, es dürften namentlich unter den bei Männern beobachteten und leichter verlaufenden Impetigo herpetiformis-Formen solche von pustulöser Psoriasis beschrieben sein, sehr wahrscheinlich nicht zu Recht besteht.

b) Beziehungen zur Psoriasis pustulosa

In der Bewertung der Beziehungen zwischen der Impetigo herpetiformis und der Psoriasis pustulosa lassen sich drei Anschauungen erkennen. Eine Gruppe hält an der von Riecke bereits formulierten Meinung fest, daß die Impetigo herpetiformis eine selbständige Krankheit darstelle, die sich morphologisch von der Psoriasis pustulosa unterscheide und durch endokrine Störungen verursacht sei, welche hauptsächlich, aber doch nicht ausschließlich von den Epithelkörperchen herstammten (Beek; Steppert; Möslein; Wolfram). Die von den Autoren angeführten morphologischen Unterschiede erscheinen aber kaum überzeugend, wie z.B. die Feststellung Mösleins, daß die Primärefflorescenz der Impetigo herpetiformis die Pustel sei, während bei der Psoriasis pustulosa die Pusteln immer sekundär aufträten.

Eine zweite Gruppe von Autoren sieht die Impetigo herpetiformis als eine durch endokrine Faktoren ausgelöste Psoriasis pustulosa an, wobei die endokrine Störung meistens, aber nicht immer, die Epithelkörperchen betreffe (BERNHARDT; VOHWINKEL; GOTTRON; KOCH; KEINING und JUNG-GRIMM; LAPIÈRE; SOLTERMANN; TIELSCH; HERRMANN und PESCH).

Die dritte Gruppe zieht die Grenzen der Impetigo herpetiformis enger als die beiden anderen Gruppen. Sie stellt die Impetigo herpetiformis der Psoriasis pustulosa morphologisch zwar gleich, ordnet aber nur solche Fälle als Impetigo herpetiformis ein, die als Zeichen einer Insuffizienz der Epithelkörperchen eine ausgesprochene Hypocalcämie sowie Anzeichen von Tetanie aufweisen, während alle Fälle, bei denen keine Insuffizienz der Epithelkörperchen besteht, als Psoriasis pustulosa angesehen werden (DANBOLT; LEONHARDI und MICHEL).

Die letztere Definition der Impetigo herpetiformis erscheint zur Zeit die beste zu sein, denn sie schafft klare Verhältnisse; denn obwohl die Impetigo herpetiformis klinisch und histologisch von der Psoriasis pustulosa nicht unterscheidbar ist, findet man bei der Psoriasis pustulosa gewöhnlich normale Calciumwerte (s. unten), ferner keine Anzeichen von Tetanie und kein Ansprechen auf AT 10.

c) Fälle von echter Impetigo herpetiformis in der Literatur

Die Zahl der unter der Diagnose Impetigo herpetiformis seit dem Erscheinen von RIECKEs Abhandlung veröffentlichten Fälle verringert sich stark, wenn das Bestehen einer Hypocalcämie und von tetanischen Anfällen zur Grundbedingung der Diagnose gemacht wird. Es qualifizieren vor allem Fälle, die nach einer Strumektomie auftraten, wie z.B. die von den folgenden Autoren mitgeteilten Fälle: BOHNSTEDT, BARTMANN, SCHUBERT, VOHWINKEL, SCHMIDT-LA BAUME, ENGFELDT und GENTELE, STEPPERT, LUTZ, GENTELE et al., LEONHARDI und MICHEL, MÖSLEIN (Fall 1 und 2) sowie WOLFRAM (Fall 1). Von Interesse ist die recht unterschiedliche Zeitspanne zwischen der Strumektomie und dem Auftreten der Hauterscheinungen, die von wenigen Monaten (LEONHARDI und MICHEL) bis zu 30 Jahren betrug (ENGFELDT und GENTELE). In mehreren Fällen, in denen ein langer Zeitunterschied bestand, setzten die pustulösen Hauterscheinungen zur Zeit des Klimakteriums ein; und bei der von BOHNSTEDT beobachteten Patientin setzten die Hauterscheinungen 10 Jahre nach der Strumektomie während einer Schwangerschaft ein.

Es steht fest, daß während der Schwangerschaft vom fünften Lunarmonat an ein Mehrbedarf an Epithelkörperchenhormon einsetzt und somit zu dieser Zeit eine latente Tetanie manifest werden kann (BARTMANN). Jedoch befinden sich nur sehr wenige Fälle in der Literatur, bei denen die Eruption von Pusteln ohne vorhergehende Strumektomie während der Schwangerschaft auftrat und dabei eine einwandfreie Hypocalcämie vorlag. Nur bei den zwei von HADIDA und TIMSIT (1956, 1961) beobachteten Schwangeren traten tetanische Anfälle auf und die Serumcalciumwerte betrugen 8,4 bzw. 4,8 mg-%. Die von SCHAUER und von KNIERER berichteten Fälle sind zweifelhaft; es bestand bei ihnen zwar eine Erniedrigung der Serumcalciumwerte zu 7,1 bzw. 7,0 mg-%, aber keine Tetanie. Sie könnten als Fälle von Psoriasis pustulosa mit sekundärer Hypocalcämie angesehen werden (s. unten).

d) Fälle in der Literatur, die nicht Impetigo herpetiformis darstellen

Bei den meisten während der Schwangerschaft auftretenden Fällen, die unter der Diagnose Impetigo herpetiformis mitgeteilt worden sind, waren die Werte für das Serumcalcium normal oder nur mäßig vermindert. Ferner blieben die pustulösen Hauterscheinungen oft nicht auf die Zeit der Schwangerschaft beschränkt, sondern bestanden entweder weiter (KOCH; TIELSCH) oder traten erneut ohne das Bestehen einer Schwangerschaft auf (TENLÉN; SCHERBER; GAUMOND; HVIDBERG; HOLLSTROM und LAGERHOLM). Bei mehreren dieser Patienten fanden sich Anzeichen einer Psoriasis vulgaris. So bestand bei dem von TIELSCH berichteten Falle (Fall 1) eine Psoriasis vulgaris seit vielen Jahren, bevor die pustulöse Eruption während der Schwangerschaft einsetzte. Bei der von KOCH beobachteten Patientin wandelten sich die Hauterscheinungen zu typischen Herden von Psoriasis vulgaris um, woraus KOCH den Schluß zog, daß die Impetigo herpetiformis, wie auch die Psoriasis pustulosa, Varianten der Psoriasis vulgaris wären; und in dem ursprünglich von TENLÉN als Impetigo herpetiformis mitgeteilten Fall änderte DANBOLT die Diagnose zu Psoriasis pustulosa um, weil die Hauterscheinungen später wiederkamen und bei Beginn der Wiederkehr einige Hautherde das Aussehen einer Psoriasis vulgaris boten, bevor sich Pusteln bildeten. Es hat also den Anschein, daß eine Schwangerschaft zu einem Ausbruch von Psoriasis pustulosa prädisponiert. So beobachteten TOLMAN und MOSCHELLA bei einer Patientin die Umwandlung einer Psoriasis vulgaris zu einer Psoriasis pustulosa während vier aufeinanderfolgenden Schwangerschaften.

Fälle, die ohne Schwangerschaft, Tetanie oder Hypocalcämie aufzuweisen, unter der Diagnose Impetigo herpetiformis mitgeteilt worden sind, können wohl ohne Zwang als Psoriasis pustulosa angesehen werden. In dieser Kategorie befinden sich z.B. die Fälle von BEEK, EBERHARTINGER, SOLTERMANN (Fall 1) und TIELSCH (Fall 2).

Bei mehreren Fällen, die ohne Strumektomie und ohne Schwangerschaft auftraten, wurde eine Erniedrigung des Serumcalciums festgestellt, besonders bei solchen, die mit schweren pustulösen Eruptionen einhergingen. Diese Erniedrigung des Calciums ist eine Sekundärerscheinung, wie sie auch beim Pemphigus vulgaris beobachtet wird (s. S. 644), hervorgerufen durch den Verlust von Calcium in dem Exsudat, das durch die stark entzündete Haut ausgeschieden wird (HERRMANN und PESCH). Die Erniedrigung des Serumcalciums läuft der Erniedrigung des Gesamteiweißes im Serum parallel und beschränkt sich fast ausschließlich auf den eiweißgebundenen Anteil des Calciums, während der ionisierte Anteil des Calciums nicht wesentlich verändert ist. Aus diesem Grunde kommt es selbst bei recht niedrigen Serumcalciumwerten nicht zu einer Tetanie. Beispiele solcher sekundärer Serumcalciumerniedrigungen sind die Fälle von SOLTERMANN, Fall 2 (Serumcalcium 7,5 mg-%), WOLFRAM (Serumcalcium 4,4 mg-%), TIELSCH, Fall 3 (Serumcalcium 7,8 mg-%) und HERRMANN und PESCH (Serumcalcium 6,6 mg-%). In dem letzteren Fall betrug der Gesamteiweißwert im Serum 3,4 mg-%. (Da bei solchen Fällen die Erniedrigung des Serumcalciums nicht durch eine Insuffizienz der Epithelkörperchen hervorgerufen ist, würde die Anwendung von AT 10 oder Vitamin D auch keine Besserung bringen.)

Es befinden sich in der Literatur recht viele unter der Diagnose Impetigo herpetiformis beschriebene Fälle, bei denen jedoch das klinische und histologische Bild und der Verlauf gegen diese Diagnose sprechen. So kann weder der von SAUER beschriebene Fall noch irgendeiner der zehn Fälle, die SAUER in der amerikanischen Literatur unter der Diagnose Impetigo herpetiformis beschrieben vorfand, einer Kritik standhalten. Bei den meisten dieser Fälle handelt es sich wohl um eine Pyodermie, und bei dem von HALL beschriebenen Patienten ist subcorneale pustulöse Dermatose die wahrscheinlichste Diagnose. Ebenfalls in die Kategorie der Pyodermien gehören wohl die zwei von TEODORESCOU und CONU (1947, 1948) als Impetigo herpetiformis beschriebenen Fälle, die unter Behandlung mit Sulfathiazol bzw. Penicillin abheilten.

e) Ätiologie

Die bei der echten Impetigo herpetiformis bestehende Insuffizienz der Epithelkörperchen stammt entweder von einer akzidentellen Entfernung der Epithelkörperchen während einer Strumektomie oder von einer Schwangerschaft, die eine latente Insuffizienz der Epithelkörperchen manifest machen kann wegen des während dieser Zeit wesentlich erhöhten Calciumbedarfs (LEONHARDI und MICHEL).

Es sollte jedoch in Betracht gezogen werden, daß eine Unterfunktion der Epithelkörperchen allein nicht zu einer Impetigo herpetiformis führt, denn nur verhältnismäßig wenige Patienten mit postoperativer Tetanie nach Strumektomie werden von einer Impetigo herpetiformis befallen; und wenn sie auftritt, geschieht dies oft erst mehrere Jahre nach dem Auftreten der Tetanie (SCHUBERT). So spielt neben der Insuffizienz der Epithelkörperchen noch ein anderer Faktor eine Rolle. Dieser Faktor ist wahrscheinlich eine Diathese zur Psoriasis pustulosa.

f) Histologie

Das histologische Bild der Impetigo herpetiformis ist dasselbe wie bei der Acrodermatitis continua (s. S. 725) und bei der Psoriasis pustulosa und zeichnet sich durch spongiforme Pustelbildung in der oberen Epidermis aus (KOGOJ; LEONHARDI und MICHEL; MÖSLEIN; HADIDA und TIMSIT 1961). Recht häufig findet man in der Pustel und in noch ausgesprochener Weise in dem Infiltrat der oberen Dermis neben zahlreichen Neutrophilen eine beträchtliche Zahl von Eosinophilen (MÖSLEIN; HADIDA und TIMSIT 1961; WOLFRAM). Jedoch ist dies nicht immer der Fall (HADIDA und TIMSIT 1956; LEONHARDI und MICHEL). Da die Gewebseosinophilie inkonstant ist und gelegentlich auch bei der Psoriasis pustulosa gefunden wird, kann sie nicht als eine spezifische Eigenschaft der Impetigo herpetiformis gelten. Im Abheilungsstadium zeigt das histologische Bild oft Ähnlichkeit mit der Psoriasis (LEONHARDI und MICHEL).

g) Behandlung

Bei der echten, mit Hypocalcämie und Tetanie einhergehenden Impetigo herpetiformis haben sich AT 10 und Vitamin D bewährt, und zwar nicht nur für die Behebung der Hypocalcämie, sondern auch für die Abheilung der Hauterscheinungen.

Das Präparat AT 10 (antitetanisches Präparat Nr. 10), das von HOLTZ erstmalig für die Behandlung der Tetanie angewandt wurde, stellt eine 0,5%ige Lösung von Dihydrotachysterin in Sesamöl dar. Sowohl das AT 10 als auch das Vitamin D_2 enthalten den sog. Calcinose-Faktor. Dabei entsprechen in ihrer Wirkung auf den Calciumstoffwechsel 1 cm³ AT 10 ungefähr 75000 Einheiten Vitamin D_2 (= 2 mg Vitamin D_2) (LEVER und TALBOTT). Auf orale Verabreichung hin verursachen sowohl AT 10 als auch Vitamin D_2 eine Mobilisierung von Calcium von den Knochen sowie eine vermehrte Resorption von Calcium vom Darm und führen auf diese Weise eine Erhöhung des Serumcalciumspiegels herbei. Sekundär kommt es zu einer vermehrten Ausscheidung von Calcium im Harn.

Die Dosierung hängt von dem Grad der Hypocalcämie und der Schwere der Tetanie ab. Wenn keine Lebensbedrohung besteht, reichen gewöhnlich zu Beginn der Behandlung 3—5 cm³ AT 10 täglich aus. Bei lebensbedrohenden Fällen sollten 30 cm³ einmal oder zweimal am ersten Tage verabreicht werden und zusätzlich Calciumgluconat (10 cm³ einer 10%igen Lösung) intravenös gegeben werden. Danach gibt man dann 3—5 cm³ AT 10 täglich. Wenn Besserung eingetreten ist und der Calciumspiegel normal ist, wird das AT 10 auf eine Erhaltungsdosis herabgesetzt, die gewöhnlich 0,5 oder 1,0 cm³ pro Tag beträgt. Zusammen mit dem AT 10 sollen 2—4 g Calciumgluconat peroral genommen werden, um die Resorption von Calcium aus dem Darm zu vermehren und somit die Resorption von den Knochen herabzusetzen.

Da die gefährlichen Seitenerscheinungen des AT 10 oder des Vitamin D_2 erst nach einer Behandlung von mehreren Wochen in Erscheinung treten können, sollte bei lebensbedrohlichen Fällen während der ersten Tage lieber zu hohe als zu niedrige Dosen gegeben werden. Die zwei Gefahren langdauernder Verabreichung hoher Dosen von AT 10 oder Vitamin D_2 sind hypercalcämisches Koma und Niereninsuffizienz. Regelmäßige Serumanalysen für Calcium und Rest-N sind daher nötig. Da jedoch ein hypercalcämisches Koma erst eintritt, wenn die Konzentration des Serumcalciums über den normalen Spiegel von ungefähr 10 mg-% auf 14—16 mg-% angestiegen ist, besteht eine recht breite Sicherheitszone. Die Niereninsuffizienz ist durch Niederschläge von Calciumsalzen in den Nierentubuli hervorgerufen. Falls die Niereninsuffizienz nicht zu schwer ist, ist sie reversibel, denn nach Absetzen der Behandlung werden die Calciumsalze allmählich ausgeschwemmt.

Die ersten Berichte über gute Erfolge mit AT 10 bei der Impetigo herpetiformis stammen von SCHUBERT im Jahre 1936 und BARTMANN im Jahre 1937. In beiden Fällen handelte es sich um nicht-schwangere Frauen, bei denen binnen weniger Tage nach einer Strumektomie Hypocalcämie und Tetanie einsetzten und mehrere Jahre später die Hauterscheinungen einer Impetigo herpetiformis auftraten. Bei beiden Patientinnen fand „überraschend schnelle", „schlagartige" Abheilung statt, obwohl die angewandten Dosen recht klein waren: SCHUBERT verabreichte zuerst 1 cm^3 AT 10 alle 2 Tage und später 2 cm^3 alle 8 Tage. BARTMANN gab 12 cm^3 AT 10 als erste Dosis und dann allmählich weniger pro Tag. LEONHARDI und MICHELS Patient zeigte Abheilung seiner Hauterscheinungen innerhalb von 3 Wochen unter Behandlung mit insgesamt 32 cm^3 AT 10. Von den zwei Patientinnen MÖSLEINS zeigte eine gute Abheilung unter AT 10 bei einer Dosierung von 6 cm^3 täglich für 7 Tage, dann 3 cm^3 täglich für 15 Tage und danach 1,5 cm^3 täglich. Bei der anderen Patientin trat unter Behandlung mit 3 cm^3 AT 10 täglich eine wesentliche Verschlechterung ein. Es wurden darauf hin an einem Tage 50 cm^3 morgens und nachmittags verabreicht, mit „schlagartiger Besserung" über Nacht. Danach erhielt die Patientin 7,5 cm^3 AT 10 einmal die Woche. In den von ENGFELDT und von GENTELE et al. berichteten Fällen trat trotz Behandlung mit AT 10 der Tod binnen weniger Tage ein; aber diese Fälle hätte eine zeitigere und vor allem höher dosierte Behandlung vielleicht retten können. ENGFELDTs Patientin hatte zwar 15 cm^3 am ersten Tag erhalten, danach aber nur 1 cm^3 täglich; und GENTELES Patientin hatte 2 cm^3 AT 10 täglich erhalten.

Vitamin D_2 ist von gleicher Wirksamkeit wie AT 10, wenn vergleichbare Dosen verabreicht werden. Die von LEONHARDI und MICHEL mitgeteilte Beobachtung, daß die Hauterscheinungen unter einer Vitamin D_2-Therapie langsamer zurückgingen als nach AT 10-Gaben, beruht wohl auf unterschiedlicher Dosierung. Bei WOLFRAMS Patientin kam es bei einer täglichen Gabe von 600000 Einheiten von Vitamin D_3 (etwa 8 cm^3 AT 10 entsprechend) zu schneller Abheilung.

Die Corticosteroide führen zwar zu einer Abheilung der Hauterscheinungen; sie haben aber, wie zu erwarten, keinen Einfluß auf die Hypocalcämie und Tetanie (GENTELE et al.; HADIDA und TIMSIT 1956, 1957). So beobachteten HADIDA und TIMSIT (1956), daß bei einer Schwangeren mit Impetigo herpetiformis unter Behandlung mit 100 mg Hydrocortison pro Tag die Hauterscheinungen abheilten; aber während noch Hydrocortison verabreicht wurde, trat Tetanie auf, die dann auf orale Dosen von AT 10 und auf intravenöse Injektionen von Calcium ansprach. Man kann daraus schließen, daß die derzeit beste Behandlung der Impetigo herpetiformis aus einer Kombination von AT 10 und Corticosteroiden besteht (WOLFRAM).

Literatur

I. Acrodermatitis continua

ANDREWS, G. C., and G. F. MACHACEK: Pustular bacterids of the hands and feet. Arch. Derm. Syph. (Chic.) **32**, 837 (1935).

BARBER, H. W.: Acrodermatitis continua vel perstans (dermatitis repens) and psoriasis pustulosa. Brit. J. Derm. **42**, 500 (1930). — BERNHARDT, R.: Psoriasis pustulosa (L. Zumbusch). Beziehungen zu der Acrodermatitis continua (Hallopeau) und der Impetigo herpetiformis (Hebra). Arch. Derm. Syph. (Berl.) **174**, 190 (1936). — BOHNSTEDT, R. M.: Morbus Reiter. In: Handbuch der Haut- und Geschlechtskrankheiten, Ergänzungswerk, hersg. von A. MARCHIONINI, Bd. 6, Teil 1, S. 931. Berlin: Springer 1964. — BRÜCK, C.: Contribution to the question of acrodermatitis continua (Hallopeau) and psoriasis pustulosa. Acta derm.-venereol. (Stockh.) **24**, 275 (1943/44).

CALKINS, E., L. REZNICK, and W. BAUER: Clinical and metabolic effects of prednisone, prednisolone and cortisone in a patient with acrodermatitis continua Hallopeau. New Engl. J. Med, **256**, 245 (1957). — CARRIÉ, C.: Zur Therapie bei Psoriasisformen („Acrodermatitis suppurativa Hallopeau") mit differential-diagnostischen Bemerkungen. Derm. Wschr. **132**, 715 (1955).

DANBOLT, N.: Kasuistischer Beitrag zur Frage Psoriasis pustulosa — Impetigo herpetiformis. Acta derm.-venereol. (Stockh.) **18**, 150 (1937). — DORE, S. E.: Notes on cases of a chronic mild localized type of acrodermatitis perstans. Brit. J. Derm. **40**, 12 (1928).

EPSTEIN, E., S. THAL, J. PONTIUS, and L. ROSS: Recalcitrant pustular eruption with generalized psoriasiform keratoderma and pseudo-arthropathy. Dermatologica (Basel) **123**, 265 (1961). — EVERALL, J.: Intractable pustular eruptions of the hands and feet. A review of 70 patients. Brit. J. Derm. **69**, 269 (1957).

FRÜHWALD, R.: Klinische Umfrage. Derm. Wschr. **102**, 322 (1936). — Acrodermatitis continua Hallopeau. Derm. Wschr. **127**, 269 (1953).

HALLOPEAU, H.: Des acrodermatites continues. Rev. gén. Clin. et Thér. **12**, 97 (1898).

INGRAM, J. T.: Pustular psoriasis. Arch. Derm. **77**, 314 (1958).

KEINING, E., u. H. JUNG-GRIMM: Über Akrodermatitis continua suppurativa Hallopeau inversa. Derm. Wschr. **136**, 900 (1957). — KOGOJ, F.: Un cas de maladie de Hallopeau. Acta derm.-venereol. (Stockh.) **8**, 1 (1927). — Acrodermatitis continua Hallopeau und Psoriasis pustulosa. Derm. Z. **75**, 252 (1937). — Die spungiforme (schwammartige) Pustel. Derm. Wschr. **107**, 1485 (1938). — Das klinische und histologische Bild der Acrodermatitis continua. Arch. Derm. Syph. (Berl.) **193**, 417 (1951). — Pustular Psoriasis. Proceed. XII. Internat. Congr. Dermatology, Bd. 1, S. 173. Amsterdam: Excerpta Medica Foundation 1962.

LANGHOF, H., H. MÜLLER, G. WOLFRAM u. R. ZABEL: Zur Pathogenese und Therapie der Psoriasis pustulosa vom Typ Hallopeau. Arch. klin. exp. Derm. **212**, 438 (1961). — LAPIÈRE, S., H. VAN RUNCKELEN et L. DUSSART: Étude de quatre cas d'acrodermatite continue pustuleuse d'Hallopeau. Arch. belges Derm. **2**, 3 (1939). — LAUSECKER, H.: Zur Kasuistik der Acrodermatitis continua Hallopeau. Hautarzt **7**, 23 (1956). — LEONHARDI, G., u. L. MICHEL: Impetigo herpetiformis, ein Symptom des Calciummangels. Arch. klin. exp. Derm. **207**, 251 (1958). — LEVER, W. F.: Acrodermatitis continua (Hallopeau). Arch. Derm. Syph. (Chic.) **49**, 273 (1944). — Histopathology of the skin, 3. Aufl., S. 121 u. 127. Philadelphia: J. B. Lippincott Co. 1961.

MATRAS, A.: Klinische Umfrage. Derm. Wschr. **102**, 322 (1936). — MILFORT, J.: Tentative de traitement de l'acrodermatite suppurative continue de Hallopeau par la cortisone. Bull. Soc. franç. Derm. Syph. **61**, 251 (1954). — MÖSLEIN, P.: Impetigo herpetiformis — Psoriasis pustulosa — Acrodermatitis continua Hallopeau. Arch. klin. exp. Derm. **208**, 410 (1959).

RAMEL, E.: Klinische Umfrage. Derm. Wschr. **102**, 322 (1936). — RIECKE, E.: Acrodermatitis continua (Hallopeau). In: Handbuch der Haut- und Geschlechtskrankheiten, hrsg. von J. JADASSOHN, Bd. 7, S. 654. Berlin: Springer 1931. — Klinische Umfrage. Derm. Wschr. **102**, 322 (1936).

SACHS, W., G. M. MACKEE, and M. J. ROTHSTEIN: Acrodermatitis pustulosa perstans (so-called pustular psoriasis). Arch. Derm. Syph. (Chic.) **56**, 766 (1947). — SACHS, W., and F. SCANNONE: So-called „pustular psoriasis". J. invest. Derm. **6**, 349 (1945). — SCHUPPENER, H. J.: Ausdrucksformen pustulöser Psoriasis. Derm. Wschr. **138**, 841 (1958). — Psoriasis mucosae. Derm. Wschr. **140**, 1029 (1959). — Das klinische Bild der Schleimhautbeteiligung bei Psoriasis pustulosa. Arch. klin. exp. Derm. **209**, 600 (1960). — SCHUPPENER, H. J., u. G. KOBER: Psoriasis pustulosa Typ Zumbusch. Derm. Wschr. **136**, 953 (1957). — SKOG, E.: Familial acrodermatitis continua (Hallopeau) — psoriasis. Acta derm.-venereol. (Stockh.) **38**, 345 (1958). — SOLTERMANN, W.: Familiäre Psoriasis pustulosa unter dem Bilde der Impetigo herpetiformis. Dermatologica (Basel) **116**, 313 (1958). — STREITMANN, B.: Beitrag zur Klinik und Histologie der Psoriasis pustulosa. Z. Haut- u. Geschl.-Kr. **19**, 65 (1955). — SULZBERGER, M. B.: Effect of treatment with sulfapyridine on acrodermatitis continua (Hallopeau). Arch. Derm. Syph. (Chic.) **40**, 853, 1019 (1939).

TYE, M. J., B. L. SCHIFF, and H. B. ANSELL: Response of psoriatic lesions to topical fluocinolone aectonide. Arch. Derm. **87**, 27 (1963).

WEINBERGER, H. W., M. W. ROPES, J. P. KULKA, and W. BAUER: Reiter's syndrome, clinical and pathologic observations. Medicine (Baltimore) **41**, 35 (1962).

II. Impetigo herpetiformis

BARTMANN, J.: Zur ätiologischen Therapie der Impetigo herpetiformis. Arch. Derm. Syph. (Berl.) **175**, 93 (1937). — BEEK, D. H.: On impetigo herpetiformis. Dermatologica (Basel) **102**, 145 (1951). — BERNHARDT, R.: Psoriasis pustulosa (L. Zumbusch). Beziehungen zu der Acrodermatitis continua (Hallopeau) und der Impetigo herpetiformis (Hebra). Arch. Derm. Syph. (Berl.) **174**, 190 (1936). — BOHNSTEDT, R. M.: Kasuistischer Beitrag zur Frage Impetigo herpetiformis und Tetanie. Arch. Derm. Syph. (Berl.) **69**, 357 (1933/34).

DANBOLT, N.: Kasuistischer Beitrag zur Frage Psoriasis pustulosa — Impetigo herpetiformis. Acta derm.-venereol. (Stockh.) **18**, 150 (1937).

EBERHARTINGER, C.: Beitrag zur Cortisontherapie der Impetigo herpetiformis. Derm. Wschr. **138**, 930 (1958). — ENGFELDT, B., and H. GENTELE: On impetigo herpetiformis and its connection with parathyroprival tetany. Acta derm.-venereol. (Stockh.) **30**, 50 (1950).

GAUMOND, E.: Recurrent impetigo herpetiformis. Brit. J. Derm. **68**, 55 (1956). — GENTELE, H., A. LODIN, and A. M. ODQUIST-NIORDSON: Impetigo herpetiformis in conjunction with parathyroprival tetany. Acta derm.-venereol. (Stockh.) **37**, 387 (1957). — GOTTRON, H.: Individualpathologie in der Dermatologie. Dtsch. med. Wschr. **72**, 580 (1947).

HADIDA, E., et E. TIMSIT: Impétigo herpétiforme de Hebra. Résultats du traitement par hydrocortisone. Bull. Soc. franç. Derm. Syph. **63**, 30 (1956). — Impétigo herpétiforme de Hebra-Kaposi. Action de la dexaméthasone et de l'hormone gonadotrope sérique. Bull. Soc. franç. Derm. Syph. **68**, 146 (1961). — HALL, A. F.: Impetigo herpetiformis in the male. Arch. Derm. Syph. (Chic.) **50**, 107 (1944). — HERRMANN, W. P., u. K. J. PESCH: Generalisierte Pustulose der Haut mit malignem Verlauf. Derm. Wschr. **149**, 369 (1964). — HOLLSTROM, E., and B. LAGERHOLM: Impetigo herpetiformis. Acta derm.-venereol. (Stockh.) **38**, 225 (1958). — HOLTZ, F., u. F. CRAMER: Wirkungsweise, Indikation und Gefahren von AT 10. Ther. d. Gegenw. **77**, 241 (1936). — HVIDBERG, E.: Impetigo herpetiformis. Report of three cases and discussion of treatment with adrenocorticotrophic hormone. A survey of 6 years' cases in the literature. Dermatologica (Basel) **114**, 337 (1957).

KEINING, E., u. H. JUNG-GRIMM: Über Akrodermatitis continua suppurativa Hallopeau inversa. Derm. Wschr. **136**, 900 (1957). — KNIERER, W.: Impetigo herpetiformis. Hautarzt **1**, 560 (1950). — KOCH, F.: Zur Frage der Identität von Impetigo herpetiformis, Psoriasis pustulosa und Psoriasis vulgaris. Hautarzt **3**, 165 (1952). — KOGOJ, F.: Die spungiforme (schwammartige) Pustel. Derm. Wschr. **107**, 1485 (1938).

LAPIÈRE, S.: A propos d'un cas d'impétigo herpétiforme. Arch. belges Derm. **14**, 146 (1958). — LEONHARDI, G., u. L. MICHEL: Impetigo herpetiformis — ein Symptom des Calciummangels. Arch. klin. exp. Derm. **207**, 251 (1958). — LEVER, W. F., and J. H. TALBOTT: Pemphigus. Further report on chemical studies of the blood serum and treatment with adrenocortical extract, dihydrotachysterol or Vitamin D. New Engl. J. Med. **231**, 44 (1944). — LUTZ, W.: Impetigo herpetiformis. Dermatologica (Basel) **110**, 369 (1955).

MÖSLEIN, P.: Impetigo herpetiformis — Psoriasis pustulosa — Acrodermatitis continua Hallopeau. Arch. klin. exp. Derm. **208**, 410 (1959).

RIECKE, E.: Impetigo herpetiformis. In: Handbuch der Haut- und Geschlechtskrankheiten, hrsg. von J. JADASSOHN, Bd. 7, Teil 2, S. 298. Berlin: Springer 1931.

SAUER, G. C., and B. J. GEHA: Impetigo herpetiformis. Arch. Derm. **83**, 119 (1961). — SCHARDORN, E.: Über Impetigo herpetiformis. Arch. Derm. Syph. (Berl.) **132**, 108 (1921). — SCHAUER, L.: Zur Pathogenese der Impetigo herpetiformis. Arch. Derm. Syph. (Berl.) **185**, 306 (1944). — SCHERBER, G.: Zur Anwendung von Parathyreoidea (G. Richter) und des Präparates A.T. 10 bei der Behandlung der Impetigo herpetiformis und der Psoriasis vulgaris pustulosa. Derm. Wschr. **106**, 391 (1938). — SCHMIDT-LA BAUME, F.: Die Bedeutung des A.T. 10 für die Dermatologie als Substitutionstherapie bei Hypocalcinosen. Med. Klin. **33**, 1590 (1937). — SCHUBERT, M.: Impetigo herpetiformis, ihre Behandlung mit A.T. 10. Derm. Wschr. **102**, 761 (1936). — SOLTERMANN, W.: Familiäre Psoriasis pustulosa unter dem Bilde der Impetigo herpetiformis. Dermatologica (Basel) **116**, 313 (1958). — STEPPERT, A.: Zur Behandlung der Impetigo herpetiformis Hebra. Hautarzt **5**, 82 (1954).

TENLÉN, S.: Successful hormone treatment of a case of impetigo herpetiformis in pregnancy. Acta derm.-venereol. (Stockh.) **18**, 165 (1937). — TEODORESCOU, S., et A. CONU: Contribution au traitement de l'impétigo herpétiforme du type Hebra-Kaposi. Ann. Derm. Syph. (Paris) VIII, **7**, 250 (1947). — Pénicilline dans l'impétigo herpétiforme de Hebra. Ann. Derm. Syph. (Paris) VIII, **8**, 149 (1948). — TIELSCH, R.: Zur Differentialdiagnose Impetigo herpetiformis — Psoriasis pustulosa. Derm. Wschr. **145**, 305 (1962). — TOLMAN, M. M., and S. L. MOSCHELLA: Pustular Psoriasis (Zumbusch). Arch. Derm. **81**, 400 (1960).

VOHWINKEL, K. H.: Psoriasis pustulosa und ihre Behandlung mit A.T. 10. Derm. Wschr. **103**, 1373 (1936).

WOLFRAM, ST.: Zur Klinik und Therapie der Impetigo herpetiformis. Hautarzt **12**, 170 (1961).

ZUMBUSCH, L. v.: Impetigo herpetiformis und Psoriasis pustulosa. Arch. Derm. Syph. (Berl.) **137**, 116 (1921).

Thermische Schädigungen

Von

Hans Kuske und **Lorenzo Zala**-Bern

Mit 13 Abbildungen (davon 8 farbige)

A. Verbrennungen und Verbrühungen

Die Pathologie der Hitzeschädigungen war in den vergangenen beiden Jahrzehnten oft Gegenstand eingehender Untersuchungen. Sowohl Chirurgen als auch Dermatologen, Internisten und Pathologen haben sich mit den verschiedenen Problemen des Schocks und der Verbrennungskrankheit befaßt. Blickt man auf die geschichtliche Entwicklung dieser Krankheitslehre zurück, so fällt auf, daß viele Fragestellungen über Jahrzehnte immer wieder auftauchen und je nach dem Stande der theoretischen Medizin oder der praktischen Therapie anders beantwortet werden. In der Beurteilung und Behandlung von Hitzeschäden spiegeln sich offenbar solche Wechsel und Wellenbewegungen der medizinischen Anschauungen besonders eindrücklich. Eine Behandlungsmethode kann in kurzer Zeit neu aufkommen und das Feld eindeutig beherrschen, bald darauf aber völlig in Vergessenheit geraten, ja sogar in Verruf kommen. Ein besonders eindrückliches Beispiel dafür ist das wechselvolle Schicksal der Tanninbehandlung der Dermatitis combustionis.

Wir sollten versuchen, die Änderungen der pathophysiologischen Anschauungen und vor allem die therapeutischen Fortschritte der letzten zwei bis drei Jahrzehnte im Überblick zusammenzufassen. Auf zwei Tatsachen sei hier nachdrücklich hingewiesen, weil sie die Bearbeitung eines solchen Ergänzungsberichtes, der einen bestimmten Umfang nicht überschreiten darf, wegleitend beeinflussen müssen. Die beiden wichtigen Tatsachen sind erstens die *Fortschritte auf dem Gebiet der Schockbekämpfung* und zweitens die Einsicht, daß die *Lokalbehandlung* zwar vernünftig und korrekt durchgeführt werden soll, daß es aber nicht eine einzige überall und immer richtige Lokalbehandlung gibt.

In den Jahren seit der Bearbeitung des Kapitels durch Ullmann sind in erster Linie in der Behandlung des Schocks und der Verbrennungskrankheit große Fortschritte erzielt worden. Wir können nicht nur über eine bessere, sondern auch über eine fast allgemein anerkannte und überall in der Welt nach gleichartigen Prinzipien erfolgende Behandlung berichten. Dieser „Konformismus" beruht auf den tatsächlich erzielten Erfolgen, und durch diese wird er gerechtfertigt. Man darf zwar noch weitere Fortschritte erwarten; das jetzige Prinzip der Allgemeinbehandlung dürfte aber unangefochten auch weiterhin bestehenbleiben.

Zweifellos haben sich in den vergangenen Dezennien mancherorts die Grundsätze über die Anwendung von lokalen Maßnahmen geändert. Aber auch hier ist man zu einer Art Übereinstimmung gelangt, wenigstens in dem Sinne, daß man kaum mehr einen Behandlungstypus als den allein richtigen herauszustellen sucht, sondern sich klargeworden ist, wie unwichtig in vielen Fällen die

Lokalbehandlung sein kann. Immerhin lassen sich auf diesem Gebiet ebenfalls einige Grundsätze aufstellen, die Anspruch auf allgemein anerkannte Gültigkeit erheben dürfen, wäre es auch nur das Gesetz des Nil nocere. Die Bedeutung der lokalen therapeutischen Maßnahmen wird teils unterschätzt, teils übertrieben. Bei allen erst- bis oberflächlich zweitgradigen Verbrennungen spielen sie sicher nur eine untergeordnete Rolle, weil solche Schäden erfahrungsgemäß in 10—20 Tagen ohnehin gut ausheilen. Bei ausgedehnten tieferen Verbrennungen sind hingegen die Rückwirkungen auf den Allgemeinzustand des Verunglückten sehr groß, und es ist darum außerordentlich wichtig, daß die Wunden durch zweckentsprechende Lokalbehandlung in einem guten Zustand erhalten werden.

Vom Bearbeiter eines Handbuchartikels erwartet man, daß er die neuere und neueste Literatur berücksichtige und verwerte. Über die Hitzeschädigung und

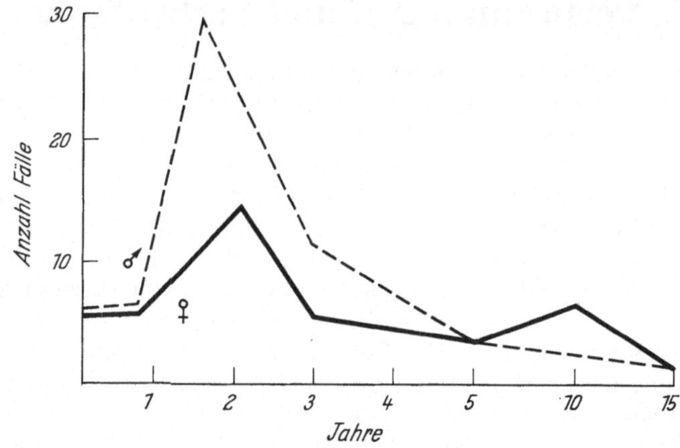

Abb. 1. Altersverteilung der Verbrennungen im Kindesalter (nach Morger, Nicole und Gayer 1962)

ihre Behandlung ist jedoch so viel geschrieben worden, daß es ganz unmöglich ist, lückenlos darüber zu berichten. Es würde ein Sammelreferat von unübersehbarer Länge entstehen. Auch im Literaturverzeichnis soll kein Anspruch auf Vollständigkeit erhoben werden. Da in den letzten Jahren wertvolle Monographien (Allgöwer, Artz und Reiss, Monsaingeon, Postnikow, Lob, Sevitt) erschienen sind, da das Thema überdies Gegenstand zahlreicher Vorträge auf Kongressen und bei Symposien bildete (Symposium on Burns 1951 und 1961), kann auf solche Veröffentlichungen verwiesen werden. Der ganze Stoff soll in vier Hauptkapitel gegliedert werden, nämlich:

I. Pathophysiologie.
II. Prognose, erste Beurteilung, Triage.
III. Behandlung des Schocks und der Verbrennungskrankheit.
IV. Lokalbehandlung.

Die enorme Bedeutung der Hitzeschäden geht aus Todesfall- und Unfallstatistiken ganz klar hervor. Es seien nur wenige Beispiele angeführt. In den spezialisierten Abteilungen der Spitäler von Birmingham wurden in $4^1/_2$ Jahren 1639 Patienten mit Verbrennungen behandelt. 70% der Fälle stammten aus dem Privathaus, 30% aus industriellen Betrieben. Mit Recht wird darauf hingewiesen, daß es nicht genügt, alle Anstrengungen zur Vervollkommnung der Behandlung der Verbrannten zu machen, wenn nicht gleichzeitig der Unfallprophylaxe viel mehr Beachtung geschenkt wird. Der Umstand, daß jetzt die meisten Verbrennungsunfälle im Haushalt erfolgen (ca. 70%, nach den Statistiken von Colebrook und von MOYER), mag damit zusammenhängen, daß die industriellen Betriebe einfacher und wirksamer gegen Verbrennungsgefährdung anzukämpfen wissen. Offene Feuerstellen, leicht entzündbare Kleiderstoffe erhöhen die Gefahren im Heim. BLECK berichtete 1955 über 344 Fälle von verbrannten Kindern. In 46% der Fälle war eine Entflammung der Kleider erfolgt. Die besondere Gefährdung des Kleinkindesalters geht übereinstimmend aus verschiedenen Arbeiten und Statistiken (Abb. 1) hervor (SLAVIK; COLEBROOK; SCHMITT; LEUTERER; MORGER u. Mitarb.; SCHWARZ). Genaue Auswertungen großer Serien von Unfällen müssen die Unterlage für eine wirksame Prophylaxe liefern. Diese Frage wurde am ersten internationalen Symposium on Burns 1961, Washington, eingehend behandelt.

Bei dieser Gelegenheit muß darauf hingewiesen werden, daß sich in vielen Ländern die Tendenz abzeichnet, die Schwerstverbrannten in ganz wenige hochspezialisierte Krankenabteilungen (Burn Units) einzuweisen und dort zu behandeln. 1952 genehmigte das britische Gesundheitsministerium offiziell die Errichtung von besonderen Behandlungszentren. Hauptursache dieser Entwicklung scheint das Bedürfnis nach größtmöglichem Schutz vor sekundärer Infektion zu sein. In großstädtischen Verhältnissen oder in der Nähe riesiger industrieller Anlagen rechtfertigt sich die Einrichtung solcher Zentren durchaus. Es besteht aber die Gefahr, daß die Lehre von der Verbrennung damit immer mehr nur als ein Grenzgebiet zwischen Chirurgie, Dermatologie und Reanimation betrachtet wird. Ausreichende Erfahrungen könnten sich dann nur relativ wenige Ärzte aneignen, und bei Brand- oder Explosionskatastrophen müßte sich das ganz nachteilig auswirken.

Natürlich sind die zweckmäßigen Lösungen für die Behandlung Schwerstverbrannter nach den örtlichen Gegebenheiten zu suchen. Dabei spielen unter anderem die Größe der Bevölkerungsagglomeration und der Grad der Industrialisierung eine wichtige Rolle (COLEBROOK). Auch der moderne Verkehr fordert immer mehr Verbrennungsopfer. Brände nach Automobilkollisionen, Explosionen von Tankwagen und Flugzeugen nehmen bedenklich zu. Es liegt ferner auf der Hand, daß solchen Spezialabteilungen im Falle kriegerischer Auseinandersetzungen besondere Bedeutung zukäme. Auch sind sie zur Forschung und zur Bewertung neuer Therapieverfahren berufen. Über die Auswirkungen von Kernwaffenexplosionen auf die Haut und die damit zusammenhängenden Probleme hat C. G. SCHIRREN 1962 eine zusammenfassende Arbeit geschrieben.

I. Pathophysiologie der Verbrennung

1. Der örtliche Wärmeschaden

Die Kenntnis der örtlichen Schäden, die im Anschluß an ein Hitzetrauma auftreten, sind grundlegend für das Verständnis der Verbrennungskrankheit.

Die erste ausführliche Beschreibung der Histologie der örtlichen Verbrennung stammt von UNNA. Die allgemeine Pathologie der Entzündung liefert uns die Voraussetzungen. Waren diese früher mehr auf morphologischer, d.h. pathologisch-anatomischer Basis erarbeitet worden, so sind sie heute stark beeinflußt von der biochemischen Arbeitsrichtung, ausgehend von MENKIN. Auf diese Arbeiten muß verwiesen werden, sowie auf die Experimente von HAM, HENRIQUES und MORITZ, SEVITT, ENTIN und BAXTER, GORDON et al., FARMER, welche die Histologie des experimentellen örtlichen Wärmeschadens mit seröser Entzündung, feinsten bis ausgedehnten Coagulationsnekrosen der Eiweißkörper in Abhängigkeit von Intensität und Dauer der thermischen Schädigung genau studiert haben.

2. Die allgemeinen Auswirkungen des Wärmeschadens (Die Verbrennungskrankheit)

Die unmittelbaren Folgen der Verbrennung auf den Gesamtorganismus und die in späteren Stadien auftretenden Veränderungen beruhen auf einer Reihe von Faktoren, deren Bedeutung zum Teil noch stark umstritten ist. Die Zusammenhänge werden dadurch noch unübersichtlicher, weil verschiedene pathogenetische Wege in gleiche Bahnen einmünden oder sich zu Circuli vitiosi schließen können. Durch diese Vorgänge im Gesamtorganismus wird das Leben des Verunfallten krisenhaft mehrmals bedroht. Es handelt sich dabei um einen mehr oder weniger gesetzmäßigen Ablauf von Krankheitszeichen und Symptomkonstellationen, so daß die heute gebräuchlich gewordene Bezeichnung „Verbrennungskrankheit" durchaus unseren modernen Vorstellungen entspricht. Es lassen sich mehrere Phasen unterscheiden, die allerdings nicht scharf voneinander abgegrenzt werden können und nur bei schwereren Fällen deutlicher hervortreten. Man spricht etwa von einer Frühphase oder einem Schockstadium, einer mittleren Phase oder Intoxikationsstadium und einer Spätphase, dem Infektionsstadium. Daß diese Einteilung, die PFEIFFER schon 1905 auf Grund von Tierexperimenten vorgeschlagen hat, nicht nur auf theoretischen Erwägungen beruht, ergibt sich nicht zuletzt aus der Tatsache, daß trotz der modernen Schocktherapie schwerere Verbrennungen immer noch eine schlechte Prognose haben: Zwar wird meist die Frühphase überstanden, aber später eingreifende Faktoren, die nicht mehr unmittelbar durch das akute volämische Kreislaufversagen bedingt sind, trüben die Prognose (s. S. 742).

a) Frühphase (Exsudationsstadium)

Im Mittelpunkt der pathogenetischen Vorgänge steht in den ersten 36—72 Std der Verbrennungsschock. Es handelt sich dabei um ein klinisches Syndrom, dem eine akute Kreislaufinsuffizienz mit ungenügender Durchblutung lebenswichtiger Körpergewebe zugrunde liegt. Hauptfaktor ist der Flüssigkeitsverlust. Es tritt ein Circulus vitiosus in Funktion, der unter Umständen zum sog. dekompensierten Schock führt und der durch folgende schematische Darstellung veranschaulicht werden kann:

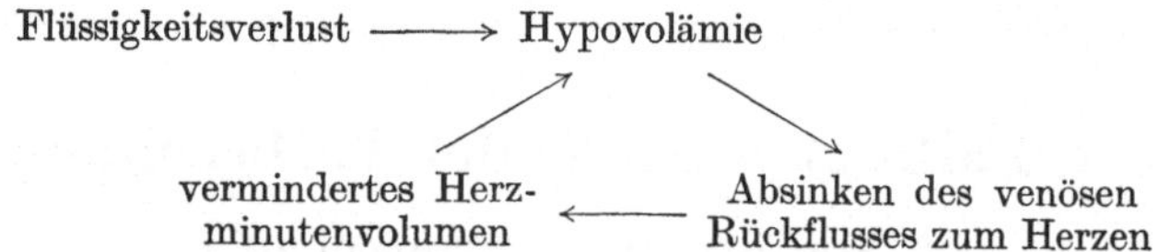

Der Flüssigkeitsverlust beginnt unmittelbar nach der Verbrennung und erfolgt vorerst in der verbrannten Zone. Diese kann geradezu als ein „Leck" bezeichnet werden, durch das zum kleineren Teil nach außen, zum größeren Teil durch Ödembildung Flüssigkeit verlorengeht. Die Ödemflüssigkeit gleicht in ihrer Zusammensetzung dem Plasma, ist also eiweißreich. Nach Beobachtungen bei Tierversuchen (SIMONART) scheint es sogar möglich, daß sofort nach der Verbrennung eine capillardilatierende Substanz resorbiert wird, die einen Wasserverlust im ganzen Körper zur Folge hätte. In der Tat findet man bei Obduktionen innerhalb der ersten Tage generalisierte Ödeme in den Lungen, in den Nieren und im Hirn (hier vor allem bei Kindern). Die Frage der Permeabilitätsstörung hat zu unzähligen Arbeiten Anlaß gegeben. (Besonders hervorzuheben sind die Experimente mit „Tracers" und Farbstoffen von COPE und MOORE und von SEVITT).

Die Einzelheiten dieses Vorgangs sind noch umstritten. Die Permeabilitätsstörungen am Verbrennungsort selber lassen sich leicht als Folge der Capillarschädigung durch Hitzewirkung erklären (DRINKER). Dabei handelt es sich zweifellos um einen primären Vorgang. Dagegen sind die genauen Ursachen der entfernt vom Verbrennungsort beobachteten Permeabilitätssteigerung noch nicht sicher bekannt.

Autolytische Vorgänge spielen sich offenbar vorwiegend in den Übergangszonen zwischen nekrotischem und weniger geschädigtem Gewebe ab, und von hier aus wird der Körper mit toxischen Eiweißabbauprodukten überschwemmt. Es ist nicht leicht, sie genau zu erfassen; sicher erscheinen im Urin vermehrt Aminosäuren (GREUER, MARGGRAF, REHN, UNGAR) und Peptide (BAAR, BALIKOV et al.). GREUER ist auch der Nachweis freier proteolytischer Fermente im Blut kurz nach Verbrennung gelungen. In parabiotischen Tierversuchen ist es möglich, durch Injektion von hitzedenaturiertem Serum in die Peritonealhöhle eindeutige Vergiftungsbilder zu erzeugen. Diese örtlich entstehenden Eiweißabbauprodukte und Entzündungssubstanzen scheinen aber nicht verbrennungsspezifisch zu sein, sondern entstehen auch bei anderen traumatischen Vorgängen und sogar unter physiologischen Bedingungen, aber in weit geringerer Quantität (KOSLOWSKI). Es scheint sich vor allem um Amine, Peptide, ferner um Histamin (ROSE und BROWNE 1938) zu handeln. Der Nachweis eines spezifischen Verbrennungstoxins ist nie gelungen. Eine Vermehrung physiologischer Eiweißabbauprodukte hatte schon BILLROTH 1878 vermutet. Das Auftreten einer starken Permeabilitätsstörung bleibt unumstößliche Tatsache; sie führt zur Verminderung des Blutvolumens und zum Ansteigen des Hämatokrits. Alle pathologisch-physiologischen Erklärungsversuche müssen zur Hauptsache von diesem Tatbestand ausgehen.

Neben der Hypovolämie durch Plasmaverlust sind zwei weitere an der Schockgenese beteiligte Vorgänge zu erwähnen: Der sog. primäre Wundschock und die Störungen der Mikrozirkulation, die als Erscheinung des „sludged blood“ bekanntgeworden sind.

Der primäre Wundschock beruht auf einer Steigerung des Sympathicotonus, die durch den Schmerzreiz ausgelöst wird. KIRCHNER hat dafür die Bezeichnung „hypertone Traumareaktion“ vorgeschlagen. Diese psychische Komponente der Schockgenese ist wohl die Erklärung dafür, daß manchmal schon bei relativ geringfügigen Verbrennungen schwerere Schockzustände auftreten können. Neuere experimentelle Arbeiten wie Tierversuche in Anaesthesie und mit Ganglienblockern (GLASSER und PAGE, LAVER, SIMONART, SANYAL) bestätigen die Bedeutung dieses Vorgangs, der zu einer Zentralisation des Kreislaufs führt und mit dem Wasserverlust zeitlich mehr oder weniger parallel geht.

Als Zentralisation des Kreislaufs wird ein regulativer Mechanismus bezeichnet, der durch Engerstellung des peripheren Kreislaufs die Blutvolumenverluste auszugleichen sucht, um wenigstens eine genügende Durchblutung der lebenswichtigsten inneren Organe zu gewährleisten. Der Verbrennungsschock ist deshalb ein tonischer Schock. Infolge der Spannung in der Peripherie bleibt der Blutdruck oft während längerer Zeit auf normalen Werten und kann daher nicht als sicheres Kriterium für die Schwere des Zustandes gelten (DUESBERG, SCHRÖDER).

„Sludged blood“ ist ein Phänomen, das schon 1—2 Std nach erfolgter Verbrennung beobachtet wird und auf einer Störung der Mikrozirkulation beruht. Die Thrombocyten werden klebrig, es kommt zur Aggregation der Erythrocyten („Geldrollenbildung“), zur Stagnation in Venolen, Capillaren, Arteriolen und zu Thrombosen (KNISELY 1945, SEVITT 1949). Die Bedeutung dieser Vorgänge für die Schockgenese ist neuerdings von JEANNET angezweifelt worden.

Die durch die geschilderten Mechanismen dem Blutvolumen entzogenen Plasmaanteile sind beträchtlich. Brooks et al. stellten bei Hundeexperimenten eine Exsudationsmenge von ungefähr 1 ml pro 1% verbrannter Körperoberfläche pro Kilogramm fest. Andere Tierexperimente ergaben bei 50% verbrannter Körperoberfläche einen Flüssigkeitsverlust von der Größenordnung des Plasmavolumens (Rossiter 1943).

Nach Allgöwer ist die Exsudationsphase nach spätestens 50 Std abgeschlossen.

Schematische Zusammenfassung der wichtigsten Vorgänge in der sog. Frühphase:

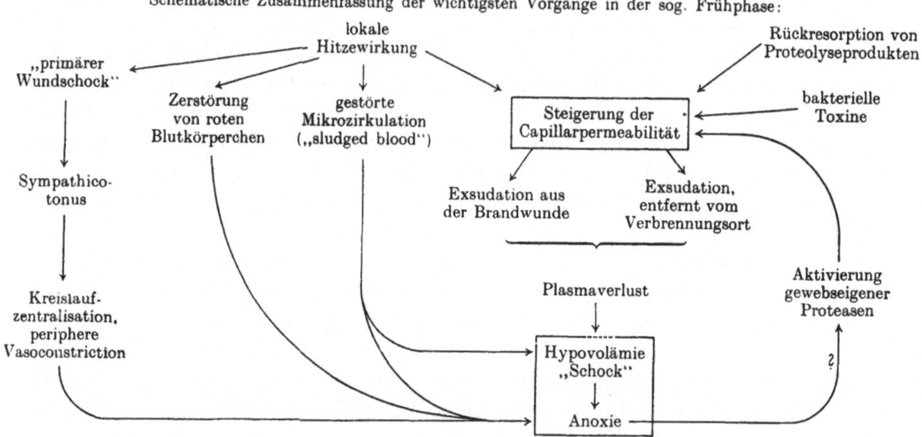

b) Mittlere Phase (Intoxikationsstadium)

Die Abgrenzung einer solchen Phase ist nicht nur im Hinblick auf die von vielen Autoren abgelehnte Intoxikationstheorie besonders problematisch, sondern auch deshalb, weil sie mit den oben beschriebenen Vorgängen eng verknüpft ist. Zeitlich umfaßt sie die ersten 5—7 Tage nach der Frühphase. Gekennzeichnet ist sie vorerst durch das Sistieren der Exsudation infolge Erholung der Capillarmembran und das Einsetzen einer oft stürmischen Ödem-Rückresorption, was sich in einer starken Polyurie äußern kann. Der Kreislauf ist nun plötzlich mit Flüssigkeit überlastet, es drohen akutes Lungenödem und Hirnödeme.

Noch wichtiger sind die Folgen der mit der Ödem-Rückresorption einhergehenden verstärkten Resorption von Eiweißzerfallsprodukten auf lebenswichtige innere Organe. Von daher ist die Bezeichnung „Intoxikationsstadium" gerechtfertigt. Die toxischen Proteolyseprodukte treffen auf Organe, die bereits durch die vorangegangene Anoxämie geschwächt sind. Als kardinal wichtige Verbrennungsfolgen gelten die Schädigungen an der Niere mit ihren klinischen Auswirkungen, die sich in Oligurie und Anurie manifestieren. Sehr viele Frühtodesfälle gehen auf Nierenversagen zurück. Schon die sog. initiale Oligurie, eine vorübergehende unmittelbare Folge der Anoxie, kann sich katastrophal auf das weitere Geschehen auswirken, obschon sie häufig nur eine relativ harmlose Episode darstellt. Noch gefürchteter ist die durch das Zusammenspiel weiterer Faktoren (z.B. Hämolyse, Myolyse) bedingte akute tubuläre Nephrose (sog. lower nephron nephrosis). Histologisch handelt es sich dabei um eine schwere seröse interstitielle Nephritis.

Auch an der Leber wirkt sich die Anoxie nachteilig aus, worunter die gerade zu diesem Zeitpunkt so dringend benötigten Entgiftungsfunktionen leiden: Bakterielle Endotoxine können nicht im üblichen Maße unschädlich gemacht werden, wodurch die Infektabwehr schwer beeinträchtigt wird. Die oft beobachteten Leberschädigungen im Verlaufe von schweren Verbrennungen waren vielleicht teilweise iatrogener Natur; vor allem ist die Tanninbehandlung angeschuldigt worden (BUIS und HARTMANN 1941, OLLINGER 1947), sehr wahrscheinlich zu unrecht (STÖR, AHNEFELD). Wie unter anderen O'BRIEN und MURRAY gezeigt haben, sind die Leberschädigungen eine Folge der umfangreichen Verbrennung selbst. Nach MCLAUGHLIN findet man bei schweren Verbrennungen vom 3. Tage an eine konstante Urobilinogenvermehrung im Urin als Zeichen der Leberschädigung. Pathologisch-anatomisch äußert sich diese in zentraler Läppchennekrose (einer typischen Anoxiefolge), ferner in Verfettung und Hämosiderose. Klinisch ist die Intoxikationsphase schon zu Beginn, also um den 2. Tag herum, durch ein Ansteigen der Körpertemperatur gekennzeichnet. Die Bedeutung dieses Temperaturanstiegs braucht noch nicht überwertet zu werden; er ist meist kein Zeichen von Infektion oder anderen Komplikationen. In Ausnahmefällen und bei sehr schweren Verbrennungen — und zwar besonders beim Kleinkind (KOCH) — steigt die Temperatur unaufhaltsam an und kann Werte über 41° C erreichen. Eine derartige Hyperthermie kann den Exitus letalis einleiten, denn die dadurch ausgelöste extreme Intensivierung der Stoffwechselvorgänge führt zu rascher Erschöpfung.

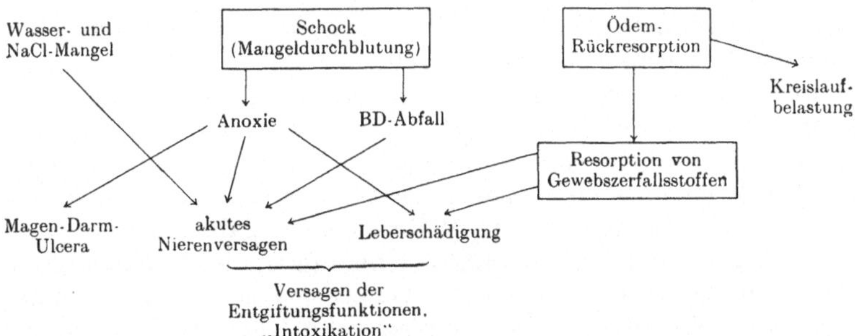

c) Spätphase (Infektionsphase)

Der Tod in der Spätphase ist nicht immer und ausschließlich durch Infektion bedingt, sondern oft auch durch einen Mangel an Regenerationsvermögen der geschädigten Organe. Es müssen auch hier sehr verwickelte pathogenetische Beziehungen postuliert werden. Die Bezeichnung als Infektionsphase ist deshalb gewiß einseitig (man hat auch von einer Phase der Reparation und Demarkation gesprochen), stellt aber dasjenige Problem in den Vordergrund, dem wir heute trotz der Antibiotica oft noch hilflos gegenüberstehen und dessen Lösung eine der wichtigsten Aufgaben für zukünftige Forschungen zur Verbrennungskrankheit darstellt. Fast alle schweren Brandwunden, gleichgültig ob sie offen oder geschlossen, mit oder ohne Antibiotica behandelt werden, besiedeln sich mit verschiedenen Bakterien. Die Infektion befällt dabei einen Organismus, dessen Resistenz für längere Zeit schwer daniederliegt. Es sind unterschiedliche Gründe, teils sichere, teils problematische aufzuführen, die für diese Abwehrschwäche verantwortlich sind. Im Vordergrund steht wohl die Anämie (s. Arbeiten von JAMES u. Mitarb.). Sie ist teils direkte Folge des Untergangs roter Blutkörperchen anläßlich der Hitzeeinwirkung. Wahrscheinlich erfolgt auch eine toxische Markschädigung durch Proteolyseprodukte. Ferner resultieren durch die Nierenschädigung eine negative Stickstoffbilanz und durch die Eiweißverluste eine Hypoproteinämie. Zu erwähnen sind hier auch die als Spätfolgen von Verbrennungen gefürchteten Magen-Darm-Ulcera, wie sie von CURLING schon im Jahre 1842 beschrieben worden sind. Sie sind meist im Magen oder Duodenum (MACFARLANE 1883) lokalisiert (LOB, ALLGÖWER). Nach tierexperimentellen Arbeiten (FRIESEN) ist der pathogenetische

Hauptfaktor eine Anoxie der Magen-Darmschleimhaut. Außer der Anämie wird auch eine mögliche Schädigung des reticuloendothelialen Systems als Ursache für die Resistenzverminderung in Erwägung gezogen, während Schädigungen der Nebennierenfunktion nicht mit Sicherheit festgestellt worden sind. Auf die Bedeutung der Leberschädigung für die Schwächung der Infektabwehr ist bereits hingewiesen worden. Besonders gefürchtet sind Infektionen mit Bact. pyocyaneus und Bact. Coli, ferner Streptokokken (Erysipel, Wundscharlach), Staphylokokken und Tetanus. Oft handelt es sich dabei um antibioticaresistente, in Krankenhäusern heimische Erreger. Relativ wenig erforscht sind die durch die Verbrennungskrankheit bedingten Schädigungen am Gehirn mit den entsprechenden Spätfolgen und Auswirkungen auf den Allgemeinzustand. Auf Hypophysenveränderungen hat speziell ZINCK hingewiesen, der ihnen eine Schlüsselstellung im ganzen pathogenetischen Ablauf der späten Stadien beimessen möchte.

II. Prognose, Beurteilung, Triage

1. Prognose

Von alters her wurde ein Zusammenhang zwischen der Größe der verbrannten Fläche und der Lebensprognose festgestellt und in ein Zahlenschema gebracht, welches Verbrennungsfläche und Überlebenszeit miteinander in Beziehung setzte (WEIDENFELD 1905—1907, RIEHL 1925, v. ZUMBUSCH 1905). In der Tat wissen wir heute, daß die dem Kreislauf verlorengehenden Flüssigkeitsmengen in einem proportionalen Verhältnis zur Flächenausdehnung und zur Schwere der Verbrennung stehen (COPE und MOORE 1947). Früher galten Verbrennungen, die mehr als ein Drittel der Körperoberfläche einnahmen, als absolut letal, und ohne Zweifel hat sich dieses alte biologische Gesetz bis zur Vervollkommnung der modernen Schockbehandlung auf eine unheimliche, tragische Weise immer wieder bestätigen lassen. Die moderne Therapie hat die Grenze für die unbedingte infauste Prognose stark verschoben. Schwerstverbrannte überstehen heute den Initialschock und die früher kritische Intoxikationsperiode zwischen dem 3. und 5. Tage nach der Verbrennung sehr viel häufiger. Leider sterben dann aber in den späteren Phasen noch immer viele Patienten. Nach wie vor muß man Verletzte, bei denen mehr als 30% der Körperoberfläche betroffen sind, als sehr schwer gefährdet betrachten, und auch heute ist es eine Ausnahme, wenn ein Verunglückter, bei dem 60—75% der Körperoberfläche schwer verbrannt wurden, mit dem Leben davonkommt. Nach BÖHLER ist die Therapie bei einer Ausdehnung bis 50% in der Regel erfolgreich, zwischen 50 und 75% nur in Ausnahmefällen (1955). Nach einer Publikation von KOSLOWSKI und GREGL aus dem Jahre 1958 haben Verbrennungen von über 40—50% trotz Schocktherapie nach wie vor eine Mortalitätsquote von gegen 100%. ALLEN (Chicago) erstellte folgende interessante Mortalitätsstatistik:

Tabelle 1

1934—1936 (Tanninära)	10% Mortalität
1937 (Tannin/Agr. nitric.)	7,3%
1939	5,8%
1941	2,7%

Auch TAPPEINER und WITTELS zeigten 1956 in Form einer Gegenüberstellung der Verbrennungsfälle der Wiener Hautklinik von 1940—1944 (also vor der Infusionsära) einerseits und von 1950—1954 andererseits, daß die Prognose wesentlich besser geworden ist. Die Mortalität ist von 19,9% auf 4,5% gefallen, also um 15,4%. Bei Verbrennungen von über 10% der Körperoberfläche betrug die Senkung der Mortalität sogar 39,6%. Die Zahl der Frühtodesfälle ließ sich dabei relativ weit mehr senken als die der Spättodesfälle. Die Überlebenszeit hat zugenommen, die Mortalität im Verhältnis weniger stark abgenommen. Jede größere und schwerere Brandkatastrophe lehrt, daß wohl fast alle Verunglückten über die erste gefährliche Zeit hinweggebracht werden können, daß sie dann aber später doch noch an Intoxikationen, Marasmus, an Infektionen und Sepsis, ja an Inanition zugrunde gehen können. Dieses Problem wird durch weitere Statistiken beleuchtet. Im *J.A.M.A.* vol. 168 (1958) erschienen folgende Zahlen aus den Spitälern von San Francisco, gewonnen an 93 Fällen mit über 20% verbrannter Körperoberfläche.

Tabelle 2

	Mortalität	In den ersten 48 Std	Später
1943—1947	40%	69%	31%
1951—1956	69%	19% (meist durch Schocktod)	81% (meist infolge Infektion)

Als Ursache der Zunahme der Gesamtmortalität wird die steigende Bedeutung der Infektionen angegeben; die Antibioticatherapie erwies sich als mehr oder weniger unwirksam (Clark und Hanson). Dzanehdze hat die Verbrennungsfälle der Leningrader Spitäler für die Jahre 1950—1951 nach Schwere und nach Flächenausdehnung zusammengestellt (s. Tabelle 3).

Tabelle 3

	Anzahl	Mortalität
Nach Schwere:		
1. Grad	14 Fälle	1 Todesfall (schwerer Sonnenbrand)
2. Grad	424 Fälle	0
3. Grad	262 Fälle	14
Nach Flächenausdehnung:		
1. weniger als 20%	642 Fälle	0,5%
2. 20—30%	22 Fälle	27,3%
3. 30—40%	10 Fälle	70,0%
4. mehr als 40%	26 Fälle	100,0%

Besondere Vorsicht in der Prognosestellung ist am Platz bei Schädigungen der Luftwege. Ihre Bedeutung wurde von Phillips und Cope (1962) besonders hervorgehoben.

Die großen Fortschritte sind darin zu sehen, daß heute die meisten derjenigen Verbrannten, die vor 20 Jahren mit 25—30% als an der kritischen Grenze angelangt betrachtet wurden, mit großer Wahrscheinlichkeit am Leben erhalten werden können. Günstige Berichte vom Überleben nach Schädigungen beispielsweise von 95% der Körperoberfläche (Hoffman und Brownell) stecken für uns ein schwer erreichbares Ziel ab. Alle derartigen Veröffentlichungen verdienen unser kritisches Interesse und fordern zu Vergleichen und eventuell zur Ergänzung und Anpassung der Behandlungsmaßnahmen auf.

2. Beurteilung der Ausdehnung einer Verbrennung

Der Beurteilung der Ausdehnung einer Verbrennung kommt eine sehr große Bedeutung zu, nicht nur im Hinblick auf die Prognose und die Beurteilung neuer Behandlungsmethoden, sondern mehr noch als Hauptkriterium für die Triage und das Aufstellen des Behandlungsplanes. Für die Berechnung der Ausdehnung einer Verbrennung in Prozenten der Körperoberfläche gibt es mehrere gangbare Möglichkeiten. Bewährt haben sich vor allem die Schemata von Berkow, besonders wenn sie für Kinder nach Lund-Browder modifiziert werden (Abb. 2).

Eine sehr gute Grundlage für die Beurteilung der Flächenausdehnung besitzen wir in der sog. Neuner-Regel (Pulaski und Tennison, Wallace). Diese Angaben

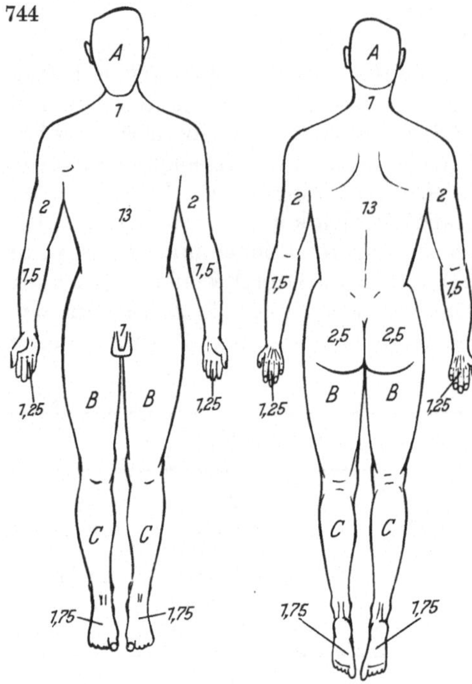

	Alter in Jahren					
	0	1	5	10	15	Erwachsener
A ½ Kopf	9,5	8,5	6,5	5,5	4,5	3,5
B ½ Oberschenkel	2,75	3,25	4	4,5	4,5	4,75
C ½ Unterschenkel	2,5	2,5	2,75	3,25	3,25	3,5

Abb. 2.
Schema von BERKOW, modifiziert nach LUND-BROWDER

können, wie jede richtige Faustregel, für die rasche Orientierung sehr empfohlen werden. Die Vereinfachung ist von großem didaktischem Wert, und das Schema bewährt sich darum besonders für den Unterricht von Ärzten und Pflegepersonal. Die Übereinstimmung mit den Zahlenangaben des Berkowschen Schemas ist sehr groß, auf jeden Fall genügend, wenn wir bedenken, daß Schätzungsfehler von $\pm 10\%$ je nach Untersucher ohnehin vorkommen werden. Auch die Neuner-Regel läßt sich für Kinder modifizieren (Abb. 3).

Für kleine Bezirke empfiehlt sich auch der Vergleich mit der Handfläche des Verletzten, die einem Prozent der Körperoberfläche entspricht. Unregelmäßig verteilte Verbrennungen oder kleine, bei schwersten Verbrennungen einzig noch intakt gebliebene Hautbezirke lassen sich mit dieser ergänzenden Regel gut abschätzen.

Immer wird man mit Vorteil die betroffenen Areale in ein Körperschema eintragen, wobei zwischen rein erstgradigen, zweitgradigen und oberflächlich oder tief drittgradigen Schädigungen womöglich unterschieden werden sollte. Es ist instruktiv, ein solches Schema beim Spitaleintritt und später, etwa am 10. bis 14. Tage nach dem Eintritt, nochmals anzufertigen. Nur so kann man sich überzeugen, wie schwierig es in den Anfangsstadien sein kann, den richtigen Grad der Tiefenausdehnung festzuhalten. Dies hat sogar dazu geführt, daß einzelne Autoren (z.B. ALLGÖWER und SIEGRIST) vorgeschlagen haben, die besonders im deutschen Sprachgebiet gebräuchliche, auf den Berner Stadtarzt FABRICIUS HILDANUS (1560—1634) zurückgehende dreistufige Beurteilung auf eine zweistufige zu reduzieren, bei der nur noch zwischen oberflächlichen und tiefen Schädigungen unterschieden würden. Andere Einteilungen dagegen, z. B. die auf DUPUYTREN zurückgehende, unterscheiden

9%
9% 9%
36%
1%
18% 18%
Erwachsener

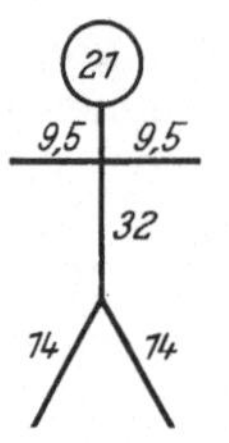

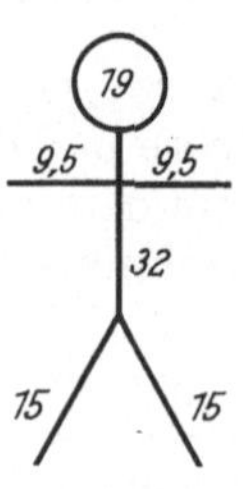

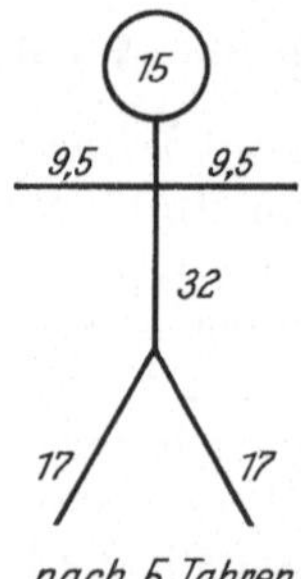

Abb. 3. Neunerregel (nach WALLACE)

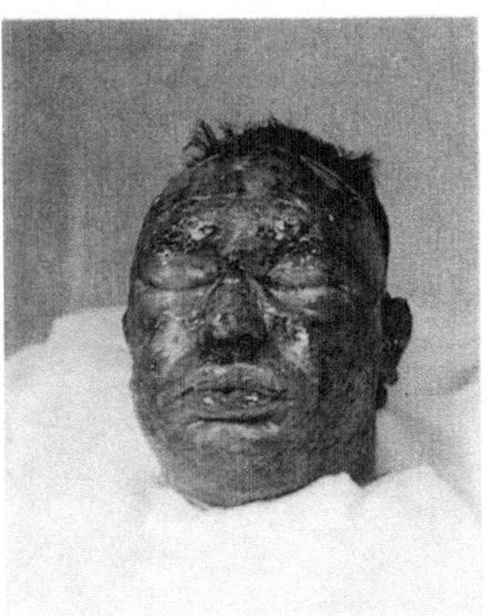

Abb. 4. Zweit- bis drittgradige Verbrennung des Gesichts, kurz nach Einlieferung in die Klinik. Durch die ödematöse Schwellung sind die Gesichtszüge bis zur Unkenntlichkeit entstellt

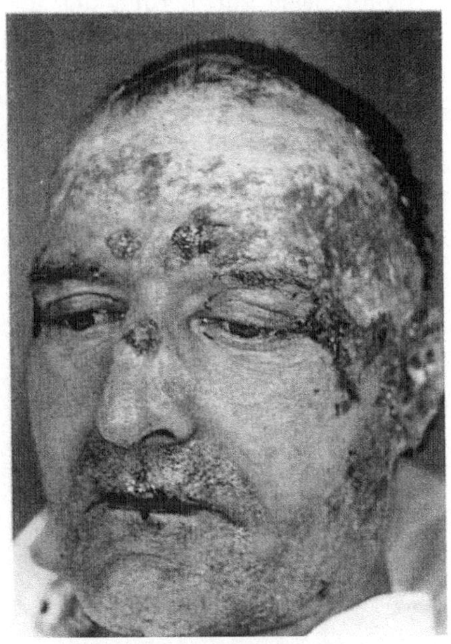

Abb. 5. Der gleiche Patient 20 Tage später

fünf oder sogar sechs Grade. Große klinische Erfahrung ist für die richtige morphologische Beurteilung der Frühstadien unerläßlich. Der Aspekt der Haut wechselt dann rasch im weiteren Verlauf, oft von Stunde zu Stunde.

Die Art der Hitzeeinwirkung — ob Verbrühung, Flamme, Strahlung, Explosion, Kontakt mit geschmolzenem Metall u.a. — kann für die prognostische Beurteilung ebenfalls ausschlaggebend werden. Die Untersuchung auf erhaltene Sensibilität ist für die Abschätzung der Tiefenausdehnung wichtig. Das Fehlen der Schmerzempfindung bei Stich mit der Nadel spricht fast immer für tief drittgradige Hitzeschädigung mit Zerstörung der sensiblen Endorgane in der Haut.

Immer ist schließlich bei der Beurteilung der Prognose daran zu denken, daß Kleinkinder und Greise besonders stark gefährdet sind. Bei Kindern kommt es offenbar besonders leicht zu Hirnödem (HUSCHKE; MORGER, NICOLE und GAYER). Konstitution, Widerstandskraft, Gesundheitszustand vor dem Unfallereignis müssen mit in Rechnung gestellt werden.

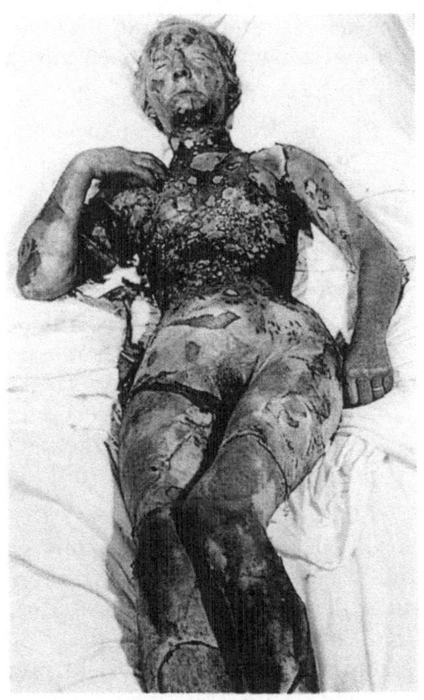

Abb. 6. Schwerste Verbrennung von fast 100% der Körperoberfläche mit ausgedehnten Verkohlungen. Die Patientin, die sich in suizidaler Absicht mit Petrol übergoß und in Brand steckte, überlebte noch 7 Std

3. Triage

Sofort nach der Beurteilung der Schwere des Falles sind die ersten Entschlüsse über die durchzuführende Schmerzstillung,

Anordnungen zur Beruhigung und für die Flüssigkeitstherapie als wichtigste Bestandteile der Schockbekämpfung zu treffen.

In Anlehnung an Schemata von Artz, Lob, Allgöwer und Koslowski treffen wir eine Unterteilung in drei Kategorien verschiedener Schweregrade, nach

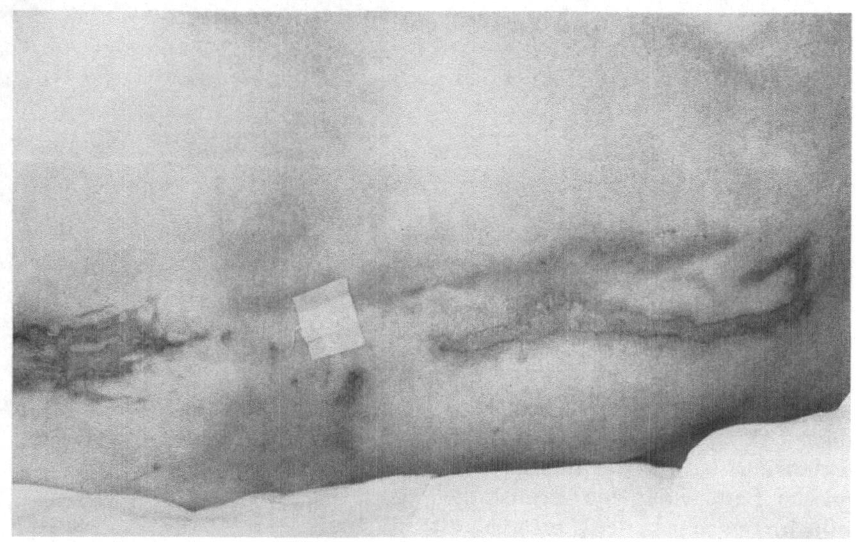

Abb. 7. Verbrennung durch Blitzschlag

welchen sich der Behandlungsplan zu richten hat (die in Klammern angeführten Prozentzahlen beziehen sich auf Kinder):

I. *Leichtere Verbrennungen — ambulante (lokale) Behandlung:*
1—15 (7)% der Körperoberfläche.

II. *Mittelschwere Verbrennungen — sofortige Schockbehandlung (Krankenhausbehandlung):*
a) Tiefe Verbrennungen von über 15 (7)% der Körperoberfläche.
b) Oberflächliche Verbrennung von über 40 (20)% der Körperoberfläche.

III. *Sehr schwere Verbrennungen — Schockbehandlungen und besondere Maßnahmen (Hibernation, Tracheotomie) (wenn möglich Behandlung in sog. Verbrennungszentren):*
a) Tiefe Verbrennungen von über 30 (20)% der Körperoberfläche.
b) Oberflächliche Verbrennungen von über 75 (50)% der Körperoberfläche.
c) Schwere Verbrennungen des Gesichtes und der oberen Luftwege.
d) Verbrennungen mit großen Weichteilwunden; schwere elektrische Verbrennungen.

Bei Katastrophenfällen mit großer Zahl von Schwerverbrannten wird man diese Schemata etwas modifizieren müssen. Schwere Verbrennungen von mehr als 40% der Körperoberfläche haben in solchen Fällen kaum Überlebenschancen (Koslowski 1964). Markley hat bei Katastrophen gute Erfahrungen mit peroralen Gaben von Elektrolytlösungen und kolloidalen Dextroselösungen gemacht. Ihre Wirksamkeit entsprach anscheinend derjenigen von Infusionen, aber nur, wenn bei Erwachsenen weniger als 50%, bei Kindern weniger als 30% der Körperoberfläche betroffen war. Auch Ahnefeld hat auf die Möglichkeit der peroralen Flüssigkeitszufuhr besonders für Katastrophenfälle hingewiesen.

III. Behandlung des Schocks und der Verbrennungskrankheit

1. Erste Hilfe am Unfallort

Schmerzstillung und Beruhigung

Bei Leuten mit entflammten Kleidern wird sofort versucht, durch Übergießen mit Wasser oder Zudecken mit Decken u. a. das Feuer zu ersticken. Die weiteren Maßnahmen am Unfallort müssen immer darauf gerichtet sein, Verschmutzung und Schmerzen möglichst zu vermeiden. Die Kleider werden nur bei Verbrühungen oder Verätzungen entfernt, in diesen Fällen aber so rasch als möglich. Anlegen von Verbänden am Unfallort ist meist unnötiger Zeitverlust. Ist der Rumpf stärker betroffen, empfiehlt sich Einwickeln in saubere Tücher. Schwerer Verbrannte müssen liegend transportiert werden. Ist die Transportstrecke nur kurz, so sollten keine Flüssigkeiten per os gegeben werden, wegen der Gefahr von Erbrechen und Aspiration.

Bei Teerverbrennungen ist es auf Grund tierexperimenteller Versuche günstiger, die Teerschicht auf der Wunde zu belassen (Nunn und Potter). Die Wundheilung wird durch die Teerschicht nicht gestört; anderseits wird das zusätzliche Trauma der meist sehr schmerzhaften Wundreinigung vermieden.

Schmerz und Schmerzäußerung gehören nicht unbedingt zum Bild der schweren Verbrennung. Man ist oft überrascht, wie verschieden sich die Verunfallten in dieser Beziehung verhalten. Offenbar sind oft leichtere ausgedehnte Verbrühungen ganz besonders schmerzhaft; jedenfalls ist bei Schmerzlosigkeit immer an tief zweitgradige oder drittgradige Schäden zu denken. Die Möglichkeit von Somnolenz und Apathie als Zeichen schon eingetretenen Schocks müssen aber dabei mitberücksichtigt werden. Der Spitalarzt hat auch immer zu bedenken, ob nicht schon vom erstbehandelnden, einweisenden Arzt Schmerzbekämpfungsmittel verabreicht worden sind. Er wird, wenn ein Einweisungszeugnis fehlt, vom Verunfallten selbst einige Angaben über die Zeitspanne seit der Einwirkung des Hitzetraumas, über schmerzstillende Injektionen, erste Lokalbehandlung, Laienhilfe usw. zu erlangen suchen und diese — neben seinen Feststellungen über die Flächenausdehnung — für die prognostische Beurteilung mitverwerten. Im Idealfall werden die Patienten rasch und ohne allgemeine oder lokale Vorbehandlung in das Krankenhaus eingeliefert. Leider wird aber gerade bei Kleinkindern oft zu lange abgewartet; in der Zwischenzeit kann sich ein schwerer Schockzustand entwickeln. Ferner bedauert man immer wieder, daß durch unzweckmäßige Laienhilfe auch die Lokalbehandlung nicht mehr frei gewählt werden kann, sondern möglicherweise schon vorbestimmt oder doch erschwert wird.

Zur Schmerzbekämpfung wird beim Erwachsenen vor allem die intravenöse Gabe von 10—15 mg Morphin empfohlen. Wenn erforderlich, dürfen die Spritzen ohne Gefahr der Kumulation wiederholt werden, während vor den intramuskulären Injektionen mit Recht immer wieder gewarnt wird. Im ausgebildeten Schock bleiben diese Morphiumdepots liegen, sie gelangen erst dann zur Resorption, wenn sich die Schockbehandlung auswirkt und den Kreislauf normalisiert. Damit entsteht die Gefahr einer kurzfristigen kumulativen Einwirkung mehrerer Morphiumgaben mit unangenehmen Rückwirkungen auf das Atemzentrum. Dies dürfte der Grund sein, weshalb sich, seit dem kritischen Einwand von Hebra, immer wieder warnende Stimmen gegen die Anwendung des Morphins (z. B. Stüttgen 1957, Bürkle de la Camp 1957, Monsaingeon 1963, Koslowský 1963) melden. Wir haben an unserer Klinik mit Morphin bzw. Morphinersatzpräparaten, nie unangenehme Zwischenfälle erlebt, auch nicht bei Kindern.

Genaue Angaben zur Schmerzstillung mit Pantopon-R und Bellafolin-R bei Säuglingen und Kleinkindern finden sich in der Arbeit von MORGER u. Mitarb. Als Vorteile der Morphinwirkung gelten die Kombination von Schmerzstillung und Euphorisierung. Beide tragen mindestens zu einer teilweisen Schockprophylaxe bei. Wenn Morphium aus irgendwelchen Gründen kontraindiziert ist — bekannt sind besonders schwerste Nausea und Erbrechen bei Überempfindlichen — kann man zur Schmerzbekämpfung intravenös Procain verabreichen; auch sprechen sich eine große Anzahl von Klinikern eher für die Anwendung von Morphium-Ersatzpräparaten (Cliradon-R, Dolantin-R, Novalgin-R) und von Barbituraten aus. Letztere haben besonders in der Kombination mit Antihistaminica und Ganglienblockern eine große Bedeutung erlangt. Im folgenden kleinen Abschnitt über die pharmakologische Hibernation wird noch davon zu reden sein.

Die *pharmakologische Hibernation* spielt in der modernen Chirurgie keine sehr große Rolle mehr, wird aber noch ab und zu für die Behandlung allerschwerster Verbrennungen (über 30% der Körperoberfläche) empfohlen. MONSAINGEON hat in seiner 1963 erschienenen Monographie ihren Wert stark angezweifelt. Man wird sie aber möglicherweise, wenn die Technik verfeinert, die Gefahren und Nachteile erkannt und vermeidbar werden, in Zukunft doch wieder häufiger zu Hilfe nehmen. Sie ist immer nur in Kombination mit der bewährten Flüssigkeitstherapie des Schocks anzuwenden, weil die zur Hibernation benötigten Phenothiazine sympathicolytisch wirken und dadurch die Kollapsgefahr erhöhen. Das Behandlungsprinzip der künstlichen Hibernation basiert zum Teil auf den Erfahrungen beim gewöhnlichen Dauerschlaf, zum Teil auf den allgemeinen Theorien der Schockentstehung und Schockbekämpfung. Der als künstlicher Winterschlaf bezeichnete Zustand wird herbeigeführt, indem durch ein Medikamentgemisch Schmerzbekämpfung, Ganglienblockade und zentralnervöse Sedation kombiniert werden (LABORIT, BÉNITTE). Als sog. lytisches Medikamentengemisch (Cocktail lytique von LABORIT) wird meist Chlorpromacin (Largactil-R), Promethacin (Phenergan-R) und Dolantin-R in der Dosierung von 50:50:100 mg alle 3—5 Std angewendet. Chlorpromacin wirkt auf Stammhirn und Ganglien, Promethacin als Antihistaminicum, und Dolantin bewirkt die zentralnervöse Sedation und die Schmerzstillung. Ferner führen physikalische Maßnahmen zu einer künstlichen Hypothermie. Die Stoffwechselintensität und der Sauerstoffverbrauch werden vermindert, Sensorium und Motorik gedämpft, man erzielt eine ruhige, langsame Atmung und erreicht eine Herabsetzung der Körpertemperatur. Die Hibernation wird in der Regel während mindestens 48 Std beibehalten. Die somnolenten Patienten können jederzeit durch Anruf geweckt werden. Ihre Überwachung durch das Pflegepersonal verlangt aber größte Sorgfalt und Aufmerksamkeit. Die Körpertemperatur muß zwischen 36 und 32° gehalten werden; keinesfalls darf sie unter 32° absinken. Auch bei der Hibernation soll die Urinausscheidung des Verbrannten nicht weniger als 40 mg pro Stunde betragen. In der Regel ist eine Tracheotomie unumgänglich.

Auch außerhalb der künstlichen Hibernation sind von vielen Autoren *Antihistaminica bzw. Phenothiazine* zur allgemeinen Behandlung von Verbrennungen empfohlen worden (GREUER, OXENIUS, LABORIT, HUGUÉNARD, ANDREESEN, KIMMIG, SCHMITT, STÜTTGEN). Neben der sedativen Wirkung dieser Medikamente wird auch eine Hemmung auf Exsudation und Ödembildung angenommen, da ja tatsächlich Histamin und histaminartige Substanzen bei der Pathogenese der Verbrennungskrankheit eine Rolle spielen. SEVITT konnte allerdings den günstigen Einfluß der Antihistaminica weder experimentell noch klinisch bestätigen.

Wenn wir die Schmerzstillung und Beruhigung an den Anfang des Kapitels über allgemeine Therapie und Schockbekämpfung gestellt haben, so bedeutet das noch nicht, daß damit die wichtigste Behandlungsmaßnahme ergriffen wäre. Die Wirkung des Schmerzes und damit eines nervösen Stresses für die Erklärung der Schockentstehung ist früher eher überwertet worden. Es gelingt aber auf experimentellem Wege lediglich über die Reizung sensibler Nerven nicht, ein Krankheitsbild zu erzeugen, das dem Schock entsprechen würde. Hingegen ist immer wieder experimentell und klinisch festgestellt worden, daß beim traumatischen Schock oder beim abundanten Blutverlust ein zusätzlicher Reiz auf das zentrale Nervensystem sehr schlimme Folgen haben kann. Die ganze Schockverhütung und -behandlung muß sich deshalb aus einer Kombination von therapeutischen Maßnahmen aufbauen. In dieser Kombination spielt dann die Schmerzbekämpfung und Beruhigung allerdings eine wichtige Rolle. Die zentrale Stellung nimmt aber der *Flüssigkeitsersatz* ein.

2. Flüssigkeitsersatz

Auf den ersten Blick mag nun die Forderung nach sofortigem und ausreichendem Ersatz des verlorengegangenen Flüssigkeitsvolumens bei einer Verbrennung als Auswirkung eines allzu mechanistischen Denkens erscheinen. Der Grundsatz gilt aber ganz allgemein für die Schockbekämpfung.

Schon vor 100 Jahren vertrat GOLTZ die Ansicht, der heilsame Effekt einer Transfusion nach einem großen Blutverlust beruhe nicht auf dem Gehalt an Ernährungsstoffen, sondern auf der Korrektur der hämodynamischen Verhältnisse. Er schlug die Verabreichung einer körperwarmen Proteinlösung vor. Die ersten, die unseres Wissens bei Verbrennungen die Durchwässerung des Organismus versucht haben, waren PONFICK (1877) und v. LESSER (1880). Ihre Idee wurde 1905 von SNEVE, ferner von WEIDENFELD und ZUMBUSCH aufgegriffen. Diese Erkenntnisse gerieten dann vorübergehend etwas in Vergessenheit; erst 1925 haben sich RAVDIN und FERGUSON (hypodermatische Infusionen), 1926 BIGGER (intravenös verabreichte NaCl-Lösung) nachdrücklich für eine reichliche Flüssigkeitszufuhr ausgesprochen.

Die Plasmainfusion wurde 1936 durch WEINER eingeführt, nachdem 1931 durch BLALOCK die Bedeutung des Flüssigkeitsverlustes bei der Schockgenese experimentell nachgewiesen worden war. Die Berechtigung dieses Behandlungsprinzips ist durch sehr viele Tierexperimente auch für die Verbrennungsfolgen eindeutig nachgewiesen worden. Wenn beispielsweise bei Verbrühungen, die regelmäßig zum Tode führen müßten, lediglich Flüssigkeitsersatz als Behandlung versucht wird, so wird schon ein beträchtlicher Teil von Tieren am Leben erhalten (BLALOCK).

Aber nicht nur die Tierexperimente, sondern vor allem klinische Erfahrungen lehren uns immer wieder, daß durch ausreichenden Ersatz des Flüssigkeitsvolumens ein schwerer Schock verhütet oder ein eingetretener schockartiger Zustand relativ rasch wieder günstig beeinflußt werden kann.

Dabei gelingt es durch frühzeitige Infusion leichter, das Auftreten eines schweren Versagens zu verhindern, als den schon eingetretenen Zustand wieder rückgängig zu machen. In diesem Sinne wäre der Lehrsatz aufzufassen, daß die Schockprophylaxe die beste Schocktherapie sei (BULL). Setzt die Flüssigkeitsbehandlung erst 2—4 Std nach dem Unfall ein, so ist schon mit irreversiblen Organschäden zu rechnen. Deshalb müssen alle schwereren und schweren Verbrennungen ohne Zeitverlust der klinischen Behandlung zugeführt werden. Bei Säuglingen und Kleinkindern ist es besonders verhängnisvoll, wenn mit der Schockbehandlung nicht früh genug begonnen werden kann.

Wenn nach der Einweisung eines verbrannten oder verbrühten Patienten durch eine erste Inspektion die Ausdehnung der Verletzung festgestellt und damit ein Urteil über die Schockgefahr möglich ist, dann wird in allen schweren Fällen eine Dauertropfinfusion vorbereitet. Als unmittelbare, erste Maßnahme wird in der Regel eine Plasmatransfusion gemacht, weil diese in modernen Spitälern neben Elektrolyt- und anderen Kolloidlösungen immer zur Verfügung stehen muß. In allen schweren Fällen empfiehlt sich auch das Einlegen eines Dauerkatheters, mindestens für die ersten 2—3 Tage. Die Messung der stündlichen Urinausscheidung ist ein zuverlässiges Kriterium für die Wirksamkeit der Infusionstherapie.

a) Die Technik der Flüssigkeitsersatz-Therapie

Den Hauptfortschritt in der Behandlung von Hitzeschädigungen sehen wir also in der nach strengen Regeln durchgeführten Flüssigkeitsersatz-Therapie. Gleiche Behandlungsprinzipien kommen auch zur Anwendung bei der Verhütung oder Beseitigung des Operationsschocks oder des Schocks bei den schweren Verwundungen des modernen Verkehrsunfalls und der Kriegsverletzungen. Allerdings stellt die therapeutische Aufgabe große Anforderungen an das Personal, an das Laboratorium und die technischen Einrichtungen. Es ist das mit ein Grund zur Tendenz, in größeren Spitalkomplexen eine spezialisierte Abteilung für die Schwerverbrannten einzurichten. Die Verbrennungstherapie war immer ein Grenzgebiet zwischen Chirurgie und Dermatologie. An vielen Orten wird sie für die schwereren Fälle ganz dem Chirurgen oder besser einem gemischten spezialisierten Behandlungsteam überlassen. Maßnahmen zur Reanimation beherrschen hier wie dort das Feld; sie sind im modernen Krankenhaus überall fast zur Selbstverständlichkeit geworden. Die eingehende Besprechung könnte darum als überflüssig erscheinen, sähe man nicht auch immer wieder Beispiele für das Versagen vor diesen schwierigen ärztlichen Aufgaben. Geht man den Ursachen fehlerhafter Behandlung nach, wird man meist feststellen müssen, daß zu spät oder zu wenig Flüssigkeit infundiert worden ist. Verstöße gegen andere Behandlungsvorschriften, z. B. ungünstiges prozentuales Verhältnis von Kolloiden und Elektrolyten bei der gewählten Infusionslösung, oder Kombination mit ungeeigneten Kreislaufmitteln, werden sich jedenfalls immer weniger schwer auswirken als verspäteter Einsatz und ungenügende Menge der Infusion.

Eine gewisse doktrinäre und schematische Handhabung der Infusionstherapie kann darum nur von Nutzen sein. Im folgenden sei auf die wichtigen *Grundregeln* für diese Behandlung kurz eingetreten. In erster Linie ist für gut funktionierende intravenöse Zufuhr zu sorgen. Oft mag anfänglich die Infusion mit der gewöhnlichen Venenpunktion genügen. Meist wird man aber einen dünnen Polyvinyl- bzw. Polyäthylen-Katheter in ein großes Gefäß einführen oder nach Freilegen einer Vene einbinden. Mit Recht wird diese therapeutische Maßnahme in der englischen Literatur als Anlegen einer „intravenösen Lebensleitung (intravenous Life-Line)“ bezeichnet.

Als ideale Lösung ist die Punktion einer Armvene mit grober Kanüle und Einführung eines dünnen Polyäthylen-Schlauches bis in die Vena subclavia anzusehen. Natürlich muß man je nach der Verteilung der Verbrennungen und nach dem Freibleiben gesunder Hautpartien anders vorgehen. Einführung der Katheter in kleinere Gefäße lohnt sich möglicherweise nicht, weil Verstopfung durch Thrombosierung in vielen Fällen nicht vermieden werden kann. Die Thrombosegefahr ist an Venen der unteren Körperhälfte größer. Aus diesem Grunde warnt Monsaingeon vor der Infusion in die Vena femoralis bzw. Cava inferior. Es wird auch empfohlen, die Tropfinfusion nicht über den 4. Tag hinaus fortzusetzen, um iatrogene Phlebitis und septische Streuung zu verhüten. Der einwandfrei funktionierende Dauereinlauf ist jedenfalls in den ersten Tagen Voraussetzung für jede wirksame Flüssigkeitstherapie. Auf die Möglichkeit einer rein oralen Flüssigkeitszufuhr wurde bereits bei der Besprechung der Triage hingewiesen. Sie eignet sich nur für leichtere Fälle; ihr größter Nachteil ist das dabei oft auftretende lästige Erbrechen.

b) Menge und Zusammensetzung der Infusionsflüssigkeit

Für die Berechnung der nötigen Infusionsmengen kann man sich von verschiedenen Regeln leiten lassen. Oberstes Gesetz bleibt: Es muß früh und viel infundiert werden. Meistens werden zur Errechnung der Menge und Zusammensetzung die Regel von EVANS oder die Brooke-Formel angewandt, wobei jede Klinik in Kleinigkeiten und Nebensächlichem von solchen Vorschriften abweichen mag; das allgemein als nötige Gesamtmenge anerkannte Volumen aber darf keinenfalls unterschritten werden, will man nicht unliebsame Erfahrungen machen.

Menge. Die Gesamtmenge berechnet sich nach folgender Formel, die neben dem Körpergewicht die prozentuale Flächenausdehnung der Verbrennung berücksichtigt:

2 cm^3 pro kg Körpergewicht × geschädigte % der Körperoberfläche (EVANS).

Andere Autoren (z. B. HARKINS, BRUNNER) geben Berechnungsmethoden an, nach denen der Plasmaverlust auf Grund der Differenz zwischen Sollhämatokrit und effektivem Hämatokrit bestimmt wird. Gegen alle diese Methoden ist einzuwenden, daß sie statisch sind: Man erfaßt damit nur das zum Zeitpunkt der Hämatokritmessung bestehende Defizit.

Für Kinder haben MORGER, NICOLE und GAYER folgendes Flüssigkeitsschema angegeben:

Tabelle 4

0—1 Jahr	132 cm^3 ± 33 cm^3 pro kg Körpergewicht
1—5 Jahre	110 cm^3 ± 33 cm^3 pro kg Körpergewicht
über 5 Jahre	88 cm^3 ± 33 cm^3 pro kg Körpergewicht

Zusammensetzung. In der Formel und Vorschrift von EVANS wird das Verhältnis von Elektrolytlösungen zu Kolloiden mit 1:1, in der Brookeschen Formel (VOGEL) mit 3:1 angegeben. Die Bezeichnung wurde nach dem Brooke-Unit gewählt (Army Surgical Research Unit, Brooke medical Center, Fort Sam Houston, Texas).

Für die Berechnung der Gesamtmenge besteht aber keine Abweichung gegenüber der Formel von EVANS. Eine sehr gute und einfache Regel ist diejenige von ALLGÖWER, der ein Vollblut-Kolloid-Elektrolytgemisch von 1:1:1 empfiehlt. Sinn der Vollbluttransfusion ist der Ersatz von geschädigten Erythrocyten, was besonders bei Verbrennungen von über 20% der Körperoberfläche wichtig ist (COLEBROOK, ABBOTT et al., EVANS). Viele Autoren haben sich gegen Bluttransfusionen im Initialstadium ausgesprochen, vor allem wegen der Kreislaufbeanspruchung (Viscositätssteigerung). Diese Einwände sind aber sicher nur berechtigt, wenn Vollblut allein gegeben wird. Ob zuerst Plasma, dann Vollblut und schließlich Elektrolytlösungen infundiert werden, ob ein Gemisch hergestellt wird oder die Reihenfolge umgestellt werden muß, kann eher als nebensächlich angesehen werden.

Zufuhr. Wichtig hingegen sind die Geschwindigkeit der Zufuhr, die Verteilung am ersten und am folgenden Tag und die zusätzliche Flüssigkeitsmenge, die per os zur Ergänzung noch gegeben wird. Man nimmt allgemein an, daß in den ersten 8 Std die Hälfte der benötigten Tagesmenge zugeführt werden soll, in den folgenden 8 Std ein Viertel und in den letzten 8 Std das restliche Viertel.

In den zweiten 24 Std der Flüssigkeitsbehandlung wird in der Regel nur die Hälfte der Infusionsmenge vom Vortag verabreicht. Wieder sollen ungefähr 2 Liter elektrolytfreier Flüssigkeit per os gegeben werden, vorausgesetzt, daß der Patient nicht erbricht und keine Magenblähung vorliegt.

Im Verlaufe der zweiten 24 Stunden ist die weitere ständige Kontrolle der stündlichen Urinausscheidung ganz besonders wichtig. In dieser Periode könnte sie plötzlich stark zurückgehen oder aber — als Zeichen zu großer Flüssigkeitszufuhr oder einsetzender Rückresorption — sehr stark überschießen.

Absinken der stündlichen Urinmenge unter 50 cm^3 beim Erwachsenen, unter 25 cm^3 beim Kinde ist ein Warnzeichen: Die Infusionsgeschwindigkeit muß erhöht werden (COLEBROOK). In diesem Zusammenhang ist die Führung eines genauen Bilanzblattes zu verlangen, mit Angaben über Blutdruck, laufende Untersuchungsbefunde, Medikation, Urinausscheidung.

Neben der ständigen Kontrolle der Urinausscheidung verwertet man zur Beurteilung der Gesamtsituation vor allem auch die klinischen Zeichen des Schocks: Blässe der Haut und der Schleimhäute, kalter Schweiß, Durstgefühl, rasche, oberflächliche Atmung oder unregelmäßige Atmung, Apathie, verhaltenes Angstgefühl, Übelkeit, jagender, fadenförmiger Puls, Kontraktion der Hautvenen, Blutdruckabfall, Oligurie bis Anurie. Fehlen von Erbrechen, von Singultus, von Somnolenz wird man als günstige Anzeichen werten. Brechreiz ist meist ein Zeichen ungenügender Schocktherapie. Von recht unbedeutenden Symptomen bis zur ominösen grauen Cyanose erstreckt sich eine ganze Stufenleiter von klinisch verwertbaren Symptomen, die alle nur durch praktische Erfahrung am Krankenbett in ihrer Bedeutung richtig erkannt und dann für die Prognose verwertet werden können.

Vom 2. Tag an sind auch häufige Kontrollen der Körpertemperatur angezeigt, vor allem bei Kindern.

Bei Verunfallten, die Rauchgase eingeatmet haben oder bei denen eine Hitzeschädigung der oberen Luftwege angenommen werden muß (Vebrennungen des Gesichts), ist das Lungenödem eine ernste Gefahr; hier ist größte Vorsicht mit der Dosierung der Infusionsmenge am Platz.

Neben der einfachen Überwachung der stündlichen Urinausscheidung und neben einer sorgfältig geführten Flüssigkeitsbilanz sind auch einige unkomplizierte Laboruntersuchungen für die Leitung der Therapie von großem Wert. Vor allem geben uns die Hämoglobin- und die Hämatokritwerte ein Bild über die Bluteindickung und ihre Bekämpfung.

Die Regulation des Elektrolythaushaltes kommt erst in zweiter Linie. Durch Natrium- und Kaliumbestimmungen sowie die Bestimmung der Alkalireserve im Blut können schwere Elektrolytverschiebungen rechtzeitig erkannt und korrigiert werden. Lungenödem, Wasservergiftung und Anurie sind als mögliche Gefahren einer übermäßigen Wasserzufuhr zu erwähnen. Im allgemeinen sind sie aber leicht vermeidbar, wenn keine groben Berechnungsfehler unterlaufen. Auch Störungen des Elektrolytgleichgewichts durch die Flüssigkeitstherapie spielen in der Regel nur eine untergeordnete Rolle. Im Zusammenhang mit der Flüssigkeitsersatztherapie wurde die Frage eines geeigneten *künstlichen Ersatzes* für die natürlichen Blutkolloide eingehend erörtert. Es ist schwierig, sich darüber schon ein abschließendes Urteil zu bilden. Meist wird man mit Humanplasma, am besten in der Form des Trockenplasmas PPL (= pasteurisiertes Plasma), um die Gefahr einer Infusions-Virushepatitis möglichst klein zu halten, ferner mit Vollblutkonserven und Elektrolytlösungen auskommen. Bei Katastrophen und im Kriegsfalle aber ist man auch auf derartige moderne Plasmaersatzstoffe (Plasmaexpander) angewiesen.

Es scheint, daß sich Dextran (Macrodex), eine Polysaccharidlösung, deren osmotischer Druck dem des Plasmas ungefähr entspricht, gut bewährt hat; von einzelnen Autoren wird es jeder Plasmatransfusion vorgezogen, weil so die Übertragung der homologen Serumhepatitis sicher vermieden werden kann (ENYART und MILLER 1955). Nach den Tierversuchen von BURRI und ALLGÖWER (1964) ist Macrodex dem Physiogel überlegen. Gegen das Dextran hat man eingewendet, daß es möglicherweise einer Staphylokokkensepsis Vorschub leisten könne (BERGENTZ u. Mitarb.). Auch Gelatinelösungen (EVANS und RAFAL) und Polyvinylpyrrolidone sind verwendet worden (CORDICE et al. 1953), ferner Periston (SCHUBERT 1949, BULL 1954), Onkotin. Die Plasmaexpander, ursprünglich aus rein hämodynamischer Überlegung eingeführt, erscheinen besonders geeignet zur Bekämpfung der Störungen der Mikrozirkulation. Das gilt aber nur für niedermolekulare Plasmaexpander wie LMD (= low molecular dextran, Rheumacrodex, spezifisches Gewicht 40000). Die hochmolekularen, wie das gewöhnliche Dextran (spezifisches Gewicht 110000), PVP und andere fördern eher die „Geldrollenbildung" der Erythrocyten (JEANNET). Trotzdem hat man sich für die hochmolekularen Stoffe entschieden, weil nur diese eine längere Verweildauer in der Blutbahn haben; die niedermolekularen verlassen das Gefäßsystem sehr rasch und leisten der Ödembildung Vorschub (SCHEGA).

Nach Untersuchungen beurteilt, die man über die Verweildauer derartiger Ersatzstoffe in der Blutbahn angestellt hat, geht einwandfrei hervor, daß einzig die Plasmainfusion ihre Wirkung länger als 4 Std aufrechterhält (HUNZINGER et al.). Bedenkt man ferner, daß in Tierversuchen nach Dextran allergische Reaktionen (MCCARTHY) und toxische Nierenschädigungen (MILLICAN) gesehen worden sind, so muß man alle Ersatzstoffe in den zweiten Rang verweisen. Ist man gezwungen, trotzdem davon Gebrauch zu machen, so wird man das Dextran dem PVP vorziehen (MCCARTHY).

Schließlich stellt sich im Zusammenhang mit der Flüssigkeitsersatztherapie noch die Frage, wie lange die Infusion beibehalten werden soll. Nach COPE und MOORE (1949) muß sie beendet werden, wenn etwa nach 48 Std das Ödem manifest geworden ist, ansonst könne es zum Lungenödem kommen. Ein interessanter Vorschlag zu diesem Problem stammt von KIRCHNER (1963). Er geht von der Tatsache aus, daß beim Verbrennungsschock eine Zentralisation des Kreislaufs mit peripherer Vasoconstriction vorliegt, wobei eventuell trotz bedrohlichem Volumenmangel normale Blutdruckwerte gemessen werden. Als diagnostisches Hilfsmittel empfiehlt nun KIRCHNER die kurzdauernde, mehrmals wiederholbare Normalisierung des Sympathicotonus mit 0,9 mg Hydergin intravenös. Absinken des Blutdrucks deutet Volumenmangel an, und es braucht nur so lange infundiert zu werden, bis der Blutdruck nach Hydergin nicht mehr abfällt.

In diesem Zusammenhang muß energisch vor der Anwendung von sog. Pressorsubstanzen (Analeptica, Sympathicomimetica) wie Noradrenalin u. a. gewarnt werden: Sie sind kontraindiziert, vor allem auch weil sie die Nierendurchblutung drosseln (KING und BALDWIN, MOORE, KIRCHNER und OEHMIG).

3. Zusätzliche Maßnahmen

a) Chemotherapie bzw. -prophylaxe, Antibiotica

Prophylaktische Verabreichung von Penicillin oder eines Penicillin-Streptomycin-Gemisches hat sich bei schweren Verbrennungen gut bewährt (LAUS-

ECKER, ALLGÖWER), wenn auch von anderer Seite der Wert einer derartigen vorbeugenden Therapie bestritten wird (HEGEMAN). Nach FINE, BENNET und CLUFF, GILBERT und anderen Autoren kommt Toxinen bakterieller Herkunft eine Rolle in der Pathogenese des Schocks zu. Über die Verhütung oder Behandlung der Wundinfektion wird in einem besonderen Abschnitt, bei der Besprechung der lokalen Maßnahmen, noch zu reden sein.

Die prophylaktische Anwendung von Sulfonamiden wird abgelehnt, weil man in schweren Fällen die zusätzliche Schädigung der Niere befürchtet.

b) Sauerstoff

Bei Verbrennungen des Gesichts und bei Einatmung von Rauchgasen besteht immer die Gefahr von Schädigungen der Luftwege (GEORGIADE et al.). In schweren Fällen kann die nasale Sauerstoffzufuhr lebensrettend sein. Sie hat so rasch als möglich zu erfolgen, unter Umständen schon am Unfallort. YASARGIL empfiehlt bei allen schwereren Schockzuständen die Sauerstoffinsufflation.

c) Tetanusprophylaxe

Die Gefahr des Wundstarrkrampfes beim Verbrennungsverletzten wird sehr unterschiedlich beurteilt. Je nachdem wird regelmäßig oder nur ausnahmsweise eine Serumprophylaxe durchgeführt. Im allgemeinen scheint man in den letzten Jahren eher von der generellen, routinenmäßigen Seruminjektion wieder abgekommen zu sein. Sicher ist die passive Immunisierung grundsätzlich unzuverlässig; auch dürfen die Risiken der Serumkrankheit für den Schwerverletzten nicht unterschätzt werden.

Bei früher aktiv Immunisierten muß die Reaktivierungs-Spritze verlangt werden, da sie völlig gefahrlos ist. In den übrigen, nicht allzu schweren Fällen gibt man, wie das auch bei anderen Verletzungen üblich ist, kleine Mengen von Tetanusserum und gleichzeitig als Beginn der aktiven Immunisierung eine Dosis von Tetanus-Toxoid.

d) Hormontherapie

In der experimentellen Schockforschung hat man durch Zufuhr von Nebennieren-Steroiden nur bei ganz speziellen Schockformen eine signifikante Schutzwirkung feststellen können. Es scheint, daß auch beim Menschen die Nebennieren durch Mangeldurchblutung nur wenig in Mitleidenschaft gezogen werden und sehr lange sekretionsfähig bleiben (FRANK et al., HUME und NELSON, MELBY und SPINK). Andererseits sind bei der Anwendung von Corticosteroiden als unerwünschte Nebenwirkungen eine Herabsetzung der Resistenz gegen Infektionen, eine Erhöhung der Thrombosegefahr und eine Hemmung der Wundheilung in Rechnung zu stellen. Deshalb ist nach unserer Auffassung in allen Verbrennungsfällen, bei denen ein normal funktionierendes Hypophysen- und Nebennierensystem vorausgesetzt werden darf, die Behandlung mit ACTH und Cortison überflüssig, als Dauerbehandlung sogar kontraindiziert.

Von einzelnen Autoren ist die Behandlung mit Hydrocortison beim sog. *irreversiblen Schock* vorgeschlagen worden. Der Ausdruck „irreversibler Schock“ stammt aus der experimentellen Schockforschung und basiert auf Ergebnissen von Tierversuchen. Es ist aber nicht sicher, ob ein irreversibler Schock in diesem Sinne beim Menschen sich überhaupt entwickeln kann. Der Kliniker verwendet besser den Ausdruck „dekompensierter Schock“ (ALLGÖWER), mit dem nur ausgesagt wird, daß beim nicht sofort und adäquat behandelten Schock rasch irreparable Schädigungen auftreten.

e) Vitamine

Vor allem braucht der Patient mit ausgedehnten Verbrennungswunden viel Ascorbinsäure, daneben auch Vitamine des B-Komplexes. Die Situation ist ähnlich wie bei andersartigen schweren Erkrankungen. Man weiß durch Untersuchungen von LUND u. Mitarb. (1947), daß der Ascorbinsäurespiegel im Plasma nach Verbrennung stark absinkt.

f) Ernährung

Bei der Festsetzung der Diät muß man berücksichtigen, daß der Bedarf an Calorien und einzelnen Nährstoffen den Normalwert um ein Vielfaches übersteigen kann. Aus Stoffwechseluntersuchungen konnte dieser Bedarf errechnet werden. Abhängig von der Ausdehnung der Verbrennungswunden ist besonders der Eiweißbedarf.

Bei Appetitlosigkeit, Übelkeit und Erbrechen ist zur *Sondenfütterung* überzugehen, denn nur so können noch größere Mengen Eiweiß und die nötigen Calorien zugeführt werden. Gefürchtet sind Inanitionszustände, erzwungen durch Nahrungsverweigerung der Patienten, besonders in der 2. und 3. Woche. Meist liegen dann ausgedehnte drittgradige Verbrennungen im Stadium der Demarkation vor. Nicht selten handelt es sich um superinfizierte, ausgedehnte Wundflächen.

In diesem Stadium beobachtet man auch ab und zu eine Vermehrung des Rest-Stickstoffes, eine Pseudourämie, die als Zeichen für stark vermehrten Eiweißabbau gewertet werden muß. Sondenkostbeispiele, z. B. der Mayo-Kliniken. finden sich bei ALLGÖWER, ferner bei COLYER et al.

g) Herztherapie

Die kardiale Insuffizienz spielt nach Verbrennungen keine wichtige Rolle. Bei tagelang anhaltenden Tachykardien von mehr als 120 Schlägen pro Minute ist die Indikation zur Verabreichung von Herzglykosiden vorhanden. Bei älteren Patienten kann prophylaktisch während der ersten Tage $^1/_8$ mg/die Strophantin verabfolgt werden.

h) Nierenschäden

Die ganze moderne Verbrennungstherapie ist darauf ausgerichtet, einen Nierenschaden gar nicht aufkommen zu lassen. Oligurie oder Anurie stellt sich nach heutiger Auffassung fast immer nur bei ungenügender Flüssigkeitstherapie ein. Die Niere ist auf vorübergehende Anoxämie außerordentlich empfindlich. Geht die Urinausscheidung trotz genügender Flüssigkeitszufuhr unter 200 cm^3 je 24 Std zurück, so ist eine Organschädigung aufgetreten. Es wurde schon erwähnt, daß die Überwachung der Flüssigkeitsbilanz und eventuell auch Elektrolytbestimmungen sehr wichtig werden können. Bei ungenügender Nierenfunktion darf kein zusätzliches Kalium zugeführt werden. Darum sind in Einzelfällen Fruchtsäfte kontraindiziert. Die Kaliämie steht vor allem mit dem Untergang zahlreicher roter Blutkörperchen im Zusammenhang. Beim akuten tubulären Syndrom kann die bedrohliche Situation eventuell durch Anwendung der *künstlichen Niere* noch beherrscht werden (REHN). Es ist jedoch schwierig, die Vor- und Nachteile gegeneinander abzuwägen. Gerade bei den schwersten Fällen erscheint die Anwendung der extrakorporalen Dialyse wegen der schlechten Zirkulationsverhältnisse oft zu riskant (TANRET, MONSAINGEON). Größere Arbeiten zu diesem Thema liegen noch nicht vor.

i) Leberschäden

Leberfunktionsproben geben klinisch wichtige Hinweise, ferner die Bestimmung des Bilirubins im Serum und Urobilinogens im Urin.

k) Gastrointestinaltrakt

Nosko und Zehetner haben durch genau dosierte Transfusionen und systematische Penicillinbehandlung die Häufigkeit der Ulcusentstehung nach Verbrennungen signifikant vermindern können. Bei massiven Darmblutungen nach Verbrennungen wird operatives Vorgehen empfohlen (Weigel et al.).

Tabelle 5. *Schematische Darstellung der Verbrennungskrankheit und ihre Behandlung*

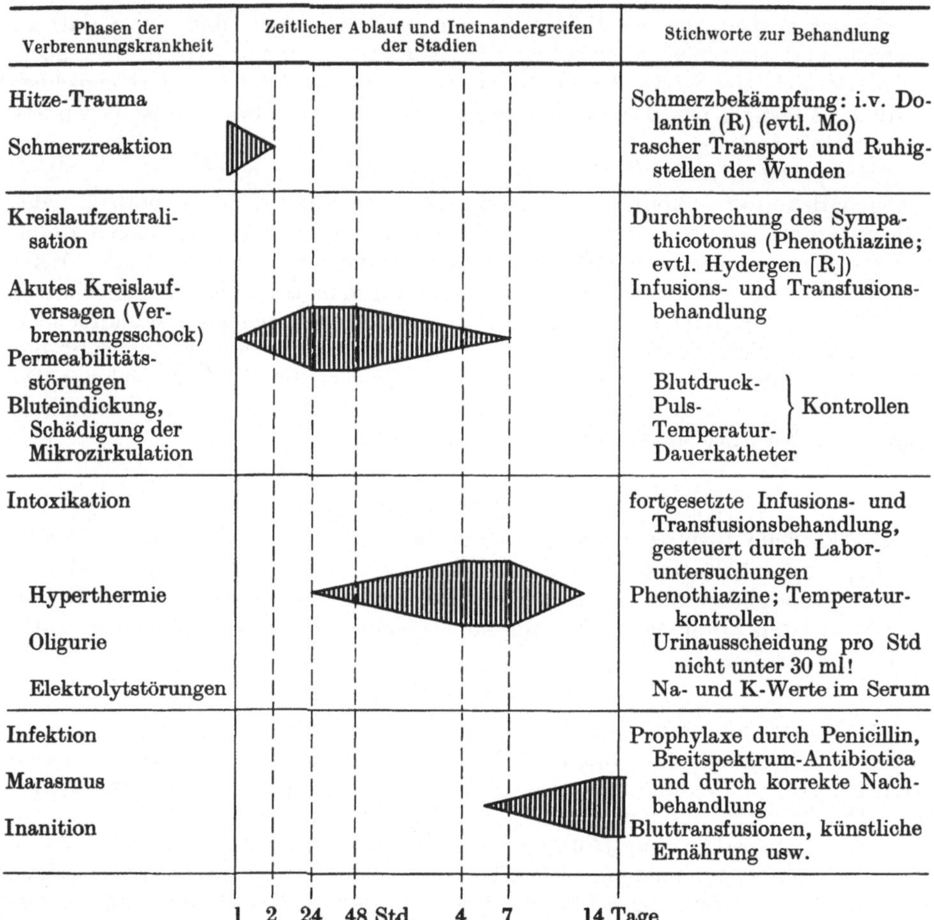

Phasen der Verbrennungskrankheit	Zeitlicher Ablauf und Ineinandergreifen der Stadien	Stichworte zur Behandlung
Hitze-Trauma Schmerzreaktion		Schmerzbekämpfung: i.v. Dolantin (R) (evtl. Mo) rascher Transport und Ruhigstellen der Wunden
Kreislaufzentralisation Akutes Kreislaufversagen (Verbrennungsschock) Permeabilitätsstörungen Bluteindickung, Schädigung der Mikrozirkulation		Durchbrechung des Sympathicotonus (Phenothiazine; evtl. Hydergen [R]) Infusions- und Transfusionsbehandlung Blutdruck-, Puls-, Temperatur-Kontrollen Dauerkatheter
Intoxikation Hyperthermie Oligurie Elektrolytstörungen		fortgesetzte Infusions- und Transfusionsbehandlung, gesteuert durch Laboruntersuchungen Phenothiazine; Temperaturkontrollen Urinausscheidung pro Std nicht unter 30 ml! Na- und K-Werte im Serum
Infektion Marasmus Inanition		Prophylaxe durch Penicillin, Breitspektrum-Antibiotica und durch korrekte Nachbehandlung Bluttransfusionen, künstliche Ernährung usw.
	1 2 24 48 Std 4 7 14 Tage	

IV. Lokalbehandlung der Dermatitis combustionis

1. Allgemeines

Schon im Eingangskapitel wurde erwähnt, daß die Methoden und Prinzipien, welche die Lokalbehandlung von Verbrennungen beherrschen, außerordentlich verschieden seien und auch periodisch immer wieder wechseln können, da sie starken Modeströmungen unterworfen sind. Die Mannigfaltigkeit lokaltherapeutischer Möglichkeiten ist derartig groß, daß jeder Versuch einer vollständigen „handbuchmäßigen" Bearbeitung kläglich scheitern müßte. Es kann sich deshalb im folgenden lediglich darum handeln, einige bewährte moderne Behandlungsprinzipien genauer zu schildern, indem Vor- und Nachteile hervorgehoben und gegeneinander abgewogen werden. In den einzelnen Behandlungszentren werden im allgemeinen gut eingeführte Verfahren, wenn sie befriedigende Erfolge bringen, über längere Zeit beibehalten. Die Auswahl und Einführung der jeweiligen Behandlungsmethode wird von den allgemein-pathologischen und pathologisch-physiologischen Auffassungen über das Verbrennungsgeschehen stark beeinflußt. Wer der Eiweißvergiftung von den Wundgebieten her große Bedeutung zumißt, wird eine entsprechende Behandlung, etwa die Gerbung oder das frühe Débridement, bevorzugen; wer in erster Linie die Bakterienbesiedlung der Wundflächen fürchtet und verhindern will, wird sich stark nach der Desinfektion hin ausrichten. Die Überlieferung in den einzelnen Krankenhäusern spielt dabei eine nicht unwichtige Rolle, und auch praktische — vor allem pflegerische — Gesichtspunkte sind bei der Auswahl und definitiven Einführung einer Methode ausschlaggebend. Eine gewisse Beweglichkeit in der Auswahl des Therapieverfahrens soll man sich schon deshalb bewahren, weil je nach der Schwere der Schädigung und je nach betroffener Körperregion einmal diese, ein andermal jene Methode geeigneter ist, so daß es falsch wäre, sich von vornherein arbiträr auf ein ganz bestimmtes Verfahren festzulegen.

Sehr oft ist aber durch die vorausgegangene Laienbehandlung oder durch die erste Hilfe des einweisenden Arztes die freie Wahl leider schon weitgehend eingeschränkt. Man sollte deshalb in Kursen für Samaritervereine, bei der Ausbildung von Gemeindekrankenschwestern oder Fabriksamaritern dahin wirken, daß schwere Verbrennungen, die ohnehin in Spitalbehandlung gehören, möglichst rasch eingeliefert werden, ohne daß mit lokalen Maßnahmen Zeit verlorengeht. Salben-, Öl-, Puder- oder Brandbindenverbände sind nicht erwünscht; sie verdecken das Erscheinungsbild. Ein lockerer, steriler, trockener Verband genügt. Der Spitalarzt kann die nicht vorbehandelten Schäden nach der Schwere und Ausdehnung besser abschätzen und danach seinen allgemeinen und lokalen Behandlungsplan aufstellen.

Die Frage nach der besten Lokalbehandlung ist in den letzten Jahrzehnten etwas weniger dringend und drängend geworden. Man strebt nicht mehr nach einer allgemein gültigen „unité de doctrine", wie dies früher, besonders in der Militärmedizin, der Fall war. Heute wird anerkannt, daß verschiedene Methoden ihre besonderen Vor- und Nachteile haben, daß alle aber vor der Wichtigkeit und Dringlichkeit der Allgemeinbehandlung in den Hintergrund treten müssen. So wie sich eine aktive oder mehr abwartende ärztliche Haltung gegenüberstehen können, so werden auch Chirurgen und Dermatologen bei der Beurteilung lokaler Behandlungsmaßnahmen in gewissen Fällen geteilter Meinung sein. In neuerer Zeit lassen sich übrigens wichtige Auseinandersetzungen zwischen Anhängern der geschlossenen oder der offenen Wundbehandlung verfolgen, und es ist vorauszusehen, daß diese Kontroverse noch über Jahre Stoff zu weiteren Diskussionen geben wird. Man wird an den langdauernden Streit um Vor- und Nachteile der gerbenden Behandlung mit Tannin erinnert, welcher erst nach mehr als einem Jahrzehnt endlich zur Ruhe kommen konnte. (Siehe PETER, Überblick über 40 Jahre Gerbstoffbehandlung in der Dermatologie.)

Rückblickend bekommt man den Eindruck, die Tanninbehandlung sei wegen falsch gedeuteter pathologisch-anatomischer Befunde an der Leber verlassen worden. Sie lebt auch in verschiedenen Formen, z. B. in Kombination mit Silbernitrat, heute noch an einzelnen Behandlungszentren weiter.

2. Beispiele für geschlossene Wundbehandlung

Die eingehendere Besprechung der dermatologischen Brandwundenbehandlung soll mit der Schilderung einiger bewährter Methoden eingeleitet werden, die alle mehr zur traditionsgebundenen, geschlossenen Wundbehandlung gehören. Als

Voraussetzung gilt, daß bei schweren Fällen die für die Schockbehandlung notwendigen Maßnahmen schon getroffen worden sind und auch zum Erfolg geführt haben. Es wäre falsch, einschneidende, psychisch noch weiter belastende Maßnahmen am unbehandelten Patienten vorzunehmen. Meist wird man die Wirkung einer intravenösen Injektion zur Schmerzbekämpfung und der Plasmainfusion vorerst abzuwarten haben. Die gewissenhafte Aufzeichnung der verschiedenartig geschädigten Hautbezirke in ein Körperschema benötigt ebenfalls einige Zeit, ferner die Aufstellung des teils darauf fußenden detaillierten Infusionsplanes für die ersten 24 Std.

Bei den stark zweitgradig geschädigten Hautregionen mit großen, prall gefüllten und teils eingerissenen Blasen stellt sich zu allererst einmal die Frage: Was soll mit den Blasen geschehen? Soll man sie entleeren und die Blasendecken entfernen, oder soll man sie ruhig belassen? Schon in diesem Punkt wird man nicht immer gleich vorgehen, dies schon deshalb, weil manchmal mit auch bakteriologisch relativ sauberen Bedingungen gerechnet werden kann, in anderen Fällen wieder eine sehr starke Verschmutzung mit Staub, Kohlenteilchen, Erde, Kleiderfetzen usw. vorliegt. Besonders bei Explosionen Verunfallte kommen oft sehr stark verschmutzt zur ersten Behandlung. Bei sauberen Verhältnissen haben wir uns zur Regel gemacht, die Blasen lediglich anzustechen, den serösen Inhalt ablaufen zu lassen und nach Pinselung oder nach Besprühung mit Mercurochromlösung (Natrium mercuridibromfluoresceinum) einen sterilen, trockenen Verband anzulegen. Es ist von besonderer Wichtigkeit, daß diese Verbände gut und ausreichend mit sekretaufnehmendem Material, steriler, hydrophiler Gaze und Watte gepolstert werden.

Abschließend verwendet man elastische Binden, die einen sanften Druck ausüben sollen. Extremitäten werden möglichst hoch gelagert, was — ähnlich wie bei Erfrierungen — als wohltuend empfunden wird. Bei diesem ersten Verband ist speziell darauf zu achten, daß vor allem die Finger in halbgebeugter Haltung und einzeln versorgt werden. Ein gut angelegter erster Verband sollte 8 Tage lang liegenbleiben, manchmal kann man ihn mit Vorteil 10—14 Tage lang ruhig belassen. Voraussetzung ist allerdings, daß der Patient nicht über Schmerzen klagt, sondern nur gut erträgliche Beschwerden äußert. Ferner ist darauf zu achten, daß die Verbände nicht vom Sekret bis nach außen durchtränkt sein dürfen. Mindestens die äußersten Schichten des durchtränkten Verbandes sind abzunehmen und durch trockene Gazeschichten zu ersetzen. Manchmal entschließen wir uns, einen neuen Verband anzulegen und dabei die Wunden zu revidieren; wenn nötig, werden sie erneut mit Mercurochromlösung behandelt. Liegenlassen eines völlig mit Wundsekret durchtränkten Verbandes wird als Kunstfehler betrachtet, denn es scheint erwiesen, daß durch einen solchen nassen Verband hindurch sehr rasch eine Besiedlung mit möglicherweise gefährlichen Keimen erfolgen kann (COLEBROOK und HOOD 1948).

Im Idealfall wird man immer streng aseptische Bedingungen für die erste Wundversorgung und für die Verbandwechsel anstreben.

Hospitalinfektionen sind in neuerer Zeit vielerorts zu einem heiklen Problem geworden. Sie bedrohen den in seiner Abwehr geschwächten Verunfallten ernstlich. Diese Infektionsgefahr ist für uns ein Grund, der geschlossenen Wundversorgung nach wirksamer Hautdesinfektion den Vorzug zu geben, obwohl allgemein anerkannt wird, daß auch auf offen und trocken gehaltenen großen Wundflächen die Gefahr der Ansiedlung gefährlicher Keime nicht viel größer sei. Schwere Verbrennungen werden — wenn immer möglich — im Einzelzimmer gepflegt; dadurch verringert sich die Gefahr gekreuzter Infektionen, die in Hautkliniken als immer latent vorhanden angenommen werden muß, ganz wesentlich. Das

Pflegepersonal sollte zur Vermeidung von Tröpfcheninfektionen Gesichtsmasken tragen. Bei der geschilderten Behandlung mit einer desinfizierenden Lösung (es braucht nicht notwendigerweise Mercurochrom zu sein, denn auch andere antibakteriell wirksame Farbstoffgemische sind mit gleichem Recht empfehlenswert) und einem lange liegenbleibenden, gut schließenden und milde komprimierenden Wundverband erwächst für den Patienten der große Vorteil, daß ein schmerzhafter Verbandwechsel in der Regel erst nach 8 Tagen notwendig wird. Für die Ärzte und das Pflegepersonal ergibt sich eine Einsparung an Arbeit; die ganze Aufmerksamkeit kann der Allgemeinbehandlung und Überwachung des Verbrennungskranken gewidmet werden. Wird im Normalfall nach ungefähr 8—10 Tagen der Verband entfernt, so ist man sehr oft völlig überrascht, wie ausgedehnte zweitgradig geschädigte Gebiete nach dieser Behandlung aussehen und schon als praktisch geheilt gelten dürfen. Tief zweitgradig bzw. oberflächlich und tief drittgradig geschädigte Hautpartien sind jetzt daran zu erkennen, daß sie noch nicht geheilt sind. Eine stärkere Wundsekretion und Zeichen der Nekrose und Demarkation haben sich in der Zwischenzeit eingestellt. Sehr oft — besonders bei den nur oberflächlich drittgradig betroffenen Bezirken — ist ein trockener, dünner, relativ elastischer Schorf entstanden, der nicht entfernt, sondern nochmals bepinselt oder besprüht und wiederum steril versorgt werden soll. Überall, wo sich unter dem primären Verband eine stärkere und anhaltende Wundsekretion eingestellt hat, ist mit schwerer geschädigten Hautpartien zu rechnen, was möglicherweise schon bei der allerersten Untersuchung wegen der fehlenden Schmerzempfindlichkeit auf Nadelstich festgestellt worden war. In diesen Gebieten verwendet man für den zweiten und die folgenden Verbände mit Vorteil desinfizierende Wundsalben. Es handelt sich dabei um eine der ältesten Behandlungsmethoden: Salbenverbände sind schon von Hippokrates bei Verbrennungen benutzt worden. Die Auswahl ist heute enorm groß, und man wird mit verschiedenen Salbentypen gute Erfahrungen machen können. Wir bevorzugen einige spezielle Verordnungen und haben die Tendenz, mit ihnen auszukommen und nicht immer wieder auf Neuheiten und Spezialitäten einzugehen.

Die bis zur Sinnlosigkeit abgewandelten, kombinierten und „verbesserten“ Fertigpräparate sind ein „Schandfleck“ auf dem heutigen Heilmittelmarkt, und die Ärzteschaft sollte gegen diese heillose Verwirrung Stellung beziehen und sich nicht immer neue und in keiner Weise bessere Therapeutica aufdrängen lassen. Einen umstrittenen Platz konnte sich vor allem die 1934 von Löhr empfohlene Lebertransalbe oder -paste behaupten. Ob sie vom Spitalapotheker nach einem bewährten Rezept selbst hergestellt wird oder ob es sich um eines der seit langem eingeführten Fertigpräparate handelt — man wird mit der Wahl einer Lebertransalbe selten fehlgehen. Wir verwenden vorwiegend Unguentolan-R, dem wir aber meist durch den Spitalapotheker entweder Aureomycin 1‰ oder Rivanol 1% (2-Äthoxy-6,9-diamino-acridinlactat) zusetzen lassen. Ausgezeichnet bewährt sich auch eine Kühlpaste mit Zusatz von 1‰ Aureomycin, Terramycin oder Neomycin. Als Nachteile der Lebertransalben-Behandlung sind zu erwähnen: die häufig beobachtete Maceration der Wundrandgebiete, eventuell eine gewisse Schmerzhaftigkeit und der von vielen Patienten als sehr abstoßend empfundene Geruch.

Verwendet man als Vehikel eine Paste, sind diese Nachteile eher kleiner. Während Lebertranpräparate praktisch kaum je allergische Überempfindlichkeitserscheinungen hervorrufen, sind solche vom Rivanol und vom Aureomycin bekannt; sie halten sich aber in einem durchaus zulässigen Prozentsatz. Sehr gute Erfahrungen sammelten wir auch mit Bepanthen-Salbe, sie gilt als besonders mild und gut verträglich. Vielleicht begünstigt sie auch die komplikationslose

Narbenbildung. Aus der Tabelle 6, S. 764, ist zu entnehmen, welche Salbentypen als besonders gut brauchbar beurteilt werden. Die Auswahl mußte nach allgemein anerkannten Gesichtspunkten streng einschränkend getroffen werden, wobei sich immer noch eine lange Liste ergibt.

Maceration und Beförderung der Wundinfektion werden immer wieder der abschließenden und fettigen Salbentherapie angekreidet. Verwendet man grobfaserigen Gittertüll als Verbandmaterial, dann fallen diese Nachteile weg. Er wird vom Kranken als angenehm empfunden, läßt Sekret austreten und gestattet einen schmerzlosen Verbandwechsel vor allem am Gesicht.

Im Bestreben, einen idealen Verband für Verbrennungswunden zu schaffen, sind Filme und Gele versucht und vorgeschlagen worden. Es liegt auf der Hand, daß man von einem epithelähnlichen, womöglich semipermeablen Membranabschluß gute Rückwirkungen auf die Wundheilung erwartet. Es ist möglich, daß sich hier eine fortschrittliche, moderne Lokalbehandlung vorbereitet.

So wurde ein eiweißhaltiger Film aus Aortenextrakt hergestellt (CHASE 1947), dem Sulfothiazol und Penicillin beigemischt wurde. Fibrinogen und Thrombin (HAWN et al. 1944), auch Kasein (CURTIS 1951) sind in der gleichen Absicht verwendet worden. Interessant sind ferner Versuche von RABINOWITZ und PELNER (1944) mit Pferdeserum. Neuerdings stehen wieder Versuche mit aufsprühbarem Polyvinyl als Lösungsmittel im Vordergrund (CHOY-WENDT). Auch über Aristamid-Gel (BENTHIEN) und mit Sulfonamiden versetztem Gel (Badional-Gel) (GLENK) wird in den letzten Jahren häufig empfehlend berichtet (JIRZIK und WARNECKE, KLEINE-NATROP und AZZOLINI). Bewährt hat sich auch die Farbstoff-Filmbehandlung nach FARGEL (KIMMIG).

Im Zusammenhang mit der geschlossenen Wundbehandlung ist noch die Anwendung von Druckverbänden zu erwähnen, die besonders von amerikanischen Autoren (ALLEN und KOCH, LEVENSON und LUND) empfohlen worden war. Man hatte sich von dieser Methode eine maßgebliche Hemmung der Ödembildung und der Exsudation versprochen. Diese Erwartungen sind nicht erfüllt worden. Auch experimentelle Arbeiten (VILAIN) haben ergeben, daß durch Anwendung von Druckverbänden die Flüssigkeitsverluste kaum vermindert werden können. Etwas ermutigendere Resultate sind in dieser Richtung mit dem sofortigen und länger dauernden Eintauchen verbrannter Körperteile in eisgekühltes Wasser erzielt worden (SHULMAN).

3. Die offene Wundbehandlung

Das Prinzip der offenen Wundbehandlung wurde mindestens für gewisse Körperregionen (Gesicht, Genital- und Analgegend) und vor allem bei wenig umfangreichen Verbrennungen ersten und zweiten Grades von jeher angewandt. Weil die Aussichten für die komplikationslose Selbstheilung dieser Schädigungsgrade besonders groß sind, hat das Verfahren sicher viel für sich. Ausgedehnte Verbrennungen bei kleinen Kindern müssen meist offen behandelt werden, weil bei entsprechender Bandagierung gefährliche Störungen der Wärmeregulation auftreten können. Sichere Vorteile der offenen Behandlung sind die Möglichkeit dauernder Beobachtung der Läsionen und des Heilungsverlaufes (ARTZ, MEADE); ferner die Einsparung an Verbandmaterial, eventuell auch die freiere Beweglichkeit der Extremitäten im Sinne einer Kontraktur-Prophylaxe. Das Verfahren wurde in den letzten Jahren stark ausgebaut und hat energische Verfechter gefunden (WALLACE, KYLE und WALLACE, BLOCKER). Die Wundflächen werden nicht bedeckt oder verbunden. Die Luft soll hinzutreten können, damit die Gebiete trocken bleiben. Die Verfechter dieser Methode sind der Ansicht, daß dabei die Infektionsgefahr eher geringer, jedenfalls nicht größer als bei der geschlossenen

Behandlung sei. Allerdings sollte die Luft möglichst keimfrei sein, was in Krankenhäusern nicht ohne weiteres zu erwarten ist. Der Zufuhr von frischer, sauberer, vorgewärmter Luft in die Krankenzimmer wird bei der Einrichtung spezialisierter Spitalabteilungen besondere Aufmerksamkeit geschenkt. Bei der offenen Wundbehandlung muß selbstverständlich auch dafür gesorgt sein, daß nicht Spitalinfektionen durch Staphylokokkenträger unter dem Behandlungspersonal vorkommen. Auch Infektionen mit Coli, Proteus und Pyocyaneus sind besonders zu fürchten. Die offene, austrocknende Wundbehandlung gelingt meist nur dann, wenn besondere Fixationsverfahren der Extremitäten angewendet werden oder wenn die Patienten z. B. bei Verletzungen an Brust und Rücken ständig umgelagert werden können. Mit modern konstruierten Drehbetten läßt sich diese Forderung erfüllen (Stryker frame).

Vor allem ist am Anfang der offenen Brandwundenbehandlung, in den ersten zweimal 24 Std, damit zu rechnen, daß die Wundflächen noch feucht sind und daß in diesem Zeitpunkt die Wahrscheinlichkeit der Infektion von außen noch groß ist. Selbst wenn sich bei drittgradigen Schädigungen durch die Expositions-Methode trockene, auf der Außenseite bakterienarme Schorfe erzielen lassen, so ist doch die Unterseite, entlang der Demarkation, meist mit pathogenen Keimen schwer infiziert, wie das auch schon bei der Tanninbehandlung festgestellt worden war. Eine wichtige Stütze, auf der die Theorie von der offenen Wundbehandlung ruhte, ist damit unseres Erachtens zusammengebrochen. Die Bedenken nehmen zu, wenn man hört, daß auch auf der Oberfläche der Wunden mehr Streptococcus pyogenes und häufiger Pseudomonas pyocyaneus gefunden wurde als in Vergleichsfällen mit geschlossener Wundbehandlung (Lowbury, Crockett, Jackson 1954). Bergamasco beobachtete bei gleichzeitiger Anwendung der offenen und geschlossenen Behandlung am gleichen Patienten, daß die geschlossen behandelten Hautbezirke rascher heilten (1958). Es scheint, daß sich die offene Behandlung ausgedehnter Verbrennungen nur in hochspezialisierten Zentren wirklich bewährt hat, aber auch dort können Infektionen nicht verhindert, sondern nur eingeschränkt werden. Am Birmingham Accident Hospital wird deshalb wieder vermehrt die geschlossene Behandlung angewandt (Colebrook).

4. Fermentative Nekrolyse. Chirurgische Versorgung (Transplantation). Behandlung von Narbenkeloiden

Vor besondere Aufgaben sieht man sich gestellt, wenn einzelne oder gar ausgedehnte Bezirke schwer drittgradig zerstört worden sind. In allen Fällen mit völligem Untergang der Hautanhangsgebilde, wenn Follikelepithel, Talg und Knäueldrüsen ganz zerstört worden sind, können sich keine Epithelinseln in den Wundflächen bilden, und es wäre mit besonders lange sich hinausziehender Wundheilung, auch in vermehrtem Maße mit Kontrakturen, mit hypertrophischen Narben und Narbenkeloiden zu rechnen. Bei der Behandlung solcher Hautbezirke ist mit speziellen Methoden dafür zu sorgen, daß die Nekrosen sich rascher abstoßen oder entfernen lassen, und sobald eine gesäuberte, frische Wundfläche erzielt ist, muß der Epithelersatz durch Transplantation angestrebt werden.

Zur Entfernung nekrotischer Wundbeläge stehen uns neuere Fermentpräparate zur Verfügung. Diesen Reinigungsprozeß der Wunden bezeichnet man vielerorts mit dem französischen Wort „Débridement“. Da der Terminus auch sonst in der Unfallchirurgie gebräuchlich ist, würde man besser von fermentativer Nekrolyse sprechen.

Sie ist vor allem in der dritten Woche nach dem Trauma aussichtsreich, dann nämlich, wenn sich ohnehin schon Zeichen der Demarkation in den Wundgebieten festellen lassen. Es können verschiedene Fermente zur Anwendung gelangen. Am ältesten sind die Versuche mit Eiweiß-Verdauungsfermenten in Form von Pankreasextrakten. Schon im Jahre 1943 hat Cooper von befriedigenden Resultaten berichtet. Es scheint aber, daß erst nach der gelungenen Reinigung und kristallinen Aufarbeitung von Trypsin wirklich empfehlenswerte Präparate erzielt worden sind. Mit Trypure Novo-R ist nach unserer Erfahrung eine fast schmerzlose fermentative Wundreinigung möglich. Der Streupuder wird auf die nekrotische Wundfläche aufgetragen, und darüber kommen feuchte Kompressen mit steriler physiologischer Kochsalzlösung. Eine weitere Anwendungsart in Spray-Form ist im Handel. Als Treibmittel und als Medikamentträger dient das nach dem Verdunsten des Lösungsmittels einen wirksamen Film erzeugende Freon.

Andere Fermente, z. B. Streptokinase-Streptodornase (Varidase-R) wirken in ähnlicher Weise auf denaturiertes Eiweiß und auf Fibrinansammlung in den Wundgebieten ein. Bei Verbrennungen dritten Grades mit Schorfen, die denaturiertes Kollagen enthalten, ist Varidase ungenügend, denn sie löst nur fibrinös-eitrige Exsudate auf, nicht aber Bindegewebe (Tillet). Möglicherweise wird sich die fermentative Wundreinigung, die sich in der Therapie chronischer Unterschenkelgeschwüre schon einen wichtigen Platz erobert hat, noch weiter ausbauen lassen. Als Nachteil sind die häufigen Verbandwechsel und die Schmerzhaftigkeit zu erwähnen. Es gibt Patienten, die diese Präparate deswegen fast nicht ertragen können und ihre weitere Anwendung ablehnen. Ältere Methoden des Débridement, etwa das Abbürsten der Wundflächen in Narkose mit Alkohol- oder Seifenlösung als erste Wundversorgung (Tschmarke und Vorläufer), sind, soviel man jedenfalls aus der neueren Literatur schließen darf, fast ganz verlassen worden. Zwei Gründe mögen dafür ausschlaggebend sein: Bei einem schwer geschädigten Verunfallten, der mit Mühe vor dem Verbrennungsschock bewahrt werden kann, ist die Narkose, auch wenn sie nach neuesten Methoden durchgeführt wird, ebenso eine zusätzliche Belastung wie der durch den Eingriff bedingte Blutverlust. Gegen das Abbürsten und auch gegen andere chirurgische Verfahren, wie Abtragen mit dem Rasiermesser, spricht auch der Umstand, daß man immer wieder erstaunt feststellt, wie oft, ausgehend von intakt gebliebenen Epithelresten in Drüsengängen und Follikeln, rasche Überhäutung erfolgt. Solche Epithelreste werden durch Bürsten oder durch chirurgisches Abtragen der Nekrosen unnötig mitentfernt.

Die sofortige chirurgische Entfernung von Nekrosen hat darum, nach unserer Ansicht, nur ein streng umschriebenes Indikationsgebiet. Dazu gehören tiefste drittgradige Verbrennungen nach Kontakt mit glühendem Metall oder nach längerer Einwirkung hoher Temperaturen auf ein kleines Hautgebiet, wie man das bei Unfällen von Epileptikern oder von Berauschten ab und zu sehen kann.

In den meisten Fällen wird man mit der fermentativen Nekrolyse auskommen können.

Die Verbrennungswunden säubern sich in der Regel zwischen dem 14. und 21. Tage nach der Hitzeeinwirkung. Es kann aber auch länger dauern; Bäder oder aktives chirurgisches Vorgehen müssen in solchen Fällen die definitive Wundreinigung möglichst rasch erzwingen.

Kontrakturen und Narbenkeloide sind vor allen Dingen dort zu fürchten, wo sich schlecht oder hypertrophisch granulierende Wundflächen einstellen.

Immer mehr setzt sich die Tendenz durch, derartige Defekte so rasch als möglich durch Epitheltransplantation zu decken. Die Forderung wird als *frühzeitiger Hautersatz* umschrieben und hat zweifellos große Berechtigung. Wir verstehen allerdings unter „frühzeitig" durchschnittlich die 3. Woche nach der Hitzeeinwirkung und nicht, wie viele moderne Autoren, die allerersten Tage. Diese zweifellos übertriebene Forderung basiert hauptsächlich auf der noch keineswegs bewiesenen Ansicht, daß ein solches Vorgehen die beste Infektionsprophylaxe darstelle, und ist mit ein Grund dafür, daß die Lehre von den Verbrennungen von einem dermatologischen teilweise zu einem chirurgischen Fachgebiet geworden ist. Da die Transplantate nur dann haften, wenn alle Nekrosen sich abgestoßen haben, bedingt ein Hautersatz innerhalb der ersten Tage immer auch ein eingreifendes chirurgisches Débridement mit entsprechenden Nachteilen und Risiken.

Die Hauttransplantation verhindert wirksamer als jedes andere Verfahren die Ausbildung von Keloiden und Narbenkontrakturen, was nicht leicht zu begründen ist, als Erfahrungstatsache aber feststeht. Am eindeutigsten wird uns die günstige Wirkung der Epitheltransplantation immer wieder vorgeführt, wenn große Wundflächen mit der sog. Briefmarkenmethode oder mit größeren dünnen Tiersch-Lappen behandelt werden: An den Grenzlinien kommt es recht oft zu ausgesprochener Keloidbildung, während unter dem transplantierten Epithel praktisch nie eine starke Bindegewebsproliferation beobachtet wird.

Ältere Verfahren, die zur Verhinderung von überschießenden Granulationen angewandt wurden — etwa die Ätzung mit dem Argent. nitric.-Stift, das Übergehen auf trockene Lokalbehandlung, z. B. das Decken mit Silberfolien oder Behandlung mit Wundpudern — haben sicher immer noch ihre Berechtigung. Über Gelenken und überall dort, wo Kontrakturen oder kosmetisch störende Keloide zu fürchten sind, gehört aber den Transplantationsmethoden der Vorrang.

Unter den Behandlungsmethoden gegen die Ausbildung von Keloiden nimmt immer noch die *prophylaktische Röntgenbestrahlung* einen wichtigen Platz ein. Es macht den Anschein, daß man in vielen Fällen die Ausbildung hypertrophischer Narben mit einer ein- bis zweimaligen Bestrahlung in vierwöchigem Abstand mit Dosen von 400 r, filtriert durch 1,0 Al. und erzeugt mit Spannungen zwischen 30—50 kV, verhindern kann (PFAHLER und KEEFER, LEVITT). Der Zeitpunkt wird verschieden gewählt. In der Regel erfolgt die erste Behandlung in der 4.—6. Woche der Verbrennungskrankheit.

Die Röntgentherapie ist auch für alle diejenigen Fälle angezeigt, bei denen es bereits zu hypertrophischen Narben und Keloiden gekommen ist. Es ist wichtig, frühzeitig nach eingetretener Keloidbildung zu bestrahlen (BRUNNER). Ausgedehnte Keloide, wie sie oft nach thermischen Schädigungen entstehen, sprechen allerdings nicht immer im gewünschten Maße auf die Röntgentherapie an (FISCHER und STORCK). Besonders über Gelenken können sie auch nach der Behandlung noch stark funktionsstörend in Erscheinung treten, so daß man zu einer Keloidexcision schreitet, die dann allerdings von einer prophylaktischen Bestrahlung gefolgt sein sollte.

Bei sehr starker Keloidbereitschaft kann es auch an den Entnahmestellen der Thiersch-Lappen zu polsterförmigen Keloiden kommen. Das gleiche gilt für die Entnahmestellen von Reverdin-Läppchen. Diese einfachste Läppchenplastik muß heute als weitgehend überholt betrachtet werden, gerade weil sowohl das eingewachsene Transplantat wie auch die Entnahmestellen wegen der Unregelmäßigkeiten, der höckerigen Oberfläche, der Keloide zwischen den eingewachsenen Läppchen, kosmetisch oft gar nicht befriedigen können. Auf der anderen Seite stellt das Verfahren keine Anforderungen an das technische Können des Arztes. Der Eingriff kann ohne Narkose in Lokalanaesthesie durchgeführt werden. Die Aussichten, daß die Läppchen selbst bei nicht ideal granulierenden Wundflächen trotzdem angehen, sind ebenfalls größer, besonders wenn man winzige Läppchen nach der Technik von BRAUN leicht schräg in die Wundflächen

Tabelle 6. *Übersicht über bewährte lokale Behandlungsmaßnahmen bei Hitzeschäden*

Behandlungsmethode	Wirksames Prinzip	Beispiele für Medikamente	Beurteilung (Besonderheiten, Vorteile, Nachteile)
Offene Wundbehandlung	Austrocknung der Wunden Bildung von Schorfen	Bei reiner offener Behandlung keine Desinficientia nötig Evtl. Waschung mit Hexachlorophenlösung	Rasch eintretende Schmerzlosigkeit, keine Verbandwechsel Seltener Superinfektion (?) Bei zirkulären Hitzeschäden allerdings Austrocknung schwer erreichbar (ständige Umlagerung, Drehbett) Bei mittelschweren Fällen personal- und zeitsparende Methode; geeignet in Katastrophenfällen
Geschlossene Wundbehandlung	a) Desinfektion mit Lösungen	Mercurochrom	Aufsaugende Verbände können ca. 1 Woche lang liegenbleiben. Bei Durchfeuchtung von innen Wechsel der äußeren Schichten. Revision, sofern die Wunden schmerzen
	b) Gerbung	Mercurochrom + Tannin + Argent. nitric.	Modifizierte Tanninbehandlung mit Vor- und Nachteilen; Retentionsabscesse unter den Schorfen als Gefahr
	c) Salben- und Pastenverbände antibakteriell und granulationsfördernd	Lebertransalben: Unguentolan R Riccovitan R, Riccomycin R Vita-Merfen R Bepanthen R	Meist nach 2—3 Tagen Verbandwechsel nötig Maceration Evtl. Entwicklung anaerober Keime auf den Wundflächen
	d) Gel	Aristamid-Gel R Badional-Gel R	Verminderung der Wundsekretion
	e) Spray f) Gittertüll	Terracortil R Tulle Gras R	Sekret kann abfließen. Ständige Desinfektion. Schmerzloser, rascher Verbandwechsel. Bewährte Wundbehandlung nach Transplantationen
	g) Fermentative Nekrolyse	Trypure Novo R	Umgehung der Nachteile des chirurgischen Débridement Bei tiefreichenden Nekrosen manchmal ungenügend. Schmerzhaftigkeit
Bädertherapie und feuchte Behandlung	Antiphlogistisches und desinfizierendes Behandlungsprinzip	Chloramin-Lösungen evtl. Kalium-Hypermanganicum-Bäder	Nur noch in wenigen Schulen üblich. Der häufige Verbandwechsel mit feuchten Kompressen verursacht Dauer-Stress. Gefahr der Wundinfektion sehr groß. Dauerbad für desperate Fälle evtl. angezeigt

einpflanzt. Trotz der kosmetischen Nachteile der Reverdin-Methode bleiben deshalb auch bei Verbrennungswunden solche, die mit diesem Verfahren gedeckt werden können. Interessant ist die Beobachtung, daß um die anwachsenden Reverdinläppchen herum die hypertrophischen Granulationen sich unter dem vorrückenden, auswachsenden Epithel abflachen. Diese Beobachtung kann als Beitrag zu dem eigenartigen Problem der Wechselwirkung zwischen Epithel und Wundfläche gelten. Sie unterstützt die Auffassung, daß nur das Decken mit Epithel die physiologisch richtige Versorgung einer Wunde sei (Abb. 8).

Ob sich in Zukunft mit Homiotransplantaten, z. B. in Form konservierter Epidermis, die nur vorübergehend anheilen können und nach durchschnittlich

4 Wochen wieder abgestoßen werden, ähnliche Resultate — nämlich Verhütung von Keloiden — erzielen lassen, erscheint noch fraglich. Bei ganz schweren Verbrennungen sind Erfolge mit Leichenhaut-Transplantaten beschrieben worden. Es soll sich um einen 1—7 Wochen haftenden „idealen" Verband handeln. Nachdem sich dann der Patient erholt hat, wird die definitive Versorgung der drittgradig geschädigten Partien mit Autotransplantaten angeschlossen. Dabei müssen die dünnen Thiersch-Lappen eventuell mehrmals von den gleichen Entnahmestellen geliefert werden (ARTZ, BECKER, SAKO, BROWNELL). In den meisten Fällen kann man ohne die Methode der homologen Transplantation, deren Bedeutung oft übertrieben worden ist, auskommen, indem man beim Patienten noch genügend zur Hautentnahme geeignete Körperstellen zur Verfügung hat. Mit der Briefmarkenmethode läßt sich durch Vergrößerung der Abstände zwischen den einzelnen Läppchen noch weiter an Deckmaterial einsparen. Jedes Epithelfetzchen ist auf diese Weise verwertbar und kann mithelfen, die Wundheilung bis zur völligen Epithelialisierung abzukürzen und Schrumpfungen zu verhüten.

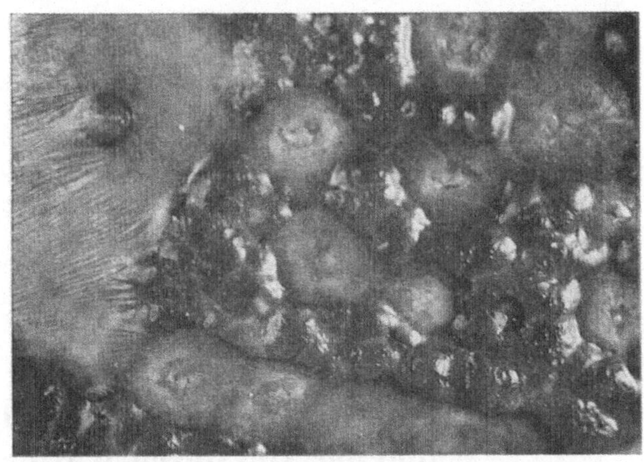
Abb. 8. Anwachsende Reverdin-Läppchen auf einer gesäuberten, drittgradigen Verbrennungswunde

Die freie Transplantation ist nicht in allen Fällen ausreichend. An mechanisch besonders exponierten Körperstellen und bei sehr tiefreichenden Defekten ist manchmal eine gestielte Hautplastik unumgänglich. Bei Narbenkontrakturen als Endzustand einer Verbrennung steht die Möglichkeit einer orthopädischen Nachbehandlung zur Verfügung.

Es dürfte auf Grund unserer Ausführungen über die allgemeine und die lokale Behandlung der Verbrennungskrankheit klargeworden sein, daß ein optimales Ergebnis nur aus der Zusammenarbeit von Dermatologen, Chirurgen und eventuell Internisten erwachsen kann.

B. Kälteschädigungen

Unter den thermischen Schädigungen können neben den Verbrennungen und Verbrühungen auch die Einwirkungen durch Wärmeentzug, als Schädigungen durch die Kälte, verstanden werden. Im Handbuchbeitrag von ULLMANN aus dem Jahre 1928 wurden diesem Kapitel 55 Seiten Text gewidmet und in einem Nachtrag von 1932 noch weitere 44 Seiten. Wir werden die Ergänzungen zu diesem Thema bewußt knapp fassen, da fast alles, was über Erfrierungen speziell im morphologisch-klinischen Gebiet in der Zeit zwischen den Weltkriegen feststand, auch jetzt noch Gültigkeit besitzt. Allerdings sind während des zweiten Weltkrieges und in den Jahren nach 1945 umfangreiche militärmedizinische Abhandlungen erschienen, die sich besonders mit der Problematik des Kältetraumas befaßt haben (STARLINGER und v. FRISCH, HAYS, COATES und McFETRIDGE). Wir werden daraus diejenigen neuen Tatsachen zur Sprache bringen, welche als Ergänzung des bisher Bekannten wertvoll sind.

Bei der Frage, wieweit der Kälteschaden ein dermatologisches Problem sei und ob nicht die Behandlung eher in den Aufgabenbereich des Chirurgen bzw. des chirurgisch orientierten Angiologen gehöre, können die Meinungen auseinandergehen. Ohne Zweifel haben sich die Grenzen eher zugunsten der Chirurgie verschoben, weil von Eingriffen am Sympathicus viel zu erwarten ist und weil Amputation und Transplantation in schweren Fällen meist nötig werden. Nach wie vor kann aber mit guten Gründen dafür eingetreten werden, daß sowohl Verbrennungs- wie Erfrierungsbehandlung im Aufgabenkreis der dermatologischen Kliniken bleiben sollten. Zusammen mit konsultierenden Chirurgen lassen sich im Teamwork die meisten Aufgaben sehr gut lösen; in anderen Fällen hat in einem späteren Zeitpunkt die Verlegung auf eine chirurgische Abteilung zu erfolgen, dann etwa, wenn nur die plastische Deckung mit schwieriger Technik die therapeutischen Probleme befriedigend lösen kann.

Schließlich sei noch erwähnt, daß gewisse dermatologische Krankheitsbilder, wie die Erythrocyanosis crurum puellarum, Urticaria e frigore, dann die Raynaudsche Krankheit, deren Einteilung bei den Kälteschäden schon immer umstritten war, heute viel eher anderen Krankheitsgruppen zugewiesen werden, nämlich den Kreislaufstörungen und den physikalischen Allergien der Haut. Die Gruppe der durch Kälte nur *mit*verursachten Schädigungen wandert ab zu denjenigen Formenkreisen, die nach wesentlicheren pathogenetischen und ätiologischen Gesichtspunkten aufgestellt worden sind. Um Wiederholungen zu vermeiden, wurde deshalb das Kapitel über Kälte als Mitursache von Dermatosen nur kurz abgehandelt.

I. Die allgemeine Unterkühlung und der Tod durch Wärmeverlust

Die allgemeine Unterkühlung und ihre Folgen sind zur Hauptsache ein militär- oder sportärztliches Problem. Mit einer Häufung von Fällen ist vor allem im Winter- und Gebirgskrieg, ferner bei Bergunfällen zu rechnen. Sehr oft kombinieren sich körperliche Erschöpfung und Auskühlung. Es wäre darum falsch, wenn man mit dem Tode durch Unterkühlung immer die Vorstellung von extrem niedrigen Temperaturen verbinden würde. Auch bei mäßigen Kältegraden ist mit fatalen Entwicklungen zu rechnen. Dabei sei besonders auch an Schiffbrüchige erinnert, die im Meer längere Zeit treiben, oder an die Flugunfälle mit Absturz ins Wasser. Unter normalen Verhältnissen kommt Tod durch Unterkühlung relativ selten vor.

Immerhin geht aus der Mortalitätsstatistik der Schweiz hervor, daß in der Zeitspanne zwischen 1942 und 1956 199 Todesfälle durch Erfrierung registriert worden sind (DREIFUSS). Sehr oft beschäftigen derartige Vorkommnisse die forensische Medizin. Besonders verhängnisvoll wirkt sich bekanntlich die allgemeine Unterkühlung beim Alkoholrausch aus, denn die normalen, sonst eine Zeitlang kompensierenden Regulationsmechanismen können dabei völlig ausfallen. Ab und zu beobachtet man die Kombination von Schlafmittelvergiftung (meist in suicidaler Absicht) mit Unterkühlung.

Die pathologische Anatomie des allgemeinen Kältetodes kann sich nicht auf spezifische Befunde stützen. Die Diagnose muß aus der Beurteilung der Leichenfund-Situation und aus den verschiedenen pathologischen Befunden durch Kombination abgeleitet werden. Als relativ verwertbar gelten immerhin: die besondere, hellere Farbe der Totenflecken, Gänsehaut, beidseitiger Hodenhochstand, Differenzen in der Blutfarbe zwischen dem Inhalt des rechten und des linken Herzens (eventuell bei gleichzeitig unterschiedlicher Senkungsgeschwindigkeit der Erythrocyten), ferner alle lokalen Erfrierungszeichen, besonders an der Haut der Ohren.

Bei Lawinenverschütteten stellt sich ab und zu die Frage des *Scheintodes durch Unterkühlung* (VOLKEN, HOSSLI). Allgemein gilt die Regel, daß eine Unterkühlung unter 22° C irreversibel sei. Mißt man im Mastdarm Temperaturen von 20° und darunter, so sind Wiederbelebungsmaßnahmen aussichtslos.

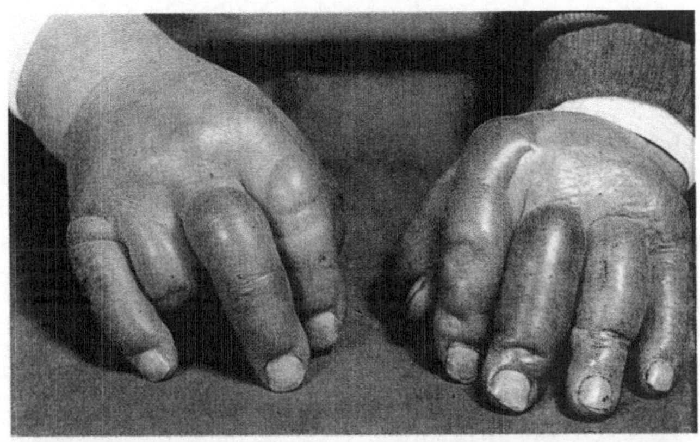

Abb. 9

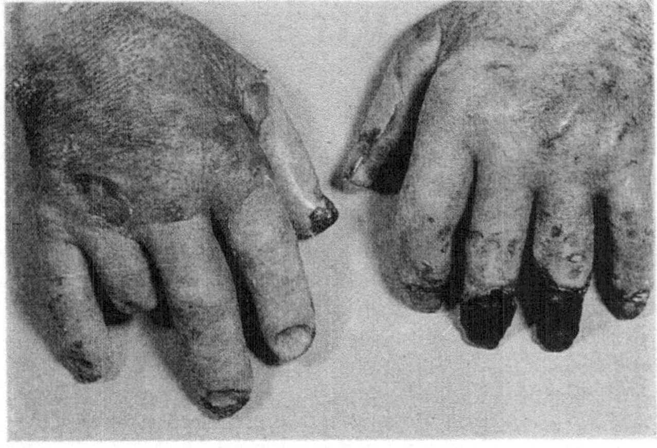

Abb. 10

Abb. 9. Erfrierung 2.—3. Grades beider Hände, nach Einschlafen im Freien bei kalter Witterung unter Alkoholeinfluß

Abb. 10. Derselbe Fall nach 4wöchiger konservativer Spitalbehandlung

II. Klinik, Ätiologie und Pathogenese der Erfrierungen

Wir verstehen unter Erfrierung den Gewebeschaden, welcher durch Gefrieren der Haut oder der subcutanen Gewebe entsteht. Die Einteilung in verschiedene Grade kann als bekannt vorausgesetzt werden:

Dermatitis congelationis erythematosa,
Dermatitis congelationis bullosa,
Dermatitis congelationis escharotica.

Sie Symptome sind normalerweise ein lokales Brennen, ein kurzdauernder Schmerz, der dann von einer stumpfen Gefühllosigkeit gefolgt wird. Besonders dieses Warnungszeichen sollte nicht übersehen werden; wenn nämlich in diesem Zustand Abwehr- oder Behandlungsmaßnahmen einsetzen, ist alles noch vollständig reversibel.

Die Haut wird grau oder weißlich, oft nimmt sie Wachsfarbe an. Das Gewebe kann enorm hart werden und ist dann eventuell unbeweglich auf der Unterlage fixiert.

Die Frage nach der Ätiologie eines Kälteschadens scheint vorerst überflüssig zu sein: Ein Umgebungsfaktor — niedrige Temperatur bzw. Kälte — löst die Störungen aus. In der Tat treten Erfrierungen vorwiegend nach länger dauerndem Kontakt mit Kältegraden beim und unter dem Nullpunkt auf. Man weiß aber aus Erfahrung, daß die Schädigung nicht immer mit den Kältegraden parallel geht. Es müssen relativ komplizierte Kombinationen von Umweltfaktoren berücksichtigt werden. Der Wärmeentzug wird durch Nässe, Luftfeuchtigkeit und Luftbewegung sehr stark gesteigert. Große Unterschiede ergeben sich auch hinsichtlich der individuellen Veranlagung (Lange); das betroffene Individuum reagiert oft mit abnormen Gefäßreaktionen. Derartige Veranlagungen können angeboren, konstitutionell verankert sein, oft sind sie aber erworben. Besonders Individuen, die schon zu einem früheren Zeitpunkt einen Frostschaden erlitten haben, ertragen in der Regel weitere Kältetraumen außerordentlich schlecht.

Zu den bei der Prophylaxe oft vernachlässigten Faktoren gehören der Kälteschutz durch richtige Bekleidung und die Möglichkeit genügender Blutzirkulation. Diese ist meist ebenfalls eine Frage zweckmäßiger Bekleidung und Beschuhung. Man wundert sich, daß die Lehren der Vergangenheit oft vergessen werden. Im zweiten Weltkrieg kam es wegen mangelhafter Prophylaxe bei den Beständen der USA-Army zu 91000 Fällen von Kälteschäden (Whaine). Über die Verluste der Deutschen Armeen in den Winterfeldzügen sind lediglich Schätzungen verhanden.

Eindrücklich ist die Erfahrung einer schweizerischen Gebirgsformation, die Debrunner mitteilt. Während eines Aufstieges von 20,5 km Länge mit 1470 m Höhenunterschied, für den 10 Std gebraucht wurden, fiel das Thermometer in den letzten Stunden des Marsches von —5° auf —18° C. Am Bestimmungsort angelangt, wiesen 27,4% der Beteiligten Kälteschäden auf, ein deutliches Beispiel für das Versagen prophylaktischer Maßnahmen und für die falsche Beurteilung der Umweltfaktoren durch die militärischen Führer.

Als weitere Faktoren sind Müdigkeit, Unterernährung und individuelle Resistenzunterschiede zu nennen. Sie spielen besonders dann eine große Rolle, wenn es sich um Kälteschäden bei Temperaturbereichen über der Nullgradgrenze handelt. Besonders gefürchtet ist der Bereich zwischen +5° und +15° C, weil sich hier, wo die Warnung durch den Kälteschmerz oft wegfällt, schleichende Schäden entwickeln können. Unter derartigen Bedingungen entsteht besonders häufig der „Schützengrabenfuß“.

Bei Schiffbrüchigen wurden sogar im Temperaturbereich des Golfstromes (15,6—21,1° C) Kälteschäden, die nach 8 Tagen bis zur Gangrän fortschritten, beobachtet. In der englischen Literatur wird für diese Schäden der Ausdruck „*Immersion foot*“ verwendet; er ist dem Begriff „Schützengrabenfuß“ nachgebildet. Hierhergehörige Beobachtungen sind vor allem auch bei Kampfhandlungen in subtropischen Gebieten gemacht worden (Brownrigg, Ungley, Blackwood, Jochim, White).

Kurze Erwähnung verdienen auch die Zirkulationsstörungen, die in England als „Schutzraum-Beine“ (Shelter legs) 1940 nach Einsetzen des Blitzkrieges beschrieben worden sind (Knight). Sie sind aber weniger als Kälteschäden denn als vorübergehende Zirkulationsstörungen und Stauungen zu deuten. Während diese beiden Faktoren beim „Schützengrabenfuß“ nur mitbeteiligt sind, waren sie bei den „Schutzraum-Beinen“ ganz im Vordergrund. Der Aufenthalt in improvisierten kalten Schutzräumen, in der Untergrundbahn, meist unbeweglich in einem mitgebrachten Faltliegestuhl, dessen Querholz in der Kniekehle vermutlich die arterielle und venöse Blutzirkulation stark beeinträchtigte, gehört zur charakteristischen Vorgeschichte. Man beobachtete diese geschwollenen Unterschenkel vorwiegend bei älteren, etwas adipösen Frauen; sie kamen aber bei beiden Geschlechtern vor. Varicosis und Herzinsuffizienz waren bei den Betroffenen nicht häufiger als bei der Normalbevölkerung vorhanden. Eine individuelle Disposition schien keine Rolle zu spielen; man muß daher annehmen, daß die Capillarwände — auch bei völlig gesunden unteren Extremitäten — ihren Tonus nicht unbeschränkt aufrechterhalten können, wenn ohne Unterbrechung durch Lagewechsel oder aktive Bewegung die Schwerkraft auf sie einwirkt.

Nach Beseitigung der Ursachen kam es in allen Fällen zu rascher Besserung der Symptome. Als Ausnahmen sind immerhin die von Simpson beschriebenen Lungenembolien zu erwähnen. Sie wurden in unmittelbarem Anschluß an Nächte, die zu den Schutzraum-Beinen geführt hatten, beobachtet. Die Thromben waren in den tibialen Venen entstanden. Nach langen Eisenbahn-, Auto- oder Flugreisen sind ähnliche Zirkulationsschäden bekanntgeworden. Auch das unbewegliche Sitzen vor dem Fernsehschirm wirkt manchmal gleichartig, so daß die Kälte vermutlich nur zusätzlich bei der Pathogenese der Schutzraum-Beine beteiligt war.

Die Frostschäden in großer Höhe, wie sie beim Flugpersonal beobachtet worden sind, unterscheiden sich nicht von sonstigen Erfrierungen, es sei denn durch ihre besondere Schweregrade (Davis et al.). Die einwirkenden Kältegrade werden mit —40 bis —52° C angegeben, wobei noch hohe Windgeschwindigkeit (200 m je sec) hinzukommen kann. Schon nach kurzdauernder Exposition kann es zu schweren Erfrierungen kommen. Undiszipliniertes Verhalten, kurzfristiges Ausziehen der Handschuhe, Versagen der Heizung in Schutzanzügen u. ä. führen zu diesen Schäden. Subjektiv stehen Parästhesien, Tage bis Wochen andauernd, im Vordergrund. Trockene oder feuchte Gangrän sind auch nach nur kurzen Expositionszeiten beobachtet worden.

III. Pathophysiologie der Erfrierungen

Die Gewebeschäden nach Kälteeinwirkung sind von der Dauer der Exposition und vom Grade der Temperaturverminderung abhängig. Es kommt aber — im Gegensatz zu den Verhältnissen bei Hitzeeinwirkung — *nicht* zu einer Eiweißkoagulation.

Über den pathophysiologischen Mechanismus des Kälteschadens sind zahlreiche neuere Arbeiten erschienen; wir erwähnen vor allem die Autoren Lewis und Kreyberg.

Lewis geht von der Beobachtung aus, daß ein warmer menschlicher Körper, der unbekleidet in einem Raum mit 16,1° C verharrt, zunehmend Wärme verliert. Als Hinweis auf die Rolle der individuellen Veranlagung beim Entstehen von Kälteschäden sei erwähnt, daß bei vielen Personen die Abkühlung schon bei 17,8° C beginnt und bei einigen sogar schon bei 20,0° C. Eine Vasoconstriction, von Kältegefühl und Kontraktion der glatten Hautmuskulatur (Gänsehaut) begleitet, ist die erste Reaktion.

Der Rückfluß von kaltem venösem Blut bewirkt eine allgemeine Abkühlung des Blutes, und diese setzt einen außerordentlich temperaturempfindlichen zentralnervösen Mechanismus in Gang. Alle Oberflächengefäße, inbegriffen Arterien, Arteriolen, Capillaren, Venolen und Venen, sind in diesen Reflexvorgang einbezogen. Im Bestreben, die allgemeine Körpertemperatur bzw. die Kerntemperatur zu erhalten, werden die subcapillären Venengeflechte — welche besonders energisch am Reflex beteiligt sind — selber geopfert. Durch diese maximale Reaktion entsteht ein starker Abfall der Extremitätentemperatur. Während sich ein Glied abkühlt, kontrahieren sich mehr und mehr die regionären Gefäße. Dieser Circulus vitiosus führt zur Angleichung der Extremitätentemperatur an die Umgebungstemperatur.

Lokale Abwehrmechanismen beobachtet man, wenn die Temperatur eines Gliedes 10° C oder weniger erreicht hat. Tast- und Schmerzempfindung sind verlorengegangen. Abwechselnde Vasoconstriction und -dilatation, wahrscheinlich auf Axonreflexen beruhend, lassen in diesem Moment die mittlere Temperatur des exponierten Körperteils nochmals um einige Grade ansteigen.

Die Kälteschädigung bewirkt nach Lewis die Ausschüttung histaminartiger Substanzen, denen eine große Bedeutung für die Auslösung der nun folgenden entzündlichen Phänomene zukomme.

Die Blutgefäße reagieren auf die frei gewordenen Substanzen mit Vasodilatation und erhöhter Capillardurchlässigkeit, also im Sinne einer beginnenden Entzündung. Die klinischen Stadien dieses entzündlichen Prozesses sind lokale Rötung, Quaddel- und Blasenbildung und Rötung der Umgebung im Sinne des Reflexerythems (sog. triple-response). Mit der Plasmatranssudation kommt es zu einer starken Verlangsamung des Blutstromes in den kleinsten Gefäßen. Bei starker Schädigung geht alles Plasma durch die Wandung hindurch verloren. Es bleiben die zelligen Elemente dicht gepackt im Lumen zurück. Sie verhindern die Bewegung wie durch einen mechanischen Verschluß. Es handelt sich anfänglich um echte Stase und nicht um intravasale Gerinnung.

Durch den Sauerstoffmangel entsteht dann Nekrose, und zwar sowohl im Gewebe wie an den in den Gefäßen steckengebliebenen Blutzellen. Prinzipiell hätten wir also eine Summationswirkung von direkter Kälteschädigung und Ischämiefolgen anzunehmen. Über die Theorie der Eiskristallbildung (Rischpler) herrscht keine Einheit; man weiß jedenfalls nicht, ob diesem Vorgang eine besondere Bedeutung zukommt.

Eine gewisse Latenzzeit bei der Manifestation von Erfrierungsschäden erklärt sich durch den Umstand, daß bei kalten Extremitäten die Reaktionen noch ausbleiben. Die biochemischen Prozesse sind verlangsamt, besonders auch weil die Arterien und Arteriolen langdauernd kontrahiert bleiben. Der Schaden entsteht somit früh, wird aber erst relativ spät, wenn sich die Temperatur wieder gehoben hat, manifest.

Die pathophysiologische Theorie von Kreyberg stimmt mit der Auffassung von Lewis überein, nur werden einzelne Etappen eingehender dargestellt und zum Teil subtile Unterschiede des Kolorits beschrieben und mit den zugehörigen pathophysiologischen Vorgängen in Parallele gesetzt.

IV. Pathologische Anatomie

Die pathologisch-anatomischen Veränderungen nach *Erfrierungen* sind besonders für die Endzustände seit langem bekannt (Marchand, Kriege, Sonnenburg und Tschmarke, Weidenfeld, Hecht). Im Anschluß an den zweiten Weltkrieg sind aber neue wichtige Arbeiten erschienen. Ihre Ergebnisse werden zur Hauptsache in der offiziellen amerikanischen Publikation „Cold Injury“ zusammengefaßt. Vor allem bot sich Gelegenheit, die frühen Veränderungen bei Schützengrabenfuß genau zu untersuchen, weil Soldaten, die aus anderen Ursachen ad exitum kamen, diese Veränderungen aufwiesen (Simeone). Man fand Ödem in Subcutis, Nerven und Muskeln, ferner verstreute Rundzelleninfiltrate in der Cutis und besonders um Arteriolen und Capillaren. Die Epidermis zeigte degenerative Veränderungen; eine Atrophie der Schweißdrüsen (cystische Erweiterung und Vacuolisierung) wird besonders hervorgehoben (ADAMS-RAY). In den subcutanen Geweben fand man eine Tendenz zum Fettschwund; in der Subcutis, um Nerven und Gefäße herum und auch in den Wandungen größerer Gefäße war das kollagene Bindegewebe vermehrt. Das elastische Gewebe war anscheinend nicht geschädigt.

In den peripheren Abschnitten der Nerven wurde die Wallersche Degeneration beobachtet. An den Muskelfasern zeigte sich früh eine Degeneration vom Zenker-Typus, die später von Atrophie und Fibrose gefolgt war.

Am Knochen fanden sich unregelmäßige Bezirke von Osteoporose und von Knochenneubildung.

FRIEDMAN berichtet über eingehende pathologisch-anatomische Untersuchungen. Die pathophysiologischen Vorstellungen, die z. T. aus Tierexperimenten gewonnen worden sind (KREYBERG), werden durch die pathologisch-anatomischen Befunde FRIEDMANs fast durchwegs bestätigt.

Besonders hervorgehoben werden von FRIEDMAN Veränderungen am subcutanen Fettgewebe und an den Blutgefäßen. Die Veränderungen am *Fettgewebe* gehören im weiteren Sinne zur Gruppe der Fettgewebsentzündung, deren Pathogenese noch unklar isr, besonders weil die Anfangsstadien nur selten zur Beobachtung gelangen. Die frühen in dieser Richtung untersuchten Erfrierungsfälle zeigten leukocytäre Infiltration, und zwar auch dann, wenn das darüberliegende Gewebe nicht betroffen schien. Es wird daraus eine besondere Empfindlichkeit des Fettgewebes gegenüber der Kälte abgeleitet. Im Hinblick auf die ausgeprägten Störungen der Blutzirkulation erscheint es gerechtfertigt, für die Fettgewebsveränderungen bei Erfrierungen eine ischämische Genese anzunehmen. Die Ischämie könnte bei der Fettgewebspathologie überhaupt eine größere Rolle spielen, als bisher angenommen wird.

An den Blutgefäßen wird in Frühfällen eine starke Füllung beobachtet, wobei es zu Extravasaten kommt. Zahlreiche Gefäße enthalten Erythrocyten-Thromben. Es waren keine sicheren Endothelläsionen anzutreffen, hingegen Entzündungszeichen innerhalb der Wandungen. Neben zahlreichen dilatierten, entzündeten oder thrombosierten Gefäßen konnte man auch maximal kontrahierte auffinden; dies war auch für die arteriellen Hauptstämme der Fall, und zwar bis weit proximal der Demarkationslinie des Kälteschadens.

In später untersuchten Fällen (z. B. 40 Tage nach dem Kältetrauma) waren alle Thromben organisiert. Endangitis obliterans war in Venen und Arterien zu finden, wieder auch in Gewebebezirken proximal der Demarkationslinie. Die Veränderungen wechselten von leichter Intimaverdickung bis zur Obliteration des Lumens und Rekanalisation. Die Tunica elastica war meist intakt geblieben. Venen waren weniger regelmäßig befallen als Arterien.

Die Veränderungen an den Muskeln, Nerven und Knochen entsprachen ungefähr denjenigen, wie sie SIMEONE beobachten konnte.

PANCHENKO, ein russischer Autor, schildert ischämische Neuritis und intensive Fibroblastenhyperplasie und -hypertrophie am perineuralen Gewebe bis ins Rückenmark und in die Medulla in denjenigen Bezirken, die dem Innervationsgebiet der geschädigten Zonen entsprachen. Die pathologisch-anatomischen Veränderungen lassen sich zusammenfassen als Störungen der Blutzirkulation bis zur Stagnation und Thrombose. Die Verschlüsse führen zur Gangrän. Das Bild erinnert ganz an die periphere ischämische Nekrose, kombiniert mit Sekundärinfektion. Gewisse ungewöhnliche Befunde sind besonders hervorzuheben: die weitverbreitete Agglutinationsthrombose, die schweren Veränderungen am Fettgewebe und die interessanten Nerven-, Muskeln- und Knochenveränderungen. Gewebsstrukturen, die stark lipoidhaltig sind (Fettgewebe und myelinisierte Nervenfasern) scheinen eine besondere Anfälligkeit gegenüber dem Kälteschaden aufzuweisen.

V. Therapie der Erfrierungen

Die Behandlung der Kälteschäden hat sich im Laufe der letzten Jahrzehnte nur wenig gewandelt. Die schweren Schäden kommen zur Hauptsache durch Verschlüsse der kleinen und größeren Blutgefäße zustande. Der Kreislauf und die Ernährung der Gewebe können sich aber oft weitgehend erholen; der Grundsatz des abwartend-konservativen Vorgehens wird darum bestehenbleiben.

Wir besprechen getrennt

1. die Sofortmaßnahmen bei der Bergung,
2. die abwartende Behandlung,
3. die chirurgischen Eingriffe,
4. neuere Behandlungsvorschläge,
   a) antikoagulierende Therapie,
   b) Eingriffe am Sympathicus,
5. Prophylaxe.

1. Die Sofortmaßnahmen bei und nach der Bergung

Es herrschte längere Zeit Unklarheit über das richtige Vorgehen beim Wiedererwärmen erfrorener Glieder. Wenn man experimentelle Untersuchungen, Gebirgs- und Kriegserfahrungen berücksichtigt, lassen sich doch allgemeingültige Regeln aufstellen.

Wenn der Gerettete seine Füße zum Überleben noch braucht — im Krieg zum Marsch in eine Deckung oder Erreichen einer Schutzhütte im Gebirge —, so dürfen die Füße vorher nicht aufgetaut werden. Ein Auftauen und erneutes Erfrieren ist unter allen Umständen zu vermeiden.

Sobald sich Gelegenheit bietet, werden erfrorene Körperteile im Wasserbad aufgetaut und erwärmt. Man beginnt bei Zimmertemperatur und erwärmt langsam. Am Schluß sollen Temperaturen über der Körpertemperatur, aber nicht wärmer als 40—42° C erreicht werden. Das früher übliche Auftauen mit Eiswasser, auch das Abreiben mit Schnee sind verlassen worden. Strahlende Wärme ist ebenfalls kontraindiziert.

Die allgemeine Unterkühlung dagegen soll, im Gegensatz zur lokalen Erfrierung, durch rasches trockenes Erwärmen behandelt werden (BINHOLD).

Früher wurde oft auf die Zerbrechlichkeit tief gefrorener Glieder hingewiesen; es scheint aber keine besondere Gefahr zu bestehen. Nur ausnahmsweise wurde das Abbrechen ganz steif gefrorener Ohren oder eines Fingers beschrieben.

2. Die abwartende Behandlung

In der zweiten Phase der Behandlung gilt es, die Erholung bzw. die Demarkation drittgradig erfrorener Gewebe abzuwarten. Blasen läßt man intakt. Grundsätzlich wendet man die offene Behandlungsmethode mit bequemer Lagerung auf Schienen an. Hochlagerung zur Bekämpfung des Ödems scheint sich sehr gut zu bewähren. Die Gelenke müssen von Anfang an viel bewegt werden. Die Finger werden in einer Mittelstellung gelagert. Bei sehr starkem Ödem wurden multiple Incisionen empfohlen (SAUERBRUCH).

Man versucht vor allem, die Infektion mit gefährlichen Keimen zu verhüten; dazu dienen Anstriche mit desinfizierenden Lösungen (Mercurochrom), Bäder mit desinfizierenden Zusätzen, ferner die offene Behandlung, weil dabei das Auftreten einer Infektion rascher erkannt wird. Partien, die vermutlich drittgradig geschädigt sind, werden mit desinfizierenden, austrocknenden Pudern behandelt. Sulfonamid-Puder, aber auch Puder mit Antibiotica-Zusätzen haben sich bewährt.

Wenn es gelingt, eine trockene Gangrän zu erhalten, wird weiterhin abgewartet, bis sich die Demarkation deutlich zeigt. Die Ablösung der Schorfe erfolgt spontan, sie darf in gewissen Stadien durch Bäder und kleinere chirurgische Maßnahmen beschleunigt werden. So lange wie möglich soll man aber die Spontanheilung mit Granulation und Epithelisierung abwarten. Sind größere Wundflächen vorhanden und ist eine spontane Epithelisation nicht zu erwarten, können dünne Hautübertragungen versucht werden.

3. Die chirurgischen Eingriffe

Wenn größere Teile, ganze Finger und Zehen dem Brand verfallen sind, versucht man, sich durch eine Röntgenaufnahme über den Zustand der Knochen ein Urteil zu bilden. Die Demarkationslinie verläuft oft mitten durch knöcherne Partien hindurch. Nach einigen Monaten schreitet man zur Amputation mit dem Ziel, möglichst belastungsfähige und gut brauchbare Stümpfe zu erhalten. Es gibt nur einen Grund zum früheren Eingreifen: die drohende Sepsis, ausgehend von Lymphangitis und septischer Thrombose. Durch die wirksamen modernen Antibiotica ist aber dieser Gefahr relativ leicht zu begegnen.

4. Neuere Behandlungsvorschläge

Weil Stase und Thrombose in der Pathogenese der Erfrierung eine so wichtige Rolle spielen, wird man — mindestens theoretisch — sowohl von einer *antikoagulierenden Behandlung* als auch von *Eingriffen am Sympathicus* etwas erwarten dürfen.

Schon LERICHE hat die günstige Wirkung der Sympathicus-Blockade bei Erfrierungen hervorgehoben. Plexusanaesthesie für den Arm und Lumbalanaesthesie für das Bein werden auch von GOLDHAHN als das beste Mittel in Feldverhältnissen gerühmt. Die Sympathektomie kann als vielversprechendes Verfahren versucht werden; ein abschließendes Urteil ist nach den bisherigen Berichten noch nicht möglich.

Wegen der starken Vasoconstriction als Antwort auf die Kälte sind ab und zu vasodilatierende Medikamente empfohlen worden. Ihre Anwendung ist aber gefährlich, weil unterkühltes Blut in die Zirkulation gelangt, das sekundär über nervöse Zentren eine verstärkte Vasoconstriction auslösen kann.

5. Prophylaxe

Aufklärung der Truppe und ständige Überwachung der prophylaktischen Maßnahmen sind wichtige Aufgaben für Truppenärzte und Gebirgsoffiziere.

In erster Linie sind genaue Instruktionen über die Pflege der Füße, des Schuhwerks und der Socken zu verlangen. Der „Schützengrabenfuß“ ist ein geeignetes Beispiel zur allgemein verständlichen Erläuterung der Entstehungsweise von Kälteschädigungen bei Temperaturen über dem Gefrierpunkt. In der amerikanischen Armee hat man mit humoristischen Zeichnungen über das richtige und falsche Verhalten des Soldaten in bezug auf Erfrierungsprophylaxe offenbar beste Erfahrungen gemacht.

C. Kälte als Mitursache von Hautkrankheiten

Bei der Besprechung der Pathophysiologie der Erfrierungsschäden wurde auf die von zahlreichen Autoren hervorgehobene Tatsache hingewiesen, daß die Reaktionen des Organismus auf Kälte stark von individuellen Faktoren abhängig sind. Sehr oft ist eine erhöhte Anfälligkeit vegetativer Dystoniker beschrieben worden. Bei den Kälteschädigungen im engeren Sinne ist aber eindeutig ein mehr oder weniger akutes Kältetrauma im Vordergrund, und der individuelle Faktor liegt noch innerhalb der Variationsbreite der Norm. Im folgenden soll kurz eine Gruppe von Krankheitsbildern besprochen werden, bei denen teils konstitutionelle, teils erworbene Faktoren eindeutig dominieren, und erst ein Terrain schaffen, das auf chronische, durch den gesunden Organismus kompensierte Kältereize mit besonderen Krankheitssymptomen reagiert. Die bereits besprochenen Krankheitsbilder Schützengrabenfuß und Eintauchfuß nehmen eine Zwischenstellung ein und können zum Teil diesem Kapitel zugerechnet werden.

I. Angiopathien

Eine erste Gruppe von Krankheitsbildern soll behelfsweise unter diesen Begriff zusammengefaßt werden. Es handelt sich im wesentlichen um Angiolopathien und Angioneurosen (nach der Einteilung von Ratschow). Sie werden ganz vorwiegend an den Extremitäten beobachtet; offenbar funktionieren dabei die physiologischen Adaptationsmechanismen auf chronische Kältereize nur ungenügend. Die ausführliche Besprechung dieser Krankheitsbilder — der Akrocyanosis, Raynaudschen Krankheit, Perniosis, Erythrocyanosis crurum puellarum und einiger seltener Formen — hat im Kapitel über periphere Zirkulationsstörungen zu erfolgen.

1. Perniosis und Erythrocyanosis crurum puellarum

Am eindeutigsten faßbar ist die ätiologische Bedeutung der Kälte bei der *Perniosis* und der *Erythrocyanosis crurum puellarum.* Die beiden Krankheitsbilder sind im Prinzip identisch (Lewis).

Die Pernionen (Frostbeulen, Chiblains) sind mit Vorliebe an den Fingern und Handrücken, ferner an den Füßen und Ohrmuscheln (Ohrperniosis von Dittrich), seltener an den Innenseiten der Knie (Beck) lokalisiert. Sie beginnen als rötliche bis cyanotische Flecken; in der Folge entwickeln sich juckende und stechende polsterförmige teigig-infiltrierte Vorwölbungen. Relativ häufig wird zentrale Ulceration beobachtet, ab und zu können auch Hyperkeratosen auftreten (Sézary, Flandin).

Der konstitutionelle Faktor tritt in einer deutlichen Disposition des weiblichen Geschlechts zutage (Jausion, Jansson).

Als typisch gilt die Exacerbation in den Übergangsmonaten zwischen warmer und kalter Jahreszeit, dann nämlich, wenn die thermoregulatorischen Funktionen am stärksten beansprucht werden. Das Vorliegen einer Zirkulationsstörung läßt sich daran erkennen, daß die Extremitäten bei befallenen Individuen eine herabgesetzte Hauttemperatur zeigen, und zwar nicht nur bei kaltem Wetter. Burckhardt fand bei experimenteller Abkühlung eine verlangsamte Wiedererwärmung, Jarret ein Ausbleiben der Vasoconstriction unter Kälteeinwirkung. Hier läßt sich auch die Beobachtung anführen, daß bei Krankheiten, die mit schlechter Blutzirkulation einhergehen, wie z. B. der Poliomyelitis und der Syringomyelie, häufig Pernionen auftreten können (Lewis, Nékám) (Abb. 11).

Abb. 11. Asymmetrische Erythrocyanosis crurum bei Status nach Poliomyelitis

Abb. 12. Erythrocyanosis crurum puellarum bei einer 25jährigen Frau. Die medialen Seiten der Knieregion sind besonders stark befallen

Abb. 13. Erythrocyanosis crurum puellarum bei einer 19jährigen Frau mit Perniosis follicularis der Oberschenkel

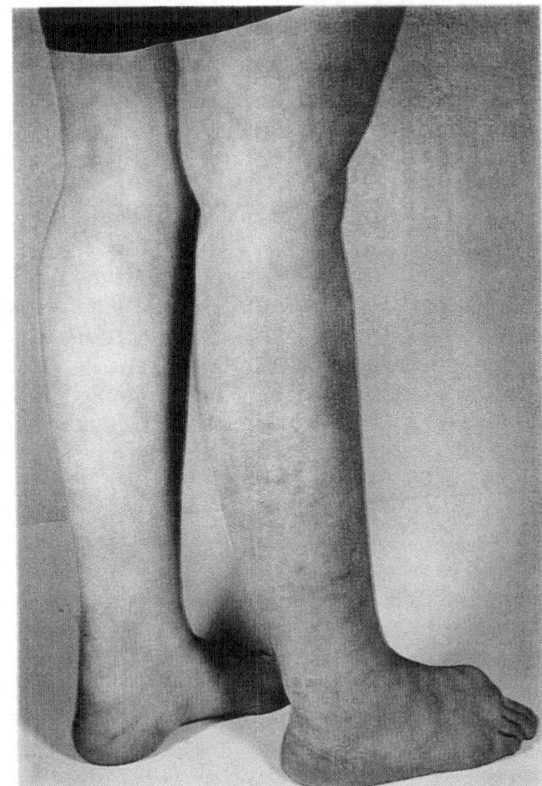

Abb. 11

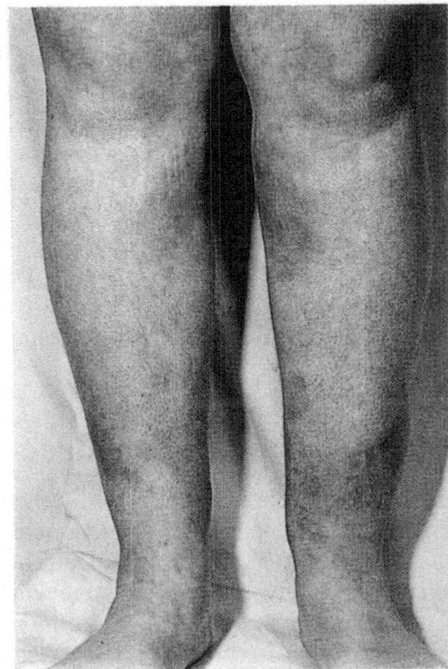

Abb. 12

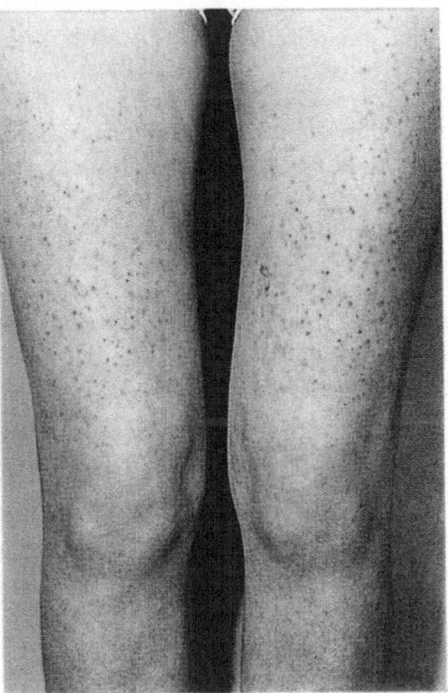

Abb. 13

Es scheint, daß der Sitz der primären Funktionsstörung im Bereich des venösen Anteils der Endstrombahn liegt (Merlen, Schoop). Die Theorie einer tuberkulösen Ätiologie der Perniosis (Stephani-Cherbuliez 1936) findet heute kaum mehr Befürworter. Im histologischen Bild dominieren Gefäßveränderungen: Vasodilation, Thrombenbildung, entzündliche Infiltration (Gans 1925). Zusätzlich können oft entzündliche oder degenerative Veränderungen am subcutanen Fettgewebe beobachtet werden (Dittrich, McGovern). Die frühesten Veränderungen treten in topographischer Beziehung zu den Follikeln auf (Pernio follicularis) (Abb. 13).

Die Erythrocyanosis crurum puellarum befällt ausschließlich Frauen jugendlichen Alters (12—25 Jahre). Der Kältefaktor wird durch die Lokalisation besonders veranschaulicht: Die Veränderungen nehmen symmetrisch die durch Kleidungsstücke kaum geschützten Teile der Unterschenkel ein, so daß man für diese Erkrankung auch die Bezeichnung „Seidenstrumpf-Dermatitis“ vorgeschlagen hat. Das Tragen von langen Hosen bringt immer eine weitgehende Besserung mit sich. Andererseits besteht eine starke Bevorzugung des adipösen Typus, was auf eine hormonelle Dysfunktion als möglichen ätiologischen Faktor hinweist.

Die klinisch wichtigsten Merkmale sind neben den bereits erwähnten eine verminderte Hauttemperatur an den befallenen Stellen und eine pastöse bis derbelastische Konsistenzvermehrung der Haut. Oft treten nach längerem Bestehen trophische Störungen in Form von Hyperkeratosis follicularis, Hypo- oder Hypertrichose hinzu.

Therapeutisch können, außer dem Tragen warmer Kleider, gefäßerweiternde Mittel (z. B. Trafuril R) und ichthyolhaltige Salben versucht werden. Als seltenes, mit der Perniosis verwandtes Krankheitsbild sei die *Induratio congelativa submentalis* (Hochsinger) erwähnt.

2. Akrocyanosis, Digitus mortuus, Raynaudsche Krankheit, Cutis marmorata

Viel umstrittener ist die Bedeutung des Faktors Kälte bei den Krankheitsbildern der *Akrocyanosis*, des *Digitus mortuus* (Reil), der *Raynaudschen Krankheit* und der sog. *Cutis marmorata e frigore* (Livedo reticularis). Sicher darf man bei diesen Formen eine gesteigerte Kälteempfindlichkeit annehmen, wie der von Kuske et al. beschriebene Fall einer Kombination von Raynaud-Krisen mit einer Perniosis zeigt, doch ist die Kälteeinwirkung hier nicht einmal mehr als auslösender Faktor im engeren Sinne zu betrachten.

Für die organischen Angiopathien ist eine ätiologische Bedeutung von chronischen thermischen Einflüssen weitgehend abzulehnen (Buerger, Hines). Dagegen können nach schweren Erfrierungen Gefäßveränderungen auftreten, die sich nicht von einer Endangitis obliterans (Winiwarter-Buerger) unterscheiden lassen (Siegmund, Stämmler).

II. Kälteurticaria und verwandte Krankheitsbilder

Duke hat 1925 den Begriff der physikalischen Allergie eingeführt. Er definiert sie als Antworten auf physikalische Noxen, die den allergischen Reaktionen auf die üblichen Antigene (wie Pollen, Arzneimittel u. a.) ähnlich sind. Die Kälteurticaria, die hier eingeordnet werden muß, war allerdings schon lange vorher bekannt. Nach örtlich begrenzter oder auch allgemeiner Abkühlung können an der Haut Erytheme, Quaddeln, Quincke-Ödem auftreten, wobei diese Erscheinungen oft auch mit schweren Störungen des Allgemeinbefindens einhergehen.

Die Temperaturschwelle, unterhalb welcher die Reaktion einsetzt, ist individuell etwas verschieden. In vitro entfalten die Kälteagglutinine ihre größte Wirksamkeit zwischen —2° und +8° C (BASSALLECK). Besonders gefährdet sind die Träger dieser Krankheit beim Baden in kaltem Wasser, weil ein „Kälteschock" mit Kollaps, Nausea, Bewußtlosigkeit und Glottisödem auftreten kann (WILDER; SAYLOR und WRIGHT).

Das hier beschriebene Krankheitsbild stellt keine nosologische Einheit dar, und man würde besser vom Symptom „Kälteurticaria" sprechen. Pathogenetisch kommen nämlich verschiedene Mechanismen in Betracht; daraus ergibt sich etwa folgende Einteilung:

a) Kälteurticaria im engeren Sinne,
b) Kryoglobulinämie und Kälteagglutininkrankheit,
c) paroxysmale Kältehämoglobinurie.

Diese Einteilung ist nur als Hilfsmittel aufzufassen und darf nicht zu streng angewandt werden; es sind öfters kombinierte Formen, z. B. Kälteurticaria mit Hämoglobinurie, beschrieben worden (HARRIS et al.).

Für die *Kälteurticaria im engeren Sinne* ist noch nicht bewiesen, daß es sich in allen Fällen um einen echten allergischen Vorgang handelt (URBACH und GOTTLIEB). Vor allem zwei Theorien werden diskutiert: Nach der einen liegt eine Reaktion auf Histamin vor (SAYLOR und WRIGHT; HEIDELMANN; GARAN et al.). Nach der anderen erfolgt eine Sensibilisierung gegen einen Wirkstoff, dessen Bildung durch die Kälteeinwirkung angeregt wird („sekundäres" Antigen).

Die passive Übertragung nach PRAUSNITZ-KÜNSTNER eines kälteaktiven Hämolysins gelingt lange nicht in allen, aber doch in vielen Fällen (WEISSENBACH; LEHNER; HARRIS et al.; STEINHARDT, SHERMAN und SEEBOHM; SAMSØE-JENSEN). Nur für diese möchte LONGHIN die Bezeichnung „essentielle Kälteurticaria" reservieren, wobei zusätzlich folgende Kriterien verlangt werden: Fehlen von Kryoglobulinen und Anfall der eosinophilen Leukocyten im Blut. Bei dem von SHELLEY und WALLACE (1962) mitgeteilten und als neues Syndrom („Cold erythema") beschriebenen Fall von ekzessiver Kälteüberempfindlichkeit konnten weder Kryoglobuline noch Agglutinine oder Hämolysine nachgewiesen werden. Nach JUHLIN und SHELLEY, die eine dominant vererbte von einer erworbenen Form unterscheiden, gelingt der passive Übertragungsversuch nur bei der zweiten. Selten wird das Auftreten einer Kälteurticaria im Zusammenhang mit Nahrungs- oder Arzneimittelallergien beobachtet (WISEMAN).

Als Behandlungsmaßnahmen werden die spezifische Desensibilisierung (DUKE; LEHNER; RAJKA; WIEST) entweder in Form von progressiv gesteigerten Kältereizen oder von Histamininjektionen (BRAY), ferner Herdsanierung, Antihistaminica (KÖLBL) und neuerdings Penicillin (OBERMAYER 1963) empfohlen.

Auch diejenigen Fälle von Kälteüberempfindlichkeit, bei denen durch die Serumuntersuchungen die Anwesenheit von Kryoproteinen oder Kälteagglutininen aufgedeckt wird, gehen mit Hauterscheinungen einher. Diese sind Folge einer intravasalen Hämagglutination und bestehen in diffusen bis retikulierten bläulichen Verfärbungen der exponierten Bezirke, namentlich der Hände und des Gesichtes. Quaddeln oder Ulcerationen (GRUMBERS; NELSON; AUPAIX; VILANOVA) treten weniger häufig auf. RODER beobachtete einen Fall von *Purpura* necroticans bei Kryoglobulinämie.

Als charakteristisches Zeichen der Dysproteinämie findet man eine extrem hohe Senkungsgeschwindigkeit der Erythrocyten. Die Kryoglobuline wandern meist mit der γ-Globulin-Fraktion. Die Kryoglobulinämie kommt entweder als idiopathische Erkrankung (McKENZIE) oder häufiger im Zusammenhang mit einer Grundkrankheit, z. B. einem Plasmacytom (LANGHOF et al.; JIRKOVA und KOUDOUSEK), einer Retikulose (JOHNSTON und WALLACE), vor. Die Kombination mit Erythematodes chronicus (CHORAZAK) ist umstritten (GENTELE et al.).

Gut bekannt ist dagegen die postinfektiös nach Viruspneumonien auftretende akute passagere Form der Kälteagglutininkrankheit. Aber auch nach anderen Virusaffektionen, z. B. nach Zoster, findet sich oft ein erhöhter Kälteagglutinin-Titer (PEIFFER).

Abdominelle Symptome (Bauchkrämpfe mit Erbrechen und Durchfall) nach Genuß kalter Getränke und Glacen sind in der Literatur mehrfach erwähnt (HADORN). Gewöhnlich wird auch eine Hämoglobinurie festgestellt. Eine sicher wirksame Behandlung ist nicht bekannt; am ehesten scheinen Corticosteroide zu nützen (WIRTSCHAFTER).

Paroxysmale Kältehämoglobinurie tritt häufig zusammen mit urticariellen Hauterscheinungen auf; dagegen fehlt die für die intravasale Agglutination charakteristische akrocyanotische Kompoente. Das verantwortliche Hämolysin reagiert, im Gegensatz zu den Antikörpern der Kryoglobulinämie und Kälteagglutininkrankheit, bithermisch, d. h. die Hämolyse erfolgt erst nach Wiedererwärmung. Die Methodik des serologischen Nachweises wurde von SCHUBOTHE ausführlich erörtert.

Die seltene Erkrankung kommt fast nur bei Syphilitikern vor, und die Penicillinbehandlung führt meist zu einer wesentlichen Besserung (CATTAN, PREBBLE).

III. Dermatosen im engeren Sinne

Eine Verschlimmerung während der kalten Jahreszeit wird häufig auch bei den folgenden Hautkrankheiten beobachtet:

Erythema induratum Bazin,
Erythematodes chronicus discoides,
Ichthyosisgruppe,
Ekzemgruppe (vor allem Handekzeme).

Literatur

A. Verbrennungen und Verbrühungen

ABBOTT, W. E., M. A. PILLING, G. E. GRIFFIN, J. W. HIRSHFELD, and F. L. MEYER: Metabolic alterations following thermal burns. V. The use of whole blood and an electrolyte solution in the treatment of burned patients. Ann. Surg. **122**, 678 (1945). — AHNEFELD, F. W.: Ist die Ablehnung der Tannintherapie bei Verbrennungen berechtigt? Mschr. Unfallheilk. **57**, 207 (1954). Zit. Zbl. Haut- u. Geschl.-Kr. **90**, 214 (1954/55). — Die Erstbehandlung von Verbrennungsschäden im Katastrophenfall. Wehrmed. Mitt. **1961**, 145. Zit. Zbl. Haut- u. Geschl.-Kr. **114**, 27 (1963). — ALLEN, H. S., and S. L. KOCH: The treatment of patients with severe burns. Surg. Gynec. Obstet. **74**, 914 (1942). Zit. Zbl. Haut- u. Geschl.-Kr. **70**, 661 (1943/44). — ALLGÖWER, M.: Pathogenese und Klinik verschiedener Schockzustände. Ther. Umsch. **2**, 70 (1960). — ALLGÖWER, M., u. J. SIEGRIST: Verbrennungen, Pathophysiologie, Pathologie, Klinik, Therapie. Berlin-Göttingen-Heidelberg: Springer 1957. — ANDREESEN, M. N., u. E. KRÜGER: Praktische Erfahrungen in der Behandlung von schweren Körperverbrennungen bei Explosionsunglücken im Bergbau. Chirurg **23**, 193 (1952). — ARTZ, C. P., J. M. BECKER, Y. SAKO, and A. W. BROWNELL: Postmortem skin homografts in the treatment of extensive burns. Arch. Surg. **71**, 682 (1955). — ARTZ, C. P., and E. REISS: The treatment burns. Philadelphia and London: W. B. Saunders Co. 1957. — ARTZ, C. P., E. REISS, J. H. DAVIS jr., and W. H. AMSPACHER: The exposure treatment of burns. Ann. Surg. **137**, 456 (1953). Zit. Zbl. Haut- u. Geschl.-Kr. **87**, 229 (1954).

BAAR, S.: Studies on urinary peptides isolated from patients suffering from burns. J. clin. Path. **9**, 144 (1956). Zit. Zbl. Haut- u. Geschl.-Kr. **96**, 296 (1956). — BALIKOV, B., R. A. CASTELLO, and E. R. LONZANO: Urinary peptide excretion in the burned patient. Clin. Chem. **3**, 217 (1957). Zit. Zbl. Haut- u. Geschl.-Kr. **100**, 311 (1957). — BÉNITTE, A.: Pharmakologische

Hybernation. Experimentelle Grundlagen. Naunyn-Schmiedebergs Arch. exp. Path. Pharmak. **222/223**, 20 (1954). — BENNETT jr., J. L., and L. E. CLUFF: Zit. nach W. W. SPINK. — BENTHIEN, C.: Klinische Erfahrungen bei der Anwendung neuer Mittel zur örtlichen Behandlung von Verbrennungen. Med. Klin. **1951**, 576. Zit. Zbl. Haut- u. Geschl.-Kr. **79**, 253 (1952). BERGAMASCO, A.: Terapia locale delle ustioni. Minerva derm. **3/4**, 276 (1958). — BERGENTZ, S. E., L. E. GELIN, C. M. RUDENSTAM, and B. ZEDERFELDT: Indications for the use of low viscous dectran in surgery. Acta chir. scand. **122**, 343 (1961). — BERKOW, S. G.: A method of estimating the extensiveness of lesions (burns and scalds) based on surface area proportions. Arch. Surg. **8**, 138 (1924). — BIGGER, J. A.: Hypertonische Na-Chloridlösung, intravenös injiziert, in der Behandlung ausgebreiteter oberflächlicher Verbrennungen. Sth. med. J. (Bgham, Ala.) **19**, 302 (1926). Zit. Zbl. Haut- u. Geschl.-Kr. **21**, 850 (1927). — BLALOCK, A.: Experimental shock. VII. The importance of the local loss of fluid in the production of the low blood pressure after burns. Arch. Surg. **22**, 610 (1931). — BLECK, E. E.: Causes of burns in children. J. Amer. med. Ass. **158**, 100 (1955). — BLOCKER jr., T. G., V. BLOCKER, S. R. LEWIS, and C. C. SNYDER: An approach to the problem of burn sepsis with the use of open-air therapy. Ann. Surg. **134**, 574 (1951). Zit. Zbl. Haut- u. Geschl.-Kr. **83**, 367 (1953). — BÖHLER, J.: Die allgemeine und öffentliche Behandlung schwerer Verbrennungen. (72. Tagg Dtsch. Ges. für Chir., München 13.—16. 4. 55.) Langenbecks Arch. klin. Chir. **282**, 116 u. Diskussion 140 (1955). Zit. Zbl. Haut- u. Geschl.-Kr. **95**, 110 (1956). — BROOKS, J. W., P. ROBINETT, T. L. LARGEN, and E. J. EVANS: A standard contact burn. Method of production and observation on the blood picture following its production in dogs. Surg. Gynec. Obstet. **93**, 543 (1951). — BRUNNER, E. P.: Hypovolämischer Schock durch internen Plasmaverlust. Inaug.-Diss. Zürich 1963. Bern: Hallwag. — BRUNNER, U.: Die Strahlentherapie der Keloide. Zürcher Erfahrungen an 104 Fällen der Jahre 1926—1955. Diss. med. Zürich 1955. — BUCHBORN, E.: Schock und Kollaps. In: Handbuch der inneren Medizin, 4. Aufl., Bd. IX/1. Berlin-Göttingen-Heidelberg: Springer 1960. — BÜRKLE DE LA CAMP, H.: Die allgemeine und örtliche Behandlung der Verbrennungskrankheit. Dtsch. med. J. **4**, 203 (1957). — BUIS, L. J., u. F. W. HARTMANN: Die Histopathologie der Leber nach oberflächlichen Verbrennungen. Amer. J. clin. Path. **11**, 275 (1941). — BULL, J. P.: Shock caused by burns and its treatment. Brit. med. Bull. **10**, 9 (1954). Zit. Zbl. Haut- u. Geschl.-Kr. **90**, 112 (1954/55). — BURRI, C., u. M. ALLGÖWER: Die Wirksamkeit zweier Plasmaexpander im experimentellen Verbrennungsschock. Schweiz. med. Wschr. **24**, 816 (1964).

CHASE, C. H.: New eschar technique for local treatment of burns. Surg. Gynec. Obstet. **85**, 308 (1947). Zit. Zbl. Haut- u. Geschl.-Kr. **72**, 129 (1948). — CHOY, D. S. J., and W. E. WENDT: A new local treatment of burns. U.S. armed Forces med. J. **3**, 1241 (1952). Zit. Zbl. Haut- u. Geschl.-Kr. **84**, 313 (1953). — CLARK, A. G., and J. H. HANSON: Mortality rates in patients with burns: A report of experience at San Francisco City and County Hospital, 1943—1956. Calif. Med. **89**, 210 (1958). Zit. J. Amer. med. Ass. **168**, 1773 (1958). — COLEBROOK, L.: Care of burned people. Plea for new policy. Lancet **1947 II**, 217. — A new approach to the treatment of burns and scalds. Fine technical publications. Cambridge 1950. — The prevention of burning accidents in England and America. Bull. N.Y. Acad. Med. **27**, 425 (1951). — Outstanding problems in the treatment of burns. Lancet **1951 II**, 273. Zit. Zbl. Haut- u. Geschl.-Kr. **80**, 163 (1952). — Die Therapie von Verbrennungen und Verbrühungen in einem modernen Behandlungszentrum. Triangel III/5, 195 (1958). — COLEBROOK, L., and V. COLEBROOK: The prevention of burns and scalds. Review of 1000 cases. Lancet **1949 II**, 181. — COLEBROOK, L., V. COLEBROOK, J. P. BULL, and D. M. JACKSON: The prevention of burning accidents. A survey of the present position. Brit. med. J. **1956 I**, 1379. — COLEBROOK, L., and A. M. HOOD: Infection through soaked dressings. Lancet **1948 II**, 682. — COLYER, B. L., J. J. COX, and E. H. VOGEL: Principles of nursing care in the management of burns. U.S. armed Forces med. J. **10**, 1428 (1959). — COOPER, G. R., G. B. HODGE, and J. W. BEARD: Enzymatic débridement in local treatment of burns, preliminary report. Amer. J. Dis. Child. **65**, 909 (1943). — COPE, O., and F. D. MOORE: A study of capillary permeability in experimental burns and burn shock using radioactive dyes in blood and lymph. J. clin. Invest. **23**, 241 (1944). — The redistribution of body water and the fluid therapy of the burned patient. Ann. Surg. **126**, 1010 (1947). — CORDICE, J., J. E. SUESS, and J. SCUDDER: Polyvinylpyrrolidone in severe burn shock. Surg. Gynec. Obstet. **97**, 39 (1953). — CURLING, TH. B.: On acute ulceration of the duodenum in cases of burns. Med. chir. transactions **25**, 250 (1842). — CURTIS, R. M., J. H. BREWER, and J. W. ROSE jr.: New technique for local treatment of burns. J. Amer. med. Ass. **147**, 741 (1951). Zit. Zbl. Haut- u. Geschl.-Kr. **81**, 299 (1952).

DRINKER, C. K.: Zit. nach MONSAINGEON. — DUESBERG, R.: Die Verbrennungskrankheit. Hefte Unfallheilk. **47**, 27 u. Diskussion 65 (1954). Zit. Zbl. Haut- u. Geschl.-Kr. **88**, 254 (1954). — DUESBERG, R., u. M. SCHRÖDER: Pathophysiologie und Klinik der Kollapszustände. Leipzig: S. Hirzel 1944. — DUPUYTREN, B. G.: Leçons orales de clinique chirurgicale «Des brûlures», article XVI, vol. 1. Paris: G. Baillière 1839. — DZANEHDZE, JU. JU.: Die Therapie der Verbrennungen. Vortrag, gehalten am allrussischen Kongr. für Unfallmedizin. Chirurgija 4, 34 (1949) [Russisch]. Zit. Zbl. Haut- u. Geschl.-Kr. **75**, 53 (1950/51).

ENTIN, M. A., and H. BAXTER: Experimental and clinical study of histopathology and pathogenesis of graduatet thermal burns in man and their clinical implication. Plast. reconstr. Surg. **6**, 1352 (1950). — ENYART, J. L., and D. W. MILLER: Treatment of burns resulting from disaster. J. Amer. med. Ass. **158**, 95 (1955). — EVANS, E., and H. S. RAFAL: Studies on traumatic shock. Treatment of clinical shock with gelatin. Ann. Surg. **121**, 478 (1945). — EVANS, E. J.: Treatment of high intensity burns. Arch. Surg. **62**, 335 (1951). Zit. Zbl. Haut- u. Geschl.-Kr. **81**, 300 (1952). — EVANS, E. J., and I. A. BIGGER: The rationale of whole blood therapy in severe burns; a clinical study. Ann. Surg. **122**, 693 (1945). — EVANS, E. J., O. J. PURNELL, P. W. ROBINETT, A. BATCHELOR, and M. MARTIN: Fluid and electrolyte requirements in severe burns. Ann. Surg. **135**, 804 (1952).

FARGEL, H.: Farbstoff-Filmbehandlung von Brandwunden. Zbl. Chir. **78**, 1569 (1953). — FARMER, A. W.: Pathology of burns. Amer. Acad. Orthop. Surg. **1943**, 182. — FISCHER, E., u. H. STORCK: Zur Röntgentherapie der Keloide. Schweiz. med. Wschr. **1957**, 1281. — FINE, J.: The infection element in shock. 1. Conf. on shock and circulatory homeostasis. New York: Josiah Macy jr. Foundation 1951. — The bacterial factor in traumatic shock. Amer. Lect. Ser. No 219. Springfield (Ill.): Ch. C. Thomas 1954. — Host resistance to bacteria and to bacterial toxins in traumatic shock. Ann. Surg. **142**, 361 (1955). — FRANK, H. A., E. D. FRANK, H. KORMAN, J. A. MACCHI, and O. HECHTER: Corticosteroid output and adrenal blood flow during hemorrhagic shock in the dog. Amer. J. Physiol. **182**, 24 (1955). — FRIESEN, S. R.: The genesis of gastroduodenal ulcer following burns; an experimental study. Surgery **28**, 123 (1950).

GEORGIADE, N. G., G. E. MATTON, and F. v. KESSEL: Facial burns. Plast. reconstr. Surg. **29**, 648 (1962). Zit. Zbl. Haut- u. Geschl.-Kr. **113**, 219 (1962/63). — GILBERT, R. P.: Mechanisms of the hemodynamic effects of endotoxin. Physiol. Rev. **40**, 245 (1960). — GLASSER, O., and I. H. PAGE: Experimental hemorrhagic shock; a study of its production and treatment. Amer. J. Physiol. **154**, 297 (1948). — GLENK, G.: Örtliche Behandlung von Verbrennungen I. und II. Grades mit Badional-Gel. Zbl. Chir. **78**, 385 (1953). Zit. Zbl. Haut- u. Geschl.-Kr. **85**, 384 (1953). — GLENN, W. W. L., D. K. PETERSON, and C. K. DRINKER: The flow of lymph from burned tissue, with particular reference to the effects of fibrin formation on lymph drainage and composition. Surgery **12**, 685 (1942). — GOLTZ, F.: Ueber den Tonus der Gefässe und seine Bedeutung für die Blutbewegung. Virchows Arch. path. Anat. **29**, 394 (1864). — GORDON, J., R. A. HALL, R. M. HEGGIE, and E. A. HORNE: Histological and bacteriological study of healing burns with enquiry into significance of local infection. J. Path. Bact. **58**, 51 (1946). — GREUER, W.: Studien zur Biologie und Therapie des Verbrennungsschadens. I. Mitt. Bruns' Beitr. klin. Chir. **177**, 213 (1948). — Über die Behandlung der Verbrennungskrankheit. Dtsch. med. Wschr. **74**, 1205 (1949). — Ist die Intoxikationstheorie der Verbrennung als widerlegt zu betrachten? Bruns' Beitr. klin. Chir. **180**, 493 (1950). — Zur Pathophysiologie und Therapie der Verbrennungskrankheit. Bruns' Beitr. klin. Chir. **198**, 257 (1959). Zit. Zbl. Haut- u. Geschl.-Kr. **104**, 239 (1959).

HAM, A. W.: Experimental study of histopathology of burns, with particular reference to sites of fluid loss in burns of different depths. Ann. Surg. **120**, 689 (1944). — HARKINS, H. N.: The treatment of burns. Springfield (Ill.): Ch. C. Thomas 1942. — HAWN, C. V., E. A. BERING jr., O. T. BAILEY, and S. H. ARMSTRONG jr.: Note on use of fibrinogen and thrombin in surface treatment of burns. J. clin. Invest. **23**, 580 (1944). — HEBRA, F. V.: Zit. nach KONRAD. — HEGEMANN, G.: Grundsätzliches zur örtlichen Behandlung von Verbrennungen. Hefte Unfallheilk. **47**, 61 (1954). Zit. Zbl. Haut- u. Geschl.-Kr. **88**, 256 (1954). — HENRIQUES jr., A. C.: Studies of thermal injury VIII. Automatic recording caloric applicator and skin-tissue and skin-surface thermocouples. Rev. Sci. Instr. **18**, 673 (1947). — HENRIQUES jr., F. C.: Studies of thermal injury V. The predictability and the significance of thermal induced rate processes leading to irreversible epidermal injury. Arch. Path. **43**, 489 (1947). — HENRIQUES jr., F. C., and A. R. MORITZ: Studies of thermal injury I. The conduction of heat to and through skin and the temperatures therein. Amer. J. Path. **23**, 531 (1947). — HOFFMAN, L., and A. W. BROWNELL: Survival after almost complete body surface burn. Relation to newer concepts of treatment and report of a case. U.S. armed Forces med. J. **2**, 577 (1951). — HUGUÉNARD, R.: Zit. nach H. WEESE. — HUME, D. M., and D. H. NELSON: Adrenal cortical function in surgical shock. Surgical Forum **5**, 568 (1955). — HUNZINGER, W., A. MEYER u. H. WILLENEGGER: Bestimmungen der Verweildauer von Plasmaersatzstoffen mit Hilfe von radioaktiven Isotopen. Communications Journées Transfusionelles Genève 1953, p. 62. — HUSCHKE, U.: Hirnschäden nach Verbrennung. Mschr. Kinderheilk. **104**, 300 (1956). Zit. Zbl. Haut- u. Geschl.-Kr. **98**, 121 (1957).

JAMES, G. W. III.: Burns anemia. Symp. on burns, 138, National research council, Washington 1951. — JAMES, G. W. III., L.-D. ABBOTT, J. W. BROOKS, and E. J. EVANS: The anemia of thermal injury III. Erythropoiesis and hemoglobin metabolism studied with

N^{15}-glycine in dog and man. J. clin. Invest. **33**, 150 (1954). — JAMES, G. W. III., O. J. PURNELL, and E. J. EVANS: The anemia of thermal injury I. Studies of pigment excretion. J. clin. Invest. **30**, 181 (1951a). — The anemia of thermal injury II. Studies of liver function. J. clin. Invest. **30**, 191 (1951b). — JEANNET, M.: "Sludged blood". A propos de l'importance de l'agrégation érythrocytaire dans la pathogenèse et le traitement des états choc. Praxis **2**, 49 (1964). — JIRZIK, H., u. K. E. WARNECKE: Zur örtlichen Behandlung der Verbrennungen. Mschr. Unfallheilk. **53**, 353 (1950).

KIMMIG, J.: Zur Therapie und Nachbehandlung der Verbrennungsschäden. Dtsch. med. J. **1954**, 660. Zit. Zbl. Haut- u. Geschl.-Kr. **92**, 316 (1955). — KING, E. S., and D. S. BALDWIN: Production of renal ischemia and proteinuria in man by the adrenal medullary hormones. Amer. J. Med. **20**, 217 (1956). — KIRCHNER, E., u. H. OEHMIG: Schock und Kollaps. In: Handbuch der gesamten Unfallheilkunde, 3. Aufl., herausgeg. von H. BÜRKLE DE LA CAMP u. M. SCHWAIGER, Bd. 1, S. 309—322. Stuttgart: Ferdinand Enke 1963. — KLEINE-NATROP, H. E., u. A. AZZOLINI: Kombinierte operativ-konservative Lokalbehandlung großflächiger Verbrennungen. Med. Kosmetik **7**, 95 (1958). Zit. Zbl. Haut- u. Geschl.-Kr. **101**, 337 (1958). — KNISELY, M. H., E. H. Bloch, T. S. ELIOT, and W. WARNER: Sludged blood. Science **106**, 431 (1947). — KNISELY, M. H., T. S. ELIOT, and E. H. BLOCH: Sludged blood in traumatic shock. Arch. Surg. **51**, 220 (1945). — KOCH, W.: Extreme Temperatursteigerung nach Verbrennung bei einem Kinde. Nord. Med. **43**, 175 (1950) [Schwedisch mit engl. Zus.fass.]. — KONRAD, J.: FERDINAND v. HEBRA und die Therapie der Verbrennungen. Wien. klin. Wschr. **1950**, 241. Zit. Zbl. Haut- u. Geschl.-Kr. **77**, 266 (1951/52). — KOSLOWSKI, L.: Die Verbrennungskrankheit. Dtsch. med. Wschr. **5**, 233 (1963). — Dringlichkeitsstufen bei Verbrennungen im Katastrophenfalle. 81. Tagg der Dtsch. Ges. für Chir. in München, 1.—4. April 1964. Münch. med. Wschr. **18**, 865 (1964). — KOSLOWSKI, L., u. A. GREGL: Verbrühungen und Verbrennungen 1945—1956. Münch. med. Wschr. **1958**, 1508. — KYLE, M. J., and A. B. WALLACE: The exposure method of treatment of burns. Brit. J. plast. Surg. **3**, 144 (1950/51).

LABORIT, H.: Réaction organique à l'agression du choc. Paris: Masson & Cie. 1952a. — Etudes de quelques travaux récent concernent les brûlures graves. Presse méd. **60**, 450 (1952b). — Potenzierte Narkose und künstlicher Winterschlaf. Naunyn-Schmiedebergs Arch. exp. Path. Pharmak. **222/223**, 41 (1954). — LAUSECKER, H.: Verbrennungsscharlach und Penicillin. Z. Haut- u. Geschl.-Kr. **21**, 149 (1956). — LAVER, M. B.: The effect of ganglion-blocking agents on survival of rats subjected to acute thermal injury. Surgery **40**, 520 (1956). LESSER, L. v.: Über die Todesursachen nach Verbrennungen. Virchows Arch. path. Anat. **79**, 248 (1880). — LEUTERER, W.: Über die Behandlung von Verbrennungen und Verbrühungen im Kindesalter. Medizinische **9**, 310 (1957). — Derm. Wschr. **1958**, 137 (615). — LEVENSON, S. M., and CH. C. LUND: The treatment of burns of the extremities with close fitting plasters of paris casts. J. Amer. med. Ass. **123**, 272 (1943). — LEVITT, W. M.: Radiotherapy in the prevention and treatment of hypertrophic scars. Brit. J. plast. Surg. **4**, 104 (1951). Zit. Zbl. Haut- u. Geschl.-Kr. **80**, 36 (1952). — LOB, A.: Mechanische, thermische und elektrische Verbrennungen. In: Handbuch der gesamten Unfallheilkunde, 3. Aufl., herausgeg. von H. BÜRKLE DE LA CAMP u. M. SCHWAIGER, Bd. 1, S. 178—243. 1963. — LÖHR, W.: Die Behandlung großer, flächenhafter Verbrennungen 1., 2. und 3. Grades mit Lebertran. Chirurg **6**, 263 (1934). Zit. Zbl. Haut- u. Geschl.-Kr. **48**, 621 (1934). — LOWBURY, E. J L., D. J. CROCKETT, and D. M. JACKSON: Bacteriology of burns treatment by exposures. Lancet **1954II**, 1151. Zit. Zbl. Haut- u. Geschl.-Kr. **92**, 54 (1955). — LUND, C. C., and N. C. BROWDER: Estimation of areas of burns. Surg. Gynec. Obstet. **79**, 352 (1944). — LUND, C. C., S. M. LEVENSON, R. W. GREEN, R. W. PAIGE, P. E. ROBINSON, M. A. ADAMS, A. H. MACDONALD, F. H. L. TAYLOR, and R. E. JOHNSON: Ascorbic acid, thiamine, riboflavine and nicotinic acid in relations to acute burns in man. Arch. Surg. **55**, 557 (1947). Zit. Zbl. Haut- u. Geschl.-Kr. **72**, 164 (1949).

MACFARLANE: Zit. nach ZINCK. — MARGGRAF, W.: Die posttraumatische intravasale Proteolyse und ihre Behandlung. Hefte Unfallheilk. **66**, 238 (1961). — MARKLEY, K.: Oral treatment of burn shock. 17. Ann. Congr. on Industr. Health, Los Angeles 1957. Arch. industr. Health **16**, 427 (1957). Zit. Zbl. Haut- u. Geschl.-Kr. **101**, 337 (1958). — MCCARTHY, M. D.: A comparison of plasma expanders with blood and plasma as a supplement to electrolyte solutions in the treatment of rats undergoing third degree burns of 50% of the body surface. Ann. Surg. **136**, 546 (1952). — MCCARTHY, M. D., and J. W. DRAHEIM: Survival of thermally injured rats infused with saline, polyvinylpyrrolidone, dextran and oxypolygelatin. Proc. Soc. exp. Biol. (N.Y.) **79**, 346 (1952). — MCLAUGHLIN jr., C. W., and D. K. NEIS: Recent advances in the management of burns. Amer. J. Surg. **83**, 746 (1952). Zit. Zbl. Haut-u. Geschl.-Kr. **83**, 365 (1953). — MEADE, R. J.: The prevention of secondary tissue destruction in burns. Plast. reconstr. Surg. **21**, 4, 263 (1958). — MELBY, J. C., and W. W. SPINK: Comparative studies on adrenal cortical function and cortisol metabolism in healthy adults and in patients with shock due to infection. J. clin. Invest. **37**, 1791 (1958). — MENKIN, V.: Dynamics of inflammation. New York: Macmillan & Co. 1940. — Newer concepts of inflammation. Springfield (Ill.): Ch. C. Thomas 1950. — MILLICAN, C. R., E. F. STOHLMAN, and R. W. MOWRY: A comparison of plasma substitutes (dextran, polyvinvylpyrrolidon-oxpolygelatine) with saline therapy in treatment of experimental burn shock in mice. Amer. J. Physiol. **170**, 173 (1952). — MILLICAN, C. R., H. TABOR, and S. M. ROSENTHAL: Traumatic shock in mice. Comparison of survival rates following therapy. Amer. J. Physiol. **170**, 179 (1952). — MONSAINGEON, A.: Les Brulés. Etudes physiopathologiques et thérapeutiques. Paris: Masson & Cie. 1963. — MOORE, F. D.: Metabolic care of the surgical patients, p. 190. Philadelphia and London: W. B. Saunders Co. 1959. — MORGER, R., R. NICOLE u. W. GAYER: Verbrennungsbehandlung im Säuglings- und Kindesalter. Ann. paediat. (Basel) **199**, 141 (1962). — MORITZ, A. R.: Studies of thermal injury III. The pathology and pathogenesis of cutaneous burns. Amer. J. Path. **23**, 915 (1947). — MORITZ, A. R., and F. C. HENRIQUES jr.: Studies of thermal injury. II. The relative importance of time and surface temperature in the causation of cutaneous burns. Amer. J. Path. **23**, 695 (1947). — The reciprocal relationship of surface temperature and time in the production of hyperthermic cutaneous injury. Amer. J. Path. **23**, 897 (1947). — MORITZ, A. R., F. C. HENRIQUES jr., F. R. DUTRA, and J. R. WEISINGER: Studies of thermal injury. IV. An exploration of the casualty-producing attributes of conflagrations; local and systemic effects of general cutaneous exposure to excessive circumambient (air) and circumambient treat of varying duration and intensity. Arch. Path. **43**, 466 (1947). — MOYER, C. A.: The sociologic aspects of trauma with particular reference to thermal injury. Amer. J. Surg. **87**, 421 (1954).

NOSKO, L., u. H. ZEHETNER: Zur Klinik und Pathogenese des Verbrennungsulcus. Hautarzt **5**, 209 (1954). Zit. Zbl. Haut- u. Geschl.-Kr. **90**, 114 (1954/55). — NUNN, J. R., and W. H. POTTER: Local treatment of burns caused by molten tar. Experimental study. Arch, Surg. **70**, 218 (1955).

O'BRIEN, G., and R. D. MURRAY: A five year report on the treatment of burns. Surgery **14**, 271 (1954). Zit. Zbl. Haut- u. Geschl.-Kr. **91**, 298 (1955). — OLLINGER, P.: Ist die Tanninbehandlung bei Verbrennungen schädlich? Chirurg **17/18**, 629 (1947). — OXENIUS, K.: Antistin bei Verbrennungen im Kindesalter; eine kurze Anregung. Kinderärztl. Prax. **18**, 29 (1950).

PETER, E. G.: Überblick über 40 Jahre Gerbstoffbehandlung in der Dermatologie. Z. Haut- u. Geschl.-Kr. **8**, 210 (1963). — PFAHLER, G. E., and G. P. KEEFER: The treatment of keloids by irradiation and electrosurgery. Amer. J. Roentgenol. **59**, 378 (1948). — PFEIFFER, H.: Experimentelle Beiträge zur Ätiologie des primären Verbrennungstodes. Virchows Arch. path. Anat. **179**, H. 3, 367 (1905). Zit. Arch. Derm. Syph. (Berl.) **77**, 309 (1905). — PHILLIPS, A. W., and O. COPE: Burn therapy. II. The relevation of respiratory tract damage as a principal killer of the burned patient. Ann. Surg. **155**, 1 (1962). Zit. Zbl. Haut- u. Geschl.-Kr. **113**, 32 (1962/63). — PONFICK, E., in: Bericht d. 50. Versammlg Dtsch. Naturforscher u. Aerzte in München 1877. München: Ackermann 1878. — POSTNIKOW, B. N.: Moderne Behandlung thermischer Verbrennungen. Berlin: VEB Verlag Volk und Gesundheit 1955. — PULASKI, E. J., and C. W. TENNISON: Zit. nach C. P. ARTZ and E. REISS, The treatment of burns. Philadelphia: W. B. Saunders Co. 1957.

RABINOWITZ, H. M., and L. PELNER: Topical application of horse serum in treatment of extensive burns. Amer. J. Surg. **64**, 55 (1944). — RAVDIN, J. S., and L. K. FERGUSON: The early treatment of superficial burns. Ann. Surg. 81, 439 (1925). — REHN, J.: Tierexperimentelle Untersuchungen zur Pathogenese der Verbrennungskrankheit. I. Arzneimittel-Forsch. **7**, 637 (1957). — Behandlung der Verbrennungen. Münch. med. Wschr. **1958 II**, 1462. — Zit. nach A. LOB. — RIEHL, G., ST. WEIDENFELD u. L. v. ZUMBUSCH: Zit. nach K. ULLMANN. — RIEHL jr., G.: Experimentelle Untersuchungen über den Verbrennungstod. Naunyn-Schmiedebergs Arch. exp. Path. Pharmakol. **135** (1928). — ROSE, B., and J. S. L. BROWNE: The distribution and rate of disappearance of intravenously injected histamine in the rat. Amer. J. Physiol. **124**, 412 (1938). — ROSSITER, R. J.: Plasma loss in burns. (Review of literature.) Bull. War Med. **4**, 181 (1943).

SANYAL, R. K.: Certain physiological changes during superficial skinburns. Med. exp. (Basel) **6**, 307 (1962). Zit. Zbl. Haut- u. Geschl.-Kr. **113**, 277 (1962/63). — SCHEGA, H. W.: Künstliche Infusionslösungen in der Therapie des Verbrennungsschocks. Chirurg **25**, 396 (1954). Zit. Zbl. Haut- u. Geschl.-Kr. **91**, 174 (1955). — SCHIRREN, C. G.: Auswirkungen von Kernwaffenexplosionen auf die Haut. In: Fortschritte der praktischen Dermatologie und Venerologie, Bd. 4. Berlin-Göttingen-Heidelberg: Springer 1962. — SCHMITT, W.: Zur Behandlung von Verbrennungen bei Säuglingen und Kleinkindern. Teil I: Zur Behandlung des Verbrennungsschocks. Ärztl. Wschr. **1956**, 649. Zit. Zbl. Haut- u. Geschl.-Kr. **97**, 43 (1957). SCHUBERT, R.: Serumsanierung mit künstlichen Kolloiden. Nicht nierenfähige Stoffe permeiren mit Kollidon die Niere. Dtsch. med. Wschr. **1949**, 1489. — SCHWARZ, F.: Tödliche Kinderunfälle. Dtsch. med. Wschr. **1956**, 730. — SEVITT, S.: Local blood-flow changes in experimental burns. J. Path. Bact. **61**, 427 (1949). — Local vascular changes in burned skin. Proc. roy. Soc. Med. **47**, 225 (1954). — Burns. Pathology and therapeutic implications.

London: Butterworth & Co. 1957. — SEVITT, S., J. P. BULL, C. N. D. CRUICKSHANK, D. M. JACKSON, and E. J. L. LOWBURY: Failure of an antihistamine drug to influence the course of experimental human burns. Brit. med. J. **1952II**, 57. — SHULMAN, A. G.: Ice water as primary treatment of burns. J. Amer. med. Ass. **173**, 1916 (1960). — SIMONART, A.: Zit. nach MONSAINGEON. — SLAVIK, J.: Verbrennungen und Verbrühungen bei Kindern. Wien. med. Wschr. **1942I**, 146. Zit. Zbl. Haut- u. Geschl.-Kr. **69**, 472 (1942/43). — SNEVE, H.: The treatment of burns and skin grafting. J. Amer. med. Ass. **45**, 1 (1905). — SPINK, W. W.: Pathogenese und Therapie des Schocks bei Infektionen: Experimentelle und klinische Untersuchungen. In: Schock, Pathogenese und Therapie; ein internat. Symp. Berlin-Göttingen-Heidelberg: Springer 1962. — STÖR, O.: Die Verbrennungskrankheit und ihre Behandlung (Vortrag a. d. prakt. Chir., H. 35). Stuttgart: Ferdinand Enke 1952. — STÜTTGEN, G.: Die heutige Behandlung schwerer Verbrennungen. Hautarzt **5**, 193 (1957). — *Symposium on burns*. National research council, national academy of science. Washington 1951.

TANRET, P.: Zit. nach MONSAINGEON. — TAPPEINER, J., u. W. WITTELS: Zur Prognose schwerer Verbrennungen; ein Vergleich der Mortalität in den Jahren 1940 bis 1944 und 1950 bis 1954. Wien. klin. Wschr. **68**, 412 (1956). — TILLET, W. S.: Early débridement of burn wounds. (Research on burns, an Amer. symp.). Lancet **1952II**, 640. — TSCHMARKE, P.: Über Verbrennungen. Dtsch. Z. Chir. **44**, 346 (1897). — TUMBUSCH, W. T., E. H. VOGEL jr., J. V. BUTKIEWICZ, C. D. GRABER, D. L. LARSON, and E. T. MITCHELL: Septicaemia in burn injury. MEDEW-RS **6** (1960).

ULLMANN, K.: Thermische Schädigungen. In: Handbuch der Haut- und Geschlechts-Krankheiten, herausgeg. von J. JADASSOHN, Bd. 4, Teil 1. Berlin: Springer 1932. — UNGAR, G., and E. DAMGAARD: Protein breakdown in thermal injury. Proc. Soc. exp. Biol. (N.Y.) **87**, 378 (1954). — UNNA, P. G.: Zit. nach GANS-STEIGLEDER.

VILAIN, R.: Zit. nach MONSAINGEON. — VOGEL, E. H.: Immediate therapy in burns. GP (Kansas City) **20**, 120 (1959).

WALLACE, A. B.: Treatment of burns. A return to basic principles. Brit. J. plast. Surg. **2**, 232 (1949). — The exposure treatment of burns. Lancet **1951I**, 109. — The treatment of burns. Practitioner **170**, 109 (1953). — WEESE, H.: „Potenzierte Narkose" und „Hibernation durch Phenothiazine". Naunyn-Schmiedebergs Arch. exp. Path. Pharmak. **222/223**, 15 (1954). — WEIDENFELD, ST.: Über den Verbrennungstod. Arch. Derm. Syph. (Berl.) **61**, 301 (1902). — WEIDENFELD, ST., u. L. v. ZUMBUSCH: Weitere Beiträge zur Pathologie und Therapie schwerer Verbrennungen. Arch. Derm. Syph. (Berl.) **76**, 77, 163 (1905). — WEIGEL, A. E., C. P. ARTZ, E. REISS, J. H. DAVIS, and W. H. AMSPACHER: Gastrointestinal ulcerations complicating burns. Surgery **34**, 826 (1953). Zit. Zbl. Haut- u. Geschl.-Kr. **90**, 24 (1954/55). — WEINER, D. O., A. P. ROWLETTE, and R. ELMAN: Significance of loss of serum protein in therapy of severe burns. Proc. Soc. exp. Biol. (N.Y.) **34**, 484 (1936). Zit. Zbl. Haut- u. Geschl.-Kr. **55**, 31 (1937).

YASARGIL, E. C.: Schockbegriff im Wandel der Zeiten und heute. III. Richtlinien zur systematischen Behandlung des Schocks und der Fettembolie. Schweiz. med. Wschr. **34**, 1165 (1964).

ZINCK, K. H.: Pathologische Anatomie der Verbrennung. Veröff. Konstit.-Wehrpath. **46**, Jena 1940. — Die Verbrennungskrankheit. 17. Tagg Dtsch. Ges. Versich.- u. Versorg.-Med. 1953. Hefte Unfallheilk. **47**, 10 (u. Diskussion 65) (1954). Zit. Zbl. Haut- u. Geschl.-Kr. **91**, 175 (1955).

B. Kälteschädigungen

ADAMS-RAY, J., and B. FALCONER: Pathologico-anatomical changes, following rapid and slow thawing, respectively, in frozen skin in man; an experimental study. Acta chir. scand. **101**, 269 (1951). — ALTENKAMP, TH.: Beitrag zur Frostschädenbehandlung durch Grenzstranganästhesie. Münch. med. Wschr. **1943**, 139.

BERGER, A.: Über Erfrierungen. Diss. Zürich 1957. — BERSON, R. C., and R. J. ANGELUCCI: Trench foot. Bull. U.S.Army med. Dep. **77**, 91 (1944). — BINHOLD, H.: Sollen Erfrierungen schnell oder langsam erwärmt werden? Dtsch. Militärarzt **8**, 491 (1942). — BLACKWOOD, W., and H. RUSSEL: Experiments in the study of immersion foot. Edinb. med. J. **50**, 385 (1943). — Studies in the pathology of human „immersion foot". Brit. J. Surg. **31**, 329 (1944). — BLAIR, J. R., R. SCHATZKI, and K. D. ORR: Sequelae to cold injury in one hundred patients. Follow-up study four years after occurrence of cold injury. J. Amer. med. Ass. **163**, 1203 (1957). — BROWNRIGG, G. M.: Frostbite in shipwrecked mariners. Amer. J. Surg. **59**, 232 (1943). — BURCH, G. H., H. L. MYERS, R. R. POTTER, and N. SCHAFFER: Objective studies on some physiologic responses in mild chronic trench foot. Bull. Johns Hopk. Hosp. **80**, 1 (1947).

Cold injury. Transactions of the second conference, nov. 1952, NewYork (Ed. M. J. FERRER). NewYork: Josiah Macy, jr. foundation 1954. — *Cold injury. Transactions of the fluid conference*, Febr. 1954, Manitoba (Ed. M. J. FERRER). NewYork: Josiah Macy, jr. foundation

1955. — Cottet, J.: Trench foot (etiology-pathology-symptomatology). War Med. (Chic.) **2**, 707 (1918/19).

Dannegger, M.: Zur Behandlung der örtlichen Erfrierungen. Münch. med. Wschr. **9**, 411 (1946). — Davis, L., J. E. Scarff, N. Rogers, and M. Dickinson: High altitude frostbite. Preliminary report. Surg. Gynec. Obstet. **77**, 561 (1943). — Debrunner, H.: Die Klinik und die Behandlung der örtlichen Erfrierungen. Bern: H. Huber 1941. — Dreifuss, H. P.: Tod durch Unterkühlung. Diss. Zürich 1958.

Fausel, E. G., and J. A. Hemphill: Study on the late symptoms of cases of immersion foot. Surg. Gynec. Obstet. **81**, 500 (1945). — Frey, S.: Die örtlichen Erfrierungen im Kriege. Med. Klin. **43**, 1009 (1942); **44**, 1036 (1942); **45**, 1067 (1942). — Friedman, N. B.: The pathology of trench foot. Amer. J. Path. **21**, 387 (1945). — The reaction of tissues to cold. Amer. J. clin. Path. **16**, 634 (1946).

Gohrbandt, E.: Wiedereinsatz Frostgeschädigter. Zbl. Chir. **70**, 1584 (1943). — Goldhahn, R.: Erfrierungen. Dtsch. med. Wschr. **3**, 58 (1940). — Goldstone, B., and H. Corbett: Etiology of "immersion foot". Brit. med. Bull. **2**, 148 (1944). — Grattan, H. W.: Trench foot. In: W. G. Macpherson, A. A. Bowlby, C. Wallace, and C. English (eds.), Official history of the war. Surgery of the war. I., p. 169. London: His Majesty's stationary office 1922. — Greene, R.: Frostbite and kindred ills. Lancet **1941 II**, 689. — The immediate vascular changes in true frostbite. J. Path. Bact. **55**, 259 (1943).

Hamilton, J.: Frost-bite. J. roy. nav. M. Serv. **29**, 225 (1943). — Häusler, H.: Das Verhalten der reaktiven Hyperämie nach Erfrierungen. Münch. med. Wschr. **1943**, 301. — Hays, S. B., J. B. Coates jr., and E. M. McFetridge: Cold injury, ground type. Office of the surgeon general department of the army. Washington, D.C. 1958. — Hecht, V.: Zur Pathologie und Therapie der Erfrierungsgangrän. Wien. med. Wschr. **65**, 1487 (1915). — Heuss, R. v.: Kriegsmedizin. — 4. Kälteschäden. Deren Entstehung, Folgen und Behandlung. Jkurse ärztl. Fortbild. **6**, 48 (1943). — Hossli, G.: Wiederbelebungsmaßnahmen bei Lawinenverschütteten. Symp. über dringliche Maßnahmen zur Rettung von Lawinenverschütteten. Davos-Weißfluhjoch Jan. 1963.

Immersion foot. Bull. U.S. Army med. Dep. **70**, 26 (1943).

Jarret, A., and M. Garretts: The effect of local cooling on the cutaneous blood flow in normal and erythrocyanotic patients. Brit. J. Derm. **71**, 66 (1959). — Jochim, K. E., and A. B. Hertzman: Vascular reactions to cold releated to the early stages of immersion foot. Proc. Fed. Amer. Soc. exp. Biol. **3**, 22 (1944).

Killian, H.: Einige neuere Anschauungen über die Kälteschäden. 45. Jahresversl. schweiz. Ges. für Chir. 1958. Schweiz. med. Wschr. **1959**, 306. — Klapp, R.: Zur Behandlung lokaler Erfrierungen. Zbl. Chir. **69**, 1794 (1942). — Knight, B. W.: „Trench foot" in civilians. Brit. med. J. **1940 II**, 610. — Kreyberg, L.: Some notes and considerations regarding injuries from cold. Report to the commanding officier, 108th United States general hospital, 12 apr. 1945. — Tissue damage due to cold. Lancet **1946 I**, 338. — Experimental immersion-foot in rabbits. Acta path. microbiol. scand. **26**, 296 (1949). — La stase et son rôle dans le développement de la nécrose. Acta path. microbiol. scand., Suppl. **91**, 40 (1950). — Kriege, H.: Über hyaline Veränderungen der Haut durch Erfrierungen. Virchows Arch. path. Anat. **116**, 64 (1889). — Kulhia, Y.: Heparin and sympathetic nerve block in frostbite. J. Amer. med. Ass. **152**, 551 (1953).

Läwen, A.: Untersuchungen über die Durchblutung des Fußes von Frontsoldaten im gesunden und kranken Zustand, namentlich bei Frostschäden. Dtsch. Militärarzt **8**, 479 (1942). — Lange, K., and L. J. Boyd: The functional pathology of experimental frostbite and the prevention of subsequent gangrene. Surg. Gynec. Obstet. **80**, 346 (1945). — Lange, K., D. Weiner, and L. J. Boyd: Frostbite, physiology, pathology and therapy. New England J. Med. **237**, 383 (1947). — Leriche, R.: A propos des gelures et de leur traitement immédiat par l'infiltration lombaire. Presse méd. **48**, 75 (1940). — Physiologie pathologique et traitement chirurgical des maladies arterielles de la vasomotricité. Paris: Masson & Cie. 1945. — Leriche, R., et J. Kunlin: Physiologie pathologique des gelures. Maladie d'abord vasomotrice, puis thrombosante. Progr. méd. Paris **68**, 169 (1940). — Lesser, A.: Report on immersion foot casualties from the battle of Attu. Ann. Surg. **121**, 257 (1944). — Lewis, T.: Observations on some normal and injurious effects of cold upon the skin and underlying tissues. I. Reactions to cold and injury of normal skin. Brit. med. J. **1941 II**a, 795. — Observation on some normal and injurious effects of cold upon the skin and underlying tissues. II. Chilblains and allied conditions. Brit. med. J. **1941 II**b, 837. — Observations on some normal and injurious effects of cold upon the skin and underlying tissues. III. Frost-bite. Brit. med. J. **1941 II**c, 869. — Lewis, T., and W. S. Love: Vascular reactions of the skin to injury. III. Some effects of freezing, of cooling and of warming. Heart **13**, 27 (1926). — Loos, H. C.: Zur Klinik und Therapie örtlicher Erfrierungen. Münch. med. Wschr. **1943**, 155. — Lutz, W.: Durch extreme physikalische und chemische Ursachen bedingte Dermatosen. Dermatologica (Basel) **95**, 129 (1948).

MARCHAND, F.: Die thermischen Krankheitsursachen: B. Die Kälte als Krankheitsursache. In: L. KREHL, u. F. MARCHAND, Handbuch der allgemeinen Pathologie. I. Allgemeine Ätiologie. Leipzig: S. Hirzel 1908. — MILLS jr., W. J.: A study of frostbite treatment. Nav. Res. Rev. march. 1962. — MÜLLER, W.: Die Todesursachen bei örtlichen Erfrierungsschäden. Dtsch. Militärarzt **1**, 16 (1943).

Nonbattle injuries. Government services. J. Amer. med. Ass. **152**, 1448 (1953).

ORR, K. D., and D. C. FAINER: Cold injuries with emphasis on frostbite. Preliminary report. U.S. armed Forces med. J. **3**, 95 (1952). — OSLER, W.: Cold bite + muscle-inertia = Trench foot. Lancet **1915 II**, 1368.

PADDOCK, F. K.: Chronic disability in mild cases of trench foot. New Engl. J. Med. **234**, 433 (1946). — PÄSSLER, H. W.: Die Behandlung von Frostspätschäden. Zbl. Chir. **70**, 1596 (1940). — PANCHENKO, D. J.: Retrograde changes in the spinal cord in frostbite of the extremities. Amer. Rev. Soviet Med. **1**, 440 (1944). — PHELAN, J. T.: Frostbite. J. int. Coll. Surg. **32**, 501 (1959). Zit. Zbl. Haut- u. Geschl.-Kr. **107**, 141 (1960). — *Prevention of trench-foot (Local frigorism)*, (editorial). Lancet **1915 II**, 1304.

RICHARDS, R. L.: Injury from exposure to low temperature; clinical features, prevention, treatment. Brit. med. Bull. **2**, 141 (1944). — RISCHPLER, A.: Über die histologischen Veränderungen nach Erfrierung. Beitr. path. Anat. **28**, 541 (1900).

SAUERBRUCH, F.: Erfrierungen. Dtsch. Militärarzt **8**, 477 (1942). — *Shelter legs* (editorial). Lancet **1940 II**, 722. — *The shelter problem* (reports of societies). Brit. med. J. **1940 II**, 801. — SHUMACKER jr., H. B., and R. E. LEMPKE: Recent advances in frostbite. With particular reference to experimental studies concerning functional pathology and treatment. Surgery **30**, 873 (1951). — SIEGMUND, H.: Pathologie allgemeiner und örtlicher Kälteschäden. Jkurse ärztl. Fortbild. **34**, 9 (1943). — SIMEONE, F. A.: Trenchfoot in the italian campaign, 1943—1945. Report to the Surgeon, Fifth U.S. Army (1945). — Trench foot. Proc. conf. Army Physicians, Central mediterranean Forces, p. 92 (1945). — SIMPSON, K.: Shelter deaths from pulmonary embolism. Lancet **1940 II**, 744. — SMITH, J. L., J. RITCHIE, and J. DAWSON: On the pathology of trench frost-bite. Lancet **1915 II**, 595. — SONNENBURG, E., u. P. TSCHMARKE: Die Verbrennungen und die Erfrierungen. Dtsch. Z. Chir. **17** (1915). — STAEMMLER, M.: Örtliche Erfrierungen, ihre pathologische Anatomie und Pathogenese. Zbl. Chir. **69**, 1757 (1942). — STARLINGER, F., u. O. v. FRISCH: Die Erfrierung als örtlicher Kälteschaden und die allgemeine Auskühlung im Kriege. Dresden u. Leipzig: Theodor Steinkopff 1944. — STUCKE, K.: Kälteschäden und Erfrierungen im Felde. Bruns' Beitr. klin. Chir. **174**, 1 (1942).

TALBOTT, J. H.: Cold exposure: Pathologic effects. In: O. GLASSER (ed.), Medical physics. Chicago: The year book publishers, Inc. 1944. — TELFORD, E. D.: Sympathectomy in treatment of the cryopathies. Brit. med. J. **1943 II**, 360.

UNGLEY, C. C.: Immersion foot and immersion hand (peripheral vasoneuropathy after chilling). Bull. War Med. **4**, 61 (1943). — UNGLEY, C. C., and W. BLACKWOOD: Peripheral vasoneuropathy after chilling. "Immersion foot and immersion hand". Lancet **1942 II**, 447.

VOLKEN, N.: Seltene Fälle aus der ärztlichen Praxis. Schweiz. med. Wschr. **75**, 353 (1945).

WEBSTER, K. R., F. M. WOLLHOUSE, and J. L. JOHNSTON: Immersion foot. J. Bone Jt Surg. (Boston) **24**, 785 (1942). — WEIDENFELD, S., and E. PULAY: Beitrag zur Pathologie der Erfrierung (Vorläufige Mitt.). Wien. med. Wschr. **65**, 349 (1915). — WHAYNE, T. F.: Cold injury in world war II — A study in the epidemiology of trauma. Doctorate thesis Harward school of public health. Boston 1950. — WHITE, J. C.: Vascular and neurologic lesions in survivors of shipwreck: immersion-foot syndrome following exposure to cold. New Engl. J. Med. **232**, 211 (1943). — WHITE, J. C., and S. WARREN: Couses of pain in feet after prolonged immersion in cold water. War Med. (Chic.) **5**, 6 (1944). — WOLL, W.: Die Thrombophlebitis purulenta nach Verletzungen und Erfrierungen an den Gliedmaßen und ihre Behandlung. Münch. med. Wschr. **1943**, 650.

C. Kälte als Mitursache von Hautkrankheiten

AUPAIX, M., et R. LELOUP: Un cas de cryoglobulinémie avec lésions cutanées. Bull. Soc. franç. Derm. Syph. **66**, 555 (1959). Zit. Zbl. Haut- u. Geschl.-Kr. **106**, 135 (1960).

BAST, G., u. S. PREUSSNER: Chronische Kälteagglutininkrankheit. Med. Bild **5**, 101 (1962). Zit. Zbl. Haut- u. Geschl.Kr. **114**, 33 (1963). — BASSALLECK, H., u. A. GALEJA: Über das Verhalten der thermischen Amplitude bei den sog. Kälteagglutininen. Klin. Wschr. **1953**, 327. Zit. Zbl. Haut- u. Geschl.-Kr. **86**, 6 (1953/54). — BAUMGARTNER, W.: Die Kälteagglutininkrankheit. Schweiz. med. Wschr. **1955**, 1157. — BECK, C. H.: Über eine eigenartige Prädilektionsstelle von Frostschäden. Dermatologica (Basel) **82**, 21 (1940). — BELL, D.: Cold urticaria. Arch. Derm. **72**, 327 (1955). — BENJAMINS, C. E.: Örtliche, passive Übertragung von Kälte-Allergie. Ned. T. Geneesk. **1934**, 5362 [Holländisch]. Zit. Zbl. Haut- u. Geschl.-Kr. **50**, 394 (1935). — BERING, FR.: Über Frostschäden. Münch. med. Wschr. **1941 I**,

123. Zit. Zbl. Haut- u. Geschl.-Kr. **67**, 346 (1941). — BERNSTEIN, F.: Zum allergischen Charakter der Kälteurticaria. Dermatologica (Basel) **64**, 242 (1932). Zit. Zbl. Haut- u. Geschl.-Kr. **43**, 281 (1933). — BLOCK, W.: Die Bedeutung des vegetativen Nervensystems beim Zustandekommen örtlicher Erfrierungen. Langenbecks Arch. klin. Chir. **204**, 64 (1942). — BLUME, H. G., u. H. LIEBESKIND: Rezidivierende Purpura bei Kryoglobulinämie. Dtsch. med. Wschr. **85**, 377 (1960). Zit. Zbl. Haut- u. Geschl.-Kr. **107**, 51 (1960). — BODENSTEIN, E.: Über Kälteurticaria. Diss. Halle a.d.S. 1943. — BRAY, G. W.: A case of physical allergy. A localized and generalized allergic type of reaction to cold. J. Allergy **3**, 367 (1932). Zit. Zbl. Haut- u. Geschl.-Kr. **43**, 282 (1933). — BREHM, G.: Zur Pathogenese der Kälteurticaria. Derm. Wschr. **136**, 1020 (1957). — BUERGER, L.: The circulatory disturbances of the extremities, including gangrene, vasomotor and trophic disorders, p. 173. Philadelphia and London: W. B. Saunders Co. 1924. — BURCKHARDT, W.: Zur Behandlung peripherer funktioneller Durchblutungsstörungen, insbesondere mit Sexualhormonen. Schweiz. med. Wschr. **1946**, 1147. — BURCKHARDT, W., et M. SCHRÖDER: Détermination du temps de réchauffement de la peau atteinte d'engelures. Dermatologica (Basel) **89**, 180 (1944). — BUTLER, K. R., and J. A. PALMER: Cryoglobulinämia in polyarteriitis nodosa with gangrene of extremities. Canad. med. Ass. J. **72**, 686 (1955). Zit. Zbl. Haut- u. Geschl.-Kr. **93**, 112 (1955/56).

CATTAN, R., P. FRUMUSAN et J. DAUSSET: Hémoglobinurie paroxystique a frigore chez un syphilitique guéri par la penicilline. Sang **26**, 714 (1955). Zit. Zbl. Haut- u. Geschl.-Kr. **95**, 156 (1956). — CHORAZAK, T.: Cryoglobulins in the chronic lupus erythematosus. Acta derm.-venereol. (Stockh.) **38**, 322 (1958). Zit. Zbl. Haut- u. Geschl.-Kr. **104**, 261 (1959).

DE NICOLÒ, F.: Contributo alla conoscenza dell'emoglobinuria parossistica «a frigore» nell'infanzia. Pediatt. Riv **41**, 854 (1933). Zit. Zbl. Haut- u. Geschl.-Kr. **46**, 507 (1933). — DIECKHOFF, J., u. C. M. ARNDTS: Zur Pathogenese der Kälteurticaria. Allergie u. Asthma **5**, 131 (1959). Zit. Zbl. Haut- u. Geschl.-Kr. **105**, 212 (1959/60). — DITTRICH, O.: Pernionen und Lichen pilaris. Zbl. Haut- u. Geschl.-Kr. **20**, 418 (1926a). — Demonstration von 4 Mikrophotogrammen typischer Pernionenbilder. Zbl. Haut- u. Geschl.-Kr. **20**, 419 (1926b). — Über Frostschäden. II. Mitt. Arch. f. Derm. u. Syph. **157**, 1 (1929). — Die Behandlung der Frostschäden (Perniosis). Ther. Gegenw. **77**, 20 (1936). Zit. Zbl. Haut- u. Geschl.-Kr. **53**, 407 (1936). — DRANT, P.: Urticaria from sensitiveness to cold. Arch. Derm. **39**, 934 (1939). Zit. Zbl. Haut- u. Geschl.-Kr. **63**, 221 (1939). — DUKE, W. W.: Urticaria caused specifically by the action of physical agents. (Light, cold, heat, freezing, burns, mechanical irritation, and physical and mental exertion.) J. Amer. med. Ass. **83**, 3 (1924). — Allergy, Asthma, hay fever, urticaria, and allied manifestations of reaction. St. Louis: C. V. Mosby Co. 1925. — DUPERRAT, B., et R. PRINGUET: Cryoglobulinémie. Bull. Soc. franç. Derm. Syph. **65**, 256 (1958). Zit. Zbl. Haut- u. Geschl.-Kr. **102**, 289 (1958/59).

FITZPATRICK, T. B.: Essential cold urticaria. Arch. Derm. **87**, 495 (1963). — FLANDIN, CH., et H. RABEAU: Dermite cyanotique des mains avec hyperkératose et ulcérations survenue pendant la saison froide. Bull. Soc. franç. Derm. Syph. **48**, 687 (1941). Zit. Zbl. Haut- u. Geschl.-Kr. **69**, 29 (1942/43). — FLECK, M.: Klinische Erscheinungsformen der Perniosis. J. med. Kosmet. **1955**, 41. Zit. Haut- u. Geschl.-Kr. **92**, 316 (1955).

GANS, O.: Histologie der Hautkrankheiten, Bd. 1, S. 175. Berlin 1925. — GARAN, R., K. ONEN et N. TUNA: A propos d'un cas d'hypersensibilité au froid. Sem. Hôp. Paris **1952**, 2433. Zit. Zbl. Haut- u. Geschl.-Kr. **85**, 309 (1953). — GENTELE, H., B. LAGERHOLM, and A. LODIN: Cryoglobulins in chronic discoid lupus erythematosus. Acta derm.-venereol. (Stockh.) **39**, 207 (1959). Zit. Zbl. Haut- u. Geschl.-Kr. **105**, 235 (1959/60). — GRUMBERS, E., M. AUPAIX et CL. FIEVEZ: Un cas de cryoglobulinémie avec lésions cutanées. Arch. belges Derm. **14**, 238 (1958). Zit. Zbl. Haut- u. Geschl.-Kr. **102**, 117 (1958/59).

HADORN, W.: Klinische Demonstrationen. Praxis **23**, 782 (1964). — HAMBRICK jr., G. W., and E. EPSTEIN: Cold urticaria. Arch. Derm. 81, 1048 (1960). — HARRIS, K. E., TH. LEWIS, and J. M. VAUGHAN: Hämoglobinuria and urticaria from cold occuring singly or in combination; observations referring especially to the mechanism of urticaria with some remarks upon Raynaud's disease. Heart **14**, 4, 305 (1929). — HAXTHAUSEN, H.: Über Arterienspasmen bei Perniosis. Finska Läk.-Sällsk. Handl. **75**, 421 (1933). Zit. Zbl. Haut- u. Geschl.-Kr. **46**, 211 (1933). — HEIDELMANN, G., E.-G. PREUSS u. W. KAISER: Zur Pathogenese und Klinik der Kälteurticaria. Dtsch. med. Wschr. **1957**, 284. Zit. Zbl. Haut- u. Geschl.-Kr. **98**, 125 (1957). — HILLENBRAND, H. J., u. N. WOLF: Endangitis und Kälteschäden. Mschr. Unfallheilk. **53**, 335 (1950). Zit. Zbl. Haut- u. Geschl.-Kr. **78**, 329 (1952). — HINES jr., E. A., and W. F. KVALE: Circulation: Effect of heat and cold, excercise and posture. In: O. GLASSER (ed.). Medical physics, p. 194. Chicago: Year Book Publ., Inc. 1944. — HOCHSINGER, K.: Induratio congelativa submentalis. Klin. Wschr. **9**, 1024 (1930). Zit. Zbl. Haut- u. Geschl.-Kr. **35**, 120 (1931).

JANSSON, H.: Über das Vorkommen von Nebenbefunden am menschlichen Hautorgan. I. Cutis marmorata, Erythrocyanose. Z. Haut- u. Geschl.-Kr. **23**, 188, 210 (1957). Zit. Zbl. Haut- u. Geschl.-Kr. **100**, 10 (1958). — JARRET, A., and M. GARRETTS: The effect of local cooling on the cutaneous blood glow in normal and erythrocyanotic patients. Brit. J. Derm. **71**, 66 (1959). Zit. Zbl. Haut- u. Geschl.-Kr. **104**, 24 (1959). — JAUSION, H., J. MEUNIER et SOMIA: Engelures et syndromes circulatoires des extrémités. Bull. Soc. franç. Derm. Syph. **48**, 227 (1941). Zit. Zbl. Haut- u. Geschl.-Kr. **68**, 21 (1942). — JIRKOVÁ, R., and R. KOUDOUSEK: Plasmocytic myeloma associated with cryoglobulinämia and dermatological symptoms. Čs. Derm. **36**, 41 (mit engl. Zus.fass.) (1961) [Tschechisch]. Zit. Zbl. Haut- u. Geschl.-Kr. **110**, 121 (1961). — JOHNSTON, E. N. M., and H. J. WALLACE: Cryoglobulinämia and reticulosis. Proc. roy. Soc. Med. **51**, 325 (1958). Zit. Zbl. Haut u. Geschl.-Kr. **102**, 289 (1958/59). — JORDAN, F. L. J., and F. G. SCHLESINGER: Red cell anomalies in paroxysmal cold hämoglobinuria of the Donath-Landsteiner (syphilitic) type. Rev. belge Path. **24**, 266 (1955). Zit. Zbl. Haut- u. Geschl.-Kr. **94**, 137 (1956). — JUHLIN, L., and W. B. SHELLEY: Role of mast cell and basophil in cold urticaria with associated systemic reactions. J. Amer. med. Ass. **177**, 371 (1961). Zit. Schweiz. med. Wschr. 8, 251 (1962).

KAISER, W., u. E. G. PREUSS: Testverfahren bei Kälteurticaria. Med. Bild **5**, 78 (1962). Zbl. Haut- u. Geschl.-Kr. **113**, 103 (1962/63). — KELLER, PH.: Zur Klinik und Therapie der Perniosis. Derm. Wschr. **1940 II**, 1041. — KELLY, F. J., and R. A. WISE: Observations on cold sensitivity. Amer. J. Med. **15**, 431 (1953). Zit. Zbl. Haut- u. Geschl.-Kr. **88**, 108 (1954). — KENEDY, D.: Influenza di stimoli meccanici e chimici sulla provocabilità del pomfo in casi di urticaria e frigore. G. ital. Derm. **79**, 99 (1938). Zit. Zbl. Haut- u. Geschl.-Kr. **59**, 596 (1938). — KIRCHDORFER, A. M., u. A. KASSIAN: Zur Therapie der Kälteurticaria. Ther. u. Gegenw. **95**, 161 (1956). Zit. Zbl. Haut- u. Geschl.-Kr. **97**, 13 (1957). — KLINGMÜLLER, V.: Pernionen. Zbl. Haut- u. Geschl.-Kr. **20**, 418 (1926). — KLINGMÜLLER, V., u. O. DITTRICH: Über Frostschäden. Derm. Z. **49**, 1 (1927). — KÖLBL, H., u. H. G. WOLF: Beitrag zur Pathogenese und Therapie der Kälteurticaria. Dtsch. med. Wschr. **1954**, 29. — KREIS, J.: Rôle pathogène du tissu conjonctiv dans la production des cyanoses et érythrocyanoses cutanées. Bull. Soc. franç. Derm. Syph. **39**, 1478 (1932). — KUSKE, H., J. M. PASCHOUD u. W. SOLTERMANN: Acrocyanosis mutilans mit Raynaud-Krisen. Dermatologica (Basel) **114**, 304 (1957).

LANGHOF, H., G. BRAUN u. H. MATZKOWSKI: Livedo reticularis durch Kältegelierung des Blutes bei Plasmozytom. Arch. klin. exp. Derm. **205**, 343 (1957). Zit. Zbl. Haut- u. Geschl.-Kr. **101**, 33 (1958). — LEHNER, J.: Kälteurticaria. Orv. Hetil. **1929 I**, 424. Zit. Zbl. Haut- u. Geschl.-Kr. **32**, 448 (1930). — LEVINE, H. D.: Urticaria due to sensibility to cold. Survey of the literature and report of a case, with experimental observations. Arch. int. Méd. exp. **56**, 498 (1935). Zit. Zbl. Haut- u. Geschl.-Kr. **53**, 39 (1936). — LEWIS, T.: Observation on some normal and injurious effects of cold upon the skin and underlying tissues. II. Chilblains and allied conditions. Brit. med. J. **1941 II**, 837. — LONGHIN, S., u. D. MURESAN: Pathogenetische Forschungen bei der Urticaria a frigore. Derm.-Vener. (Buc.) **7**, 493 (1962) [Rumänisch]. Zit. Zbl. Haut- u. Geschl.-Kr. **115**, 233 (1964).

MCGOVERN, T., I. S. WRIGHT, and E. KRUGER: Pernio: a vascular disease. Amer. Heart J. **22**, 583 (1941). — MCKENZIE, A. W., J. H. O. EARLE, E. LOCKEY, and G. B. MITCHELL-HEGGS: Essential cryoglobulinämia. Brit. J. Derm. **73**, 22 (1961). Zit. Zbl. Haut- u. Geschl.-Kr. **109**, 286 (1961). — MERLEN, J. F.: Le problème etiopathogénique de l'acrocyanose. Angéologie, N.S. **7**, 6 (1955). Zit. Zbl. Haut- u. Geschl.-Kr. **95**, 380 (1956). — MIDANA, A., e F. FRANCHI: Sul meccanismo etiopatogenetico dell'urticaria factitia e da freddo. Dermosifilografo **9**, 614 (1934). Zit. Zbl. Haut- u. Geschl.-Kr. **50**, 498 (1935). — MIKHAILOV, P., and N. BEROVA: Cold agglutinins and cryoglobulins in dermatoses associated with the effect of cold. Vestn. Vener. Derm. **36**, 14 (mit engl. Zus.fass.) (1962) [Russisch]. Zit. Zbl. Haut- u. Geschl.-Kr. **112**, 205 (1962). — MISCALL, L.: Frost-bite. Surg. Clin. N.Amer. **17**, 303 (1937). — MULLER, S. A.: Urticarial sensitivity to cold in the tropics. A report of 2 cases. Arch. Derm. **83**, 930 (1961).

NÉKAM jr., L.: Auf einen hemiatrophischen Unterschenkel beschränkte Perniosis. Sitzg ungar. derm. Ges. 1940. Zit. Zbl. Haut- u. Geschl.-Kr. **65**, 9 (1940). — NELSON, C. T.: Leg ulcer associated with cryoglobulinemia. Arch. Derm. **76**, 150 (1957). — NÖDL, F.: Purpura bei essentieller Kryoglobulinämie. Arch. klin. exp. Derm. **210**, 76 (1960). Zit. Zbl. Haut- u. Geschl.-Kr. **107**, 51 (1960).

OBERMAYER, E.: Treatment of cold urticaria with penicillin. Arch. Derm. **87**, 269 (1963).

PFEIFFER, K.: Über das Vorkommen von Kälteagglutininen in verschiedenen Lebensaltern. Z. Alternsforsch. **6**, 231 (1952). Zit. Zbl. Haut- u. Geschl.-Kr. **88**, 108 (1954). — PREBBLE, E. E.: Syphilitic paroxysmal cold hämoglobinuria. A case report. Brit. J. vener. Dis. **37**, 197 (1961). Zit. Zbl. Haut- u. Geschl.-Kr **111**, 250 (1961/62).

RAJKA, E.: Allergie und allergische Erkrankungen, Bd. II, S. 607. Budapest 1959. — RATSCHOW, M.: Die peripheren Durchblutungsstörungen, 5. Aufl. Dresden u. Leipzig: Theodor Steinkopff 1953. — RODER, H.: Rheumatische Purpura necroticans bei Kryoglobulinämie. Zit. Zbl. Haut- u. Geschl.-Kr. **30**, 148 (1961). — ROGGENSTROH, D.: Die dicken Beine. V. Mitt. Kälteschäden: Erfrierung, Pernio und Erythrocyanosis crurum. J. med. Kosmet. **1956**, 61.

SAMSØE-JENSEN, T.: Cold urticaria. Report of a case. Passive transfer and in vitro experiments with skin cells. Acta derm.-venereol. (Stockh.) **35**, 107 (1955). Zit. Zbl. Haut- u. Geschl.-Kr. **93**, 296 (1955/56). — SAYLOR, L. L., and P. S. WRIGHT: Studies on two cases of urticaria from cold sensitivity and of the effect of histamin treatment. Amer. J. med. Sci. **192**, 388 (1936). Zit. Zbl. Haut- u. Geschl.-Kr. **55**, 293 (1937). — SCHNEIDER, W.: Kälteschäden der Haut. Dtsch. med. Wschr. **83**, 2172 (1958). — SCHNEIDER, W., u. R. HATTON: Über Pathogenese, Prophylaxe und Therapie der Kälteschäden der Haut. Dtsch. med. Wschr. **1954**, 223. Zit. Zbl. Haut- u. Geschl.-Kr. 88, 257 (1954). — SCHOOP, W., u. H. MARX: Experimentelle Untersuchungen bei der Akrocyanose. Nordwestdtsch. Ges. inn. Med. 1955, S. 15. Zit. Zbl. Haut- u. Geschl.-Kr. **97**, 102 (1957). — SCHUBOTHE, H.: Die Serologie der Kältehämolysine. 5. Kongr. Europ. Ges. Hämatol. 1956, S. 781. Zit. Zbl. Haut- u. Geschl.-Kr. **99**, 13 (1957/58). — SÉZARY, A., et R. RABUT: Engelures ponctuées et engelures kératosiques. Bull. Soc. franç. Derm. Syph. **47**, 402 (1940). Zit. Zbl. Haut- u. Geschl.-Kr. **67**, 257 (1941). — SHELLEY, W. B., and W. A. CARO: Cold erythema. A new hypersensitivity syndrome. J. Amer. med. Ass. **180**, 639 (1962). Zit. Zbl. Haut- u. Geschl.-Kr. **113**, 163 (1962/63). — SHERMAN, W. B., and P. M. SEEBOHM: Passive transfer of cold urticaria. J. Allergy **21**, 414 (1950). — SIEGMUND, H.: Pathologisch-anatomische Befunde bei örtlichen Kälteschädigungen mit Berücksichtigung der Spätschäden. Zbl. Chir. **70**, 1558 (1943). — STÄMMLER, M.: Örtliche Erfrierungen, ihre pathologische Anatomie und Pathogenese. Zbl. Chir. **69**, 1757 (1942). — STEINHARDT, M. J., and G. S. FISHER: Cold urticaria and purpura as allergic aspects of cryoglobulinämia. J. Allergy **24**, 335 (1953). Zit. Zbl. Haut- u. Geschl.-Kr. **87**, 41 (1954). — STEPHANI-CHERBULIEZ, J.: Les engelures, une forme atténuée de tuberculose. Rev. Tuberc. (Paris) **2**, 277 (1936). Zit. Zbl. Haut- u. Geschl.-Kr. **54**, 348 (1937). — STORCK, H.: Multiple Granulomata annularia bei ausgesprochener Akrocyanose. Dermatologica (Basel) **112**, 569 (1956). — Urticaria pigmentosa mit Urticaria factitia und Kälteurticaria. Dermatologica (Basel) **112**, 571 (1956).

TELFORD, E. D.: Sympathectomy in treatment of the cryopathies. Brit. med. J. **1943 II**, 360. — TÉMIME, P.: Rôle favorisant du froid sur une récidive ulcéreuse de lupus tuberculeux ancien. Bull. Soc. franç. Derm. Syph. **63**, 299 (1956).

URBACH, E., and P. M. GOTTLIEB: Allergy. New York: Grune & Stratton, Inc. 1946.

VILANOVA, X., J. PIÑOL AGUADÉ y J. M. DE MORAGAS: Crioglobulinemia esencial con lesiones cutáneas ulcerosas y gangrenosas. Arch. argent. Derm. **8**, 267 (1958). Zit. Zbl. Haut- u. Geschl.-Kr. **105**, 35 (1959/60).

WAGNER, K., u. B. SCHREINER: Symmetrische periphere Durchblutungsstörungen durch Kälteisohämagglutinine bei Virusinfekt. Wien. med. Wschr. **111**, 340 (1961). Zit. Zbl. Haut- u. Geschl.-Kr. **110**, 213 (1961). — WATSON, K. C., and W. LAURIE: Syphilitic cold haemoglobinuria. S.Afr. Med. **1956**, 1001. Zit. Zbl. Haut- u. Geschl.-Kr. **97**, 365 (1957). — WEISSENBACH, R. J.: A propos de l'érythème pernio papuleux dit encore engelures papuleuses ou froidures papuleuses. Bull. Soc. franç. Derm. Syph. **47**, 410 (1940). Zit. Zbl. Haut- u. Geschl.-Kr. **67**, 347 (1941). — WEISSENBACH, R. J., et J. P. BRISSET: Etude biologique d'un cas d'urticaire a frigore. Crise hémoclasique et épreuve de Prausnitz-Küstner positives. Arm. Méd. **32**, 333 (1932). Zit. Zbl. Haut- u. Geschl.-Kr. **43**, 748 (1933). — WIEST, E.: Urticaire par le froid traitée par la methode de désensibilisation. Bull. Soc. franç. Derm. Syph. **47**, 26 (1940). Zit. Zbl. Haut- u. Geschl.-Kr. **65**, 556 (1940). — WILDER, J.: Kälteurticaria mit schweren Allgemeinerscheinungen. Wien. klin. Wschr. **1932 II**, 1458. Zit. Zbl. Haut- u. Geschl.-Kr. **44**, 680 (1933). — WIRTSCHAFTER, Z. T., E. C. GAULDEN, and D. W. WILLIAMS: Cold allergy associated with cryoproteinemia. Arch. Derm. **74**, 302 (1956). Zit. Zbl. Haut- u. Geschl.-Kr. **97**, 260 (1957). — WISEMAN, R. D., and D. K. ADLER: Acetic acid sensitivity as a cause of cold urticaria. J. Allergy **27**, 50 (1956). Zit. Zbl. Haut- u. Geschl.-Kr. **95**, 340 (1956).

Namenverzeichnis

Die *kursiv* gesetzten Seitenzahlen beziehen sich auf die Literatur

Sachverzeichnis